Diagnostic Soft Tissue Pathology

Diagnostic Soft Tissue Pathology

MARKKU MIETTINEN, MD
Chairman, Department of Soft Tissue Pathology
Armed Forces Institute of Pathology
Washington, DC

CHURCHILL LIVINGSTONE
An Imprint of Elsevier Science
New York Edinburgh London Philadelphia

CHURCHILL LIVINGSTONE
An Imprint of Elsevier Science

The Curtis Center
Independence Square West
Philadelphia, Pennsylvania 19106

DIAGNOSTIC SOFT TISSUE PATHOLOGY ISBN 0-443-06611-6

Notice

Medicine is an ever-changing field. Standard safety precautions must be followed, but as new research and clinical experience broaden our knowledge, changes in treatment and drug therapy may become necessary or appropriate. Readers are advised to check the most current product information provided by the manufacturer of such drug to be administered to verify the recommended dose, the method and duration of administration and contraindications. It is the responsibility of the treating physician, relying on experience and knowledge of the patient, to determine dosages and the best treatment for each individual patient. Neither the Publisher nor the author assume any liability for any injury and/or damage to persons or property arising from this publication.

The Publisher

Library of Congress Cataloging-in-Publication Data

Miettinen, Markku
Diagnostic soft tissue pathology / Markku Miettinen.—1st ed.
p.; cm
Includes bibliographical references.
ISBN 0-443-06611-6
1. Soft tissue tumors—Pathophysiology. 2. Soft tissue tumors—Diagnosis. I. Title
[DNLM: 1. Soft Tissue Neoplasms—diagnosis. 2. Soft Tissue Neoplasms—pathology.
WD 375 M632d 2003]
RC280.S66 M545 2003
616.99'2075—dc21 2002073672

Acquisitions Editor: Natasha Andjelkovic

PIT/DNP

Printed in Hong Kong.

Last digit is the print number: 9 8 7 6 5 4 3 2 1

Contributors

John K. C. Chan, MD
Queen Elizabeth Hospital
Department of Pathology
Kowloon
Hong Kong

Julie C. Fanburg-Smith, MD
Armed Forces Institute of Pathology
Department of Soft Tissue Pathology
Georgetown University Hospital
Department of Pathology
Washington, DC
Uniformed Services University of the Health Sciences
Department of Pathology
Bethesda, MD

Mark J. Kransdorf, MD
Mayo Clinic
Department of Radiology
Jacksonville, FL

Jerzy Lasota, MD, PhD
Armed Forces Institute of Pathology
Department of Soft Tissue Pathology
Washington, DC

Mark D. Murphey, MD
Armed Forces Institute of Pathology
Department of Radiologic Pathology
Washington, DC
Uniformed Services University of the Health Sciences
Departments of Radiology and Nuclear Medicine
Bethesda, MD
University of Maryland School of Medicine
Department of Radiology
Baltimore, MD

David M. Parham, MD
Chief, Pediatric Pathology
Arkansas Children's Hospital
Department of Pathology
Vice-Chair, Pathology
University of Arkansas for Medical Sciences
Little Rock, AR

Van H. Savell, Jr., MD
Driscoll Children's Hospital
Department of Pathology
Corpus Christi, TX

Preface

This book is intended primarily for diagnostic, investigative and teaching pathologists, although those who review topics related to soft tissue tumor diagnosis, classification, and biology will also find it useful. The concept of soft tissue tumors is understood broadly here. Based on our experience in consultation practice, a wide variety of reactive and neoplastic lesions beyond sarcomas and other traditional soft tissue tumors can form a soft tissue mass. Therefore, this book also includes tumors such as metastatic melanomas, metastatic carcinomas, and hematopoietic and histiocytic processes.

The new understanding of tumor pathology provided by advances in genetics, molecular genetics, and tumor immunohistochemistry is covered in two dedicated chapters as well as integrated in other chapters where relevant. Many specific genetic alterations have become proven or provisional diagnostic markers. This knowledge can also have treatment implications, as has been seen recently with the gastrointestinal stromal tumors. Hopefully the day when our knowledge on specific pathogenesis may help in tumor prevention is not far off; this hope should be an encouragement for all of us to incorporate molecular medicine as a part of our practice.

The many contributions of the staff of the Department of Soft Tissue Pathology of the Armed Forces Institute of Pathology to this book are gratefully acknowledged. The expert advice and comments of Drs. Julie C. Fanburg-Smith and Jerzy Lasota, who also contributed chapters to the book, Drs. John F. Fetsch, Mohammad Nadjem, Sumitra Parekh, and Fabrizio Remotti are greatly appreciated. My thanks also go to Dr. Franz M. Enzinger, the Emeritus Chairman of our department, who continues to inspire all of us in the study of soft tissue tumors. I also want to thank the leadership of the Institute for creating a conducive and productive environment for studying the tumors in the context of modern medicine.

This book would not have been possible without an outstanding group of specialists who kindly contributed chapters to it. Drs. Mark Murphey, Mark Kransdorf, Van Savell, David Parham, and John K. C. Chan all made an outstanding effort to provide the best possible coverage of their topics. The photographic support of Anthony Shirley and the laboratory support of Virginia Achstetter and Wanda King are also greatly appreciated.

Finally, my sincerest thanks go to the editors Marc Strauss and Natasha Andjelkovic from Elsevier Science for their continuous encouragement and guidance, to Nancy Lombardi and Joan Sinclair for smooth editing and production, and to my family for their understanding and patience.

Markku Miettinen, MD

Contents

Overview of Soft Tissue Tumors

CHAPTER 1

Definition, classification, histogenesis, epidemiology, etiology, grading, staging, evaluation of soft tissue tumor specimen, tissue procurement for special studies, and electron microscopy are reviewed here. Radiologic evaluation, immunohistochemistry, and genetics are discussed separately (see Chapters 2, 3, and 4, respectively).

Definition

Soft tissue tumors are generally defined as tumors of connective tissues, and among cancers they include most nonosseous sarcomas. They are usually considered to include tumors of the extremities, trunk wall, intra-abdominal and intrathoracic space, and head and neck, although definitions vary. Generally excluded are nonmesenchymal tumors of the skin, cutaneous melanoma, most primary epithelial tumors, and brain and bone tumors.

In this book, the concept of soft tissue is understood broadly to include any important tumors of nonbony tissues of the extremities, trunk wall, retroperitoneum, mediastinum, and head and neck, except organ-specific tumors. However, gastrointestinal and gynecologic stromal tumors are included because similar tumors occur elsewhere in the abdomen. Metastatic epithelial tumors and melanoma are included because of their importance as soft tissue lesions (Table 1–1). As a subspecialty, soft tissue pathology has relations to almost every other subspecialty of pathology.

Classification

The purpose of classification is to link together similar tumors for creating an understanding of tumor behavior for treatment and follow-up and to help to investigate the biology of tumors. The ultimate goal is to discover the pathogenesis, devise biology-based treatments, and perhaps learn to prevent the tumors altogether.

Soft tissue tumors continue to be classified according to the cell type they resemble or have been thought to resemble. The clinical correlations already obtained by the present classifications are so numerous that the basis of this classification will probably remain, although it continues to be refined by cytogenetic, molecular genetic, and gene expression studies. However, reaching an ideal classification that would be simple, highly reproducible and clinically most informative at the same time is not easy for this complex group of tumors.

By tumor type, soft tissue tumors comprise a diverse group of benign, malignant, and borderline malignant (intermediate malignant) tumors. Most of them arise from (or show differentiation toward) mesenchymal cells, but some are of neuroectodermal (e.g., Schwann cell tumors), epithelial (metastatic carcinomas), or hematolymphatic (extranodal lymphoid and histiocytic infiltrates and lymphomas) origin (Table 1–2). The generally accepted basis for soft tissue tumor classification is the system of the World Health Organization.[1]

Table 1-1. A Definition/Summary of Soft Tissue Tumors

Primary tumors of different locations
Extremities
Trunk wall
External genitalia
Body cavities, including retroperitoneum and mediastinum
Head and neck
Mesenchymal tumors of the gastrointestinal tract
Other organ-based connective tissue tumors
Tumors of different categories
Benign mesenchymal tumors (e.g., lipoma)
Benign neuroectodermal tumors (e.g., neurofibroma)
Sarcomas
Metastatic carcinomas
Metastatic melanoma
Hematolymphatic neoplasms
Miscellaneous tumors and reactive conditions

Malignant mesenchymoma is the designation for a sarcoma that displays differentiation toward more than one specific line, except the fibroblastic one. This designation is rarely applied today because many tumors formerly classified as mesenchymoma are now preferably diagnosed as liposarcomas or nerve sheath tumors with heterologous differentiation.

Benign tumors generally show the greatest similarity to the normal cell counterparts. For example, lipoma is histologically indistinguishable from normal adipose tissue, and leiomyoma cells greatly resemble normal smooth muscle cells.

Sarcoma cells show varying resemblance to the normal cell types depending on their degree of differentiation. For example, well-differentiated liposarcoma cells greatly resemble fat cells, whereas pleomorphic ones contain more limited numbers of cells with specific fat differentiation. Some sarcoma types, such as synovial sarcoma, epithelioid sarcoma, and alveolar soft part sarcoma, do not have normal cell counterparts.

Histogenesis

According to the present understanding, all tumors are derived from multipotential precursor cells (stem cells) that are preprogrammed to differentiate into various mature cell types. The tumors do not arise of mature cells, such as skeletal muscle and mature adipocytes, because such cells are terminally differentiated and not capable of cellular division.

The preprogrammed nature of many stem cells explains why some sarcomas closely resemble the mature cell types. For example, the cells of leiomyosarcoma have a close similarity to smooth muscle cells. However, some tumors contain cellular components that have no resemblance to normal cell types of that location. For example, metaplastic or neoplastic cartilage components can be present in different sarcomas. Also, origin of benign rhabdomyoma as a polyp in the vaginal mucosa and rhabdomyosarcoma of the urinary bladder cannot be understood based on the normal cells types present in these locations.

The tissue origin of soft tissue stem cells is not fully clear. It seems likely that many of them come from the local, organ-specific pools of stem cells. However, new data indicate that some soft tissue components are replenished from stem cells of bone marrow origin; these cells could also be the origin for some soft tissue tumors. For example, some regenerating skeletal muscle cells have been shown to be of bone marrow origin,[2] and a portion of endothelial progenitor cells are of bone marrow origin.[3]

The histogenesis of sarcomas with no known normal cell counterparts may reflect the unique genetic makeup that has created unprecedented tumor phenotypes not comparable to those of any normal tissues.

Epidemiology

There were 8700 new cases of soft tissue sarcomas in the United States in 2001 (fewer than 1% of all cancers), and 4400 people died of these tumors, according to the American Cancer Society estimates.[4] However, the total incidence of sarcomas is higher and may be close to double, if organ-based tumors are included; in the current statistics they are pooled together with carcinomas in organ-specific locations. Many sarcomas are more common in men, although leiomyosarcomas more often occur in women.

Sarcomas are rare tumors, and their incidence is only about 5% of that of each of the most common carcinomas (prostate, breast, and lung), half of that of brain tumors, and similar to that of acute myeloid leukemia.[4] The relative rarity of soft tissue sarcomas may be explained by the location of the mesenchymal cells behind protective epithelial barriers.

Based on the preceding data, the approximate incidence of sarcomas in the United States is approximately 3.3/100,000, similar to that obtained in the Survey of Epidemiology and End Results (SEERS)

Table 1-2. Simplified Chart of the Major Types of Primary Soft Tissue Tumors (Grouped According to the Cell Types They Resemble)

Cell Type	Benign Tumor*	Malignant Tumor
Fibroblast, including myofibroblast	Fibroma, myxoma	Fibrosarcoma, malignant fibrous histiocytoma
Adipocyte	Lipoma	Liposarcoma
Smooth muscle cell	Leiomyoma	Leiomyosarcoma
Skeletal muscle cell	Rhabdomyoma	Rhabdomyosarcoma
Endothelial cell	Hemangioma	Angiosarcoma, Kaposi sarcoma
Schwann cell	Schwannoma, neurofibroma	Some malignant peripheral nerve sheath tumors
Cartilage cell	Chondroma	Chondrosarcoma
Interstitial cell of Cajal of intestines	Gastrointestinal stromal tumors (benign and malignant)	
Histiocyte	Juvenile xanthogranuloma Tenosynovial giant cell tumor? Rosai-Dorfman disease	True histiocytic lymphoma (sarcoma)
Lymphoid cells	Benign lymphoid hyperplasia	Extranodal lymphomas in soft tissues
No known normal cell or benign counterparts		Ewing family tumors Synovial sarcoma Epithelioid sarcoma Alveolar soft part sarcoma

*Intermediate categories between benign and malignant tumors are excluded for simplicity.

program based on a sample population of the United States, where the overall incidence of soft tissue sarcomas was approximately 4/100,000 if excluding Kaposi sarcoma.[5] According to the SEERS data, the incidence of soft tissue sarcomas has increased from the 1960s, although some studies have attributed this increase solely to Kaposi sarcoma epidemics.[6]

Global differences in sarcoma incidence may exist according to data from different cancer registries. For example, the incidence per 100,000 was only 0.8 in Osaka, Japan, 1.4 in Bombay, India, and 2.4 in Shanghai, China.[7] These figures are less than reported for United States and Europe, where the incidence is between 3 and 4/100,000. Moderate male predominance of soft tissue sarcoma patients is shown by all registries;[7] however, some specific tumor types have a female predominance. The apparent variances in incidence may result from differences in diagnosis and classification.

Like most other cancers, the majority of soft tissue sarcomas occur in older adults, who have higher age-specific incidence of these tumors.[7,8] However, important subgroups of soft tissue tumors occur predominantly or exclusively in children (neuroblastoma, embryonal rhabdomyosarcoma, angiomatoid fibrous histiocytoma) and young adults (Ewing family tumors, alveolar rhabdomyosarcoma, and synovial sarcoma).

The incidence of benign soft tissue tumors is impossible to accurately determine, because benign tumors are underrepresented in hospital materials and are generally not included in tumor registries. However, as surgical specimens, benign soft tissue tumors outnumber the malignant ones at least by a margin of 100:1.

Etiology

The etiologic agents for soft tissue sarcomas are relatively poorly understood and apply only to a small portion of these tumors, much less than for many other cancers that are more clearly related to environmental carcinogenesis, for example, lung cancer.

The known etiologic factors for soft tissue sarcomas most importantly include ionizing radiation, oncogenic viruses, and chemicals. The role of trauma is questionable although anecdotal cases seem to support it.

All tumors are believed to arise as a result of acquired genetic alterations that lead to abnormal quality or quantity of proteins that control the cellular proliferation and differentiation. The known etiologic environmental factors, radiation, certain viruses, and chemicals, are known as capable of causing genetic alterations that can lead to tumorigenesis.

A small percentage of sarcomas arise on the basis of host factors. Among them, the most important are hereditary genetic alterations (tumor syndromes), of which the most common by far is neurofibromatosis type 1 (see Chapters 4 and 15). Rarely, other host factors are involved, such as immunosuppression and chronic lymphedema.

Radiation

Radiation-induced sarcomas develop in a small minority of patients (<1%) who have undergone therapeutic irradiation, typically 5 to 10 or more years after the radiation. Such postirradiation sarcomas most commonly include undifferentiated tumor types such as fibrosarcomas and malignant fibrous histiocytoma (MFH) and osteosarcoma and rarely angiosarcoma and malignant peripheral nerve sheath tumors (MPNSTs).[9–11] The most common scenarios of postirradiation sarcoma are lower abdominal wall and pelvic tumors of women treated for gynecologic cancer, and sarcomas in the chest wall in women having radiation for breast carcinoma.

Thorotrast, colloidal thorium-oxide containing radioactive radiologic contrast medium, was used until the 1940s, especially for angiographic studies. This material was permanently deposited to the reticuloendothelial cell system, especially in the liver, and some patients subsequently developed angiosarcoma of the liver or more commonly hepatic carcinoma or leukemia.[12]

Viruses

Oncogenic viruses introduce new genomic material, which encode for oncogenic proteins that disrupt the regulation of cellular proliferation. These genes are read and proteins made by the host, on which the viruses parasitize. Two DNA viruses have been linked to specific types of soft tissue sarcomas: human herpesvirus 8 (HHV8) to Kaposi sarcoma,[13] and Epstein-Barr virus (EBV) to certain leiomyosarcomas.[14] In both instances, the virus-sarcoma connection is more common in immunosuppressed patients.

Most if not all Kaposi sarcomas contain HHV8 sequences. This gammaherpesvirus is parenterally or sexually transmitted and is believed to be etiologically significant for the development of Kaposi sarcoma and explaining its epidemic nature in populations infected with human immunodeficiency virus (HIV) and higher prevalence in populations with higher prevalence of HHV8 infection.[13]

The EBV-associated leiomyosarcomas occur in immunodeficient or immunosuppressed patients, especially in children with HIV infection. Some have been seen in patients under chronic medically induced immunosuppression.[14]

Chemicals

Epidemiologic studies have linked phenoxyacetic acid herbicides to increased incidence of peripheral soft tissue sarcomas in some studies, although others have not confirmed this association. The carcinogenicity of these herbicides has been suspected to have resulted from dioxins that have been present as impurities in some commercial preparations of 2,4,5-T ("agent orange") and MCPA phenoxyherbicides.[5]

Sarcomas have developed around permanently retained metal objects, such as shrapnel and implanted surgical devices. These tumors have been mainly angiosarcomas and malignant fibrous histiocytomas.[15] Experimental studies support the capability of implanted metal or plastic objects to cause sarcomas. Several types of plastics and metals chronically implanted in tissues were shown to induce local formation of a sarcoma, most commonly MFH or fibrosarcoma in rats. Proliferative mesenchymal lesions possibly representing preneoplastic changes were also observed.[16]

Epidemiologic studies have failed to show association of soft tissue sarcomas with smoking, alcohol use, and exposure to organic solvents.[5,8]

Hepatic angiosarcoma is an exceptional sarcoma, which more commonly than any other sarcoma is associated with specific chemical agents. According to a large epidemiologic study, such factors were present in approximately 25% of patients with these sarcomas, and included vinyl chloride (used in plastic manufacturing), inorganic arsenic (used as a pesticide or historically as a syphilis medicine), Thorotrast, and androgenic anabolic steroids, the latter used medicinally or for doping purposes.[17]

Host Factors

Immunosuppression is known to be associated with sarcomas with viral connection, but it may also cause other sarcomas, although less commonly than observed for non-Hodgkin lymphomas.[5] Hereditary or acquired (infection-associated or iatrogenic) lymphedema is a rare cause for extremity-based angiosarcomas, of which postmastectomy angiosarcoma in the lymphedematous arm is the most common example.

Grading

The grade is an arbitrary estimate for the degree of malignancy. The grading of soft tissue sarcomas by histologic parameters is to provide guidance for prognostic prediction and treatment, especially in relation to the need for adjuvant therapy. Important other factors independent of grade are tumor size, completeness of the surgical excision, and the overall clinical situation.

In general, low-grade sarcomas are locally aggressive but have a very low metastatic potential and generally good prognosis. Consequently, they are usually treated with a wide surgical excision whenever possible. High-grade sarcomas have a high risk for both local recurrence and metastasis, and radiation and chemotherapy are used as adjuvant or as the main mode of treatment for some high-grade tumors (especially childhood rhabdomyosarcoma, Ewing family tumors) and as a possible adjuvant therapy for adult soft tissue sarcomas.

Grading is also an element in the current staging systems. None of the grading systems replace histologic typing, which is of great importance whenever type can be specified. In fact, the prevalent grading systems include histologic type as a grading variable. Two excellent reviews on sarcoma grading are recommended.[18,19]

Table 1–3. Grading System* of the French Federation of Cancer Centers

	Score
Tumor differentiation (per Table 1–4)	1–3
Well-differentiated tumors	1
Defined histogenetic types	2
Poorly differentiated tumors and undefined histogenetic types	3
Mitotic count	
0–9/10 HPF	1
10–19/10 HPF	2
≥20/20 HPF	3
Tumor necrosis	
None	0
<50%	1
>50%	2
Histologic grade	Sum of the preceding scores
1	2 or 3
2	4 or 5
3	6, 7, or 8

*This grading system formulates the overall grade based on total points of scores from tumor differentiation, mitotic rate, and tumor necrosis.
HPF, high power field.
(Based on Guillou et al.[22])

Grading Systems

The most extensively documented and widely used grading system for adult soft tissue sarcomas is the one developed by the French Federation of Cancer Centers (FFCC).[20–22] This grading system has been evolving during the past 15 years and has been specifically validated for spindle cell sarcomas.[21] This system uses the parameters of tumor differentiation, necrosis, and mitotic activity; the two latter parameters were used differently in the previously introduced grading system of the National Cancer Institute.[23] A comparative study suggested that the FFCC system may result in a more informative grade, a higher number of high-grade tumors, a lesser number of intermediate-grade tumors, and a higher prognostic predictive value.[22]

The current FFCC system is based on score points obtained as a sum of three factors: differentiation, mitotic rate, and tumor necrosis (Table 1–3). Each soft tissue sarcoma type has a differentiation score assigned based on the histologic type (Table 1–4). In some cases, the assignment is subjective, for example, when based on identification of "conventional" examples of certain tumor types.

The Pediatric Oncology Group grading system is applicable to nonrhabdomyosarcomatous soft tissue sarcomas of children. It significantly relies on the histologic type as the basis of the grade, especially for the low-grade (grade 1) and high-grade (grade 3) tumors. It also incorporates necrosis and mitotic activity as grading parameters for some histologic types.[24] This system has been summarized in Table 1–5.

A four-tiered system dividing both low- and high-grade tumors into two grades has also been suggested.[25] Another grading system was suggested mainly based on mitotic activity.[26]

Limitations of Grading

The grading applies best to an excision specimen. Limited sampling (e.g., needle biopsy) can give a minimum grade only. Preoperative treatments, such as radiation, chemotherapy, and embolization commonly induce tumor necrosis and variable tumor abolition and can make grading inapplicable.

Table 1–4. Tumor Differentiation Score (According to the Updated Version of the French Federation of Cancer Centers Grading System)

- Differentiation score 1
  - Well-differentiated sarcoma (fibro-, lipo-, leiomyo-, chondro-)
  - Well-differentiated MPNST (neurofibroma with malignant transformation)
- Differentiation score 2
  - Conventional fibrosarcoma
  - Myxoid sarcomas (MFH, liposarcoma, chondrosarcoma)
  - Storiform-pleomorphic MFH
  - Conventional leiomyosarcoma
  - Conventional angiosarcoma
  - Conventional MPNST
- Differentiation score 3
  - Poorly differentiated fibrosarcoma
  - Giant cell and inflammatory MFH
  - Round cell liposarcoma
  - Pleomorphic sarcomas (liposarcoma, leiomyosarcoma)
  - Rhabdomyosarcoma (except spindle cell and botryoid)
  - Poorly differentiated and epithelioid angiosarcoma
  - Triton tumor, epithelioid MPNST
  - Extraskeletal mesenchymal chondrosarcoma
  - Osteosarcoma
  - Ewing family tumors
  - Synovial sarcoma
  - Clear cell sarcoma
  - Epithelioid sarcoma
  - Alveolar soft part sarcoma
  - Malignant rhabdoid tumor
  - Undifferentiated sarcoma

(Modified from Guillou et al.[22])

Table 1–5. The Pediatric Oncology Group Grading System for Nonrhabdomyosarcomatous Soft Tissue Sarcomas of Children

- Grade 1
  - Dermatofibrosarcoma protuberans, deep
  - Infantile fibrosarcoma, well-differentiated (children not over age 4 years)
  - Infantile hemangiopericytoma, well-differentiated
  - Well-differentiated and myxoid liposarcoma
  - Well-differentiated MPNST
  - Extraskeletal myxoid chondrosarcoma
  - Angiomatoid (malignant) fibrous histiocytoma
- Grade 2
  - Sarcomas not included in grades 1 and 3 with <15% of necrosis with no more than 5 mitoses/10 HPF
  - No marked atypia, no markedly high cellularity
  - Includes noninfantile fibrosarcomas, poorly differentiated infantile fibrosarcomas, leiomyosarcomas, and MPNSTs fitting these criteria
- Grade 3
  - Round cell and pleomorphic liposarcoma
  - Mesenchymal chondrosarcoma
  - Extrasekeletal osteosarcoma
  - Malignant Triton tumor
  - Alveolar soft part sarcoma
  - Sarcomas not included in grade 1 with >15% of necrosis, or with over 5 mitoses/10 HPF

Marked atypia and cellularity may also result in assignment into grade 3.

HPF, high power field.
(Modified and adapted from Parham et al.[24])

The impact of histologic grading is diluted by the nearly automatic high-grade assignment for some tumor types, because all examples of such entities would result in a high-grade scoring, and lack of grading principles for some tumor types, as pointed out by the Association of Directors of Anatomic and Surgical Pathology.[27] Even the best grading systems include an element of subjectivity in the assessment of tumor differentiation, mitosis counting, and evaluation of the amount of necrosis. The reliability of grading is likely greater for the more common tumor types, and, conversely, the grading systems for rare tumor types have been often assessed for a very limited number of cases. Clinicopathologic analyses of large series of all specific sarcoma types should be performed to specifically validate grading for these tumors.

Staging

The stage is an estimate for the extent or dissemination of tumor, and in the current system includes tumor grade as a component. Stage is an important characterization of a tumor for formulation of the treatment, cooperative clinical trials, and clinicopathologic studies on tumor behavior. It is based on clinical and radiologic evaluation of the tumor. There is an illustrative review on sarcoma staging systems.[28]

The most widely used staging system is the Union Internationale Contre le Cancer (UICC) tumor-node-metastasis (TNM) system,[29] whose current version has merged with the American Joint Committee of Cancer staging system.[30] These two identical systems classify the tumors into stages I to IV where a low stage represents a small local tumor and stage IV metastatic disease (Table 1–6). All low-grade tumors are stage IA or IB depending on the tumor size. Nonmetastatic high-grade tumors are divided into stages II and III, where the latter is assigned to deep large tumors (>5 cm). This system excludes visceral sarcomas and certain cutaneous tumors such as Kaposi sarcoma and dermatofibrosarcoma protuberans. Also angiosarcoma has been excluded because its common multifocal nature makes the evaluation of size and metastasis problematic.

The current UICC-TNM staging system has developed on the basis of previous systems, especially the one originally suggested by the task force on Soft Tissue Sarcoma of the American Joint Committee for Cancer Staging and End Results Reporting.[31] This system incorporated histologic grade into the final stage and was based on evaluation of 1215 cases of 13 types of soft tissue sarcomas, mainly from the extremities. The study documented the value of stage toward prediction of survival.[31]

The surgical staging system developed by Enneking and colleagues[32] is mainly applicable to extremity sarcomas. Like UICC-TNM, it also incorporates grade as a factor, but it subdivides the stages by the relationship of the tumor to the compartments of the extremities, instead of tumor size. In this system, low-grade tumors are stage I, high-grade nonmetastatic tumors are stage II, and metastatic tumors are stage III. Further summary on the radiologic aspects of staging systems is shown in Chapter 2.

Evaluation of Soft Tissue Tumor Specimen

The nature of a specimen varies from punch and needle biopsies to open biopsies, piecemeal excisions, and complete resection specimens.

Table 1–6. Summary of the Current TNM or the American Joint Committee for Cancer Staging System for Soft Tissue Sarcomas

Stage	Histologic Grade (G)	Primary Tumor	Lymph Node Status (N)	Distant Metastasis (M)
I–IV	*Low or High*	*T1 or T2*	*Negative/Positive*	*Absent/Present*
IA	Low	T1a or T1b	Negative	Absent
IB	Low	T2a or T 2b	Negative	Absent
IIA	High	T1a or T1b	Negative	Absent
IIB	High	T2a	Negative	Absent
III	High	T2b	Negative	Absent
IV	Any	Any	Positive	Absent
	Any	Any	Negative or positive	Present

Grade (G): An arbitrary determination based on current grading systems. In a three-tier system, intermediate grade (G 2 of 3) is merged with high grade.

T Maximum diameter of tumor T1 = ≤5 cm T2 = >5 cm

Tumors of each T group are subclassified based on depth or anatomic location or both:
- a = Superficial tumors of the trunk and extremities not invading the superficial fascia
- b = Deep tumors invading, permeating, or located below the superficial fascia, or tumors in intra-abdominal, retroperitoneal, and intrathoracic location

(Modified from Sobin and Wittekind.[29])

A trend toward minimally invasive diagnostic procedures has led to an increased volume of small specimens, such as needle biopsies. Diagnostic specimens from internal sites, such as intra-abdominal and intrathoracic tumors, are commonly needle biopsies. Ultrasound or other radiologically guided procedures have increased the accuracy of lesional sampling.

Definitive diagnosis and tumor typing is variably successful on needle biopsies. Abdominal tumors that can often be reliably diagnosed on needle biopsy include diffuse large cell lymphoma, well-differentiated liposarcoma, leiomyosarcoma, gastrointestinal stromal tumor, schwannoma, and solitary fibrous tumor. However, a small biopsy cannot rule out a malignant or high-grade component and can underestimate the potential of the tumor. Definitive diagnosis of reactive conditions and low-grade lymphomas is often impossible.

Open Biopsy and Resection Specimen

Ideally, all tumor specimens should be received fresh immediately from the surgery without fixation because this increases the options for special studies and scientific evaluation. However, needle biopsies may be exempted, because the material is limited and optimal fixation may be best ensured if the biopsy is immediately placed in the fixative.

Steps that can be taken for the comprehensive analysis of a soft tissue tumor are listed in Table 1–7. These steps depend on the clinical environment and the scope of the studies planned in the future. High-quality clinicopathologic evaluation with thorough gross description, evaluation of margins, and histologic sampling has to be performed in every case.

If the diagnosis is unknown when the specimen is received, frozen section is useful for triage purposes to guide the pathologist to the optimal selection of special studies. In some centers, frozen section is also used as a primary diagnostic mode and can be highly accurate with a large volume of tumors and experienced pathology staff.

Grossing

Small specimens should usually be inked universally and large specimens selectively in the areas closest to the tumor. Then the specimen should be sliced with 1-cm intervals and the tumor measured in three dimensions. The margins are usually best evaluated by sections perpendicular to specimen surface closest to the tumor. Possible satellite nodules outside the main tumor mass should also be recorded. The percentage of gross necrosis should be estimated. Other features to be recorded include color, consistency, and the presence of hemorrhage, calcification, ossification, cysts, and grossly different tumor components. Representative sections should be documented and sampled for microscopy, and small tumors should be submitted entirely (1–2 cm or less). A minimum sampling should include 1 section per each 1 cm of tumor diameter, unless the tumor is very large (>20 cm, in which case half of that is sufficient). Photocopying the tumor slices (with plastic protective sheet) gives a documentation of tumor measurements and allows for annotation of histologic sampling.

A peculiar diagnostic pitfall is missing a lipomatous component in dedifferentiated liposarcoma; therefore surrounding fat should be included in sampling of a sarcoma, especially of a retroperitoneal one.

Although smaller tumors can be submitted for tissue processing the same day the specimen is received, larger tumors and all lipomatous tumors should be

Table 1–7. Steps and Parameters in a Comprehensive Analysis of a Soft Tissue Tumor Specimen

Gross examination
1. Gross photography (preferably fresh tissue, possibly also fixed)
2. Evaluation and inking of margins
3. Gross description and tumor measurements
4. Sampling of tumor and margins for histology (perpendicular recommended)
5. Frozen section for diagnostic or triaging purposes

Sampling of fresh tissue for further analysis*
1. Frozen tissue procurement (frozen, in special preservatives) for RNA, DNA, fluorescence in situ hybridization, proteomics, chemical, and immunohistochemical analysis
   Formalin-fixation of adjacent tissues for morphologic documentation of the selections
2. Submission of material for cytogenetics or assessment of chemosensitivity for initiation of a short-term cell culture and a possible continuous cell line
3. Sampling in special fixatives (alcohol, Carnoy's B5) for further studies
4. Sampling for glutaraldehyde fixation for electron microscopy

*Fresh tissue sampling should be performed as soon as possible, preferably first.

allowed to fix overnight to improve tissue processing and quality of tissue sections.

Gross Photography

This is an excellent permanent document of the tumor. The ideal photographic documentation includes intact and sliced tumor with overview and close-up views, some of them with a metric scale.

Reporting

As suggested by the Association of the Directors of Anatomic and Surgical Pathology,[27] the surgical pathology report should accurately document the tumor site, histologic type, grade, tumor size, status or margins, percentage of necrosis, lymph node status, and a number of other factors (Table 1–8).

Tissue Procurement for Special Studies

This is an important part of specimen handling, especially in academic centers, and can usually be easily accommodated without interfering with the diagnostic sampling and evaluation of the margins. It not only relates to scientific studies but also allows for the optimal use of advanced diagnostic modalities.

Table 1–8. Suggested Parameters to Be Included in the Surgical Pathology Report of a Sarcoma

Final report

1. Tumor site, type of excision
2. Depth of the tumor
3. Tumor type, possibly variant
4. Grade, if possible
5. Tumor size (maximum diameter in cm), plus possible presence of satellite nodules
6. Status of margins (minimal distance to margins) and lymph node status if present
7. Microscopic quantitation of necrosis
8. Vascular invasion (if present)

Addendum report or reports (if studies cannot be completed by the issue of final report)

1. Immunohistochemistry
2. Electron microscopy
3. Cytogenetics

(Modified and adapted from parameters suggested by the Association of the Directors of Anatomic and Surgical Pathology.[27])

Frozen Tissue

Freezing of tissue is clinically indicated to help more easily or reliable perform molecular genetic assays, and it is also scientifically indicated to build the knowledge on genetic and biochemical changes in tumors, in comparison to normal tissue.

Frozen tissue is required for optimal and more effective analysis of nucleic acids. High-molecular-weight DNA and RNA can be generally obtained only from fresh and not from formaldehyde-fixed tissue. Similarly, native proteins can be reliably obtained only from fresh or frozen tissue for proteomics, biochemical microanalysis of the spectrum of cell signaling, and other functionally important proteins.

Freezing in liquid nitrogen is optimal, and long term storage in −70°C freezer or liquid nitrogen are both adequate, but well-organized storage compartments and accounting systems are required for optimal retrieval. Liquid nitrogen storage has the advantage of being independent of electric power and protects the tissue bank from power outages. For liquid nitrogen tanks, automatic refilling systems are available.

Ideally, aliquots of both tumor and normal tissue should be sampled separately. The best way to store the tissue is to freeze small pieces separately in liquid nitrogen bath, and transfer them to the cryovial (allowing the nitrogen to evaporate in −20°C cryostate to prevent cap-popping of the vial). Such separately frozen "pearls" of tissue are easy to pour out from the cryovial and use one at the time or as needed.

Cytogenetics and Cell Culture

Cytogenetic studies are diagnostically indicated in tumors with specific translocations or other chromosomal morphologic changes (see Chapter 4). They are also indicated scientifically to build knowledge on previously uncharacterized tumor types.

Cytogenetic specimens can be sent to the laboratory in a culture medium and should be preserved in a sterile manner. A very thin slice of well-preserved, nonnecrotic tumor tissue should be submitted.

Short-term cultures needed for karyotyping are obtained with a high success rate of malignant tumors, but benign tumors may be difficult to grow. Such cultures can also be used for in vitro testing of chemosensitivity of a tumor.

Long-term cultures and establishing a cell line from a tumor are more challenging and the success rate is only modest, even with highly experienced investigators. However, long-term cultures offer priceless dynamic models for investigating cell biologic, biochemical, and pharmacologic characteristics of the tumor.

Special Fixatives

Fixation in special fixatives is often indicated in the optimal evaluation of tumors expected to be diagnostically problematic.

The tissue aliquots should have small dimensions, not exceeding the thickness of a standard coin to allow the penetration of the fixative prior to autolysis.

Alcohol (absolute ethanol)-fixed tissue can be saved for further studies, such as RNA, DNA, and protein extraction or they can be embedded in paraffin for tissue section-based studies. Alcohol-fixed tissue may be advantageous for immunohistochemical analysis of some antigens. It may also be suitable for Western blotting analysis of proteins and obtaining high-molecular-weight nucleic acids.

Carnoy's fixative is a modified alcohol fixation, added with glacial acetic acid in a ratio of 1:4. Methacarn is an alcoholic fixative where methanol is used instead of ethanol.

Heavy metal-containing formalin fixative (B5 solution containing mercury chloride) yields superior nuclear detail and is often used for hematopoietic neoplasia. Zinc salts can be used for a similar purpose as less toxic and more environmentally friendly alternatives.

A small aliquot of viable tumor, or if necessary, samples of several different areas should be sampled in 2.5% buffered glutaraldehyde for electron microscopy. The easiest way to prepare a sample is to first cut a thin slice, then section this further to a rod, and then mince this to cubes not exceeding 1 mm in greatest dimension.

Electron Microscopy

Electron microscopy is very rarely mandatory, but it can add diagnostic information and should be part of tissue procurement program in unusual tumors. The processed tissue may be saved for future studies, if analysis is not desired for immediate diagnostic use. The most fruitful applications of electron microscopy are on those soft tissue tumors that have highly distinctive ultrastructural features (Table 1–9).

The ultrastructural details at a magnification ranging from 3000 to 50,000 can give valuable diagnostic information for selected soft tissue tumors.[33,34]

Table 1–9. Frequent Distinctive Electron Microscopic Findings in Selected Soft Tissue Tumors

Tumor Type	Diagnostic Features
Fibroblastic neoplasms	Variable myofibroblastic differentiation found in subsets of tumor cells
Desmoid, fibrosarcoma, MFH	Fibroblast-like cells with scattered bundles of actin filaments
Smooth muscle tumors, glomus tumor	Cytoplasmic bundles of actin filaments, attachment plaques, basal lamina
Rhabdomyosarcoma	Ribosome myosin complexes, collections of thin and thick filaments, possible sarcomeres and Z-bands
Angiosarcoma	Weibel-Palade bodies (predominantly in well-differentiated tumor cells)
Schwannoma	Spindle cells, complex interdigitating cell processes, and prominent basal laminas
Perineurial cell tumors	Spindle cell with long cytoplasmic processes, prominent intermediate filaments, frequent pinocytic vesicles, basal laminas
Melanoma	Melanosomes. Can be sparse and difficult to find in some melanomas
Paraganglioma	Dense core granules of variable size and morphology, typically abundant
Neuroendocrine carcinoma	Membrane bound dense core granules of 100–400 nm in diameter, typically abundant
Rhabdoid tumor, sarcomas with rhabdoid cytologic features	Spherical collections of cytoplasmic intermediate filaments displacing the cytoplasmic organelles
Alveolar soft part sarcoma	Cytoplasmic rhomboid crystals with 70 Å periodicity
Mesothelioma, differentiated	Long, slender microvilli that are typically 15 times longer than their width
Dendritic reticulum cell sarcoma	Desmosomes

However, for many groups of tumors, such as lymphomas, melanoma, and undifferentiated tumors, immunohistochemistry has largely replaced electron microscopy as a diagnostic method, and for others it is only infrequently used because of its labor-intense nature and cost.

Although glutaraldehyde fixation is optimal for preserving the cytoplasmic details, fixation in buffered formalin is also adequate. However, cytoplasmic texture and many membranous structures deteriorate during routine formalin-fixation and can be lost during tissue processing and paraffin embedding.

Currently electron microscopy is extensively practiced by a small group of dedicated investigators who continue to make interesting ultrastructural observations related to tumor cell differentiation and histogenesis.

REFERENCES

1. Weiss SW, Sobin LH: Histological Typing of Soft Tissue Tumors, 2nd ed. WHO Histological Classification of Tumors. Berlin, Springer Verlag, 1994.
2. Ferrari G, Cusella-De Angelis G, Coletta M, et al: Muscle regeneration by bone marrow-derived myogenic progenitors. Science 1998;279:1528–1530.
3. Asahara T, Masuda H, Takahashi T, et al: Bone marrow origin of endothelial progenitor cells responsible for postnatal vasculogenesis in physiological and pathological neovascularization. Circ Res 1999;85: 221–228.
4. Greenlee RT, Hill-Harmon MB, Murray T, Thun M: Cancer statistics, 2001. CA Cancer J Clin 2001;51:15–36.
5. Zahm SH, Fraumeni JF: The epidemiology of soft tissue sarcoma. Semin Oncol 197:24:504–514.
6. Ross JA, Severson RK, Davis S, Brooks JJ: Trends in the incidence of soft tissue sarcomas in the United States from 1973 through 1987. Cancer 1993;72:486–490.
7. Clemente C, Orazi A, Rilke F: The Italian registry of soft tissue tumors. Appl Pathol 1988;6:221–240.
8. Olsson H: A review of the epidemiology of soft tissue sarcoma. Acta Orthop Scand (suppl 285) 1999;70: 8–19.
9. Laskin WB, Silverman TA, Enzinger FM: Postirradiation soft tissue sarcomas. An analysis of 53 cases. Cancer 1988;62:2230–2240.
10. Wiklund TA, Blomqvist CP, Raty J, Elomaa I, Rissanen P, Miettinen M: Postirradiation sarcoma. Analysis of a nationwide cancer registry material. Cancer 1991;68: 524–531.
11. Mark RJ, Poen J, Tran LM, Fu YS, Selch MT, Parker RG: Postirradiation sarcomas. A single-institution study and review of the literature. Cancer 1994;73:2653–2662.
12. Stover BJ: Effect of Thorothrast in humans. Health Phys 1983;44(suppl 1):253–257.
13. Boshoff C, Chang Y: Kaposi's sarcoma-associated herpesvirus: A new DNA tumor virus. Annu Rev Med 2001; 52:453–470.
14. Hsu JL, Glaser SL: Epstein-Barr virus-associated malignancies: Epidemiologic patterns and etiologic implications. Crit Rev Oncol Hematol 2000;34:27–53.
15. Jennings TA, Peterson L, Axiotis CA, Friedlaender GE, Cooke RA, Rosai J: Angiosarcoma associated with foreign body material. A report of three cases. Cancer 1988;62:2436–2444.
16. Kirkpatrick CJ, Alves A, Köhler H, et al: Biomaterial-induced sarcoma. A novel model to study preneoplastic change. Am J Pathol 2000;156:1455–1467.
17. Falk H, Thomas LB, Popper H, Ishak KG: Hepatic angiosarcoma associated with androgenic-anabolic steroids. Lancet 1979;2:1120–1123.
18. Kilpatrick SE: Histologic prognostication in soft tissue sarcomas: Grading versus subtyping or both? A comprehensive review of the literature with proposed practical guidelines. Ann Diagn Pathol 1999;3:48–61.
19. Oliveira AM, Nascimento AG: Grading in soft tissue tumors: Principles and problems. Skeletal Radiol 2001; 30:543–559.
20. Trojani M, Contesso G, Coindre JM, et al: Soft-tissue sarcomas of adults: Study of pathological prognostic variables and definition of a histopathological grading system. Int J Cancer 1984;33:37–42.
21. Coindre JM, Bui NB, Bonichon F, de Mascarel I, Trojani M: Histopathologic grading in spindle cell soft tissue sarcomas. Cancer 1988;61:2305–2309.
22. Guillou L, Coindre JM, Bonichon F, et al: Comparative study of the National Cancer Institute and French Federation of Cancer Centers Sarcoma Group grading systems in a population of 410 adult patients with soft tissue sarcoma. J Clin Oncol 1997;15:350–362.
23. Costa J, Wesley RA, Glatstein E, Rosenberg SA: The grading of soft tissue sarcomas. Results of a clinicohistopathologic correlation in a series of 163 cases. Cancer 1984;53:530–541.
24. Parham DM, Webber BL, Jenkins JJ, Cantor AB, Maurer HM: Nonrhabdomyosarcomatous soft tissue sarcomas of childhood: Formulation of a simplified system for grading. Mod Pathol 1995;8:705–710.
25. Markhede G, Angervall L, Stener B: A multivariate analysis of the prognosis after surgical treatment of malignant soft tissue tumors. Cancer 1982;49:1721–1733.
26. Myhre-Jensen O, Kaae S, Madsen EH, Sneppen O: Histopathological grading in soft tissue tumours. Relation to survival in 261 surgically treated patients. Acta Pathol Microbiol Scand A 1983;91:145–150.
27. Association of the directors of anatomic and surgical pathology: Recommendations for the reporting of soft tissue sarcomas. Mod Pathol 1998;11:1257–1260.
28. Peabody TD, Gibbs CP, Simon MA: Evaluation and staging of musculoskeletal neoplasms. J Bone Joint Surg 1998;80A:1204–1218.
29. Sobin LH, Wittekind C: TNM classification of malignant tumors. UICC, Wiley-Liss, 2002.
30. Greene FL, Page D, Morrow M, Balch C, Haller D, Fritz A, Fleming I, eds. AJCC Cancer Staging Manual, 6th ed. New York, Springer, 2002.
31. Russell WO, Cohen J, Enzinger F, Hajdu SI, et al: A clinical and pathological staging system for soft tissue sarcomas. Cancer 1977;40:1562–1570.

32. Enneking WF, Spanier SS, Goodman MA: A system for the surgical staging of musculoskeletal tumors. Orthop Rel Res 1980;153:106–120.
33. Erlandson RA, Woodruff JM: Role of electron microscopy in the evaluation of soft tissue neoplasms, with emphasis on spindle cell and pleomorphic tumors. Hum Pathol 1998;29:1372–1981.
34. Ordonez MG, Mackay B: Electron microscopy in tumor diagnosis: Indications for its use in the immunohistochemical era. Hum Pathol 1998;29:1403–1411.

Mark D. Murphey
Mark J. Kransdorf

Radiologic Evaluation of Soft Tissue Tumors

CHAPTER 2

Introduction

The ultimate goal of imaging of soft tissue tumors remains threefold: (1) detecting lesions, (2) identifying a specific diagnosis or reasonable differential diagnosis, and (3) staging lesions. The radiologic evaluation of soft tissue tumors to achieve these goals has markedly evolved, improved, and expanded with the advent of computed tomography (CT) and magnetic resonance imaging (MRI). Indeed, CT and, particularly more recently, MRI allow lesion detection and staging by delineating anatomic extent in essentially all cases and relatively specific diagnosis in approximately 25% to 50% of soft tissue tumors.[1–7] We would suggest that evaluation of soft tissue tumors is now similar to bone tumors in that pathologic diagnosis should incorporate the imaging findings in the vast majority of cases. This is particularly true in large tumors where only a small amount of tissue may be available for histologic review initially and the question arises as to the true representation of the entire lesion. Also similar to bone tumors, this requires a close working relationship among three groups of physicians: the pathologist, the radiologist, and the orthopedic oncologist. The purpose of this chapter is to provide a framework for the use of radiologic evaluation of soft tissue tumors. Although our approach reviews multiple imaging modalities, we emphasize MRI because it is generally considered the optimal radiologic tool in evaluation of soft tissue tumors.

The annual incidence of benign soft tissue tumors has been estimated at 300/100,000 people leading to an estimated 750,000 to 800,000 lesions in the United States.[8,9] Thus, benign soft tissue tumors are relatively common lesions and outnumber malignant soft tissue tumors by a ratio of 100 to 150:1.[8,9] Soft tissue sarcomas are relatively infrequent, although increasing in incidence, representing approximately 1% of all malignant tumors.[10,11] The American Cancer Society figures of 2000 reveal 8100 soft tissue malignancies annually in the United States accounting for 4100 deaths.[12]

Radiologic Evaluation

In our opinion, the radiologic evaluation of a soft tissue tumor should *always* begin with radiographs. Although not helpful in a high percentage of lesions, certain features may be diagnostic and more difficult to appreciate on advanced imaging (CT and MRI). Unfortunately, in this age of "high tech" imaging this simple inexpensive step is frequently forgotten and may lead to disastrous results. Radiographs may reveal that an apparent soft tissue mass is related to an underlying osseous lesion such as an osteochondroma or posttraumatic deformity. Calcification of a soft tissue mass significantly restricts reasonable diagnostic considerations and may be pathognomonic in hemangioma, synovial chondromatosis, or heterotopic bone formation (myositis ossificans)[8,13]

(Fig. 2–1). Calcification may also be nonspecific in appearance on radiographs. However, nonspecific mineralization is frequently associated with extraskeletal chondrosarcoma or osteosarcoma and synovial sarcoma. Finally, radiographs allow detection of underlying bone involvement in the form of periosteal reaction or cortical destruction and marrow invasion.[8,13] In our experience, the common soft tissue sarcomas to reveal bone invasion are synovial sarcoma and malignant fibrous histiocytoma (MFH).

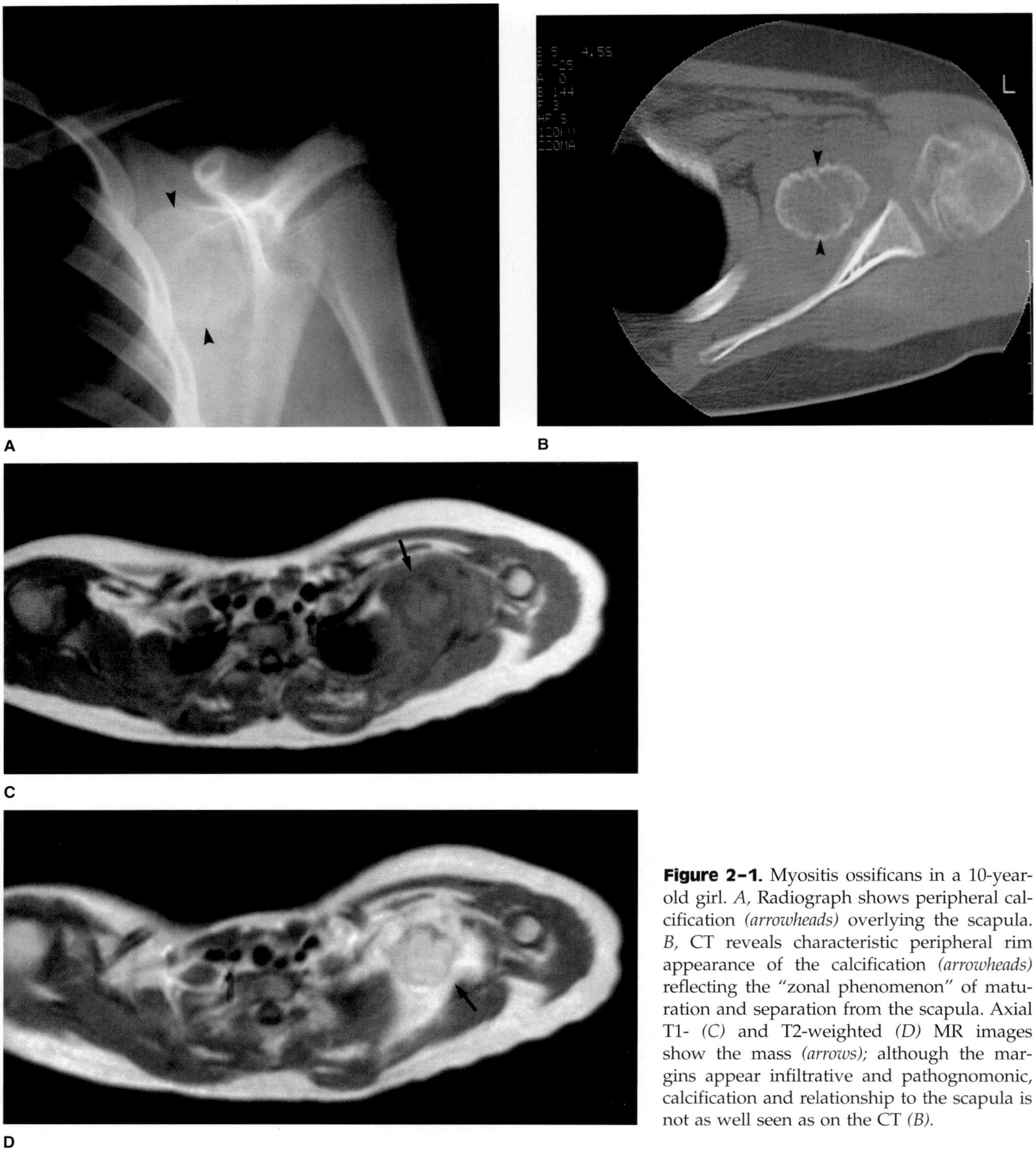

Figure 2–1. Myositis ossificans in a 10-year-old girl. *A,* Radiograph shows peripheral calcification *(arrowheads)* overlying the scapula. *B,* CT reveals characteristic peripheral rim appearance of the calcification *(arrowheads)* reflecting the "zonal phenomenon" of maturation and separation from the scapula. Axial T1- *(C)* and T2-weighted *(D)* MR images show the mass *(arrows);* although the margins appear infiltrative and pathognomonic, calcification and relationship to the scapula is not as well seen as on the CT *(B).*

Nuclear Medicine

Scintigraphic evaluation does not play a primary role in evaluation of soft tissue tumors. Both benign and malignant soft tissue tumors, particularly more vascularized lesions, often reveal mild increased uptake of radionuclide on bone scintigraphy because of increased blood flow. In addition, lesions with mineralization may show more extensive radiotracer activity from the increased turnover of calcium and phosphate. Gallium scanning has been advocated, although evaluation has included only small numbers of patients, to distinguish benign peripheral nerve sheath tumors (BPNSTs) from malignant peripheral nerve sheath tumor (MPNSTs).[14–16] Specifically, prominent gallium uptake is seen in MPNSTs in contradistinction to BPNSTs (neurilemoma or neurofibroma) that demonstrate limited or no uptake.[14–16] Thallium and positron emission tomographic studies have been used to assess response to therapy (radiation therapy or chemotherapy or both) as well evaluate possible recurrent tumor after surgical resection, although an in-depth discussion of this topic is beyond the scope of this chapter.

Angiography

In the past, angiographic evaluation of soft tissue tumors, particularly sarcomatous lesions, was relatively common to assess the degree of vascularity and serve as a vascular road map during surgery. In addition, angiography was often used to evaluate the effect of preoperative therapy depicted as decreased vascularity usually as a result of hemorrhage or necrosis. However, angiography has largely been supplanted by other imaging modalities such as CT or MRI and magnetic resonance angiography.[17] Embolization of soft tissue neoplasms may be performed via angiographic access as a method to decrease blood loss at surgical resection in lesions with prominent vascularity. Angiomatous lesions, particularly when diffuse or extensive (angiomatosis), may be embolized as the sole method of treatment.

CT, MRI, and Ultrasound

The advantages of these three-dimensional imaging modalities in comparison to radiographs in evaluation of soft tissue tumors is primarily a function of their superior contrast resolution. Although not universally accepted, in our opinion and experience, MRI is generally far superior to CT in radiologic evaluation of soft tissue tumors owing to its marked improvement in contrast resolution and multiplanar capabilities (ability to image in any plane desired)[1–7,18–28] (see Fig. 2–1). MRI may be contraindicated, and thus CT preferred, for a variety of reasons including severe claustrophobia and the presence of a cardiac pacemaker or metallic foreign bodies (including recent surgery with clips in anatomically sensitive areas such as the brain). CT may also be preferable in certain anatomic regions such as the periscapular area or chest or abdominal wall where motion artifact can be a problem with MRI (see Fig. 2–1). In addition, CT is the imaging modality of choice to both detect and characterize calcification (chondroid or osteoid) in soft tissue tumors in cases where radiographs are inadequate owing to their subtle nature or obscuration by complex anatomy particularly overlying osseous structures (i.e., pelvis) (see Fig. 2–1). Although newer studies would suggest that CT and MRI are equivalent for identification of bone involvement by soft tissue tumors, in our opinion, CT remains preferable for this assessment particularly when subtle or affecting a small osseous structure such as the fibula or scapula.

Placement of a marker over the soft tissue lesion is helpful with both CT and MRI. This is particularly important for superficial lipomas, which may be obscured by the surrounding subcutaneous fat (Fig. 2–2). Patient positioning may also be important with both modalities, particularly again in superficial lesions so that the lesion is not compressed. This may require prone positioning in patients with superficial paraspinal lesions or buttock or posterior extremity masses.

Although an extensive review of technical factors to optimize MRI in evaluation of soft tissue tumors is beyond the scope of this chapter, a few basic concepts are essential. As a general rule it is essential to obtain MRI in two orthogonal planes. The axial plane is usually optimal for evaluation and both T1-weighted and T2-weighted MRI should be obtained. Technical factors and the appearance of different musculoskeletal tissues are listed in Table 2–1 for standard T1- and T2-weighted MRI. In general, T1-weighted images are used for anatomic delineation of structures (spatial resolution), whereas T2-weighted sequences are used to differentiate normal from abnormal tissue such as tumor (contrast resolution). A second plane of imaging should also be performed either coronal (best for masses located medial or lateral in a compartment) or sagittal (best for masses located in anterior or posterior in a compartment). Fat suppression T2-weighted sequences (essentially subtracting fat making its signal null and black) are often used in the second plane to increase the conspicuity of signal (high signal intensity; white in appearance) of tumors.[29–32]

Intravenous (IV) contrast material can be administered for either CT (iodinated material) or MRI (para-

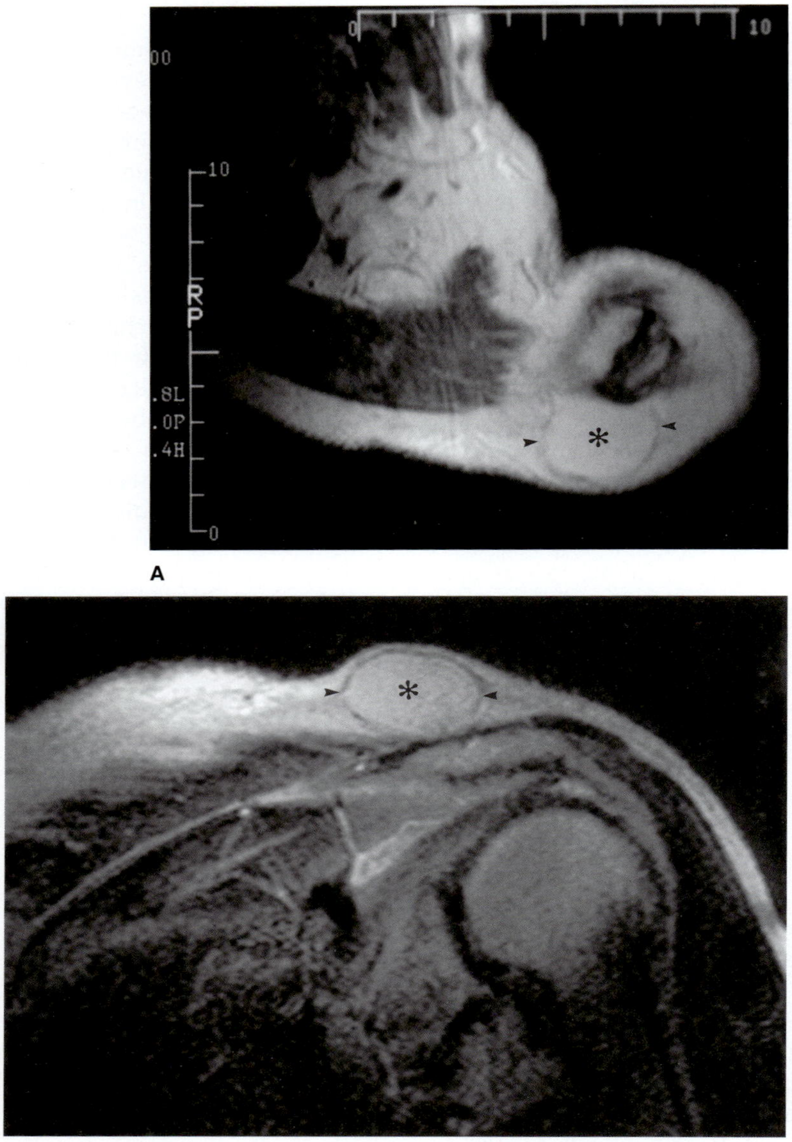

A

B

Figure 2–2. Subcutaneous lipoma about the shoulder in a 50-year-old woman. Axial T1- *(A)* and coronal T2-weighted *(B)* MR images show a subcutaneous lipoma (*) isointense to subcutaneous fat on both pulse sequences. Distinction from the surrounding fat is seen as a low signal peripheral capsule-like lining *(arrowheads)*.

magnetic substance, gadolinium) in an attempt to improve the contrast resolution in evaluation of soft tissue tumors. In general, contrast is much more important for CT in differentiating soft tissue tumors from surrounding muscle owing to its inferior contrast resolution. In contradistinction, lesion detection and delineation is typically easily evaluated on MRI without IV contrast. However, an exception to this is encountered with neoplasms that are highly necrotic, hemorrhagic, or myxomatous (Fig. 2–3). In these cases IV contrast can be very informative for identifying areas of enhancing solid and cellular tissue[33–44] (see Fig. 2–3). This becomes vitally important in directing biopsy to these areas that harbor diagnostic tissue for histologic evaluation as opposed to nondiagnostic regions of hemorrhage, necrosis, and nonspecific myxoid tissue.

Ultrasound (US) is another imaging modality that can be used in the evaluation of soft tissue tumors. Advantages of sonography include its low cost, real-time scanning, lack of ionizing radiation, and no use of IV contrast. Lesions of subcutaneous location are often best evaluated by US because of their superficial location.[45,46] Perhaps the most important use of US is in distinguishing a solid from cystic mass.[47,48] This distinction is important in differential diagnosis and US is quite adept at identifying truly cystic structures, which are anechoic with posterior acoustic enhancement (Fig. 2–4). These cystic lesions include ganglion, synovial cyst, bursa, and abscess (see Fig. 2–4). In contradistinction, US demonstrates the solid consistency with internal echoes of other soft tissue

Table 2–1. MRI Signal Intensity of Various Tissues

Tissue Type	T1 Signal Intensity	T2 Signal Intensity
Fat	High	Intermediate
Bone marrow (yellow)	High	Intermediate
Tumor*	Intermediate	High
Muscle	Intermediate	Low
Hyaline cartilage	Intermediate	High
Water	Very low	Very high
Tendons/ligaments	Very low	Very low
Cortex	Very low	Very low
Fibrocartilage	Very low	Very low
Fibrous tissue	Low to intermediate	Variable†
Blood‡	Variable	Variable

High, bright (white); intermediate, gray; low, dark (black).
*Tumor: majority of lesions.
†Highly collagenized low signal, more cellular high signal.
‡Dependent on components of methemoglobin, hemosiderin, oxyhemoglobin, deoxyhemoglobin, frequently heterogeneous with areas of high signal on both T1- and T2-weighting except hemosiderin, which is low signal on all pulse sequences.

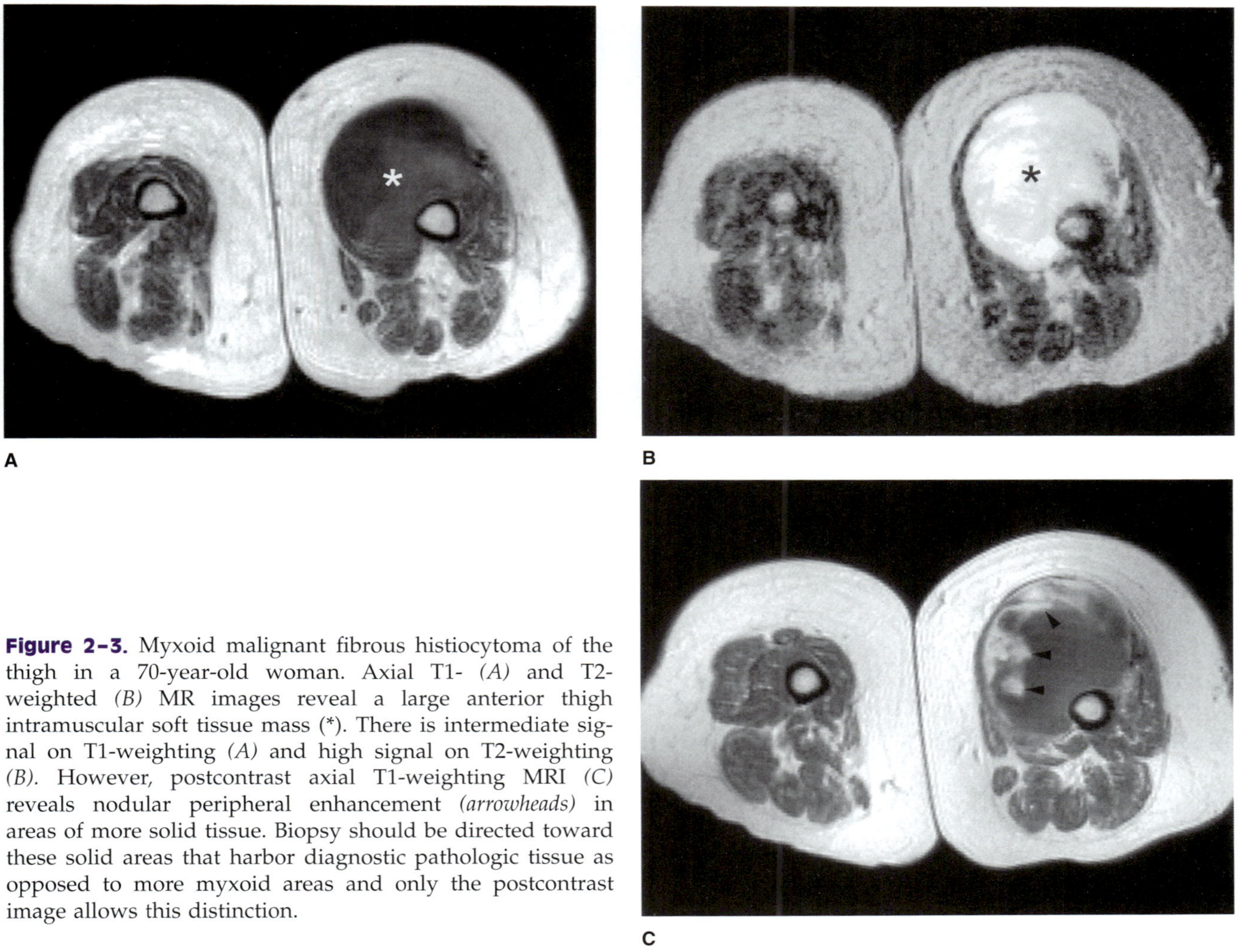

Figure 2–3. Myxoid malignant fibrous histiocytoma of the thigh in a 70-year-old woman. Axial T1- *(A)* and T2-weighted *(B)* MR images reveal a large anterior thigh intramuscular soft tissue mass (*). There is intermediate signal on T1-weighting *(A)* and high signal on T2-weighting *(B)*. However, postcontrast axial T1-weighting MRI *(C)* reveals nodular peripheral enhancement *(arrowheads)* in areas of more solid tissue. Biopsy should be directed toward these solid areas that harbor diagnostic pathologic tissue as opposed to more myxoid areas and only the postcontrast image allows this distinction.

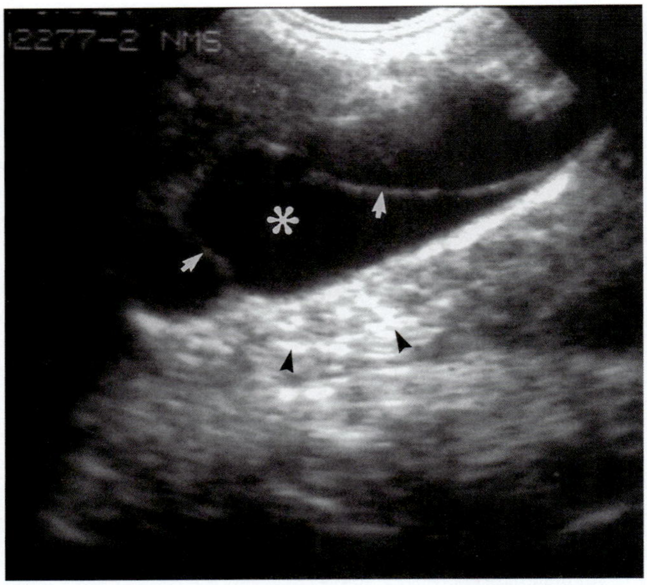

Figure 2–4. Ultrasound of a popliteal (Baker) cyst in the posterior knee of a 50-year-old woman. Sonogram shows an anechoic mass (*) with posterior acoustic enhancement *(arrowheads)* typical of a fluid-filled mass. Several thin septations are also seen *(arrows)*.

tumors including myxomas and myxoid neoplasms (i.e., myxoid liposarcoma), which on CT or MRI may simulate a cyst owing to the high intrinsic water content (Fig. 2–5). Doppler assessment can also be applied with US to evaluate lesion vascularity and response of neoplasm to preoperative chemotherapy and radiation therapy.[49]

Despite these many advantages of US, there are also many disadvantages. This modality is very operator dependent and relatively unusual examinations, such as musculoskeletal tumors, often require physician scanning, which involves a significant amount of time. Additionally, the field of view is often limited and large lesions may be difficult to entirely assess. Although US is adept at evaluating superficial lesions, deep-seated lesions, particularly in complex areas of anatomy such as the pelvis, may be obscured by overlying structures including bone, bowel, and excessive fat. The contrast resolution of sonography is also inferior to that of MRI.

Staging

Several staging systems (Tables 2–2, 2–3, and 2–4) are used for evaluating soft tissue tumors.[50–52] However, all have in common the need for a close working relationship among the orthopedic oncologist, musculoskeletal radiologist, and pathologist to appropriately stage lesions and guide treatment options. Limb salvage is the surgical treatment of choice for the vast majority of soft tissue sarcomas.[53–56] Much of the information necessary, particularly the lesion extent and involvement of adjacent structures, to stage soft tissue tumors is obtained by imaging. Important features to assess include lesion extent (does the tumor cross a major fascial plane to involve more than one compartment), size (is the lesion >5 cm), and involvement of adjacent bone, joint, or neurovascular structures.[57] Again, the multiplanar capabilities and superior contrast resolution of MRI make this modality the technique of choice in the assessment of most soft tissue tumors (particularly deep-seated lesions).

Lesion Specificity by Imaging

Relatively specific diagnosis by imaging characteristics has been reported in 20% to 50% of soft tissue tumors.[1–7] In our opinion, this percentage will gradually increase with more experience and description of specific characteristics, particularly on MRI, although likely not beyond approximately 70% to 80% of soft tissue masses. The imaging characteristics that allow specific diagnosis include lesion location (i.e., lesion deep to scapular tip for elastofibroma; Fig. 2–6), lesion shape or morphology (i.e., fusiform shape in neurogenic tumor with entering and exiting nerve), and intrinsic appearance (i.e., presence of fat for lipomatous lesions). Soft tissue masses that can frequently be diagnosed with imaging alone include lipomatous lesions, angiomatous lesions, neurogenic tumors, elastofibroma, intra-articular masses (pigmented villonodular synovitis, synovial chondromatosis), cystic lesions (ganglion, synovial cysts), and occasionally fibrous masses such as fibromatosis and nodular fasciitis.

Lipomatous Lesions

Soft tissue tumors containing significant amounts of fat are usually easily detected on CT (low attenuation or density) or MRI (high signal on T1-weighting and intermediate signal on T2-weighting) because their intrinsic appearance is identical to subcutaneous fat (see Figs. 2–2 and 2–7). These lesions include lipoma, lipoblastoma, hibernoma, liposarcoma, and hemangioma.

Imaging of lipomas typically reveals a mass with homogeneous adipose tissue reflecting its monotonous

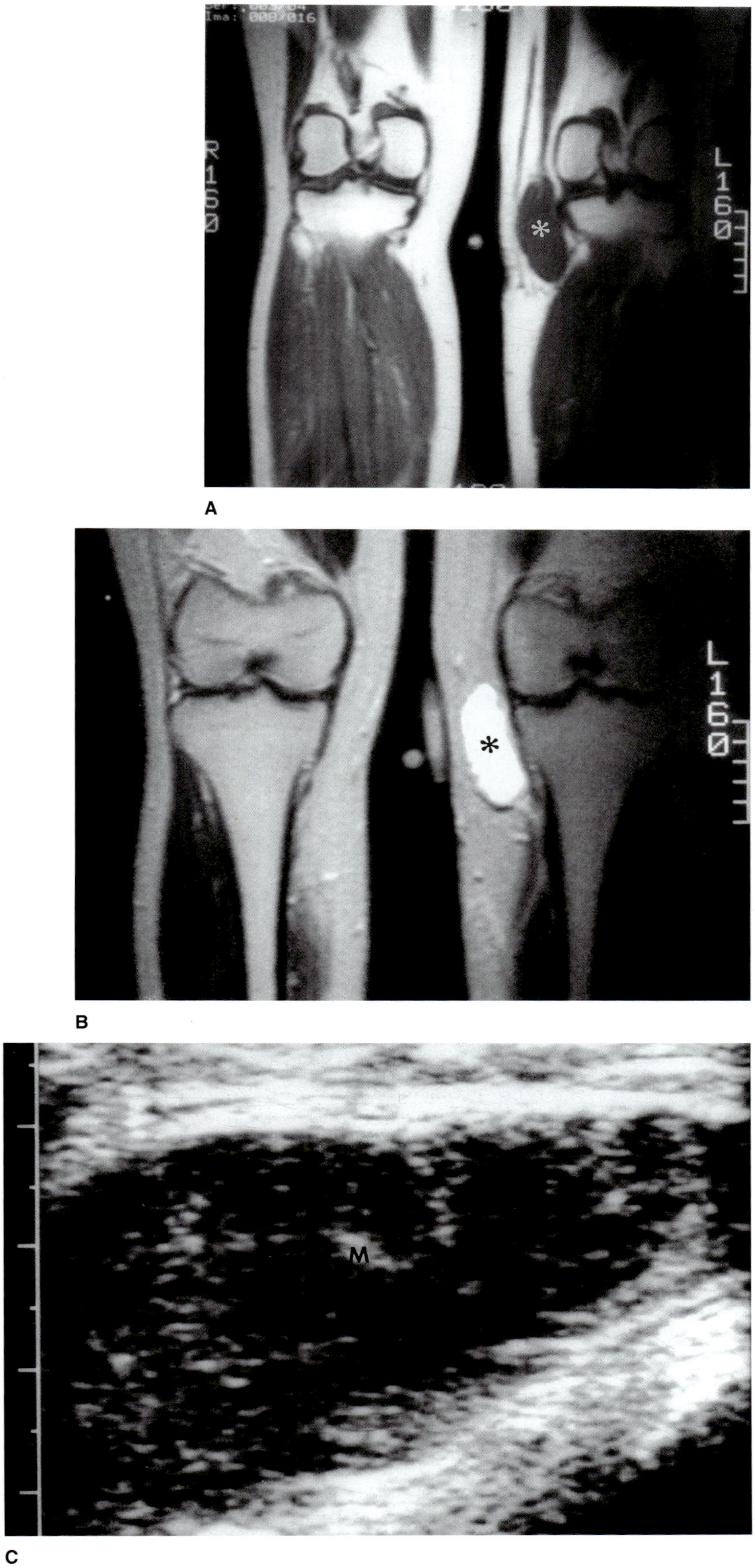

Figure 2–5. Myxoid liposarcoma medial to the knee in a 45-year-old woman simulating a cyst. Coronal T1-weighted *(A)* and T2-weighted *(B)* MR images show a soft tissue mass (*). There is homogeneous low signal on T1-weighting and high signal on T2-weighting simulating a cyst, although the unusual location should raise doubts as to this diagnosis. Sonogram *(C)* clearly demonstrates the hypoechoic but solid (not anechoic; see Fig. 2–4) internal consistency of the mass (M). Resection revealed myxoid liposarcoma, accounting for the MRI appearance.

Table 2–2. Enneking Staging of Sarcomas of Soft Tissue and Bone

Stage	Grade	Extent	Metastasis
IA	G1	T1	M0
IB	G1	T2	M0
IIA	G2	T1	M0
IIB	G2	T2	M0
III	G1–G2	T1	M1
	G1–G2	T2	M1

Histologic grade: G1, low risk of metastasis, <25%; G2, high risk of metastasis, >25%.
Site: T1, intracompartmental; T2, extracompartmental.
Metastasis: M0, no regional or distant metastases; M1, regional or distant metastases.
(Modified from Enneking et al.[50])

Table 2–3. Hajdu Classification

Stage	Size (cm)	Site	Grade
0	<5	S	L
1A	<5	S	H
1B	<5	D	L
1C	>5	S	L
IIA	<5	D	H
IIB	>5	S	H
IIC	>5	D	L
III	>5	D	H

Site: S, superficial (subcutaneous) to fascia; D, deep to fascia.
Histologic grade: L, low; H, high.
(Modified from Hajdu.[51])

pathologic appearance.[58–65] Intramuscular and intermuscular lesions are easily differentiated from surrounding tissue[58–60] (see Fig. 2–7). However, subcutaneous lipomas can be difficult to detect because of their location in surrounding adipose tissue with which they have an identical appearance (see Fig. 2–2). Identification of a thin surrounding pseudocapsule is necessary to distinguish these lesions from the background of subcutaneous fat (see Fig. 2–2). This capsule is of low signal intensity on all MRI

Table 2–4. American Joint Commission Staging Protocol for Sarcoma of Soft Tissue

Histiologic Grade (G)	Primary Tumor (T)	Regional Lymph Nodes (N)	Distant Metastasis (M)
G1 well differentiated	T1 tumor 5 cm or less in greatest dimension	N0 no regional lymph node metastasis	M0 no distant metastasis
G2 moderately well differentiated	T2 tumor more than 5 cm in greatest dimension	N1 regional lymph node metastasis	M1 distant metastasis
G3 poorly differentiated			
G4 undifferentiated			

Stage	G	T	N	M
1A	1	1	0	0
1B	1	2	0	0
IIA	2	1	0	0
IIB	2	2	0	0
IIIA	3–4	1	0	0
IIIB	3–4	2	0	0
IVA	1–4	1–2	1	0
IVB	1–4	1–2	0–1	1

(Modified from Russell et al.[52])

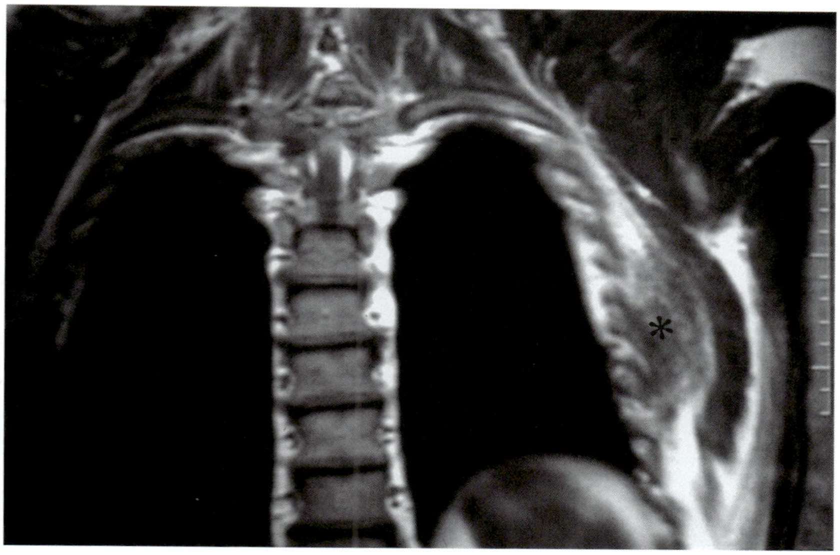

A

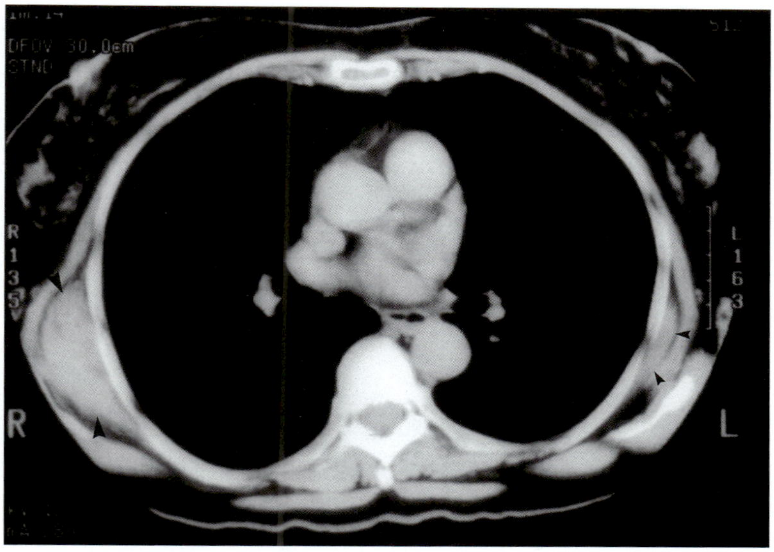

B

Figure 2–6. Elastofibroma in two different patients. *A,* Coronal T1-weighted MRI shows a chest wall mass (*). *B,* CT reveals a soft tissue mass deep to the right scapular tip *(large arrowheads)* and a smaller elastofibroma lesion on the left *(small arrowheads).*

pulse sequences and of muscle density on CT. Nonlipomatous mesenchymal components in lipomas are occasionally seen typically as small inconspicuous septa (see Fig. 2–7). Contrast enhancement is only minimal in lipomas usually in the nonlipomatous components. Lipomas can be multiple in 5% to 15% of cases and may also be infiltrative in cases of lipomatosis.[61–66]

Lipoblastomas and the diffusely infiltrative lipoblastomatosis usually reveal a predominantly fat-containing mass.[67,68] However, particularly in very young patients, myxoid components predominate with only small elements of adipose tissue.[67,68] These largely nonlipomatous lesions can simulate liposarcoma by imaging although the young age of the patient should make this diagnosis untenable.

Hibernoma, reflective of its pathology composed of brown fat, images in most patients like tissue similar to but not identical to fat.[69,70] These lesions are generally more vascular than lipomas and can reveal prominent enhancement after IV contrast by CT or MRI.[70]

Liposarcomas show a varying imaging appearance dependent on their histologic subtype.[71–75] Well-differentiated liposarcomas reveal extensive areas identical to subcutaneous fat by CT and MRI[71,72] (Fig. 2–8). In fact, differentiation from lipoma, similar to pathologic evaluation, can be difficult. In general, well-differentiated liposarcoma demonstrates more nonlipomatous components particularly prominent septa both in number and thickness.[71,72] Focal areas of mineralization (calcification or ossification) have been reported in

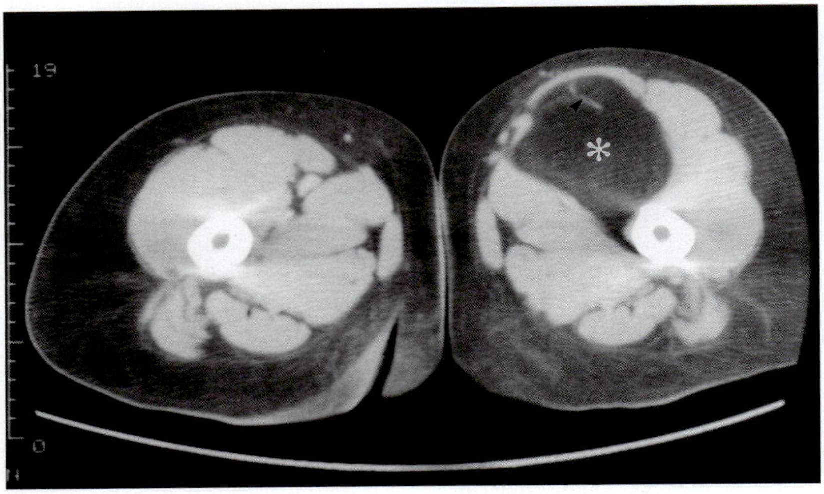

A

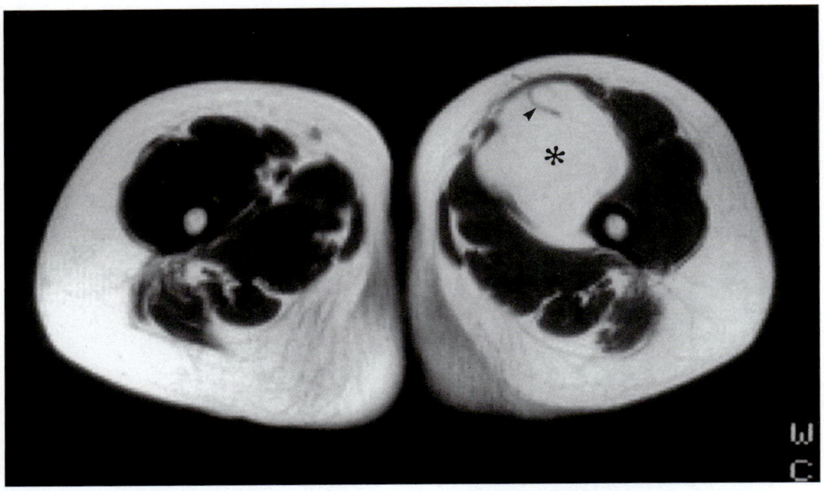

B

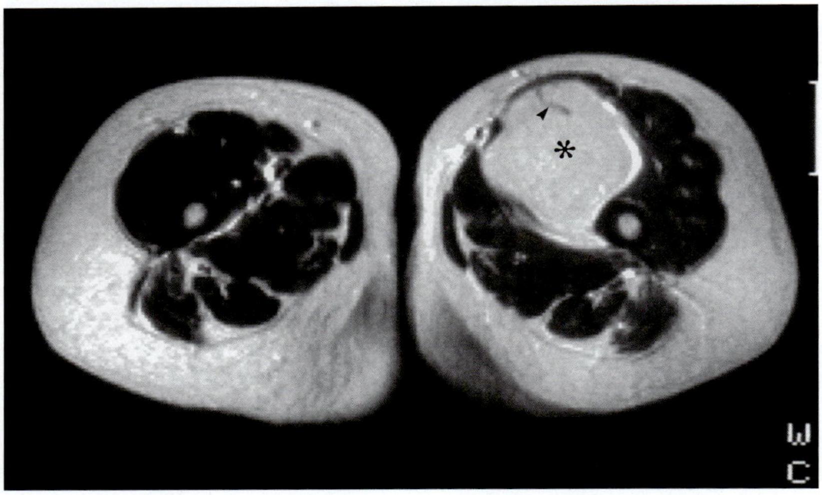

C

Figure 2–7. Lipoma of the thigh in a 54-year-old woman. All imaging studies including CT *(A)*, T1-weighted MRI *(B)*, and T2-weighted MRI *(C)* show the soft tissue mass (*) with intrinsic characteristics identical to subcutaneous fat. A single thin, small fibrous septation is seen anteriorly *(arrowheads)*.

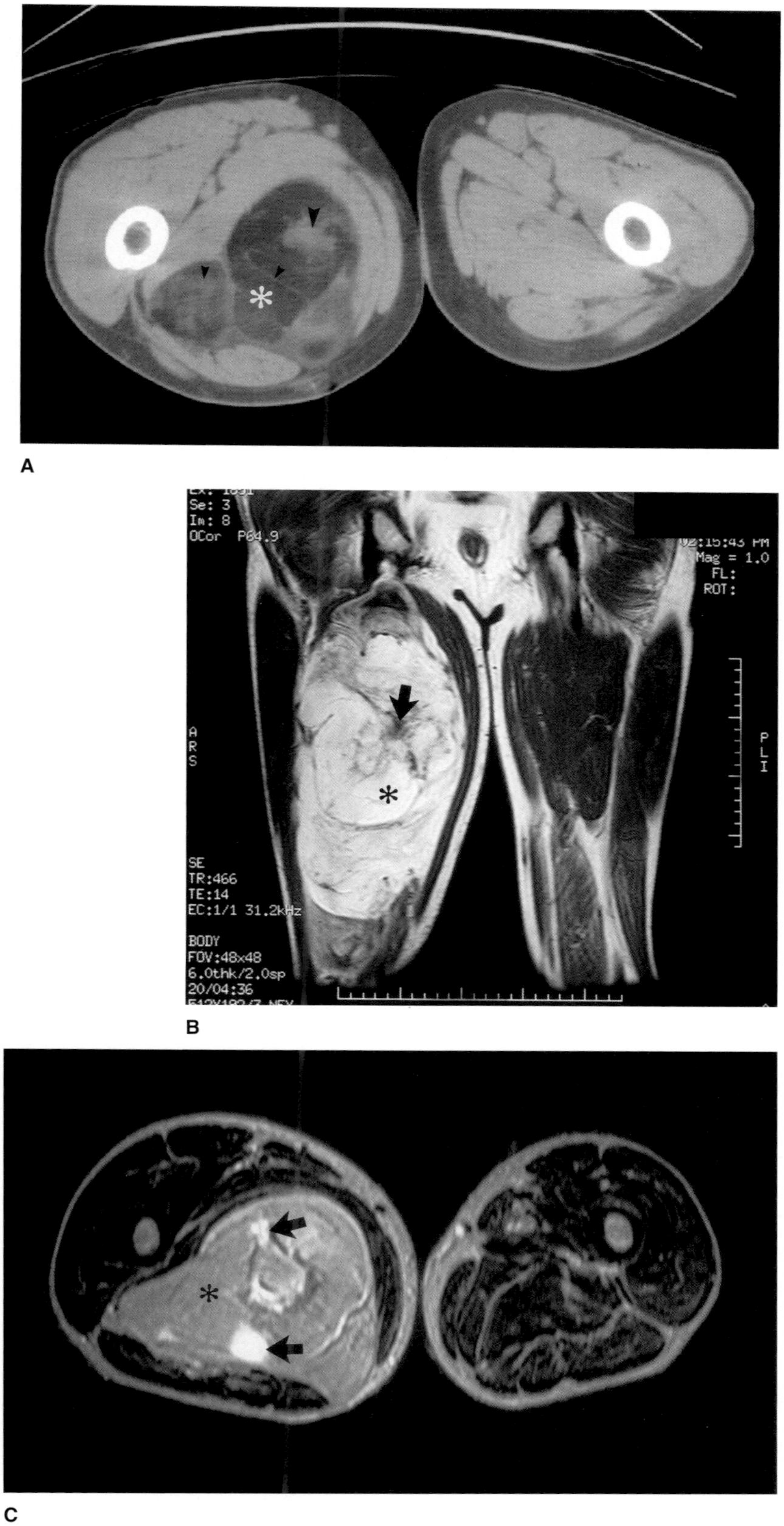

Figure 2–8. Well-differentiated liposarcoma of the thigh in a 68-year-old man. *A,* CT shows a heterogeneous mass in the posterior thigh with areas of fat (*) and multiple septae and regions of soft tissue density *(arrowheads).* Coronal T1-weighted *(B)* and axial T2-weighted *(C)* MR images also reveal the mass to contain large areas of fat (*) and prominent nonlipomatous nodules and septae *(arrows).*

up to 10% of cases.[17] Higher grade liposarcomas (myxoid, round cell, and pleomorphic), reflecting more anaplasia, reveal a less lipomatous imaging appearance.[73,74] However, in our experience, focal areas of fat (usually <10% of the tumor by volume) are seen in the vast majority of lesions (90–95%) by MRI (superior to CT) suggesting the diagnosis[75] (Fig. 2–9). Myxoid liposarcomas are usually intermuscular lesions and their high water content histologically is reflected in much of the lesion showing a "cyst-like" appearance. In our experience, 5% to 10% of cases of myxoid liposarcoma may suggest an entirely cystic lesion on CT and MRI although IV contrast demonstrates more diffuse or peripheral nodular enhancement and US also reveals evidence of a solid not cystic mass[75] (see Fig. 2–5). Round cell and pleomorphic liposarcoma, though high-grade lesions, also usually demonstrate focal areas of identifiable fat particularly by MRI.

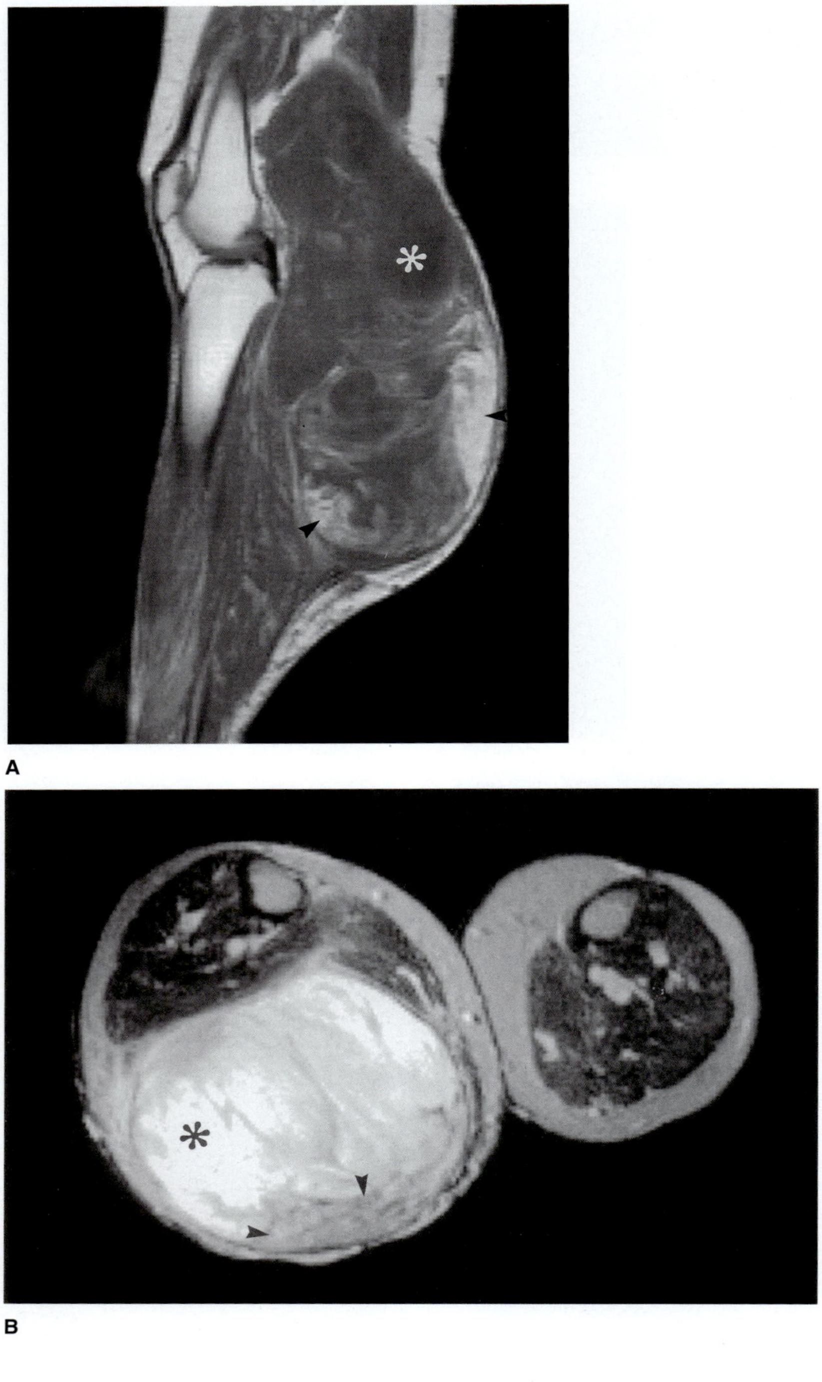

A

B

Figure 2–9. Myxoid liposarcoma of the popliteal fossa in a 60-year-old woman. Sagittal T1-weighted *(A)* and axial T2-weighted *(B)* MR images show a large soft tissue mass with a high water content myxoid component (*) and other areas containing fat *(arrowheads)*. The myxoid regions are low signal on T1-weighting and high signal on T2-weighting, whereas the fat areas are isointense on both pulse sequences to subcutaneous adipose tissue.

Dedifferentiated liposarcomas usually arise in an otherwise well-differentiated liposarcoma and are most common in the retroperitoneum.[73] These lesions are often quite large in size with only a relatively small focus of dedifferentiation. Imaging by CT or MRI typically depicts this small focus of nonlipomatous solid tissue as distinctly different from the surrounding adipose tissue. These imaging features allow biopsy to be directed to the dedifferentiated focus as well as to lipomatous regions. Similarly, either percutaneous needle or open biopsy can be directed by imaging in other high-grade liposarcomas (myxoid, round cell, or pleomorphic) to more lipomatous and nonlipomatous solid areas of tumor and away from nondiagnostic regions of hemorrhage or necrosis. This is extremely helpful, particularly in large heterogeneous tumors, to improve the ease and accuracy of pathologic diagnosis and certainly has implications in patient management and prognosis.

Angiomatous Lesions

Angiomatous lesions include hemangioma, lymphangioma, angiomatosis (and angiomatous syndromes), and the more aggressive vascular neoplasms hemangioendothelioma, hemangiopericytoma, and angiosarcoma. Hemangioma is the most frequent angiomatous lesion and accounts for 7% of all benign soft tissue tumors.[8,17] Hemangioma represents the most common neoplasm in infancy and childhood.

Imaging of hemangioma is partially dependent on the histologic type of lesion, specifically, the size of the vascular channels comprising the majority of the lesion (capillary, cavernous, arteriovenous, or venous). Radiographs may be normal, reveal a nonspecific soft tissue mass, or show characteristic calcification in the form of phleboliths (particularly in cavernous lesions, 30–50%).[17,76] Nonspecific calcification may also be seen. Bone scintigraphy frequently is normal or reveals only mild increased uptake of radionuclide. Angiography commonly shows enlarged feeding vessels and staining. Venous hemangiomas may require venography or direct puncture with injection of contrast for detection. US examination demonstrates large vascular channels and spaces (cavernous and venous lesions) with low vascular resistance and forward flow in both systole and diastole.[77,78] On the other hand, high-flow arteriovenous lesions reveal a high vascular resistance arterial Doppler signal.

Evaluation by CT requires IV contrast for optimal detection of enhancing serpentine vascular channels and spaces[78,79] (Fig. 2–10). Areas of calcification are usually easily detected on radiographs. However, very small phleboliths or location in a complex area of anatomy with overlying osseous structures such as the pelvis may obscure these diagnostic calcifications on radiographs as opposed to CT that allows identification.

An MRI of hemangioma is frequently diagnostic in appearance. In fact, in our opinion and experience, hemangiomas often reveal pathognomonic characteristics that make biopsy unnecessary unless surgical resection is warranted clinically. Cavernous hemangiomas are most frequently evaluated radiologically because they present as nonspecific palpable deep soft tissue masses and are usually intramuscular.[80–83] MRI signal intensity is typically very heterogeneous on all pulse sequences related to the intermixture of fat and vascular components (Fig. 2–11). Recognition of the morphologic shape of the vascular elements with serpentine vascular channels and spaces as well as the fat overgrowth in adjacent muscle is diagnostic of hemangioma (see Fig. 2–11). We believe that the presence of fat in muscle adjacent to the vascular

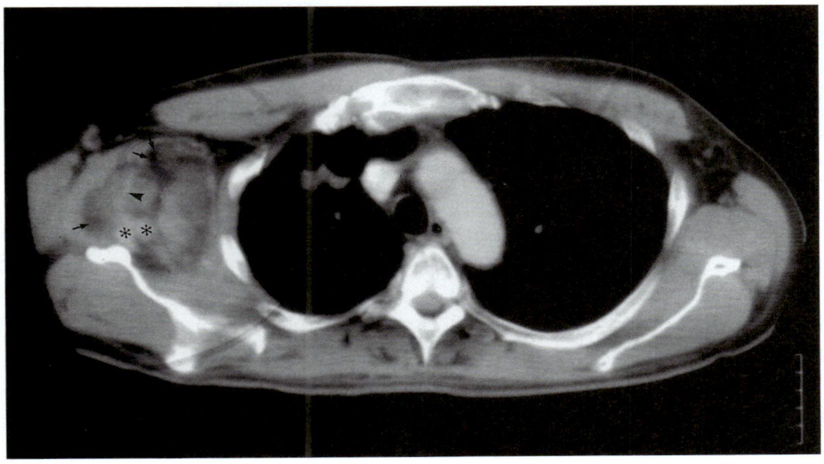

Figure 2–10. Intramuscular cavernous hemangioma about the shoulder in a 43-year-old man. CT after intravenous contrast shows the heterogeneous mass with serpentine *(arrowhead)* and circular (*) enhancing regions representing cavernous vascular structures and low density periphery *(arrows)* caused by secondary fat atrophy of muscle.

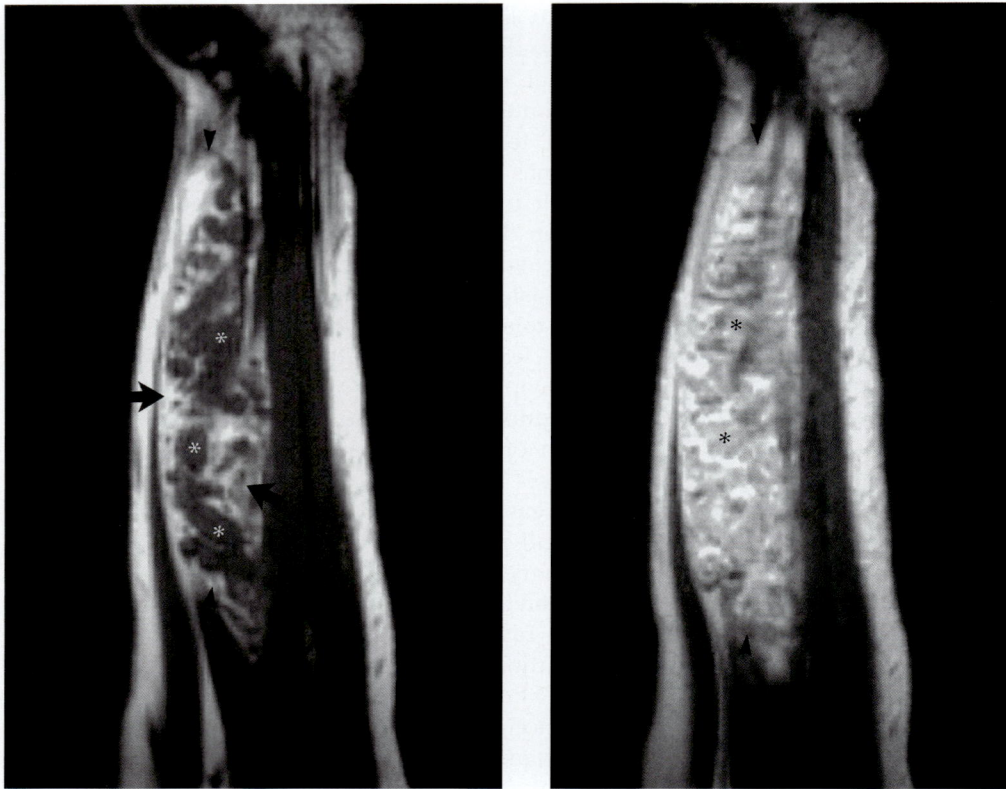

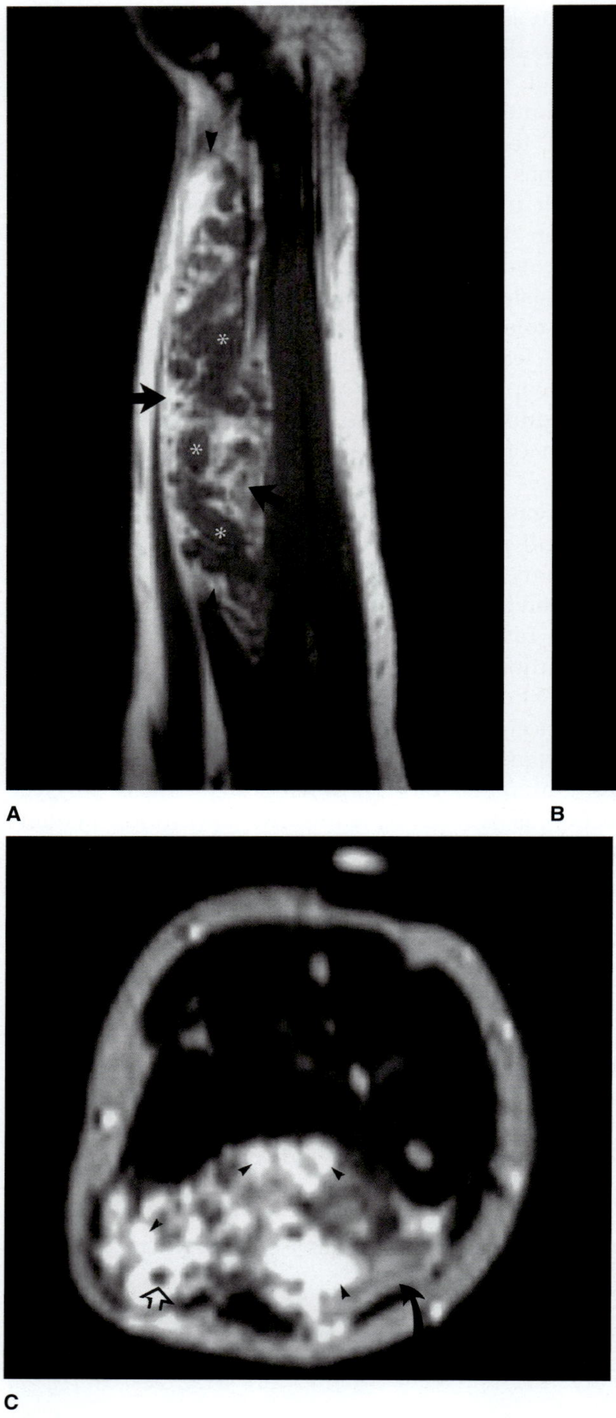

Figure 2–11. Intramuscular cavernous hemangioma of the forearm in a 24-year-old woman. Sagittal T1-weighted MRI before *(A)* and after *(B)* intravenous contrast show a large heterogeneous volar compartment mass *(large arrowheads)* composed of low signal serpentine vascular channels and spaces *(white *)* with associated fat overgrowth *(arrows)*. Enhancement of these vascular areas are seen after contrast *(B, black *)*. T2-weighted MRI *(C)* reveals high signal in the slow flowing circular vascular channels and spaces *(small arrowheads)* resulting in the "spot and dot" appearance, whereas fat becomes lower signal *(curved arrow)* and phlebolith is low signal *(open arrow)*.

channels and spaces represents atrophy resulting from chronic ischemia.[76] This essentially represents a vascular steal phenomenon and interestingly clinical history of pain with exercise is not infrequent in these patients likely corresponding to this occurrence. In our experience visualization of one or both of these MRI features is present in 90% to 95% of cavernous hemangiomas.[84]

The vascular channels or spaces in cavernous hemangiomas show low to intermediate intensity on T1-weighting and become very high signal on T2-weighted MRI reflecting the slow blood flow in these lesions (see Fig. 2–11). The vascular channels and spaces appear circular when seen *en face* as opposed to linear and often serpentine when depicted longitudinally. This often creates multiple circular foci of high signal on T2-weighted MRI and we often refer to them as the "spot and dot" appearance (see Fig. 2–11). Phleboliths remain low signal intensity on all MRI pulse sequences but are better identified by radiographs or CT.

Arteriovenous hemangiomas (often referred to as arteriovenous malformations) may demonstrate high or low flow in the serpentine vascular channels and are generally devoid of larger cavernous spaces; this affects the imaging appearance. High-flow lesions reveal persistent low signal intensity on all MRI pulse sequences owing to the lack of mobile protons in rapidly moving blood. Doppler US shows these vascular structures as vessels of high resistance. Low-flow arteriovenous hemangiomas show similar intrinsic characteristics on MRI and US as seen with cavernous lesions. Perhaps the most important feature in distinguishing high-flow arteriovenous lesions is in the recognition of the potential for bleeding during biopsy or surgical resection. It may be impossible to obtain vascular stasis after biopsy of deep-seated lesions such as in the retroperitoneum and cases of death by exsanguination have been reported.

Capillary hemangiomas are probably the least common to be imaged although they are the most frequently encountered clinically (1/200 births).[8,17] These lesions are often located in the superficial subcutaneous tissues and are easily clinically evaluated. The diagnosis is usually obvious, related to the apparent bluish skin discoloration or "strawberry" nevus of a patient in the first few years of life. In addition, 75% to 90% of juvenile capillary hemangiomas involute by age 7 and therefore patients are not typically surgical candidates.[8,17,76] For these reasons, similar to other subcutaneous lesions, imaging is infrequently performed. Interestingly, the imaging appearance of these hemangiomas is often nonspecific, reflecting their underlying histology. In our opinion and experience, the high degree of cellularity and small size of the vascular channels accounts for the nonspecific imaging appearance of a soft tissue mass seen on CT and MRI. Fat overgrowth is usually not identified in these superficial lesions. The extent of the capillary hemangioma and effect on adjacent structures is well evaluated by imaging, which fortunately is the clinical question because the diagnosis is generally already known, as previously described.

Hemangiomas involving the synovium are unusual and account for less than 1% of all lesions.[8] The imaging appearance is identical to that already described. However, in addition, repetitive episodes of hemarthrosis may result in associated synovitis and subsequent joint destruction. The appearance of the synovial thickening may simulate that of hemophiliac arthropathy except that synovial hemangioma is a monoarticular disease. On MRI, the synovial thickening remains low signal intensity on all pulse sequences identical to pigmented villonodular synovitis (PVNS).

Lymphangiomas are generally cavernous lesions present at birth or discovered in the first 2 years of life (50–90%) affecting the head, neck, or axilla.[8,17] Imaging by CT, MRI, or US reveals these large cystic spaces either unilocular but more frequently multilocular. Admixture with a hemangiomatous component or hemorrhage may be associated with a more complex appearance from bleeding and recognized as fluid–fluid levels.

Angiomatosis and angiomatous syndromes (Maffucci, Osler-Weber-Rendu, Klippel-Trenaunay-Weber, etc.) represent diffuse infiltration of either one tissue plane (bone, subcutaneous, muscle, or viscera) or more commonly multiple tissue planes by hemangiomatous and lymphangiomatous lesions. Individual lesions appear identical to those previously described for solitary lesions but are much more extensive. Imaging is frequently performed to evaluate for visceral involvement, which when present is associated with a worsened prognosis.[17,76]

The more aggressive vascular lesions, hemangioendothelioma, hemangiopericytoma, and angiosarcoma, are uncommon lesions and frequently show a nonspecific imaging appearance. However, identification of a soft tissue mass with serpentine vascular channels with high flow should suggest the diagnosis of a more aggressive vascular neoplasm. Unlike hemangiomas these lesions do not demonstrate fat overgrowth and in addition are usually intermuscular in location (not intramuscular as with hemangiomas). Interestingly, the majority of other soft tissue sarcomas do not generally reveal identifiable vessels on MRI. In our opinion this reflects the small size of the vascular channels feeding most soft tissue sarcomas below the spatial resolution of MRI. The differential diagnosis of a soft tissue lesion with prominent identifiable vascular channels includes synovial sarcoma (unusual pattern), alveolar soft part sarcoma, rhabdomyosarcoma, and extraskeletal Ewing sarcoma or primitive neuroectodermal tumor (PNET) in addition to the aggressive vascular lesions.[17]

Neurogenic Tumors

Neurogenic tumors include traumatic neuroma, Morton neuroma, neurilemoma (schwannoma), neurofibroma, and MPNSTs. Advanced imaging (CT, US, or MRI) of these lesions is frequently diagnostic. Important features are typically either location (Morton or traumatic neuroma) or characteristic morphology and relationship to a known nerve distribution (BPNST or MPNST).

Radiographs of neurogenic tumors are usually normal or reveal only a nonspecific soft tissue mass. Calcification of the lesions is unusual. Bone overgrowth is rarely associated with neurogenic neoplasms, particularly in patients with neurofibromatosis type 1 (NF1).[85]

Similar to radiographs, bone scintigraphy and angiography usually reveal nonspecific features in evaluation of neurogenic tumors. Peripheral nerve sheath tumors generally show mild increased radionuclide uptake on bone scintigraphy. Angiography reveals a variable degree of staining with neurogenic neoplasms although MPNSTs typically show more prominent vascularity.[17,85]

Advanced imaging (US, CT, or MRI) more clearly depicts location and intrinsic characteristics of these lesions. Neurogenic tumors are often fusiform in shape, representing the entering and exiting nerve at the lesion margins (Figs. 2–12 and 2–13). This morphologic appearance is well seen by US, CT, or MRI and should always suggest the diagnosis of neurogenic tumor because it is unusual in other soft tissue masses.[85–90] MRI and US are often superior to CT (limited to the axial plane) because of their ability to image in any plane particularly along the long axis of the tumor (see Figs. 2–12 and 2–13).

Traumatic neuromas are usually seen in association with amputation (traumatic or surgical) and are typically painful. A palpable mass may also be present. Imaging of traumatic neuromas of larger nerve trunks typically reveals a thickened tubular structure ending in a bulbous mass.[91,92] No exiting nerve is seen in cases related to amputation. In contradistinction, traumatic neuromas related to chronic irritation (spindle neuromas) may reveal focal nerve thickening with both entering and exiting nerve. Traumatic neuromas of small superficial nerves may show entirely nonspecific imaging findings of only a round or oval soft tissue mass.

Morton neuromas are usually diagnosed because of their characteristic location. These nonneoplastic masses are related to the plantar digital nerve between the third and fourth metatarsals or less commonly the second and third metatarsals.[8,17] MRI and US are the best radiologic methods to detect Morton neuroma and demonstrate small focal masses centered in the neurovascular bundle location.[93–95] The small, round or oval mass represents perineural fibrosis of the plantar nerve, which is typically not well seen owing to its small size. Morton neuromas that are smaller than 5 mm in size may be difficult to detect on US.[94] Lesions are low to intermediate signal

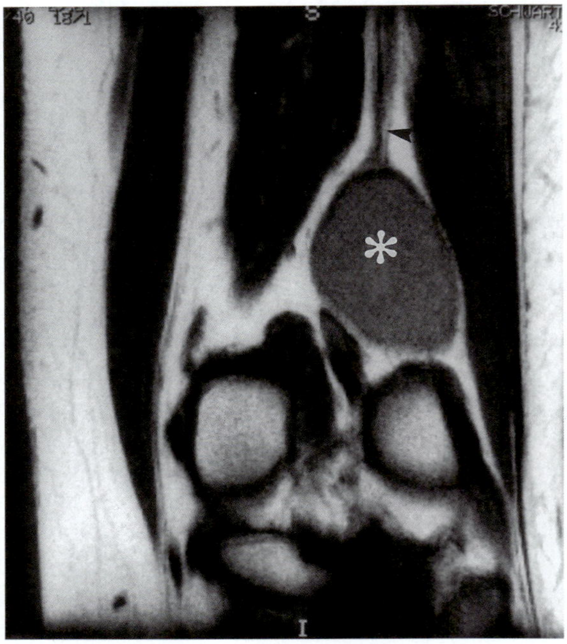

A

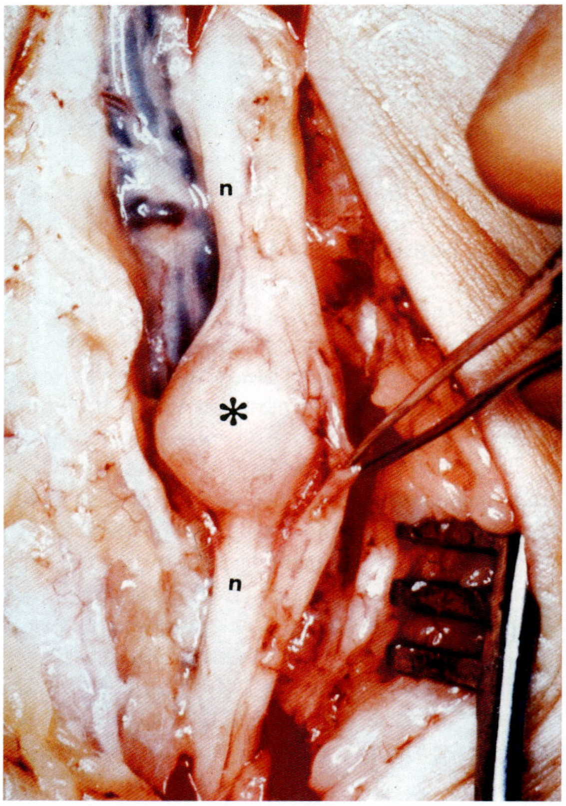

B

Figure 2–12. Neurilemoma of the popliteal fossa in a 49-year-old woman. *A,* Coronal T1-weighted MRI shows linear tube representing the sciatic nerve *(arrowhead)* entering the mass (*). *B,* Intraoperative photograph reveals the entering and exiting nerve (n) relationship to the mass (*), and the cause of the MRI appearance.

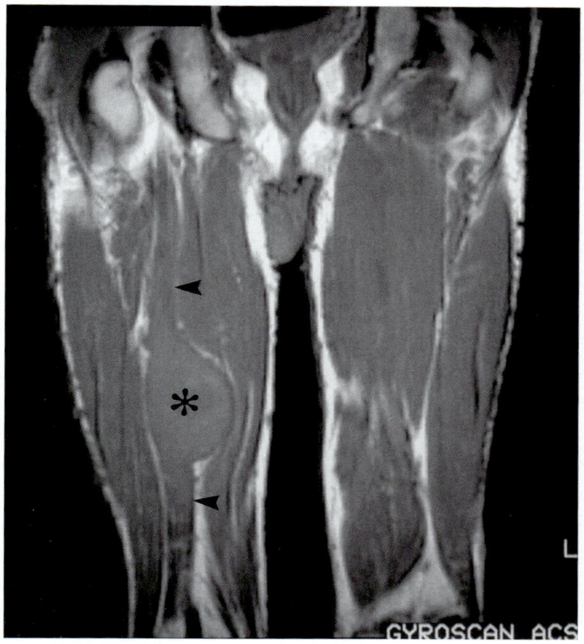

A

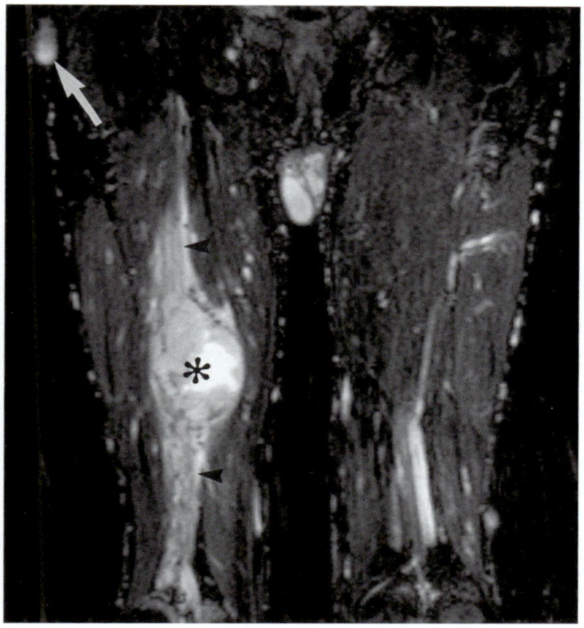

B

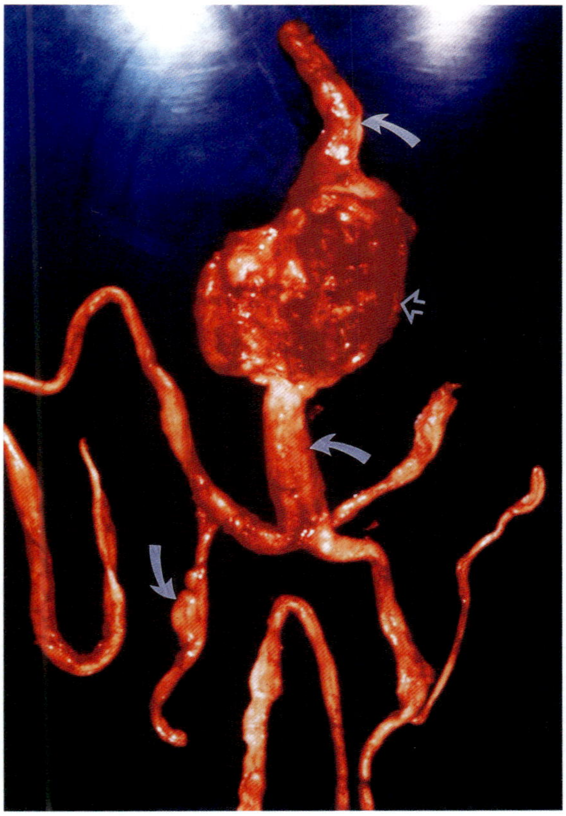

C

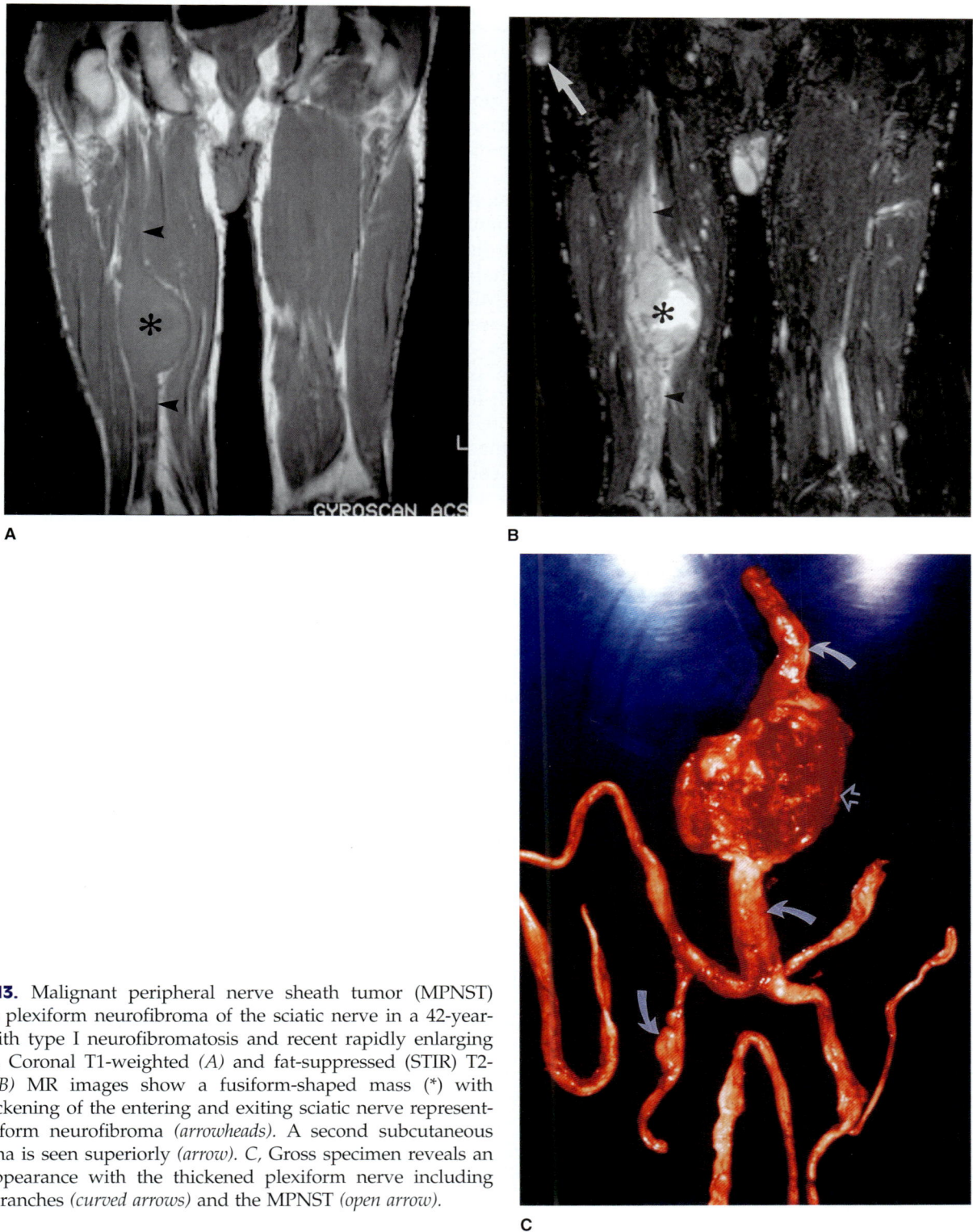

Figure 2–13. Malignant peripheral nerve sheath tumor (MPNST) arising in a plexiform neurofibroma of the sciatic nerve in a 42-year-old man with type I neurofibromatosis and recent rapidly enlarging thigh mass. Coronal T1-weighted *(A)* and fat-suppressed (STIR) T2-weighted *(B)* MR images show a fusiform-shaped mass (*) with marked thickening of the entering and exiting sciatic nerve representing a plexiform neurofibroma *(arrowheads)*. A second subcutaneous neurofibroma is seen superiorly *(arrow)*. *C,* Gross specimen reveals an identical appearance with the thickened plexiform nerve including the sciatic branches *(curved arrows)* and the MPNST *(open arrow)*.

on T1-weighted MRI and unlike many other tumors do not typically show high signal on T2-weighting. For this reason they are more conspicuous on T1-weighted MRI. Lesions usually enhance, often intensely following IV MR contrast. Associated intermetatarsal bursal fluid is also a common feature. It has recently been reported that asymptomatic Morton neuromas may be relatively common (30% in a group of 70 volunteers) and clinical correlation to symptoms is as always important.[95]

Neurogenic neoplasms include benign lesions (BPNSTs), neurilemoma (schwannoma), and neurofibroma as well as MPNSTs. As previously discussed, these lesions demonstrate a fusiform shape with entering and exiting nerves best seen on MRI or US particularly when involving large nerves (see Figs. 2–12 and 2–13). Other imaging features of neurogenic neoplasms include low attenuation on CT, target sign (MRI), fascicular sign (MRI), split-fat sign (CT, MRI), and associated muscle atrophy (CT, MRI). [85–90] The low attenuation (density) of these lesions on CT is likely related to a high water content or the lipid contained in the myelin.[86] The target sign on T2-weighted MRI represents low signal centrally (fibrous tissue with higher collagen content) and high signal peripherally (more myxoid areas with higher water content).[85,88] This sign is suggestive of a neurogenic neoplasm and is more common with neurofibroma. The fascicular sign is seen on MRI (best on T2-weighted images) as multiple ringlike structures in the lesion.[85] We believe this corresponds to fascicular bundles seen pathologically in neurogenic neoplasms. The split-fat sign represents a rim of fat about neurogenic neoplasms as a result of these lesions arising from an intermuscular location about the neurovascular bundle.[85] This structure is normally surrounded by fat and as these neoplasms slowly enlarge a rim of fat is maintained. It is best seen by MRI followed by CT. Finally, associated fat atrophy of surrounding muscle is seen in up to 23% of cases related to nerve involvement and is relatively uncommon in association with other soft tissue masses.[87]

Differentiation of neurilemoma (nerve eccentric to the mass) and neurofibroma (nerve inseparable from the mass) should be possible by the relationship of the soft tissue masses to the entering and exiting nerve. Cerofolini and coworkers believed they could differentiate these lesions in two thirds of cases.[89] In our experience, however, this distinction is extremely difficult except in lesions of very large nerves.

Neurofibromas may also be multiple or plexiform in association with NF1 (see Fig. 2–12). The imaging of plexiform neurofibromas identically reflects their pathologic appearance of a serpentine "bag of worms."[8,17,85] There is diffuse nerve thickening and nodularity and the target sign is frequently seen on T2-weighted MRI. Diffuse neurofibromas typically involve the subcutaneous tissue and demonstrate a reticulated branching appearance on MRI or CT along the connective tissue septa.

The distinction of BPNST from MPNST by imaging is often difficult or impossible. Imaging features that suggest MPNST include size greater than 5 cm, infiltrative margins, central necrosis, rapid growth, and increased uptake on gallium nuclear medicine studies[17,85] (see Figs. 2–12 and 2–13). In addition, MPNSTs less commonly reveal the target sign, fascicular sign, and split-fat sign, reflecting their higher degree of anaplasia and more aggressive growth.

Cystic Masses

Soft tissue masses that typically have an imaging appearance of cysts include synovial cyst, bursal fluid collection, ganglion, perilabral or meniscal cyst, hematoma, abscess, and myxomatous neoplasms. These lesions can all have a similar intrinsic appearance on noncontrast CT on MRI. CT shows low attenuation and MRI reveals low signal intensity on TI-weighting and very high signal on T2-weighting. US demonstrates an anechoic lesion with posterior acoustic enhancement in truly cystic masses (see Fig. 2–4). Clinical history and lesion location are helpful in distinguishing these lesions.

Synovial cysts represent an extension of the joint usually a result of chronic effusion from mechanical internal derangement or arthropathy (particularly rheumatoid arthritis).[96,97] These lesions are lined by synovium and the most common is the popliteal cyst (Baker cyst). A Baker cyst is typically easily diagnosed by its location and identifying the narrow neck of communication to the joint from the gastrocnemius-semimembranosus bursa (Fig. 2–14). Septations, osteochondral fragments, and nodules of synovitis may be seen in synovial cysts. Popliteal cysts may rupture and dissect (complicated Baker cyst) into the calf, simulating deep venous thrombosis clinically. Imaging reveals this dissection as a fusiform shape and the often prominent resulting surrounding edema caused by tissue irritation. The shape and surrounding edema usually allow distinction from other causes of popliteal soft tissue masses despite the fact that complicated Baker cysts may show solid regions resulting from hemorrhage.

Ganglia are not true cysts but are lined by fibrous tissue. These lesions more frequently involve the wrist (70%) and less commonly affect the foot, ankle,

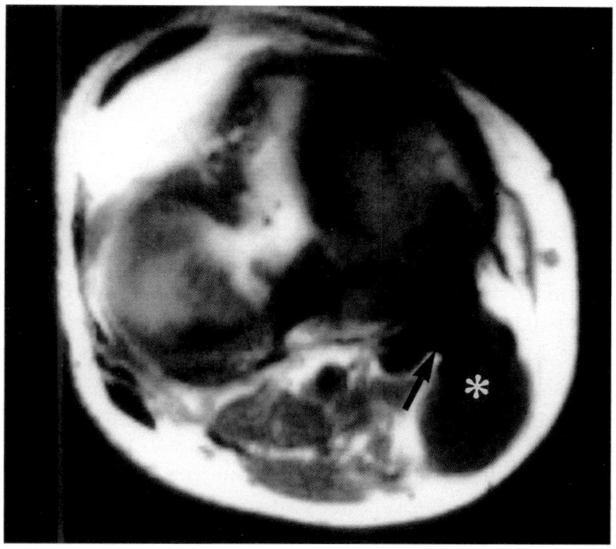

A

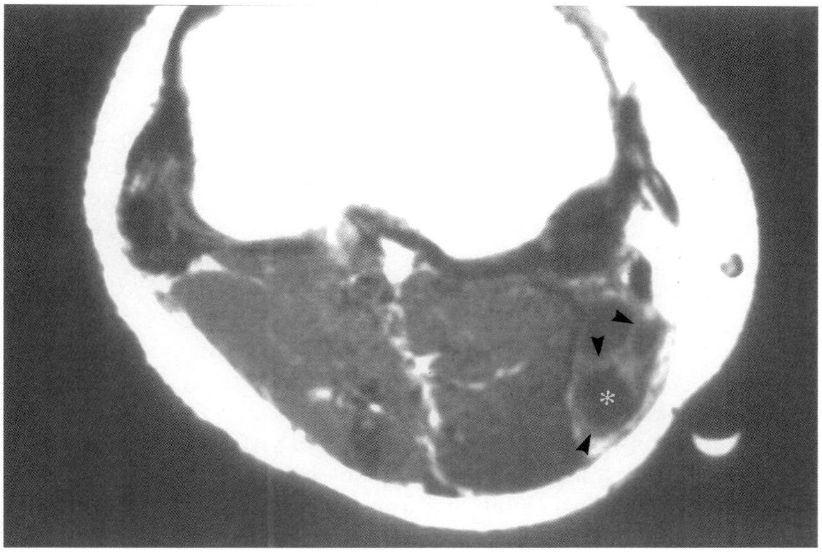

B

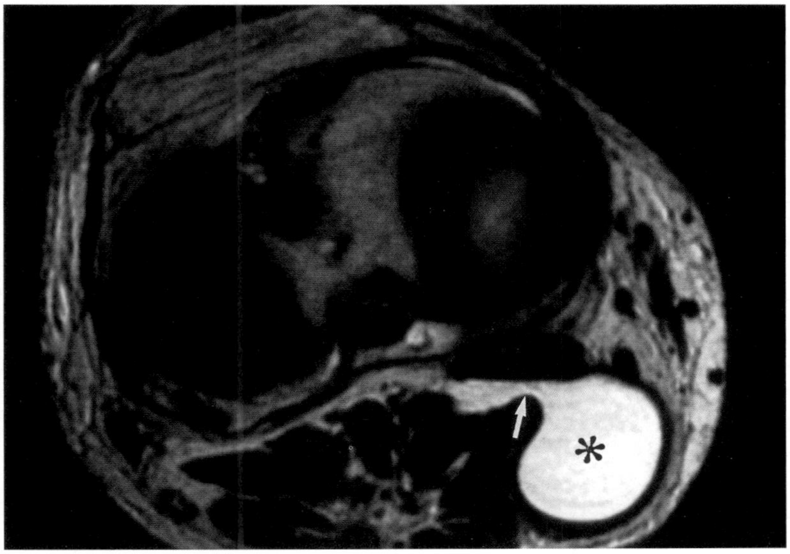

C

Figure 2–14. Popliteal cyst in a 40-year-old man. Axial T1-weighted MRI before *(A)* and after intravenous contrast *(B)* and T2-weighted image *(C)* show a homogeneous cystic mass (low intensity on T1-weighting and very high signal on T2-weighting) (*) and a neck extending back toward the joint *(arrows)*. After contrast, thin peripheral and septal enhancement is seen *(arrowheads)* confirming the cystic consistency of the lesion.

knee, shoulder, and hip.[98-100] Ganglia are typically near but not in joints, although more recently intra-articular lesions have been recognized.[100] Ganglia are usually small (1–3 cm) lesions that show fluid characteristics on CT, MRI, and US and may be multilocular. US is often the quickest and least expensive method to image and diagnose a ganglion.

Focal fluid collections adjacent to menisci and labral cartilage have been referred to as ganglia and juxta-articular myxomas in the past. However, it is now recognized that many of these lesions, in fact, result from tears of these fibrocartilaginous structures with fluid extending through these injuries and accumulating in an adjacent "cyst." These perilabral or meniscal cysts are thus a result of trauma and do not represent ganglia or myxomas.[101-103] This has treatment implications in that these lesions are likely to recur if the underlying cartilaginous damage is not repaired. Although CT and US can identify these "cysts," MRI is the modality of choice because of its ability to detect the associated internal joint derangement. The cyst may be complex and not contain purely fluid related to associated debris. Extrinsic erosion of bone rarely occurs particularly with lesions of the hip and acetabular labral tears.

Liquified hematoma and abscess formation may also cause "cystic" soft tissue masses.[17] Clinical history and associated inflammation are helpful in diagnosis. Imaging typically reveals a much thicker and irregular wall about these lesions as compared to other cystic masses. Abscess formation may also reveal attempts at linear extension representing a sinus tract.

Myxomatous neoplasms include myxoma, neurogenic neoplasm, liposarcoma, malignant fibrous histiocytoma, and extraskeletal chondrosarcoma.[8,17,104,105] These lesions may simulate cystic masses on noncontrast CT and MRI reflecting their intrinsic high water content. However, after IV contrast peripheral nodular of mild diffuse enhancement is apparent in distinguishing these lesions from a ganglion, synovial cyst, abscess, or hematoma, which demonstrates peripheral or septal enhancement (see Fig. 2–14). US can also distinguish these lesions because myxomatous lesions, though having a high water content, are still solid lesions and are hypoechoic but not anechoic as in cystic masses.

Other Lesions with Specific Imaging Appearances

Elastofibroma represents a reactive process that can usually be diagnosed by its specific location of a mass deep to the scapular tip (see Fig. 2–6). It is a common lesion that can be recognized on 2% of CT chest examinations.[106] Small streaks of fat may be seen on both CT and MRI and lesions typically show intermediate signal intensity on all MR pulse sequences.[106-108]

Pigmented villonodular synovitis (PVNS) represents a benign proliferative lesion of the synovium. Both the diffuse intra-articular form and localized usually extra-articular form (giant cell tumor of tendon sheath [GCTTS]) often show characteristic imaging findings.[109-111]

Radiographs of GCTTS may show only a nonspecific soft tissue mass most commonly involving the hand or wrist (65–89% of lesions).[110] Extrinsic erosion of underlying bone is apparent in about 15% to 21% of cases.[110] Calcification has been reported in 6% of lesions.[110] Radiographs of the diffuse form of PVNS typically reveal only evidence of effusion or a nonspecific soft tissue mass or both. Extrinsic erosion of bone has been described in 50% of cases, affecting both sides of the joint.[109-111] However, this finding is dependent on the joint involved, specifically the size of the articulation. Small capacity joints such as the hip (second most commonly involved joint) almost invariably (93%) demonstrate erosion, whereas the knee (most frequently affected joint) with its large size only reveals erosion in 26% of cases.[109-111]

Hemosiderin deposition in PVNS may allow more definitive imaging diagnosis on CT or more commonly MRI (Fig. 2–15). CT reveals extrinsic erosion of bone and the accompanying soft tissue mass may have increased attenuation (density) resulting from the hemosiderin. MRI more clearly shows lesion extent and the hemosiderin effect causing marked decreased signal intensity on T2-weighting (see Fig. 2–15). Focal areas of effusion are common and reveal high signal intensity on T2-weighted MRI. The degree of hemosiderin deposition is usually prominent in the diffuse form of PVNS although GCTTS often reveals a more variable degree of pigment deposition. This variation is reflected in the MRI appearance and lesions with little or no hemosiderin, particularly GCTTS, may show nonspecific higher signal intensity on T2-weighting MRI.

Synovial chondromatosis also represents a synovially based process that frequently shows a characteristic imaging appearance. Radiographs classically reveal multifocal (often innumerable) areas of calcification (up to 70% of cases) frequently with a typical chondroid appearance (rings and arcs) scattered throughout the articulation.[112-115] Enchondral ossification may also occur in these cartilaginous nodules. Similar to PVNS, other nonspecific radiographic changes include a soft tissue mass, effusion, extrinsic erosion of bone, and secondary osteoarthritis.

Computed tomography is the best imaging modality to detect calcification in the areas of

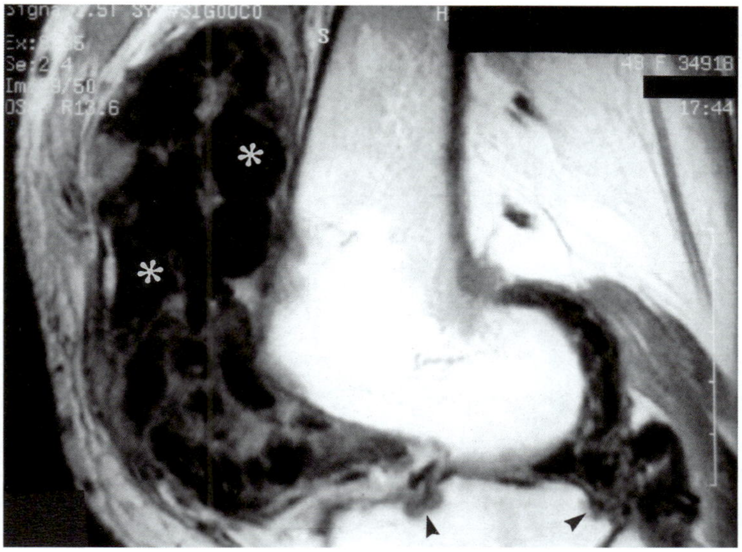

Figure 2-15. Pigmented villonodular synovitis of the knee in a 34-year-old woman with joint pain. Sagittal T2-weighted MRI shows extensive abnormal tissue in the knee joint (*) remaining low signal intensity as a result of hemosiderin deposition. Subtle bone erosion of the tibia is also seen *(arrowheads)*.

chondroid synovial metaplasia particularly if the calcification is small or involves complex areas of anatomy such as the hip (Fig. 2–16). The calcifications are often very similar in size and shape. MRI shows diffuse synovial abnormality with intermediate signal on T1-weighting. However, the high water content of hyaline cartilage (75–80%) shows high signal on T2-weighted MRI similar to effusion.[17,112–115] Areas of calcification remain low signal on all MRI pulse sequences. However, small calcifications are often difficult or impossible to detect on MRI as compared to CT or radiographs (see Fig. 2–16). Synovial chondromatosis usually affects joints (knee in 50% of cases), but tendon sheaths (tenosynovial chondromatosis) or bursa (bursal chondromatosis) may also be affected with identical imaging appearances.[8,17]

Multiple various forms of fibromatosis can involve the musculoskeletal system including aggressive infantile, extra-abdominal desmoid, palmar, and myofibromatosis.[8,17,116–120] Although an extensive discussion of these lesions individually is beyond the scope of this chapter, as a group these lesions often show characteristic MRI findings suggesting the diagnosis. The fibromatoses commonly affect the foot, hand, shoulder (Fig. 2–17), chest wall, and paraspinal areas.[8,17] Highly collagenized lesions frequently reveal marked areas of diffuse low signal intensity of T2-weighted MRI (see Fig. 2–17). On the other hand, less collagenized and more cellular lesions may show nonspecific high signal on T2-weighted MRI. However, even these latter lesions often show collagenized low signal intensity bands[116–118] (see Fig. 2–17). In addition, the growth pattern frequently reveals tails of extension along fascial planes (see Fig. 2–17), which is an unusual growth patterns in other neoplasms except nodular fascitis and dermatofibrosarcoma protuberans.[117] In our opinion and experience, fibromatosis with predominant low signal intensity on T2-weighted MRI is less likely to recur or grow significantly. In patients treated with radiation, tumor response can also be assessed by MRI. Good response to radiation is reflected as increasing collagenization pathologically and progressive low signal intensity (by MRI) and decreased mass size.

Nonspecific Soft Tissue Masses

Soft tissue masses with a nonspecific imaging appearance should be assessed for extent and stage.[121,122] Imaging features of small size (<5 cm), defined margins, homogeneity, and lack of neurovascular encasement suggest a more benign process.[123–126] In contradistinction, large size (>5 cm), ill-defined margins, heterogeneity, and neurovascular or bone involvement suggest a malignant (aggressive) process.[123–126] However, in our opinion, *differentiation of benign versus malignant cannot be made with enough confidence to alter the need for biopsy.* Benign lesions that can reveal aggressive characteristics simulating malignancy include hematoma, fibromatosis, reactive lymph nodes, abscess, and myositis ossificans. Malignant lesions that at times reveal indolent features simulating benign disease include synovial sarcoma and myxoid liposarcoma.[17]

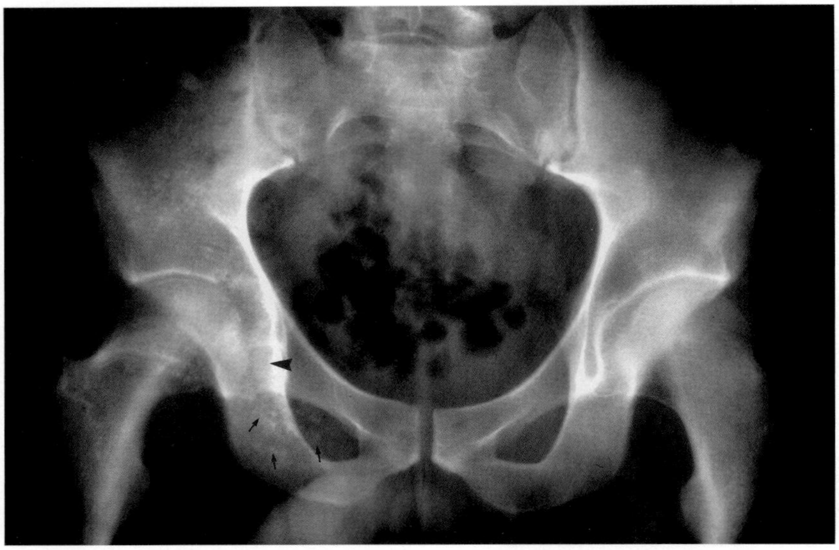

A

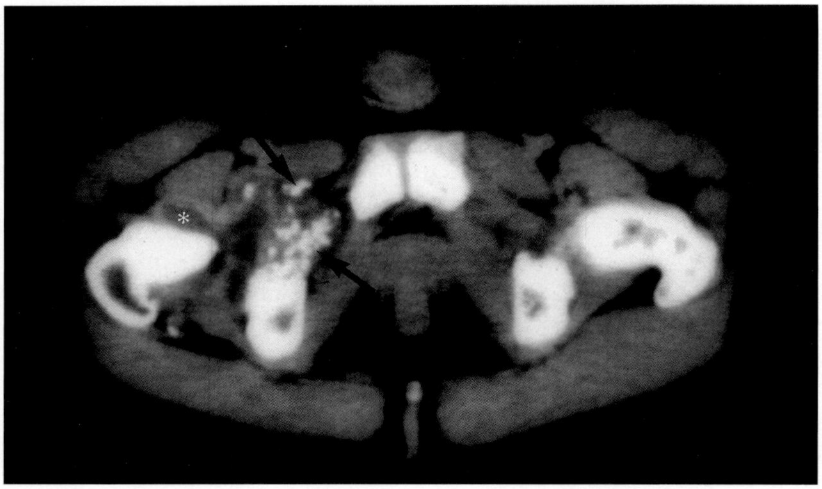

B

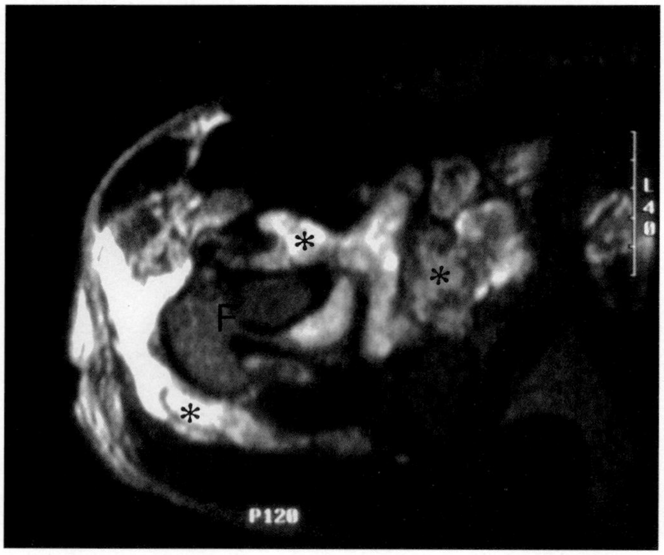

C

Figure 2-16. Synovial chondromatosis of the hip in a 27-year-old man with joint pain. *A,* Pelvis radiograph shows widening of the right hip joint *(large arrowhead)* with subtle calcifications *(small arrows)*. *B,* CT easily reveals multiple small calcifications *(large arrows)* and joint effusion *(white *)*. Axial T2-weighted MRI *(C)* shows a marked degree of abnormal tissue (*black* *) in the hip joint about the proximal femur (F) although the calcification allowing diagnosis is not readily apparent.

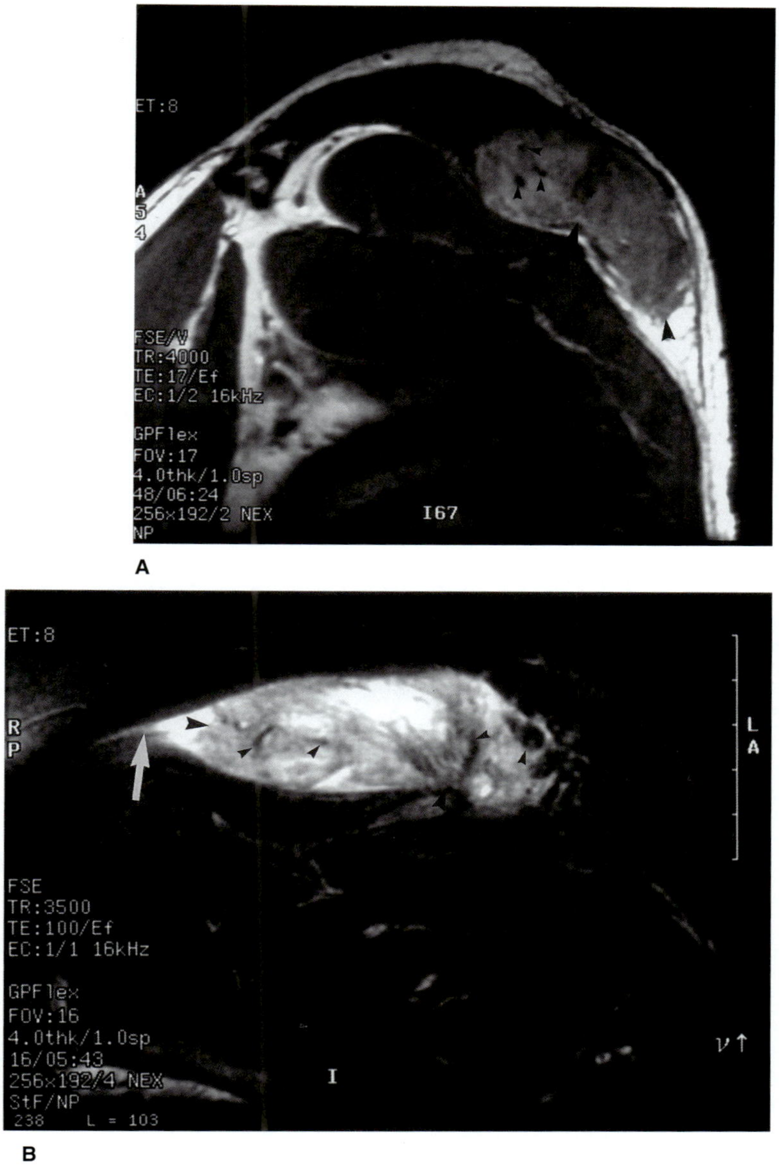

Figure 2–17. Extra-abdominal desmoid of the shoulder in a 32-year-old man. Sagittal T1-weighted *(A)* and coronal T2-weighted *(B)* MR images show a large mass *(large arrowheads)* about the shoulder. Intrinsic signal characteristics of low to intermediate signal intensity on T1-weighting and high signal on T2-weighting are nonspecific. Low signal intensity bands *(small arrowheads)*, fascial extension *(arrow)* as well as lesion location suggest the diagnosis.

Conclusion

In summary, the role of imaging in evaluation of soft tissue tumors has markedly improved because of the advent of CT, US, and more recently MRI. Indeed the latter modality has particularly improved the goal of imaging that includes lesion detection, characterization, and staging. Relatively specific histologic diagnosis can be made by imaging characteristics in 25% to 50% of lesions. We believe this will gradually increase over time with continuing experience. Soft tissue masses that often reveal pathognomonic imaging appearance include lipomatous lesions, angiomatous lesions, neurogenic tumors, "cystic" masses, elastofibroma, PVNS, synovial chondromatosis, and the fibromatoses. In imaging evaluation of soft tissue tumors with a nonspecific imaging appearance, lesion extent remains a vital role of radiologic assessment but distinction of benign from malignant lesions is fraught with uncertainty. These nonspecific masses require biopsy to direct definitive treatment. Clinical evaluation and treatment of soft tissue masses must emphasize a team approach incorporating the combined skills of radiologists, pathologists, and orthopedic oncologists with the ultimate goal of improving patient management and outcome.

Acknowledgments

The authors gratefully acknowledge the support of Linda C. Wilkins for manuscript preparation and Janeth Amarillo for photographic preparation. In addition, we thank the residents who attend the Armed Forces Institute of Pathology's radiologic-pathology courses for their contribution to our series of patients and without whom this project would not have been possible.

REFERENCES

Introduction

1. Weekes RG, McLeod RA, Reiman HM, Pritchard DJ: CT of soft-tissue neoplasms. AJR Am J Roentgenol 1985;144: 355–360.
2. Sundaram M, McGuire MH, Herbold DR: Magnetic resonance imaging of soft tissue masses: An evaluation of fifty-three histologically proven tumors. Magn Reson Imaging 1988;6:237–248.
3. Petasnick JP, Turner DA, Charters JR, Gitelis S, Zacharias CE: Soft-tissue masses of the locomotor system: Comparison of MR imaging with CT. Radiology 1986;160:125–133.
4. Totty WG, Murphy WA, Lee JKT: Soft-tissue tumors: MR imaging. Radiology 1986;160:135–141.
5. Kransdorf MJ, Jelinek JS, Moser RP, et al: Soft-tissue masses: Diagnosis using MR imaging. AJR Am J Roentgenol 1989;153:541–547.
6. Berquist TH, Ehman RL, King BF, Hodgman CG, Ilstrup DM: Value of MR imaging in differentiating benign from malignant soft tissue masses: Study of 95 lesions. AJR Am J Roentgenol 1990;155: 1251–1255.
7. Crim JR, Seeger LL, Yao L, Chandnani V, Eckardt JJ: Diagnosis of soft-tissue masses with MR imaging: Can benign masses be differentiated from malignant ones? Radiology 1992;185:581–586.
8. Weiss SW, Goldblum JR: General considerations. In Enzinger FM, Weiss SW, (eds): Soft Tissue Tumors, 4th ed, St. Louis, CV Mosby, 2001, 1–19.
9. Mettlin C, Priore R, Rao U, Gamble D, Lane W, Murphy GP: Results of the national soft-tissue sarcoma registry. Analysis of survival and prognostic factors. J Surg Oncology 1982;19:224–227.
10. Angervall L, Kindblom LG: Principles for pathologic-anatomic diagnosis and classification of soft-tissue sarcomas. Clin Orthop 1993;289:9–18.
11. Baldursson G, Agnarsson BA, Benediktsdottir KR, Hrafnkelsson J: Soft tissue sarcomas in Iceland 1955–1988. Acta Oncol 1991;30:563–568.
12. Greenlee RT, Taylor M, Bolden S, Wingo PA: Cancer statistics 2000. CA Cancer J. Clin 2000;50:7–33.

Radiologic Evaluation

13. Kransdorf MJ, Murphey MD: Radiologic evaluation of soft tissue masses: A current perspective. AJR Am J Roentgenol 2000;175:575.

Nuclear Medicine

14. Levine E, Huntrakoon M, Wetzel LH: Malignant nerve sheath neoplasms in neurofibromatosis: Distinction from benign tumors by using imaging techniques. AJR Am J Roentgenol 1987;149:1059–1064.
15. Hammond JA, Driedger AA: Detection of malignant change in neurofibromatosis (von Recklinghausen's disease) by gallium-67 scanning. Can Med Assoc J 1978;119:252–253.
16. Kaplan IL, Swayne LC, Baydin IA: Uptake of Ga-67 citrate in a benign neurofibroma. Clin Nucl Med 1989; 14:224–227.

Angiography

17. Kransdorf MJ, Murphey MD (eds): Imaging of Soft Tissue Tumors. Philadelphia, WB Sanders, 1997.

CT, MRI, and Ultrasound

18. Panicek DM, Gatsonis C, Rosenthal DI, et al: CT and MR imaging in the local staging of primary malignant musculoskeletal neoplasms: Report of the Radiology Diagnostic Oncology Group. Radiology 1997;202: 237–246.
19. Dalinka MK, Zlatkin MD, Chao P, Kricun ME, Kressel HY: The use of magnetic resonance imaging in the evaluation of bone and soft tissue tumors. Radiol Clin North Am 1990;28:461–470.
20. Pettersson H, Gillespy T, Hamlin DJ, et al: Primary musculoskeletal tumors: Examination with MR imaging compared with conventional modalities. Radiology 1987;164:237–241.
21. Tehranzadeh J, Mnaymneh W, Ghavam C, Morillo G, Murphy BJ: Comparison of CT and MR imaging in musculoskeletal neoplasms. J Comput Assist Tomogr 1989;13:466–472.
22. Aisen AM, Martel W, Braunstein EM, McMillin KI, Phillips WA, Kling TF: MRI and CT evaluation of primary bone and soft-tissue tumors. AJR Am J Roentgenol 1984;146:749–756.
23. Chang AE, Matory YL, Dwyer AJ, et al: Magnetic resonance imaging versus computed tomography in the evaluation of soft tissue tumors of the extremities. Ann Surg 1987;205:340–348.
24. Demas BE, Heelan RT, Lane J, Marcove R, Hajdu S, Brennan MF: Soft-tissue sarcomas of the extremities: Comparison of MR and CT in determining the extent of disease. AJR Am J Roentgenol 1988;150:615–620.
25. Hudson TM, Hamlin DJ, Enneking MD, Pettersson H: Magnetic resonance imaging of bone and soft-tissue tumors: Early experience in 31 patients compared with computed tomography. Skeletal Radiol 1985;13: 134–146.
26. Weekes RG, Berquist TH, McLeod RA, Zimmer WD: Magnetic resonance imaging of soft-tissue tumors: Comparison with computed tomography. Magn Reson Imaging 1985;3:345–352.
27. Bloem JL, Taminiau AHM, Eulderink F, Hermans J, Pauwels EK: Radiologic staging of primary bone sar-

coma: MR imaging, scintigraphy, angiography, and CT correlated with pathologic examination. Radiology 1988;169:805–810.
28. Rubin DA, Kneeland JB: MR imaging of the musculoskeletal system: Technical considerations for enhancing image quality and diagnostic yield. AJR Am J Roentgenol 1994;163:1155–1163.
29. Mirowitz SA: Fast scanning and fat-suppression MR imaging of musculoskeletal disorders. AJR Am J Roentgenol 1993;161:1147–1157.
30. Fujimoto H, Murakami K, Ichikawa T, et al: MRI of soft-tissue lesions: Opposed-phase T2*-weighted gradient-echo images. J Comput Assist Tomogr 1993; 17:418–424.
31. Shuman WP, Baron RL, Peters MJ, Tazioli PK: Comparison of STIR and spin-echo MR imaging at 1.5T in 90 lesions of the chest, liver and pelvis. AJR Am J Roentgenol 1989;152:853–859.
32. Dwyer AJ, Frank JA, Sank VJ, Reinig JW, Hickey AM, Doppman JL: Short-Tau inversion-recovery pulse sequence: Analysis and initial experience in cancer imaging. Radiology 1988;168:827–836.
33. Beltran J, Chandnani V, McGhee RA, Kursungoglu-Brahme S: Gadopentetate dimeglumine-enhanced MR imaging of the musculoskeletal system. AJR Am J Roentgenol 1991;156:457–466.
34. Verstraete KL, De Deene Y, Roels H, Dierick A, Uyttendaele D, Kunnen M: Benign and malignant musculoskeletal lesions: Dynamic contrast-enhanced MR imaging-parametric "first pass" images depict tissue vascularization and perfusion. Radiology 1994;192: 835–843.
35. Benedikt RA, Jelinek JS, Kransdorf MJ, Moser RP, Berrey BH: MR imaging of soft-tissue masses: Role of gadopentetate dimeglumine. J Magn Reson Imaging 1994;4:485–490.
36. Takebayashi S, Sugiyama M, Nagase M, Matsubara S: Severe adverse reaction to IV gadopentetate dimeglumine. AJR Am J Roentgenol 1993;160:659.
37. Tardy B, Guy C, Barral G, Page Y, Ollagnier M, Bertrand C: Anaphylactic shock induced by intravenous gadopentetate dimeglumine. Lancet 1992; 339:494.
38. Tisher S, Hoffman JC: Anaphylactoid reaction to IV gadopentetate dimeglumine. AJNR Am J Neuroradiol 1990;174:17–23.
39. Omohundro JE, Elderbrook MK, Ringer TV: Laryngospasm after administration of gadopentetate dimeglumine. J Magn Reson Imaging 1992;2: 729–730.
40. Shellock FG, Hahn HP, Mink JH, Itskovich E: Adverse reaction to intravenous gadoteridol. Radiology 1993; 189:151–152.
41. Jordan RM, Mintz RD: Fatal reaction to gadopentetate dimeglumine. AJR Am J Roentgenol 1995;164: 743–744.
42. Harkens KL, Moore TE, Yuh WTC, et al: Gadolinium-enhanced MRI of soft-tissue masses. Australas Radiol 1993;37:30–34.
43. Seeger LL, Widoff BE, Bassett LW, Rosen G, Eckardt JJ: Preoperative evaluation of osteosarcoma: Value of gadopentitate dimeglumine-enhanced MR imaging. AJR Am J Roentgenol 1991;157:347–351.
44. Kransdorf MJ, Murphey MD: The use of gadolinium in the MR evaluation of soft tissue tumors. Semin Ultrasound CT MR 1997;18:251–268.
45. Lin J, Jacobson JA, Fessell DP, Weadock WJ, Hayes CW: An illustrated tutorial of musculoskeletal sonography: Part 4, musculoskeletal masses, sonographically guided interventions, and miscellaneous topics. AJR Am J Roentgenol 2000;175:1711–1719.
46. Fornage BD, Tassin GB: Sonographic appearances of superficial soft-tissue lipomas. J Clin Ultrasound 1991;19:215–220.
47. Lin J, Fessell DP, Jacobson JA, Weadock WJ, Hayes CW: An illustrated tutorial of musculoskeletal sonography. 1. Introduction and general principles. AJR Am J Roentgenol 2000;175:637–645.
48. Loyer EM, DuBrow RA, David CL, Coan JD, Eftekhari F. Imaging of superficial soft-tissue infections: Sonographic findings in cases of cellulitis and abscess. AJR Am J Roentgenol 1996;166:149–152.
49. Choi H, Varma DG, Fornage BD, Kim EE, Johnston DA: Soft-tissue sarcoma: MR imaging vs. sonography for detection of local recurrence after surgery. AJR Am J Roentgenol 1991;157:353–358.

Staging

50. Enneking WF, Spanier SS, Goodman MA: A system for the surgical staging of musculoskeletal sarcoma. Clin Orthop 1980;153:106–120.
51. Hajdu SI: Pathology of Soft Tissue Tumors. Philadelphia, Lea & Febiger, 1979.
52. Russell WO, Cohen J, Edmonson JH, et al: Staging system for soft tissue sarcoma. Semin Oncol 1981; 8:156–159.
53. McDonald DJ: Limb-salvage surgery for treatment of sarcomas of the extremities. AJR Am J Roentgenol 1994;163:509–513.
54. Myhre-Jensen O: A consecutive 7-year series of 1331 benign soft tissue tumors. Clinicopathologic data. Comparison with sarcomas. Acta Orthop Scand 1981;52:287–293.
55. Rydholm A: Management of patients with soft-tissue tumors. Strategy developed at a regional oncology center. Acta Orthop Scand Suppl 1983;203:13–77.
56. Peabody TD, Simon MA: Principles of staging of soft-tissue sarcomas. Clin Orthop 1993;289:19–31.
57. Anderson MW, Temple HT, Dussault RG, Kaplan PA: Compartmental anatomy: Relevance to staging and biopsy of musculoskeletal tumors. AJR Am J Roentgenol 1999;173:1663–1671.

Lesion Specificity by Imaging

Lipomatous Lesions

58. Osment LS: Cutaneous lipomas and lipomatosis. Surg Gynecol Obstet 1968;127:129–132.
59. Leffert RD: Lipomas of the upper extremity. J Bone Joint Surg Am 1972;54-A:1262–1266.

60. Rydholm A, Berg NO: Size, site and clinical incidence of lipoma. Factors in the differential diagnosis of lipoma and sarcoma. Acta Orthop Scand 1983; 54:929–934.
61. Dooms GC, Hricak H, Sollitto RA, Higgins CB: Lipomatous tumors and tumors with fatty component: MR imaging potential and comparison of MR and CT results. Radiology 1985;157:479–483.
62. Kransdorf MJ, Moser RP, Meis JM, Meyer CA: Fat containing soft tissue masses of the extremities. RadioGraphics 1991;11:81–106.
63. Hunter JC, Johnston WH, Genant HK: Computed tomography evaluation of fatty tumors of the somatic soft tissues: Clinical utility and radiographic-pathologic correlation. Skeletal Radiol 1979;4:79–91.
64. Dolph JL, Demuth RJ, Miller SH: Familial multiple lipomatosis. Plast Reconstr Surg. 1980;66:620–622.
65. Barkhof F, Melkert P, Meyer S, Blomjous CEM: Derangement of adipose tissue: A case report of multicentric retroperitoneal liposarcomas, retroperitoneal lipomatosis and multiple subcutaneous lipomas. Eur J Surg Oncol 1991;17:547–550.
66. Leffell DJ, Braverman IM: Familial multiple lipomatosis. Report of a case and a review of the literature. J Am Acad Dermatol 1986;15:275–279.
67. Chung EB, Enzinger FM: Benign lipoblastomatosis: An analysis of 35 cases. Cancer 1973;32:482–492.
68. Jimenez JF: Lipoblastoma in infancy and childhood. J Surg Oncol 1986;32:238–244.
69. Lateur L, Van Ongeval C, Samson I, et al: Case report 842. Benign hibernoma. Skeletal Radiol 1994;23:306–309.
70. Seynaeve P, Mortelmans L, Knockx M, et al: Case report 813. Hibernoma of the left thigh. Skeletal Radiol 1994;23:137–138.
71. Jelinek JS, Kransdorf MJ, Shmookler BM, et al: Liposarcoma of the extremities: MR and CT findings of the histologic subtypes. Radiology 1993;186:455–459.
72. London J, Kim EE, Wallace S, et al: MR imaging of liposarcomas: Correlation of MR features and histology. J Comput Assist Tomogr 1989;15:832–835.
73. Kransdorf MJ, Meis JM, Jelinek JS: Dedifferentiated liposarcoma of the extremities: Imaging findings in four patients. AJR Am J Roentgenol 1993;161:127–130.
74. Sundaram M, Baran G, Merenda G, McDonald DJ: Myxoid liposarcoma: Magnetic resonance imaging appearances with clinical and histological correlation. Skeletal Radiol 1990;19:359–362.
75. Murphey MD, Flemming DJ, Jelinek JS, Temple HT, Levinc A, Torop AH: Imaging of higher grade liposarcoma with pathologic correlation. Radiology 1997; 205(P):332.

Angiomatous Lesions

76. Murphey MD, Fairbairn KJ, Parman LM, et al: Musculoskeletal angiomatous lesions: Radiologic-pathologic correlation. RadioGraphics 1995;15:893–917.
77. Derchi LE, Balconi G, De Flaviis L, et al: Sonographic appearances of hemangiomas of skeletal muscle. J Ultrasound Med 1989;8:263–267.
78. Greenspan A, McGahan JP, Vogelsang P, Szabo RM: Imaging strategies in the evaluation of soft tissue hemangiomas of the extremities: Correlation of the findings of plain radiography, angiography, CT, MRI, and ultrasonography in 12 histologically proven cases. Skeletal Radiol 1992;21:11–18.
79. Hawnaur JM, Whitehouse RW, Jenkins JPR, Isherwood I: Musculoskeletal hemangiomas: Comparison of MRI with CT. Skeletal Radiol 1990;19:251–258.
80. Buetow PC, Kransdorf MJ, Moser RP, et al: Radiologic appearance of intramuscular hemangioma with emphasis on MR imaging. AJR Am J Roentgenol 1990; 154:563–567.
81. Yuh WTC, Kathol MH, Sein MA, et al: Hemangiomas of skeletal muscle: MR findings in five patients. AJR Am J Roentgenol 1987;149:765–768.
82. Cohen EK, Kressel HY, Perosio T, et al: MR imaging of soft-tissue hemangiomas: Correlation with pathologic findings. AJR Am J Roentgenol 1988;150:1079–1081.
83. Nelson MC, Stull MA, Teitelbaum GP et al: Magnetic resonance imaging of peripheral soft-tissue hemangiomas. Skeletal Radiol 1990;19:447–482.
84. McRae GA, Murphey MD, Temple HT, Torop AH, Fanburg-Smith J: Imaging of soft tissue hemangioma with pathologic correlation. Radiology 1997; 205(P):449.

Neurogenic Tumors

85. Murphey MD, Smith WS, Smith SE, Kransdorf MJ, Temple HT: Imaging of musculoskeletal neurogenic tumors: Radiologic-pathologic correlation. RadioGraphics 1999;19:1253–1280.
86. Suh JS, Abenoza P, Galloway HR, Everson LI, Griffiths HJ: Peripheral (extracranial) nerve tumors: Correlation of MR imaging and histologic-findings. Radiology 1992;183:341–346.
87. Kumar AJ, Kuhajda FP, Martinez CR, Fishman EK, Jezic DV, Siegelman SS: Computed tomography of extracranial nerve sheath tumors with pathologic correlation. J Comput Assist Tomogr 1983;7:857–865.
88. Stull M, Moser RP, Kransdorf MJ, Bogumill GP, Nelson MC: Magnetic resonance appearance of peripheral nerve sheath tumors. Skeletal Radiol 1991;20:9–14.
89. Cerofolini E, Landi A, DeSantis G, Mairorana A, Canossi G, Romagnoli R: MR of benign peripheral nerve sheath tumors. J Comput Assist Tomogr 1991;15: 593–597.
90. Cohen LM, Schwartz AM, Rockoff SD: Benign schwannomas: Pathologic basis for CT inhomogeneities. AJR Am J Roentgenol 1983;147:141–143.
91. Singson RD, Feldman F, Slipman CW, Gonzalez E, Rosenberg ZS, Kiernan H: Postamputation neuromas and other symptomatic stump abnormalities: Detection with CT. Radiology 1987;162:743–745.
92. Boutin RD, Pathria MN, Resnick D: Disorders in the stumps of amputee patients: MR imaging. AJR Am J Roentgenol 1998;171:497–501.
93. Zanetti M, Ledermann T, Zollinger H, Hodler J: Efficacy of MR imaging in patients suspected of having

Morton's neuroma. AJR Am J Roentgenol 1997; 168:529–532.
94. Redd RA, Peters VJ, Emery SF, Branch HM, Rifkin MD: Morton neuroma: Sonographic evaluation. Radiology 1989;171:415–417.
95. Zanetti M, Strehle JK, Zollinger H, Hodler J: Morton neuroma and fluid in the intermetatarsal bursae on MR images of 70 asymptomatic volunteers. Radiology 1997;203:516–520.

Cystic Masses

96. Feldman F, Singson RD, Staron RB: Magnetic resonance imaging of para-articular and ectopic ganglia. Skeletal Radiol 1989;18:353–358.
97. Schwimmer M, Edelstein G, Heiken JP, Gilula LA: Synovial cysts of the knee: CT evaluation. Radiology 1985;154:175–177.
98. Haller J, Resnick D, Greenway G, et al: Juxtaacetabular ganglionic (or synovial) cysts: CT and MR features. J Comput Assist Tomogr 1989;13: 976–983.
99. DeFlaviis L, Nessi R, Del Bo P, et al: High-resolution ultrasonography of wrist ganglia. J Clin Ultrasound 1987;15:17–22.
100. Recht MP, Applegate G, Kaplan P, et al: The MR appearance of cruciate ganglion cysts: A report of 16 cases. Skeletal Radiol 1994;23:597–600.
101. Burk DL Jr, Dalinka MK. Kanal E, et al: Meniscal and ganglion cysts of the knee: MR evaluation. AJR Am J Roentgenol 1988;150:331–336.
102. Schuldt DR, Wolfe RD. Clinical and athrographic findings in meniscal cysts. Radiology 1980;134:49–52.
103. Tyson LL, Daughters TC Jr, Ryu RKN, Crues JV III: MRI appearance of meniscal cysts. Skeletal Radiol 1995;24:421–424.
104. Sundaram M, McDonald DJ, Merenda G: Intramuscular myxoma: A rare but important association with fibrous dysplasia of bone. AJR Am J Roentgenol 1989;153:107–108.
105. Wirth WA, Leavitt D, Enzinger FM. Multiple intramuscular myxomas: Another extraskeletal manifestation of fibrous dysplasia. Cancer 1971;27:321–340.

Other Lesions with Specific Imaging Appearances

106. Brandser EA, Goree JC, El-Khoury GY: Elastofibroma dorsi: Prevalence in an elderly patient population as revealed by CT. AJR Am J Roentgenol 1998;171: 977–980.
107. Kransdorf MJ, Meis JM, Montgomery E: Elastofibroma: MR and CT appearance with radiologic pathologic correlation. AJR Am J Roentgenol 1992;159: 575–579.
108. Bui-Mansfield LT, Chew FS, Stanton CA: Elastofibroma dorsi of the chest wall. AJR Am J Roentgenol 2000;175:244.
109. Cotten A, Flipo RM, Chastanet P, et al: Pigmented villonodular synovitis of the hip: Review of radiographic features in 58 patients. Skeletal Radiol 1995;24:1–6.
110. Jelinek JS, Kransdorf MJ, Shmookler BM, et al: Giant cell tumor of tendon sheath: MR imaging in nine cases. AJR Am J Roentgenol 1994;162:919–922.
111. Jelinek JS, Kransdorf MJ, Utz JA, et al: Imaging of pigmented villonodular synovitis with emphasis on magnetic resonance imaging. AJR Am J Roentgenol 1989;152:337–342.
112. Milgram JW: Synovial osteochondromatosis. A histopathological study of thirty cases. J Bone Joint Surg 1977;59A:792–801.
113. Blandino A, Salvi L, Chirico G, et al: Synovial chondromatosis of the ankle: MR findings. Clin Imaging 1992;16:34–36.
114. Sundaram M, McGuire MH, Fletcher J, et al: Magnetic resonance imaging of lesions of synovial origin. Skeletal Radiol 1986;15:110–116.
115. Kramer J, Recht M, Deely DM, et al: MR appearance of idiopathic synovial osteochondromatosis. J Comput Assist Tomogr 1993;17:772–776.
116. Rock MG, Pritchard DJ, Reiman HM, Soule EH, Brewster RC: Extra-abdominal desmoid tumors. J Bone Joint Surg Am 1984;66-A:1369–1374.
117. Sundaram M, Duffrin H, McGuire MH, Vas W: Synchronous multicentric desmoid tumors (aggressive fibromatosis) of the extremities. Skeletal Radiol 1988;17:16–19.
118. Kransdorf MJ, Jelinek JS, Moser RP, et al: MR appearance of fibromatosis: A report of 14 cases and review of the literature. Skeletal Radiol 1990;19:495–499.
119. Quinn SF, Erickson SJ, Dee PM, et al: MR imaging in fibromatosis: Results in 26 patients with pathologic correlation. AJR Am J Roentgenol 1991;156:539–542.
120. Sundaram M, McGuire MH, Schajowicz F: Soft tissue masses: Histologic basis for decreased signal (short T2) on T2-weighted MR images. AJR Am J Roentgenol 1987;148:1247–1250.

Nonspecific Soft Tissue Masses

121. Kransdorf MJ: Malignant soft-tissue tumors in a large referral population: Distribution of diagnoses by age, sex and location. AJR Am J Roentgenol 1995;164: 129–134.
122. Kransdorf MJ:. Benign soft-tissue tumors in a large referral population: Distribution of diagnoses by age, sex and location. AJR Am J Roentgenol 1995;164: 395–402.
123. Beltran J, Simon DC, Katz W, Weis LD: Increased MR signal intensity in skeletal muscle adjacent to malignant tumors: Pathologic correlation and clinical relevance. Radiology 1987;162:251–255.
124. Hanna SL, Fletcher BD, Parham DM, Bugg MF: Muscle edema in musculoskeletal tumors: MR imaging characteristics and clinical significance. J Magn Reson Imaging 1991;1:441–449.
125. Mirowitz SA, Totty WG, Lee JKT: Characterization of musculoskeletal masses using dynamic Gd-DTPA enhanced spin-echo MRI. J Comput Assist Tomogr 1992;16:120–125.
126. DeSchepper A, Ramon F, Degryse H: Statistical analysis of MRI parameters predicting malignancy in 141 soft tissue masses. Rofo Fortschr Geb Rontgenstr Neuen Bildgeb Verfahr 1992:156:587–591.

Immunohistochemistry of Soft Tissue Tumors

CHAPTER 3

This chapter outlines the biologic background and the distribution of the most significant immunohistochemical markers in normal and neoplastic soft tissues. Tumor type-specific applications are detailed with the specific tumors in Chapters 5 through 21, and markers for lymphomas are found in Chapter 21. There are several review articles on this topic.[1-7]

The most important cell-type markers are grouped under subheadings of endothelial, muscle cell, neural and neuroendocrine, melanoma and histiocytic markers, keratins, other epithelial and mesothelial markers, other cell type markers, and cell cycle markers. These markers and their main diagnostic targets have been listed in Table 3–1.

Immunohistochemistry is the most practical way to evaluate the presence of certain protein and carbohydrate epitopes on tissue sections, and evaluation of cell- or tumor-type specific or cell cycle related markers is often of high diagnostic and differential diagnostic significance, although very few markers are totally specific for one tumor type, and no cell cycle marker is able to separate benign and malignant tumors.

Complete knowledge of antigen expression of different tumors is also important for understanding the biology of tumors. There are an estimated 30,000 to 50,000 genes, many of which are yet to be discovered. Undoubtedly, some of their products will prove to be important markers in the evaluation of soft tissue and other tumors. The advances in epitope retrieval, especially by heat (by microwave, heating, or steaming) has made many antibodies available in paraffin sections that were previously thought to perform on fresh or specially fixed tissue only.

There is voluminous literature on diagnostic immunohistochemistry, sometimes with contradictory information. This partly results from the use of different and sometimes incompletely characterized antibodies, variations in detection methods, and progressive improvement in epitope retrieval that makes some older findings outdated. Many markers have not yet been critically evaluated with large panels of tumors and nonneoplastic tissues; such studies will likely settle many existing controversies and uncertainties.

The most useful markers represent cell surface and cell membrane antigens, structural proteins, secretory products, cytoplasmic antigens, and nuclear antigens (cell cycle and transcriptional regulators), as shown in Table 3–2. Many antigens are classified as leukocyte antigens with a cluster of differentiation (CD) number, and their expression in mesenchymal cells is sometimes highly diagnostic. The use of leukocyte-specific antigens in the diagnosis of lymphoid and histiocytic lesions of soft tissues is discussed in Chapter 21.

Use of well-documented specific antibodies, good detection systems, clean quality of staining, validation of positive and negative controls, thorough knowledge on the distribution of various antigens in different tissues and tumors, and experience in the interpretation are the key elements in successful application of immunohistochemistry. Diagnostic immunohistochemistry has to be understood as an

Table 3–1. Main Groups of Immunohistochemical Cell Differentiation Markers, with Selected Single Markers and Their Most Important Applications in Soft Tissue Tumors

Group of Markers	Useful in the Diagnosis of/Positive in
Endothelial markers	
CD31	Angiosarcoma, Kaposi sarcoma
CD34	Kaposi sarcoma, many vascular fibroblastic and some other tumors
vWF	Angiosarcoma, hemangioendothelioma (especially epithelioid)
Ulex europaeus/BNH9	Angiosarcoma, many carcinomas
VEGFR-3	Kaposi sarcoma, many angiosarcomas and hemangiomas
Podoplanin	Kaposi sarcoma, many angiosarcomas
Thrombomodulin (CD141)	Variable in angiosarcoma, positive also in mesothelioma, squamous carcinoma
Fli-1	Angiosarcomas, Ewing sarcoma
Muscle cell markers	
Actins: Common muscle	Smooth and skeletal muscle tumors, myofibroblastic tumors
Smooth muscle	Smooth muscle and myofibroblastic tumors
Sarcomeric	Skeletal muscle and rhabdomyosarcoma
Desmin	Smooth and skeletal muscle tumors, some others
HCD	Smooth muscle and its tumors, myoepithelia, GI stromal tumors
Calponin	Smooth muscle, myofibroblasts, myoepithelia Synovial sarcoma (often)
MyoD1, myogenin	Rhabdomyosarcoma (reactive skeletal muscle)
Myoglobin	Rhabdomyosarcoma (differentiated)
Myosins	Isoforms for smooth and skeletal muscle tumors
Neural and neuroendocrine-specific markers	
Synaptophysin	Neuroblastoma, paraganglioma, neuroendocrine carcinomas
Chromogranin	Paraganglioma, neuroendocrine carcinoma (especially low-grade)
NSE	General neuroendocrine marker, specificity not good
NF proteins	Neuroblastoma, paraganglioma, Merkel cell carcinoma
α-Internexin	Same as NFs
S-100 protein and other multispecific neural markers	
S-100 protein	Melanocytic, schwannian, chondroid, Langerhans cell
Nerve growth factor receptor p75	Dermatofibrosarcoma protuberans, many other sarcomas Nerve sheath tumors
CD56 (NCAM)	Neuroendocrine carcinomas, rhabdomyosarcoma, many other sarcomas
CD57	Nerve sheath tumors, also synovial sarcoma, leiomyosarcoma, relatively nonspecific
Melanoma markers other than S-100 protein	
HMB45	Melanoma, clear cell sarcoma, angiomyolipoma
Tyrosinase	Nevi, melanoma
Melan A	Nevi, melanoma, angiomyolipoma
Microphthalmia	Melanoma, osteoclastic giant cells
CD63	Melanoma, some carcinomas, alveolar soft part sarcoma
Histiocytic markers	
Lysozyme	Histiocytes, myelomonocytic cells
AAT	Histiocytes, many tumors of any lineage
AACT	Histiocytes, many tumors of any lineage
Factor XIIIa	Histiocytes, especially dendritic ones

Table continued on following page

Table 3–1. Main Groups of Immunohistochemical Cell Differentiation Markers, with Selected Single Markers and Their Most Important Applications in Soft Tissue Tumors *continued*

Group of Markers	Useful in the Diagnosis of/Positive in
CD68	Histiocytes and any lysosome-rich cells of any derivation, melanoma, paraganglioma, schwannoma, granular cell tumor
CD163	Histiocytes, seems highly specific, experience limited
Keratins	Carcinomas, synovial and epithelioid sarcoma, chordoma, sporadically in many other sarcomas and metastatic melanoma (see separate tables)
Other epithelial and mesothelial markers with variable specificities	
EMA	Epithelial tumors in general, perineurial tumors, some others Synovial sarcoma, epithelioid sarcoma
B72.3	Many adenocarcinomas, epithelioid angiosarcoma
BerEp4	Many adenocarcinomas, biphasic synovial sarcoma
Cadherins	Complex distribution in epithelial and some nonepithelial tumors
Calretinin	Mesothelioma, some carcinomas, synovial sarcoma (often)
CEA	Many adenocarcinomas, biphasic synovial sarcomas?
Desmoplakins	Epithelial tumors in general, meningioma, Ewing sarcoma
HBME-1	Mesothelioma, some adenocarcinomas, synovial sarcoma chordoma, chondrosarcoma
Mesothelin	Mesothelioma, ovarian serous carcinoma, some other adenocarcinomas, biphasic synovial sarcoma
MOC31	Most adenocarcinomas, rare mesotheliomas
TTF-1	Carcinomas of thyroid and pulmonary (adeno, small cell) origin, small cell carcinomas of many organs (not Merkel cell carcinoma)
Villin	GI and renal carcinomas, some carcinoids
WT protein	Small round cell desmoplastic tumor, mesothelioma, ovarian serous carcinoma and related tumors
Other important tumor type markers	
ALK	Large cell anaplastic lymphoma (variable), IMT (variable) Basement membrane proteins, Schwann cell tumors, angiosarcoma
Bcl-2	Widespread
CD10	Endometrial stromal sarcoma
CD99	Ewing sarcoma, widespread in different tumors
CD117	GI stromal tumor, mast cell neoplasms, angiosarcoma, Ewing sarcoma, neuroblastoma, seminoma/dysgerminoma, some melanomas and clear cell sarcomas, adenoid cystic carcinoma, few other carcinomas
ERs and PR	Carcinomas of breast, endometrium, and ovaries (some) Most uterine and retroperitoneal leiomyomas (in women) Angiomyofibroblastoma, aggressive angiomyxoma
GFAP	Glial tumors, schwannomas, myoepithelial tumors
Inhibin	Granulosa cell tumor, adrenal cortical carcinoma Granular cell tumor
Osteocalcin	Osteosarcoma, osteoid material
Vimentin	Widespread in mesenchymal tumors, many poorly differentiated carcinomas highlighted as negative, but many are variably positive
Cell cycle markers	
Ki67 analogs (MIB-1)	
Cyclins	
p53 (TP53)	
p16	
p21	
p27	
MDM2	
RB1	

Table 3–2. Examples of Classes of Proteins by Location or Function, Used as Cell-Type or Diagnostic Markers in Immunohistochemistry of Soft Tissue Tumors

Cell Membrane Proteins	Organelle-Specific Proteins	Cytoplasmic Proteins	Cytoskeletal Proteins	Nuclear Proteins
CD10	Lysosomes	S-100 protein	Intermediate filament proteins	Transcriptional regulators
CD31		AAT		
CD34	CD68	NSE	Vimentin	ER
CD117 (KIT)			Keratins	PR
Ber-EP4			Desmin	Myogenic regulators
EMA	Mitochondria		GFAP Neurofilaments	TTF-1
	bcl-2			Cell cycle regulators
			Microfilament proteins	
	Melanocytes			
			Actins	Ki67 analogs p21, p27, p53, RB1
	HMB45, tyrosinase			
	Microvesicles: Synaptophysin			
	Neuroendocrine granules: Chromogranin			

adjunct test, to be interpreted in the context of histology and clinicopathologic situation. The technical aspects of immunohistochemistry will be discussed in the end of the chapter.

Endothelial Markers

A number of cellular antigens are typical constitutional components of endothelial cells, and some of them are useful in the evaluation of endothelial cell differentiation of tumors, helping in the differential diagnosis of vascular tumors, especially Kaposi sarcoma and angiosarcoma. None of these antigens is entirely endothelial cell specific, and their use in combination is recommended in problem cases. The most useful endothelial markers are summarized in Table 3–3.

In addition, many other endothelial (and leukocyte) antigens are produced by endothelial cells in a cytokine-dependent manner, giving the modified endothelia different functional properties. So far, these antigens have not been proven significant in tumor diagnosis.

CD31

CD31 is platelet endothelium cell adhesion molecule 1, (PECAM-1). This transmembrane glycoprotein of 130 kd has six extracellular immunoglobulin-like loops and homology to other cell adhesion molecules, such as the carcinoembryonic antigen (CEA). CD31 is constitutively expressed in most endothelial cells and associates internally with catenin family proteins.[8,9] In hematopoietic cells, CD31 is present in a subset of myeloblasts, platelets, megakaryocytes, sinus histiocytes of lymph nodes, some lymphoid cells, and some histiomonocytic cells.[10] A distinctive membrane staining pattern is typically observed in positive cells. Platelet aggregates and areas of thrombosis and hemorrhage are typically positive. Inflammatory infiltrates often contain positive cells, which should not be confused with tumor cell reactivity.

Most data published on CD31 in pathology literature are based on the use of monoclonal antibody JC/70, with enzymatic predigestion. CD31 is nearly consistently present in benign and malignant vascular tumors including hemangiomas, epithelioid hemangioendothelioma, angiosarcomas, and Kaposi

Table 3–3. Overview of Endothelial Cell Markers

CD31	PECAM-1	All endothelia	Most angiosarcomas Kaposi sarcoma
CD34	Hematopoietic progenitor cell antigen	All endothelia	50% of angiosarcomas All Kaposi sarcomas
vWF	Factor VIII-related antigen	Most endothelia	
CD141	Thrombomodulin	Endothelia and mesothelia, squamous and some other carcinomas	
VEFGR-3	flt-4	Lymphatics, fenestrated endothelia, neovascular endothelia	
Fli-1		Endothelia	All angiosarcomas?

sarcoma.[10–12] Many angiosarcomas show a distinct membrane staining pattern, which is more distinct in epithelioid vascular tumors. Although positivity in carcinoma or mesothelioma has been occasionally reported, this appears to be rare (<1%) based on a large series.[13] No significant reactivity has been reported in melanoma and nonvascular sarcomas.

This marker is probably closest to the immunohistochemical gold standard for the definition of an endothelial neoplasm; without a positive result for CD31 it might be difficult to verify a tumor as an angiosarcoma. In addition, CD31 is variably expressed in blasts of extramedullary myeloid tumors.

CD34 (Hematopoietic Progenitor Cell Antigen)

This heavily glycosylated transmembrane glycoprotein of 115 kd is a sialomucin of an unknown, possibly receptor-related function, but no ligands have been identified.[14] CD34 is expressed in early hematopoietic blasts, virtually all endothelial cells, and subsets of fibroblasts. In the skin, the positive fibroblasts are located especially periadnexally and perivascularly, and in different organs they are commonly seen in septal structures and around blood vessels.[15,16] Superficial stroma of the uterine cervix and vagina are also positive. Positive spindle cells usually show an apparently cytoplasmic staining pattern, whereas a distinct membrane staining is seen especially in large cytoplasmic cells.

Two monoclonal antibodies to CD34 are commonly used in formalin-fixed and paraffin-embedded tissue: QBEND10 and My10/HPCA1, both following enzyme pretreatment of heat-induced epitope retrieval. CD34 is useful in the evaluation of vascular and spindle cell, especially fibroblastic tumors. The differential diagnostic applications have been listed in Table 3–4.

Kaposi sarcoma is a consistently positive vascular tumor (100%). Angiosarcomas of different types and epithelioid hemangioendotheliomas are variably positive in approximately 50% of the cases, although some early reports showed 100% positivity, and others suggested positivity for CD34 to differentiate Kaposi sarcoma from angiosarcoma.[17–19] The contrast between CD34$^-$ spindle cell hemangioma and positive Kaposi sarcoma can be diagnostically useful (Fig. 3–1).

Several spindle cell-fibroblastic tumors are consistently positive for CD34. These include dermatofibrosarcoma protuberans.[20–22] However, tumors with fibrosarcomatous transformation may be less uniformly positive or occasionally even CD34$^-$.[23] CD34 is useful in the differential diagnosis of dermatofibrosarcoma protuberans (DFSP) and benign fibrous histiocytoma, because the latter is almost always negative.

Solitary fibrous tumors and hemangiopericytomas of different locations are equally positive,[15,24,25] but desmoplastic mesotheliomas[26] and synovial sarcomas are usually negative. A small subset of true meningiomas are variably CD34$^+$; this is more common in fibroblastic variants, in our experience.

Of tumors of adipose tissue, spindle cell lipomas are consistently positive, and many well-differentiated and some dedifferentiated liposarcomas contain CD34$^+$ tumor cells.[27]

The CD34$^+$ fibroblastic component is typically present in neurofibromas, often in a netlike pattern.[28,29] In our experience, loss of the CD34$^+$ cell

Table 3-4. Differential Diagnostic Applications of CD34 in Immunohistochemical Analysis of Soft Tissue Tumors: Examples of Tumors with Contrasting Patterns of Immunoreactivity

CD34⁺ Tumors	Typically CD34⁻ Tumors
DFSP	Cellular fibrous histiocytoma, benign fibrous histiocytoma
Solitary fibrous tumor	Desmoid, fibrosarcoma, sarcomatous mesothelioma, synovial sarcoma
Hemangiopericytoma	Meningioma (<10% positive)
Kaposi sarcoma (spindle cells)	Spindle cell hemangioma (spindle cells)
GISTs (70%)	GI leiomyomas and schwannomas Leiomyosarcoma (20–30% variably positive)
Angiosarcoma (50%)	Metastatic carcinoma, primary squamous cell carcinoma
Epithelioid sarcoma (50%)	
Neurofibroma (a CD34⁺ component)	Schwannoma (few CD34⁺ cells) MPSNT

population may be a helpful feature in evaluation transformation of neurofibroma into a malignant peripheral nerve sheath tumor (MPNST).

Gastrointestinal (GI) stromal tumors (defined as KIT⁺ tumors) are CD34⁺ in (70%) of cases, including both spindle cell and epithelioid variants. More consistently positive are esophageal, gastric, and rectal tumors, whereas small intestinal ones express CD34 in 50% of the cases; the positivity does not appear to vary by tumor malignancy. GI leiomyomas and schwannomas are negative.[30] However, typical leiomyosarcomas, especially the retroperitoneal and uterine ones, are variably CD34⁺ in 20% to 30% of cases.[12,30,31]

Other positive tumors include epithelioid sarcoma (50%), which is diagnostically useful considering the very rare CD34 positivity of carcinomas.[19] In hematopoietic tumors, CD34 is essentially limited to primitive leukemias and blastic extramedullary myeloid tumors.

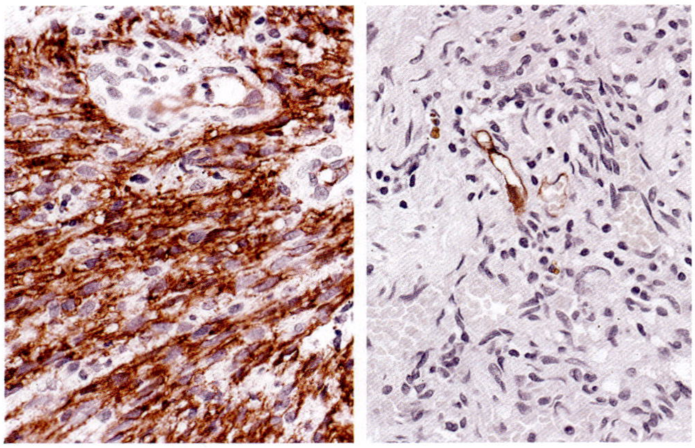

Figure 3-1. Kaposi sarcoma spindle cells are strongly positive for CD34 (*left*). Negativity for this marker in spindle cell hemangioma, except in capillary endothelia, can be diagnostically helpful (*right*).

von Willebrand Factor (vWF, Factor VIII-Related Antigen)

This structurally complex polymeric glycoprotein is composed of monomers of 270 kd, is noncovalently bound to factor VIII, and acts in the coagulation system.[32] It is synthesized and expressed in megakaryocytes and vascular endothelial cells, which also secrete it into the circulating blood and subendothelial matrix. Vascular endothelia of different types are positive, except some capillaries, liver sinusoids, and lymphatics may be negative.[10] Immunostaining often reveals granular cytoplasmic positivity reflecting the subcellular location in the Weibel-Palade bodies of endothelial cells.

The vWF was the first marker to be used for the identification of neoplastic endothelial cells.[33] Although consistently present in benign endothelia, this antigen is inconsistently expressed in transformed endothelia and angiosarcomas, although its endothelial specificity is high. It is more often present in well-differentiated angiosarcomas, often only focally.[12,34] Epithelioid hemangioendotheliomas often show luminal and cytoplasmic staining, which helps to differentiate them from carcinomas.

This marker is best used together with other endothelial markers, especially CD31. Necrotic and hemorrhagic tissue shows a high biologic background due to the content of this antigen in the serum; this may make the staining uninterpretable.

Ulex europaeus I Lectin and BNH9 Monoclonal Antibody

Ulex europaeus I lectin (UEAI) and the BNH9 monoclonal antibody recognizing the H and Y blood group antigens bind to certain fucosyl sugar residues on the surface glycocompounds of endothelial and many epithelial cells.[35] They have a similar distribution except UEAI binds only to blood group O erythrocytes, whereas BNH9 recognizes all erythrocytes.

All endothelia are positive, and benign vascular tumors and angiosarcomas are consistently and Kaposi sarcomas variably positive. The UEAI/BNH9 positivity of many epithelia and epithelial tumors (squamous carcinomas, many adenocarcinomas, synovial sarcoma epithelium) limits the diagnostic utility of these markers in vascular tumors.[12,35]

Other Potential Endothelial Markers

Vascular endothelial growth factor receptor type 3 (VEGFR-3, formerly named Flt-4) is a transmembrane receptor tyrosine kinase specific for subsets of endothelia and trophoblast. The receptor is constitutively expressed in lymphatics and certain capillary endothelia, especially in the fenestrated endothelia in the renal glomeruli, endocrine organs, and nasal mucosa. Its ligands are vascular endothelial growth factors C and D (VEGFC and VEGFD). The growth factors themselves are produced by different cell types, VEGFD by the cells of the dispersed endocrine system.[36]

VEGFR3 is expressed in 100% of Kaposi sarcomas.[37,38] A majority of angiosarcomas (80%) of different sites are positive, but those with epithelioid cytology, including epithelioid hemangioendotheliomas, are less often positive (40–50%). Also endothelia of neovascular capillaries in carcinomas and sarcomas are often positive. Limited review of nonvascular tumors has shown them negative, suggesting that this marker may be useful in the separation of malignant vascular tumors from the nonvascular ones.[38]

Podoplanin is a membrane protein present in podocytes of renal glomeruli. It is also expressed in lymphatic vessels and in a subset of angiosarcomas. Positive tumors have been hypothesized to display dual lymphatic endothelial-like differentiation.[39]

Thrombomodulin (CD141) is a thrombin-binding and thrombolysis-activating antithrombotic protein of 75 kd, constitutively expressed in endothelia, trophoblast, and mesothelial cells.[40] Although original studies suggested a good diagnostic value,[41,42] thrombomodulin in our experience is variably and inconsistently expressed in hemangiomas, hemangioendotheliomas, and angiosarcomas. In our experience, some synovial sarcomas and epithelioid sarcomas also demonstrate positivity, the former usually in the spindle cell components. The common CD141 expression in mesothelioma versus rare expression in pulmonary and other adenocarcinomas has made thrombomodulin a commonly used marker for the immunohistochemical differential diagnosis for mesothelioma.[43]

Freund's leukemia integration site *(Fli-1)* gene encodes for a transciptional regulator protein consistently expressed in the nuclei of endothelial cells, lymphocytes, and Ewing sarcoma cells. The *Fli-1* gene is a partner in the t(11;22) translocation in Ewing sarcoma. In one study, normal vascular endothelia, all 9 conventional and 11 of 13 epithelioid angiosarcomas and all 12 Kaposi sarcomas were immunohistochemically Fli-1^+ and 68 nonvascular tumors negative.[441]

Muscle Cell Markers

Smooth muscle, skeletal muscle, and myofibroblastic differentiation can be evaluated with a number of markers (Table 3–5). They are mostly cytoskeletal or cytoskeleton-associated proteins. Actins are a family of microfilament (6-nm) proteins, desmin is the intermediate filament (10-nm) protein typical of muscle cells, and calponin and heavy-caldesmon are actin-binding, cytoskeleton associated proteins of smooth muscle cells.

Transcriptional regulators of the skeletal muscle, MyoD1 and myogenin, are new specific nuclear markers for skeletal muscle differentiation and rhabdomyosarcoma.

An important problem and diagnostic pitfall in all muscle cell markers is the presence of entrapped or reactive muscle cells or myofibroblasts between the tumor cells; in some instances the nature of these components is difficult to determine, and this can lead to misidentification of a tumor as a myoid one.

Actins

The microfilament (diameter 6 nm) cytoskeleton composed actin is ubiquitous in all types of cells, but it is abundant and bundled into myofilaments in muscle cells. There are at least six different, highly homologous actin isoforms of 43 kd, originally discovered by 2-dimensional gel electrophoresis and found to have different cell type specificities. There are three α-actins specific for smooth, skeletal, and

Table 3–5. Overview of the Most Widely Used Muscle Cell Markers and Their Application in Muscle Cell and Other Tumors

Marker	Antibody Clone	Normal Distribution	Tumors
Muscle specific actin	HHF35	Smooth and skeletal muscle Myoepithelia	Myofibroblastic (nodular fasciitis) Leiomyoma, leiomyosarcoma Rhabdomyoma, rhabdomyosarcoma Some myoepithelial cell tumors
α-SMA	1A4	Smooth muscle, myoepithelia	Myofibroblastic (nodular fasciitis) Leiomyoma, leiomyosarcoma Rare cells in rhabdomyosarcoma Some myoepithelial cell tumors
Desmin	D33	Smooth muscle (most) Skeletal muscle Some mesothelial cells (reactive) Myoid cells of lymph nodes	Some myofibroblastic tumors Leiomyoma, leiomyosarcoma (70%) Rhabdomyosarcoma Angiomatoid fibrous histiocytoma (50%) Mesothelioma (rare) Desmoplastic small round cell tumor Aggressive angiomyxoma Angiomyofibroblastoma
Calponin		Myofibroblasts, smooth muscle	Myofibroblastic tumors Smooth muscle tumors, synovial sarcoma
HCD		Smooth muscle	Leiomyomas, leiomyosarcoma GISTs
MyoD1, myogenin		Skeletal muscle (fetal and reactive)	Rhabdomyosarcoma, heterologous skeletal muscle differentiation in any tumor
Myoglobin	Polyclonal	Skeletal muscle (more when regenerative)	Well-differentiated cells in rhabdomyosarcoma and tumors with heterologous skeletal muscle differentiation

cardiac muscle, respectively, a smooth muscle-specific γ-actin, and a ubiquitous β-actin.[45] Actin cytoskeleton is not only related to cell contraction and motility, but is also linked to numerous membrane and cytoplasmic cytoskeletal and cytoskeleton-associated proteins with complex interactions and functions.[46]

The antibodies HHF35 and 1A4 perform well in formalin-fixed tissue without epitope retrieval.

HHF-35 (Muscle-Specific Actin)

This antibody identifies smooth and skeletal muscle-specific α- and γ-actins and has been widely used in diagnostic immunohistochemistry.[47] In normal tissues, it reacts with subsets of myoepithelial cells of complex glands, vascular and parenchymal smooth muscle, pericytes, and skeletal muscle cells.[47,48]

Skeletal muscle tumors are typically positive for HHF35 including rhabdomyosarcomas of all types.[45,46] The previous notion that HHF35 is more sensitive than desmin was partly based on historical difficulties in consistent demonstration of desmin in formalin-fixed tissue.

Smooth muscle tumors, leiomyomas, leiomyosarcomas, and glomus tumors are consistently positive and hemangiopericytomas are typically negative representing a clinically useful contrasting pattern.[48] Leiomyosarcomas typically show higher numbers of HHF35$^+$ cells than observed in desmin immunostaining.

Some myofibroblastic lesions, such as nodular fasciitis, are strongly HHF35$^+$,[49] which should not lead to misdiagnosis of leiomyosarcoma. Other myofibroblastic tumors, for example, desmoids, have only scattered HHF35$^+$ cells. Myofibroblasts in the desmoplastic stroma of carcinomas are more often positive for HHF35 than desmin.[50] Malignant fibroblastic tumors (fibrosarcomas, malignant fibrous histiocytomas [MFHs]) often have HHF35$^+$ cells, reflecting the presence of a neoplastic (or sometimes reactive?) myofibroblastic component.[48,50]

Alpha Smooth Muscle Actin (SMA)

Antibodies specific to this actin subset (e.g., the widely used 1A4) have otherwise similar reactivities in normal tissues as HHF35, except that they do not react with skeletal muscle cells. In neoplastic smooth muscle and myofibroblastic tissues, they are relatively similar to HHF35. For example, leiomyomas, leiomyosarcomas, and glomus tumors are positive and hemangiopericytomas negative for SMA.[51–53] SMA antibodies generally do not stain rhabdomyosarcomas, although occasional tumors have been focally positive.[54]

The best documented SMA (and MSA) positive carcinomas are perhaps myoepithelial carcinomas, which have been reported positive in 50% and 31% for these markers.[55] It is not well understood whether the SMA$^+$ cells in other spindle cell carcinomas represent true myoid differentiation, myofibroblastic interstitial components, or perhaps are a reflection of multipotential mesenchymal differentiation.

Sarcomeric Actin

Antibodies to sarcomeric actin are expected to react with skeletal muscle and rhabdomyosarcomas. Although well-differentiated rhabdomyosarcomas have shown consistent expression, poorly differentiated ones have been variably positive, and occasional leiomyosarcomas have also been positive.[54,56] Our experience has been disappointing on the specificity of the commercially available antibodies for sarcomeric actin.

Desmin

Biology and Normal Distribution

This essentially muscle-specific intermediate filament protein (molecular weight [MW] 53 kd) binds the myofilaments together as bundles in both smooth and skeletal muscle, and is one of the oldest markers for myogenic sarcomas. Desmin is present in some but not all vascular and all parenchymal smooth muscle cells and cardiac and skeletal muscle cells.[57] Aortic vascular smooth muscle has been specifically reported as desmin negative,[58] whereas the smooth muscle cells of most small veins and arteries are positive. Desmin is also present in subsets of interstitial reticulum cells in the paracortex of lymph nodes.[59]

Desmin positivity in reactive mesothelial cells is a diagnostic pitfall potentially leading to a misdiagnosis of rhabdomyosarcoma. Transient desmin expression has been described in fetal mesothelial cells,[60] and some adult mesothelial cells may also be desmin positive.[60–62] The presence of desmin in reactive mesothelial cells in effusions has been confirmed by Western blotting.[62]

Soft Tissue Tumors

All rhabdomyomas and nearly all rhabdomyosarcomas are positive, and this includes differentiated rhabdomyoblasts, as well as varying numbers of small undifferentiated cells.[47,48,54] Desmin is also useful to highlight the heterologous skeletal muscle components in Triton tumor, endometrial carcinosarcoma, and dedifferentiated liposarcoma (Fig. 3–2).

Of smooth muscle tumors, practically all leiomyomas and 70% of leiomyosarcomas are positive. The negative subset is not only an artifact of formalin-fixed tissue, because lack of desmin expression has also been observed in frozen sections of ultrastructurally documented leiomyosarcomas.[51] Whether the desmin negativity reflects loss of antigen in less-differentiated cells or origin from a desmin-negative subset of smooth muscle is not known.

In the GI tract, desmin is useful in separating leiomyomas from GI stromal tumors (GISTs), because the latter, the CD117 (KIT$^+$) GISTs, are almost always negative (<5% are desmin positive).

Some myofibroblasts in fibrous tumors are desmin positive, for example, subsets of tumor cells in desmoids. Some specific female genital stromal tumors, angiomyofibroblastoma,[63] and aggressive angiomyxoma,[64] are typically desmin positive, although they are not believed to be tumors of ordinary smooth muscle, but rather myofibroblastic ones. Desmin-positive tumor cells may also be present in typical myxoid[65] and sometimes in well-differentiated liposarcomas and in pleomorphic MFH; in the

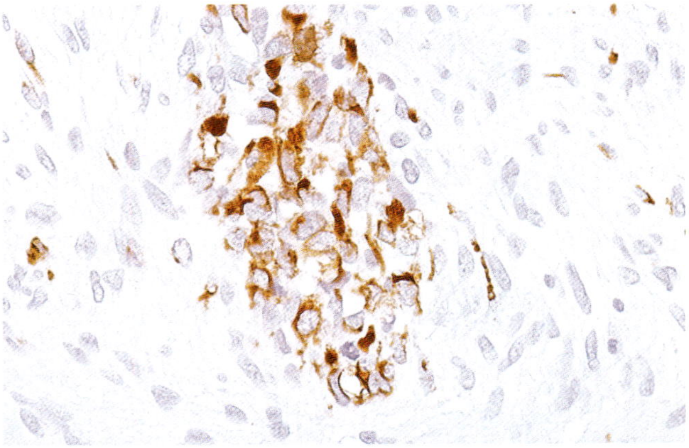

Figure 3–2. Desmin immunostaining highlights the rhabdomyoblastic component in dedifferentiated liposarcoma.

latter they probably represent desmin-positive myofibroblasts.

Approximately 50% of angiomatoid (malignant) fibrous histiocytomas,[66,67] and 30% to 50% of alveolar soft part sarcomas are also desmin positive.[68,69] In desmoplastic small round cell tumors, desmin is typically coexpressed with keratins, often showing a dot-like cytoplasmic pattern.[70] It has been occasionally reported in rare examples of Ewing family tumors, primitive neuroectodermal tumors (PNETs),[71] including one cytogenetically verified case.[72]

A minority of malignant mesotheliomas have been desmin positive, similar to some reactive mesothelial cells.[61,62,73,74] Desmin has also been commonly detected in the blastemal component of Wilms' tumors, which have been negative for other muscle cell markers.[75] Large desmin-positive cells with dendritic processes of unknown significance have been identified in tenosynovial giant cell tumors.[76]

Heavy Caldesmon (HCD)

The heavy molecular weight isoform of caldesmon (HCD) is an actin, Ca^{++}, and calmodulin binding cytoskeleton-associated protein of 34 kd involved in the regulation of smooth muscle contraction. This protein is highly expressed in smooth muscle and myoepithelial cells, but not in myofibroblasts.[77–79]

Heavy caldesmon is consistently present in leiomyomas, most glomus tumors (Fig. 3–3), and nearly in all leiomyosarcomas, but poorly differentiated ("dedifferentiated") areas of the latter may be negative.[80–83] It is absent in rhabdomyosarcomas.[80,81] Interestingly, most GISTs are also positive, indicating traits of smooth muscle differentiation in these tumors.[81]

Heavy caldesmon may be used as a supplemental marker in the diagnosis of smooth muscle tumors and to separate myofibroblastic tumors from smooth muscle tumors, because the former are typically negative. The significance of the focal HCD positivity in MFH remains to be determined.[81,82]

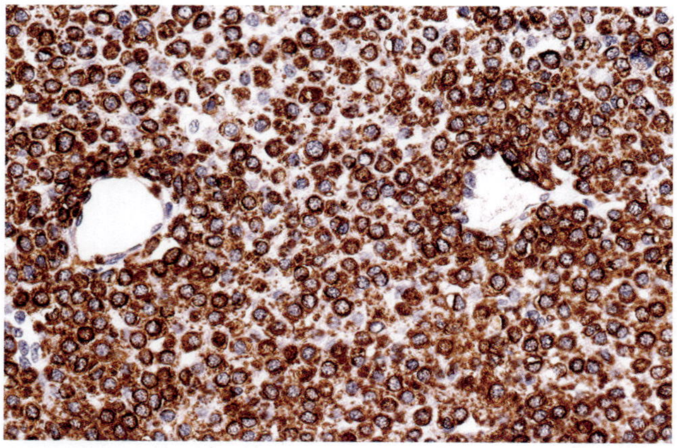

Figure 3–3. Glomus tumor cells are positive for HCD.

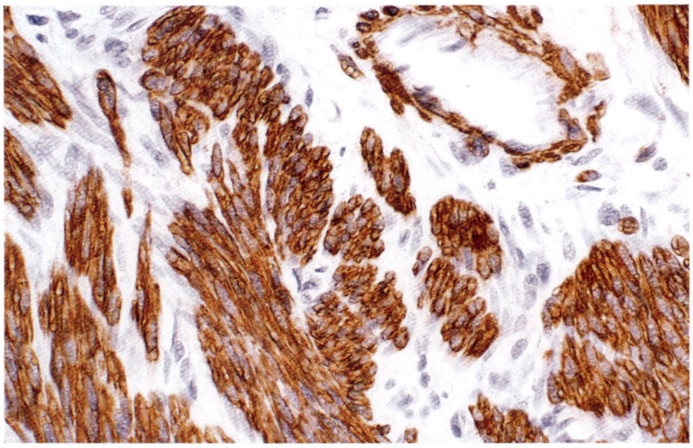

Figure 3–4. A retroperitoneal leiomyoma is strongly positive for calponin.

Calponin

This is an F-actin- and tropomyosin-binding, cytoskeleton-associated protein considered important in the regulation of smooth muscle contraction. It is highly expressed in smooth muscle, myoepithelial cells, and myofibroblasts.[84] The desmoplastic stroma of many carcinomas is positive, as are tumor cells in leiomyomas (Fig. 3–4) and leiomyosarcomas.[79] The majority of GISTs are negative. Myofibroblastic tumors such as nodular fasciitis are often positive. Synovial sarcomas often show positivity in spindle cell components.[81]

Myogenic Regulatory Factors MyoD1 and Myogenin (MYF4 Antibody)

These transciptional regulators (transcription factors) of the MyoD/Myf (myogenic determination/myogenic factor) family are DNA-binding nuclear proteins with c-myc homologous helix-loop-helix (HLH) regions.[85–87] They regulate expression of the skeletal muscle-specific proteins and are lineage specific. MyoD1 (46 kd) determines the commitment to skeletal muscle differentiation, and myogenin (32 kd) is responsible for the terminal differentiation of myotubes and maintenance of skeletal muscle phenotype.[87] Both proteins are expressed in the nuclei of fetal (Fig. 3–5*A*) and regenerating but not in normal adult skeletal muscle cells or other mesenchymal cells.[84–88] Only nuclear positivity should be considered, and cytoplasmic positivity should be discounted.

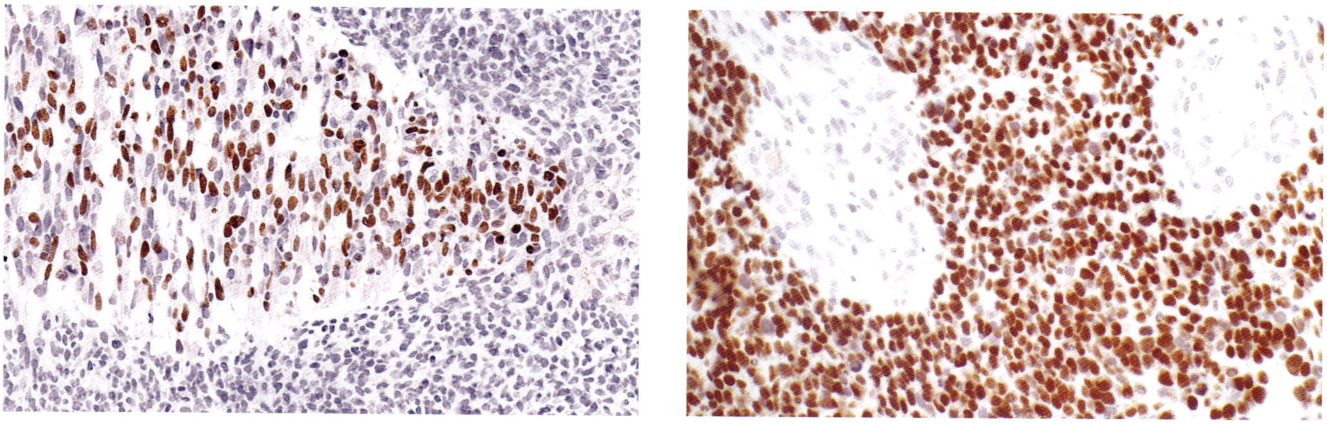

A B

Figure 3–5. *A*, MyoD1 immunostaining in fetal mesenchyme shows nuclear positivity in the whole somite developing into skeletal muscle. *B*, Embryonal rhabdomyosarcoma cells are strongly MyoD1$^+$ with purely nuclear staining. Note that the vascular component is negative.

Both MyoD1 and myogenin are expressed in a great majority of rhabdomyosarcomas of different types (90%), and only nuclear positivity should be counted as positive (Fig. 3–5*B*). Myogenin has been most commonly detected with Myf4 antibody. The expression is higher in less differentiated rhabdomyosarcoma cells, and these markers may be undetectable in differentiating rhabdomyoblasts in postchemotherapy specimens.[89–92] Alveolar rhabdomyosarcoma has been reported as more strongly myogenin positive.[93,94] Both markers appear highly specific for skeletal muscle tumors and have not been found expressed in other small, round cell tumors and nonrhabdomyosarcoma spindle cell sarcomas with very rare exceptions; such ones include Wilms' tumor with myogenous differentiation.[91]

The expression of MyoD1/myogenin in reactive skeletal muscle in the periphery of any muscle infiltrating tumors should not lead to misdiagnosis of rhabdomyosarcoma. Cytoplasmic MyoD1 positivity may be present in nonmuscle tumors, for example, in alveolar soft part sarcoma, where this pattern of immunoreactivity has an unknown significance.[95,96]

Myoglobin

This oxygen-transporting hemoprotein is present in skeletal and cardiac muscle and is somewhat useful in the diagnosis of rhabdomyosarcoma.[97–99] Most currently used antibodies are polyclonal, and background problems are common, which reduces the value of these reagents. Myoglobin antibodies should be used only to test if desmin-positive large cytoplasmic cells are rhabdomyoblasts, which typically show diffuse cytoplasmic staining. This marker is generally not useful in the diagnosis of poorly differentiated rhabdomyosarcomas, including most alveolar ones. Acquired, phagocytosed myoglobin can give positive staining in histiocytes, which can be a diagnostic pitfall.[100]

Myosins

Together with actins, myosins form the ubiquitous microfilament cytoskeleton composed of 6-nm filaments, and several isoforms have been recognized. The smooth muscle isoform of myosin shows a tissue distribution generally similar to that of α-SMA. Most smooth muscle tumors are positive. Of GISTs, approximately 30% are positive in our experience, similar to SMA.

Noncommercial slow and fast myosin antibodies have been tested in rhabdomyosarcomas. In one study, reactivity for the latter was present in 10 of 15 cases, and the former in 6 of 15 cases.[101] Fetal heavy myosin, normally expressed in embryonal skeletal muscle, was detected in 11 of 14 embryonal and 5 of 6 alveolar rhabdomyosarcomas in another study, indicating oncofetal expression.[102]

Neural and Neuroendocrine-Specific Markers

The most important applications are listed in Table 3–6. Chromogranin and synaptophysin are important in the diagnosis of paraganglioma and primary and metastatic neuroendocrine carcinoma. Synaptophysin and NB84 are used to separate the

Table 3–6. Applications of Neural and Neuroendocrine Markers in Soft Tissue Tumors

	Synaptophysin	Chromogranin	NSE	NF Proteins	Keratins
Neuroblastoma	+	+/−	+	+	−
Paraganglioma	+	+	+	+*	−/(+)
Low-grade neuroendocrine carcinomas (carcinoids)	+	+	+	−/+*	+
Merkel cell carcinoma	+/−	−	+	+	+
High-grade neuroendocrine carcinomas, lung	+	−/+	+/−	−/+*	+/(−)
Adenocarcinomas	−/(+)	−/(+)	−/+	−	+

*Neurofilament positivity limited to NF68.
−, negative; + positive; +/(−), generally positive, rarely negative; +/−, variable (approximately equally often positive as negative); −/+, positive in a minority of cases; −/(+), generally negative, rarely positve, usually focally.

neuroblastoma group of tumors from other small, round cell tumors.

Synaptophysin

This acidic, 38-kd transmembrane glycoprotein of the small presynaptic vesicles has been shown as a membrane channel protein.[103,104] In peripheral tissues, it is expressed in neural and neuroendocrine cells, such as ganglion cells, axons, paraganglia, and most cells of the dispersed neuroendocrine system.[105,106]

Neuroblastomas, including a majority of the poorly differentiated ones, are positive for synaptophysin, the latter ones often only focally (Fig. 3–6). Well-differentiated tumors are more consistently positive, and in ganglioneuroma, the ganglion cells and stromal axons are positive.[107,108] Synaptophysin is also detectable in medulloblastoma, "central PNET,"[109] and in most estesioneuroblastomas.[110]

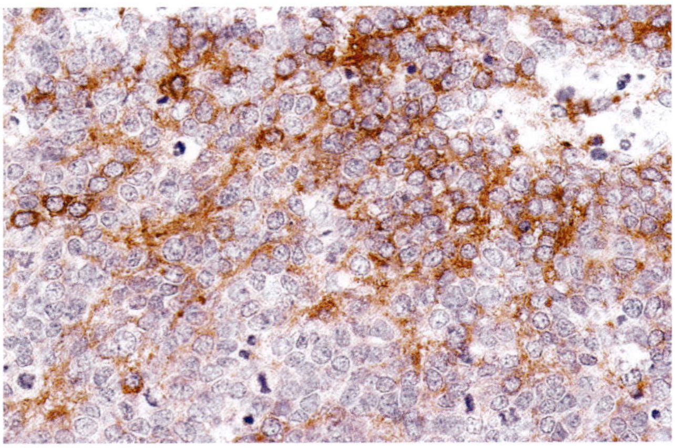

Figure 3–6. Primitive neuroblastoma shows focal cytoplasmic synaptophysin positivity.

The Ewing family of tumors, "peripheral PNETs," have been sometimes reported as synaptohysin-positive, and positivity for this and other neuroendocrine markers has been considered evidence for the diagnosis of PNET, as opposed to typical Ewing sarcoma.[111] Typical Ewing sarcomas are usually synaptophysin negative or only rarely positive.[112,113] In our experience, synaptophysin is rarely immunohistochemically demonstrable in any type of Ewing family of tumors. A recent series concluded that PNET-like differentiation with neuroendocrine markers does not have adverse prognostic significance.[114]

Paragangliomas of all types contain synaptophysin in the chief cells in 100% of cases.[115–117] Both primary and metastatic low- and high-grade epithelial neuroendocrine tumors (carcinoids and small cell carcinomas, including Merkel cell carcinoma) are almost invariably synaptophysin positive, although high-grade tumors may show limited positivity;[115,116] this is especially true in paraffin-embedded tissue.

Synaptophysin is particularly helpful in distinguishing spindled neuroendocrine tumors (carcinoid, medullary thyroid carcinoma), from mesenchymal spindle cell neoplasms. High-grade neuroendocrine carcinomas, such as small cell carcinoma, tend to be more consistently positive for synaptophysin than for chromogranin.

Recently, synaptophysin positivity was reported in 87% of extraskeletal myxoid chondrosarcomas (ESMCs) in a series of 15 cases. Neuroendocrine granules were also demonstrated by electron microscopy and verified by immunoelectron microscopy. Neuron-specific enolase (NSE) was demonstrated in all cases.[118] The significance of these observations is unclear at the present, but they have been suggested to indicate neural/neuroendocrine differentiation in ESMCs.[118]

Malignant melanomas are synaptophysin negative, but there is an exceptional report on lymph node metastasis of a cutaneous melanoma with focal ganglioneuroblastic differentiation having synaptophysin and chromogranin positivity in the neuronal component.[119]

Chromogranin A

Chromogranin A is an acidic, glutamic-acid rich, calcium-binding soluble protein of the dense core granules of neural and neuroendocrine cells.[120] It is widely used as an immunohistochemical marker, and most data are based on this chromogranin. Other chromogranins (secretogranins) are less known as immunohistochemical markers due to lack of established reagents.

Chromogranin A is present in paraganglia, pheochromocytes (chromaffin cells) of the adrenal medulla, and epithelial neuroendocrine cells in the respiratory and GI tracts, thyroid, and pituitary.[121]

In soft tissue tumors, chromogranin has a limited distribution. It is expressed in most neuroblastomas, although it may be absent in some primitive examples.[108,122] Paragangliomas, pheochromocytomas, and metastatic neuroendocrine carcinomas are chromogranin positive.[117,121] Low-grade tumors, such as carcinoids, are more consistently positive, whereas high-grade tumors, such as Merkel cell carcinoma often show limited positivity (25% of tumor cells), and small carcinomas may have even fewer positive cells (<1% or are negative), reflecting their low content of dense core granules.[121]

Chomogranin A has a very limited distribution in soft tissue sarcomas. Glandular MPNSTs were reported chromogranin positive in 5 of 8 cases, and neuropeptides (serotonin, pancreatic polypeptide, and gastrin) were also detected, indicating neuroendocrine epithelial differentiation in these exceedingly rare tumors, which may histologically have colon carcinoma-like columnar epithelial differentiation.[123] Ewing family tumors (PNETs especially) have been found almost invariably chromgranin negative, although they may have other neuroendocrine markers.[111-113] Secretogranin II, a protein of the chromogranin family, has been detected in Ewing sarcoma.[124]

Neuron-Specific Enolase (NSE)

The γ-γ homodimer of the enzyme enolase of the glycolytic pathway has been named neuron-specific enolase. It is highly expressed in most neural and neuroendocrine cells.[125] However, NSE has also been demonstrated in smooth muscle cells, including myometrium, prostate stroma, and GI smooth muscle, and in skeletal muscle.[126]

Neural and neuroendocrine cells and tumors, such as paragangliomas, carcinoid, and neuroendocrine carcinomas, have been consistently positive with polyclonal antisera.[127,128] Also melanomas are commonly positive,[129] although they are negative for chromogranin and synaptophysin.

In childhood small round cell tumors, NSE has been demonstrated in all neuroblastomas,[108,130,131] but also in some rhabdomyosarcomas.[130] Ewing family of tumors are commonly positive, and the positivity does not seem to be limited to tumors with PNET-like morphology.

The nonneural tumors reported as positive for NSE with a significant frequency with older polyclonal antisera include fibroadenoma (epithelia), ductal carcinomas of breast, renal cell carcinomas, tenosynovial giant cell tumor[132] and leiomyosarcomas and angiosarcomas.[133]

Some monoclonal NSE antibodies were originally suggested to be more specific but somewhat less sensitive for neural and neuroendocrine tumors.[134,135] Our experience indicates that even monoclonal NSE antibodies significantly react with nonneural cells and tumors. NSE has been largely replaced by synaptophysin and chromogranin, which are more specific and approximately equally sensitive markers for neural and neuroendocrine tumors.

Neurofilament (NF) Proteins

The intermediate filament cytoskeleton of neurons and their axons contain NF proteins as a major component. Aberrant organization or accumulation of NFs are likely central events in the pathogenesis of certain neurodegenerative diseases.[136] There are three NF forms: the low-molecular-weight NF68 (68 kd), medium-weight NF160 (160 kd), and high-molecular-weight NF200 (200 kd), also referred to as NFL, NFM, and NFH, respectively. These forms are differentially expressed in different types of neurons and are developmentally regulated.[137]

Neurofilaments have a very restricted distribution in normal tissues. In addition to neurons, they are present in adrenal medulla,[138] but not in normal epithelial or neuroendocrine cells.

Neurofilaments in Soft Tissue Tumors

In soft tissue tumors, demonstration of NF in Merkel cell carcinoma, often with a perinuclear dotlike pattern, has a great diagnostic value;[139] most other carcinomas are negative.

Neuroblastomas are almost invariably NF$^+$, based on frozen sections studies. All subunits have been detected, but NF68 is expressed with the highest frequency.[122,131,139]

Adrenal pheochromocytomas are consistently and globally NF$^+$,[139,140] similar to paragangliomas of head and neck.[139] However, this can only be demonstrated with antibodies that react with NF68.

Epithelial neuroendocrine tumors with NF$^+$ cells, other than Merkel cell carcinoma, include pancreatic islet cell tumors,[141] and bronchial carcinoids.[142]

Neurofilament proteins have been reported in different sarcomas, including Ewing sarcoma,[143] metastatic epithelioid sarcoma,[144] poorly differentiated synovial sarcoma,[145] and embryonal rhabdomyosarcoma; the latter contained NF68$^+$ cells.[146] The diagnostic and biologic significance of these observations is unknown.

The presence of axons can often be demonstrated with NF antibodies in neurofibroma, whereas axons are generally not present in schwannoma (except possibly focally in the periphery at the nerve junction); this may have some differential diagnostic value.

α-Internexin

This NF-related 66-kd intermediate filament protein (previously also called NF66) is present in neural cells and often but not always in neuroblastomas.[147,148] This NF-related marker may be a useful marker for neural and neuroendocrine tumors, because our experience has shown consistently positive results in paraganglioma and pheochromocytoma and some epithelial neuroendocrine tumors.

NB84 (Neuroblastoma Marker)

The monoclonal antibody NB84 raised to neuroblastoma cells detects a biochemically uncharacterized 57-kd protein.[149] Immunohistochemically, it shows a cytoplasmic staining pattern (Fig. 3–7). The antibody consistently reacts with neuroblastomas irrespective of their level of differentiation.[149–151] About a third of Ewing sarcomas also show positive cells, where positivity in other small, round cell tumors is limited, but has occasionally reported in rhabdomyosarcoma, Wilms' tumor, and small cell osteosarcoma.[150,151]

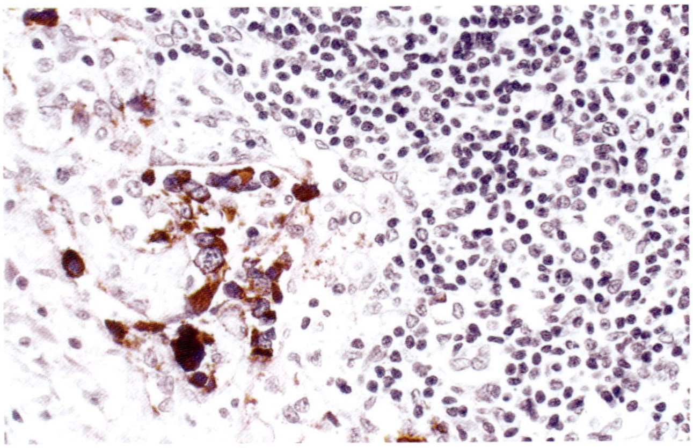

Figure 3–7. NB84 immunostaining highlights a micromestasis of neuroblastoma in a lymph node sinus.

S-100 Protein and Other Multispecific Neural Markers

S-100 protein, low-affinity nerve growth factor receptor p75, CD56 (neural cell adhesion molecule [NCAM]), and CD57 (Leu7) have schwannian or neural specificities, but all of these markers react with many other cell types as well.

Although S-100 protein has a moderately wide distribution in normal and neoplastic tissues, it remains a clinically useful marker because of its contrasting patterns of reactivity in morphologically similar tumors, and because it has been well studied. The diagnostic applications of S-100 protein are listed in Table 3–7.

Nerve growth factor receptor p75 is broadly distributed in neural and mesenchymal tissues, but its ability to separate DFSP (positive) from dermatofibroma (negative) may be a diagnostic application.

CD56 and CD57 are leukocyte antigens of natural killer cell lineage, which are also expressed in many other tissues, including neural and neuroendocrine ones. In soft tissue tumors, they have limited applications.

S-100 Protein

S-100 protein is a small acidic calcium-binding protein (MW 21 kd) that belongs to the family of EF-hand proteins. It was originally isolated in bovine brain extract, and named so by its solubility to saturated ammonium sulfate; most other proteins precipitate.[152] S-100 protein has multiple extracellular and intracellular functions related to regulation of Ca^{++} homeostasis, enzymatic activities, and cell prolifera-

Table 3–7. Distribution of S-100 Protein in Nonneoplastic and Neoplastic Soft Tissues (Selected Most Important Applications)

Normal Cell	Tumor
Melanocyte	Nevi, malignant melanoma, all types
Schwann cell	Schwannoma, neurofibroma True nerve sheath myxoma
Cartilage	Chondroma (Extraskeletal myxoid chondrosarcoma <30%)
Adipocyte	Liposarcoma (variable)
Regenerating skeletal muscle	Rhabdomyosarcoma (variable)
Myoepithelial cells	Myoepithelioma, mixed tumor
Langerhans cell/ Interdigitating reticulum cell	Rosai-Dorfman disease Langerhans cell histiocytosis Interdigitating reticulum cell sarcoma
Tumors with unknown normal cell counterpart	Ossifying fibromyxoid tumor (>50%) Synovial sarcoma (20–30%)

tion and differentiation.[153] There are two types of subunits: S-100A and S-100B, which are differentially expressed. The immunostaining patterns of the commonly used polyclonal antisera largely reflect the distribution of S-100B.[154]

S-100 protein is expressed in a variety of cell types that include melanocytes, schwann cells and sustentacular cells of paraganglia, chondrocytes, adipocytes, myoepithelial cells of various glands, and Langerhans cells of the skin and the related interdigitating reticulum cells. Positive cells typically have both cytoplasmic and nuclear staining.[155]

Melanocytes and Their Tumors

Normal and neoplastic melanocytes are consistently positive, and S-100 protein is present in virtually all benign and malignant melanocytic tumors.[155–158] It is expressed in primary as well as metastatic melanomas; only 1% to 2% of the latter are negative. Melanoma is by far the most common malignant, strongly S-100 protein-positive tumor, and this diagnosis has to be always ruled out, whenever such an epithelioid or spindled mesenchymal-appearing tumor is being examined. Despite its lack of tumor-specificity, S-100 protein remains an important screening marker in the identification of metastatic melanoma.[158]

Clear cell sarcoma of tendons and aponeurosis is a S-100 protein positive tumor that is distinct from melanoma,[159,160] although it also is HMB45$^+$.

Schwann Cells and Their Tumors

Schwann cells are the strongly S-100 protein positive components in peripheral nerves. Benign schwann cell tumors, including the cellular "Antoni-A" areas of conventional as well as cellular schwannomas are strongly positive; the latter is often useful in the differential diagnosis from smooth muscle tumors and neurogenic sarcomas, which are much less often positive. Neurofibromas have a relatively smaller number of S-100 protein-positive cells, but some elements in these tumors, especially the Meissner-like bodies and tumor cells with epithelioid morphology, are strongly positive.[156,159]

Almost all granular cell tumors are positive, with the notable exception of those in the newborn; the latter represent a distinct histogenetically unrelated tumor category. Additionally, in adults there are rare granular cell neoplasms that are rather fibroblastic/ fibrohistiocytic tumors; to date these tumors remain poorly characterized.

The MPNSTs are only inconsistently and variably S-100 protein positive. In published series they have shown positivity in 50% to 60% of cases.[161,162] In our experience, the S-100 protein positivity in MPNSTs has the following two aspects. First, in many tumors, preexistent neurofibroma elements are seen as S-100 protein-positive cells intermingling with the S-100 protein-negative tumor cells. Secondly, approximately one third of MPNSTs have schwannian or melanocytic-like differentiation and are S-100 protein positive; the latter group includes most epithelioid MPNSTs.

Normal paraganglia and most paragangliomas contain a pericompartmental sheath of slender, S-100 protein-positive Schwann cell-like cells, the sustentacular cells.[155] Their numbers vary in paragangliomas, and low number or absence of such cells is more commonly seen in malignant than benign tumors.[163,164]

Cartilage and Bone Tumors

Normal cartilage cells are S-100 protein positive, but osteoblasts are negative. Well-differentiated cartilaginous tumors, such as chondromas and low-grade hyaline cartilage-type chondrosarcomas are positive.

Islands of differentiated cartilage are highlighted as S-100 protein positive in mesenchymal chondrosarcoma.[165,166] However, extraskeletal myxoid chondrosarcomas are variably positive in 30% of cases; S-100 protein has limited value in their diagnosis. Chordomas are often S-100 positive, similar to their ancestral notochord cells,[167] although to variable degree.

Fat and Its Tumors

Normal adipocytes are variably positive, and S-100 protein has been suggested useful in highlighting lipoblasts in liposarcomas and revealing adipocyte differentiation in poorly differentiated myxoid (round cell) liposarcomas, and in the distinction between myxoid liposarcoma and myxoid MFH, the latter being negative.[168,169] In our experience, S-100 protein positivity is variable in all types of liposarcomas, especially the pleomorphic ones, and dedifferentiated tumors are usually negative, but it can be useful in the diagnosis of poorly differentiated round cell liposarcomas.

Other Mesenchymal Tumors with S-100 Protein Positivity

Ossifying fibromyxoid tumor is a distinctive soft tissue tumors of unknown histogenesis, which shows S-100 protein positivity in over 50% to 70% of cases.[170] Approximately 20% to 30% of synovial sarcomas contain S-100 protein-positive cells, some of them extensively. Positivity may be seen in both spindle cell and epithelial areas and both biphasic and monophasic tumors.[171]

Although generally negative for S-100 protein, many other sarcomas and benign mesenchymal tumors can have sporadic S-100 protein-positive tumor cells. Rhabdomyosarcomas may be S-100 protein positive; this may reflect the fact that regenerative, although not normal, skeletal muscle may also be S-100 protein positive.[172] KIT^+ GISTs, especially those of the small intestine, are S-100 protein positive in 10% to 15% of cases, and these tumors may also coexpress smooth muscle actins.[30]

Epithelial Cells and Carcinomas

Among benign epithelial cells, myoepithelial cells of sweat glands, salivary glands, and other complex epithelia are typically S-100 protein positive.[155]

Positivity for S-100 protein is typically seen in myoepithelial tumors, and it is not infrequent in carcinomas, which can represent a diagnostic pitfall. In two studies, 12% and 42% of primary and metastatic carcinomas of the breast and other sites had S-100 protein-positive tumor cells.[173,174] Carcinomas reported S-100 protein positive with a 50% to 60% frequency include carcinomas of eccrine sweat glands, salivary glands, and breast,[173,174] and some report metastatic renal, endometrial, and ovarian carcinomas positive with a frequency of 66% to 87%.[174]

Histiocyte-Related Cells

The cutaneous Langerhans cells[175] and their analogs in lymphoid tissues, the interdigitating reticulum cells, are S-100 protein positive,[176] and varying numbers of similar cells with dendritic processes are seen in almost all reactive and neoplastic soft tissues. These cells serve as a good universal internal control for S-100 protein immunostaining. The large epithelioid histiocytes in Rosai-Dorfman disease (sinus histiocytosis with massive lymphadenopathy) are strongly S-100 positive,[177,178] which is diagnostically helpful. Langerhans cell histiocytosis cells in bone and nodal lesions are strongly positive.[155]

Interdigitating reticulum cell sarcomas are extremely rare S-100 protein-positive malignant hematopoietic tumors. This diagnosis of a nodal lesion with no apparent primary is often considered. In our experience, a great majority of tumors initially suspected as such prove to be metastatic malignant melanomas, and interdigitating reticulum cell sarcoma should be a diagnosis only made after careful exclusion of melanoma, supported by other more specific markers, such as CD1a, or electron microscopy.

Nerve Growth Factor Receptor (Low-Affinity), p75

This receptor protein of 75 kd is expressed in many cell types, including schwann cells, dendritic reticulum cells, certain basal epithelia, and myoepithelia. Its shows extensive reactivity with fetal fibroblasts and focal perivascular positivity in adult fibroblasts.[179–182]

Benign and malignant nerve sheath tumors such as schwannomas, neurofibromas, and MPNSTs are positive. Among other sarcomas, synovial sarcoma and rhabdomyosarcoma are also usually positive. Because DFSP is almost always strongly positive and benign fibrous histiocytomas are negative, this marker may be useful in the differential diagnosis of these tumors.[182] Its role in the differential diagnosis of sarcomas seems limited because the expression pattern is wide. Dendritic reticulum cell sarcoma has also been shown to be positive, indicating its phenotypic similarity with the normal cell counterpart.[183]

CD56 (NCAM)

This cell adhesion molecule with five immunoglobulin-like extracellular loops is important in homotypic cell adhesion during morphogenesis.[184] It is expressed in killer lymphocytes and a subset of lymphomas with natural killer cell phenotype. Peripheral nerves and neuroendocrine cells and tumors, such as small cell carcinomas, are positive.[185,186]

Older information on soft tissue tumors was based on application on small numbers of fresh-frozen tumors. Neural and neuroectodermal tumors such as neuroblastoma, paraganglioma, and schwannoma and MPNSTs are positive. Many nonneural tumors are positive as well, including synovial sarcoma (especially the spindle cells), rhabdomyosarcomas, some leiomyosarcomas, and fibrosarcomas. Ewing family of tumors are typically negative.[187–189]

Recently, monoclonal antibodies performing in formalin-fixed tissue have become available. They have given similar immunostaining patterns as seen in previous frozen section studies and will allow further delineation of the possible clinical applications.[190]

CD57 (Myelin-Associated Glycoprotein, Leu7 HNK1 Antibodies)

This leukocyte antigen is a 110-kd membrane glycoprotein. Leu7 antibody was raised to a membrane antigen of a T-cell line, and it recognizes killer lymphocytes[191] and also reacts with myelin-associated glycoprotein.[192] In normal tissues, subsets of lymphocytes (natural killer cells), schwann cell components of nerves, perivascular mesenchymal cells, and prostatic epithelium are positive. Also neuroendocrine tumors are variably positive.[193]

Of soft tissue tumors, schwannomas are consistently positive, and MPNSTs are positive in 75% of cases. However, a significant portion of synovial sarcomas (40%) and leiomyosarcomas (16%) are also positive.[193,194] In our experience, additional positive soft tissue elements include perivascular mesenchyme and chondroid matrix. Practical application in soft tissue diagnosis is limited.

Melanoma Markers, Other than S-100 Protein

HMB45, tyrosinase, melan A (MART-1), microphthalmia transcription factor, and CD63 are the most important melanoma markers. All of them have additional specificities that are sometimes diagnostically useful and at times may be confusing (Table 3–8).

HMB45

This monoclonal antibody was raised to pigmented metastatic melanoma by Gown and coworkers and so named after the immunogen, "human melanoma, black."[195] It recognizes an oncofetal 100-kd glycoprotein gp100 present in the immature but not mature melanosomes and is believed to be an organelle-

Table 3–8. Summary of Melanocyte-Specific Markers and Their Reactivities

	HMB45	Tyrosinase	Melan A	MITF
Normal melanocytes	−	+/−	+	+
Activated melanocytes	+	+	+	+
Primary melanoma	+	+	+	+
Metastatic melanoma	+/(−)	+/(−)	+/(−)	+/(−)
Desmoplastic melanoma	−	−	−	−
Clear cell sarcoma	+	+/−	+/−	+/−
Angiomyolipoma	+	−/(+)	+	−/+
Lymphangiomyoma	+	−	−/+	−/+
Adrenal cortical carcinoma	−	−	+	−
Metastatic carcinomas, other	−	−	−	−
Osteoclast-like giant cells	−	−	−	+

Information based on references 196–225.
−, negative; +, positive; +/(−), generally positve rarely negative; +/−, variable (approximately equally often positive as negative); −/+, positive in a minority of cases; −/(+), generally negative, rarely positive, usually focally.

specific marker.[196] Fetal and activated, junctional adult melanocytes are positive, whereas the resting adult melanocytes and intradermal nevus cells and melanophages are negative. Blue nevi of conventional and cellular types and primary melanomas are consistently positive.

Several studies have shown primary melanomas to be positive in 90% to 100% of cases but spindle cell melanomas may be negative.[197,198] Metastatic melanomas are positive with a slightly lower frequency varying from 70% to 90%.[197–200] The number of positive cells vary and may be limited to a few cells. Heat-induced epitope retrieval may improve the detection of this antigen.[199] Desmoplastic melanomas are HMB45$^-$ in more than 90% of the cases.[200,201]

Clear cell sarcoma of tendons and aponeuroses is a tumor with melanocytic differentiation, and it is consistently HMB45$^+$.[160] Sometimes this tumor has a stronger reactivity for HMB45 than for S-100. Generally, MPNSTs are negative for HMB45, which is useful in separating them from metastatic melanoma. However, rare pigmented nerve sheath tumors with a melanocytic component may be HMB45-positive. Of these, pigmented neurofibroma has scattered HMB45-positive cells,[202] and psammomatous melanotic schwannoma can be also be positive.

Angiomyolipoma[203–205] and the closely related lymphangiomyoma(tosis)[205] are unique nonmelanocytic renal, hepatic, retroperitoneal, or pulmonary tumors that contain HMB45$^+$ cells in 90% to 100% of cases. The number of positive cells is highly variable. The positive cells often have epithelioid morphology and often show granular cytoplasmic immunostaining. Sugar tumor of the lung and some recently described similar extrarenal tumors, designated as perivascular epithelioid cell tumors, "PEComas" or myomelanocytic tumors, are HMB45$^+$ angiomyolipoma-related tumors that usually coexpress smooth muscle actins and variably desmin.[206]

HMB45 is believed to be a highly specific lineage marker for melanocytic differentiation, but it does not distinguish malignant lesions from the benign ones. A spectrum of carcinomas, sarcomas, and lymphomas has been consistently negative. The previously reported positivity in primary and metastatic carcinomas is now believed to have resulted from impure antibody preparations at least in most cases.[196]

Tyrosinase

This enzyme glycoprotein of 75 kd catalyzes the two earliest steps of tyrosine incorporation into melanin pigment.[207] It has been identified as a target for melanoma immunotherapy, for which monoclonal antibodies were initially raised.[208] Later these antibodies have been applied for diagnostic immunohistochemistry.

Based on several studies, tyrosinase has been suggested as an excellent marker for metastatic melanoma, which shows diffuse cytoplasmic staining in 80% to 90% of cases.[199,200,209–211] However, desmoplastic melanomas are almost invariably negative.[200,211] In cutaneous pigmented nevi, the superficial components are more tyrosinase positive than the deeper ones. Clear cell sarcomas are also often positive,[200] whereas carcinomas, other sarcomas, and lymphomas have been consistently negative.[199] Renal angiomyolipoma is only rarely positive for this melanocytic marker.[212]

In our experience, tyrosinase is a more sensitive marker for metastatic melanoma than HMB45, especially because a larger number of tumor cells tend to be positive (Fig. 3–8).

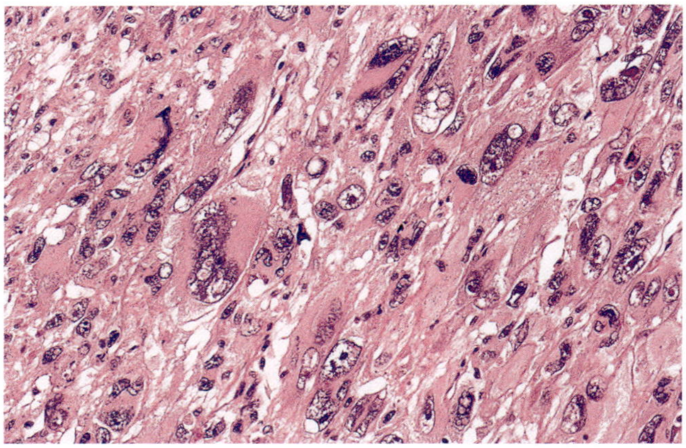

A

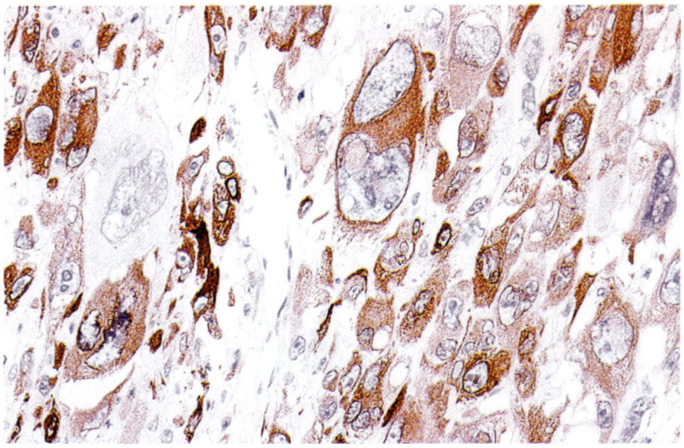

B

Figure 3–8. *A,* This pleomorphic malignant neoplasm in the small intestine does not have diagnostic histologic features. *B,* Tyrosinase immunostaining is strongly positive, supporting the diagnosis of metastatic melanoma.

Melan A

Melan A or melanoma antigen recognized by T lymphocytes (MART-1) was originally identified as a target for T-cell immunologic response to melanoma. The gene was cloned and simultaneously identified as MART-1[213] and melan A.[214] The antigen is closely related to the gp100 recognized by HMB45 monoclonal antibody, and has been identified as an antigen recognized by autologous T lymphocytes in an immune response leading to tumor lysis.[215] The melan A protein is believed to be restricted to melanocytes[213] and is expressed in all normal melanocytes.[216]

Melan A antibody has been shown useful immunohistochemical marker for melanoma. Based on two large series, melan A is present in all primary melanomas, and 81% to 88% of metastatic conventional melanomas, but desmoplastic melanomas have been generally negative.[200,216] Mucosal melanomas have also been positive.[217]

Angiomyolipomas are positive for melan A, typically more homogeneously than for HMB45, and melan A transcript has also been demonstrated.[218] Lymphangiomyomas have been variably positive.[219]

Melan A positivity has also been detected in steroid cell tumors, including adrenal cortical adenomas and carcinomas, and in ovarian and testicular Leydig cell tumors with A103 antibody to melan A. Because carcinomas of other organs have been melan A negative, this marker has been suggested useful in the identification of carcinomas of adrenal cortical origin.[220]

Microphtalmia Transcription Factor (MITF)

This nuclear protein is a transcriptional regulator for key melanocyte genes, such as tyrosinase.[221,222] It is also expressed in osteoclasts and functionally important there, because MITF-deficient mice develop osteopetrosis.[223]

This protein is expressed in melanocytes (Fig. 3–9), primary melanomas, and a majority of metastatic malignant melanomas, typically with the majority of tumor cells showing nuclear positivity.[200,224,225] Clear cell sarcomas are also often but not always positive.[200] MITF may be a useful adjunct for diagnosis of metastatic melanomas. However, some histiocytes, especially osteoclastic giant cells and epithelioid histiocytes granulomas, are also positive.

Three series have found desmoplastic melanomas essentially negative for MITF,[200,211,226] and one showed 50% of these variants to be positive.[227] This antigen has been variably detected in angiomyolipoma from

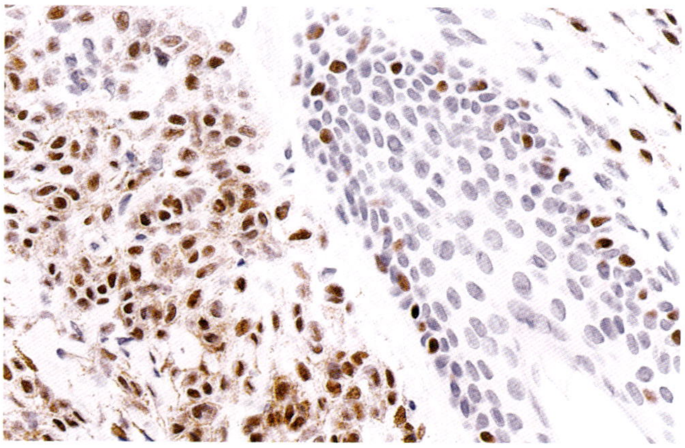

Figure 3–9. Hair shaft melanocytes and nevus cells are selectively positive for MITF with nuclear staining.

20% to 70%.[200,212] Reported positivity in mononuclear histiocytes[200] and smooth muscle and leiomyosarcoma[211] require caution in its diagnostic use and require additional studies on specificity.

CD63 (NK1C3)

This membrane-spanning lysosomal glycoprotein of 30 to 60 kd has been identified as melanoma-associated antigen ME491[228] and subsequently as a platelet antigen.[229]

CD63 is recognized by a monoclonal antibody NKI/C3, which was available already in the mid 1980s. Immunohistochemical studies[230,231] showed consistent expression in primary and metastatic melanoma, and somewhat variable expression in melanocytic nevi. However, various carcinomas (4 of 21, 19%) can also be positive.[230] Our experience indicates that specificity to malignant melanoma is low. Experience in other soft tissue tumors is limited, but alveolar soft part sarcomas are strongly positive.[69]

Histiocytic Markers

These markers identify subsets of myeloid and histiomonocytic cells, and true histiomonocytic tumors, which are very few: extramedullary myeloid tumors, very rare true histiocytic lymphomas, and juvenile xanthogranuloma; they do not include MFH. Hardly any of the histiocytic markers are truly histiocyte specific, and some "histiocytic" antigens are widely expressed. The histiocytic markers discussed here are lysozyme, α_1-antitrypsin (AAT) and α_1-antichymotrypsin (AACT), factor XIIIa, CD68, and

Table 3–9. Summary of Reactivity for Histiocytic Markers in Tumor Cells in Various Lesions

	Histiocytic Specificity	Positive Tumors
Lysozyme	High	Juvenile xanthogranuloma Myelomonocytic leukemias and extramedullary myeloid tumors
Factor XIIIa	High	Juvenile xanthogranuloma Infiltrating histiocytes in fibrous histiocytomas and many sarcomas
CD68	Low	Histiocytic, schwannian, melanocytic tumors Granular cell tumor Some carcinomas
CD163	High	True histiocytic tumors Mononuclear histiocytes positive Osteoclasts negative
AAT	Low	Histiocytes, carcinomas, melanoma, lymphomas
AACT	Low	Histiocytes, carcinomas, melanoma, lymphomas

All markers also detect tumor infiltrating histiocytes or dendritic histiocytes.

CD163. Their diagnostic applications have been listed in Table 3–9.

Lysozyme (Muramidase)

This bacteriolytic enzyme lytic to bacterial cell wall is highly expressed in leukocytes of granulocyte and monocyte/histiocyte series. Some epithelia and their secretions (lacrimal glands, tears) are also positive.[232,233] True histiocytic differentiation by lysozyme positivity can be verified in lesional cells of juvenile xanthogranuloma,[234,235] Langerhans cell histiocytosis, and in giant cells of multicentric reticulohistiocytosis.[235] All extramedullary myeloid tumors with any differentiation are positive with a cytoplasmic staining pattern,[236,237] but purely blastic variants may be negative in half of the cases.[236] Rare examples of true histiocytic lymphomas typically show cytoplasmic staining for lysozyme.[238] However, in fibrohistiocytic tumors, such as benign and malignant fibrous histiocytomas, only tumor infiltrating histiocytes are positive indicating lack for true histiocytic differentiation in these lesions.[234,239] Solar elastotic fibers in the dermis are lysozyme positive for some reason, and this can facilitate the identification of these structures.[240]

AACT (MW 68 kd) and AAT

These serine protease inhibitors (SERPINs) are so called acute phase proteins that are synthesized in the liver. They are homologous products of the same gene family.[241] Both proteins are also present in histiocytes, and antibodies to them identify tumor infiltrating histiocytes. Positive cells display a diffuse cytoplasmic staining pattern.

Although initially believed useful in the diagnosis of fibrohistiocytic tumors,[242] subsequent studies have demonstrated AAT^{+} and $AACT^{+}$ tumor cells in a wide variety of malignant neoplasms (sarcomas, lymphomas, carcinomas, melanomas, Fig. 3–10) obliterating the value of these antigens as histiocyte-specific markers[238,243,244] and suggesting that these acute phase proteins are expressed by a wide variety of malignant tumors. AACT and AAT also have no value in the identification of MFH, which is a nonhistiocytic tumor, often with high content of reactive histiocytes.

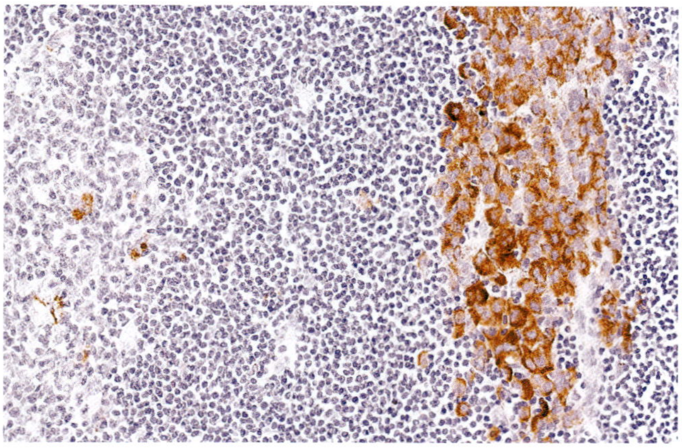

Figure 3–10. Metastatic melanoma in a lymph node is strongly positive for AAT. Some histiocytes are also positive.

Factor XIIIa (FXIIIa)

This enzyme protein, a protransglutaminase, operates in the late stages of blood coagulation in the formation of the fibrin clot.[245] This immunohistochemical marker selectively identifies subsets of dendritic histiocytes in lymph nodes[246] and skin, where these cells have been called "dermal dendrocytes" and were once thought to be the origin for Kaposi sarcoma spindle cells.[247]

FXIIIa immunostaining is mainly used in dermatopathologic lesions, and it has now been realized that the FXIIIa$^+$ cells mostly represent nonneoplastic infiltrating cells. These cells are prominent in benign fibrous histiocytomas, but scant in DFSP, which may have some diagnostic value.[21] FXIII$^+$ stromal histiocytes are abundant in MFHs, but may also be present in other tumors, such as leiomyosarcoma, and therefore their demonstration does not have a significant value in tumor typing.[248] The lesional cells of juvenile xanthogranuloma are positive, and in this instance the positivity reflects true histiomonocytic differentiation.[249,250]

CD68

This lysosomal protein of 110 kd can be detected in formalin-fixed and paraffin-embedded tissue with the KP1 and PG-M1 antibodies.[251–253] CD68 is a lysosomal, not a histiocyte-specific marker, and this explains its expression in many nonhistiocytic lysosome-rich cells and tumors, such as granular cell tumor and schwann cell neoplasms[254,255] and metastatic melanoma and paraganglioma.[256] In epithelial tumors, positivity has been noted especially in renal adenocarcinoma.[252,256,257] Although some MFHs show tumor cell immunoreactivity, this finding does not indicate histiocytic differentiation, and it has no specific diagnostic value,[256,258] in view of common staining in definitely nonhistiocytic cells.

CD68 is highly expressed in histiomonocytic cells, such as tumor infiltrating mononucleated and multinucleated histiocytes including osteoclasts, and a cytoplasmic staining pattern is observed; its demonstration may have some value in their evaluation. Juvenile xanthogranuloma and tenosynovial giant cell tumors are CD68$^+$ true histiocytic tumors.

CD163

This antigen is an erythrocyte scavenger receptor and is expressed in histiocytes in a cytokine-dependent manner.[259] In our experience, it seems to be an excellent histiocytic marker in paraffin-embedded and formalin-fixed tissue. Most mononuclear histiocytes are positive (Fig. 3–11). However, the majority of

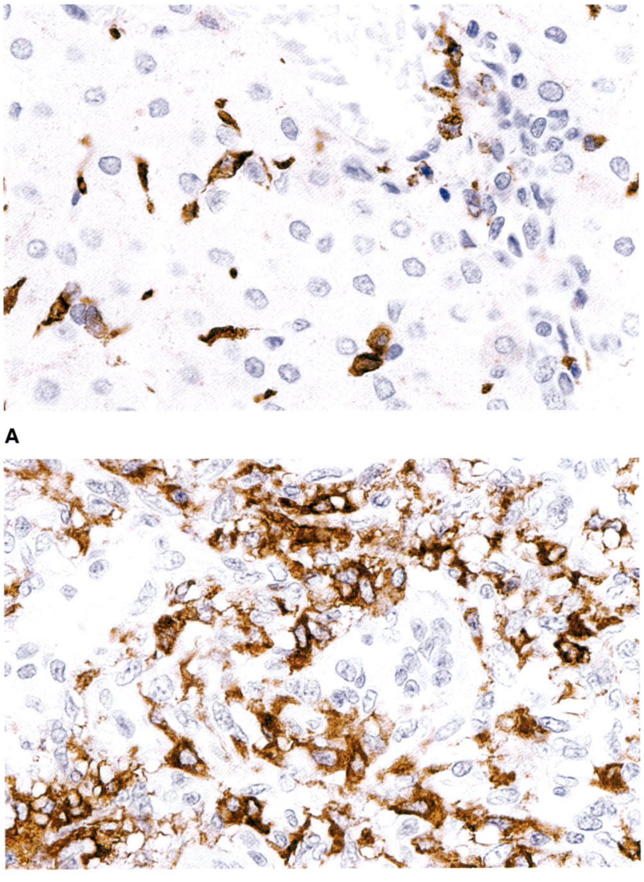

Figure 3–11. *A,* Only Kupfer cells are CD163$^+$ in the normal liver. *B,* Most mononuclear cells in the tenosynovial giant cell tumor are CD163$^+$. Note that this histiocytic marker does not react with the osteoclastic giant cells.

epithelioid cells of granulomas and multinucleated histiocytic giant cells, such as osteoclasts, are negative. CD163 is more histiocyte specific than CD68; melanomas and granular cell tumors are CD163$^-$, whereas they are usually CD68$^+$.

Keratins (Cytokeratins)

Keratins form the intermediate filament cytoskeleton typical of, but not restricted to, epithelial cells and their tumors. Epithelial keratins (cytokeratins, soft keratins) form a group of proteins of two multigene families. In addition, there are additional keratins restricted to hair and nail. They are called hard keratins and are not discussed here.

The individual epithelial keratins are relevant to pathologists because antibodies to most of them are now applicable in formalin-fixed tissue, and diagnostic patterns of their distribution have emerged. The knowledge on the individual keratins also makes it easier to understand the results obtained with keratin cocktails. Although keratins are filaments, the positivity is typically seen as diffuse cytoplasmic immunostaining. Their filamentous nature can often be seen in immunofluorescence staining, especially in cytologic specimens, or by confocal microscopy.

History

The 20 different epithelial keratins were originally identified biochemically by two-dimensional gel electrophoresis by Franke et al.[260] and numbered by Moll et al.[261,262] and Sun et al.[263–265] In the two-dimensional system, the keratins are first solubilized with high molar urea. Then they are separated first by isoelectric properties (isoelectric focusing or nonequilibirium pH gradient electrophoresis [NEPHGE]), and thereafter by molecular weights under denaturing conditions (sodium dodecyl sulfate-polyacrylamide gel electrophoresis [SDS-PAGE]). Keratins were identified in most carcinomas, but not in mesenchymal cells in general.[261,264]

In soft tissues, keratins were first identified by polyclonal epidermal keratin antibodies in synovial sarcoma,[266] epithelioid sarcoma,[267] chordoma,[268] and normal myometrium.[269] These results have been subsequently confirmed with monoclonal antibodies and some by Western blotting, and detailed analysis of keratin subsets has been performed on many tumor types.

Keratins (especially keratins 8 and 18), have also been reported in many other sarcomas complicating the separation of epithelial and mesenchymal tumors by keratin immunohistochemistry.[270] The imunohistochemical as well as biochemical demonstration of keratins in fetal mesenchymal cells[60] and cultured fibroblasts[271] forms a rational basis for their presence in various mesenchymal tumors.

Overview of Keratins

The individual keratins (abbreviated here by K followed by the number) and their main normal distribution are summarized in Table 3–10. Their distribution in mesenchymal cells, carcinomas, and soft tissue tumors is summarized in Tables 3–11 through 3–13.

Keratins of type I (type A, with acidic isoelectric points) are numbered 9 through 20. They constitute a spectrum from low- (K19: 40 kd) to high-molecular-weight keratins (K9: 58 kd)[261–264] and are encoded by genes clustered in 17q suggesting evolution by gene duplication.[272,273] Keratins of type II (type B, with basic isoelectric properties) are numbered 1 through 8. They also constitute a spectrum from low (K8, 52 kd) to higher molecular weights (K1, 67 kd), and are encoded by a cluster of genes in 12q.[273,274]

Keratin filaments are formed as heteropolymers of at least one type I and at least one type II keratin. The pair forming type II keratin is typically 8 kd larger than the corresponding type I keratin. Based on this principle, all epithelial cells contain at least two different keratins. For example, hepatocytes contain two keratins (K8 and K18), whereas epidermal keratinocytes have a complex constellation of 6 to 10 keratin polypeptides.[261,263,264]

The lowest molecular weight keratins in each group are typically expressed in simple, nonstratified, noncomplex epithelia (such as GI epithelia and mesothelia), whereas the others are present in complex glandular, ductal, and stratified squamous and transitional cell epithelia. The keratins of simple epithelia are often called "low-molecular weight keratins." This is partly misleading, because type II keratins of the lowest molecular weight have higher molecular weights than some of the higher molecular weight keratins of the type I keratins.

The keratins will be discussed later in their order of relative importance. Keratins of simple epithelia are the ones most commonly detected in carcinomas and sarcomas, but extensive studies have shown stratified and even keratinizing epithelial keratins to a surprising degree in mesenchymal cells and tumors.

Table 3–10. Summary of the Epithelial Keratins and Their Most Important Distribution Patterns

Type II (Basic, B) Keratins			Type I (Acidic, A) Keratins	
		Soft epithelia of palms and soles	K9	64 kd
K1	67 kd	Keratinizing epithelia of skin Some endothelia (K1 only)	K10	56–57 kd
		Keratinizing epithelia of skin	K11	56 kd
K2	65 kd	Some keratinizing epithelia		
K3	63 kd	Restricted to corneal epithelium	K12	55 kd
K4	59 kd	Cells other than basal layer of internal squamous epithelia. Urothelial cells	K13	51 kd
K5	58 kd	Basal cells of glandular and some squamous epithelia, including myoepithelial cells Upper layers of some squamous epithelia	K14	50 kd
		Some skin adnexal epithelia Especially hair shaft basal cells	K15	50 kd
K6	56 kd	Hyperproliferative epidermis, some skin adnexa (sweat glands, subsets of hair shaft epithelia)	K16	48 kd
		Myoepithelia, basal cells of complex glandular epithelia, subsets of hair shaft epithelia	K17	46 kd
K7	54 kd	Respiratory and upper GI epithelia, mesothelia, some basal cells, complex glandular epithelia, some endothelial cells		
K8	52 kd	Most types of simple epithelia + mesothelia Superficial layer of urothelia Some endothelial cells (K18 only)	K18	45 kd
		Most types of simple epithelia and mesothelia. Absent in hepatocytes, some renal tubules and normal thyroid follicles Complex distribution in internal squamous epithelia Absent in normal epidermis	K19	40 kd
		Lower GI tract epithelia, urothelia, Merkel cells	K20	46 kd

Keratins typically expressed as a pair are shown on the same line, and those with less known pairing patterns are shown singly on a line.

Table 3–11. Immunohistochemical Distribution of Keratins in Normal Mesenchymal Cells

	K8	K18	K19	K7	K1
Myometrium	(+)	(+)	(+)	–	–
Other smooth muscle	(+)	(+)	(+)	occasional	–
Capillary endothelia	–	(+)	–	(+)	(+)
Interstitial reticulum cells of lymphoid tissue	+	+	–	–	–

+, consistently positive; (+), variably positive; –, negative

Table 3–12. Expected Results of Immunostainings for Different Keratin Polypeptides in Selected Carcinomas

	K7	K8	K13	K14	K17	K18	K19	K20
Metastatic adenocarcinoma from								
Breast	+	+	−/(+)	−/+	−/(+)	+	+	−/(+)
Lung	+	+	−/(+)	−/(+)	−/(+)	+	+	−/(+)
Stomach	+/(−)	+	−	−	−	+	+	+/−
Pancreas	+	+	−	+/−	+/−	+	+	+/−
Colon	−/(+)	+	−	−	−	+	+	+/(−)
Kidney	−/(+)	+	−	−	−	+	+/−	−
Prostate	−/(+)	+	−	−	−	+	+	−/(+)
Squamous cell carcinoma	+/−	+/−	+/−	+	+	+/−	+	−
Transitional cell carcinoma	+	+	+/−	−/+	+/−	+	+	+/−
Small cell carcinoma, lung origin	+	+/(−)	−	−	−	+/(−)	+	−
Merkel cell carcinoma	−/(+)	+	−	−	−	+	+	+

Note that results represent typical cases, and aberrations are possible.
−, negative; +, positive; +/(−), generally positive, rarely negative; +/−, variable (approximately equally often positive as negative); −/+, positive in a minority of cases; −/(+), generally negative, rarely positive, usually focally.
(Based on references 261–265 and 270, and author's unpublished results.)

Table 3–13. Expected Results from Immunostainings for Different Keratin Polypeptides in Selected Soft Tissue Tumors

	K7	K8	K13	K14	K17	K18	K19	K20
Malignant mesothelioma, epithelial	+	+	−	+/−	−/(+)	+	+	−
Synovial sarcoma, biphasic, epithelia	+	+	−/+	+	−/+	+	+	−/+
Synovial sarcoma, monophasic	+	+	−	−/(+)	−	+	+	−
Epithelioid sarcoma	−/(+)	+	−	−/+	−	+	+/−	−
Epithelioid hemangioendothelioma	+/−	−/(+)	−	−	−	+	−	−
Epithelioid angiosarcoma	−/+	−/+	−	−	−	+/−	−/(+)	−
Angiosarcoma, non-epithelioid	−/(+)	−/(+)	−	−	−	−/+	−	−
Ewing family of tumors	−	−/(+)				−/(+)	−	−
Desmoplastic small round cell tumor	−	+	−	−	−	+	+/−	−
Chordoma	−/(+)	+	−	−	−	+	+	−/(+)
Leiomyosarcoma	−	−/+	−	−	−	−/+	−	−
Melanoma metastasis	−	−/+	−	−	−	−/+	−	−

Note that results represent typical cases, and aberrations are possible.
−, negative; +, positive; +/(−), generally positive, rarely negative; +/−, variable (approximately equally often positive as negative);−/+, positive in a minority of cases; −/(+), generally negative, rarely positive, usually focally.
(Based on references 270, 275–290, 293, 296, and author's unpublished results.)

Keratins of Simple, Nonstratified Epithelia: K8 and K18

K8 (52 kd) and K18 (45 kd) are the evolutionarily oldest keratins and are present already in the earliest embryonal stages. They are widely expressed and generally codistributed in practically all simple epithelia of all organs, including mesothelia.[261,275] In normal undisturbed hepatocytes and some renal tubular cells they are the only keratins present. In many complex glandular epithelia, they are preferentially expressed in the luminal epithelial cells and are absent in most normal squamous epithelia. In the epidermis, they are only present in Merkel cells. In the urothelium, they are limited to the uppermost cell layer, the umbrella cells.[276,277]

K8 and K18 are present in most nonsquamous cell carcinomas and absent in most well-differentiated squamous cell carcinomas of skin, but are variably expressed in poorly differentiated cutaneous and many internal organ squamous cell carcinomas.[278,279]

K8 and K18 in Mesenchymal Cells and Soft Tissue Tumors

In mesenchymal cells, reactivity to K8 or K18 antibodies or both has been demonstrated in smooth muscle cells,[280–282] where their presence has also been demonstrated by Western blotting.[282] These keratins can also be expressed in developing myocardium (Fig. 3–12*A*), whereas they are absent from adult heart.[60,283] In our experience, myometrial smooth muscle often shows dotlike immunoreactivity, and GI, prostatic, and vascular smooth muscle cells can also be positive.

K18 but not K8 is expressed in some capillary endothelial cells.[284,285] Both K8 and K18 are present in interstitial reticulum cells of lymph nodes (Fig. 3–12*B*), a subset of paracortical spindle cells.[286]

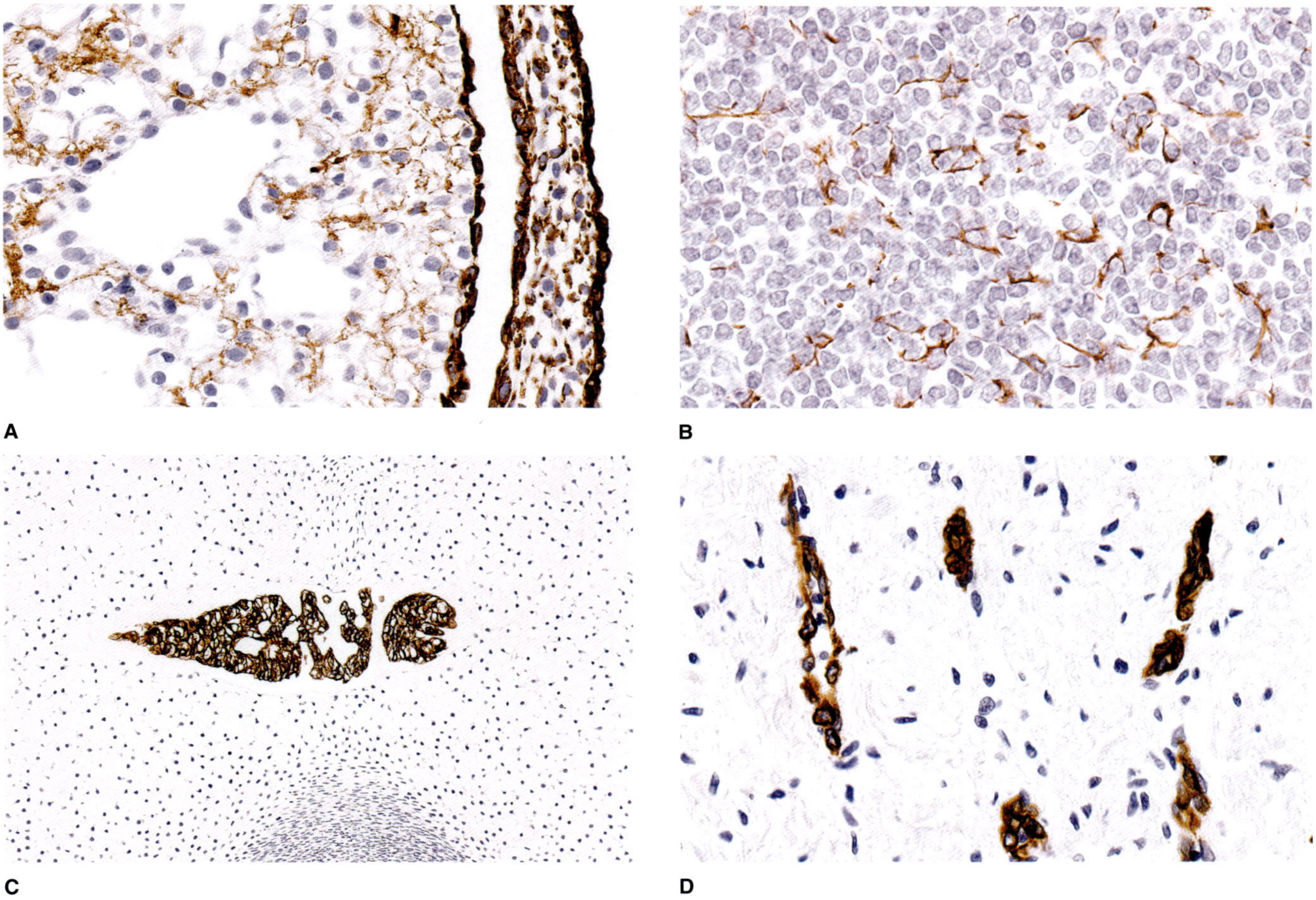

Figure 3–12. *A,* Keratin 18 immunostaining is seen in fetal myocardium, as well as pericardial mesothelium. *B,* Interstitial reticulum cells of lymph node paracortex are positive for K8. *C,* Fetal notochord is K18$^+$, but the cartilage is negative. *D,* Capillary endothelial cells in the esophageal submucosa are K7$^+$, but fibroblasts are negative.

Expression of K8 and K18 in virally transformed fibroblasts has been shown by multiple methods. Such expression is believed to indicate a relaxed control of K8 and K18 expression in transformed mesenchymal cells,[287] and could explain the presence of these keratins in some sarcomas and other nonepithelial tumors. Nearly ubiquitous expression of keratin 8 and 18 transcripts has been demonstrated by reverse transcription-polymerase chain reaction (RT-PCR) in various nonepithelial tissues.[288]

In epithelial soft tissue tumors, K8 and 18 are expressed in the epithelia of biphasic synovial sarcoma, and in scattered cells in monophasic and some poorly differentiated synovial sarcomas.[289,290] Epithelioid sarcoma[291–293] and normal notochord (Fig. 3–12C) and chordoma[294–296] are usually positive, although one study found K18 only in half of the chordomas.[295] Merkel cell carcinoma and the vast majority of all metastatic carcinomas are positive.

K8 and K18 are present in reactive submesothelial spindle cells, along with other simple epithelial keratins.[297]

Subsets of angiosarcomas have been shown to be variably keratin-positive with antibodies recognizing K8 and K18.[298] Epithelioid hemangioendotheliomas are typically K18$^+$, but negative for K8, and over 50% of angiosarcomas are K18$^+$ and K8$^+$; this probably represents neoexpression in transformed cells, because normal endothelial cells are K8$^-$.[284,285]

Leiomyosarcomas are K8$^+$ or K18$^+$ in 20% to 30% of cases,[281,299] and positivity has been seen in other types of sarcomas such as MFH[300–302] and MPNST.[289] Some rhabdomyosarcomas may also contain K8$^+$ cells.[146,172] In our experience, GISTs, especially the malignant ones, are K18$^+$ in 20% to 30% of cases, but they are rarely K8$^+$.

Ewing family of tumors commonly have scattered K8$^+$ and K18$^+$ cells, often in a starry-sky–like random pattern.[143]

Other nonepithelial malignant tumors with K8 or K18 expression include 10% to 20% of metastatic melanomas[303] and occasional B-cell lymphomas, mostly the plasmacytoid ones,[304,305] and some large cell anaplastic lymphomas.[306]

Keratins of Simple, Nonstratified Epithelia: K19

K19 (40 kd) is the lowest molecular weight keratin. It is normally present in most simple epithelia, including mesothelia, but normal hepatocytes and some renal tubular cells are negative.[261] K19 is widely expressed in complex glandular epithelia, especially in the luminal cells. K19 is absent in the epidermis, but it is present in skin adnexa and basal cells of internal squamous epithelia of esophagus and cervix and in other layers with a complex, variable distribution pattern.[307]

K19 in Mesenchymal Cell and Soft Tissue Tumors

In mesenchymal cells, K19 can be expressed as myometrium, which often shows dotlike cytoplasmic positivity. However, leiomyosarcomas are generally negative.[289] Submesothelial spindle cells are positive, and endothelia are negative.

Most types of primary and metastatic carcinomas are positive, except some hepatocellular, renal, and adrenal cortical carcinomas.[278]

The epithelial cells in biphasic synovial sarcoma and small numbers of spindle cells in most monophasic synovial sarcomas are positive.[289,290] K19 can be demonstrated in 70% to 80% of epithelioid sarcomas[293] and virtually all chordomas.[294–296] K19 is very rarely present in malignant epithelioid vascular tumors, and therefore antibodies to it or multispecific antibodies that do not recognize K18 or K8, such as AE1 antibody, are suitable in the differential diagnosis of malignant epithelioid vascular tumors and carcinomas.[285]

Keratins of Simple, Nonstratified Epithelia: K7

K7 (54 kd) is a simple epithelial keratin with a moderately wide distribution in simple and complex glandular epithelia, such as breast, respiratory tract, upper GI tract, mesothelia, and urogenital tract epithelia.[261,308,309] In breast epithelia, it shows a predominantly luminal distribution, whereas in the prostate it marks selectively basal cells. K7 is absent in colorectal epithelium (except for neuroendocrine cells). In squamous epithelia, K7 is absent in the epidermis, but is variably present in internal squamous epithelia of the esophagus and larynx.

K7 in Soft Tissue Tumors

Carcinomas generally show a similar distribution as seen in the normal tissues. Typically positive are adenocarcinomas of breast, lung, hepatobiliary and urogenital tracts, uterus, and ovaries. Typically negative are colorectal, prostatic, and hepatocellular carcinomas, although minor subsets of these tumors are positive.[310–313] Merkel cell carcinomas are usually negative, but can be focally positive.[314]

In mesenchymal cells, K7 is often present in endothelia of venules and lymphatics (Fig. 3–12*D*). In vascular tumors, K7 is present in lymphangioma, epithelioid hemangioendothelioma (50%), and in 10% to 20% of angiosarcomas.[285] It also seems to be present in some but not all smooth muscle cells.

In sarcomas, K7 is strongly expressed in the epithelial cells of biphasic synovial sarcoma, and it is probably the most prevalent keratin present in monophasic synovial sarcoma with positive foci in most cases,[290] and has been found useful to separate poorly differentiated synovial sarcoma from MPNSTs and Ewing family tumors, which are negative.[289,315]

Epithelioid sarcomas show limited K7 reactivity, usually focal, in 30% of cases.[293] Chordomas are focally positive in 10% to 20% of cases.[296]

Keratins of Simple, Nonstratified Epithelia: K20

K20 (46 kd), originally discovered as "protein IT,"[262] is expressed in GI epithelia, urothelia, and Merkel cells of skin.[262,316] Of soft tissue tumors Merkel cell carcinomas are consistently positive showing variably perinuclear dotlike or diffuse cytoplasmic positivity.[316] Biphasic synovial sarcomas commonly have focal positivity in the glandular epithelium,[290] but monophasic tumors and epithelioid sarcomas are negative. Metastatic carcinomas from colorectal and urothelial and to lesser degree of other GI origin are positive, whereas carcinomas of pulmonary, breast, prostatic, and renal origin are generally negative, with possible sporadic positive cells.[312,313,316,317]

Keratins of Basal Cells of Complex Epithelia: K5 and K14

K5 (58 kd) and K14 (50 kd) are present in basal cells of squamous and other complex epithelia, including the myoepithelial cells and tumors derived thereof.[261,263,273,313,318–320] Mutations in basal cell keratins of skin seem causative to diseases such as epidermolysis bullosa simplex.[321] Although normally present only in the basal cells of squamous epithelia, these keratins are typically present in most cells of squamous cell carcinomas. In addition, they are variably expressed in subsets of adenocarcinomas and ductal carcinomas, which may represent clinically aggressive tumors as shown in breast.[314,315] K5 is typical of mesothelioma,[322] often detected with K5/6 antibody, and has been considered one of the most useful markers in the differential diagnosis between mesothelioma and adenocarcinoma, because the adenocarcinomas are usually negative.[323] A study of paraffin-embedded carcinomas suggested that K14 antibody may be useful in demonstrating squamous differentiation of carcinomas.[324] However, focal positivity in ductal adenocarcinomas of various organs is possible.

In soft tissue tumors, K14 is typically extensively expressed in the epithelia of most biphasic synovial sarcomas, but is rarely present in monophasic and poorly differentiated tumors.[290] It is also present in some epithelioid sarcomas, usually focally.[293] K14 expression is usually only focal in mesothelioma.[297]

K5 (often studied with an antibody that reacts with both K5 and K6) is less prominently expressed in synovial sarcoma than K14; however, foci of positive cells are seen in most biphasic tumors and in about half of the monophasic tumors.

Keratins of Basal Cells of Complex Epithelia: K17

K17 (46 kd) is present in myoepithelia, basal cells of many glandular complex epithelia (such as respiratory epithelia), and in subsets of hair shaft epithelia.[325,326] Although not present in normal squamous epithelia, it may be expressed in hyperplastic ones.

In soft tissue tumors K17 is often present focally in the glandular epithelia of biphasic synovial sarcoma but is absent in monophasic tumors and almost always absent in epithelioid sarcoma. Squamous carcinomas are usually positive, and some adenocarcinomas, especially those of pancreatic origin, show variable positivity.[327,328]

Keratins of Internal Squamous Epithelia and Urothelium: K4 and K13

K4 (60 kd) and K13 (52 kd) are present and coexpressed in all but basal cells of internal squamous epithelia (mouth, esophagus, cervix, vagina) and in the urothelium.[273,274] Differentiated urothelial and squamous carcinomas of internal squamous epithelia are typically positive, whereas this marker is generally lost in the poorly differentiated carcinomas. Focal positivity is rare in adenocarcinomas of different organs.[278,329,330]

In soft tissue tumors, focal K13 reactivity occurs in the epithelia of some biphasic synovial sarcomas,[290] but K4 is rarely demonstrable in our experience.

Keratins of Keratinizing Stratified Epithelia: K1

K1 is the highest molecular weight keratin (67 kd). In normal epithelia it is selectively expressed in keratinizing squamous epithelia, and in the epidermis except in the basal layer. Keratinizing squamous carcinomas show variable positivity, but nonkeratinizing squamous and other carcinomas are negative.[278,331]

Recently, K1 has also been reported as a kininogen receptor in endothelial cells.[332] It can be immunohistochemically demonstrated in many but not all normal endothelia. Some vascular tumors, such as epithelioid hemangioendotheliomas, are consistently positive. Variably positive are hemangiomas and angiosarcomas, the epithelioid one being more commonly positive. Focal expression may also been seen in the spindle cell components of biphasic synovial sarcoma, epithelioid sarcoma, and schwannoma.[331]

Keratins of Keratinizing Stratified Epithelia: K10

Of the other keratins of stratified epithelia, experience is more extensive on K10, to which antibodies reactive in formalin-fixed tissue have been available for a longer time. This keratin is quite specific for squamous differentiation in carcinomas.[333] In soft tissue tumors, reactivity is limited to rare cells in those biphasic synovial sarcomas that have squamous differentiation,[290] and to subsets of keratinizing squamous cell carcinomas. Although expected to be the pair for K1, K10 cannot be equally demonstrated in endothelial and mesenchymal tumors.[331]

Other Keratins

K2, K9, and K11 are the other high-molecular-weight keratins. They are believed to be limited to keratinizing squamous epithelia. Of these, K9 appears to be limited to the epithelia of soles and palms.[261,263,264,334] Because antibodies have not been widely available, experience remains limited.

K6 (56 kd) and K16 (48 kd) are present in hyperproliferative keratinocytes of the skin and in subsets of hair shaft epithelia.[263,264] These keratins are only sporadically expressed in the epithelia of biphasic synovial sarcoma and are not present in epithelioid sarcoma. Distribution in carcinomas is essentially limited to those with squamous differentiation.

K15 (50 kd) is present in certain skin adnexa. It is also recognized by a monoclonal antibody to CD8, which cross-reacts with this keratin.[335] In our experience, expression is very limited in soft tissue tumors.

K3 (62 kd) and K12 (54 kd) are a keratin pair believed to be restricted to the corneal epithelium of the eye.[263,264] There are no data on soft tissue tumors.

Multispecific Keratin Antibodies and Keratin Cocktails

Patterns of reactivities of some commonly used monoclonal keratin antibodies and cocktails in soft tissue tumors are summarized in Table 3–14.

Monoclonal antibodies AE1-AE3 used as a cocktail have reactivity with most keratins except K18 and K20.[263] This cocktail shows positivity with nearly all synovial sarcomas, epithelioid sarcomas, and chordomas. Vascular endothelia of some venules and lymphatics are also positive, probably reflecting their reactivity with K7. Almost all carcinomas are positive, except some hepatocellular and adrenal cortical carcinomas.

Monoclonal antibody CAM 5.2 reacts with K8 based on immunoblotting,[280] and its patterns of reactivity seem to correspond to those of other K8 antibodies. For example, it does not react with normal endothelia.[281,282]

Most synovial sarcomas, epithelioid sarcomas, and chordomas are positive. Most carcinomas are positive, except well-differentiated and some moderately differentiated squamous cell carcinomas, whereas the poorly differentiated ones commonly reacquire simple epithelial keratins.

Monoclonal antibodies PKK1 and MNF11 react with combinations of simple epithelial keratins 8, 18, and 19 (said to react with all of them). Therefore, most synovial sarcomas, epithelioid sarcomas, chordomas, and carcinomas would be expected to be positive in most cases.

Table 3–14. Patterns of Keratin Reactivities of Selected Monoclonal Antibodies

Monoclonal Antibody	Keratins Recognized	Reference
AE1	K9–K17, K19	263
AE3	K1–K8	263
CAM5.2	K8	283
34βE12	K1, K10, K5, K14	—
MNF11	K8, K18, K19	—

Monoclonal antibody 34βE12 reacts with a combination of keratins 1, 5, 10, and 14. Based on this, it shows reactivity with epidermis and other squamous epithelia, myoepithelial cells, and basal cells of various ductal epithelia (such as prostatic basal epithelia). In soft tissue tumors, biphasic synovial sarcoma shows variable epithelial positivity. Monophasic synovial sarcomas and epithelioid sarcoma commonly show focal reactivity. Chordoma is also variably positive.

Tissue Polypeptide Antigen

Tissue polypeptide antigen (TPA), expressed in epithelial cells and present in serum of many carcinoma patients, has been shown to represent degradation products of simple epithelial keratins.[336]

Other Epithelial and Mesothelial Markers with Variable Specificities

The application of these epithelial and mesothelial markers is related to differential diagnosis between carcinoma and mesothelioma (Table 3–15), prediction of primary site for a carcinoma of an unknown origin (Table 3–16), and to some degree, to establish the diagnosis of an epithelial tumor. Primary soft tissue tumors, especially synovial sarcoma, epithelioid sarcoma, and chordoma are positive for some of these antigens.

Epithelial Membrane Antigen

Epithelial membrane antigen (EMA) is a highly glycosylated integral membrane glycoprotein of over 200 kd. Its protein has been recognized as a *MUC1* gene product, and it belongs to the family of polymorphic epithelial mucins.[337] EMA was initially referred to as human milk fat globule protein (HMFG), based on the immunogen used to generate the first antibodies.[338]

Epithelial membrane antigen is expressed on many epithelial cell membranes. EMA is present in the luminal aspect of most glandular and secretory epithelia. In nonepithelial cells, EMA is also detectable in perineurial and meningeal cells and plasma cells. The positive staining may appear in the membrane or be apparently cytoplasmic.[339–341]

Soft tissue tumors positive for EMA include synovial sarcoma (glandular lumina in biphasic tumors, spindle cell foci in monophasic tumors), epithelioid sarcoma, chordoma, and metastatic carcinomas except hepatocellular and adrenal cortical

Table 3–15. Immunohistochemical Markers Useful in the Differential Diagnosis of Adenocarcinoma and Mesothelioma

	Mesothelioma	Pulmonary Adenoca	Ovarian Serous Ca
B72.3	−/(+)	+/(−)	+/(−)
BerEp4	−/(+)	+	+
CEA	−	+	−/+
CD15 (LeuM1)	−/(+)	+/−	+/−
E-cadherin	−/(+)	+	+
N-cadherin	+/−	−	−
Calretinin	+	−/(+)	−
HBME-1	+	−/+	+
Mesothelin	+	−/+	+
MOC-31	−	+	+
Thrombomodulin	+	−/(+)	?
WT1	+	−	+
Keratin 5	+/(−)	−/(+)	−/(+)

(Based on references 347–373 and 389.)

Table 3–16. Immunohistochemical Markers That May Help to Determine Primary Origin for Metastatic Carcinoma

BCA225	Breast (lung)
CA19-9	Upper GI tract, including pancreas (ovary, breast, lung)
CA-125	Ovary (breast, lung, upper GI tract)
ERs and PRs	Breast, endometrium, ovary
K7	Widespread, absent in most colonic and kidney carcinomas
K17	Pancreatic carcinoma among upper abdominal carcinomas
K20	GI and urothelial and Merkel cell carcinomas (others may have focal positivity)
PSA, PSAP	Prostate, some carcinoid-type neuroendocrine tumors?
TTF-1	Thyroid, lung, small cell carcinomas of various locations (not Merkel cell carcinoma)
Villin	GI tract, kidney (lung)
WT1	Ovarian serous carcinoma and related tumors

PSA, prostate-specific antigen; PSAP, prostate-specific acid phosphatase

carcinomas. Detection of EMA is often useful in the diagnosis of meningioma (most cases positive) and is of central importance in the recognition of many types of perineurial cell tumors and perineuriomas.[342–344]

Epithelial membrane antigen may be focally detectable in some other sarcomas such as leiomyosarcomas, angiosarcomas, and extraskeletal myxoid chondrosarcomas.[299,345] We have also detected it variably in fibroblastic tumors raising a caution in interpretation of positive results, for example, in the diagnosis of perineurial cell tumors.

The antigen is also expressed in 50% to 65% of large cell anaplastic lymphomas and is most common in those anaplastic lymphomas that express T-cell markers. It is rare in Hodgkin disease, except the lymphocytic predominance, which is positive in 60% of cases.[346]

Although initially believed to be useful in the differential diagnosis of carcinoma and mesothelioma, cumulative experience indicates highly overlapping patterns and lack of diagnostic utility in mesothelioma.[347]

B72.3

The antigen recognized by this antibody has been called tumor-associated glycoprotein (TAG). It is expressed in 80% to 95% of pulmonary and most other adenocarcinomas and, but it is present in only 5% of mesotheliomas.[347–350] B72.3 immunoreactivity has also been detected in malignant epithelioid vascular tumors, but not in epithelioid sarcoma.[351] However, before using this marker to detect an epithelioid vascular tumor, poorly differentiated carcinoma has to be ruled out.

BerEp4

The BerEP4 monoclonal antibody recognizes epithelial glycoproteins of 34 and 39 kd. These proteins are expressed in the membranes of most glandular and some basal epithelial cells, but not in the mesothelia.[352] BerEP4 has been used in the distinction of mesothelioma and adenocarcinoma; the latter are typically positive with membrane staining, whereas the mesotheliomas are only rarely positive (10–15%) showing occasional focal staining.[353]

BerEP4 positivity is seen in 90% of biphasic synovial sarcomas in the glandular epithelia, but rarely (6–7%) in monophasic and poorly differentiated tumors.[354]

Cadherins

This is a family of large (120–140 kd) calcium-dependent cell adhesion molecules that maintain the integrity of epithelial and some nonepithelial tissues by homotypic cell adhesion. E-cadherin is expressed in nearly all normal epithelia, N-cadherin in neural tissues and mesothelia, P-cadherin in placental trophoblast, and VE-cadherin in vascular endothelia and perineurial cells.[355,356]

In soft tissue tumors, E-cadherin has been reported in epithelial cells in biphasic synovial sarcoma, but rarely in epithelioid sarcoma. It is commonly present in clear cell sarcoma,[357] and metastatic melanoma.[358] One study found VE-cadherin in 5 of 7 epithelioid sarcomas.[359] Malignant mesotheliomas are more commonly positive for N-cadherin, and negative for E-cadherin, whereas many carcinomas have the opposite patterns.[360] However, ovarian serous carcinomas may also express N-cadherin.[347]

Our experience suggests the following diagnostically useful, contrasting patterns in E- and N-cadherin expression. Epithelioid sarcomas are negative for E-cadherin in 90% of cases, whereas squamous carcinomas are always positive. Chordoma is positive for N-cadherin, but conventional and myxoid chondrosarcomas are negative.[361]

Calretinin

This calcium-binding protein belongs to the E-hand proteins that are related to S-100 protein and regulate intracellular calcium levels. Calretinin is expressed in normal mesothelial cells, mast cells, and fat cells, which show cytoplasmic and often also nuclear positivity.[362] Calretinin has been proven a useful although not fully specific marker for malignant mesothelioma. Most mesotheliomas of all types are positive, whereas most adenocarcinomas are negative. In several studies, only rare pulmonary, breast, and ovarian adenocarcinomas have been positive.[362–364] Calretinin positivity has also been reported in some colon carcinomas and colon carcinoma cell lines[365] and in ameloblastomas of the jaw.[366]

Among soft tissue tumors, the majority of synovial sarcomas are calretinin positive. In biphasic tumors, positivity in the spindle cell component is more common, but it may also occur in the epithelial component. Also monophasic and poorly differentiated synovial sarcomas often contain calretinin-positive tumor cells. Calretinin positivity is rare in other sarcomas, but may occur in some MPNSTs. Therefore, calretinin may be a useful marker in the differential diagnosis of synovial sarcoma.[353]

A subset of myofibroblastic neoplasms also contain calretinin positive lesional cells, especially proliferative fasciitis, and to lesser degree nodular fasciitis and desmoid.

CEA

Applications are limited in soft tissue tumors. Polyclonal antibodies have given staining in the epithelial component of biphasic synovial sarcoma,[367] but in our experience, such staining is not commonly obtained with monoclonal CEA antibodies.

Carcinoembryonic antigen is usually expressed in pulmonary adenocarcinoma but not in mesothelioma and is useful in distinguishing these tumors. However, ovarian and peritoneal serous carcinomas are often CEA$^-$.[347]

Combined patterns of CEA (upper GI tract, colon) and carcinoma antigen expression CA19-9 (pancreatic, upper GI tract), CA-125 (ovary), and BCA225 (breast, lung, ovary) have also been suggested useful in determining primary origin for metastatic adenocarcinomas.[368]

Desmoplakins

Desmoplakin proteins of the desmosome junctions are widely expressed in epithelial cells and their tumors. Presence has also been demonstrated in other tumors with desmosome-like junctions, such as meningioma and Ewing sarcoma.[369] Lack of antibodies reactive in formalin-fixed tissue has inhibited the practical use of these markers. A small series of sarcomas studied in frozen sections showed desmoplakin in synovial sarcoma epithelium, but not in MPNST and leiomyosarcoma.[289]

HBME1

This monoclonal antibody raised by Hector Battifora to mesothelioma cells (HBME1) recognizes an unknown membrane antigen on mesothelial and some epithelial cells. In normal tissue, HBME1 positivity is seen in normal mesothelia and bronchial and endocervical epithelia, and cartilage.[370]

Malignant mesotheliomas typically show strong membrane staining, but sarcomatoid mesotheliomas are generally negative. Adenocarcinomas of lung are variably positive in 50% of cases, but typically more focally than mesothelioma.[364,370] Ovarian serous carcinomas and thyroid papillary carcinomas are strongly positive. Because normal thyroid and goiter are generally negative, this antibody may be useful in the identification foci of thyroid papillary carcinoma.[370]

Positive soft tissue tumors are synovial sarcoma, which shows luminal epithelial staining in 100% biphasic tumors and focal positivity in 40% monophasic tumors,[290] and chordomas and chondrosarcomas.[296]

Mesothelin (K1 Monoclonal Antibody)

This membrane antigen of 40 kd was originally known as CAK1 antigen. It is a membrane antigen highly expressed in mesothelial cells and coelomic epithelia. It is present in mesotheliomas and also in ovarian serous carcinomas, but was originally reported absent in pulmonary adenocarcinomas.[371] In our experience, many adenocarcinomas of different locations are positive, including those of pulmonary, gastric, and pancreatic origin. Biphasic synovial sarcoma epithelium is positive, and epithelioid sarcomas are negative.

MOC-31

This monoclonal antibody originally raised to small cell carcinoma of lung reacts with a 41-kd cell membrane glycoprotein.[372] A great majority of adenocarcinomas of different origins (60–100%) but only 5% of mesotheliomas are positive.[373] This marker has been considered highly useful in the distinction of mesothelioma and adenocarcinoma.[347]

Thyroid Transcription Factor (TTF-1)

This nuclear protein is a transcriptional regulator present in thyroid and pulmonary epithelium and subsets of cells in the diencephalon.[374]

Differentiated thyroid carcinomas and their differentiated metastases are positive, but anaplastic thyroid carcinomas are typically negative.[375,376] Approximately 60% of pulmonary adenocarcinomas and 80% to 90% of small cell carcinomas are positive, and TTF-1 may be a useful marker to pinpoint pulmonary origin of metastatic adenocarcinoma.[377,378] Although pulmonary small cell carcinomas are typically positive,[379] one study found 80% of nonpulmonary small cell carcinomas have also been positive,[380] indicating limited value in determining the primary site for a small cell carcinoma. However, Merkel carcinomas seem to be consistently negative.[381]

Villin

Villin is a 95-kd actin cytoskeleton-associated protein typical of GI epithelial and renal proximal tubular brush border.[382] Its presence in metastatic adenocarcinoma may be useful to establish the renal[382] or GI origin[383] (Fig. 3–13). Also a subset of pulmonary bronchioloalveolar carcinomas,[382,383] endometrial and ovarian adenocarcinomas (and small cell carcinomas of lung[384] may be villin positive, whereas carcinomas of the breast and lung are generally negative. Synovial and epithelioid sarcomas have been negative in our experience.

The GI carcinoids have very commonly (83%), and pulmonary carcinoids less often (40%) villin positivity, more often focally. Small cell carcinomas are usually negative.[385]

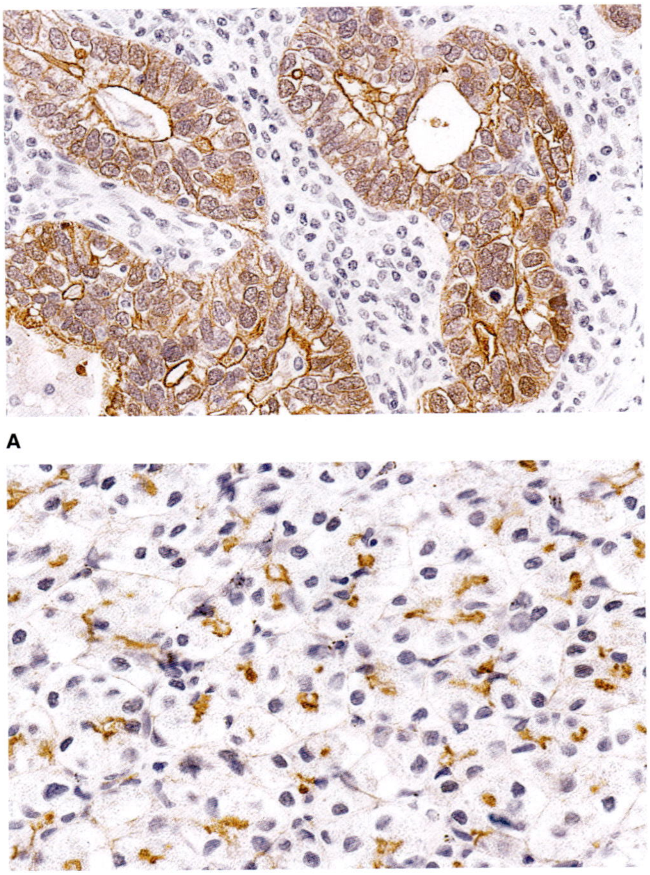

A

B

Figure 3–13. *A*, Villin positivity in poorly differentiated metastatic colon carcinoma. *B*, Subtle luminal villin positivity is present in renal cell carcinoma.

Wilms' Tumor Protein (WT1)

This nuclear protein is a transcriptional regulator (transcription factor). It is expressed in developing glomerular epithelia of the kidney (Fig. 3–14*A*), mesothelial cells, and müllerian epithelia.[386]

Positive tumors include Wilms tumor and (intra-abdominal) desmoplastic small round cell tumor (Fig. 3–14*B*).[387] This marker has been suggested useful in the differential diagnosis of small, round cell tumors, because other tumors of this group have been found negative.[388]

In epithelial tumors WT1 is expressed in the majority of malignant mesotheliomas but may be lost in less differentiated tumors.[347,389] WT1 seems to be selectively expressed in carcinomas of müllerian origin (ovarian surface epithelial and related tumors) and it

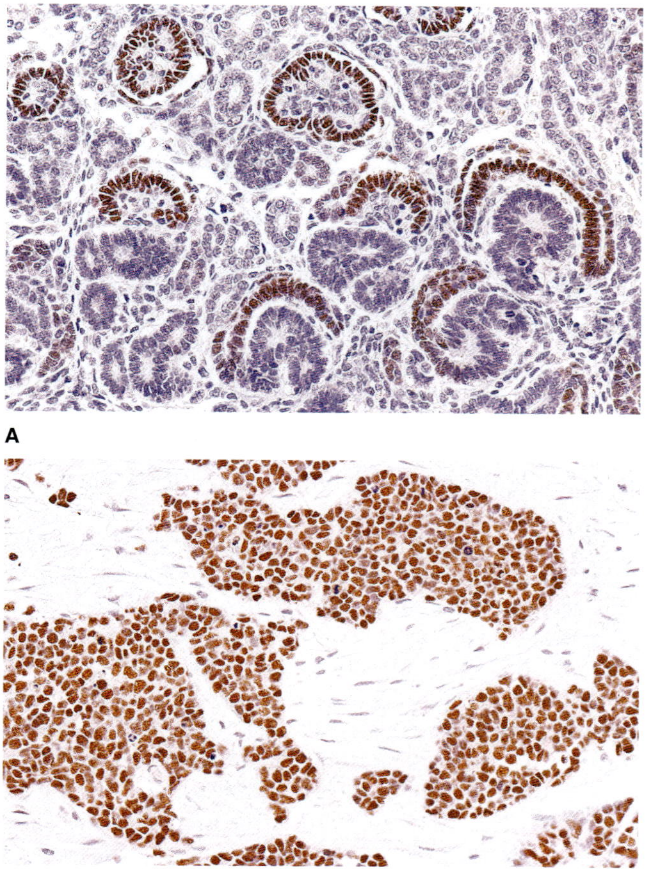

Figure 3-14. *A,* WT1 immunostaining in the developing kidney shows nuclear staining in the comma-shaped developing glomeruli. *B,* Desmoplastic small round cell tumor shows nuclear positivity for WT1.

may be useful in evaluating the müllerian epithelial origin of metastatic carcinomas, or in the diagnosis of primary peritoneal müllerian serous carcinomas.[328,390]

Oher Important Tumor-Type Markers (Alphabetically Arranged)

Anaplastic Lymphoma Kinase

The anaplastic lymphoma kinase *ALK* gene located in 2p23 is rearranged and overexpressed in large cell anaplastic lymphoma. Recently, its involvement has also been demonstrated in inflammatory myofibroblastic tumors (IMT), in which the plump spindle cells often demonstrate strong cytoplasmic ALK positivity.[391-393] However, similar reactivity may be seen in a variety of nonneoplastic and neoplastic fibroblastic lesions, calling for caution in the use of this marker for IMT.

Basement Membrane Proteins

Laminin

This high-molecular-weight basement membrane protein (900 kd) is composed of several subunits (chains). Laminin is present in most basement membrane-invested epithelial and mesenchymal cells with a generally similar distribution as observed with collagen IV (see the following discussion). Soft tissue tumors showing pericellular positivity in a network-like pattern include schwannomas, glomus tumors, and well-differentiated smooth and skeletal muscle tumors.[394-396] The α chain of laminin (merosin) shows a narrower distribution, but schwannomas show focal positivity.[397]

Collagen Type IV

This basement membrane collagen is present on the basal aspect of basal epithelial cells and vascular endothelia. Normal smooth muscle and skeletal muscle cells are typically surrounded by a basement membrane, whereas fibroblasts are not. Of soft tissue tumors, schwannomas with complex cell processes show apparently diffuse positivity, whereas well-differentiated smooth and skeletal muscle tumors typically show pericellular positivity in a network-like pattern.[396,398] The staining pattern is generally similar to that observed with antibodies to laminin. Collagen type VII is another basement membrane collagen shown to have a relatively similar distribution as collagen type IV.[399] Specific experience in soft tissue tumors is limited.

Bcl-2

The *bcl2* gene product is a 25-kd protein in the mitochondrial, microsomal, and some inner membranes. It has an apoptosis preventing function and has complex interactions with other apoptosis-modulating proteins.[400] This gene for *bcl2* was originally known from follicular lymphoma, where it is overexpressed as a result of the t(14;18) translocation, which causes juxtaposition of the *bcl2* gene with the promoter of the immunoglobulin heavy chain gene.[401] Bcl2 is constitutively expressed in many long-lived cell types, such as neurons.[402]

Of soft tissue tumors, bcl2 has been widely expressed in the tested tumors. Strongly positive are Kaposi sarcoma, GISTs, solitary fibrous tumor, synovial sarcoma (especially spindle cell components), whereas nodular fasciitis and desmoid and GI leiomyomas are negative. These findings may be of some differential diagnostic value.[403,404]

Although there are indications for the use of bcl2 as a prognostic/biologic potential marker for breast and some other carcinomas, no such applications have been validated for soft tissue tumors.

CD10

CD10, also called common acute lymphoblastic leukemia antigen (CALLA), is a cell surface aminopeptidase.[405,406] It is expressed in follicular lymphocytes, some epithelial surfaces (small intestine), and some fibroblasts, and has been used as a marker for common acute lymphoblastic lymphomas and follicular lymphomas. In mesenchymal tissues, subsets of fibroblasts and endometrial stromal cells are positive.

Endometrial stromal sarcomas are commonly strongly CD10$^+$, but uterine smooth muscle tumors are negative, and this feature has been shown useful in the differential diagnosis of endometrial stromal sarcoma and cellular smooth muscle tumors.[407–409]

CD99 (MIC-2 Gene Product, Protein p30/32)

This antigen, originally discovered in T lymphoblasts, can be detected with monoclonal antibodies E12, HBA71, and O13. CD99 is widely expressed in different tissues at a low level, but diagnostically useful is the consistent, high expression in Ewing sarcoma and related tumors (PNETs), which typically show a distinctive membrane staining.[410–412] T-lymphoblastic lymphomas are also strongly positive. However, such reactivity is not specific, because strong immunoreactivity can be seen in other tumors such as neuroendocrine carcinomas, synovial sarcoma, hemangiopericytoma, and meningioma.[412,413] Also endothelial cells and fibroblasts are often positive, especially after microwave epitope retrieval.

CD117 (KIT, Stem Cell Factor/Mast Cell Growth Factor Receptor)

This transmembrane protein is a growth factor receptor, which is type III receptor tyrosine kinase with five immunoglobulin-like extracellular loops. It is homologous to the feline Hardy-Zuckerman sarcoma retroviral oncoprotein.[414]

KIT is constitutionally expressed in early hematopoietic cells, mast cells (Fig. 3–15*A*), germ cells, melanocytes and interstitial cell of Cajal, the GI pacemaker cells in and around the myenteric plexus (Fig. 3–15*B*). Certain epithelial cells that are KIT$^+$ include breast lobular epithelium and some basal cells of skin and hair shafts.[415–417] The positive staining usually appears as distinctive membrane staining in normal cells and as diffuse cytoplasmic staining in Golg zone, or membrane staining in neoplastic cells with KIT expression.

The GISTs with Cajal cell-like differentiation are CD117$^+$, and the positivity is now considered a major definitional feature for GISTs, which separates the GISTs from true smooth muscle tumors and schwannomas.[30,418–420] Mast cell tumors mastocytoma, mastocytoma, and urticaria pigmentosa,[417] many myeloid leukemias, and extramedullary myeloid tumors are

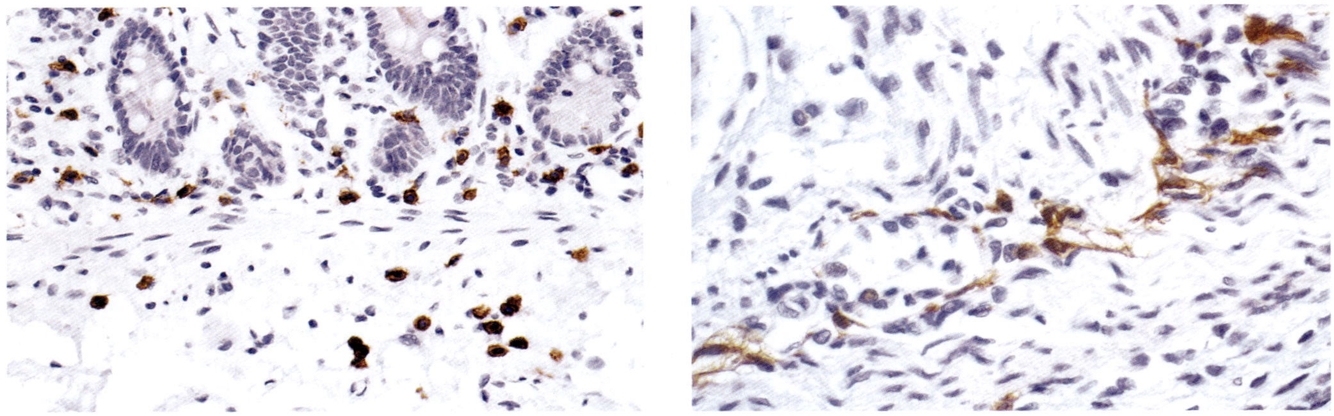

A B

Figure 3–15. *A*, Mast cells are an excellent positive control for KIT (CD117) immunostaining, which should be present in any valid staining. *B*, The interstitial cells of Cajal are KIT$^+$ elements around the myenteric plexus of fetal intestine.

positive.[421] Seminomas are positive,[415] but other germ cell tumors are typically negative.

Approximately 50% of angiosarcomas, Ewing sarcomas, and clear cell sarcomas (20–45%) are also positive.[30,422] KIT expression has been noted to decrease in melanoma progression. Nevertheless, up to 50% of metastatic melanomas are KIT$^+$.[419,423] Most other soft tissue tumors are negative, but sporadic cells in other tumors and neovascular endothelia can be positive.[30]

Activating (gain-of-function) type of c-kit gene mutations have been found in GISTs (exons 9, 11, and 13) and mastocytomas (exon 17). There is considerable interest in tumors with a KIT-activation mechanism, because a new KIT tyrosine kinase inhibitor drug imatinib has shown promise in early clinical trials in GIST (see Chapters 4 and 11).

Estrogen and Progesterone Receptors

Like many other steroid hormone receptors, estrogen and progesterone receptors (ERs and PRs) are nuclear transcriptional regulator proteins for a number of hormone-dependent genes. ER and PR are expressed in female sex hormone-sensitive epithelia of the breast and endometrium, and in endometrial stromal cells and myometrium.

In soft tissue tumors, especially uterine smooth muscle tumors, and subsets of similar abdominal and retroperitoneal tumors, uterine-type leiomyomas in women (Fig. 3–16) are positive.[30] However, uterine leiomyosarcomas can also be positive. Other positive mesenchymal tumors are female genital stromal tumors such as endometrial stromal sarcoma, aggressive angiomyxoma of the pelvis, and angiomyofibroblastoma of the vulva. Evaluation of ERs and PRs can be useful in the diagnosis of these entities.

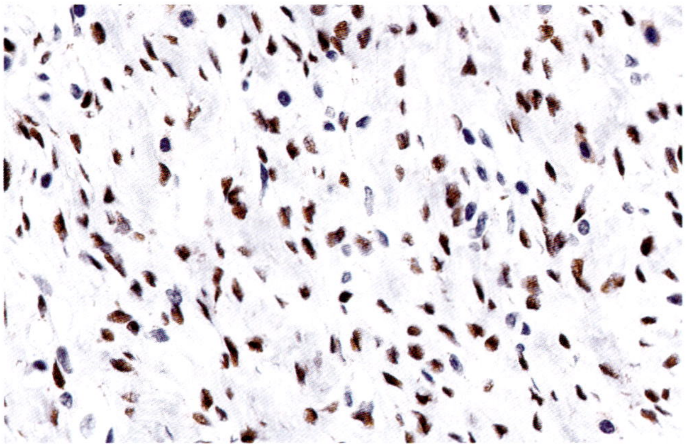

Figure 3–16. Most retroperitoneal leiomyomas show nuclear positivity for estrogen receptor, similar to uterine leiomyomas.

The PRs may be present in a broader spectrum of tumors as ERs, and therefore be less specific for true hormonally sensitive tumors. Both receptors should be evaluated together.

The ER positivity of a metastatic carcinoma may pinpoint to mammary (or uterine/ovarian) origin. In a large study, 66% of ductal and 88% of lobular mammary carcinomas were positive, whereas all of 500 pulmonary and GI carcinomas were negative.[424]

Fli-1

The gene encoding for this nuclear protein belongs to the ETS family of transcriptional regulators and is a partner in the most common types of Ewing family translocations.[425] Nuclear expression of Fli-1 protein has been detected in 60% of Ewing sarcomas and suggested as a useful marker. However, positivity also occurs in endothelial cells and some lymphocytes, necessitating caution in interpretation.[426] Use for identification of angiosarcomas has also been suggested.[44]

Glial Fibrillary Acidic Protein

The intermediate filaments of glial cells, especially astrocytes and some ependymal cells, contain glial fibrillary acidic protein (GFAP, MW 51 kd). Some myoepithelial cells of salivary gland, breast, and skin also express GFAP, but otherwise this protein has a restricted distribution.[427] Although most peripheral nerve Schwann cells are negative, increased GFAP expression has been observed in reactive Schwann cells in axonal neuropathies.[428]

This protein is present in most astrocytic and ependymal glial tumors and is a marker for myxopapillary ependymomas.

In the peripheral nervous system, it is present in 30% to 50% of schwannomas,[429–432] and in true nerve sheath myxomas, but it is generally absent in MPNSTs. In our experience, a majority of GI schwannomas are positive, whereas GISTs are negative representing a useful discriminating parameter.

Myoepitheliomas and mixed tumors of salivary glands and skin adnexa often contain GFAP$^+$ epithelial cells, consistent with their myoepithelial-like differentiation.[427]

Inhibin

Inhibin is a growth factor of the transforming growth factor-β superfamily. It was originally identified as a gonadal peptide that inhibited or stimulated the release of pituitary follicle-stimulating hormones (FSHs). Inhibin is consistently present in granulosa cell tumor[433,434] but not in surface epithelial tumors. It is also present in adrenal cortical carcinomas (Fig. 3–17) but rarely in pheochromocytomas,[435,436] and may have value in the identification of these tumors in unusual locations or their atypical variants. Recently, inhibin was reported in granular cell tumor of the hepatobiliary three.[437] Our experience indicates common presence of inhibin in granular cell tumors, but not in peripheral nerve sheath tumors, such as schwannomas and neurofibromas. Other soft tissue tumors are negative.

Osteocalcin

This protein of the bone matrix is present in osteoid and bone and has a great specificity for osteoid.[438] In soft tissue diagnosis, this marker may be useful in highlighting true osteoid in the diagnosis of extraskeletal osteosarcoma.[439]

Vimentin

The intermediate filaments in most mesenchymal cells (fibroblasts, endothelial cells, cartilage, histiocytes, lymphoid cells) are predominantly or exclusively composed of vimentin (MW 57 kD), which is the name given by Franke et al. to this intermediate filament protein.[440] Among mesenchymal cells, vimentin is specifically absent in most mature smooth and skeletal muscle cells. Certain epithelial cells (thyroid follicle cells, endometrial glands, mesothelia, and ovarian surface epithelial cells) also contain vimentin, often in the basal aspect of the cytoplasm.[441]

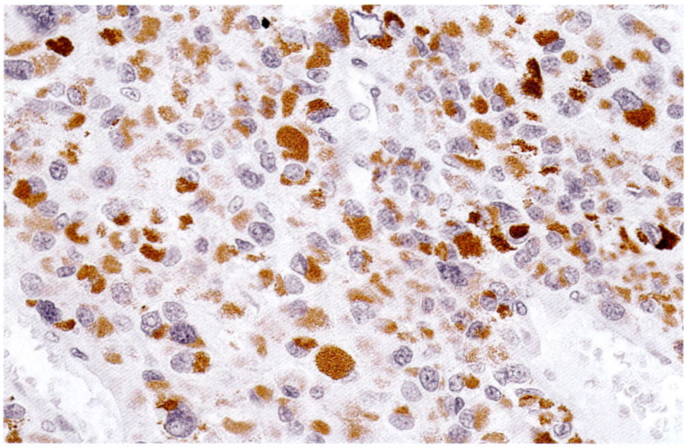

Figure 3–17. Cytoplasmic melan A positivity in metastatic adrenal cortical carcinoma.

Vimentin is widely expressed in mesenchymal and neuroectodermal tumors, including most sarcomas and malignant melanoma, but it is absent in some leiomyomas. Of carcinomas, many renal, thyroid, ovarian, and endometrial carcinomas, and small portions of others, are variably positive. Poorly differentiated carcinomas are variably and sarcomatoid carcinomas typically vimentin positive.

Vimentin has limited application in the differential diagnosis of soft tissue tumors because of its widespread tissue distribution, but its absence in the tumor cells of many poorly differentiated carcinomas (with the presence of internal control) may be diagnostically useful. Once thought to be a marker for antigen preservation,[442] vimentin positivity can now be consistently demonstrated after heat-induced epitope retrieval, virtually independent of fixation parameters. Therefore, vimentin has lost its value to monitor the antigen preservation.

Cell Cycle Markers

Cell cycle regulators are nuclear proteins that work in a highly orchestrated manner in regulatory pathways. Aberrations in the cell cycle are considered among the most fundamental and functionally most relevant alterations in cancer.[443,444] This rapidly advancing field is in its early stages of application. Numerous cell cycle regulators have been evaluated in soft tissue tumors. In some cases, immunohistochemical detection or lack of detection has been found to give prognostically useful information. However, static analysis of formalin-fixed tissue only gives limited information toward functional understanding of the cell cycle aberrations. It is likely that analysis of some proteins could give meaningful information at the immunohistochemical level, whereas analysis of some parameters has to be based on molecular genetic studies. Studies that address the regulatory pathways in specific tumor entities are needed to gather systematic information.

The most widely applied cell cycle markers are proliferation markers, Ki67-analogs, of which MIB-1 is probably the most widely used in formalin-fixed tissue. p53 (TP53) has also been analyzed extensively, whereas the information of many other regulators, such as the cyclins, cyclin-dependent kinases, and their inhibitors, is more limited. Examples of

Table 3–17. Examples of Studies on Selected Cell Cycle Control Proteins in Soft Tissue Sarcomas

Cyclin-Dependent Kinase Inhibitors	Findings in Soft Tissue Tumors	References
p16	Loss of expression in some sarcomas	459
	Homozygous loss and loss of expression in MPNST arising in neurofibroma	460, 461
p21	Widely expressed in different sarcomas, no clear correlations in a small study	462
p27	Loss found as an adverse prognostic sign in synovial sarcoma	463
	Loss not found prognostically significant in synovial sarcoma	455
p53	Overexpression found to be common and a prognostically adverse sign in various sarcomas	454, 455
	Overexpression found not significant in MFH	456
Cyclins		
Cyclin A	Expression found to correlate with tumor aggressiveness	464
Cyclin D1	Overexpression associated with poor prognosis in extremity tumors	465
Cyclin E	Found in leiomyosarcoma but not in leiomyoma	466
MDM2	High expression found in some sarcomas	467
RB1	Loss of protein in subsets of sarcomas, especially in high-grade ones	453

some of other cell cycle markers have been listed in Table 3–17.

Ki67 and Analogs

A cell cycle stage-related nuclear protein identified with the Ki-67 monoclonal antibody is selectively expressed in cells that have entered in the cell cycle and are other than G_0.[445] The original antibody only reacted in frozen sections, and the percentage of nuclear positivity (Ki-67 score) was found to correlate with malignancy grade; benign soft tissue tumors usually have a low score.[446] Subsequently other Ki-67 analog antibodies raised to bacterially expressed Ki-67 peptide sequences were introduced that performed well in formalin-fixed tissue, and the most important of them is MIB-1.[447] Others, such as Ki-S11, have also been suggested useful.[448]

Numerous studies have evaluated MIB-1 immunostaining in different types of sarcomas. Higher score has generally correlated with tumor grade, and many studies have concluded that MIB-1 score offers statistically significant prognostic predictive information.[449–452] A cut-off value of 20% of positive nuclei has been suggested giving statistically significant, independent prognostic information predictive of metastasis and tumor-related death in high-grade sarcomas of the extremities.[451,452]

p53 (TP53)

This cell cycle regulator is a nuclear protein of 53 kd. It has been studied extensively, and there is a general assumption that most normal and benign cells do not show detectable expression, and that its detected expression is abnormal. Some studies have documented that immunohistochemically detected p53 expression has prognostic value in soft tissue sarcomas,[453–455] but some studies, for example on MFH, have found no prognostic significance.[456] Also, p53 immunoreactivity has been detected in some benign soft tissue tumors.[457,458]

Use of p53 as an immunohistochemical marker of malignancy and prognosis requires caution and further studies, and more studies are needed to validate this marker in specific types of soft tissue sarcomas. p53 is affected by complex genetic mutations in almost any type of cancer, and there is no clear correlation between mutation and immunohistochemically detected expression. There has been an assumption that high p53 expression results from abnormal accumulation of p53. The gene is discussed in Chapter 4.

Other Cell Cycle Control Proteins

Selected examples of studies in soft tissue sarcomas have been summarized in Table 3–17. The loss of cyclin dependent kinase inhibitors p16 (CKND2), p21 WAF1, and p27 KIP or overexpression of cyclins, their kinases, or MDM2 can be factors that lead to uncontrolled cell proliferation.[455,459–467]

Retinoblastoma gene product p110RB is a nuclear protein that acts as a cell cycle regulator. Loss of this protein is the cause of hereditary bilateral retinoblastoma. Somatic loss of p100RB has been evaluated in soft tissue sarcomas. One study found such loss in 5 of 7 intermediate- or high-grade MFHs and less commonly in other sarcomas. Concern of reproducibility of detection in paraffin-embedded tissue has been also raised.[450]

Technical Considerations for Immunohistochemistry

Optimal technique is crucially important for the successful application of immunohistochemistry. Fixation, epitope retrieval, optimization, automation and standardization, and interpretation of immunostains will be briefly commented on here.

Fixation

The complex biochemical events occurring during formaldehyde fixation are not completely known, but they include cross-linking of proteins.[468] Formalin-fixation time influences immunoreactivity and ideally should be 8 to 24 hours. A shorter fixation may lead to unoptimal fixation and loss of sections during heat-induced epitope retrieval. Longer fixation times may cause permanent loss of antigenicity,[469] or necessitate the use of a more effective epitope retrieval mode.

Alcohol fixation (absolute ethanol) may be advantageous for some markers (especially structural antigens). It also offers easily storable tissue that is superior for genetic analysis, compared to formalin-fixed tissue. Many commercial nonformalin fixatives contain alcohol(s) as essential components. Note that alcohol-fixed tissue does not need (and it does not withstand) the enzymatic digestion and microwave epitope retrieval often necessary for formalin-fixed tissue.[469]

Epitope Retrieval

The two principal methods are enzyme digestion and heat-induced epitope retrieval. The optimal retrieval modality for each antibody should be determined but is usually suggested by the manufacturer or vendor. Note that the optimization parameters for different antibodies to the same antigen can vary.

Enzyme digestion is the best modality for a minority of antibodies, including, for example many keratin antibodies,[470] such as AE1, K7, and K20. Digestion may not be necessary for tissues with a very short fixation time (<4 hours), whereas those with a longer fixation time may need a longer digestion. At least to some degree, longer fixation time can be compensated with an extended digestion.[471,472]

Approximately 60% to 70% of the most common antibodies generally used in diagnosis benefit from heat-induced epitope retrieval. Studies examining large numbers of antibodies have found that very few antibodies perform less well with such a retrieval prompting near to universal use. Initially performed by microwave heat, epitope retrieval is now often carried out with alternative methods such as a vegetable steamer or pressure cooker, which are easier to standardize.[473–476] The solutions initially used included heavy metal solutions, but one study showed that for most antibodies, 1 mM/L EDTA solution of pH 8.0 gave excellent results and was superior to 10 mM/L citrate buffer of pH 6.0.[476] This is also supported by our experience.

Immunostaining for some markers (e.g., for p53) has been found to be less satisfactory in stored slides,[477] and the same can be true for some other antigens. However, microwave epitope retrieval can compensate for the loss of p53 antigenicity in stored slides.[478] Similarly, optimization of epitope retrieval has been found to compensate a similar loss observed for other antigens, and storage of unstained slides in cold temperature has also been suggested.[479]

Optimization, Automation, and Standardization of Immunohistochemistry

It is advantageous to test the pattern of tissue reactivities of all antibodies used in one's own laboratory, to ascertain that previously well-documented patterns of reactivities are obtained. This can be accomplished by using a panel of normal and neoplastic tissues on one or a few slides generated from

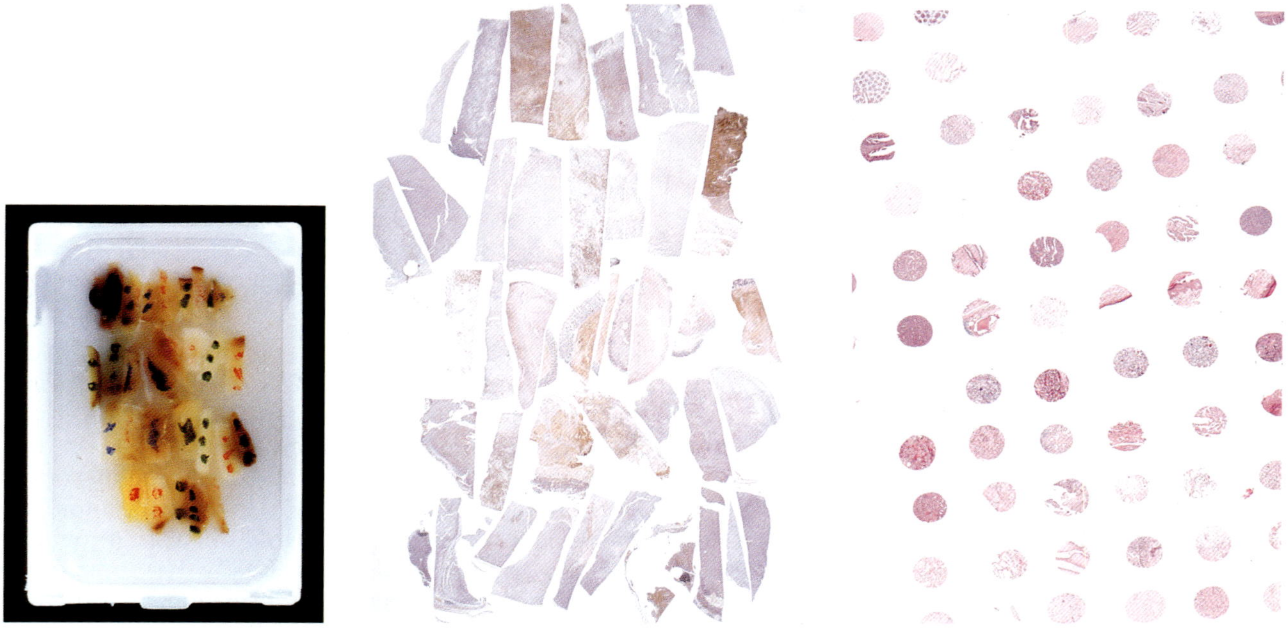

A B C

Figure 3-18. Examples of multitumor blocks and slides derived from them. *A,* Face of an uncut block containing 35 different tissues. The tissue profiles have been marked for identification to validate the embedding order prior to the cutting. *B,* Slide derived from a similar block immunostained for desmin highlighting true smooth muscle tumors among the negative GISTs. *C,* Hematoxylin and eosin-stained slide from a tissue array using 0.6-mm punch biopsies of blocks.

multitissue blocks (tumor array blocks). Several methods for making such blocks have been published and reviewed.[480-482] A range of 10 to 500 different tissues can be fit in a single block, depending on the size of tissue used (Fig. 3-18).

All antibodies should be optimized for dilution. Although this measure is often more related to antibody economy in the case of monoclonal antibodies, the optimal dilution is critical for polyclonal antisera to reduce background staining. All antibodies should be evaluated on a panel of control tissues, whether heat-induced epitope retrieval with a citrate buffer (pH 6.8), EDTA buffer (pH 8.0), or enzymatic digestion gives the optimal results.

Several types of automation are available.[483,484] Their use typically saves technical time and standardizes the procedure, but increases the reagent cost, as compared with manual staining. The suitability of automated conditions, for example, elevated temperature of incubations, should be tested for each antibody, because for some antibodies, this reduces staining optimality.

Standardization of the interpretation is only starting to evolve.[485,486] It includes elements such as ensuring appropriate localization of immunostaining, monitoring the effects of fixation and processing in immunoreactivity, and developing criteria and cut-off for interpretation. Standardization is especially critical when using tests that are quantitated (e.g., MIB-1, p53).

Interpretation of Immunostains

Monitoring the presence of endogenously positive tissue components in tumor samples as internal controls helps to validate the antibody performance on each tissue and is always more relevant than an external positive control, which only controls the antibody and the technique. Such a positive control is almost always available for S-100 protein (dendritic cells or nerves), muscle actins (pericytes, vascular smooth muscle), CD34 (endothelial cells), and vimentin (most mesenchymal cells).

Staining unrelated to specific antigen content can be caused by avidin binding because of endogenous biotin content (especially liver, adrenal, oncocytic cells, nuclei in certain tissues, after heat-induced epitope retrieval). This was initially observed in frozen sections,[487] but paraffin sections were shown to reacquire biotin reactivity following heat epitope retrieval.[488] This can be countered with avidin biotin block (several kits commercially available), and such block is recommended if heat induced epitope retrieval is used.

Diffuse presence of the antigen in the tissue can cause background problems. Examples of this include the immunoglobulin heavy and light chains and vWF, which as serum proteins are inevitably present in necrotic tissue or sites of exudation. This unavoidable presence of certain circulating antigens has to be considered when interpreting the results.

Contamination of the tumor specimen by extraneous material may cause difficulties in interpretation. Although this is often obvious (placental villi, pieces of villous adenoma), epithelial tumor cells may be smeared in the periphery of specimens (cutting board metastasis). Human epithelial dust easily contaminates section surfaces, and such epithelial contaminants become visible in immunostaining for epithelial markers (e.g., keratins).

Separation of normal and neoplastic components may be difficult but is important for the interpretation. For example, entrapped skeletal muscle should not be confused with skeletal muscle differentiation. Such cells are often present in the periphery of tumors, and are seen "streaming" into the tumor from periphery. Similarly, ubiquitous tumor-infiltrating histiocytes and Langerhans cells interdigitating reticulum cells should not be confused with tumor components. For some lesions with heterogeneous cellular composition, it is difficult to determine which lesional cells are neoplastic and which are reactive (e.g., fibrous histiocytomas).

Other Methods for Demonstrating Protein/Gene Expression

The validity of a positive immunohistochemical result depends on the specificity of the antibody and the technique used. Also, a positive result does not prove that the protein has been manufactured on that site, because proteins can be absorbed or transported from another source. Although, in general, immunohistochemical results are highly reliable (provided that the specificity of the antibody has been adequately proven), scientific confirmation of results is often desirable, although generally is not necessary in clinical practice. Other methods to detect gene expression are listed in Table 3–18. Systematic information is available in laboratory manuals.[489]

Table 3–18. Different Methods for Evaluation of Gene Expression

Method	Description	Requirements, Comments
Immunohistochemistry	Recognizes variably molecule-specific epitopes with antibodies	Frozen or formalin-fixed tissue Specific antibody required
SDS-PAGE and Western blotting	Sorting of proteins by molecular masses, electrotransfer onto membrane and probing of the membrane with antibody	Fresh/frozen, possibly alcohol-fixed tissue Can confirm the presence of immunoreactive protein of the expected molecular weight Specific antibody required Tissue topography is lost
mRNA in situ hybridization	Demonstrates transcript on tissue sections	Fresh, frozen, possibly formalin-fixed tissue Specific probes required Observes tissue topography
RT-PCR	Reverse transcription to cDNA, DNA amplification, preferably quantitatively	Preferably fresh or frozen tissue Thermal cycler, or quantitative PCR system (light cycler/real-time PCR) No topographic correlation
cDNA microarray analysis	Hybridization of tumor c-DNA onto filters or slides and simultaneous screening of potentially thousands of transcripts	Specifically prepared filters/slides with probes, hybridization, and filter reader are required No topographic correlation
Serial analysis of gene expression	New technique, experience very limited	

Immunoblotting (Western Blotting)

This method implies immunostaining of a protein of certain size on a membrane with an antibody on a membrane. The application preferably requires fresh or frozen tissue, but in some instances, alcohol-fixed tissue is also suitable. The steps include (1) extraction and solubilization of the desired protein fraction (membrane, cytosolic, cytoskeletal residue), (2) size separation by PAGE, (3) electric transfer onto membrane, and (4) immunostaining the membrane or membrane strip with the desired antibody. Positive results support that the positive immunohistochemical finding indeed reflects the presence of a certain protein.

Analysis of Messenger RNA

Gene expression can be measured directly by demonstrating the specific messenger RNA (mRNA) sequences. This can be accomplished by: (1) in situ hybridization on a tissue section using a specific complementary DNA (cDNA) probe, (2) RT-PCR, (3) Northern blotting, or (4) membrane hybridization on cDNA-tag filter in a cDNA microarray. The latter method allows for analysis of a large number of genes simultaneously (see Chapter 4).

The results obtained by RNA demonstration are not always comparable to protein demonstration of a several reasons. These include inherent differences of assay sensitivities, variations of mRNA half-life in tissue versus protein half-life.

REFERENCES

Reviews, General

1. Miettinen M: Immunohistochemistry of soft-tissue tumors. Possibilities and limitations in surgical pathology. Pathol Annu 1990;25(Part 1):1–36.
2. Swanson PE, Wick MR: Soft tissue tumors. In Colvin RB, Bhan AK, McCluskey RT (eds): Diagnostic Immunopathology. New York, Raven Press, 1995: 599–631.
3. Brooks JSJ: Immunohistochemistry in the differential diagnosis of soft tissue tumors. Monogr Pathol 1996; 38:65–128.
4. Ordonez NG. Application of immunocytochemistry in the diagnosis of soft tissue sarcomas: A review and update. Adv Anat Pathol 1998;5:67–85.
5. Miettinen M: Immunohistochemistry of soft tissue tumors. J Histotechnol 1999;22:219–227.
6. Folpe AL, Gown AM: Immunohistochemistry for analysis of soft tissue tumors. In Weiss SW, Goldblum JR (eds). Soft Tissue Tumors, 4th ed. Mosby, St Louis, 2001.
7. Nagle RB: Intermediate filaments: A review of the basic biology. Am J Surg Pathol 1988;12(Suppl 1):4–16.

Endothelial Cell Markers, Including CD34

8. Newman PJ, Berndt MC, Gorski J, et al: PECAM-1 (CD31) cloning and relation to adhesion molecules of the immunoglobulin gene superfamily. Science 1990; 247:1219–1222.
9. Ilan N, Cheug L, Pinter E, Madri JA: Platelet-endothelial cell adhesion molecule-1 (CD31), a scaffolding molecule for selected catenin family members whose binding is mediated by different tyrosine and serine/threonine phosphorylation. J Biol Chem 2000;275:21435–21443.
10. Kuzu I, Bicknell R, Harris AL, Jones M, Gatter KC, Mason DY: Heterogeneity of vascular endothelial cells with relevance to diagnosis of vascular tumours. J Clin Pathol 1992;45:143–148.
11. de Young BR, Wick MR, Fitzgibbon JF, Sirgi KE, Swanson PE: CD31: An immunospecific marker for endothelial differentiation in human neoplasms. Appl Immunohistochem 1993;1:97–100.
12. Miettinen M, Lindenmayer AE, Chaubal A: Endothelial cell markers CD31, CD34, and BNH9 antibody to H- and Y-antigens. Evaluation of their specificity and sensitivity in the diagnosis of vascular tumors and comparison with von Willebrand's factor. Mod Pathol 1994;7:82–90.
13. De Young BR, Frierson HF Jr, Ly MN, Smith D, Swanson PE: CD31 immunoreactivity in carcinomas and mesotheliomas. Am J Clin Pathol 1998;110:374–377.
14. Lanza F, Healy L, Sutherland DR: Structural and functional features of the CD34 antigen: An update. J Biol Regul Homeostat Agents 2001;15:1–13.
15. van de Rijn M, Rouse RV: CD34. A review. Appl Immunohistochem 1994;2:71–80.
16. Nickoloff BJ: The human progenitor cell antigen (CD34) is localized on endothelial cells, dermal dendritic cells, and perifollicular cells in formalin-fixed normal skin, and on proliferating endothelial cells and stromal spindle-shaped cells in Kaposi's sarcoma. Arch Dermatol 1991;127:523–529.
17. Ramani P, Bradley NJ, Fletcher CDM: QBEND/10, a new monoclonal antibody to endothelium: Assessment of its diagnostic utility in paraffin sections. Histopathology 1990;17:237–242.
18. Sankey EA, More L, Dhillon AP: QBEnd/10: A new immunostain for the routine diagnosis of Kaposi's sarcoma. J Pathol 1990;161:267–271.
19. Traweek ST, Kandalaft PL, Mehta P, Battifora H: The human hematopoietic progenitor cell antigen (CD34) in vascular neoplasia. Am J Clin Pathol 1991;96:25–31.
20. Aiba S, Tabata N, Ishii H, Ootani H, Tagami H: Dermatofibrosarcoma protuberans is a unique fibrohistiocytic tumor expressing CD34. Br J Dermatol 1992;127: 79–84.
21. Abenoza P, Lillemoe T: CD34 and factor XIIIa in the differential diagnosis of dermatofibroma and der-

matofibrosarcoma protuberans. Am J Dermatopathol 1993;15:429–434.
22. Cohen PR, Rapini RP, Farhood AI: Expression of the human hematopoietic progenitor cell antigen CD34 in vascular and spindle cell tumors. J Cutan Pathol 1993;20:15–20.
23. Goldblum JR: CD34 positivity in fibrosarcomas which arise in dermatofibrosarcoma protuberans. Arch Pathol Lab Med 1995;119:238–241.
24. Westra WH, Gerald WL, Rosai J: Solitary fibrous tumor. Consistent CD34 immunoreactivity and occurrence in the orbit. Am J Surg Pathol 1994;18:992–998.
25. Hanau CA, Miettinen M: Solitary fibrous tumor. Histological and immunohistochemical spectrum of benign and malignant variants presenting at different sites. Hum Pathol 1995;26:440–449.
26. Flint A, Weiss SW: CD34 and keratin expression distinguishes solitary fibrous tumor (fibrous mesothelioma) of pleura from desmoplastic mesothelioma. Hum Pathol 1995;26:428–431.
27. Suster S, Fisher C: Immunoreactivity for the human hematopoietic progenitor cell antigen (CD34) in lipomatous tumors. Am J Surg Pathol 1997;21:195–200.
28. Weiss SW, Nickoloff BJ: CD34 is expressed by a distinctive cell population in peripheral nerve, nerve sheath tumors, and related lesions. Am J Surg Pathol 1993;17:1039–1045.
29. Chaubal A, Paetau A, Zoltick P, Miettinen M: CD34 immunoreactivity in nervous system tumors. Acta Neuropathol 1994; 88:454–458.
30. Miettinen M, Sobin LH, Sarlomo-Rikala, M: Immunohistochemical spectrum of GISTs at different sites and their differential diagnosis with other tumors with a reference to CD117 (KIT). Mod Pathol 2000;13: 1134–1142.
31. Rizeq MN, van de Rijn M, Hendrickson MR, Rouse RV: A comparative immunohistochemical study of uterine smooth muscle neoplasms with emphasis on the epithelioid variant. Hum Pathol 1994;25:671–677.
32. Ruggeri ZM: Structure and function of von Willebrand factor. Thomb Hemost 1999;82:576–584.
33. Burgdorf WHC, Mukai K, Rosai J: Immunohistochemical identification of factor VIII-related antigen in endothelial cells of cutaneous lesions of alleged vascular nature. Am J Clin Pathol 1981;75:167–171.
34. Leader M, Collins M, Patel J, Henry K: Staining for Factor VIII related antigen and *Ulex europaeus* agglutinin I (UEA I) in 230 tumors. An assessment of their specificity for angiosarcoma and Kaposi's sarcoma. Histopathology 1986;10:1153–1162.
35. Aziza J, Mazerolles C, Selves J, et al: Comparison of the reactivities of monoclonal antibodies QBEND10 (CD34) and BNH9 in vascular tumors. Appl Immunohistochem 1993;1:51–57.
36. Partanen TA, Arola J, Saaristo A, et al: VEGF-C and VEGF-D expression in neuroendocrine cells and their receptor, VEGFR-3, in fenestrated blood vessels in human tissues. FASEB J 2000;14:2087–2096.
37. Jussila L, Valtola R, Partanen A, et al: Lymphatic endothelium and Kaposi's sarcoma spindle cells detected by antibodies against the vascular endothelial growth factor receptor-3. Cancer Res 1998;58: 1599–1604.
38. Partanen TA, Alitalo K, Miettinen M: Lack of lymphatic vascular specificity of vascular endothelial growth factor receptor 3 in 185 vascular tumors. Cancer 1999;86:2406–2412.
39. Breiteneder-Geleff S, Soleiman A, Kowalski H, et al: Angiosarcomas express mixed endothelial phenotypes of blood and lymphatic capillaries: Podoplanin as a specific marker for lymphatic endothelium. Am J Pathol 1999;154:385–394.
40. Esmon CT, Esmon NL, Harris KW: Complex formation between thrombin and thrombomodulin inhibits both thrombin catalyzed fibrin formation and factor V activation. J Biol Chem 1982;257:7944–7947.
41. Yonezawa S, Maruyama I, Sakae K, Igata A, Majerus PW, Sato E: Thrombomodulin as a marker for vascular tumors. Comparative study with factor VIII and Ulex europaeus lectin. Am J Clin Pathol 1987;88: 405–411.
42. Appleton MA, Attanoos RL, Jasani B: Thrombomodulin as a marker for vascular and lymphatic tumours. Histopathology 1996;29:153–157.
43. Collins CL, Ordonez NG, Schaefer R, et al: Thrombomodulin expression in malignant pleural mesothelioma and pulmonary adenocarcinoma. Am J Pathol 1992;141:827–833.
44. Folpe AL, Chand EM, Goldblum JR, Weiss SW: Expression of Fli-1, a nuclear transcription factor, distinguishes vascular neoplasms from potential mimics. Am J Surg Pathol 2001;25:1061–1066.

Muscle Cell Markers

45. Vandekerckhove J, Weber K: At least six different actins are expressed in higher mammals: An analysis based on the amino acid sequence of the amino terminal tryptic peptide. J Mol Biol 1978;126:783–802.
46. Small JV: Structure-function relationships in smooth muscle: The missing links. Bioessays 1995;17:785–792.
47. Tsukada T, McNutt MA, Ross R, Gown AM: HHF35, a muscle actin-specific monoclonal antibody. II. Reactivity in normal, reactive and neoplastic human tissues. Am J Pathol 1987;127:389–402.
48. Miettinen M: Antibody specific for muscle actin in the diagnosis and classification of soft tissue tumors. Am J Pathol 1988; 130:205–215.
49. Montgomery EA, Meis JM: Nodular fasciitis. Its morphologic spectrum and immunohistochemical profile. Am J Surg Pathol 1991;15:942–948.
50. Rangdaeng S, Truong LD: Comparative immunohistochemical staining for desmin and muscle-specific actin: A study of 576 cases. Am J Clin Pathol 1991;96:32–45.
51. Schurch W, Skalli O, Seemayer TA, Gabbiani G: Intermediate filament proteins and actin isoforms as markers for soft tissue tumor differentiation and origin. I. Smooth muscle tumors. Am J Pathol 1987;128:91–103.
52. Schurch W, Skalli O, Lagace R, Seemayer TA, Gabbiani G: Intermediate filament proteins and actin iso-

forms as markers for soft tissue tumor differentiation and origin. III. Hemangiopericytomas and glomus tumors. Am J Pathol 1990;136:771–786.
53. Roholl PJM, Elbers HRJ, Prinsen I, Claessens JAJ, van Unnik JAM: Distribution of actin isoforms in sarcomas: An immunohistochemical study. Hum Pathol 1990;21:1269–1274.
54. Skalli O, Gabbiani G, Babai F, Seemayer TA, Pizzolato G, Schurch W: Intermediate filament proteins and actin isoforms as markers for soft tissue tumor differentiation and origin. II Rhabdomyosarcomas. Am J Pathol 1988;130:515–531.
55. de Jong ASH, van Raamsdonk W, van Kessel-van Vark M, Voute PA, Albus-Lutter CE: Skeletal muscle actin as tumor marker in the diagnosis of rhabdomyosarcoma in childhood. Am J Surg Pathol 1986;10:467–474.
56. Savera AT, Sloman A, Huvos AG, Klimstra DS: Myoepithelial carcinoma of the salivary glands: A clinicopathologic study of 25 patients. Am J Surg Pathol 2000;24:761–774.
57. Franke WW, Schmid E, Schiller DL, et al: Differentiation-related patterns of expression of proteins of intermediate-size filaments in tissues and cultured cells. Cold Spring Harb Symp Quant Pathol 1982; 46(Pt 1):431–453.
58. Frank ED, Warren L: Aortic smooth muscle cells contain vimentin instead of desmin. Proc Natl Acad Sci USA 1981;78:2020–2024.
59. Toccanier-Pelte MF, Skalli O, Kapanci Y, Gabbiani G: Characterization of stromal cells with myoid features in lymph nodes and spleen in normal and pathologic conditions. Am J Pathol 1987;129:109–118.
60. van Muijen GNP, Ruiter DJ, Warnaar SO: Coexpression of intermediate filament polypeptides in human fetal and adult tissues. Lab Invest 1987;57:359–369.
61. Hurlimann J: Desmin and neural markers in mesothelial cells and mesotheliomas. Hum Pathol 1994;25:753–757.
62. Ferrandez-Izquierdo A, Navarro-Fos S, Gonzalez-Devesa M, Gil-Benso R, Llombart-Bosch A: Immunocytochemical typification of mesothelial cells in effusions: In vivo and in vitro models. Diagn Cytopathol 1994;10:256–262.
63. Fletcher CDM, Tsang WYW, Fisher C, Lee KC, Chan JKC: Angiomyofibroblastoma of the vulva. A benign neoplasm distinct from aggressive angiomyxoma. Am J Surg Pathol 1992;16:373–382.
64. Fetsch JF, Laskin WB, Lefkowitz M, Kindblom LG, Meis-Kindblom JM: Aggressive angiomyxoma: A clinicopathologic study of 29 female patients. Cancer 1996;78:79–90.
65. Gibas Z, Miettinen M, Limon J, et al: Cytogenetic and immunohistochemical profile of myxoid liposarcoma. Am J Clin Pathol 1995;103:20–26.
66. Fletcher CD: Angiomatoid "malignant fibrous histiocytoma": An immunohistochemical study indicative of myoid differentiation. Hum Pathol 1991;22:563–568.
67. Fanburg-Smith JC, Miettinen M: Angiomatoid "malignant" fibrous histiocytoma: A clinicopathologic study of 158 cases and further exploration of the myoid phenotype. Hum Pathol 1999;30:1336–1343.
68. Persson S, Willems JS, Kindblom LG, Angervall L: Alveolar soft part sarcoma. An immunohistochemical, cytologic and electron-microscopic study and a quantitative DNA analysis. Virchows Arch A Pathol Anat Histopathol 1988;412:499–513.
69. Miettinen M, Ekfors T: Alveolar soft part sarcoma. Immunohistochemical evidence for muscle cell differentiation. Am J Clin Pathol 1990;93:32–38.
70. Gerald WL, Miller HK, Battifora H, Miettinen M, Silva EG, Rosai J: Intra-abdominal desmoplastic small, round cell tumor: Report of 19 cases of a distinctive type of high grade polyphenotypic malignancy affecting young individuals. Am J Surg Pathol 1991;15:499–513.
71. Parham DM, Dias P, Kelly DR, Rutledge JC, Houghton PJ: Desmin-positivity in primitive neuroectodermal tumors of childhood. Am J Surg Pathol 1992;16:483–492.
72. Thorner P: Intra-abdominal polyphenotypic tumor. Pediatr Pathol Lab Med 1996;16:161–169.
73. Truong LD, Rangdaeng S, Cagle P, Ro JY, Hawkins H, Font RL: The diagnostic utility of desmin: A study of 584 cases and review of the literature. Am J Clin Pathol 1990;93:305–314.
74. Mayall FG, Goddard H, Gibbs AR: Intermediate filament expression in mesotheliomas: Leiomyoid mesotheliomas are not uncommon. Histopathology 1992; 21:453–457.
75. Folpe AL, Patterson K, Gown AM: Antibodies to desmin identify the blastemal component of nephroblastoma. Mod Pathol 1997;10:896–900.
76. Folpe AL, Weiss SW, Fletcher CD, Gown AM: Tenosynovial giant cell tumors: Evidence for a desmin-positive dendritic cell subpopulation. Mod Pathol 1998;11:939–944.
77. Takahashi K, Hiwada K, Kokubu T: Isolation and characterization of a 34.000 dalton calmodulin- and F-actin binding protein from chicken gizzard smooth muscle. Biochem Biophys Res Commun 1986;141:20–26.
78. Sobue K, Sellers JR: Caldesmon, a novel regulatory protein in smooth muscle and nonmuscle actomyosin systems. J Biol Chem 1990;266:12115–12118.
79. Lazard D, Sastre X, Frid MG, Glukhova MA, Thiery JP, Koteliansky VE: Expression of smooth muscle-specific proteins in myoepithelium and stromal myofibroblasts of normal and malignant human breast tissue. Proc Natl Acad Sci USA 1993;90:999–1003.
80. Watanabe K, Kusakabe T, Hoshi N, Saito A, Suzuki T: h-Caldesmon in leiomyosarcoma and tumors with smooth muscle cell-like differentiation: Its specific expression in the smooth muscle cell tumor. Hum Pathol 1999;30:392–396.
81. Miettinen M, Sarlomo-Rikala M, Kovatich AJ, Lasota J: Calponin and h-caldesmon in soft tissue tumors: Consistent h-caldesmon immunoreactivity in gastrointestinal stromal tumors indicates traits of smooth muscle differentiation. Mod Pathol 1999;12:756–762.

82. Ceballos KM, Nielsen GP, Selig MK, O'Connell JX: Is anti-h-caldesmon useful for distinguishing smooth muscle and myofibroblastic tumors? An immunohistochemical study. Am J Clin Pathol 2001;14:746–753.
83. Hisaoka M, Wei-Qi S, Jian W, Morio T, Hashimoto H: Specific but variable expression of h-caldesmon in leiomyosarcomas: An immunohistochemical reassessment of a novel myogenic marker. Appl Immunohistochem Mo1 Morphol 2001;9:302–308.
84. Gimona M, Herzog M, Vandekerckhove J, Small JV: Smooth muscle specific expression of calponin. FEBS Lett 1990;274:159–162.
85. Weintraub H: The MyoD family and myogenesis: Redundancy, networks and thresholds. Cell 1993;75: 1241–1244.
86. Dias P, Dilling M, Hougton P: The molecular basis of skeletal muscle differentiation. Semin Diagn Pathol 1994;11:3–14.
87. Rudnicki MA, Jaenisch R: The MyoD family of transcription factors and skeletal myogenesis. Bioessays 1995;17:203–209.
88. Parham DM, Dias P, Bertorini T, von Wronski MA, Horner L, Houghton P: Immunohistochemical analysis of the distribution of MyoD1 in muscle biopsies of primary myopathies and neurogenic atrophy. Acta Neuropathol 1994;87:605–611.
89. Dias P, Parham DM, Shapiro DN, Tapscott SJ, Houghton PJ: Monoclonal antibodies to the myogenic regulatory protein MyoD1 epitope mapping and diagnostic utility. Cancer Res 1992;52:6431–6439.
90. Tallini G, Parham DM, Dias P, Cordon-Cardo C, Houghton PJ, Rosai J: Myogenic regulatory protein expression in adult soft tissue sarcomas: A sensitive and specific marker of skeletal muscle differentiation. Am J Pathol 1994;144:693–701.
91. Wang NP, Marx J, McNutt MA, Gown AM: Expression of myogenic regulatory proteins (myogenin and MyoD1) in small blue round cell tumors of childhood. Am J Pathol 1995;147:1799–1810.
92. Cui S, Hano H, Harada T, Takai S, Masui F, Ushigome S: Evaluation of new monoclonal anti-MyoD1 and anti-myogenin antibodies for the diagnosis of rhabdomyosarcoma. Pathol Int 1999;49:62–68.
93. Kumar S, Perlman E, Harris CA, Raffeld M, Tsokos M: Myogenin is a specific marker for rhabdomyosarcoma: An immunohistochemical study in paraffin-embedded tissues. Mod Pathol 2000;13:988–993.
94. Dias P, Chen B, Dilday B, et al : Strong immunostaining for myogenin in rhabdomyosarcoma is significantly associated with tumors of the alveolar subclass. Am J Pathol 2000;156:399–408.
95. Wang NP, Bacchi CE, Jiang JJ, McNutt MA, Gown AM: Does alveolar soft-part sarcoma exhibit skeletal muscle differentiation? An immunocytochemical and biochemical study of myogenic regulatory protein expression. Mod Pathol 1996;9:496–506.
96. Gomez JA, Amin MB, Ro JY, Linden MD, Lee MW, Zarbo RJ: Immunohistochemical profile of myogenin and Myo D1 does not support skeletal muscle lineage in alveolar soft part sarcoma. A study of 19 tumors. Arch Pathol Lab Med 1999;123:503–507.
97. Mukai K, Rosai J, Hallaway BE: Localization of myoglobin in normal and neoplastic human skeletal muscle cells using an immunoperoxidase method. Am J Surg Pathol 1979;3:373–376.
98. Corson JM, Pinkus GS: Intracellular myoglobin: A specific marker for skeletal muscle differentiation in soft tissue sarcomas. Am J Pathol 1980;103:384–389.
99. Brooks JJ: Immunohistochemistry of soft tissue tumors: Myoglobin as a tumor marker for rhabdomyosarcoma. Cancer 1982;50:1757–1763.
100. Eusebi V, Bondi A, Rosai J: Immunohistochemical localization of myoglobin in nonmuscular cells. Am J Surg Pathol 1984;8:51–55.
101. Eusebi V, Ceccarelli C, Gorza L, Schiffiano S, Bussolati G: Immunocytochemistry of rhabdomyosarcoma. The use of four different markers. Am J Surg Pathol 1986;10:293–299.
102. Eusebi V, Rilke F, Ceccarelli C, Fedeli F, Schiffiano S, Bussolati G: Fetal heavy chain skeletal myosin. An oncofetal antigen expressed in rhabdomyosarcoma. Am J Surg Pathol 1986;10:680–686.

Neural and Neuroendocrine Markers

Synaptophysin

103. Wiedenmann B, Franke WW: Identification and localization of synaptophysin, an integral membrane glycoprotein of Mr 38,000 characteristic of presynaptic vesicles. Cell 1985;41:1017–1028.
104. Thomas L, Hartung K, Langosch D, et al: Identification of synaptophysin as a hexameric channel protein of the synaptic vesicle membrane. Science 1988;242: 1050–1052.
105. Wiedenmann B, Franke WW, Kuhn C, Moll R, Gould VE: Synaptophysin: A marker protein for neuroendocrine cells and neoplasms. Proc Natl Acad Sci USA 1986;83:3500–3504.
106. Wiedenmann B, Huttner WB: Synaptophysin and chromogranins/secretogranins: Widespread constituents of distinct types of neuroendocrine vesicles and new tools in tumor diagnosis. Virchows Arch B Cell Pathol 1989;58:95–121.
107. Miettinen M, Rapola J: Synaptophysin: An immunohistochemical marker for childhood neuroblastoma. Acta Pathol Microbiol Scand A 1987;95:167–170.
108. Hachitanda Y, Tsuneyoshi M, Enjoji M: Expression of pan-neuroendcorine proteins in 53 neuroblastic tumors. Arch Pathol Lab Med 1989;113:381–384.
109. Schwechheimer K, Wiedenmann B, Franke WW: Synaptophysin: A reliable marker for medulloblastomas. Virchows Arch A Pathol Anat Histol 1987; 411:53–59.
110. Frierson HF, Ross GW, Mills SE, Frankfurter A: Olfactory neuroblastoma. Additional immunohistochemical characterization. Am J Clin Pathol 1990;94:547–553.
111. Cavazzana AO, Ninfo V, Roberts J, Triche TJ: Peripheral neuroepithelioma: A light microscopic, immunocytochemical, and ultrastructural study. Mod Pathol 1992;5:71–78.
112. Ladanyi M, Heinemann FS, Huvos AG, Rao PH, Chen QG, Jhanwar SC: Neural differentiation in small

round cell tumors of bone and soft tissue with the translocation t(11l22)(q24;q12): An immunhistochemical study of 11 cases. Hum Pathol 1990;21:1245–1251.
113. Amann G, Zoubek A, Salzer-Kuntschik M, Windhager R, Kovar H: Relation of neurological marker expression and EWS gene fusion types in MIC2/CD99-positive tumors of the Ewing family. Hum Pathol 1999;30:1058–1064.
114. Parham DM, Hijazi Y, Steinberg SM, et al: Neuroectodermal differentiation in Ewing's sarcoma family of tumors does not predict tumor behavior. Hum Pathol 1999;30:911–918.
115. Gould VE, Wiedenmann B, Lee I, et al: Synaptophysin expression in neuroendocrine neoplasms as determined by immunocytochemistry. Am J Pathol 1987;126:243–257.
116. Miettinen M: Synaptophysin and neurofilament proteins as markers for neuroendocrine tumors. Arch Pathol Lab Med 1987;111:813–818.
117. Johnson TL, Zarbo RJ, Lloyd RV, Crissman JD: Paragangliomas of the head and neck: Immunohistochemical neuroendocrine and intermediate filament typing. Mod Pathol 1988;1:216–223.
118. Goh YW, Spagnolo DV, Platten M, et al: Extraskeletal myxoid chondrosarcoma: A light microscopic, immunohistochemical, ultrastructural, and immuno-ultrastructural study indicating neuroendocrine differentiation. Histopathology 2001;39:514–524.
119. Banerjee SS, Menasce LP, Eyden BP, Brain AN: Malignant melanoma showing ganglioneuroblastic differentiation: Report of a unique case. Am J Surg Pathol 1999;23:582–588.

Chromogranin A

120. O'Connor DT, Mahata SK, Taupenot L, et al: Chromogranin A in human disease. Adv Exp Med Biol 2000; 482:377–388.
121. Lloyd RV: Immunohistochemical localization of chromogranin in normal and neoplastic endocrine tissues. Pathol Annu 1987;22(Part 2):69–90.
122. Molenaar WM, Baker DL, Pleasure D, Lee VMY, Trojanowski JQ: The neuroendocrine and neural profiles of neuroblastomas, ganglioneuroblastomas, and ganglioneuromas. Am J Pathol 1990;136:375–382.
123. Christensen WN, Strong EW, Bains MS, Woodruff JM: Neuroendocrine differentiation in the glandular peripheral nerve sheath tumor. Pathologic distinction from the biphasic synovial sarcoma with glands. Am J Surg Pathol 1988;12:417–426.
124. Pagani A, Fischer-Colbrie R, Sanfilippo B, Winkler H, Cerrato M, Bussolati G: Secretogranin II expression in Ewing's sarcomas and primitive neuroectodermal tumors. Diagn Mol Pathol 1992;1:165–172.

NSE

125. Marangos PJ, Schmechel DE: Neuron specific enolase, a clinically useful marker for neurons and neuroendocrine cells. Annu Rev Neurosci 1987;10:269–295.
126. Haimoto H, Takahashi Y, Koshikawa T, Nagura H, Kato K: Immunohistochemical localization of gamma-enolase in normal human tissues other than nervous and neuroendocrine tissues. Lab Invest 1985;52:257–263.
127. Wick MR, Scheithauer BW, Kovacs K: Neuron-specific enolase in neuroendocrine tumors of the thymus, bronchus, and skin. Am J Clin Pathol 1983;79:703–707.
128. Iwanaga T, Takahashi Y, Fujita T: Immunohistochemistry of neuron-specific and glia-specific proteins. Arch Histol Cytol 1989;52(Suppl):13–24.
129. Rode J, Dhillon AP: Neuron-specific enolase and S100 protein as possible prognostic indicators in melanoma. Histopathology 1984;8:1041–1052.
130. Triche TJ, Tsokos M, Linnoila RI, Marangos PJ, Chandra R: NSE in neuroblastoma and other round cell tumors of childhood. Prog Clin Biol Res 1985;175: 295–317.
131. Osborn M, Dirk T, Kaser H, Weber K, Altmannsberger M: Immunohistochemical localization of neurofilaments and neuron-specific enolase in 29 cases of neuroblastoma. Am J Pathol 1986;122:433–442.
132. Vinores SA, Bonnin JM, Rubinstein LJ, Marangos PJ: Immunohistochemical demonstration of neuron-specific enolase in neoplasms of the CNS and other tissues. Arch Pathol Lab Med 1984;108:536–540.
133. Leader M, Collins M, Patel J, Henry K: Antineuron specific enolase staining reactions in sarcomas and carcinomas: Its lack of neuroendocrine specificity. J Clin Pathol 1986;39:1186–1192.
134. Thomas P, Battifora H, Manderino GL, Patrick J: A monoclonal antibody against neuron-specific enolase. Immunohistochemical comparison with a polyclonal antiserum. Am J Clin Pathol 1987;88:146–152.
135. Seshi B, True L, Carter D, Rosai J: Immunohistochemical characterization of a set of monoclonal antibodies to human neuron-specific enolase. Am J Pathol 1988; 131:258–269.

Neurofilament and Related IFS

136. Lee MK, Cleveland DW: Neuronal intermediate filaments. Annu Rev Neurosci 1996;19:187–217.
137. Dahl D: Immunohistochemical differences between neurofilaments in perikarya, dendrites and axons. Immunofluorescence study with antisera raised to neurofilament polypeptides (200K, 150K, 70K) isolated by anion exchange chromatography. Exp Cell Res 1983;149:397–408.
138. Gould VE, Moll R, Moll I, Lee I, Franke WW: Neuroendocrine (Merkel) cells of the skin: Hyperplasias, dysplasias, and neoplasms. Lab Invest 1985;52:334–353.
139. Mukai M, Torikata C, Iri H, et al: Expression of neurofilament triplet proteins in human neural tumors. An immunohistochemical study of paraganglioma, ganglioneuroma, ganglioneuroblastoma and neuroblastoma. Am J Pathol 1986;122:28–35.
140. Miettinen M, Lehto VP, Virtanen I: Immunofluorescence microscopic evaluation of the intermediate filament expression of the adrenal cortex and medulla and their tumors. Am J Pathol 1985; 118:360–366.

141. Miettinen M, Lehto VP, Dahl D, Virtanen I: Varying expression of cytokeratin and neuro-filaments in neuroendocrine tumors of human gastrointestinal tract. Lab Invest 1985; 52:429–436.
142. Lehto VP, Miettinen M, Virtanen I: A dual expression of cytokeratin and neurofilaments in bronchial carcinoid cells. Int J Cancer 1985; 35:421–425.
143. Moll R, Lee I, Gould VE, Berndt R, Roessner A, Franke WW: Immunocytochemical analysis of Ewing's tumors. Patterns of expression of intermediate filaments and desmosomal proteins indicate cell-type heterogeneity and pluripotential differentiation. Am J Pathol 1987;27:288–304.
144. Gerharz CD, Moll R, Meister P, Knuth A, Gabbert H: Cytoskeletal heterogeneity of an epithelioid sarcoma with expression of vimentin, cytokeratins, and neurofilaments. Am J Surg Pathol 1990;14:274–283.
145. Folpe AL, Gown AM: Poorly differentiated synovial sarcoma: Immunohistochemical distinction from primitive neuroectodermal tumors and high grade malignant peripheral nerve sheath tumors. Am J Surg Pathol 1998;22:673–682.
146. Miettinen M, Rapola J: Immunohistochemical spectrum of rhabdomyosarcoma and rhabdomyosarcoma-like tumors. Expression of cytokeratin and the 68 kD neurofilament protein. Am J Surg Pathol 1989; 13:120–132.
147. Foley J, Witte D, Chiu FC, Parysek LM: Expression of the neural intermediate filament proteins peripherin and neurofilament-66/alpha-internexin in neuroblastoma. Lab Invest 1994;71:193–199.
148. Kaplan MP, Chin SS, Fliegner KH, Liem RK: Alpha-internexin, a novel neuronal intermediate filament protein, precedes the low molecular weight neurofilament protein (NF-L) in the developing rat brain. J Neurosci 1990;10:2735–2748.

NB84

149. Thomas JO, Nijjar J, Turley H, Micklem H, Gatter KC: NB84: A new monoclonal anti-body for the recognition of neuroblastoma in routinely processed material. J Pathol 1991;163:69–75.
150. Miettinen M, Chatten J, Paetau A, Stevenson AJ: Monoclonal antibody NB84 in the differential diagnosis of neuroblastoma and other small round cell tumors. Am J Surg Pathol 1998;22:327–332.
151. Folpe AL, Patterson K, Gown AM: Antineuroblastoma antibody NB-84 also identifies a significant subset of other small blue round cell tumors. Appl Imunohistochem 1997;5:239–245.

S-100 Protein and Other Broadly Specific Neural Markers

S-100

152. Moore BW: A soluble protein characteristic of the nervous system. Biochem Biophys Res Commun 1965;19:739–744.
153. Donato R: S100: A multigenic family of calcium-modulated proteins of the EF-hand type with intracellular and extracellular functional roles. Int J Biochem Cell Biol 2001;33:638–668.
154. Takahashi K, Isobe T, Ohtsuki Y, Akagi T, Sonobe H, Okuyama T: Immunhistochemical study on the distribution of alpha and beta subunits of the S-100 protein in human neoplasms and normal tissues. Virchows Arch B Cell Pathol 1984;45:385–396.
155. Nakajima T, Watanabe S, Sato Y, Kameya T, Hirota T, Shimosato Y: An immunoperoxidase study of S-100 protein distribution in normal and neoplastic tissues. Am J Surg Pathol 1982;6:715–727.
156. Stefansson K, Wollmann R, Jerkovic M: S100 protein in soft tissue tumors derived from Schwann cells and melanocytes. Am J Pathol 1982;106:261–268.
157. Kahn HJ, Marks A, Thom H, Baumal R: Role of antibody to S100 protein in diagnostic pathology. Am J Clin Pathol 1983;79:341–347.
158. Cochran AJ, Lu HF, Li PX, Saxton R, Wen DR: S-100 protein remains a practical marker for melanocytic and other tumours. Melanoma Res 1993;3:325–330.
159. Weiss SW, Langloss JM, Enzinger FM: Value of S-100 protein in the diagnosis of soft tissue tumors with particular reference to benign and malignant Schwann cell tumors. Lab Invest 1983;49:299–308.
160. Swanson PE, Wick MR: Clear cell sarcoma: An immunohistochemical analysis of six cases and comparison with other epithelioid neoplasms of soft tissue. Arch Pathol Lab Med 1989;113:55–60.
161. Daimaru Y, Hashimoto H, Enjoji M: Malignant peripheral nerve sheath tumors (malignant schwannomas): An immunohistochemical study of 29 cases. Am J Surg Pathol 1985;9:434–444.
162. Wick MR, Swanson PE, Scheithauer BW, Manivel JC: Malignant peripheral nerve sheath tumors: An immunohistochemical study of 62 cases. Am J Clin Pathol 1987:87:425–433.
163. Kliewer KE, Wen DR, Cancilla PA, Cochran AJ: Paragangliomas. Assessment of prognosis by histologic, immunohistochemical, and ultrastructural techniques. Hum Pathol 1989;20:29–39.
164. Achilles E, Padberg BC, Holl K, Klöppel G, Schröder S: Immunocytochemistry of paragangliomas: Value of staining for S-100 protein and glial fibrillary acid protein in diagnosis and prognosis. Histopathology 1991;18:453–458.
165. Nakamura Y, Becker LE, Marks A: S-100 protein in tumors of cartilage and bone. Cancer 1983;52: 1820–1824.
166. Okajima K, Honda I, Kitagawa T: Immunohistochemical distribution of S-100 protein in tumors and tumor-like lesions of bone and cartilage. Cancer 1988;61:792–799.
167. Nakamura Y, Becker LE, Marks A: S100 protein in human chordoma and human and rabbit notochord. Arch Pathol 1983;107:118–120.
168. Hashimoto H, Daimaru Y, Enjoji M: S-100 protein distribution in liposarcoma. An immunoperoxidase study with special reference to the distinction of

liposarcoma from myxoid malignant fibrous histiocytoma. Virchows Arch A 1984;405:1–10.
169. dei Tos A, Wadden C, Fletcher CDM: S-100 protein staining in liposarcoma. Its diagnostic utility in the high-grade myxoid (round-cell) variant. Appl Immunohistochem 1996;4:95–101.
170. Enzinger FM, Weiss SW, Liang CY: Ossifying fibromyxoid tumor of soft parts. A clinicopathological analysis of 59 cases. Am J Surg Pathol 1989;13:817–827.
171. Guillou L, Wadden C, Kraus MD, Dei Tos AP, Fletcher CDM: S-100 protein reactivity in synovial sarcomas: A potentially frequent diagnostic pitfall. Immunohistochemical analysis of 100 cases. Appl Immunohistochem 1996;4:167–175.
172. Coindre JM, de Mascarel A, Trojani M, de Mascarel I, Pages A: Immunohistochemical study of rhabdomyosarcoma: Unexpected staining with S100 protein and cytokeratin. J Pathol 1988;155:127–132.
173. Drier JK, Swanson PE, Cherwitz DL, Wick MR: S100 protein immunoreactivity in poorly differentiated carcinomas. Immunohistochemical comparison with malignant melanoma. Arch Pathol Lab Med 1987; 111:447–452.
174. Herrera GA, Turbat-Herrera EA, Lott RL: S-100 protein expression by primary and metastatic carcinomas. Am J Clin Pathol 1988;89:168–176.
175. Cocchia D, Michetti F, Donato R: Immunochemical and immuno-cytochemical localization of S-100 antigen in normal human skin. Nature 1981;294:85–87.
176. Takahashi K, Yamaguchi H, Ishizeki J, Nakajima T, Nakazato Y: Immunohistochemical and immunoelectron microscopic localization of S-100 protein in the interdigitating reticulum cells of the human lymph node. Virchows Arch [Cell Pathol] 1981;37:125–135.
177. Aoyama K, Terashima K, Imay Y, et al: Sinus histiocytosis with massive lymphadenopathy. A histogenetic analysis of histiocytes found in the fourth Japanese case. Acta Pathol Jpn 1984;34:375–388.
178. Eisen RN, Rosai J: Immunohistochemical characterization of sinus histiocytosis with massive lymphadenopathy (Rosai-Dorfman disease). Semin Diagn Pathol 1990;7:74–82.

NGFR p75

179. Perosio PM, Brooks JJ: Expression of nerve growth factor receptor in paraffin-embedded soft tissue tumors. Am J Pathol 1988;132:152–160.
180. Garin-Chesa P, Rettig WJ, Thomson TM, Old LJ, Melamed MR: Immunohistochemical analysis of nerve growth factor receptor expression in normal and malignant human tissues. J Histochem Cytochem 1988;36:383–389.
181. Thompson SJ, Schatteman GC, Gown AM, Bothwell M: A monoclonal antibody against nerve growth factor receptor. Immunohistochemical analysis of normal and neoplastic human tissue. Am J Clin Pathol 1989;92:415–423.
182. Fanburg-Smith JF, Miettinen M: Low-affinity nerve growth factor receptor in dermatofibrosarcoma protuberans and other non-neural tumors. A study of 1150 tumors and fetal and adult normal tissues. Hum Pathol 2001;32:873–879.
183. Dorfman DM, Chan JKC, Fletcher CDM: Dendritic reticulum cell (DRC) sarcomas are immunoreactive for low-affinity nerve growth factor receptor (LNGFR). Appl Immunohistochem 1996;4:249–258.

CD56

184. Cunningham BA, Hemperly JJ, Murray BA, Prediger EA, Brackenbury R, Edelman GM: Neural cell adhesion molecule: Structure, immunoglobulin-like domains, cell surface modulation, and alternative RNA-splicing. Science 1987;236:799–806.
185. Mechtersheimer G, Staudter M, Moller P: Expression of the natural killer cell-associated antigens, CD56 and CD57 in human neural and striated muscle cells and their tumors. Cancer Res 1991;51:1300–1307.
186. Jin L, Hemperly JJ, Lloyd RV: Expression of neural cell adhesion molecule in normal and neoplastic human neuroendocrine tissues. Am J Pathol 1991;138:961–969.
187. Garin-Chesa P, Fellinger EJ, Huvos AG, et al: Immunohistochemical analysis of neural cell adhesion molecules. Am J Pathol 1991;139:275–286.
188. Miettinen M, Cupo W: Neural cell adhesion molecule distribution in soft tissue tumors. Hum Pathol 1993; 24:62–66.
189. Molenaar WM, Muntinghe FLH: Expression of neural cell adhesion molecules and neurofilament protein isoforms in Ewing's sarcoma of bone and soft tissue sarcomas other than rhabdomyosarcoma. Hum Pathol 1999;30:1207–1212.
190. Shipley WR, Hammer RD, Lennington WJ, Macon WR: Paraffin immunohistochemical detection of CD56, a useful marker for neural adhesion molecule (NCAM), in normal and neoplastic tissues. Appl Immunohistochem 1997;5:87–93.

CD57

191. Abo T, Balch CM: A differentiation antigen of human NK and K cells identified by a monoclonal antibody (HNK-1). J Immunol 1981;127:1024–1029.
192. McGarry RC, Helfand SL, Quarles RH, Roder JC: Recognition of myelin-associated glycoprotein by the monoclonal antibody HNK-1. Nature 1983;306:376–378.
193. Arber DA, Weiss LM: CD57: A review. Appl Immunohistochem 1995;3:137–152.
194. Swanson PE, Manivel JC, Wick MR: Immunoreactivity for Leu-7 in neurofibrosarcomas and other spindle cell sarcomas of soft tissue. Am J Pathol 1987;126: 546–560.

Melanocytic Markers, Other than S-100 Protein

195. Gown AM, Vogel AM, Hoak D, Gough F, McNutt MA: Monoclonal antibodies specific for melanocytic tumors distinguish subpopulations of melanocytes. Am J Pathol 1985;123:195–203.

196. Bacchi CE, Bonetti F, Pea M, Martignoni G, Gown AM: HMB-45: A review. Appl Immunohistochem 1996;4: 73–85.
197. Wick MR, Swanson PE, Rocamora A: Recognition of malignant melanoma by monoclonal antibody HMB-45. An immunohistochemical study of 200 paraffin-embedded cutaneous tumors. J Cutan Pathol 1988;15:201–207.
198. Ordonez NG, Ji XL, Hickey RC: Comparison of HMB-45 monoclonal antibody and S100 protein in the immunohistochemical diagnosis of melanoma. Am J Clin Pathol 1988;90:385–390.
199. Kaufmann O, Koch S, Burghardt J, Audring H, Dietel M: Tyrosinase, Melan-A and KBA62 as markers for the immunohistochemical identification of metastatic amelanotic melanomas. Mod Pathol 1998;11:740–746.
200. Miettinen M, Fernandez M, Franssila K, Gatalica Z, Lasota J, Sarlomo-Rikala M: Microphthalmia transcription factor in the immunohistochemical diagnosis of metastatic melanoma. Comparison with four other melanoma markers. Am J Surg Pathol 2001;25:205–211.
201. Longacre TA, Egbert BM, Rouse RV: Desmoplastic and spindle-cell malignant melanoma. An immunohistochemical study. Am J Surg Pathol 1996;20:1489–1500.
202. Fetsch JF, Michal M, Miettinen M: Pigmented (melanotic) neurofibroma: A clinicopathologic and immunohistochemical analysis of 19 lesions from 17 patients. Am J Surg Pathol 2000;24:331–343.
203. Pea M, Bonetti F, Zamboni G, et al: Melanocyte marker HMB-45 is regularly expressed in angiomyolipoma of the kidney. Pathology 1991;23:185–188.
204. Ashfaq R, Weinberg A, Albores-Saavedra J: Renal angiomyolipomas and HMB-45 reactivity. Cancer 1993;71:3091–3097.
205. Chan JK, Tsang WY, Pau M, Tang MC, Pang SW, Fletcher CD: Lymphangiomyomatosis and angiomyolipoma: Closely related entities characterized by hamartomatous proliferation of HMB-45 positive smooth muscle. Histopathology 1993;22:445–455.
206. Bonetti F, Pea M, Mortignoni G, et al: Clear cell ("sugar") tumor of the lung is a lesion strictly related to angiomyolipoma: The concept of a family of lesions characterized by the presence of the perivascular epithelioid cells (PEC). Pathology 1994;26:230–236.
207. Kwon BS: Pigmentation genes: The tyrosinase gene family and the Pmel 17 family. J Invest Dermatol 1993;100(2 Suppl):134S–140S.
208. Chen YT, Stockert E, Tsang S, Coplan KA, Old LJ: Immunophenotyping of melanomas for tyrosinase: Implications for vaccine development. Proc Natl Acad Sci USA 1995;92:8125–8129.
209. Hofbauer GF, Kamarashev J, Geertsen R, Boni R, Dummer R: Tyrosinase immunoreactivity in formalin-fixed, paraffin embedded primary and metastatic melanoma: Frequency and distribution. J Cutan Pathol 1998;25:204–209.
210. Jungbluth AA, Iversen K, Coplan K, et al: T311: An anti-tyrosinase monoclonal antibody for the detection of melanocytic lesions in paraffin-embedded tissues. Path Res Pract 2000;196:235–242.
211. Busam KJ, Iversen K, Coplan KC, Jungbluth AA: Analysis of microphthalmia transcription factor expression in normal tissues and tumors, and comparison of its expression with S-100 protein, gp100, and tyrosinase in desmoplastic malignant melanoma. Am J Surg Pathol 2001;25:197–204.
212. Zavala-Pompa A, Folpe AL, Jimenez RE, et al: Immunohistochemical study of microphthalmia transcription factor and tyrosinase in angiomyolipoma of the kidney, renal cell carcinoma, and renal and retroperitoneal sarcomas. Am J Surg Pathol 2001; 25: 65–70.
213. Kawakami Y, Eliyahu S, Delgado CH, et al: Cloning of the gene coding for a shared human melanoma antigen recognized by autologous T-cells infiltrating into tumor. Proc Natl Acad Sci USA 1994;91:3515–3519.
214. Coulie PG, Brichard V, van Pel A, et al: A new gene coding for a differentiation antigen recognized by autologous cytolytic T lymphocytes on HLA-A2 melanomas. J Exp Med 1994;180:35–42.
215. Kawakami Y, Eliyahu S, Delgado CH, et al: Identification of a human melanoma antigen recognized by tumor-infiltrating lymphocytes associated with in vivi tumor rejection. Proc Natl Acad Sci USA 1994; 91:6458–6462.
216. Jungbluth AA, Busam KJ, Gerald WL, et al: A103: An anti melan-A monoclonal antibody for the detection of malignant melanoma in paraffin embedded tissues. Am J Surg Pathol 1998;22:595–602.
217. Orosz Z: Melan-A/MART-1 expression in various melanocytic lesions and in non-melanocytic soft tissue tumours. Histopathology 1999;34:517–525.
218. Jungbluth AA, Iversen K, Coplan K, et al: Expression of melanocyte-associated markers gp-100 and Melan-A/MART-1 in angiomyolipomas. An immunohistochemical and RT-PCR analysis. Virchows Arch 1999; 434:429–435.
219. Fetsch PA, Fetsch JF, Marincola FM, Travis W, Batts KP, Abati A: Comparison of melanoma antigen recognized by T-cells (MART-1) to HMB-45: Additional evidence to support a common lineage for angiomyolipoma, lymphangiomyomatosis and clear cell sugar tumor. Mod Pathol 1998;11:699–703.
220. Busam KJ, Iversen K, Coplan KA, et al: Immunoreactivity for A103, an antibody to melan-A (Mart-1), in adrenocortical and other steroid tumors. Am J Surg Pathol 1998:22:57–63.
221. Yasumoto K, Yokoyama K, Shibata K, Tomita Y, Shibahara S: Microphthalmia-associated transcription factor as a regulator for melanocyte-specific transcription of the human tyrosinase gene. Mol Cell Biol 1994;14:8058–8070.
222. Hemesath TJ, Steingrimsson E, McGill G, et al: Microphthalmia, a critical factor in melanocyte development, defines a discrete transcription factor family. Genes Dev 1994; 8:2770–2780.
223. Weilbacher KN, Hershey CL, Takemoto CM, et al: Age-resolving osteopetrosis: A rat model implicating microphthalmia and the related transcription factor TEF3. J Exp Med 1998;187:775–785.

224. King R, Weilbaecher KN, McGill G, Cooley E, Mihm M, Fisher DE: Microphthalmia transcription factor. A sensitive and specific melanocytic marker for melanoma diagnosis. Am J Pathol 1999;155:731–738.
225. King R, Googe PB, Weilbaecher KN, Mihm MC, Fisher DE: Microphthalmia transcription factor expression in cutaneous benign, malignant melanocytic, and nonmelanocytic tumors. Am J Surg Pathol 2001;25:51–57.
226. Granter SR, Weilbaecher KN, Quigley C, Fletcher CDM, Fisher DE: Microphthalmia transcription factor. Not a sensitive or specific marker for the diagnosis of desmoplastic melanoma and spindle cell (nondesmoplastic) melanoma. Am J Dermatopathol 2001; 23:185–189.
227. Koch MB, Shih IM, Weiss SW, Folpe AL: Microphthalmia transcription factor and melanoma cell adhesion molecule expression distinguish desmoplastic/spindle cell melanoma from morphologic mimics. Am J Surg Pathol 2001;25:58–64.
228. Hotta H, Ross AH, Huebner K: Molecular cloning and characterization of an antigen associated with early stages of melanoma tumor progression. Cancer Res 1988;48:2955–2962.
229. Metzelaar MJ, Winjngaard PL, Peters PJ, Sixma JJ, Niewenhuis HK, Clevers HC: CD63 antigen. A novel lysosomal membrane glycoprotein, cloned by a screening procedure for intracellular antigens in eukaryotic clels. J Biol Chem 1991;266:3239–3245.
230. MacKie R, Campbell I, Turbitt ML: Use of NK1 C3 monoclonal antibody in the assessment of benign and malignant melanocytic lesions. J Clin Pathol 1984;37:367–372.
231. Barrio MM, Bravo AI, Portela P, Hersey P, Mordoh J: A new epitope on human melanoma-associated antigen CD63/ME491 expressed by both primary and metastatic melanoma. Hybridoma 1998;17:355–364.

Histiocytic Markers

232. Mason DY, Taylor CR: The distribution of muramidase (lysozyme) in human tissues. J Clin Pathol 1975; 28:124–132.
233. Pinkus GS, Said JW: Profile of intracytoplasmic lysozyme in normal tissues, myeloproliferative disorders, hairy cell leukemia, and other pathologic processes. Am J Pathol 1977;106:351–366.
234. Burgdorf WHC, Duray P, Rosai J: Immunohistochemical identification of lysozyme in cutaneous lesions of alleged histiocytic nature. Am J Clin Pathol 1981;75:162–167.
235. Sonoda T, Enjoji M: Juvenile xanthogranuloma. Clinicopathological analysis and immunohistochemical study of 57 patients. Cancer 1985;56:2280–2286.
236. Traweek ST, Arber DA, Rappaport H, Brynes RK: Extramedullary myeloid tumors. An immunohistochemical and morphologic study of 28 cases. Am J Clin Pathol 1993;17:1011–1019.
237. Hudock J, Chatten J, Miettinen M: Immunohistochemical evaluation of myeloid leukemia infiltrates (granulocytic sarcomas) in formaldehyde-fixed, paraffin-embedded tissue. Am J Clin Pathol 1994;102:55–60.
238. Copie-Bergman C, Wotherspoon AC, Norton AJ, Diss TC, Isaacson PG: True histiocytic lymphoma. A morphologic, immunohistochemical, and molecular genetic study of 13 cases. Am J Surg Pathol 1998; 22:1386–1392.
239. Soini Y, Miettinen M: Alpha-1-antitrypsin and lysozyme. Their limited significance in fibrohistiocytic tumors. Am J Clin Pathol 1989;91:515–521.
240. Albrecht S, From L, Kahn HJ: Lysozyme in abnormal elastic fibers of cutaneous aging, solar elastosis and pseudoxanthoma elasticum. J Cutan Pathol 1990;18:75–80.
241. Potempa J, Korzus E, Travis J: The serpin superfamily of proteinase inhibitors: Structure, function, and regulation. J Biol Chem 1994;269:15957–15960.
242. Kindblom LG, Jacobsen GK, Jacobsen M: Immunohistochemical investigations of tumors of supposed fibroblastic-histiocytic origin. Hum Pathol 1982;13: 834–840.
243. Leader M, Patel J, Collins M, Henry K: Alpha-1-antichymotrypsin staining of 194 sarcomas, 38 carcinomas and 17 malignant melanomas. Am J Surg Pathol 1987;11:133–139.
244. Soini Y, Miettinen M: Widespread immunoreactivity for alpha-1-antichymotrypsin in different types of tumors. Am J Clin Pathol 1988;90:131–136.
245. Ichinose A: Physiopathology and regulation of factor XIII. Thomb Hemost 2001;86:57–65.
246. Nemes Z, Thomazy V, Adany L, Muszbek L: Identification of histiocytic reticulum cells by the immunohistochemical demonstration of factor XIII (F-XIIIa) in human lymph nodes. J Pathol 1986;149:121–132.
247. Nickoloff BJ, Griffiths CEM: Factor XIIIa-expressing dermal dendrocytes in AIDS-associated cutaneous Kaposi's sarcomas. Science 1989;243:1736–1737.
248. Nemes Z, Thomazy V: Factor XIIIa and the classic histiocytic markers in malignant fibrous histiocytoma: A comparative immunohistochemical study. Hum Pathol 1988;19:822–829.
249. Misery L, Boucheron S, Claudy AL: Factor XIIIa expression in juvenile xanthogranuloma. Acta Dermatovenerol 1994;74:43–44.
250. Kraus MD, Haley JC, Ruiz R, Essary L, Moran CA, Fletcher CDM: "Juvenile" xanthogranuloma. An immunophenotypic study with reappraisal of histogenesis. Am J Dermatopathol 2001;23:104–111.
251. Pulford KAF, Rigney EM, Jones M, et al: KP1: A new monoclonal antibody detecting a monocyte/macrophage associated antigen in routinely processed tissue sections. J Clin Pathol 1989;42:414–421.
252. Weiss LM, Arber DA, Chang KL: CD68: A review. Appl Immunohistochem 1994;2:2–8.
253. Warnke RA, Pulford KAF, Pallesen G, et al: Diagnosis of myelomonocytic and macrophage neoplasms in routinely processed tissue biopsies with monoclonal antibody KP1. Am J Pathol 1989;135:1089–1095.
254. Tsang WY, Chan JK: KP1 (CD68) staining of granular cell neoplasms: Is KP1 a marker for lysosomes rather

than the histiocytic lineage? Histopathology 1992;21: 84–86.
255. dei Tos A, Doglioni C, Laurino L, Fletcher CDM: KP1 (CD68) expression in benign neural tumours. Further evidence of its low specificity as a histiocytic/myeloid marker. Histopathology 1993;23:185–187.
256. McHugh M, Miettinen M: CD68: Its limited specificity for histiocytic tumors. Appl Immunohistochem 1994; 2:186–190.
257. Cassidy M, Loftus B, Whelan A, Sabt B, Hickey D, Henry K, Leader M: KP-1: Not a specific marker. Staining of 137 sarcomas, 48 lymphomas, 28 carcinomas, 7 malignant melanomas and 8 cystosarcoma phyllodes. Virchows Arch 1994;424:635–640.
258. Binder SW, Said JW, Shintaku IP, Pinkus GS: A histiocyte-specific marker in the diagnosis of malignant fibrous histiocytoma. Use of monoclonal antibody KP-1 (CD68). Am J Clin Pathol 1992;97:759–763.
259. Buechler C, Ritter M, Orso E, Langmann T, Klucken J, Schmitz G: Regulation of scavenger receptor CD163 expression in human monocytes and macrophages by pro- and antiinflammatory stimuli. J Leukoc Biol 2000;67:97–103.

Keratins

260. Franke WW, Schiller DL, Moll R, et al: Diversity of cytokeratins. Differentiation specific expression of cytokeratin polypeptides in epithelial cells and tissues. J Mol Biol 1981;153:933–959.
261. Moll R, Franke WW, Schiller DL, Geiger B, Krepler R: The catalog of human cytokeratins: Patterns of expression in normal epithelia, tumors and cultured cells. Cell 1982;31:11–24.
262. Moll R, Schiller DL, Franke WW: Identification of protein IT of the intestinal cytoskeleton as a novel type I cytokeratin with unusual properties and expression patterns. J Cell Biol 1990;111:567–580.
263. Sun T-T, Eichner R, Schermer A, Cooper D, Nelson WG, Weiss RA: Classification, expression and possible mechanisms of evolution of mammalian epithelial keratins: A unifying model. In Levine AJ, van de Voude GF, Topp WC, Watson JD (eds): Cancer Cell I/The Transformed Phenotype. Cold Spring Harbor, NY, Cold Spring Harbor Laboratory, 1985:169–176.
264. Cooper D, Schermer A, Sun TT: Biology of disease. Classification of human epithelia and their neoplasms using monoclonal antibodies to keratins: Strategies, applications and limitations. Lab Invest 1985;52:243–256.
265. Eichner R, Bonitz P, Sun TT: Classification of epidermal keratins according to their immunoreactivity, isoelectric point, and mode of expression. J Cell Biol 1984;98:1388–1396.
266. Miettinen M, Lehto VP, Virtanen I: Keratin in the epithelial-like cells of classical biphasic synovial sarcoma. Virchows Arch [Cell Pathol] 1982; 40:157–161.
267. Chase DR, Enzinger FM, Weiss SW, Langloss JM: Keratin in epithelioid sarcoma. An immunohistochemical study. Am J Surg Pathol 1984;8:435–441.
268. Miettinen M, Lehto VP, Dahl D, Virtanen I: Differential diagnosis of chordoma, chondroid, and ependymal tumors as aided by anti-intermediate filament antibodies. Am J Pathol 1983;112:160–169.
269. Huitfeldt HS, Brandtzaeg P: Various keratin antibodies produce immunohistochemical staining of human myocardium and myometrium. Histochemistry 1985;83: 381–389.
270. Miettinen M: Keratin immunohistochemistry—Update of applications and pitfalls. Pathol Annu 1993; 24(part 2):113–143.
271. von Koskull H, Virtanen I: Induction of cytokeratin expression in human mesenchymal cells. J Cell Physiol 1987;133:321–329.
272. Rosenberg M, Ray Chaudhury A, Shows TB, et al: A group of type I keratin genes on human chromosome 17: Characterization and expression. Mol Cell Biol 1988;8:722–736.
273. Romano V, Bosco P, Rocchi M, et al: Chromosomal assignments of human type I and type II cytokeratin genes to different chromosomes. Cytogenet Cell Genet 1988;48:148–151.
274. Rosenberg M, Fuchs E, Le Beau MM: Three epidermal and one simple epithelial type II keratin genes map to chromosome 12. Cytogenet Cell Genet 1991; 57:33–38.
275. Blobel GA, Moll R, Franke WW, Kayser KW, Gould VE: The intermediate filament cytoskeleton of malignant mesotheliomas and its diagnostic significance. Am J Pathol 1985;121:235–247.
276. Moll R, Achstatter T, Becht E, Balcarova-Stander J, Ittensohn M, Franke WW: Cytokeratins in normal and malignant transitional epithelium. Maintenance of expression of urothelial differentiation features in transitional cell carcinomas and bladder carcinoma cell culture lines. Am J Pathol 1990;132:123–144.
277. Schaafsma HE, Ramaekers FC, van Muijen GN, et al: Distribution of cytokeratin polypeptides in human transitional cell carcinomas, with special emphasis on changing expression patterns during tumor progression. Am J Pathol 1990;136:329–343.
278. Moll R: Cytokeratins as markers of differentiation in the diagnosis of epithelial tumors. Subcell Biochem 1998;31:205–262.
279. Markey AC, Lane EB, Churchill LJ, McDonald DM, Leigh IM: Expression of simple epithelial keratins 8 and 18 in epidermal neoplasia. J Invest Dermatol 1991;97:763–770.
280. Brown DC, Theaker JM, Banks PM, Gatter KC, Mason DY: Cytokeratin expression in smooth muscle and smooth muscle tumours. Histopathology 1987; 11:477–486.
281. Norton AJ, Thomas JA, Isaacson PG: Cytokeratin-specific monoclonal antibodies are reactive with tumours of smooth muscle derivation. An immunocytochemical and biochemical study using antibodies to intermediate filament cytoskeletal proteins. Histopathology 1987;11:487–499.
282. Gown AM, Boyd HC, Chang Y, Ferguson M, Reichler B, Tippens D: Smooth muscle cells can express cyto-

keratins of "simple" epithelium. Immunocytochemical and biochemical studies in vitro and in vivo. Am J Pathol 1988;132:223–232.
283. Kuruc N, Franke WW: Transient coexpression of desmin and cytokeratins 8 and 18 in developing myocardial cells of some vertebrate species. Differentiation 1986;38:177–193.
284. Jahn L, Fouquet B, Rohe K, Franke WW: Cytokeratins in certain endothelial and smooth muscle cells of two taxonomically distant vertebrate species, *Xenopus laevis* and man. Differentiation 1987;36:234–254.
285. Miettinen M, Fetsch JF: Distribution of keratins in normal endothelial cells and a spectrum of vascular tumors: Implications in tumor diagnosis. Hum Pathol 2000;31:1062–1067.
286. Franke WW, Moll R: Cytoskeletal components of lymphoid organs. I. Synthesis of cytokeratins 8 and 18 and desmin in subpopulations of extrafollicular reticulum cells of human lymph nodes, tonsils and spleen. Differentiation 1987;36:145–163.
287. Knapp AC, Franke WW: Spontaneous losses of control of cytokeratin gene expression in transformed, non-epithelial human cells occurring at different levels of regulation. Cell 1989;59:67–79.
288. Traweek ST, Liu J, Battifora H: Keratin gene expression in non-epithelial tissues. Detection with polymerase chain reaction. Am J Pathol 1993;142:1111–1118.
289. Miettinen M: Keratin subsets in spindle cell sarcomas. Keratins are widespread but synovial sarcoma contains a distinctive keratin polypeptide pattern and desmoplakins. Am J Pathol 1991;138:505–513.
290. Miettinen M, Limon J, Niezabitowski A, Lasota J: Patterns of keratin polypeptides in 110 biphasic, monophasic and poorly differentiated synovial sarcomas. Virchows Arch 2000;437:275–283.
291. Manivel JC, Wick MR, Dehner LP, Sibley RK: Epithelioid sarcoma. An immunohistochemical study. Am J Clin Pathol 1987;87:319–326.
292. Daimaru Y, Hashimoto H, Tsuneyoshi M, Enjoji M: Epithelial profile of epithelioid sarcoma. An immunohistochemical analysis of six cases. Cancer 1987;59:34–41.
293. Miettinen M, Fanburg-Smith JC, Virolainen M, Shmookler BM, Fetsch JF: Epithelioid sarcoma: An immunohistochemical analysis of 112 classical and variant cases and a discussion of the differential diagnosis. Hum Pathol 1999;30:934–942.
294. Heikinheimo K, Persson S, Kindblom LG, Morgan PR, Virtanen I: Expression of different cytokeratin subclasses in human chordoma. J Pathol 1991;164:145–150.
295. Naka T, Iwamoto Y, Shinohara N, Chuman H, Fukui M, Tsuneyoshi M: Cytokeratin subtyping in chordoma and the fetal notochord: An immunohistochemical analysis of aberrant expression. Mod Pathol 1997;10:545–551.
296. O'Hara BJ, Paetau A, Miettinen M: Keratin subsets and monoclonal antibody HBME-1 in chordoma: Immunohistochemical differential diagnosis between tumors simulating chordoma. Hum Pathol 1998;29:119–126.
297. Bolen JW, Hammar SP, McNutt MA: Reactive and neoplastic serosal tissue. A light microscopic, ultrastructural, and immunocytochemical study. Am J Surg Pathol 1986;10:34–47.
298. Gray MH, Rosenberg AE, Dickersin GR, Bhan AK: Cytokeratin expression in epithelioid vascular neoplasms. Hum Pathol 1990;21:212–217.
299. Miettinen M: Immunoreactivity for cytokeratin and epithelial membrane antigen in leiomyosarcoma. Arch Pathol Lab Med 1988; 112:637–640.
300. Miettinen M, Soini Y: Malignant fibrous histiocytoma. Heterogeneous patterns of inter-mediate filament proteins by immunohistochemistry. Arch Pathol Lab Med 1989; 113:1363–1366.
301. Rosenberg AE, O'Connell JX, Dickersin GR, Bhan AK: Expression of epithelial markers in malignant fibrous histiocytoma of the musculoskeletal system: An immunohistochemical and electron microscopic study. Hum Pathol 1993;24:284–293.
302. Litzky LA, Brooks JJ: Cytokeratin immunoreactivity in malignant fibrous histiocytoma and spindle cell tumors: Comparison between frozen and paraffin-embedded tissues. Mod Pathol 1992;5:30–34.
303. Zarbo RJ, Gown AM, Nagle RB, Visscher DW, Crissman JD: Anomalous cytokeratin expression in malignant melanoma: One- and two-dimensional Western blot analysis and immunohistochemical survey of 100 melanomas. Mod Pathol 1990;3:494–501.
304. Wotherspoon AC, Norton AJ, Isaacson PG: Immunoreactive cytokeratins in plasmacytomas. Histopathology 1989;14:141–150.
305. Lasota J, Hyjek E, Koo C, Blonski J, Miettinen M: Cytokeratin-positive B-cell lymphomas: Verification by polymerase chain reaction. Am J Surg Pathol 1996;20:346–354.
306. Gustmann C, Altmannsberger M, Osborn M, Griesser H, Feller AC: Cytokeratin expression and vimentin content in large cell anaplastic lymphomas and other non-Hodgkin's lymphomas. Am J Pathol 1991;138: 1413–1422.
307. Bartek J, Vojtesek B, Staskova Z, et al: A series of 14 new monoclonal antibodies to keratins: Characterization and value in diagnostic histopathology. J Pathol 1991;164:215–224.
308. Ramaekers F, Huysmans A, Schaart G, Moesker O, Vooijs P: Tissue distribution of keratin 7 as monitored by a monoclonal antibody. Exp Cell Res 1987;170: 235–249.
309. van Niekerk CC, Jap PH, Ramaekers FC, van de Molengraft F, Poels LG: Immunohistochemical demonstration of keratin 7 in routinely fixed paraffin-embedded human tissues. J Pathol 1991;165:145–152.
310. Osborn M, van Lessen G, Weber K, Kloppel G, Altmannsberger M: Differential diagnosis of gastrointestinal carcinomas by using monoclonal antibodies specific for individual keratin polypeptides. Lab Invest 1986;55:497–504.
311. Ramaekers F, van Niekerk C, Poels L, et al: Use of monoclonal antibodies to keratin 7 in the differential diagnosis of adenocarcinomas. Am J Pathol 1990;136: 641–655.

312. Wang NP, Zee S, Zarbo RJ, Bacchi CE, Gown AM: Coordinate expression of cytokeratins 7 and 20 defines unique subsets of carcinomas. Appl Immunohistochem 1995;3:99–107.
313. Chu P, Wu E, Weiss LM: Cytokeratin 7 and cytokeratin 20 expression in epithelial neoplasms: A survey of 435 cases. Mod Pathol 200;13:962–972.
314. Jensen K, Kohler S, Rouse RV: Cytokeratin staining in Merkel cell carcinoma: An immunohistochemical study of cytokeratins 5/6, 7, 17, and 20. Appl Immunohistochem Mol Morphol 200;8:310–315.
315. Folpe AL, Schmid RA, Chapman D, Gown AM: Poorly differentiated synovial sarcoma: Immunohistochemical distinction from primitive neuroectodermal tumors and high-grade malignant peripheral nerve sheath tumors. Am J Surg Pathol 1998;22:673–682.
316. Moll R, Lowe A, Laufer J, Franke WW: Cytokeratin 20 in human carcinomas. A new histodiagnostic marker detected by monoclonal antibodies. Am J Pathol 1992;140:427–447.
317. Miettinen M: Keratin 20: Immunohistochemical marker for gastrointestinal, urothelial, and Merkel cell carcinomas. Mod Pathol 1995;8:384–388.
318. Purkis PE, Steel JB, Mackenzie IC, Nathrath WB, Leigh IM, Lane EB: Antibody markers of basal cells in complex epithelia. J Cell Science 1990;97:39–50.
319. Wetzels RHW, Kuijpers HJH, Lane EB, et al: Basal cell-specific and hyperproliferation-related keratins in human breast cancer. Am J Pathol 1991;138:751–763.
320. Malzahn K, Mitze M, Thoenes M, Moll R: Biological and prognostic significance of stratified epithelial cytokeratins in infiltrating ductal breast carcinomas. Virchows Arch 1988;433:119–129.
321. Irvine AD, McLean WH: The human keratin diseases: The increasing spectrum of disease and subtlety of the phenotype-genotype correlation. Br J Dermatol 1999;140:815–828.
322. Moll R, Dhouailly D, Sun TT: Expression of keratin 5 as a distinctive feature of epithelial and biphasic mesotheliomas. An immunohistochemical study using monoclonal antibody AE14. Virchows Arch B Cell Pathol 1989;58:129–145.
323. Ordonez NG: Value of cytokeratin 5/6 immunostaining in distinguishing epithelial mesothelioma of the pleura from lung adenocarcinoma. Am J Surg Pathol 1998;22:1215–1221.
324. Chu PG, Luda MH, Weiss LM: Cytokeratin 14 expression in epithelial neoplasms: A survey of 435 cases with emphasis on its value in differentiation squamous carcinomas from other epithelial tumours. Histopathology 2001;39:9–16.
325. Troyanovsky SM, Guelstein VI, Tchipysheva TA, Krutovskikh VA, Bannikov GA: Patterns of expression of keratin 17 in human epithelia: Dependency on cell position. J Cell Sci 1989;93:419–426.
326. Troyanovsky SM, Leube RE, Franke WW: Characterization of the human gene encoding cytokeratin 17 and its expression pattern. Eur J Cell Biol 1992;59:127–137.
327. Miettinen M, Nobel MP, Tuma BT, Kovatich AJ: Keratin 17. Immunohistochemical mapping of its distribution in human epithelial tumors and its potential applications. Appl Immunohistochem 1997;5:152–159.
328. Goldstein NS, Bassi D, Uzieblo A: WT1 is an integral component of an antibody panel to distinguish pancreaticobiliary and some ovarian epithelial neoplasms. Am J Clin Pathol 2001;116:246–252.
329. Moll R, Krepler R, Franke WW: Complex cytokeratin polypeptide patterns observed in certain human carcinomas. Differentiation 1983;23:256–269.
330. van Muijen GNP, Ruiter DJ, Franke WW: Cell-type heterogeneity of cytokeratin expression in complex epithelia and carcinomas as demonstrated by monoclonal antibodies specific for cytokeratins 4 and 13. Exp Cell Res 1986;62:97–113.
331. Remotti F, Fetsch JF, Miettinen M: Keratin 1 expression in endothelia and mesenchymal tumors. Immunohistochemical analysis of normal and neoplastic tissues. Hum Pathol 2001;32:873–879.
332. Hasan AAK, Zisman T, Schmaier AH: Identification of cytokeratin 1 as a binding protein and presentation receptor for kininogens on endothelial cells. Proc Natl Acad Sci USA 1998;95:3615–3620.
333. Ivanyi D, Ansink A, Groeneweld E, Hageman PC, Mooi WJ, Heinz AP: New monoclonal antibodies recognizing epidermal differentiation-associated keratins in formalin-fixed, paraffin-embedded tissue. Keratin 10 expression in carcinoma of the vulva. J Pathol 1989;159:7–12.
334. Knapp AC, Franke WW, Heid H, Hatzfeld M, Jorcano JL, Moll R: Cytokeratin no. 9, an epidermal type I keratin characteristic of a special program of keratinocyte differentiation displaying body site specificity. J Cell Biol 1986;103:657–667.
335. Jih DM, Lyle S, Elenitsas R, Elder DE, Cotsarelis G: Cytokeratin 15 expression in trichoepitheliomas and a subset of basal cell carcinomas suggests they originate from hair follicle stem cells. J Cutan Pathol 1999;26:113–118.
336. Weber K, Osborn M, Moll R, Wiklund B, Luning B: Tissue polypeptide antigen (TPA) is related to the non-epidermal keratins 8, 18 and 19 typical of simple and non-squamous epithelia: Re-evaluation of a human tumor marker. EMBO J 1984;3:2707–2714.

Other Epithelial and Mesothelial Markers

EMA

337. Gendler SJ: MUC1, the renaissance molecule. J Mammary Gland Biol Neoplasia 2001;6:339–353.
338. Sasaki M, Peterson JA, Wara WM, Ceriani RL: Human mammary epithelial antigens (HME-Ags) in the circulation of nude mice implanted with a breast tumor and non-breast tumors. Cancer 1981;48:2204–2210.
339. Sloane JP, Ormerod MG: Distribution of epithelial membrane antigen in normal and neoplastic tissues and its value in diagnostic tumor pathology. Cancer 1981;47:1786–1795.
340. Pinkus GS, Kurtin PJ: Epithelial membrane antigen: A diagnostic discriminant in surgical pathology; immunohistochemical profile in epithelial, mesenchymal,

and hematopoietic neoplasms using paraffin sections and monoclonal antibodies. Hum Pathol 1985;16:929–940.
341. Heyderman E, Strudley I, Powell G, Richardson TC, Cordell JL, Mason DY: A new monoclonal antibody to epithelial membrane antigen (EMA)-E29. A comparison of its immunocytochemical reactivity with polyclonal anti-EMA antibodies and with another monoclonal antibody, HMFG-2. Br J Cancer 1985;52:355–361.
342. Ariza A, Bilbao JM, Rosai J: Immunohistochemical detection of epithelial membrane antigen in normal perineurial cells and perineurioma. Am J Surg Pathol 1988;12:678–683.
343. Theaker JM, Fletcher CDM: Epithelial membrane antigen expression by the perineurial cell: Further studies on peripheral nerve lesions. Histopathology 1989;14: 581–588.
344. Fetsch JF, Miettinen M: Sclerosing perineurioma. A clinicopathologic study of 19 cases of a distinctive soft tissue lesion with a predilection for the fingers and palms of young adults. Am J Surg Pathol 1997;21:1433–1442.
345. Swanson PE, Manivel JC, Scheithauer BW, Wick MR: Epithelial membrane antigen reactivity in mesenchymal neoplasms: An immunohistochemical study of 306 soft tissue sarcomas. Surg Pathol 1989;2:313–322.
346. Chittal, S, Al Saati T, Delsol G: Epithelial membrane antigen in hematolymphoid neoplasms. A review. Appl Immunohistochem 1997;5:203–215.
347. Ordonez NG: Role of immunohistochemistry in differentiating epithelial mesothelioma from adenocarcinoma. Am J Clin Pathol 1999;112:75–89.

B72.3

348. Warnock ML, Stoloff A, Thor A: Differentiation of adenocarcinoma of the lung from mesothelioma. Periodic acid-Schiff, monoclonal antibodies B72.3 and LeuM1. Am J Pathol 1988;133:30–38.
349. Kokoulis GK, Radosevich JA, Warren WH, Rosen ST, Gould VE: Immunohisto-chemical analysis of pulmonary and pleural neoplasms with monoclonal antibodies B72.3 and CSLEX-1. Virchows Arch B Cell Pathol 1990;58:427–433.
350. Wick MR, Loy T, Mills SE, Legier JF, Manivel JC: Malignant epithelioid pleural mesothelioma versus peripheral pulmonary adenocarcinoma: A histochemical, ultrastructural, and immunohistologic study of 103 cases. Hum Pathol 1990;21:759–766.
351. Sirgi KE, Wick MR, Swanson PE: B72.3 and CD34 immunoreactivity in malignant epithelioid soft tissue tumors. Adjuncts in the recognition of endothelial neoplasms. Am J Surg Pathol 1993;17:179–185.

BerEp

352. Latza U, Niedobitek G, Schwarting R, Nekarda H, Stein H: Ber-EP4: New monoclonal antibody which distinguishes epithelia from mesothelial cells. J Clin Pathol 1990;43:213–219.
353. Sheibani K, Shin SS, Kezirian J, Weiss LM: Ber-Ep4 antibody as a discriminant in the differential diagnosis of malignant mesothelioma versus adenocarcinoma. Am J Surg Pathol 1991;15:779–784.
354. Miettinen M, Limon J, Niezabitowski A, Lasota J: Calretinin and other mesothelioma markers in synovial sarcoma: Analysis of antigenic similarities and differences with malignant mesothelioma. Am J Surg Pathol 2001;25:610–617.

Cadherins

355. Angst RD, Marcozzi C, Magee AI: The cadherin superfamily. J Cell Sci 2001;114:625–626.
356. Smith MEF, Pignatelli M: The molecular histology of neoplasia: The role of the cadherin/catenin complex. Histopathology 1997;31:107–111.
357. Sato H, Hasegawa T, Abe Y, Skai H, Hirohashi S: Expression of E-cadherin in bone and soft tissue sarcoma. A possible role in epithelial differentiation. Hum Pathol 1999;30:1344–1349.
358. Danen EH, de Vries TJ, Morandini R, Ghanem GG, Ruiter DJ, van Muijen GN: E-cadherin expression in human melanoma. Melanoma Res 1996;6:127–131.
359. Smith ME, Brown JI, Fisher C: Epithelioid sarcoma: Presence of vascular-endothelial cadherin and lack of epithelial cadherin. Histopathology 1998;33: 425–431.
360. Han AC, Peralta-Soler A, Knudsen KA, Wheelock MJ, Johnson KR, Salazar H: Differential expression of N-cadherin in pleural mesotheliomas and E-cadherin in lung adenocarcinomas in formalin-fixed, paraffin-embedded tissues. Hum Pathol 1997;28: 641–645.
361. Laskin WB, Miettinen M: Epithelial-type and neural-type cadherin expression in malignant noncarcinomatous neoplasms with epithelioid features that involve the soft tissues. Arch Pathol Lab Med. 2002;126:425–431.

Calretinin

362. Dei Tos AP, Doglioni C: Calretinin: A novel tool for diagnostic immunohistochemistry. Adv Anat Pathol 1998;5:61–66.
363. Ordonez NG: Value of calretinin immunostaining in differentiating epithelial mesothelioma from lung adenocarcinoma. Mod Pathol 1998;11:929–933.
364. Riera, JR, Astengo-Osuna C, Longmate JA, Battifora H: The immunohistochemical diagnostic panel for epithelial mesothelioma. A reevaluation after heat-induced epitope retrieval. Am J Surg Pathol 1997;21: 1409–1419.
365. Gotzos V, Wintergrest ES, Musy JP, Spichtin HP, Genton CY: Selective distribution of calretinin in adenocarcinomas of the human colon and adjacent tissues. Am J Surg Pathol 1999;23:701–711.
366. Altini M, Coleman H, Doglioni C, Favia G, Maiorano E: Calretinin expression in ameloblastomas. Histopathology 2000;37:27–32.

Carcinoembryonic Antigen (CEA)

367. Corson JM, Weiss LM, Banks-Schlegel SP, Pinkus GS: Keratin protein and carcinoembryonic antigen in synovial sarcomas: An immunohistochemical study of 24 cases. Hum Pathol 1984;15:615–621.
368. Brown RW, Campagna LB, Dunn JK, Cagle PT: Immunohistochemical identification of tumor markers in metastatic adenocarcinoma: A diagnostic adjunct in the determination of primary site. Am J Clin Pathol 1997:107:12–19.

Desmoplakin

369. Moll R, Cowin P, Kapprell HP, Franke WW: Desmosomal proteins: New markers for identification and classification of tumors. Lab Invest 1986;54:4–25.

HBME1

370. Miettinen M, Kovatich AJ: HBME-1: A monoclonal antibody useful in the differential diagnosis of mesothelioma, adenocarcinoma, and soft tissue and bone tumors. Appl Immuno-Histochem 1995;3:115–122.

Mesothelin

371. Chang K, Pai LH, Pass H, et al: Monoclonal antibody K1 reacts with epithelial mesothelioma but not with lung adenocarcinoma. Am J Surg Pathol 1992;16: 259–268.

MOC-31

372. de Leij L, Helrich W, Stein R, Mattes MJ: SCLC-cluster-2 antibodies detect pancarcinoma/epithelial glycoprotein EGP-2. Int J Cancer Suppl 1994;8:60–63.
373. De Young BR, Wick MR: Immunohistologic evaluation of metastatic carcinomas of unknown origin: An algorithmic approach. Semin Diagn Pathol 2000;17: 184–193.

Thyroid Transcription Factor TTF1

374. Bingle CD: Thyroid transcription factor-1. Int J Biochem Cell Biol 1997;29:1471–1473.
375. Fabbro G, Di Loreto C, Beltrami CA, Belfiore A, Di Lauro R, Damante G: Expression of thyroid-specific transcription factors TTF-1 and PAX-8 in human thyroid neoplasms. Cancer Res 1994;54:4744–4749.
376. Miettinen M, Franssila K: Variable expression of keratin and nearly uniform lack of thyroid transcription factor in anaplastic thyroid carcinoma. Hum Pathol 2000;31:1139–1145.
377. Holzinger A, Dingle S, Bejarano PA, et al: Monoclonal antibody to thyroid transcription factor-1: Production, characterization, and usefulness in tumor diagnosis. Hybridoma 1996;15:49–53.
378. Bejarano PA, Baughman RP, Biddinger PW, et al: Surfactant proteins and thyroid transcription factor-1 in pulmonary and breast carcinomas. Mod Pathol 1996; 9:445–452.
379. Folpe AL, Gown AM, Lamps LW, et al: Thyroid transcription factor-1: Immunohistochemical evaluation in pulmonary neuroendocrine tumors. Mod Pathol 1999;12:5–8.
380. Kaufmann O, Dietel M: Expression of thyroid transcription factor-1 in pulmonary and extrapulmonary small cell carcinomas and other neuroendocrine carcinomas of various primary sites. Histopathology 2000;36:415–420.
381. Byrd-Gloster AL, Khoor A, Glass LF, et al: Differential expression of thyroid transcription factor I in small cell lung carcinomas and Merkel cell tumor. Hum Pathol 2000;31:58–62.

Villin

382. Grone HJ, Weber K, Helmchen U, Osborn M: Villin: A marker of brush border differentiation and cellular origin in human renal cell carcinoma. Am J Pathol 1986;124:294–302.
383. Bacchi CE, Gown AM: Distribution and pattern of expression of villin, a gastrointestinal-associated cytoskeletal protein, in human carcinomas: A study employing paraffin-embedded tissue. Lab Invest 1991; 64:418–424.
384. Sharma S, Tan J, Sidhu G, Wieczorek R, Miller DC, Cassai ND: Lung adenocarcinomas metastatic to the brain with and without ultrastructural evidence of rootlets: An electron microscopic and imunohistochemical study using cytokeratin 7 and 20 and villin. Ultrastruct Pathol 1998;22:385–391.
385. Zhang PJ, Harris KR, Alobeid B, Brooks JJ: Immunoexpression of villin in neuroendocrine tumors and its diagnostic implications. Arch Pathol Lab Med 1999; 123:812–816.

WT1

386. Scharnhorst V, van der Eb AJ, Jochemsen AG: WT1 proteins: Functions in growth and differentiation. Gene 2001;273:141–161.
387. Ordonez NG: Desmoplastic small round cell tumor. II: An ultrastructural and immunohistochemical study with emphasis on new immunohistochemical markers. Am J Surg Pathol 1998;22:1314–1327.
388. Barnoud R, Sabourin J, Pasquier D, et al: Immunohistochemical expression of WT1 by desmoplastic small round cell tumor: A comparative study with other small round cell tumors. Am J Surg Pathol 2000; 24:830–836.
389. Amin KM, Litzky LA, Smythe WR, et al: Wilms' tumor 1 susceptibility (WT1) gene products are selectively expressed in malignant mesothelioma. Am J Pathol 1995;146:344–356.
390. Shimizu M, Toki T, Takagi Y, Konishi I, Fujii S: Immunohistochemical detection of the Wilms' tumor gene (WT1) in epithelial ovarian tumors. Int J Gynecol Pathol 2000;19:158–163.

Other Markers

Anaplastic Lymphoma Kinase (ALK)

391. Coffin CM, Patel A, Perkins S, Elenitoba-Johnson KS, Perlman E, Griffin CA: ALK1 and p80 expression and

chromosomal rearrangements involving 2p23 in inflammatory myofibroblastic tumor. Mod Pathol 2001; 14:569–576.

392. Chan JK, Cheuk W, Shimizu M: Anaplastic lymphoma kinase expression in inflammatory pseudotumors. Am J Surg Pathol 2001;25:761–768.
393. Cook JR, Dehner LP, Collins MH, et al: Anaplastic lymphoma kinase (ALK) expression in the inflammatory myofibroblastic tumor: A comparative immunohistochemical study. Am J Surg Pathol 2001;25: 1364–1371.

Basement Membrane Proteins

394. Miettinen M, Foidart JM, Ekblom P: Immunohistological demonstration of laminin, the major glycoprotein of basement membranes, as an aid in the diagnosis of soft tissue tumors. Am J Clin Pathol 1983;79:306–311.
395. Autio-Harmainen H, Apaja-Sarkkinen M, Martikainen J, Taipale A, Rapola J: Production of basement membrane laminin and type IV collagen by tumors of striated muscle: An immunohistochemical study of rhabdomyosarcomas of different histologic types and a benign vaginal rhabdomyoma. Hum Pathol 1986; 17:1218–1224.
396. Leong ASY, Vinyuvat S, Suthipintawong C, Leong FJ: Patterns of basal lamina immunostaining in soft tissue and bony tumors. Appl Immunohistochem 1997; 5:1–7.
397. Leivo I, Engvall E, Laurila P, Miettinen M: Distribution of merosin, a laminin-related tissue-specific basement membrane protein in human Schwann cell neoplasms. Lab Invest 1989;61:426–432.
398. Ogawa K, Oguchi M, Yamabe H, Nakashima Y, Hamashima Y: Distribution of collagen type IV in soft tissue tumors. An immunohistochemical study. Cancer 1986;58:269–277.
399. Wetzels RH, Robben HC, Leigh IM, Schaafsma HE, Vooijs GP, Ramaekers FC: Distribution patterns of type VII collagen in normal and malignant human tissues. Am J Pathol 1991;139:451–459.

bcl2

400. Hockenberry DM: bcl-2, a novel regulator of cell death. Bioessays 1995;17:631–638.
401. Tsujimoto Y, Croce CM: Analysis of the structure, transcripts, and protein products of bcl-2, the gene involved in human follicular lymphoma. Proc Natl Acad Sci USA 1986;83:5214–5218.
402. LeBrun DP, Warnke RA, Cleary ML: Expression of bcl-2 in fetal tissues suggests a role in morphogenesis. Am J Pathol 1993;142:743–753.
403. Suster S, Fisher C, Moran CA: Expression of bcl-2 oncoprotein in benign and malignant spindle cell tumors of soft tissue, skin, serosal surfaces, and gastrointestinal tract. Am J Surg Pathol 1998;22:863–872.
404. Miettinen M, Sarlomo-Rikala M, Kovatich AJ: Cell-type and tumor-type related bcl-2 reactivity in mesenchymal cells and soft tissue tumors. Virchows Arch 1998;433:255–260.

CD10

405. Mechtersheimer G, Moller P: Expression of the common acute lymphoblastic leukemia antigen (CD10) in mesenchymal tumors. Am J Pathol 1989;134: 961–965.
406. Chu P, Arber DA: Paraffin-section detection of CD10 in 505 nonhematopoietic neoplasms. Frequent expression in renal cell carcinoma and endometrial stromal sarcoma. Am J Clin Pathol 2000;113:374–382.
407. Agoff SN, Grieco VS, Garcia R, Gown AM: Immunohistochemical distinction of endometrial stromal sarcoma and cellular leiomyoma. Appl Immunohistochem Mol Morphol 2001;9:164–169.
408. Chu PG, Arber DA, Weiss LM, Chang KL: Utility of CD10 in distinguishing between endometrial stromal sarcoma and uterine smooth muscle tumors: An immunohistochemical comparison of 34 cases. Mod Pathol 2001;14:465–471.
409. McCluggage WG, Sumathi VP, Maxwell P: CD10 is sensitive and diagnostically useful immunohistochemical marker of normal endometrial stroma and of endometrial stromal neoplasms. Histopathology 2001;39:273–278.

CD99

410. Ambros JM, Ambros PF, Strehl J, et al: MIC2 is a specific marker for Ewing's sarcoma and peripheral neuroectodermal tumors: Evidence for a common histogenesis of Ewing's sarcoma and peripheral primitive neuroectodermal tumors from MIC2 expression and common chromosome aberration. Cancer 1991; 67:1886–1893.
411. Fellinger EJ, Garin-Chesa P, Triche TJ, Huvos AG, Rettig WJ: Immunohistochemical analysis of Ewing's sarcoma cell surface antigen $p30/32^{MIC2}$ Am J Pathol 1991;1139:317–325.
412. Stevenson AJ, Chatten J, Bertoni F, Miettinen M: CD99 (p30/32 -MIC2) neuroectodermal/Ewing sarcoma antigen as an immunohistochemical marker. Review of more than 600 tumors and the literature experience. Appl Immunohistochem 1994;2:231–240.
413. Renshaw AA: O13 (CD99) in spindle cell tumors. Reactivity with hemangiopericytoma, solitary fibrous tumor, synovial sarcoma, and meningioma but rarely with sarcomatoid mesothelioma. Appl Immunohistochem 1995;3:250–256.

CD117 (KIT)

414. Kitamura Y, Hirota S, Nishida T: Molecular pathology of c-kit proto-oncogene and development of gastrointestinal stromal tumors. Ann Chir Gyn 1998;87: 282–286.
415. Tsuura Y, Hiraki H, Watanabe K, et al: Preferential localization of c-kit product in tissue mast cells, basal cells of skin, epithelial cells of breast, small cell lung carcinoma and seminoma/dysgerminoma in human: Immunohistochemical study of formalin-fixed, paraffin-embedded tissues. Virchows Arch 1994;424:135–141.

416. Lammie A, Drobnjak M, Gerald W, Saad A, Cote R, Cordon-Cardo C: Expression of c-kit and kit ligand proteins in normal human tissues. J Histochem Cytochem 1994;42:1417–1425.
417. Arber DA, Tamayo R, Weiss LM: Paraffin section detection of the c-kit gene product (CD117) in human tissues: Value in the diagnosis of mast cell disorders. Hum Pathol 1998;29:498–504.
418. Kindblom LG, Remotti HE, Aldenborg F, Meis-Kindblom JM: Gastrointestinal pacemaker cell tumor (GIPACT): Gastrointestinal stromal tumors show phenotypic characteristics of the interstitial cells of Cajal. Am J Pathol 1998;152:1259–1269.
419. Sarlomo-Rikala M, Kovatich AJ, Barusevicius A, Miettinen M: CD117: A sensitive marker for gastrointestinal stromal tumors that is more specific than CD34. Mod Pathol 1998;11:728–734.
420. Sircar K, Hewlett BR, Huizinga JD, Chorneyko K, Berezin I, Riddell RH: Interstitial cells of Cajal as precursors for gastrointestinal stromal tumors. Am J Surg Pathol 1999;23:377–389.
421. Chen J, Yanuck RR 3rd, Abbondanzo SL, Chu WS, Aguilera NS: c-kit (CD117) reactivity in extramedullary myeloid tumor/granulocytic sarcoma. Arch Pathol Lab Med 2001;125:1448–1452.
422. Miettinen M, Sarlomo-Rikala M, Lasota J: KIT expression in angiosarcomas and in fetal endothelial cells. Lack of c-kit mutations in exon 11 and 17 of c-kit. Mod Pathol 2000;13:536–541.
423. Montone KT, van Belle P, Elenitsas R, Elder DE: Protooncogene c-kit expression in malignant melanoma: Protein loss with tumor progression. Mod Pathol 1997;10:939–944.

Estrogen and Progesterone Receptors

424. Deamant FD, Pombo MT, Battifora H: Estrogen receptor immunohistochemistry as a predictor of site of origin in metastatic breast cancer. Appl Immunohistochem 1993;1:188–192.

Fli-1

425. Truong AH, Ben-David Y: The role of Fli-1 in normal cell function and malignant transformation. Oncogene 2000;18:6482–6489.
426. Folpe AL, Hill CE, Parham DM, O'Shea PA, Weiss SW: Immunohistochemical detection of Fli-1 protein expression: A study of 132 round cell tumors with emphasis on CD99-positive mimics of Ewing sarcoma/primitive neuroectodermal tumor. Am J Surg Pathol 2000;24:1657–1662.

Glial Fibrillary Acidic Protein (GFAP)

427. Achstatter T, Moll R, Anderson A, et al: Expression of glial filament protein (GFP) in nerve sheaths and non-neural cells re-examined using monoclonal antibodies, with special emphasis on the co-expression of GFP and cytokeratins in epithelial cells of human salivary gland and pleomorphic adenomas. Differentiation 1986;31:206–227.
428. Mancardi GL, Cadoni A, Tabaton M, et al: Schwann cell GFAP expression increases in axonal neuropathies. J Neurol Sci 1991;102:177–183.
429. Memoli VA, Brown EF, Gould VE: Glial fibrillary acidic protein (GFAP) immunoreactivity in peripheral nerve sheath tumors. Ultrastruct Pathol 1984;7:269–275.
430. Gould VE, Moll R, Moll I, Lee I, Schwechheimer K, Franke WW: The intermediate filament complement of the spectrum of nerve sheath neoplasms. Lab Invest 1986;55:463–474.
431. Kawahara E, Oda Y, Ooi A, Katsuda S, Nakanishi I, Umeda S: Expression of glial fibrillary acidic protein (GFAP) in peripheral nerve sheath tumors. A comparative study of immunoreactivity of GFAP, vimentin, S100-protein and neurofilament in 38 schwannomas and 18 neurofibromas. Am J Surg Pathol 1988;12:115–120.
432. Gray MH, Rosenberg AE, Dickersin GR, Bhan AK: Glial fibrillary acidic protein and keratin expression by benign and malignant nerve sheath tumors. Hum Pathol 1989;20:1089–1096.

Inhibin

433. Flemming P, Wellmann A, Maschek H, Lang H, Georgii A: Monoclonal antibodies against inhibin represent key markers of adult granulosa cell tumors of the ovary even in their metastases. A report of three cases with late metastases, being previously interpreted as hemnagiopericytoma. Am J Surg Pathol 1995;19:927–933.
434. Rishi M, Howard LN, Bratthauer GL, Tavassoli FA: Use of monoclonal antibody against human inhibin as a marker for sex cord-stromal tumors of the ovary. Am J Surg Pathol 1997;21:583–589.
435. Chivite A, Matias-Guiu X, Pons C, Algaba F, Prat J: Inhibin A expression in adrenal neoplasms. A new immunohistochemical marker for adrenocortical tumors. Appl Immunohistochem 1998;6:42–49.
436. McCluggage WG, Burton J, Maxwell P, Sloan JM: Immunohistochemical staining of normal, hyperplastic, and neoplastic adrenal cortex with a monoclonal antibody against alpha-inhibin. J Clin Pathol 1998;51: 114–116.
437. Murakata LA, Ishak KG: Expression of inhibin-alpha by granular cell tumors of the gallbladder and extrahepatic bile ducts. Am J Surg Pathol 2001;25:1200–1203.

Osteocalcin

438. Fanburg JC, Rosenberg AE, Weaver DL, et al: Osteocalcin and osteonectin immunoreactivity in the diagnosis of osteosarcoma. Am J Clin Pathol 1997;108: 464–473.
439. Fanburg-Smith JF, Bratthauer GL, Miettinen M: Osteocalcin and osteonectin immunoreactivity in extraskeletal osteosarcoma: A study of 28 cases. Hum Pathol 1999;30:32–38.

Vimentin

440. Franke WW, Schmid E, Osborn M, Weber K: Different intermediate-sized filaments distinguished by immunofluorescence microscopy. Proc Natl Acad Sci USA 1978;75:5034–5038.
441. Azumi N, Battifora H: The distribution of vimentin and keratin in epithelial and nonepithelial neoplasms. A comprehensive immunohistochemical study on formalin- and alcohol-fixed tumors. Am J Clin Pathol 1987;88:286–296.
442. Battifora H: Assessment of antigen damage in immunohistochemistry. The vimentin internal control. Am J Clin Pathol 1991;96:669–671.

Cell Cycle Markers

443. Sherr CJ: Cancer cell cycles. Science 1996;274: 1672–1677.
444. Bartek J, Lukas J, Bartkova J: Perspective: Defects in cell cycle control and cancer. J Pathol 1999;187:95–99.
445. Gerdes J, Li L, Schlueter C, et al: Immunobiochemical and molecular biologic characterization of the cell proliferation-associated nuclear antigen that is defined by monoclonal antibody Ki-67. Am J Pathol 1991:138:867–873.
446. Swanson SA, Brooks JJ: Proliferation markers Ki-67 and p105 in soft tissue lesions. Correlation with DNA flow cytometric characteristics. Am J Pathol 1990;137:1491–1500.
447. Key G, Becker MH, Baron B, et al. New Ki-67 equivalent murine monoclonal antibodies (MIB 1-3) generated against bacterially expressed parts of the Ki-67 cDNA containing three 62 base pair repetitive elements encoding for the Ki-67 epitope. Lab Invest 1993;68:629–636.
448. Rudolph P, Kellner U, Chassevent A, et al: Prognostic relevance of a novel proliferation marker, Ki-S11, for soft-tissue sarcoma. Am J Pathol 1997;150:1997–2007.
449. Choong PF, Akerman M, Willen H, et al: Prognostic value of Ki-67 expression in 182 soft tissue sarcoma. Proliferation—A marker of metastasis? APMIS 1994;102:915–924.
450. Huuhtanen RL, Blomqvist CP, Wiklund TA, et al: Comparison of the Ki67-score and S-phase fraction as prognostic variables in soft-tissue sarcoma. Br J Cancer 1999;79:945–951.
451. Heslin MJ, Cordon-Cardo C, Lewis JJ, Woodruff JM, Brennan MF: Ki-67 detected by MIB-1 predicts distant metastasis and tumor mortality in primary, high grade extremity sarcomas. Cancer 1998;83:490–497.
452. Hoos A, Stojadonovic A, Mastorides S, et al: High Ki-67 proliferative index predicts disease specific survival in patients with high-risk soft tissue sarcomas. Cancer 2001;92:869–874.
453. Wang J, Coltrera MD, Gown AM: Abnormalities of p53 and p110^{RB} tumor suppressor gene expression in human soft tissue tumors: Correlations with cell proliferation and tumor grade. Mod Pathol 1995;8: 837–842.
454. Wurl P, Taubert H, Meye A, et al: Prognostic value of immunohistochemistry for p53 in primary soft-tissue sarcomas: A multivariate analysis of five antibodies. J Cancer Res Clin Oncol 1997;123:502–508.
455. Antonescu CR, Leuang DH, Dudas M, et al: Alterations of cell cycle regulators in localized synovial sarcoma: A multifactorial study with prognostic implications. Am J Pathol 2000;156:977–983.
456. Yang P, Hirose T, Hasegawa T, Seki K, Sano T, Hizawa K: Prognostic implication of the p53 protein and Ki-67 antigen immunohistochemistry in malignant fibrous histiocytoma. Cancer 1995;76: 618–625.
457. Soini Y, Vahakangas K, Nuorva K, Kamel D, Lane DP, Paakko P: p53 immunohistochemistry in malignant fibrous histiocytomas and other mesenchymal tumours. J Pathol 1992;168:29–33.
458. Dei Tos AP, Doglioni C, Laurino L, Barbareschi M, Fletcher CD: p53 protein expression in non-neoplastic lesions and benign and malignant neoplasms of soft tissues. Histopathology 1993;22:45–50.
459. Cohen JA, Geradts J: Loss of RB and MTS1/CDKN2 (p16) expression in human sarcomas. Hum Pathol 1997;28:893–898.
460. Kourea HP, Orlow I, Scheithauer BW, Cordon-Cardo C, Woodruff JM: Deletions of the *INK4A* gene occur in malignant peripheral nerve sheath tumors but not in neurofibromas. Am J Pathol 1999;155: 1855–1860.
461. Nielsen GP, Stemmer-Rachamimov AO, Ino Y, Moller MB, Rosenberg AE, Louis DN: Malignant transformation of neurofibromas in neurofibromatosis 1 is associated with CDKN2A/p16 inactivation. Am J Pathol 1999;155:1879–1884.
462. Pindzola JA, Palazzo JP, Kovatich AJ, Tuma B, Nobel M: Expression of p21 WAF1/CIP1 in soft tissue sarcomas: A comparative immunohistochemical study with p53 and Ki-67. Path Res Pract 1998;194:685–691.
463. Kawauchi S, Goto Y, Liu XP, et al: Low expression of p27(Kip1), a cyclin-dependent kinase inhibitor, is a marker of poor prognosis in synovial sarcoma. Cancer 2001;91:1005–1012.
464. Huuhtanen RL, Blomqvist CP, Bohling TO: Expression of cyclin A in soft tissue sarcomas correlates with tumor aggressiveness. Cancer Res 1999;59: 2885–2890.
465. Kim SH, Lewis JJ, Brennan MF, Woodruff JM, Dudas M, Cordon-Cardo C: Overexpression of cyclin D1 is associated with poor prognosis in extremity soft-tissue sarcomas. Clin Cancer Res 1998;4:2377–2382.
466. Noguchi T, Dobashi Y, Minehara H, Itoman M, Kameya T: Involvement of cyclins in cell proliferation and their clinical implications in soft tissue smooth muscle tumors. Am J Pathol 2000;156:2135–2147.
467. Stefanou DG, Nonni AV, Agnantis NJ, Athanassiadou SE, Brassoulis E, Pavlidis N: p53/MDM-2 immunohistochemical expression correlated with proliferative activity in different subtypes of human sarcomas:

A ten-year follow-up study. Anticancer Res 1998;18: 4673–4681.

Technical Considerations

468. Mason JT, O'Leary TJ: Effects of formaldehyde fixation on protein secondary structure: A calorimetric and infrared spectroscopic investigation. J Histochem Cytochem 1991;39:225–229.
469. Werner M, Chott A, Fabiano A, Battifora H: Effect of formalin tissue fixation and processing in immunohistochemistry. Am J Surg Pathol 2000;24:1016–1019.
470. Pinkus GS, O'Connor EM, Etheridge CL, Corson JM: Optimal immunoreactivity of keratin proteins in formalin-fixed, paraffin-embedded tissue requires preliminary trypsinization. An immunoperioxidase study of various tumors using polyclonal and monoclonal antibodies. J Histochem Cytochem 1985;33:465–473.
471. Battifora H, Kopinski M: The influence of protease digestion and duration of fixation on the immunostaining of keratins. J Histochem Cytochem 1986;34: 1095–1100.
472. Miettinen M: Immunostaining of intermediate filament proteins in paraffin sections. Evaluation of the optimal protease treatment to improve the immunoreactivity. Pathol Res Pract 1989; 184:431–436.
473. Cattoretti G, Suurmeijer AJH: Antigen unmasking on formalin-fixed paraffin-embedded tissues using microwaves: A review. Adv Anat Pathol 1995;2:2–9.
474. Gown AM, de Wever N, Battifora H: Microwave-based antigenic unmasking. A revolutionary new technique for routine immunohistochemistry. Appl Immunohistochem 1993;1:256–266.
475. Shi SR, Cote RJ, Chaiwun B, et al: Standardization of immunohistochemistry based on antigen retrieval technique for routine formalin-fixed tissue sections. Appl Immunohistochem 1998;6:89–96.
476. Pileri SA, Roncador G, Ceccarelli C, et al: Antigen retrieval techniques in immunohistochemistry: Comparison of different methods. J Pathol 1997;83:116–123.
477. Prioleau J, Schnitt SJ: p53 antigen loss in stored paraffin slides. N Engl J Med 1995;332:1521–1522.
478. Shin HJ, Kalapurakal SK, Lee JJ, Ro JY, Hong WK, Lee JS: Comparison of p53 immunoreactivity in fresh-cut versus stored slides with and without microwave heating. Mod Pathol 1997;10:224–230.
479. Wester K, Wahlund E, Sundstrom C, et al: Paraffin section storage and immunohistochemistry. Effects of time, temperature, fixation, and retrieval protocol with emphasis on p53 protein and MIB1 antigen. Appl Immunohistochem Molec Morphol 2000;8:61–70.
480. Battifora H: The multitumor (sausage) tissue block. Novel method for immunohistochemical antibody testing. Lab Invest 1986;55:244–248.
481. Miller RT, Groothuis CL: Multitumor "sausage" blocks in immunohistochemistry. Simplified method preparation, practical uses, and roles in quality assurance. Am J Clin Pathol 1991;96:228–232.
482. Kallioniemi OP, Wagner U, Kononen J, Sauter G: Tissue microarray technology for high-throughput molecular profiling of cancer. Hum Mol Genet 2001;10: 657–662.
483. Grogan TM: Automated immunohistochemical analysis. Am J Clin Pathol 1992;98(4 suppl 1):S35–38.
484. Moreau A, Le Neel T, Joubert M, Trouchaud A, Laboisse C: Approach to automation in immunohistochemistry. Clin Chim Acta 1998;278:177–184.
485. Seidal T, Balaton AJ, Battifora H: Interpretation and quantification of immunostains. Am J Surg Pathol 2001;25:1204–1207.
486. Wick MR, Mills SE: Consensual interpretive guidelines for diagnostic immunohistochemistry. Am J Surg Pathol 2001;25:1208–1210.
487. Wood GS, Warnke R: Suppression of endogenous avidin-binding activity in tissues and its relevance to biotin-avidin detection systems. J Histochem Cytochem 1981;29:1196–1204.
488. Rodriguez-Soto J, Warnke RA, Rouse RV: Endogenous avidin-binding activity in paraffin-embedded tissue after microwave treatment. Appl Immunohistochem 1997;5:59–62.
489. Harlow E, Lane D: Antibodies. A Laboratory Manual. Cold Spring, NY, Cold Spring Harbor Laboratory, 1988.

Jerzy Lasota

Genetics of Soft Tissue Tumors

CHAPTER 4

Introduction

Over the past several years, intensive studies on the human cancer genome have identified numerous cancer-specific genetic alterations. Some of them, like chromosomal numerical changes, translocations, large deletions, and gene amplifications are already seen at the cytogenetic level of resolution. Other subtle changes, such as single base pair substitutions, small deletions, or a few nucleotide insertions, require molecular genetic detection.

It is now widely accepted that accumulation of these genetic changes destabilizes cellular growth control mechanisms, promotes uncontrolled clonal proliferation, and results in development of benign and malignant tumors. However, benign tumors compared to malignant ones most likely develop based on subtle genetic changes.

Many genetic alterations affect the function of growth-controlling genes, often called human oncogenes and tumor suppressor genes. Gain of function of oncogenes and loss of function of tumor suppressor genes are among the major molecular events in the development of human cancer. Identification of structural changes in the cancer genome and understanding of their functional consequences are leading to the development of new diagnostic approaches and better treatment strategies targeting the affected gene products and their signaling pathways.

The ongoing "genetic revolution" has already had an impact on surgical pathology of soft tissue tumors (STTs). Detection of specific translocations or translocation gene fusion products can be used as disease-specific markers to improve the diagnosis of STTs. Expression of different variants of the gene fusion products may have prognostic implications. Other genetic alterations can also correlate with favorable or poor clinical outcome. Finally, specific genetic changes can be used in the molecular staging of disease by screening of peripheral blood, bone marrow, or other fluids for minimal residual disease or micrometastases.

Integration of genetics into surgical pathology of STTs is expanding. Genetic studies will add new diagnostic and prognostic assays and define new markers to guide the optimal treatment. Collection of fresh or frozen tumor tissue will expedite the progress in the genetic studies and enable utilization of a wider spectrum of techniques. Incorporation of the new information into diagnostic pathology requires continuing education for the surgical pathologist in molecular genetics.

Oncogenes in STTs

Proto-oncogenes are human cellular genes often involved in cellular growth and differentiation, and many of them are growth factor receptors. Some of these genes show sequence homology to known retroviral oncogenes.

Gain-of-function genetic mutations can change proto-oncogenes into active oncogenes, which are presumed to lead to uncontrolled cell growth and development of cancer.

Gene transfer assays were the first in vitro experiments that provided strong evidence of existence of oncogenes in human cancer. In these assays, human cancer DNA transferred into mouse recipient cells induced neoplastic transformation. Following gene transfer experiments, a number of human oncogenes have been identified. Progress in cancer cytogenetics and positional cloning of genetic alterations led to the identification of other human proto-oncogenes activated by translocations, amplifications, or subtle molecular genetic mutations.[1]

RAS Gene Family

The first human oncogene ever identified, HRAS, was discovered, cloned, and sequenced following a gene transfer experiment in which DNA extracted from a human bladder carcinoma cell line was transferred to mouse NIH3T3 cells and induced neoplastic transformation.[2,3] Comparison of the nucleotide sequences of normal *HRAS* proto-oncogene and oncogene revealed a G-to-T mutation at codon 12 causing replacement of one amino acid in the encoded protein as the sole difference. This proved that subtle molecular changes can alter gene function and be responsible for neoplastic transformation.[4] In subsequent studies, other members of the RAS family have been identified.[5]

Gain-of-function *RAS* mutations occurring in a few mutational "hot spots" (amino acids 12, 13, 59, and 61) are among the most common genetic changes identified in human cancer. However, the incidence of *RAS* gene mutations varies widely in different types of tumors.[6]

In sarcomas, *RAS* mutations have been reported in subsets of embryonal rhabdomyosarcomas,[7] malignant fibrous histiocytomas,[8,9] liposarcomas (LSs),[9] and leiomyosarcomas/gastrointestinal stromal tumors (GISTs),[10] and in sporadic or thorium dioxide or vinyl chloride exposure-associated hepatic angiosarcomas.[11,12]

Distinct but closely related proteins encoded by genes belonging to the RAS family play a central role in signal transduction leading to cell proliferation or apoptotic cell death. Activation of RAS, the 21-kd protein, which is localized on the inner surface of the cell membrane, occurs through the signaling initiated by growth factor binding to the membrane tyrosine kinase receptors. Activated RAS-GTP protein, in turn, starts signaling cascades leading to cell growth and differentiation.[13] Recent studies have shown that blocking of the pathologically activated RAS signaling pathways could be a rational anticancer therapy.[14,15]

Oncogenic Protein Tyrosine Kinase Receptors and Their Therapeutic Inhibition

Protein tyrosine kinases (PTKs) are important regulators of signal transduction pathways. More than 90 genes have been identified in the human genome to encode either receptor or cytoplasmic nonreceptor PTKs.[16] Structural or functional alterations of PTKs can result in dominant oncogenic activity causing malignant transformation in hematopoietic, mesenchymal, and epithelial cells.[17]

KIT proto-oncogene, the human homolog of v-kit (segment of Hardy-Zuckerman 4 feline sarcoma virus), is mapped to 4q11-q12. It encodes a PTK receptor for stem cell factor.[18] Gain-of-function KIT mutations leading to oncogenic activation of the gene have been reported in familial and sporadic GISTs.[19,20] Most of these mutations have been documented in the juxtamembrane domain (exon 11) of the gene, but extracellular (exon 9) and tyrosine kinase domains (exons 13 and 17) can also be mutated (see Chapter 11). Successful inhibition of the oncogenic KIT activity in metastatic GISTs using tyrosine kinase inhibitor imatinib mesylate (STI571/Gleevec, Novartis Pharmaceuticals, East Hanover, NJ) is the first example of this type of therapy in sarcomas.[21,22] However, a response to the tyrosine kinase inhibitor-based therapy might vary by the type of *KIT* mutation.[23]

Among other targets for this type of therapy can be dermatofibrosarcoma protuberans (DFSP). This tumor is characterized by a specific t(17;22)(q22;q13.1) chromosome translocation or supernumerary ring chromosome derived from t(17;22).[24,25] As a result of this translocation, the *COL1A1* gene, mapped to 17q22, encoding component of type I collagen and plated-derived growth factor, β chain (*PDGFB*) gene, a human homologue of v-sis oncogene, are rearranged and fused.[26]

COL1A1-PDGFB gene fusion results in production of mature PDGFB and leads to autocrine growth stimulation through the PDGF receptor. Expression of COL1A1-PDGFB fusion protein increases growth rate of transfected cells and causes their morphologic transformation. Moreover, expression of this oncoprotein is tumorigenic in nude mice.[27,28] Recent studies showed that treatment with STI571, a tyrosine kinase inhibitor, causes growth inhibition of DFSP-derived cell cultures and mouse tumors, apparently by its ability to inhibit PDGFR.[29]

Targeting the pathologically activated PTK receptors with tyrosine kinase inhibitors is a new, biology-based therapeutic strategy for subsets of human sarcomas whose proliferation is driven by oncogenetically activated PTK receptors.[30–32]

Translocations and Oncogenic Gene Fusions

Translocations are common primary cytogenetic aberrations in human cancer. They form abnormal chromosomes containing genetic material from two or more chromosomes. A reciprocal translocation generates two translocated chromosomes by a reciprocal exchange of chromosomal material. A nonreciprocal translocation refers to the situation when only one translocated chromosome is present.

Translocations variably lead to recombination of regulatory or coding sequences of different genes. Replacement of regulatory sequences results in abnormal expression of a normal protein, such as BCL-2 or BCL-1. These translocations are typical of specific types of lymphomas, such as follicular and mantle cell ones, and are not common in sarcomas. Recombination of coding sequences of different genes leads to the formation of pathologic fusion genes and expression of the pathologic gene fusion products. These translocations are typical of specific types of sarcomas and some types of hematopoietic malignancies, such as chronic myeloid leukemia.

Gene fusion proteins are believed to act like oncoproteins promoting uncontrolled cell growth and tumor formation. The normal function of many of the genes targeted by translocations and the biologic effects of translocation-related oncoproteins are not fully understood, despite intensive studies. However, many of the involved genes encode for transcriptional regulators and for other signaling proteins. Identification of genes directly or indirectly targeted by the oncoproteins and understanding of the biochemical events caused by the oncoproteins are important steps toward the development of new therapeutic strategies targeting the pathologically activated cell signaling pathways.

Because the translocations in general are specific for particular types of tumors, they are useful diagnostic markers, as detected cytogenetically or by gene fusion assays. However, different members of a gene family can be involved in tumor-specific translocations, and different fusions may occur between the fused genes. This contributes to structural and possibly functional diversity among the gene fusion products, which in some cases, may have a prognostic significance.[33–37] Examples of STT-specific chromosome translocations and other rearrangements leading to gene fusions and oncogenic activation of proto-oncogenes are shown in Table 4–1.

Translocations and Gene Fusions Involving *EWS* and Related Genes

The first cytogenetically and molecular genetically characterized translocation in STTs was a t(11;22)(q24;q12) chromosome translocation specific for Ewing sarcoma.[38,39] Subsequently, the same translocation was identified in peripheral neuroepithelioma and Askin tumor,[40,41] suggesting that these tumors are phenotypic variants and belong to the Ewing sarcoma family.

The t(11;22) translocation rearranges and fuses *EWS* and *FLI1* genes.[42,43] The genomic breakpoints are dispersed and several types of EWS-FLI1 fusion transcripts have been identified.[44] Presence of the so-called type I EWS-FLI1 fusion transcript characterized by the fusion of *EWS* exon 7 and *FLI1* exon 6 is a prognostically favorable variant.[45]

Subsequently, other rare Ewing sarcoma-specific translocations were identified and several new fusion genes were cloned. All these fusions involved the *EWS* gene and genes *ERG, ETV1, ETV4, FEV,* or *ZSG* belonging to the ETS transcription factor gene family, like FLI1.[46–51] The second most frequent gene fusion in Ewing sarcoma is *EWS-ERG*. Presence of the EWS-FLI1 (without subtyping of the fusions) or EWS-ERG fusion transcripts showed no difference in clinical behavior.[52]

Detection of the EWS-FLI1 and EWS-ERG fusions in more than 80% of Ewing sarcomas creates a basis for a sensitive and specific molecular genetic diagnosis for these tumors.[34] Occasionally, EWS-FLI1 fusion transcripts have been reported in other childhood sarcomas with polyphenotypic, myogenic, or neural differentiation.[53–55] Whether these tumors represent a separate entity or are related to the Ewing sarcoma family should be investigated. Also, this provides a further argument that diagnosis and classification of tumors should be based on both molecular genetic and morphologic perspective. Unexpected detection of the EWS-FLI1 transcripts in olfactory neuroblastoma[56] and more recently in giant cell tumor of bone[57] raised new controversies, because their presence could not be confirmed by others.[58–60]

Molecular genetic studies of other STT-specific translocations revealed that *EWS* gene and other members of TET family are often fused with genes belonging to the ETS family. EWS was found to be a fusion partner to the *ATF-1* gene in t(12;22)(q13;q12) specific for clear cell sarcoma,[61] to the *WT-1* gene in t(11;22)(p13;q12) specific for desmoplastic round cell tumor,[62,63] to the *CHN* gene in the t(9;22)(q22;q12) specific for myxoid chondrosarcoma,[64,65] and to the *CHOP* gene in t(12;16)(q13;p11) specific for myxoid liposarcoma.[66]

Table 4–1. Examples of Chromosomal Translocations and Other Rearrangements Leading to Formation of Oncogenic Gene Fusions or Overexpression of Normal Genes

Tumor	Aberration	Affected Gene	Reference
Aggressive angiomyxoma	t(8;12)(p12;q15)	*HMGIC*	486
Alveolar soft part sarcoma	t(X;17)(p11;q25)	*ASPL-TFE3*	160, 161
Angiomatoid fibrous histiocytoma*	t(12;16)(q13;p11)	*FUS-ATF1*	95
Chondrosarcoma, extraskeletal myxoid	t(9;22)(q22;q12) t(9;17)(q22;q11) t(9;15)(q22;q21)	*EWS-CHN* *TAF15-CHN* *TCF12-CHN*	64, 65, 69, 70, 71, 495
Clear cell sarcoma	t(12;22)(q13;q12)	*EWS-ATF1*	61
Desmoplastic small round cell tumor	t(11;22)(p13;q12)	*EWS-WT1*	62, 63
Dermatofibrosarcoma protuberans	t(17;22)(q21;q13)	*COL1A1-PDGFB*	24, 25
Endometrial stromal sarcoma	t(7;17)(p15;q21)	*JAXF1-JJAZ1*	487
Ewing's sarcoma/Primitive neuroectodermal tumor	t(11;22)(q24;q12) t(21;22)(q22;q12) t(7;22)(p22;q12) t(17;22)(q12;q12) t(2;22)(q33;q12) 22q12 rearrangement t(1;16)(q21;q13)†	*EWS-FLI1* *EWS-ERG* *EWS-ETV1* *EWS-ETV4* *EWS-FEV* *EWS-ZSG* ?	38–43, 46–51, 491
Fibrosarcoma, infantile Cellular mesoblastic nephroma	t(12;15)(p13;q25)	*ETV6-NTRK3*	148, 155, 156
Hemangioendothelioma, epithelioid*	t(1;3)(p36.3;q25)	?	488
Hemangiopericytoma*	t(12;19)(q13;q13)	?	489
Inflammatory myofibroblastic tumor	2p23 rearrangements	*TPM3-ALK* *TPM4-ALK* *CLTC-ALK*	146, 147
Leiomyoma, uterine	t(12;14)(q15;q24)	*RAD51B-HMGIC*	490
Lipoblastoma	8q12 rearrangements	*PLAG1* *HAS2-PLAG1* *COL1A2-PLAG1*	492–494
Lipoma	t(3;12)(q27;q14-q15) t(12;13)(q13-q15;q12-q14) 6p23-21 rearrangements 12q14-15 rearrangements	*HMGIC-LPP* *HMGIC-LHPF* *HMGIY* *HMGIC*	78, 173, 174
Liposarcoma, myxoid/round cell	t(12;16)(q13;p11) t(12;22)(q13;q12)	*FUS-CHOP* *EWS-CHOP*	66–68, 83
Rhabdomyosarcoma, alveolar	t(2;13)(q35;q14) t(1;13)(p36;q14)	*PAX3-FKHR* *PAX7-FKHR*	101–104
Synovial sarcoma	t(X;18)(p11;q11)	*SYT-SSX1* *SYT-SSX2* *SYT-SSX4*	135–138

*Small number of cases analyzed
†Secondary nonrandom translocation, all cases also contain the t(11;22)

The *FUS* gene of the TET family was shown to be fused to *CHOP* in t(12;16)(q13;p11) of myxoid liposarcoma,[67,68] *TAFII68* and *TCF12* to *CHN* in t(9;17)(q22;q11) and t(9;15)(q22;q21) of the myxoid chondrosarcoma-specific translocations.[69–71]

Translocations rearranging the TET and ETS families seem to represent molecular events highly specific for certain types of STTs. However, a t(16;21)(p11;q22) chromosome translocation, reported in a subset of acute myeloid leukemias, results in gene fusion between the *TLS* and *ERG* members of the TET and ETS families.[72,73]

The TET family is characterized by a putative RNA binding domain at the C-terminus and a glutamine rich N-terminus, whereas the ETS family is defined by a specific DNA-binding domain and flanking protein-protein interaction domains. Products of TET-ETS fusion consist of an N-terminal portion of TET and DNA-binding domain of ETS. Functions of these fusion proteins are not fully known. Based on studies on EWS-FLI1, it seems likely that these fusion proteins act like aberrant transcription factors targeting a network of genes normally modulated by the ETS family transcription factors. However, the EWS-FLI1 fusion protein may also act as an aberrant TET factor and interfere with the normal RNA processing.[34,74,75] Gene fusions involving the ETS transcription factor family are shown in Table 4–2.

The cytogenetic hallmark of myxoid LS is a t(12;16)(q13;p11) chromosome translocation,[76,77] present in more than 90% of cases.[78] This translocation leads to the rearrangement and fusion of the *FUS/TLS* gene, mapped to 16p11 and the *CHOP* gene, mapped to12q13.[67,68]

FUS (for fusion), also called TLS (for translocated in liposarcoma), encodes for a nuclear RNA-binding protein and shares extensive sequence homology with *EWS*.[79] *CHOP* (for C/EBP homologous protein), also referred to as GADD153 or DDIT3, is a member of leucine zipper transcription factor family[67,68] and plays a role in adipocyte differentiation and growth arrest.[80,81] *FUS-CHOP* fusion consists of the N-terminus of *FUS* and DNA binding and leucine zipper dimerization domain of *CHOP*.[67,68] The FUS-CHOP oncoprotein can inhibit adipocyte differentiation.[82]

A t(12;22)(q13;q12) chromosome translocation, cytogenetic variant of t(12;16), involves the *EWS* and *CHOP* genes. In this translocation, the N-terminus of EWS, a functional equivalent of FUS, is fused to CHOP.[66,83] Expression of FUS-CHOP and EWS-CHOP in murine cells revealed transforming activity. In both cases, the oncogenic effect was related to the FUS or EWS component of the fusion protein and could not be fully substituted by fusion of other activators with the CHOP.[84,85] In nude mice, TLS/FUS-CHOP induced formation of tumors analogous to human myxoid liposarcomas.[84]

Identification of t(12;16) and FUS-CHOP fusion transcripts in the round cell component of myxoid LS and in pure round cell LS supported the notion that myxoid and round cell LS represent a phenotypic spectrum of one genetically related disease.[86–88] Of the two common variants of *FUS-CHOP* gene fusion, types I and II, the latter is more frequent.[86–89]

Table 4–2. Oncogenic Fusion Involving Gene Encoding for Transcription Factors

<table>
<tr><th colspan="2">Fusion gene</th><th>Sarcoma</th><th>Leukemia/Lymphoma</th><th>Carcinoma</th></tr>
<tr><td>TCF12</td><td>CHN</td><td rowspan="3">Extraskeletal myxoid chondrosarcoma</td><td rowspan="14"></td><td rowspan="15"></td></tr>
<tr><td>TAF15</td><td>CHN</td></tr>
<tr><td rowspan="10">EWS</td><td>CHN</td></tr>
<tr><td>FLI1</td><td rowspan="6">Ewing/PNET</td></tr>
<tr><td>ERG</td></tr>
<tr><td>ETV1</td></tr>
<tr><td>ETV4</td></tr>
<tr><td>FEV</td></tr>
<tr><td>ZSG</td></tr>
<tr><td>WT1</td><td>Desmoplastic small round cell tumor</td></tr>
<tr><td>ATF1</td><td>Clear cell sarcoma</td></tr>
<tr><td>CHOP</td><td rowspan="2">Myxoid liposarcoma</td></tr>
<tr><td rowspan="3">FUS</td><td>CHOP</td></tr>
<tr><td>ATF1</td><td>Angiomatoid fibrous histiocytoma</td></tr>
<tr><td>ERG</td><td></td><td>Acute myeloid leukemia</td></tr>
<tr><td>ASPL</td><td>TFE3</td><td>Alveolar soft part sarcoma</td><td rowspan="3"></td><td rowspan="3">Renal cell carcinoma</td></tr>
<tr><td>PRCC</td><td>TFE3</td><td rowspan="2"></td></tr>
<tr><td>SFPQ</td><td>TFE3</td></tr>
</table>

However, identification of fusion type seems to have no prognostic value.[90]

Three different types of previously reported FUS-CHOP fusion transcripts and two new variants were detected in 1 of 3 well-differentiated and in 4 of 14 pleomorphic LSs in one study,[91] but these findings were not confirmed in other reverse transcription-polymerase chain reaction (RT-PCR) studies.[86–88] In addition, neither t(12;16) nor CHOP or FUS rearrangements have been reported in well-differentiated or pleomorphic LS.[92–94] Thus, this translocation and its gene fusion products should be considered diagnostic of myxoid LS.

A t(12;16)(12q13;16p11.2) leading to the rearrangement of TET and ETS family genes has been described in a case of angiomatoid fibrous histiocytoma (see Chapter 20). Using an RT-PCR approach, the *FUS-ATF1* gene fusion product was identified in this tumor.[95] However, more cases should be evaluated to confirm that the *FUS-ATF1* gene fusion is specific for this tumor.

Translocations and Gene Fusions Involving *PAX* and *FKHR* Genes

Alveolar rhabdomyosarcoma (ARMS) is characterized by two tumor-specific chromosomal translocations: t(2;13)(q35;q14) and t(1;13)(p36;q14).[96–100] These translocations result in fusions of the *PAX3* or *PAX7* genes, mapped to 2q35 and 1p36, with the *FKRH* gene mapped to 13q14.[101–104]

PAX3 and *PAX7* genes are members of the PAX (paired box) transcription factor gene family and show high structural and sequence similarities. *PAX* genes are involved in embryogenesis, and expression of murine PAX3 and PAX7 homologues was documented during the development of nervous and muscular systems.[105–107]

Loss-of-function *PAX3* mutations have been implicated in congenital neural and muscular anomalies seen in mice (splotch mouse) and humans (Waardenburg type I–III and craniofacial-deafness-hand) malformation syndromes.[108–113]

FKHR (forkhead-related), also called *FOXO1A*, belongs to one of the FOX gene subfamilies, members of which encode a transcription factor with a highly conserved DNA-binding motif related to the *Drosophila* region-specific homeotic gene "forkhead."[114] *FKHR* and other subfamily members, *AFX* and *FKHRL1*, play a role in insulin-signaling pathways regulating apoptosis.[115–117]

PAX3-FKRH and *PAX7-FKRH* fusion genes contain highly homologous PAX3- and PAX7-derived N-terminal DNA-binding domains fused to the activating, COOH-terminal domain of the *FKHR* gene. Expression studies in ARMS showed that fusion proteins are overexpressed, compared to wild-type *PAX* gene expression. Overexpression of PAX7-FKHR results from a secondary genetic event, amplification of the *PAX7-FKHR* fusion gene. Overexpression of PAX3-FKHR is believed to result from a higher transcriptional rate of the pathologic fusion gene, compared to that of the wild-type *PAX3*.[118–121]

Oncogenic PAX3-FKRH fusion protein acts as a strong transcriptional activator and shows transforming ability when introduced into cell culture.[122,123] Murine cells with the PAX3-FKRH expression construct revealed activation of genes involved in the myogenic pathways.[124]

Chromosome translocations t(2;13) and t(1;13) and their gene fusion products represent highly specific and sensitive genetic markers useful in the molecular diagnosis of ARMS, seen in approximately 80% of cases.[104] Correlation between the type of gene fusion and the clinical features has been identified. PAX7-FKHR tumors often represent extremity lesions, have a more limited pattern of metastatic disease, and have a longer disease-free survival than the PAX3-FKHR tumors, which have an adverse prognosis with more extensive metastasis.[125,126] In an ARMS cell line, PAX3-FKHR fusion protein increased in vitro proliferative rate and promoted cell growth in the absence of added growth factors,[127] and showed increased cell cycle deregulation, as compared with the PAX7-FKHR$^+$ tumors; this may contribute to a poorer prognosis.[128]

Synovial Sarcoma-Specific t(X;18) Translocation and *SYT-SSX* Gene Fusions

Synovial sarcoma-specific t(X;18)(p11;q11) was first described in 1986 as a cytogenetic observation.[129] A t(X;18) and its rare variant translocations are synovial sarcoma-specific and have not been reported in other cancers.[130–132] This translocation involves the *SYT* gene on chromosome 18 and one of the *SSX* genes on chromosome X, leading to the functional *SYT-SSX* fusion.[133]

Five different *SSX* genes have been identified,[134] of which *SSX1* and *SSX2* are common fusion partners with *SYT*.[135,136] However, two cases of a rare *SYT-SSX4* fusion were recently reported.[137,138] SSX1 and SSX2 genomic sequences and the encoded proteins are highly homologous. Thus, the SYT-SSX1 and SYT-SSX2 fusion junctions are almost identical. Heterogeneity within the fusion junctions is rare, although variants of nonrecurrent fusions with different junctions and with the insertions of additional genetic material have been described.[135,136,139]

Both the normal SYT and SSX proteins and the SYT-SSX fusion protein are localized in the nucleus, where SYT interacts with BRM proteins and SSX with a polycomb group of proteins. Normal SYT and SSX proteins appear to be involved in transcriptional regulation, SYT as an activator and SSX as repressor of transcription. The function of the SYT-SSX fusion protein and the possible interaction between the SYT-SSX and the normal SYT and SSX targets are not fully understood.[132,140] Ongoing studies may soon define a molecular genetic model for the complex interactions between the normal SYT and SSX and the SYT-SSX fusion proteins.

Detection of SYT-SSX fusion transcripts by RT-PCR is a highly specific and sensitive genetic marker for the diagnosis of synovial sarcoma.[132,140] Clinicopathologic studies have shown a correlation between the clinical behavior and the type of SYT-SSX fusion. The presence of the SYT-SSX1 type of fusion correlates with a higher rate of proliferation and a shorter metastasis-free survival, whereas SYT-SSX2 is a favorable prognostic factor for overall survival and is seen almost exclusively in tumors with monophasic spindle cell morphology.[141,142] SYT-SSX fusions have been detected in both the spindle cell and epithelioid components of biphasic tumors.[143–145]

Translocations and Gene Fusions Involving PTK Receptors

Anaplastic lymphoma kinase (ALK) and neurotrophic tyrosine kinase receptor, type 3 (NTRK3), 2 of the 58 known human transmembrane PTK receptors, have been shown to be pathologically activated in STTs by chromosome translocations. ALK is involved in inflammatory myofibroblastic (IMF) tumors by oncogenic fusions to the *TPM3*, *TPM4*, and *CLTC* genes,[146,147] and NTRK3 in infantile fibrosarcoma by oncogenic fusion to the *ETV6* gene.[148]

The *ALK* gene was first identified as a fusion partner of nucleophosmin (*NPM1*) gene in the t(2;5)(p23;q35), the main chromosomal translocation in anaplastic large cell lymphoma. The *ALK* gene, mapped to 2p23, encodes for a transmembrane receptor PTK and has a structure typical of a PTK receptor with a large extracellular domain, a transmembrane segment, and a tyrosine kinase domain. *NPM*, mapped to 5q35, encodes for a 38-kd nucleolar phosphoprotein.[149]

The NMP-ALK fusion protein consists of an N-terminus of NPM containing an oligomerization motif and a cytoplasmic tyrosine kinase domain of ALK. The NPM-mediated oligomerization leads to the constitutive activation of NPM-ALK tyrosine kinase function. A strong NPM promoter results in a high level of expression of the NPM-ALK fusion protein. This fusion oncoprotein shows a strong in vitro transforming potential in both hematopoietic and fibroblastic cell lines. Molecular mechanisms leading to NPM-ALK–mediated oncogenic transformation can involve the activation of several pathways including *RAS*, PLC-γ, PI-3 kinase and STAT3.[150,151]

Several variants of ALK fusions including TPM3-ALK[152,153] and CLTC-ALK[154] have been identified in anaplastic large cell lymphoma over the past few years. In all these fusions, the NPM N-terminus with the oligomerization motif is replaced by other proteins containing functionally similar motifs leading to the activation of ALK kinase domain.[150,151]

A nonrandom t(12;15)(p13;q25) chromosomal translocation leads to the fusion of the *ETV6* and *NTRK3* genes in infantile fibrosarcoma. This gene fusion represents another example of pathologic activation of a PTK receptor.[148] An identical t(12;15) translocation associated with the *ETV-NTRK3* gene fusion was also found in the "cellular" form of congenital mesoblastic nephroma.[155] Morphologic and genetic similarity between congenital mesoblastic nephroma and infantile fibrosarcoma suggest that both lesions represent a single neoplastic entity in either renal or soft tissue locations.[155,156] The ETV6-NTRK3 chimeric transcript consists of helix-loop-helix dimerization domain of ETV6 (ETS variant gene 6 also known as TEL) fused to the protein tyrosine kinase domain of NTRK3. ETV6-NTRK3 oncoprotein expressed in NIH3T3 cells deregulates NTRK3 signaling pathways, leads to high constitutive expression of cyclin D1 and an aberrant cell cycle progression.[157,158] A t(12;15)(p13;q25) chromosomal translocation and the resulting *ETV6-NTRK3* gene fusion have also been reported in a case of acute myeloid leukemia.[159]

Presence of similar gene fusions in tumors derived from different cell lineages, hematopoietic and mesenchymal, suggests that oncogenic activation of PTK receptors and deregulations of PTK signaling pathways may represent a universal oncogenic mechanism.[150] Gene fusions involving PTK receptors are shown in Table 4–3.

ASPL-TFE3 Gene Fusion in Alveolar Soft Part Sarcoma and Renal Tumors

Recently, a t(X;17)(p11.2;q25) chromosomal translocation was identified in a case of alveolar soft part sarcoma.[160] As a result of this translocation, the *ASPL* gene mapped to 17q25 is fused in-frame to the *TFE3* gene mapped to Xp11.2. The *ASPL-TFE3* gene fusion consists of N-terminus of *ASPL* and *TFE3* DNA-binding domain. Using an RT-PCR assay, ASPL-TFE3

Table 4–3. Oncogenic Fusion Involving Gene Encoding for Protein Tyrosine Kinase Receptors

Fusion gene		Sarcoma	Leukemia/Lymphoma
NPM	ALK		Anaplastic large cell lymphoma
CLTC		Inflammatory myofibroblastic tumor	
TPM3			
TPM4			
ETV6	NTRK3	Infantile fibrosarcoma Cellular mesoblastic nephroma	Acute myeloid leukemia

fusion transcripts were consistently detected in all 12 alveolar soft part sarcomas analyzed.[161]

ASPL, also called *ASPSCR1* (for alveolar soft part sarcoma chromosome region, candidate 1), is a newly identified human gene. The function of the corresponding protein is unknown.[161]

The *TFE3* gene is a member of the helix-loop-helix family of transcription factors and was identified as a fusion partner in the t(X;1)(p11;q21), t(X;1)(p11.2;p34) and t(X;17)(p11.2;q25) translocations in papillary renal cell carcinoma. These translocations result in fusions of *PRCC*, *SFPQ*, and *RCC17* gene sequences to the TFE3 DNA-binding domain. Replacement of the N-terminus and retention of the TFE3 DNA-binding domain implicate transcriptional deregulation as a possible tumorigenic mechanism.[162–164]

Subsequent studies identified RCC17 as *ASPL* gene and confirmed the presence of ASPL-TFE3 fusion products in a subset of renal cell carcinomas in children and young adults. This tumor may be a distinctive entity sharing genetic features with alveolar soft part sarcoma.[165]

Translocations and Other Rearrangements Involving the *HMGIC* Gene

Genetic alterations of the 12q13-15 have been extensively documented in a variety of malignant and benign STTs.[78] Amplification of 12q13-15 was reported in a subset of sarcomas. *CHOP* and *ATF1* genes involved in myxoid LS and clear cell sarcoma-specific translocations were mapped to this region. Rearrangements of 12q13-15 were also reported in a variety of benign tumors including lipomas, uterine leiomyomas, pulmonary chondroid hamartomas, aggressive angiomyxomas, pleomorphic adenomas of the salivary gland, fibroadenomas, and adenolipomas of the breast.[166–168] A typical feature of the 12q13-15–related translocations is participation of different chromosome partners. For example, in lipomas, at least 10 different chromosomes have been indicated as the partners of translocations involving the 12q13-15 region.[78] The most common of these are t(3;12) and t(12;13).

Subsequent molecular studies identified the *HMGIC* gene, mapped to 12q15, as the gene playing a critical role in the alterations involving 12q13-q15.[167] HMGIC encodes for a protein that consists of three DNA-binding domains (AT-hook domains) and an acidic C-terminal tail. HMGIC protein belongs to the HMG family.[169] Three spliced forms of HMGI(Y) proteins are the other members of this family.[170] HMGI proteins are involved in the regulation of chromatin structure and function.[171]

Cloning of the t(3;12)(q27;q14-q15) chromosomal translocation revealed a gene fusion involving *HMGIC* and a novel member of LIM protein family, *LPP* (lipoma preferred partner) gene.[172] However *HMGIC-LPP* fusion is frequent among lipomas, is not lipoma specific, and was also detected in pulmonary chondroid hamartomas.[173] HMGIC-LPP fusion protein consists of three HMGIC DNA-binding domains and three LPP LIM domains.[166,172]

HMGIC-LHFP fusion protein resulting from t(12;13)(q13-q15;q12-q14) translocation similarly to HMGIC-LPP consists of three DNA-binding domains of HMGIC and an ectopic sequence, representing 69 amino acids encoded by a frameshifted LHFP (lipoma HMGIC fusion partner) sequence.[174] Thus, the fusion mechanisms underlying HMGIC rearrangements, consistently separate HMGIC DNA binding domains from the C-terminal region and fuse to ectopic sequences from other genes.[166,167] Fused ectopic sequences can include only a few amino acids.[175,176] In some cases, ectopic sequences were identified to be located within the fourth HMGIC intron and may represent abnormal splicing induced by genetic mutations in the vicinity of the gene.[177]

Similar types of *HMGIC* gene rearrangements were found in human sarcomas including well-differentiated liposarcomas. HMGIC truncation often coexists with gene amplification and overexpression, which may contribute to tumorigenesis of well-differentiated liposarcomas.[178,179]

Expression of truncated HMGIC in murine fibroblasts was shown to induce in vitro neoplastic transformation. However, acquisition of ectopic sequences does not increase the transforming potential of the truncated HMGIC indicating that the specific truncation of the gene rather than its fusion with other genes is responsible for the oncogenic potential.[180]

Transgenic mice carrying a truncated HMGIC were shown to develop a giant phenotype with predominantly abdominal and pelvic lipomatosis[181] and had increased incidence of lipomas.[182] In contrast, HMGIC null mice showed a pygmy phenotype and reduced body weight with a decrease in body fat.[183]

HMGI(Y) gene, mapped to 6p21, was identified as a possible target of chromosome rearrangements involving this region in benign tumors, including lipomas.[184–186] HMGI(Y) intragenic deletions were demonstrated in two cases of lipoma.[187] Recent studies showed that the HMGI(Y) proteins, similar to the HMGIC protein, can play an important role in adipocytic growth and differentiation. Suppression of the HMGI(Y) expression in vitro in mouse 3T3-L1 preadipocytic murine cells increased the growth rate and prevented terminal adipocyte differentiation suggesting that HMGI(Y) proteins may regulate adipocyte growth.[171,188]

Detection of Translocations and Gene Fusion Products

Specific translocations, gene fusions, and gene fusion products can be detected using a spectrum of cytogenetic, molecular cytogenetic, and molecular genetic techniques. Combined use of the cytogenetic and molecular genetic assays can be helpful in eliminating false-negative results in some cases, although this may not be realistic in a clinical setting. Critical evaluation of unexpectedly negative or positive results of genetic assays and use of negative and positive controls should be always included as quality control measures (see "Techniques for Genetic Analysis" in this chapter).

Some pathologic fusion transcripts have been detected in tumors without specific chromosome translocations, including some with normal karyotypes.[54,70,189–191] The presence of pathologic fusion transcripts in these cases is most likely the result of cytogenetically undetectable cryptic rearrangements.[54,70] A good example of such a cryptic rearrangement is the recently reported subtle chromosome aberration, inversion of 5′ portion of EWS, and insertion into chromosome 21, which created *EWS-ERG* gene fusion typical of the t(22;21) chromosome translocation seen in some Ewing sarcomas.[192]

The presence of some gene fusion sequences in normal human cells has been documented using PCR-based assays. Genomic sequences of t(14;18) translocation, and *BCR-ABL* and *NPM-ALK* gene fusion transcripts have been detected in peripheral blood of healthy individuals.[193–195] However, so far STT-specific fusion transcripts have not been shown in normal tissues or peripheral blood of healthy individuals.

DNA Amplification in STTs

DNA amplification means multiplication of genes located in the amplified region (amplicon), and as a consequence leads to the overexpression of their protein products. Amplified DNA is associated with two cytogenetically detectable abnormalities, extrachromosomal double minutes (dmin) and intrachromosomal, homogenous staining regions (hsr). The dmins and hsrs are interchangeable forms of amplified DNA. The hsrs can become detached and be excised from the chromosome and form dmins, and dmins can be integrated into another chromosome and form hsrs. Amplicons can be demonstrated by a spectrum of cytogenetic and molecular genetic techniques. These include karyotyping, fluorescence in situ hybridization (FISH), comparative genomic hybridization (CGH), Southern blot hybridization (SBH), and assays based on PCR amplification. However, interphase FISH may be the most practical method for the clinical testing of DNA amplification.[1,35,36,78,196]

The *MYC* gene, located on the chromosome band 8q24, was the first cellular oncogene shown to be amplified in human cancer.[197,198] Amplification of *MYC* was found in primary aggressive and metastatic tumors.[199] Four- to sevenfold amplification of *MYC* was demonstrated in a subset of high-grade soft tissue sarcomas.[200] Subsequently, *MYCN*, the other member of the MYC oncogene family (helix-loop-helix leucine zipper class of transcription factors) was identified[201] and mapped to the chromosome 2p24.[202] High-level MYCN amplification and up to 100-fold overexpression was reported in childhood neuroblastoma cell lines and clinically aggressive neuroblastomas with poor clinical outcome.[203,204] Evaluation of *MYCN* status in neuroblastoma is now considered a useful clinical test important for the design of the appropriate therapy.[205]

Amplification of the 12q13-15 region is a common event in human brain tumors and STTs. This region is frequently rearranged in a variety of benign and malignant STTs.[78] Several genes including *GLI*, *MDM2*, *CHOP*, *CDK4*, *SAS*, and *HMGIC* have been mapped to the 12q13-15 (http://www.ncbi.nlm.nih.gov/). However, the molecular structure of this amplicon is complex and not entirely known.[206] Two amplification units, one including CDK4/SAS and another MDM2, have been identified.[207–209] However, more amplification units may exist.[207] These units can either be coamplified or amplified separately.[208] In some cases, other genes (*CHOP*, *GLI*, *RAP1B*, *LRP1*, and *IFNG*) located in the 12q13-15 region have been found to be coamplified but not consistently expressed.[209] Functional consequences of these complex genetic changes are still under investigation.

The *MDM2* ("murine double minute") gene is a human homolog of the evolutionarily highly conserved gene, initially identified in the 3T3DM mouse cell line.[210] The *MDM2* gene encodes for a 90-kd zinc finger protein that contains a TP53 binding site.[211] *MDM2* regulates TP53 actions either through inhibiting the transactivating function of TP53 in the nucleus or by targeting TP53 degradation in the cytoplasm.[212] MDM2 interacts with the retinoblastoma (RB) protein and can inhibit its growth regulatory capacity.[213] Thus, the overexpression of the MDM2 oncoprotein promotes cell survival and cell cycle progression leading to deregulated cell proliferation, which is a fundamental event in tumorigenesis.

Different amplification patterns have been reported in various types of sarcomas. Amplification of *MDM2* alone has been observed in soft tissue but not bone sarcomas. The opposite, namely, amplification of CDK4 without MDM2 amplification, was observed only in osteosarcomas and chondrosarcomas.[214] This may reflect the primary involvement of two different pathways, MDM2-TP53 in soft tissue sarcomas versus CDK4-RB in bone tumors. Among fatty tumors, amplification of 12q13-15 was seen almost exclusively in well-differentiated LSs and atypical lipomas, but not in other subtypes.[215] Supernumerary ring and giant rod marker chromosomes are characteristic cytogenetic features of these tumors and carry amplified 12q13-21 sequences and multiplied copies of MDM2.[216,217] Based on CGH studies, overrepresentation of 12q13-21 was suggested to be useful in separating lipoma-like LSs from lipomas.[218] Lack of MDM2 immunoreactivity in lipomas[219] seems to confirm the diagnostic significance of this observation.

Tumor Suppressor Genes

Extensive genetic studies of inherited cancer syndromes resulted in the identification of genes, now called tumor suppressor genes, whose inactivation by genetic mutations promotes development of inherited forms of cancer. Further studies indicated that somatic inactivation of these genes can also play an important role in development of sporadic tumors. Since the retinoblastoma gene (*RB1*), the first human tumor suppressor gene, was identified, the list of tumor suppressor genes has extended rapidly. Some of these genes are important cell cycle regulators. Physiologic function of other suppressor genes is not well characterized and understood. Here, we present examples of hereditary cancer syndromes and tumor suppressor genes whose inactivation is fundamental for the development of these syndromes and related soft tissue tumors. They include *RB1*, *TP53*, *CHK2*, *CDKN2A*, *WT1*, *SMARCB1*, *NF1*, *NF2*, and *APC* (Table 4–4).

Retinoblastoma Gene *(RB1)*

Hereditary retinoblastoma (RB) occurs in young children and usually develops by the age of 3 years. The disease is also characterized by special predisposition to developed radiation treatment-related and nonrelated osteosarcomas.

In the early 1970s, Alfred Knudson formulated a hypothesis explaining the genetic mechanism of cancer development in hereditary RB by inactivation of the hypothetical "retinoblastoma gene," based on epidemiologic studies of familial and sporadic RBs. Knudson assumed that for tumor formation both alleles of the gene had to be inactivated by mutations in a tumor cell.[220,221]

This indeed turned out to be the case. In familial RB, one mutated copy of the gene is inherited, and the second copy is mutated somatically. Because all cells of the body are carrying one inherited mutated allele, the chances of tumor development at an early age are very high. In sporadic tumors, both copies of the gene have to be randomly mutated in one cell, and the probability for such an event is many times lower.

The hypothetical RB gene (*RB1*) has been mapped to 13q14 and subsequently molecularly cloned. The *RB1* gene extends over 200 kb of genomic DNA and consists of 27 exons.[222–224]

Deletions in *RB1* and loss-of-function mutations have been extensively documented in familial and sporadic RB and in RB-related and sporadic osteosarcomas. The majority of mutations are non-

Table 4-4. Examples of Familial Cancer Syndromes, Inherited and Sporadic Tumors, and Affected Gene/Pathways

Inherited Cancer Syndrome	Inherited Tumor	Sporadic Tumor	Affected Gene/Pathway
Familial adenomatous polyposis Familial infiltrative fibromatosis Hereditary desmoid disease	Desmoid	Desmoid	*APC* (5q21)/ *CTNNB1* (3p22)
Familial melanoma/neurofibroma	Neurofibroma	Ewing's sarcoma MFH MPNST	*CDKN2A* (9p21)
Familial retinoblastoma	Retinoblastoma Osteosarcoma	Retinoblastoma	*RB1* (13q14)
Familial Wilms tumor WAGR syndrome Denys-Drash syndrome	Wilms' tumor	Wilms tumor Mesothelioma	*WT1* (11p13)
Li-Fraumeni familial cancer syndrome	Soft tissue and bone sarcomas (rhabdomyosarcoma)	Spectrum of sarcomas	*TP53* (17p13) *CHK2* (22q12)
Neurofibromatosis type 1	Neurofibroma	Neurofibroma MPNST	*NF1* (17q11)
Neurofibromatosis type 2	Meningioma Schwannoma	Meningioma Schwannoma Perineurioma	*NF2* (22q12)
Rhabdoid predisposition syndrome	Malignant rhabdoid tumor	Malignant rhabdoid tumor	*SMARCB1* (22q11)

MFH, malignant fibrous histiocytoma; MPNST, malignant peripheral nerve sheath tumor; WAGR, Wilms tumor, aniridia, genitourinary abnormalities, and mental retardation.

sense mutations creating premature termination codons and leading to inactivation of the RB1 protein. Nonsense mutations and in-frame deletions are rarely reported.[225,226] Alterations of the RB1 pathway have been reported in other than RB or osteosarcoma sporadic human cancers including sarcomas.[227,228] However, frequency of mutational inactivation of the *RB1* gene in soft tissue sarcomas appears to be low.[229,230]

The *RB1* gene, an important cell cycle regulator, encodes for a 105-kd nuclear phosphoprotein, whose phosphorylation status is controlled by enzymatic activity of cyclin-dependent protein kinase (Cdk) complexes. Underphosphorylated RB, an active form of the protein, binds to the transcription regulators and prevents the cell from progressing through the G_1 phase of the cell cycle. Phosphorylated protein allows cell progression into the late G_1 phase and the rest of the cycle. Alteration of *RB1* or its pathway can lead directly to abnormal cell proliferation and development of cancer.[231,232]

In vitro experiments have demonstrated that introduction of a functional *RB1* gene suppresses tumorigenicity of a tumor cell line with an inactivated endogenous *RB1* gene.[233,234]

Thus, *RB1* has become a prototype tumor suppressor gene, which can inhibit tumor formation acting as a negative regulator of cell proliferation. Subsequently, alterations of more tumor suppressor genes, including *TP53* and *CDKN2* involved in the cell cycle regulation, were discovered in inherited and noninherited, sporadic human cancers.

Tumor Protein p53 Gene *(TP53)*

The *TP53* (p53) gene was the second tumor suppressor gene identified in human cancers. This gene was named after the 53-kd cellular protein isolated from SV40 virus-transformed cells that bound to the large T antigen of SV40 T.[235,236] Detection of increased TP53 expression in SV40-transformed cells, low level of expression in normal cells, and transforming activity of TP53 molecular clones in gene transfer experiments, initially suggested that TP53 may act like an oncogene.[237,238] However, cloning and use of the wild-type TP53 in subsequent gene transfer studies showed that *TP53* rather was a tumor suppressor gene inhibiting cell transformation.[239,240]

The normal TP53 protein consists of 393 amino acids and acts as a transcription factor activating the expression of genes that inhibit cell growth. The terms "guardian of the genome" or "cellular gatekeeper for growth and division" were applied to stress the importance of TP53 function in cell cycle control.[241,242]

DNA damage or other cellular stress factors can induce expression of TP53. This protein functions by binding to the CDKN1A (p21) regulatory elements and activates its expression. The CDKN1A protein inhibits Cdk activity preventing phosphorylation of Cdk substrates (RB protein) and blocking cell cycle progression. Cells arrested in G_1 undergo repair of DNA damage before replication. Unsuccessful repair of DNA damage directs a cell into apoptosis. Interruptions of the TP53 pathway promote unregulated cellular growth and prevent cells from entering apoptosis.[231,232,243]

Several mechanisms lead to inactivation of *TP53*. Genetic mutations include deletions of one or both alleles, nonsense or splice site mutations resulting in protein truncation, and missense mutations resulting in the expression of an active dysfunctional mutant TP53 protein. In addition, *TP53* can be inactivated by interactions with viral proteins (SV40 large T antigen, the adenovirus E1B protein, and the human papilloma virus E6 protein) and by the MDM2 cellular protein, frequently overexpressed in human brain tumors and sarcomas due to *MDM2* gene amplification.[244]

The *TP53* gene has been mapped to chromosome 17p13.1.[245,246] Since the first TP53 mutation studies,[247,248] hundreds of *TP53*-inactivating mutations have been documented in a variety of human cancers. The majority of mutations are missense and most of them cluster in the central part of the gene, which encodes for the DNA-binding domain. The most commonly mutated TP53 codons, 175, 245, 248, 249, and 273, have been designated as the mutational hotspots.[249] TP53 mutation databases listing thousands of somatic and more than 100 germline mutations are available online at the European Bioinformatics Institute (EBI, http://www.ebi.ac.uk/) and the International Agency for Research and Cancer (IARC, http://www.iarc.fr/.).

Studies based on TP53 transgenic mice models have also implicated TP53 in tumorigenesis. Transgenic mice carrying a high number of copies of mutated TP53 and a normal wild-type allele developed multiple tumors including osteosarcomas, lung adenocarcinomas, and lymphomas. Transgenic mice homozygous null for TP53 developed tumors and died earlier than mice with heterozygous null/wild-type genotype.[250–253]

Additional evidence confirming that inactivation of TP53 plays an important role in promoting cancer came from the studies on the rare, hereditary Li-Fraumeni syndrome (LFS) characterized by significantly increased frequency of cancer.[254,255] Children and young adults from the LFS families developed a spectrum of tumors including soft tissue and bone sarcomas, brain tumors, adrenocortical tumors, acute leukemias, and premenopausal breast cancers. Some of the families that do not fulfill all classic epidemiologic criteria of LFS are often diagnosed with Li-Fraumeni-like syndrome (LFL). Molecular studies revealed germline *TP53* mutations in the majority of LFS and in some LFL families.[256,257] In addition, loss of heterozygosity (LOH) at the TP53 locus was documented in approximately 50% of tumors from LFS families.[258] Detection of germline (inherited) mutation in one TP53 allele and loss of the second TP53 allele in tumor fulfils Knudson's criteria for tumor suppressor gene. Lack of TP53 mutations in some of LFS or LFL families may suggest that another tumor suppressor gene is involved in those cases.

Checkpoint Kinase 2 Gene *(CHK2)*

This mammalian homolog of yeast Rad53 and cds1+ protein kinases is a cell cycle regulator required for DNA damage and replication checkpoints.[259–261] The CHK2 protein regulates cell cycle interacting with CDC25C and TP53 proteins.[259,262,263] CHK2-deficient mouse embryonic stem cells failed to maintain DNA damage-induced arrest in the G_2 phase and CHK2-deficient thymocytes were resistant to DNA damage-induced apoptosis. In two of three recently published studies, CHK2 heterozygous germline mutations have been identified in the LFS and LFL families.[264,265] These observations provide strong evidence that the *CHK2* gene functionally related to the cell cycle is another tumor suppressor gene.

Cyclin-Dependent Kinase Inhibitor-2A Gene *(CDKN2A)*

Involvement of 9p21 in a spectrum of chromosomal aberrations including inversions, translocations, and deletions has been described in a variety of human cancers, implicating the presence of an important, target locus in this region.[78] The putative tumor suppressor gene found in this region[266,267] and initially called multiple tumor suppressor-1 (*MTS1*) has been shown to encode the previously identified p16(INK4) protein.[268] The CDKN2A name replaced MTS1 because MTS1 had been designated for another gene, malignant transformation suppression-1 gene, located on chromosome 1p.

Subsequent studies have shown that the *CDKN2A* gene encodes two unrelated proteins, p16(INK4) and p19(ARF), by alternative splicing of unique exons, 1α and 1β, to the common exons 2 and 3. While the 1αβ-2-3 transcript encodes p16(INK4), the 1β-2-3 transcript encodes p19(ARF) through an alternative reading frame. p16(INK4a) inhibits phosphorylation of the RB protein and induces a G_1 cell cycle arrest through the interaction with CDK4 and CDK6. The p19(ARF) protein binds to the MDM2 protein and promotes its rapid degradation. Degradation of MDM2 leads to stabilization and accumulation of TP53. The functional consequence of this interaction is restoration of G_1 cell cycle arrest. Thus, genetic mutations involving the 9p21 region and the *CDKN2A* gene region simultaneously affect two different INK4-cyclin D/CDK4-RB and ARF-MDM2-p53 cell cycle-related suppression pathways.[231,232,243,269]

Homozygous deletions affecting the CDKN2A locus have been found in different human cancers including sarcomas.[270,271] Germline mutations affecting p16(INK4A) have been well documented in inherited human malignant melanoma syndromes.[272,273]

De novo methylation of the 5′CpG islands in the CDKN2A promoter region, which causes a complete transcriptional block, has been discovered in cancer but not in normal cells and represents another common mechanism of tumor suppressor gene inactivation.[274]

Another member of the so-called INK4 protein family, p15(INK4B), has been isolated and designated as *CDKN2B*.[275] This gene was mapped adjacent to *CDKN2A* on chromosome 9p21. *CDKN2B* has been shown to be codeleted with *CDKN2A* in cancer cell lines and in primary tumors.[265,267,275,276] However, no mutations selectively affecting *CDKN2B* have been identified in human tumors. Also, mice deficient for the p15(INK4B) do not develop cancer.[271] In contrast, deletion of p16(INK4A)/p19(ARF) or p19(ARF) alone leads to tumorigenesis in mice and gives rise to different types of cancers, including sarcomas.[277,278]

Wilms Tumor Gene *(WT1)*

Inherited Wilms tumor, already reported in 1955,[279] is one of the more extensively studied inherited cancers.[280] Early cytogenetic and restriction fragment-length polymorphism-based studies revealed that both familial and sporadic Wilms tumors show losses on chromosome 11 often involving 11p13.[281–284] Introduction of normal chromosome 11 into a Wilms tumor cell line suppressed the ability of the cell line to form tumors in nude mice.[285] A candidate Wilms tumor suppressor gene, *WT1*, was identified and cloned.[286,287] Subsequently, gene transfer experiments confirmed that the normal *WT1* gene can suppress the growth of Wilms tumor cell lines,[288] and that the dominant-negative mutant of *WT1* can induce transformation by suppressing the function of the wild-type WT1 protein.[289]

The *WT1* gene spans about 50 kb and contains 10 exons, 2 of which (exon 5 and 9) are alternatively spliced. Alternative splicing involving exon 9 creates two forms of the WT1 messenger RNA with three amino acids inserted (+KTS) or absent (−KTS) between zinc fingers III and IV. Four WT1 protein isoforms, created through the alternative splicing, function mainly as transcription factors. However WT1 isoforms containing the KTS insert can also be involved in postranscriptional processing of RNA.[290–293]

WT1 plays a crucial role in normal genitourinary development. Patients with Denys-Dash syndrome, WAGR, and Frasier syndrome, characterized by genitourinary abnormalities, carry germline *WT1* mutations.[294–296] Also WT1 null mice failed to develop kidneys and gonads.[297] In addition to affecting the urogenital system, WT1 is expressed during embryonal development of the central nervous system (CNS), limbs, epicardium, mesothelium, and spleen.[298–300]

Intragenic *WT1* mutations have been reported in nonasbestosis-related mesothelioma[301,302] and acute myeloid leukemia[303] but not in human neural tumors.[304]

In desmoplastic small round cell tumor, the *WT1* gene is altered by reciprocal t(11;22)(p13;q12) translocation involving the *EWS* gene. In this oncogenic translocation, the N-terminal domain of the *EWS* gene is fused to the last three zinc fingers of the *WT1* gene. The *EWS-WT1* gene fusion product is represented by two isoforms, EWS-WT1 (+KTS) and EWS-WT (-KTS) due to the retained alternative splicing of the *WT1* gene.[62,63] Introduction of EWS-WT1 (-KTS) into NIH3T3 cells causes their tumorigenic transformation, whereas EWS-WT1 (+KTS) shows no tumorigenic potential.[305]

SMARCB1

The SWI/SNF-related, matrix-associated, actin-dependent regulator of chromatin, subfamily B, member 1, is also known as the *hSNF5* or *INI1* gene.

Malignant rhabdoid tumor (MRT) is an early childhood cancer, originally classified as a sarcomatous variant of Wilms tumor[306] and subsequently reported in extrarenal locations, including the CNS.[307] Genetic studies on MRT showed monosomy of chromosome 22 and losses of 22q11.2,[308,309] which turned to harbor the "rhabdoid tumor locus."[310] Molecular genetic studies identified the *hSNF5/INI1* gene, mapped to 22q11, as the rhabdoid tumor suppressor gene. Inactivation of the *hSNF5/INI1* gene by association of deletions and frameshift mutations, fully consistent with the Knudson's two-hit hypothesis of tumor suppressor gene inactivation, was commonly seen in sporadic MRTs.[311] Subsequently, loss-of-function mutations of the *hSNF5/INI1* gene were reported in the constitutional DNA from the families with a predisposition to develop extrarenal MRTs and tumors of the CNS, including choroid plexus carcinoma, medulloblastoma, and central primitive neuroectodermal tumor.[312–314] This further supported the hypothesis that *hSNF5/INI1* acts as a tumor suppressor gene.

Neurofibromatosis Type 1 Gene *(NF1)*

Neurofibromatosis type 1 is an autosomal dominant disorder caused by genetic alterations of the *NF1* gene[315,316] (see Chapter 15). The *NF1* gene is mapped to 17q11.2 and encodes for a protein designated neurofibromin.[317,318] The function of neurofibromin is not fully understood. However, strong evidence indicates that neurofibromin, which shows high homology to the GTPase-activating proteins, is involved in the RAS oncogene pathway and negatively regulates RAS product p21ras.[316,318–320]

Germline *NF1* mutations have been extensively documented in patients with neurofibromatosis type 1,[316] and these data are available at the Human Gene Mutation Database (HGMD, htpp://www.uwcm.ac.uk/uwcm/mg/search/120231.html) and Human Genome Organization (HUGO, htpp://www.nf.org/nf1gene/nf1.gene.home.html).

Losses of heterozygosity at the NF1 locus and inactivating mutations in the *NF1* gene have been shown in different types of neurofibromatosis type 1-associated malignancies.[321–335] However, the frequency of detected mutations has appeared to be low in some of these studies. This can be related to the cellular heterogeneity of the samples composed of neoplastic cells carrying mutated NF1 and non-neoplastic cells with NF1 in germline configuration. Furthermore, the large size of the gene, which spans over 350 kb of genomic DNA and contains 60 exons, and the presence of several pseudogenes makes the PCR-based screening for mutations difficult especially in partially degraded DNA extracted from formaldehyde-fixed, paraffin-embedded (FFPE) tissues due to the coamplification of NF1-homologous sequences.[336]

Mice carrying a truncated NF1 allele were cancer prone and developed pheochromocytomas and leukemias but not neurofibromas.[337] However, chimeric mice partially composed of cells with both NF1 alleles inactivated developed neurofibromas with plexiform histology.[338] Thus, the *NF1* gene can be considered a recessive tumor suppressor gene in the sense of the Knudson's "two-hit" hypothesis.

Neurofibromatosis Type 2 Gene *(NF2)*

Neurofibromatosis type 2 is an autosomal dominant disorder caused by genetic alterations of the *NF2* gene.[339] *NF2* gene is mapped to 22q12.2 and encodes for an intracellular cytoskeleton-associated protein, designated as merlin or schwannomin, which is involved in the regulation of cell proliferation and may play a role in integrating multiple cell-signaling pathways.[340,341]

Inactivating mutations of *NF2* have been observed in 34% to 66% of the patients screened for neurofibromatosis type 2.[342,343] These mutations are nonsense, frameshift, or spliced donor site mutations, all of which result in a nonfunctional, truncated protein. Example of a missense NF2 mutation is shown in Figure 4–1. More recently, large deletions in the *NF2* genes were found in NF2 patients, raising the frequency of detectable NF2 alterations in this population to 84%.[344] NF2 mutation databases are available on line at HGMD (htpp://www.uwcm.ac.uk/uwcm/mg/search/120232.html) and HUGO (htpp://neuro-www2mgh.harvard.edu/nf2).

Bilateral vestibular schwannomas and other hereditary brain tumors are a typical diagnostic feature of neurofibromatosis type 2 (see Chapter 15). In these tumors both NF2 alleles are altered by deletions or point mutations as predicted by Knudson's two-hit hypothesis of recessive tumor suppressor gene inactivation.

Monosomy of chromosome 22,[78] LOH at NF2 locus, and inactivating NF2 mutations have been documented in different type of STTs including mesotheliomas,[345,346] schwannomas,[347–349] and perineuriomas.[350] A reduced expression or absence of merlin, the functional consequence of mutational NF2 inactivation, has been shown in schwannomas and meningiomas.[351–353] More recently, increased proteolytic degradation of merlin by calpain was

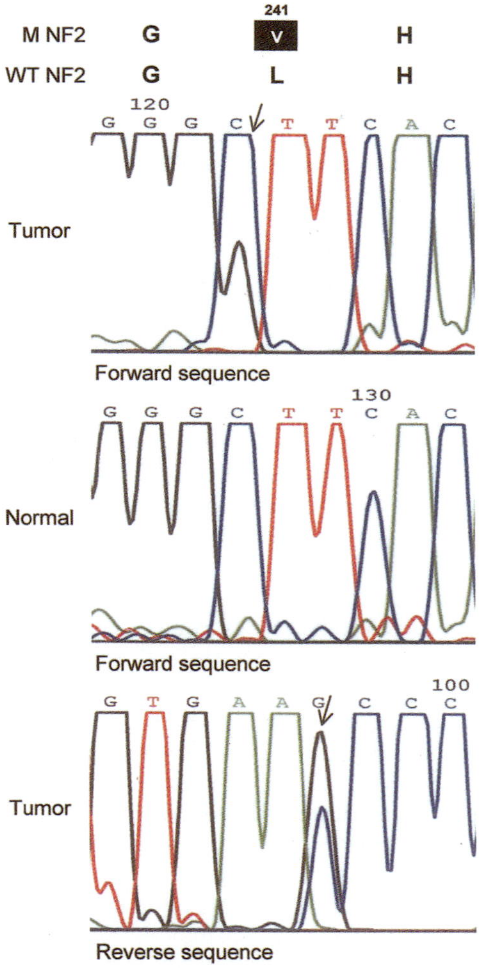

Figure 4-1. Example of missense mutation in *NF2* gene. A single nucleotide replacement CTT to GTT affects codon 241 causing a change of the NF2 protein amino acid sequence. Arrows and black square indicate mutation. M, mutant; WT, wild-type; L, leucine; V, valine.

shown in meningiomas and schwannomas without detected *NF2* gene alterations.[354] This may explain the functional inactivation of the NF2 protein in the tumors without allelic losses or mutations.

Adenomatous Polyposis Coli *(APC)* and β-Catenin *(CTNNB1)* Genes

Familial adenomatous polyposis (FAP) of the colon is an inherited disease, which typically presents in an early adult age with colon polyposis and predisposition to develop colon cancer and other extraintestinal malignancies. Following extensive genetic studies, the FAP locus was linked to the chromosome 5q21 and a specific gene, mutated in FAP patients, was simultaneously cloned by two different groups of investigators. Subsequently, losses and mutations of the *APC* gene have been documented in a majority of familial and sporadic colorectal tumors.[355–358]

An increased frequency of desmoid tumors is one of the clinical features of FAP.[359,360] As predicted by Knudson's two-hit hypothesis, somatic *APC* mutations were documented in desmoid tumors in patients with FAP.[361] Germline *APC* mutations were found in the hereditary desmoid disease[362] and familial infiltrative fibromatosis (FIF) suggesting that FAP and FIF can be different clinical manifestations of the same genetic syndrome.[363] Subsequently, *APC* mutations were also documented in sporadic desmoid tumors.[364]

Germline mutations at the 3′ end of the *APC* gene result in a severe desmoid phenotype and overexpression of the β-catenin (CTNNB1) protein in FAP-related desmoid tumors.[365] A high expression of CTNNB1 and possibly activating mutations were also documented in sporadic desmoid tumors.[366] This suggests that both the APC and the CTNNB1 protein, which links the cytoskeleton to the cadherin family of cell adhesion molecules,[367] targeted by different types of mutations may play an essential role in promoting cellular proliferation by deregulation of the APC/CTNNB1/Tcf pathway.

Unlike some other tumor suppressor genes, the *APC* gene can act as a tumor suppressor gene in nonclassical fashion. A slightly lower level of APC expression without detectable structural changes was associated with predisposition to hereditary tumors.[368,369] Also, the site of a germline *APC* mutation can determine the site of the second-hit mutation and the severity of the disease.[370]

Detection of Minimal Residual Disease

The PCR and RT-PCR amplification assays have been proven useful in the detection and monitoring of a minimal residual disease (MRD) in cancer. Occult cancer cells can be detected by PCR amplification out of millions of normal cells. However, tumor-specific markers are required for such assays. Altered DNA or RNA molecules (specific gene fusion transcripts, genomic breakpoint sequences of chromosome translocations, and tumor-specific somatic mutations) in the tumor cells have been commonly used as MRD markers.

In sarcoma patients, the method of choice for MRD monitoring is based on RT-PCR detection of tumor cell-specific pathologic gene fusion transcripts.[371–380] A nested PCR approach based on amplification of genomic breakpoint sequences has also been used to identify myxoid LS cells circulating in peripheral blood.[381] The presence of neoplastic cells was documented in peripheral blood and bone marrow or in bone marrow alone at the time of operation and during the progression of Ewing sarcoma,[371–376,380] alveolar rhabdomyosarcoma, and desmoplastic small round cell tumor.[380] However, the clinical significance of these observations is unknown.

Detection of MRD in peripheral blood and bone marrow is expected to be an important criterion for molecular staging of the disease and might be used to identify patients who could benefit from tumor-specific therapy before a clinically diagnosed relapse. Targeting gene fusion transcripts might be one of such therapeutic options. However, more studies are needed to determine the clinical significance of the molecularly detectable MRD in soft tissue sarcomas.

Autologous reinfusion of peripheral blood stem cells (PBSCs) is part of the therapeutic treatment protocol of high-risk childhood sarcomas. Evaluation of PBSC samples for the presence of specific fusion transcripts can prevent reinfusion of PBSCs contaminated by tumor cells.[382,383]

Tumor-specific alterations of DNA microsatellite markers,[384–389] tumor-specific messenger RNAs (mRNA),[390] and somatic mutations in tumor mitochondrial DNA[391] were detected using assays based on PCR and RT-PCR in plasma, serum, and peritoneal fluid from patients with various cancers. These findings have opened new prospects for early detection, staging, and monitoring of cancer. This approach can be applicable in molecular evaluation of those STTs that lack tumor-specific translocations and gene fusion transcripts.

Detection of MyoD1 mRNA based on RT-PCR has been suggested to be a highly sensitive and specific marker useful for the differential diagnosis and detection of MRD in rhabdomyosarcoma.[392] However, specificity of this assay has been recently vigorously discussed, and instead, detection of the acetylcholine receptor mRNA has been suggested as a more specific and sensitive marker for the identification of MRD in those rhabdomyoscarcomas that lack tumor-specific translocations.[393,394]

Assessment of Clonality Using Chromosome X Inactivation Assays

Analysis of the clonal nature of a lesion is rarely diagnostically important in soft tissue tumors, but it is often used as an investigational measure to examine the nature of a cellular proliferation on an assumption that clonal proliferations are neoplastic. Consistent nonrandom chromosomal aberrations like translocations, large deletions, amplifications, numerical changes, and molecular genetic changes like single base pair substitutions, deletions, insertions of a few nucleotides and gene fusion transcripts represent relevant markers confirming the clonal nature of a given lesion. These markers can be specific for a particular tumor type or case.

However, tumor-specific markers are not always easy to identify and other more universal approaches have to be applied to confirm the clonal nature of the proliferating tumor cells. According to Lyon's hypothesis, one of the copies of the X chromosome is inactivated in each somatic cell of an adult female.[395] Inactivation occurs randomly at an early stage of embryogenesis and results in a cellular mosaic pattern with either the maternal or paternal chromosome X inactivated.[396] Polyclonal cells extracted from normal tissue contain equal numbers of maternally and paternally derived chromosome X. In contrast, monoclonal proliferation has only one type of inactivated chromosome X of paternal or maternal origin, transmitted from its progenitor cell. By the nature of this phenomenon, assays can be performed in tissue from female patients only.

Various polymorphic genes on the X chromosome have been used in clonality studies based on Lyon's hypothesis. The initial studies were focused on the expression pattern of glucose-6-phospate dehydrogenase (G6PD) isoenzyme.[397,398] Females heterozygous for G6PD polymorphism express Gd^B and variants Gd^A or GD^{A-} in normal tissue but only one isoenzyme in each individual cell. In a G6PD assay, monoclonal proliferation expresses a single G6PD phenotype and polyclonal proliferation a double G6PD phenotype. However, this assay was limited by a very low informativeness.[399] Next generation, DNA-based clonality assays examine the methylation pattern of the chromosome X polymorphic loci (phosphoglycerate kinase [*PGK*] gene, hypoxanthine phosphoribosyl transferase [*HPRT*] gene, and hypervariable DXS255 locus [M27β]) using methylation sensitive restriction endonucleases.[400–403] Tumor and normal tissue DNA samples obtained from the same individual are cleaved with methylation-sensitive restriction endonucleases and analyzed by SBH or PCR amplification. Monoclonal samples show different hybridization or amplification patterns from normal tissue controls. Major limitations of these methylation-based clonality assays are relatively low informativeness of PGK and HPRT polymorphisms and incomplete methylation at the M27β locus.[404]

Finally, an assay based on amplification of the short tandem trinucleotide (CAG) repeat (STR) polymorphism, identified in the coding region of the first exon of human androgen-receptor gene and closely located to methylation-sensitive restriction enzyme sites (*Hhp*II and *Hha*I), has been developed. Human androgen-receptor assay (HUMARA) shows a reliable methylation pattern and is highly informative;[405,406] however, its use is limited by several technical factors and valid interpretation may be impossible without appropriate controls.[407] More recently, an expression (mRNA)-based HUMARA assay has been developed, but usefulness of this assay may be limited by the level of expression of the androgen receptor in different tumors.[408] A number of benign soft tissue lesions were evaluated for clonality status using HUMARA. A monoclonal pattern supporting neoplastic rather than hyperplastic, reactive proliferation has been identified in fibrous histiocytoma,[409] desmoid tumor,[410,411] and angiomyolipoma.[412,413]

Genetic Instability

Genetic instability is a common feature of human cancer and can be seen on either the chromosomal (cytogenetic) or nucleotide (molecular genetic) level. Numerical changes, losses, and gains of the parts of the entire chromosome represent chromosome instability (CIN). Dysfunction of cellular processes involved in the replication and segregation of the chromosomes during mitosis is believed to be responsible for CIN. Structural and functional alterations of human homologous of yeast *BUB* and *MAD* genes controlling mitotic checkpoints have been shown in a subset of human cancers.[414–416]

A "microsatellite instability" (MIN), widespread sequence length alterations within repeated sequences, has been identified in human cancers.[417,418] Repetitive DNA sequences arranged as short tandem repeats (STRs), also known as microsatellites, are present in the human genomes. Microsatellites are unique to an individual and highly conserved through the generation. A hypothesis that MIN can result from the defective function of the mismatch repair (MMR) system was subsequently confirmed by showing mutational inactivation of hMSH2 and hMSH1, human homologues of yeast *MMR* genes in hereditary nonpolyposis colorectal cancer exhibiting MIN phenotype.[415,419–421]

In STTs, a high frequency of MIN has been reported in NF1-related neurofibromas[422] and sporadic cardiac myxomas[423] and a low incidence or lack of MIN in neuroblastomas,[424–426] clear cell sarcomas,[427] LSs,[428,429] and other sarcomas.[430] However, some of these investigations were based on a relatively small number of cases and a larger histologic homogeneous group of STTs should be analyzed to assess the frequency and significance of MIN in STTs. Also, the genetic basis of CIN and MIN in STTs remains to be investigated.

Techniques for Genetic Analysis

Since the discovery of the Philadelphia chromosome (Ph1), the first consistent chromosomal abnormality in human cancer, many clonal genetic aberrations have been documented in benign and malignant tumors.[78] These aberrations can be detected on the cytogenetic or molecular genetic level. Over the past two decades, the spectrum of cytogenetic, molecular cytogenetic, and molecular genetic techniques have been developed and successfully applied in genetic evaluation of STTs. Examples of these techniques in the context of specific applications and the required cell/tissue material necessary for the optimal performance are shown in Table 4–5.

Cytogenetics

Despite the development of new molecular genetic techniques, classical karyotyping supplemented by molecular cytogenetic techniques still plays a central role in ongoing genetic studies of STTs. Detection of tumor-specific morphologic chromosome aberrations is an important early step leading to the identification of genes involved in tumorigenesis. Routine karyotyping of soft tissue tumors, especially sarcomas, should be a common diagnostic practice. However, it is still often limited by the difficulty in obtaining fresh tissue and availability of cytogenetic laboratories.

Classical karyotyping requires fresh viable tumor cells. Sterile collection of pure tumor tissue and use of an appropriate shipping buffer or culture medium are crucial first steps in establishing the cell culture. Highly malignant sarcomas with mitotic activity require a shorter cell culture time than benign tumors with low mitotic indexes. Cell culture is necessary for obtaining neoplastic cells undergoing divisions. The goal is to arrest neoplastic cells at the stage of metaphase, when the individual chromosomes are highly contracted and the different chromosomes dispersed. Harvested metaphase spreads of chromosomes are stained with a special dye. Staining generates banding patterns unique for each chromosome, which enables the identification of the individual chromosomes and chromosome regions involved in genetic aberrations.[78,431,432] Commonly used Giemsa dye or related staining solutions generate the so-called G-banding pattern. Each metaphase chromosome has two arms, a short arm (p) and a long arm (q), divided by a centromere (cen). The ends of chromosome arms are called telomeres (tel). Specific regions consisting of one or more bands are defined on both arms. Each region and each band within the region is numbered in consecutive order starting from the centromere. For

Table 4–5. Techniques Used to Detect Cytogenetic and Molecular Genetic Aberrations and the Required Tissue or Cell Material

	Techniques							
	Cytogenetics	*Molecular Cytogenetics*				*Molecular Genetics*		
Genetic Aberrations	**Karyotyping**	**Methaphase FISH**	**Interphase FISH**	**SKY**	**CGH**	**SBH**	**NBH**	**PCR**
Chromosomal abnormalities	Cell culture	Cell culture	—	Cell culture	—	—	—	—
Translocations	Cell culture	Cell culture	Fresh, fixed	Cell culture	—	—	—	—
Gene fusions	—	—	—	—	—	Fresh	—	Fresh, fixed
Gene fusion products	—	—	—	—	—	—	Fresh	Fresh, fixed
Large amplicons	Cell culture	Cell culture	Fresh, fixed	Cell culture	Fresh, fixed	Fresh	Fresh	—
Amplified genes	Cell culture	Cell culture	Fresh, fixed	—	Fresh, fixed	Fresh	Fresh	Fresh, fixed
Large deletions	Cell culture	Cell culture	—	Cell culture	Fresh, fixed	Fresh	Fresh	Fresh, fixed
Subtle changes Point mutations Small deletions Small insertions	—	—	—	—	—	—	—	Fresh, fixed

example, 8q24 will refer to the fourth band in the second region of the q arm of chromosome 8, and 1p36 will refer to the sixth band of the third region of the p arm of chromosome 1. The International System for Human Cytogenetic Nomenclature (ISCN) provides recommendations for karyotype description and uniform cytogenetic terminology.[433] Cytogenetic abbreviations used in this book are explained in Table 4–6.

Tumor karyotypes vary from almost diploid ones with a single cytogenetic aberration to extremely complex ones with multiple chromosomal aberrations and bizarre marker chromosomes of uncertain origin. Complexity of such karyotypes cannot be understood based on the classical karyotyping and G-banding alone.

Molecular Cytogenetics

Fluorescent in situ hybridization (FISH) combines molecular genetic and cytogenetic approaches. FISH relies on hybridization of the metaphase or interphase cells with fluorescence-labeled probes.[434,435] A major advantage of interphase FISH compared to classical karyotyping is that it does not require cell culture. Instead, touch preparations from fresh tissue, isolated nuclei from fresh or FFPE tissue and routine histologic sections from paraffin blocks can be used. Since FISH was introduced, a variety of probes have been developed. Whole chromosome "painting" probes and sequence- and gene-specific probes can be used to detect chro-

Table 4–6. Commonly Used Cytogenetic Abbreviations

Abbreviation	Meaning
add	Additional material of unknown origin
cen	Centromere
del	Deletion
der	Derivative chromosome
dmin or dm	Double minute chromosome
dup	Duplication
hsr	Homogeneously staining region
i	Isochromosome
ins	Insertion
inv	Inversion
mar	Marker chromosome
p	Short arm of a chromosome
q	Long arm of a chromosome
r	Ring chromosome
t	Translocation
+	When before chromosome number indicates an additional chromosome
–	When before chromosome number indicates a missing chromosome

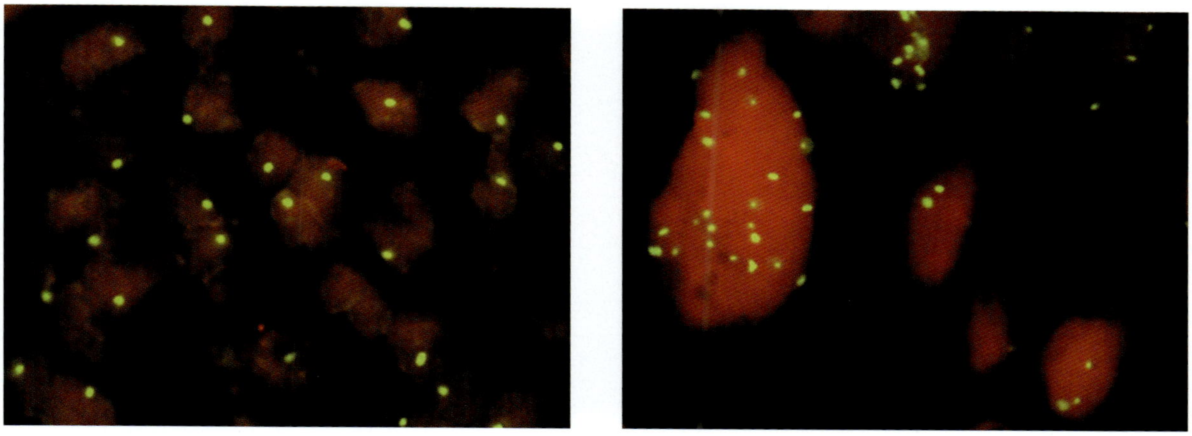

A B

Figure 4-2. Examples of chromosome numerical changes identified by interphase FISH with centromeric probes. *A*, Monosomy of chromosome 18 in malignant GIST. *B*, Polysomy of chromosome X in leiomyosarcoma.

mosome numerical (Fig. 4-2) and other structural changes. Introduction of multicolor FISH detection systems allows identification of more than one target sequence simultaneously.[436] A number of clinically useful FISH-based tests (some of them approved by the Food and Drug Administration and commercially available) for the detection of STT-specific chromosome abnormalities have been developed.[437]

Multicolor spectral karyotyping (SKY) is a newly emerging molecular cytogenetic technology. Simultaneous hybridization of the 24 fluorescently labeled chromosome painting probes allows for the definitive identification of all human chromosomes and material derived from them. SKY is a valuable technique in defining the origin of complex or subtle chromosome rearrangements, which may be undetectable or difficult to diagnose by classical karyotyping.[438,439] Recently, the SKY approach was successfully used to characterize complex abnormalities in STTs, human neuroblastomas,[440] and atypical DFSP.[441]

Comparative genomic hybridization (CGH) is a method to study gains and losses of DNA copy numbers, but balanced translocations or polyploidy cannot be detected. Differentially labeled tumor DNA and normal reference DNA are hybridized simultaneously to normal human metaphase chromosomes. The intensity of the hybridization is measured and the ratio between reference, normal DNA (labeled red) and tumor DNA (labeled green) indicates DNA copy number changes.[442-444] CGH is a powerful screening procedure allowing detection of total gains and losses in a large number of archival cases. These data provide a critical initial step for further molecular genetic studies in the identification of genes that are amplified or lost in a particular tumor. CGH databases are available online (http://www.ncbi.nlm.nih.gov/sky, http://www.helsinki.fi~lgl_www/CMG.html). However, combining the data obtained by different investigators may be limited by the technical differences between CGH studies.[445] Analysis of CGH data with clinical outcome may help to identify patterns of gains and losses correlating with malignant or benign clinical outcome as documented in GISTs.[446] However, the prognostic value of CGH data has not been yet clearly established for STTs.

Molecular Genetics

Southern blot hybridization (SBH) analysis was first described by E. M. Southern in 1975.[447] The assay is based on DNA digestion with enzymes, restriction endonucleases, which recognize specific DNA sequences (restriction sites) as cleavage points. The assay requires high-molecular DNA, which has to be extracted from fresh or frozen tissue. Digested DNA is separated by gel electrophoresis, denatured, and transferred onto a membrane. The membrane is hybridized with DNA or complementary DNA (cDNA) probes, specific for the genes or loci of interest. Detection of new larger or smaller than expected DNA fragments is related to the genetic alterations that rearrange positions of specific restriction endonuclease cleavage sites (Fig. 4-3).

The SBH analysis was adapted to evaluate RNA and called *Northern blot hybridization (NBH)* analysis, as a pun on Dr. Southern's name. Extracted RNA is size fractionated using gel electrophoresis, transferred to the membranes, and hybridized with specific probes. NBH can be used to detect normal or pathologically altered RNA and to evaluate its quantity. Although SBH and NBH are well known molecular genetic techniques, their use in molecular diagnostic pathology of STTs is limited, largely because of the difficulty in obtaining fresh tissue for DNA and RNA extraction.

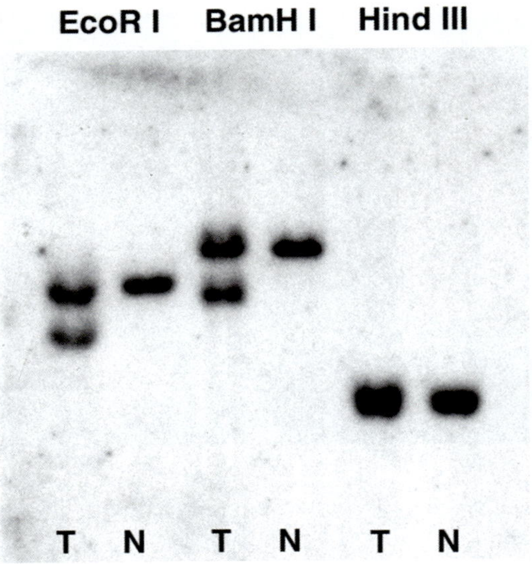

Figure 4–3. Example of radioactive Southern blot hybridization. T and N refer to tumor and normal genomic DNA. Specific restriction endonucleases used for the DNA digestion are shown above. Tumor DNA fragments of different length than ones seen in normal control indicate gene rearrangement.

Polymerase chain reaction (PCR) amplification is a technique that allows automated, enzymatic in vitro synthesis of target DNA sequence in millions of copies for subsequent sequence analysis. The method was invented by Kary Mullis,[448] for which he received the 1993 Nobel Prize in chemistry. It was initially applied to amplify the human β-globin gene for the prenatal diagnosis of sickle cell anemia.[449–451] A standard PCR contains template (double-stranded DNA), primers (oligonucleotides complementary to the sequences flanking the target of amplification), enzyme (Taq DNA polymerase), a mixture of nucleotides (dNTPs-A,C,G,T), and a reaction buffer. Amplification of the target sequence occurs through the cycling (approximately 25 to 40 cycles), and each cycle consists of three steps. In the first step, the template DNA is denatured (separated into single strands) by heating the reaction to the 98°C temperature. In the second, annealing step, primers complementary to the opposite strands of DNA bind to the specific sites. In the third elongation step, Taq DNA polymerase initiates synthesis of the target sequence directionally from the 5′ ends.

Since the PCR technique was introduced, a large number of new applications and modifications of this technique have been developed. PCR-based techniques have had an enormous impact on the basic molecular biology and have contributed to the rapid development of molecular diagnostic pathology.

Reverse transcription-polymerase chain reaction (RT-PCR) allows for the amplification of mRNA. First, mRNA is converted to cDNA using reverse transcriptase reaction. Next, the cDNA is used as a template for PCR amplification as in regular PCR. RT-PCR can detect small quantities of transcripts undetectable by less sensitive methods. Fusion transcripts resulting from the chromosome translocations in STTs are very good targets for RT-PCR amplification.

Long-distance PCR is a technique developed to amplify large fragments of DNA.[452] This technique can be used to amplify unique genomic breakpoints, dispersed over several kilobases.[453,454] However, the translocation breakpoints can be dispersed over several hundred kilobases, beyond the present capacity of long-range PCR technology.[455]

Multiplex PCR allows for the amplification of several target sequences simultaneously. In STT pathology multiplex PCR amplification may be a method of choice in screening samples for several different gene fusion transcripts or in identifying fusion transcript variants of the gene fusions characterized by multiple variants.[456]

Nested PCR is a modified PCR technique, which allows for effective amplification of low copy number templates. In this technique, PCR products from the first, standard PCR amplification are used as a template for the second (nested) PCR amplification. Nested PCR is an extremely useful method for a wide spectrum of applications in diagnostic molecular pathology.[457] The method has been used successfully to amplify target sequences from severely degraded DNA and RNA obtained from FFPE tissues.[458] However, use of this technique carries a serious danger of random contamination, which is difficult to monitor. Cross-contamination of the studied samples with PCR products positive for a particular PCR test is one of the major problems preventing the introduction of the nested PCR technique in diagnostic pathology. To avoid cross-contamination, precautions including use of disposable labware, gloves, and lab coats at all stages and extensive cleaning of all work areas after each experiment is required. Physical isolation of the template preparation area from the PCR preparatory and PCR product amplification analysis areas is also crucial. In addition, use of already premixed reagents for a single PCR experiment and use of multiple negative controls at all stages of nested PCR can help to identify and eliminate random contamination.[458,459]

Strategies for PCR product analysis vary and depend on the primary goal of amplification. A spectrum of molecular techniques including different types of gel electrophoresis, radioactive or nonradioactive hybridization with specific probes, and direct sequencing can be used to evaluate and identify PCR products. Examples of different PCR product analyses are shown in Figure 4–4.

Detection of unknown germline and somatic mutations requires sequencing of the specific PCR products.

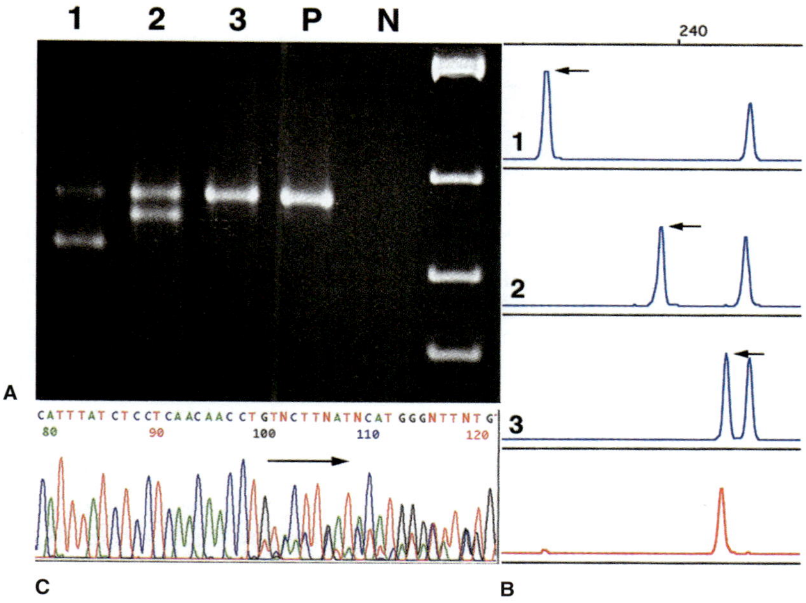

Figure 4–4. Examples of PCR amplification product analysis. *A*, Standard nondenaturing polyacrylamide gel electrophoresis of PCR products. Lines 1 to 3 represent PCR products amplified from tumor DNA samples; P and N refer to positive and negative control of PCR amplification. Additional PCR products seen in lines 1 and 2 indicate deletions. *B*, More sensitive capillary gel electrophoresis has revealed deletions in all three cases. Arrows indicate peaks representing PCR products with deletion. *C*, Identification of deletion by direct sequencing of PCR product. A shift of sequence marked by horizontal arrow indicates deletion.

However, this becomes labor intensive and relatively expensive when large numbers (thousands) of samples are analyzed. Scanning of the PCR products with a high-throughput system is necessary to separate mutated sequences from the wild-type ones. Several methods have been developed to scan DNAs for polymorphisms and mutations.[460] Denaturing gradient gel electrophoresis (DGGE) and single-strand conformation polymorphism (SSCP) assay are two conventional methods commonly used to prescreen PCR products for the mutations. DGGE is based on differential melting of double-stranded DNA molecules during the electrophoresis in the gel with an increasing concentration of denaturing agent. The melting behavior is sequence dependent and allows separation of the fragments differing by a single nucleotide.[461,462] SSCP assay is based on different, sequence-related mobility of denatured single-stranded DNA molecules in nondenaturing polyacrylamide gel. Single nucleotide substitutions, losses, or insertions of a few nucleotides change conformation of the single-stranded DNA molecule and shift its position during the electrophoresis, compared to the wild-type sequence.[463,464]

More recently, denaturing high performance liquid chromatography (DHPLC) has been used to analyze DNA fragments and was applied for mutation analysis.[465] The method showed high sensitivity and specificity in detection of germline and somatic mutations.[466,467] Other major advantages of DHPLD include use of automated instrumentation, a high throughput (time of single analysis about 5 minutes), and ability to evaluate relatively large (up to 1.5 kb) DNA fragments.

PCR amplification of microsatellite markers is used to detect either LOH or MIN in cancer. Microsatellite markers consist of numbers of repeats of two to seven nucleotides and are dispersed throughout the genome mostly outside of the coding sequences. Genetic mutations can lead to the loss of one allele (LOH) or to the appearance of multiple new alleles (instability) at a microsatellite locus. Status of highly polymorphic microsatellite markers is evaluated by the comparison of capillary gel electrophoresis of PCR products amplified from normal and tumor DNA obtained from the same individual (Fig. 4–5).

Sample preparation for molecular genetic studies requires careful evaluation of the tissue material. Cross-contamination of tumor samples with normal tissue and vice versa can influence the results of the molecular genetic assays and lead to false-negative or false-positive results. Morphologic verification of frozen or FFPE tissue before submitting for the nucleic acid extraction should always be performed. Normal tissue, surrounding or trapped inside the tumor, has to be precisely dissected out, using a laser-based capture microdissection technique if necessary (Fig. 4–6).

Extraction of DNA and RNA from FFPE tissues is particularly important in the molecular testing and research of STTs. Despite the progress in understanding a need to perform molecular genetic testing, tumor samples are not consistently freeze-preserved and therefore the molecular genetic studies have to rely on nucleic acids recovered from the FFPE tissues. Also, research of new genetic markers requires testing of well-characterized cases, with long-term follow-up. This cannot be easily achieved in prospective studies and analysis of the tumors retrieved from the archival files is helpful. Partially degraded but amplifiable DNA or RNA can be recovered from FFPE tissues and different extraction procedures have been

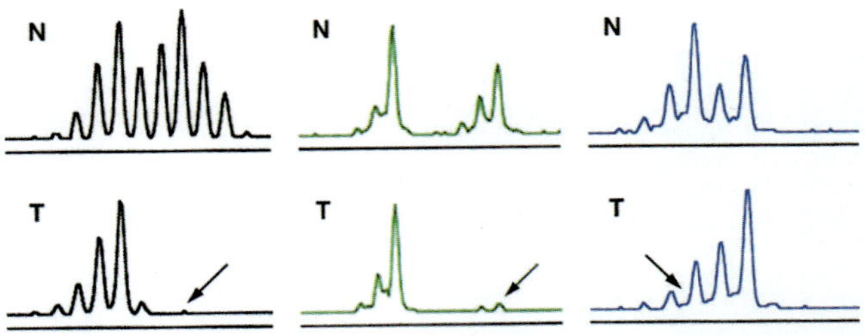

Figure 4-5. Examples of LOH detected in tumor DNA using PCR amplification of microsatellite markers and capillary gel electrophoresis. N and T refer to normal and tumor DNA. Arrows indicate lost alleles in tumors.

described.[468,469] Based on our experience, optimal recovery can be achieved by using acid-phenol chloroform extraction following extended proteinase K digestion.[470] The quality of the recovered nucleic acids can vary between the samples. This depends on the type of fixative used and time of fixation, which can influence the degradation of the nucleic acids and affect recovery of the DNA and RNA from FFPE tissue.[470–472] In some cases, neither DNA nor RNA can be successfully extracted. The effect of fixatives on DNA preservation and PCR amplification is shown in Table 4–7. Suboptimal PCR amplification of low quantity and quality templates can generate a false pattern of LOH, MIN, and mutation artifacts with a relatively higher frequency. Repeated analysis of independent amplification products can help to distinguish true mutations and true microsatellite patterns from PCR artifacts.[473,474] In general, if successful DNA or RNA extraction is achieved, fragments below 200 bp are relatively easy targets for PCR amplification, but fragments larger than 300 bp are difficult to amplify. RT-PCR amplification of low-level expression transcripts can be difficult to achieve and negative results should be always evaluated in the context of amplification quality of other transcripts. Real-time PCR can be helpful in such cases because of highly specific detection and direct quantitation of the amplified sequences.

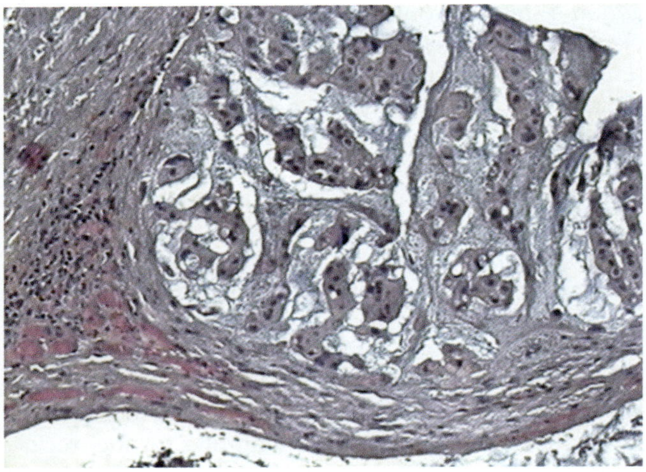

A

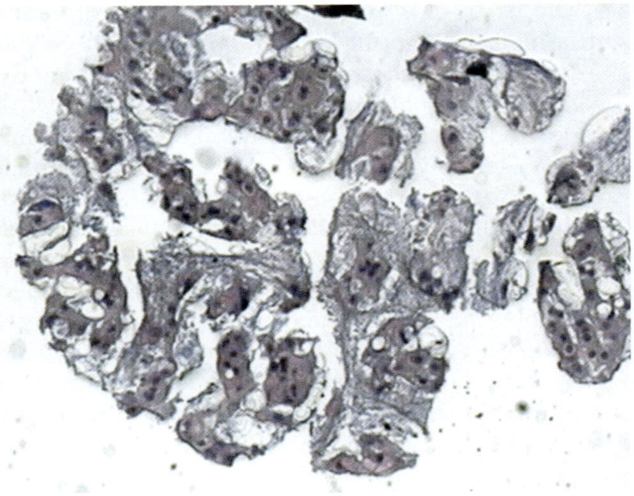

B

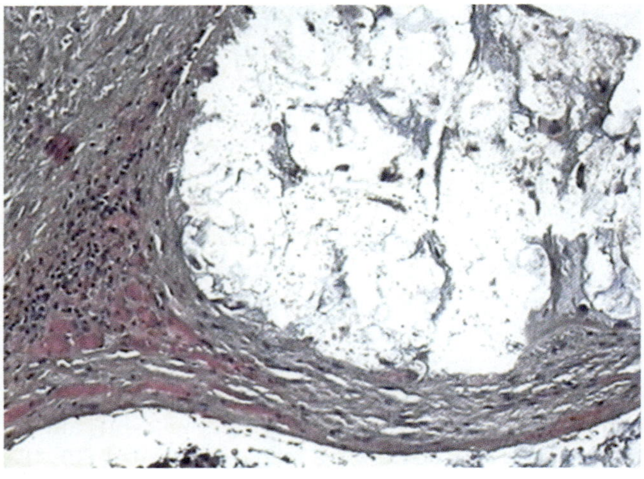

C

Figure 4-6. Example of laser-based capture microdissection of tumor tissue (chordoma). *A*, Sample before dissection. *B*, Captured tumor tissue. *C*, Sample after dissection.

Table 4–7. Fixatives and Preservation of DNA for PCR Amplification[469–471]

Fixative	PCR Amplification
Acetone	Very good
Alcohol	Very good
Formalin	Good
B-5	Unsatisfactory
Bouin	Unsatisfactory
Carnoy	Variable (contradictory results reported)
Zenker	Unsatisfactory

New Molecular Technologies

Real-time PCR is a new rapid-temperature cycling and fluorescence detection-based analysis technique allowing the amplification and reliable quantitation of PCR products. Oligonucleotide fluorogenic probe 5′ labeled with a reporter dye and 3′ labeled with a quencher dye anneals specifically to the template between forward and reverse primers. During the PCR amplification, Taq polymerase cleaves the probe between reporter and quencher and releases a fluorescent reporter due its 5′/3′ nucleotidase activity. PCR products are measured in "real-time" at each cycle during the extension phase of amplification, by quantitation of the fluorescence, which increases proportionally to the amount of amplified product.[475] Monitoring the fluorescence during the temperature change allows for the identification of the PCR products by their melting temperatures and serves as an indirect measure of sequence alterations. Multiple targets might be amplified at the same time using different oligonucleotide probes labeled with different fluorescent dyes. Simple, rapid real-time PCR-based clinical assays detecting simultaneously multiple STT-specific gene fusion products have been developed recently.[476,477] The method allows for quantitative and reproducible detection of low copy number DNA or RNA targets and has been shown to be useful in monitoring MRD.[478,479] Because the quantitation of the PCR product occurs in "real time," there is no need for post-PCR processing of the PCR products. This substantially reduces the chance of cross-contamination of the samples.

The *cDNA microarrays*, also known as DNA chips or gene arrays, represent a new generation of assays, developed to simultaneously analyze large numbers of genes or transcripts. Gene sequences on the chip are represented by homologous cDNAs, oligonucleotides, or more recently by peptide nucleic acid (PNA) probes. Hundreds or thousands of probes attached to the chip are hybridized with RNA from tumor and normal tissue. Comparison of the hybridization signal between the normal and tumor RNA shows up-regulated and down-regulated genes.[480,481]

Identification of tumor-specific gene expression profiles is expected to define new diagnostic and prognostic markers.[482] However, application of this technology in the pathology of STTs is still on the level of early scientific experiments.[483] In soft tissue pathology, obstacles include lack of normal RNA counterpart to the tumor RNA, lack of availability of fresh-frozen tissue necessary to extract a large amount of RNA, and complex cytologic composition of the lesions. The need to meticulously verify the target sequence on the chip adds to the technical challenge of this procedure. Laser-based capture, microdissection of neoplastic and normal cells, and development of new methods for RNA extraction from FFPE tissues will help to develop these applications.

Gene Nomenclature

According to the Human Genome Project, approximately 30,000 to 40,000 genes will be gradually identified in the human genome.[484,485] Also cloning of new tumor-specific, primary or secondary genetic aberrations leading to creation of the pathologic fusion genes will continue to progress and add new members to the family of "pathologic genes."

Uniform genetic nomenclature, which will ensure proper communication among molecular biologists, pathologists, and clinicians, is extremely important.

Unfortunately, some of the genes are recognized by more than one name or the same name has been given to different genes. This may be confusing for those who did not follow the history of genetic discoveries and do not know that some of the genes were cloned simultaneously by different groups of investigators or were found to be altered in different diseases and initially called by different names.

These names circulate in the scientific literature and will continue to be used for some time before internationally recognized uniform genetic nomenclature will be widely accepted.

In Table 4–8, we have listed all genes cited in this book; their full names and alternative symbols are provided based on the data available online at Online Mendelian Inheritance in Man (OMIM), Johns Hopkins University, Baltimore, MD, (http://www.ncbi.nlm.nih.gov/omim/).

Table 4-8. Nomenclature of Genes Cited in Text (Including Alternative Symbols)

Symbol	Full Name	Chromosomal Location	Alternative Names and Symbols	Book Chapter
ALK	Anaplastic lymphoma kinase (Ki-1)	2p23		4, 6
APC	Adenomatosis polyposis coli	5q21-q22		4, 5, 18
ASPL	See ASPSCR1			
ASPSCR1	Alveolar soft part sarcoma chromosome region, candidate 1	17q25	ASPL; RCC17	4, 20
ATF1	Activating transcription factor 1	12q13.1-q13.2		4, 16
BCL2	B-cell CLL/Lymphoma 2	18q21.3		13
CCND1	Cyclin D1	11q13		10, 19
CDK4	Cyclin-dependent kinase 4	12q14	Cell division kinase 4; CMM4	4, 9, 18
CDKN2A	Cyclin-dependent kinase inhibitor 2A	9p21	CDKN2; CDK4 inhibitor; TP16; p16(INK4); p16(INK4A); p14(ARF); Multiple tumor suppressor 1 (MTS1)	4, 7, 18
CHN	see NR4A3; CHN1 has been used for chimerin 1 gene (2q31-q32.1)			
CHOP	see DDIT3			
CLTC	Clathrin, heavy polypeptide	17q11-qter		4
COL1A1	Collagen type I alpha-1	17q21.31-q22		4, 7
COL1A2	Collagen type I alpha-2	7q22.1		4
COL4A5	Collagen type IV alpha-5	Xq22.3		10
COL4A6	Collagen type IV alpha -6	Xq22.3		10
CTNNB1	Catenin, beta-1	3p22-p21.3	Cadherin-associated protein, beta (CTNNB)	4, 5
DDIT3	DNA-damage-inducible transcript 3	12q13	GADD153; CCAAT/enhancer-binding protein homologous protein (CHOP)	4, 9
ERG	v-ets avian erythroblastosis virus E26 oncogene like (avian)	21q22.3		4, 18
ETV1	ETS variant gene 1	7p22		4, 18
ETV4	ETS variant gene 4	17q21	E1A enhancer binding protein; E1AF	4, 18
ETV6	ETS variant gene 6	12p13	TEL oncogene (for translocation, ETS, leukemia)	4, 6
EWSR1	Ewing sarcoma breakpoint region 1	22q12	EWS, ES	4, 9, 16, 17, 18

Symbol	Full Name	Chromosomal Location	Alternative Names and Symbols	Book Chapter
FEV	Fifth Ewing variant	22q		4, 18
FLI1	Friend leukemia virus integration 1	11q24		4, 18
FKHR	See FOXO1A			
FOXO1A	Forkhead box O1A	13q14.1	Forkhead in rhabdomyosarcoma (FKHR)	4, 13
FUS	Fusion, derived from t(12;16)	16p11.2	Translocated in liposarcoma (TLS)	4, 9
GLI	Glioma-associated oncogene homolog	12q13.2-q13.3	Oncogene GLI; GLI1	4
HAS2	Hyaluronan synthase 2	8q24.12		4
HMGIC	High mobility group protein isoform I-C	12q15	High mobility group protein HMGIC breakpoint associated with benign lipoma, (BABL)	7, 8, 17
HMGIY	High mobility group protein isoforms I and Y	6p21		4
HRAS	V-HA-RAS Harvey rat sarcoma viral oncogene homolog	11p15.5	HRAS1; RASH1	4
IGF2	Insulin-like growth factor II	11p15.5		13
IFNG	Interferon, gamma	12q14	IFG; IFI	4
INI1	see SMARCB1			
JAZF1	Zinc finger gene	7p15		4, 12
JJAZ1	Zinc finger gene	17q21		4, 12
KIT	V-KIT Hardy-Zuckerman 4 feline sarcoma viral oncogene homolog	4q12		4, 11
LHFP	Lipoma HMGIC fusion partner	13q12		4, 8
LPP	LIM domain-containing preferred translocation partner in lipoma	3q28	Lipoma preferred partner	4
LRP1	Lipoprotein receptor-related protein	12q13.1-q13.3	Alpha-2-macroglobulin receptor (A2MR)	4
MDM2	Mouse double minute 2 homolog	12q14.3-q15		4, 7, 9, 18
MEN1	Multiple endocrine neoplasia, type I	11q13		8
MFHAS1	Malignant fibrous histiocytoma-amplified sequence 1	8p23.1	Malignant fibrous histiocytoma-amplified sequences with leucine-rich tandem repeats 1, (MASL1)	7
MYC	v-myc avian myelocytomatosis viral oncogene homolog	8q24.12-q24.13		4, 18

Table continued on following page

Table 4–8. Nomenclature of Genes Cited in Text (Including Alternative Symbols) *continued*

Symbol	Full Name	Chromosomal Location	Alternative Names and Symbols	Book Chapter
MYCN	v-myc avian myelocytomatosis viral related oncogene, neuroblastoma derived	2p24.1		4, 13, 18
MYF5	Myogenic factor 5	12q21		13
MYF6	Myogenic factor 6	12q21	Muscle regulatory factor 4; Herculin; Becker muscular dystrophy modifier, (MRF4)	13
MYOD1	Myogenic differentiation antigen 1	11p15.4	MYOD; Myogenic factor 3	4, 13
MYOG	Myogenic factor 4	1q31-q41	MYF4; Myogenin	13
NF1	Neurofibromatosis type 1	17q11.2		4, 16
NF2	Neurofibromatosis type II	22q12.2		4, 14
NTRK1	Neurotrophic tyrosine kinase, receptor, type 1	1q21-q22	Tyrosine kinase receptor, (TRK)	18
NTRK3	Neurotrophic tyrosine kinase, receptor, type 3	15q25	Tyrosine kinase receptor C; Neurotrophin 3 receptor	4, 6
PAX3	Paired box gene 3	2q35	Waardenburg syndrome type I (WS1); Paired domain gene HUP2	4, 13
PAX7	Paired box gene 7	1p36.2-p36.12	Paired domain gene HUP1	4, 13
PDGFB	Platelet-derived growth factor, beta polypeptide	22q12.3-q13.1	V-SIS platelet-derived growth factor, beta polypeptide; Oncogene SIS; SSV simian sarcomaviral oncogene homolog	4, 7
PGL2	Paraganglioma or familial glomus tumors 2	11q13.1		16
PLAG1	Pleomorphic adenoma gene 1	8q12		8
PRCC	Renal cell carcinoma, papillary, 1 gene	1q21	RCCP1	4
PRKAR1A	Protein kinase, cAMP-dependent, regulatory, type I, alpha	17q23-q24	Tissue specific extinguisher 1, (TSE1); PTC2 chimeric oncogene	5
RAP1B	RAS-related protein RAP1B	12q14		4
RAD51L1	S. cerevisiae RAD51-like 1	14q23.3-q24	RAD51B; REC2; RAD51 homolog 2 (R51H2)	
RB1	Retinoblastoma	13q14.1-q14.2	p105-Rb	7, 10
RCC17	see ASPSCR1			
RET	RET protooncogene	10q11.2		16
SAS	Sarcoma amplified sequence	12q13-q14		4, 9
SDHC	Succinate dehydrogenase complex, subunit C, Integral membrane protein	1q21	PGL3	16

Symbol	Full Name	Chromosomal Location	Alternative Names and Symbols	Book Chapter
SDHD	Succinate dehydrogenase complex, subunit D, Integral membrane protein	11q23	PGL; PGL1; Succinate dehydrogenase 4, Integral membrane protein	16
SFPQ	Splicing factor, proline- and glutamine-rich	1p34	PSF; PTB-associated splicing factor	4
SMARCB1	SWI/SNF-related, matrix-associated, actin-dependent regulator of chromatin, subfamily B, member 1	22q11	SNF5 homolog of yeast SNF5; INI1 integrase interactor 1	4, 18
SNF5	see SMARCB1			
SSX	Sarcoma, synovial, X breakpoint	Xp11.2		4, 19
SS18	Synovial sarcoma, translocation, chromosome 18	18q11.2	SYT, synovial sarcoma translocated to X chromosome	4, 19
SYT	see SS18			
TAF15	TAF15 RNA polymerase II, TATA Box-binding protein-associated factor, 68 kd	17q11.1-q11.2	TATA Box-binding protein-associated factor (TAF2N); RNA binding protein 56 (RBP56); TAFII68	4, 17
TCF12	Transcription factor 12	15q21	Helix-loop-helix transcription factor 4 (HTF4)	4 ,17
TEC	see NR4A3; TEC has been used for TEC protein tyrosine kinase (4p12)			
TFE3	Transcription factor for immunoglobulin heavy-chain enhancer 3	Xp11.22		20
TGF-beta	Transforming growth factor beta			5
TP53	Tumor protein p53	17p13.1	P53; Transformation related protein 53	4, 10, 13, 18
TPM3	Tropomyosin 3	1q22-q23	Alpha-Tropomyosin 3; Alpha-Tropomyosin, slow skeletal	4, 6
TPM4	Tropomyosin 4	19p13.1		4, 6
TSC2	Tuberous sclerosis 2 gene	16p13.3	Tuberous sclerosis 4 gene (TSC4)	8, 10
VHL	Von Hippel-Lindau Syndrome	3p26-p25		16
WT1	Wilms tumor 1	11p13		18
ZSG	Zinc finger sarcoma gene	22q12		4

REFERENCES

Oncogenes in Soft Tissue Tumors

1. Cooper GM: Oncogenes, 2nd ed. Boston, Jones and Bartlett, 1995.

Ras Gene Family

2. Der CJ, Krontiris TG, Cooper GM: Transforming genes of human bladder and lung carcinoma cell lines are homologous to the ras genes of Harvey and Kiristen sarcoma viruses. Proc Natl Acad Sci USA 1982; 79:3637–3640.
3. Parada LF, Tabin CJ, Shih C, Weinberg RA: Human EJ bladder carcinoma oncogene is homologue of Harvey sarcoma virus ras gene. Nature 1982;297: 474–478.
4. Reddy EP, Reynolds RK, Santos E, Barbacid M: A point mutation is responsible for the acquisition of transforming properties by the T24 human bladder carcinoma oncogene. Nature 1982;300:149–152.
5. Barbacid M: Ras genes. Annu Rev Biochem 1987; 56:779–827.
6. Bos JL: Ras oncogenes in human cancer: A review. Cancer Res 1989;49:4682–4689.
7. Stratton MR, Fisher C, Gusterson BA, Cooper CS: Detection of point mutations in N-ras and K-ras genes of human embryonal rhabdomyosarcomas using oligonucleotide probes and the polymerase chain reaction. Cancer Res 1989;49:6324–6327.
8. Bohle RM, Brettreich S, Repp R, Borkhardt A, Kosmehl H, Altmannsberger HM: Single somatic ras gene point mutation in soft tissue malignant fibrous histiocytomas. Am J Pathol 1996;148:731–738.
9. Yoo J, Robinson RA, Lee JY: H-ras and K-ras gene mutations in primary human soft tissue sarcomas: Concomitant mutations of the ras genes. Mod Pathol 1999;12:775–780.
10. Hill MA, Gong C, Casey TJ, et al: Detection of K-ras mutations in resected primary leiomyosarcoma. Cancer Epidemiol Biomarkers Prev 1997;6: 1095–1100.
11. Marion MJ, Froment O, Trepo C: Activation of Ki-ras gene by point mutation in human liver angiosarcoma associated with vinyl chloride exposure. Mol Carcinog 1991;4:450–454.
12. Przygodzki RM, Finkelstein SD, Keohavong P, et al: Sporadic and Thorotrast-induced angiosarcomas of the liver manifest frequent and multiple point mutations in K-ras-2. Lab Invest 1997;76:153–159.
13. Rebollo A, Martinez-A C: Ras proteins: Recent advances and new functions. Blood 1999;94:2971–2980.
14. Reuter CW, Morgan MA, Bergmann L: Targeting the Ras signaling pathway: A rational, mechanism-based treatment for hematologic malignancies? Blood 2000; 96:1655–1669.
15. Adjei AA: Blocking oncogenic Ras signaling for cancer therapy. J Natl Cancer Inst 2001;93:1062–1074.

Inhibition of Oncogenic PTKs

16. Robinson DR, Wu YM, Lin SF: The protein tyrosine kinase family of the human genome. Oncogene 2000; 19:5548–5557.
17. Blume-Jensen P, Hunter T: Oncogenic kinase signalling. Nature 2001;411:355–365.
18. Taylor ML, Metcalfe DD: KIT signaling transduction. Hematol Oncol Clin North Am 2000;14:517–535.
19. Hirota S, Isozaki K, Moriyama Y, et al: Gain-of-function mutations of c-kit in human gastrointestinal stromal tumors. Science 1998;279:577–580.
20. Nishida T, Hirota S, Taniguchi M, et al: Familial gastrointestinal stromal tumours with germline mutation of the KIT gene. Nat Genet 1998;19:323–324.
21. Joensuu H, Roberts PJ, Sarlomo-Rikala M, et al: Effect of the tyrosine kinase inhibitor STI571 in a patient with metastatic gastrointestinal stromal tumor. N Engl J Med 2001;344:1052–1056.
22. van Oosterom AT, Judson I, Verweij J, et al: Safety and efficacy of imatinib (STI571) in metastatic gastrointestinal stromal tumorous: A phase I study. Lancet 2001;358:1421–1423.
23. Longley BJ, Reguera MJ, Ma Y: Classes of c-KIT activating mutations: Proposed mechanisms of action and implications in disease classification and therapy. Leuk Res 2001;25:571–576.
24. Pedeutour F, Simon MP, Minoletti F, et al: Translocation, t(17;22)(q22;q13), in dermatofibrosarcoma protuberans: A new tumor-associated chromosome rearrangement. Cytogenet Cell Genet 1996;72:171–174.
25. Kiuru-Kuhlefelt S, El-Rifai W, Fanburg-Smith J, Kere J, Miettinen M, Knuutila S: Concomitant DNA copy number amplification at 17q and 22q in dermatofibrosarcoma protuberans. Cytogenet Cell Genet 2001; 92:192–195.
26. Simon MP, Pedeutour F, Sirvent N, et al. Deregulation of the platelet-derived growth factor B-chain gene via fusion with collagen gene COL1A1 in dermatofibrosarcoma protuberans and giant-cell fibroblastoma. Nat Genet 1997;15:95–98.
27. Shimizu A, O'Brien KP, Sjoblom T, et al: The dermatofibrosarcoma protuberans-associated collagen type Iα1/platelet-derived growth factor (PDGF) B-chain fusion gene generates a transforming protein that is processed to functional PDGF-BB. Cancer Res 1999;59:3719–3723.
28. Simon MP, Navarro M, Roux D, Pouyssegur J: Structural and functional analysis of a chimeric protein COL1A1-PDGFB generated by the translocation t(17;22)(q22;q13.1) in dermatofibrosarcoma protuberans (DP). Oncogene 2001;20:2965–2975.
29. Sjoblom T, Shimizu A, O'Brien KP, et al: Growth inhibition of dermatofibrosarcoma protuberans tumors by the platelet-derived growth factor receptor antagonist STI571 through induction of apoptosis. Cancer Res 2001;61:5778–5783.
30. Morin MJ: From oncogene to drug: Development of small molecule tyrosine kinase inhibitors as antitumor and anti-angiogenic agents. Oncogene 2000;19: 6574–6582.

31. Demetri GD: Targeting c-kit mutations in solid tumors: Scientific rationale and novel therapeutic options. Semin Oncol 2001;28:19–26.
32. Tuveson DA, Fletcher JA: Signal transduction pathways in sarcoma as targets for therapeutic intervention. Curr Opinon Oncol 2001;13:249–255.

Translocation and Oncogenic Gene Fusion

33. Rabbitts TH: Chromosomal translocation in human cancer. Nature 1994;372:143–149.
34. Ladanyi M: The emerging molecular genetics of sarcoma translocation. Diagn Mol Pathol 1995;4:162–173.
35. Fletcher JA: Cytogenetic analysis of soft tissue tumors. In Weiss SW, Goldblum JR (eds): Enzinger and Weiss's Soft Tissue Tumors, 4th ed. St. Louis, MO, Mosby-Year Book, 2001.
36. Meltzer PS: Molecular genetics of soft tissue tumors. In Weiss SW, Goldblum JR (eds): Enzinger and Weiss's Soft Tissue Tumors, 4th ed. St. Louis, MO, Mosby-Year Book, 2001.
37. Rabbitts TH: Chromosomal translocation master genes, mouse models and experimental therapeutics. Oncogene 2001;20:5763–5777.

Translocations and Gene Fusion Involving *EWS* and Related Genes

38. Aurias A, Rimbout C, Buffe D, Zucker J-M, Mazabraud A: Translocation involving chromosome 22 in Ewing's sarcoma: A cytogenetic study of four fresh tumors. Cancer Genet Cytogenet 1984;12:21–25.
39. Turc-Carel C, Philip I, Berger M-P, Philip T, Lenoir GM: Chromosomal translocations 11;22 in cell lines of Ewing's sarcoma. N Engl J Med 1983;309:497–498.
40. Whang-Peng J, Triche TJ, Knutsen T, Miser J, Douglass EC, Israel MA: Chromosome translocation in peripheral neuroepithelioma. N Engl J Med 1984;311: 584–585.
41. Whang-Peng J, Triche TJ, Knutsen T, et al: Cytogenetic characterization of selected small round cell tumors of childhood. Cancer Genet Cytogenet 1986; 21:185–208.
42. Delattre O, Zucman J, Plougastel B, et al: Gene fusion with an ETS DNA binding domain caused by chromosome translocation in human tumorous. Nature 1992;359:162–165.
43. Zucman J, Delattre O, Desmaze C, et al: Cloning and characterization of the Ewing's sarcoma and peripheral neuroepithelioma t(11;22) translocation breakpoints. Genes Chromosomes Cancer 1992;5: 271–277.
44. Zoubek A, Dockhorn-Dworniczak B, Delattre O, et al: Does expression of different EWS chimeric transcripts define clinically distinct risk groups of Ewing tumors patients? J Clin Oncol 1996;14:1245–1251.
45. de Alava E, Kawai A, Healey JH, et al: EWS-FLI1 fusion transcript structure is an independent determinant of prognosis in Ewing's sarcoma. J Clin Oncol 1998;16:1248–1255.
46. Zucman J, Melot T, Desmaze C, et al: Combinatorial generation of variable fusion proteins in Ewing family of tumors. EMBO J 1993;12:4481–4487.
47. Sorensen PH, Lessnick SL, Lopez-Terrada D, Liu XF, Triche TJ, Denny CT: A second Ewing's sarcoma translocation, t(21;22), fuses the EWS gene to another ETS-family transcription factor, ERG. Nat Genet 1994;6:146–151.
48. Jeon IS, Davis JN, Braun BS, et al: A variant Ewing's sarcoma translocation t(7;22) fuses the EWS gene to the ETS gene ETV1. Oncogene 1995;10:1229–1234.
49. Kaneko Y, Yoshida K, Handa M, et al: Fusion of an ETS-family gene, EIAF, to EWS by t(17;22)(q12;q12) chromosome translocation in an undifferentiated sarcoma of infancy. Genes Chromosomes Cancer 1996;15: 115–121.
50. Peter M, Couturier J, Pacquement H, et al: A new member of the ETS family fused to EWS in Ewing tumors. Oncogene 1997;14:1159–1164.
51. Mastrangelo T, Modena P, Tornielli S, et al: A novel zinc finger gene is fused to EWS in small round cell tumor. Oncogene 2000;19:3799–3804.
52. Ginsberg JP, de Alava E, Ladanyi M, et al: EWS-FLI1 and EWS-ERG gene fusions are associated with similar clinical phenotypes in Ewing's sarcomas. J Clin Oncol 1999;17:1809–1814.
53. Sorensen PH, Shimada H, Liu XF, Lim JF, Thomas G, Triche J: Biphenotypic sarcomas with myogeneic and neural differentiation express the Ewing's sarcoma EWS/FLI1 fusion gene. Cancer Res 1995;55:1385–1392.
54. Thorner P, Squire J, Chilton-MacNeill S, et al: Is the EWS/FLI-1 fusion transcript specific for Ewing sarcoma and peripheral primitive neuroectodermal tumor? A report of four cases showing this transcript in a wider range of tumor types. Am J Pathol 1996; 148:1125–1138.
55. Burchill SA, Wheeldon J, Cullinane C, Lewis IJ: EWS-FLI1 fusion transcripts identified in patients with typical neuroblastoma. Eur J Cancer 1997;33:239–243.
56. Sorensen PB, Wu JK, Berean KW, et al: Olfactory neuroblastoma is a peripheral primitive neuroectodermal tumor related to Ewing sarcoma. Proc Natl Acad Sci USA 1996;93:1038–1043.
57. Scotlandi K, Chano T, Benini S, et al: Identification of EWS/FLI-1 transcripts in giant-cell tumor of bone. Int J Cancer 2000;87:328–335.
58. Argani P, Perez-Ordoñez B, Xiao H, Caruana SM, Huvos AG, Ladanyi M: Olfactory neuroblastoma is not related to the Ewing family of tumors: Absence of EWS/FLI1 gene fusion and MIC expression. Am J Surg Pathol 1998;22:391–398.
59. Mezzelani A, Tornielli S, Minoletti F, Pierotti MA, Sozzi G, Pilotti S: Esthesioneuroblastoma is not a member of the primitive peripheral neuroectodermal tumour-Ewing's group. Br J Cancer 1999;81:586–591.
60. Panagopoulos I, Mertens F, Domanski HA, et al: No EWS/FLI1 fusion transcripts in giant-cell tumors of bone. Int J Cancer 2001;93:769–772.

61. Zucman J, Delattre O, Desmaze C, et al.: EWS and ATF-1 gene fusion induced by t(12;22) translocation in malignant melanoma of soft parts. Nat Genet 1993;4:341–345.
62. Ladanyi M, Gerald WL: Fusion of the EWS and WT1 genes in the desmoplastic small round cell tumor. Cancer Res 1994;54:2837–2840.
63. Gerald WL, Rosai J, Ladanyi M: Characterization of the genomic breakpoint and chimeric transcripts in the EWS-WT1 gene fusion of desmoplastic small round cell tumor. Proc Natl Acad Sci USA 1995;14: 1028–1032.
64. Clark J, Benjamin H, Gill S, et al: Fusion of the EWS gene to CHN, a member of the steroid/thyroid receptor gene superfamily, in a human myxoid chondrosarcoma. Oncogene 1996;12:229–235.
65. Labelle Y, Zucman J, Stenman G, et al: Oncogenic conversion of the novel orphan nuclear receptor by chromosome translocation. Hum Mol Genet 1995;4: 2219–2226.
66. Panagopoulos I, Höglund M, Mertens F, Mandahl N, Mitelman F, Åman P: Fusion of EWS and CHOP genes in myxoid liposarcoma. Oncogene 1996;12: 489–494.
67. Crozat A, Åman P, Mandahl N, Ron D: Fusion of CHOP to a novel RNA-binding protein in human myxoid liposarcoma. Nature 1993;363:640-644.
68. Rabbitts TH, Forster A, Larson R, Nathan P: Fusion of the dominant negative transcription regulator CHOP with a novel gene FUS by translocation t(12;16) in malignant liposarcoma. Nat Genet 1993;4:175–180.
69. Attwooll C, Tariq M, Harris M, Coyne JD, Telford N, Varley JM: Identification of a novel fusion gene involving hTAFII68 and CHN from a t(9;17)(q22;q11.2) translocation in an extraskeletal myxoid chondrosarcoma. Oncogene 1999;18:7599–7601.
70. Sjögren H, Meis-Kindblom J, Kindblom LG, Åman P, Stenman G: Fusion of the EWS-related gene TAF2N to TEC in extraskeletal myxoid chondrosarcoma. Cancer Res 1999;59:5064–5067.
71. Sjögren H, Wedell B, Kindblom JM, Kindblom LG, Stenman G: Fusion of the basic helix-loop-helix protein TCF12 to TEC in extraskeletal myxoid chondrosarcoma with translocation t(9;15)(q22;q21). Cancer Res 2000;60:6832–6835.
72. Panagopoulos I, Aman P, Fioretos T, et al: Fusion of the FUS gene with ERG in acute myeloid leukemia with t(16;21)(p11;q22). Genes Chromosomes Cancer 1994;11:256–262.
73. Ichikawa H, Shimizu K, Hayashi Y, Ohki M: An RNA-binding protein gene, TLS/FUS, is fused to erg in human myeloid leukemia with t(16;21) chromosomal translocation. Cancer Res 1994;54:2865–2868.
74. Truong AH, Ben-David Y: The role of Fli-1 in normal cell function and malignant transformation. Oncogene 2000;19:6482–6489.
75. Arvand A, Denny CT: Biology of EWS/ETS fusions in Ewing's family tumors. Oncogene 2001;20:5747–5754.
76. Turc-Carel C, Limon J, Dal Cin P, Rao U, Karakousis C, Sandberg AA: Cytogenetic studies of adipose tissue tumors. II. Recurrent reciprocal translocation t(12;16)(q13;p11) in myxoid liposarcomas. Cancer Genet Cytogenet 1986;23:291–299.
77. Åman P, Ron D, Mandahl N, et al: Rearrangement of the transcription factor gene CHOP in myxoid liposarcomas with t(12;16)(q13;p11). Genes Chromosomes Cancer 1992;5:278–285.
78. Heim S, Mitelman F: Cancer Cytogenetics. Chromosomal and Molecular Genetic Aberrations of Tumor Cells. New York, Wiley, 1976.
79. Åman P, Panagopoulos I, Lassen C, et al: Expression patterns of the human sarcoma-associated genes FUS and EWS and the genomic structure of FUS. Genomics 1996;37:1–8.
80. Ron D, Brasier AR, McGehee RE Jr, Habener JF: Tumor necrosis factor-induced reversal of adipocytic phenotype of 3T3-L1 cells in preceded by a loss of nuclear CCAAT/enhancer binding protein (C/EBP). J Clin Invest 1992;89:223–233.
81. Ron D, Habener JF: CHOP: A novel developmentally regulated nuclear protein that dimerizes with transcription factors C/EBP and LAP and functions as a dominant negative inhibitor of gene transcription. Genes Dev 1992;6:439–453.
82. Adelmant G, Gilbert JD, Freytag SO: Human translocation liposarcoma-CCAAT/enhancer binding protein (C/EBP) homologous protein (TLS-CHOP) oncoprotein prevents adipocyte differentiation by directly interfering with C/EBPbeta function. J Biol Chem 1998;273:15574–15581.
83. Dal-Cin P, Sciot R, Panagopoulos I, et al: Additional evidence of a variant translocation t(12;22) with EWS/CHOP fusion in myxoid liposarcoma: Clinicopathological features. J Pathol 1997;182:437–441.
84. Kuroda M, Ishida T, Takanashi M, Satoh M, Machinami R, Watanabe T: Oncogenic transformation and inhibition of adipocytic conversion of preadipocytes by TLS/FUS-CHOP type II chimeric protein. Am J Pathol 1997;151:735–744.
85. Zinszner H, Albalat R, Ron D: A novel effector domain from the RNA-binding protein TLS or EWS is required for oncogenic transformation by CHOP. Genes Dev 1994;8:2513–2526.
86. Knight JC, Renwick PJ, Dal Cin P, Van Den Berghe H, Fletcher CDM: Translocation t(12;16)(q13;p11) in myxoid liposarcoma and round cell liposarcoma: Molecular and cytogenetic analysis. Cancer Res 1995;55:24–27.
87. Kuroda M, Ishida T, Horiuchi H, et al: Chimeric TLS/FUS-CHOP gene expression and heterogeneity of its junction in human myxoid and round cell liposarcoma. Am J Pathol 1995;147:1221–1227.
88. Hisaoka M, Tsuji S, Morimitsu Y, et al: Detection of TLS/FUS-CHOP fusion transcripts in myxoid and round cell liposarcomas by nested reverse transcription-polymerase chain reaction using archival paraffin-embedded tissues. Diagn Mol Pathol 1998;7:96–101.
89. Panagopoulos I, Mandahal N, Ron D, et al: Characterization of the CHOP breakpoints and fusion transcripts in myxoid liposarcomas with the 12;16 translocation. Cancer Res 1994;54:6500–6503.
90. Antonescu CR, Tschernyavsky SJ, Decuseara R, et al: Prognostic impact of P53 status, TLS-CHOP fusion

transcript structure, and histological grade in myxoid liposarcoma: A molecular and clinicopathologic study of 82 cases. Clin Cancer Res 2001;7:3977–3987.
91. Willeke F, Ridder R, Mechtersheimer G, et al: Analysis of FUS-CHOP fusion transcripts in different types of soft tissue liposarcoma and their diagnostic implications. Clin Cancer Res 1998;4:1779–1784.
92. Tallini G, Akerman M, Dal Cin P, et al: Combined morphologic and karyotypic study of 28 myxoid liposarcomas: Implications for a revised morphologic typing (a report from the CHAMP Group). Am J Surg Pathol 1996;20:1047–1055.
93. Fletcher CD, Akerman M, Dal Cin P, et al: Correlation between clinicopathological features and karyotype in lipomatous tumors: A report of 178 cases from the Chromosome and Morphology (CHAMP) Collaborative Study Group. Am J Pathol 1996;148:623–630.
94. Antonescu CR, Elahi A, Humphrey M, et al: Specificity of TLS-CHOP rearrangement for classic myxoid/round cell liposarcoma: Absence in predominantly myxoid well-differentiated liposarcomas. J Mol Diagn 2000;2:132–138.
95. Waters BL, Panagopoulos I, Allen EF: Genetic characterization of angiomatoid fibrous histiocytoma identifies fusion of the FUS and ATF-1 genes induced by a chromosomal translocation involving bands 12q13 and 16p11. Cancer Genet Cytogenet 2000;121:109–116.

Translocations and Gene Fusion Involving *PAX* and *FKHR* Genes

96. Seidal TM, Mark J, Hagmar B, Angervall L: Alveolar rhabdomyosarcoma: A cytogenetic and correlated cytological and histological study. Act Pathol Microbiol Immunol Scand Sect A 1982;90:345–354.
97. Turc-Carel C, Lizard-Nacol S, Justrabo E, Favrot M, Philip T, Tabone E: Consistent chromosomal translocation in alveolar rhabdomyosarcoma. Cancer Genet Cytogenet 1986;19:361–362.
98. Biegel JA, Meek RS, Parmiter AH, Conrad K, Emanuel BS: Chromosomal translocation t(1;3)(p36;q14) in a case of rhabdomyosarcoma. Genes Chromosomes Cancer 1991;3:483–484.
99. Dal Cin P, Brock P, Aly MS, et al: A variant (2;13) translocation in rhabdomyosarcoma. Cancer Genet Cytogenet 1991;55:191–195.
100. Douglass EC, Rowe ST, Valentine M, et al: Variant translocations of chromosome 13 in alveolar rhabdomyosarcoma. Genes Chromosomes Cancer 1991;3:480–482.
101. Barr FG, Galili N, Holick J, Biegel JA, Rovera G, Emanuel BS: Rearrangement of the PAX3 paired box gene in the paediatric solid tumour alveolar rhabdomyosarcoma. Nat Genet 1993;3:113–117.
102. Galili N, Davis RJ, Fredericks WJ, et al: Fusion of a fork head domain gene to PAX3 in the solid tumour alveolar rhabdomyosarcoma. Nat Genet 1993;5:230–235.
103. Davis RJ, D'Cruz CM, Lovell MA, Biegel JA, Barr FG: Fusion of PAX7 to FKHR by the variant t(1;3)(p36;q14) translocation in alveolar rhabdomyosarcoma. Cancer Res 1994;54:2869–2872.
104. Barr FG: Gene fusions involving PAX and FOX family members in alveolar rhabdomyosarcoma. Oncogene 2001;20:5736–5746.
105. Tremblay P, Gruss P: Pax: Genes for mice and men. Pharmacol Ther 1994;61:205–226.
106. Underhill DA: Genetic and biochemical diversity in the Pax gene family. Biochem Cell Biol 2000;78:629–638.
107. Chi N, Epstein JA: Getting your Pax straight: Pax proteins in development and disease. Trends Genet 2002;18:41–47.
108. Epstein DJ, Vekemans M, Gros P: Splotch (Sp-2H), a mutation affecting development of the mouse neural tube, shows a deletion within the paired homeodomain of Pax-3. Cell 1991;67:767–774.
109. Baldwin CT, Hoth CF, Amos JA, da-Silva EO, Milunsky A: An exonic mutation in the HuP2 paired domain gene causes Waardenburg's syndrome. Nature 1992;355:637–638.
110. Tassabehji M, Read AP, Newton VE, et al: Waardenburg's syndrome patients have mutations in the human homologue of the PAX-3 paired box gene. Nature 1992;355:635–636.
111. Tassabehji M, Read AP, Newton VE, et al: Mutations in the PAX3 gene causing Waardenburg syndrome type 1 and type 2. Nat Genet 1993;3:26–30.
112. Hoth CF, Milunsky A, Lipsky N, Sheffer R, Clarren SK, Baldwin CT: Mutations in the paired domain of the human PAX3 gene cause Klein-Waardenburg syndrome (WS-III) as well as Waardenburg syndrome type I (WS-I). Am J Hum Genet 1993;52:455–462.
113. Asher JH Jr, Sommer A, Morell R, Friedman TB: Missense mutation in the paired domain of PAX3 causes craniofacial-deafness-hand syndrome. Hum Mutat 1996;7:30–35.
114. Kaufmann E, Knochel W: Five years on the wings of fork head. Mech Dev 1996;57:3–20.
115. Durham SK, Suwanichkul A, Scheimann AO, et al: FKHR binds the insulin response element in the insulin-like growth factor binding protein-1 promoter. Endocrinology 1999;140:3140–3146.
116. Guo S, Rena G, Cichy S, He X, Cohen P, Unterman T: Phosphorylation of serine 256 by protein kinase B disrupts transactivation by FKHR and mediates effects of insulin on insulin-like growth factor-binding protein-1 promoter activity through a conserved insulin response sequence. J Biol Chem 1999;274:17184–17192.
117. Brunet A, Bonni A, Zigmond MJ, et al: Akt promotes cell survival by phosphorylating and inhibiting a forkhead transcription factor. Cell 1999;96:857–868.
118. Barr FG, Nauta LE, Davis RJ, Schafer BW, Nycum LM, Biegel JA: In vivo amplification of the PAX3-FKHR and PAX7-FKHR fusion genes in alveolar rhabdomyosarcoma. Hum Mol Genet 1996;5:15–21.
119. Davis RJ, Barr FG: Fusion genes resulting from alternative chromosomal translocations are overexpressed by gene-specific mechanisms in alveolar rhabdomyosarcoma. Proc Natl Acad Sci USA 1997;94:8047–8051.
120. Weber-Hall S, McManus A, Anderson J, et al: Novel formation and amplification of the PAX7-FKHR fusion gene in a case of alveolar rhabdomyosarcoma. Genes Chromosomes Cancer 1996;17:7–13.

121. Fitzgerald JC, Scherr AM, Barr FG: Structural analysis of PAX 7 rearrangements in alveolar rhabdomyosarcoma. Cancer Genet Cytogenet 2000;117:37–40.
122. Fredericks WJ, Galili N, Mukhopadhyay S, et al: The PAX3-FKHR fusion protein created by the t(2;13) translocation in alveolar rhabdomyosarcomas is a more potent transcriptional activator than PAX3. Mol Cell Biol 1995;15:1522–1535.
123. Scheidler S, Fredericks WJ, Rauscher FJ III, Barr FG, Vogt PK: The hybrid PAX3-FKHR fusion protein of alveolar rhabdomyosarcoma transforms fibroblasts in culture. Proc Natl Acad Sci USA 1996;93:9805–9809.
124. Khan J, Bittner ML, Saal LH, et al: cDNA microarrays detect activation of a myogenic transcription program by the PAX3-FKHR fusion oncogene. Proc Nat Acad Sci USA 1999;96:13264–13269.
125. Anderson J, Gordon T, McManus A, et al: Detection of the PAX3-FKHR fusion gene in paediatric rhabdomyosarcoma: A reproducible predictor of the outcome? Br J Cancer 2001;85:831–835.
126. Kelly KM, Womer RB, Sorensen PH, Xiong QB, Barr FG: Common and variant gene fusions predict distinct clinical phenotypes in rhabdomyosarcoma. J Clin Oncol 1997;15:1831–1836.
127. Anderson J, Ramsay A, Gould S, Pritchard-Jones K: PAX3-FKHR induces morphological change and enhances cellular proliferation and invasion in rhabdomyosarcoma. Am J Pathol 2001;159:1089–1096.
128. Collins MH, Zhao H, Womer RB, Barr FG: Proliferative and apoptotic differences between alveolar rhabdomyosarcoma subtypes: A comparative study of tumors containing PAX3-FKHR gene fusions. Med Pediatr Oncol 2001;37:83–89.

Synovial Sarcoma-Specific t(X;18) Translocation and *SYT-SSX* Gene Fusions

129. Limon J, Dal Cin P, Sandberg AA: Translocations involving the X chromosome in solid tumors: Presentation of two sarcomas with t(X;18)(q13;p11). Cancer Genet Cytogenet 1986;23:87–91.
130. Turc-Carel C, Dal Cin P, et al: Involvement of chromosome X in primary cytogenetic change in human neoplasia: Nonrandom translocation in synovial sarcoma. Proc Natl Acad Sci USA 1987;84:1981–1985.
131. Dal Cin P, Rao U, Jani-Sait S, Karakousis C, Sandberg AA: Chromosomes in the diagnosis of soft tissue tumors. I. Synovial sarcoma. Mod Pathol 1992;5:357–362.
132. dos Santos NR, de Bruijn DR, van Kessel AG: Molecular mechanisms underlying human synovial sarcoma development. Genes Chromosomes Cancer 2001;30: 1–14.
133. Clark AJ, Rocques PJ, Crew AJ, et al. Identification of novel genes, SYT and SSX, involved in the t(X;18)(p11.2;q11.2) translocation found in human synovial sarcoma. Nat Genet 1994;7:502–508.
134. Gure AO, Türeci Ö, Sahin U, et al. SSX: A multigene family with several members transcribed in normal testis and human cancer. Int J Cancer 1997;72:965–971.
135. Crew AJ, Clark J, Fisher C, et al: Fusion of SYT to two genes, SSX1 and SSX2, encoding proteins with homology to the Kruppel-associated box in human synovial sarcoma. EMBO J 1995;14:2333–2340.
136. Fligman I, Lonardo F, Jhanwar SC, Gerald WL, Woodruff J, Ladanyi M: Molecular diagnosis of synovial sarcoma and characterization of a variant SYT-SSX2 fusion transcript. Am J Pathol 1995;147: 1592–1599.
137. Skytting B, Nilsson G, Brodin B, et al: A novel fusion gene, SYT-SSX4, in synovial sarcoma. J Natl Cancer Inst 1999;91:974–975.
138. Mancuso T, Mezzelani A, Riva C, et al: Analysis of SYT-SSX fusion transcripts and bcl-2 expression and phosphorylation status in synovial sarcoma. Lab Invest 2000;80:805–813.
139. Safar A, Wickert R, Nelson M, Neff JR, Bridge JA: Characterization of a variant SYT-SSX1 synovial sarcoma fusion transcript. Diagn Mol Pathol 1998;7: 283–287.
140. Ladanyi M: Fusions of the SYT and SSX genes in synovial sarcoma. Oncogene 2001;20:5755–5762.
141. Kawai A, Woodruff J, Healey JH, Brennan MF, Antonescu CR, Landanyi M: SYT-SSX fusion as a determinant of morphology and prognosis in synovial sarcoma. N Engl J Med 1998;338:153–160.
142. Nilsson G, Skytting B, Xie Y, et al: The SYT-SSX1 variant of synovial sarcoma is associated with a high rate of tumor cell proliferation and poor clinical outcome. Cancer Res 1999;59:3180–3184.
143. Hiraga H, Nojima T, Abe S, et al: Diagnosis of synovial sarcoma with the reverse transcriptase-polymerase chain reaction: Analyses of 84 soft tissue and bone tumors. Diagn Mol Pathol 1998;7:102–110.
144. Birdsall S, Osin P, Lu YJ, Fisher C, Shipley J: Synovial sarcoma specific translocation associated with both epithelial and spindle cell components. Int J Cancer 1999;82:605–608.
145. Kasai T, Shimajiri S, Hashimoto H: Detection of SYT-SSX fusion transcripts in both epithelial and spindle cell areas of biphasic synovial sarcoma using laser capture microdissection. Mol Pathol 2000;53:107–110.

Translocations and Gene Fusions Involving PTK Receptors

146. Lawrence B, Perez-Atayde A, Hibbard MK, et al: TPM3-ALK and TPM4-ALK oncogenes in inflammatory myofibroblastic tumors. Am J Pathol 2000;157: 377–384.
147. Bridge JA, Kanamori M, Ma Z, et al: Fusion of the ALK gene to the clathrin heavy chain gene, CLTC, in inflammatory myofibroblastic tumor. Am J Pathol 2001;159:411–415.
148. Knezevich SR, McFadden DE, Tao W, Lim JF, Sorensen PH: A novel ETV6-NTRK3 gene fusion in congenital fibrosarcoma. Nat Genet 1998;18:184–187.
149. Morris SW, Kirstein MN, Valentine MB, et al: Fusion of a kinase gene, ALK to a nucleolar protein gene,

NPM, in non-Hodgkin's lymphoma. Science 1994;263: 1281–1284.
150. Ladanyi M: Aberrant ALK tyrosine kinase signaling. Different cellular lineages, common oncogenic mechanisms? Am J Pathol 2000;157:341–345.
151. Duyster J, Bai R-Y, Morris SW: Translocations involving anaplastic lymphoma kinase (ALK). Oncogene 2001;20:5623–5637.
152. Lamant L, Dastugue N, Pulford K, Delsol G, Mariame B: A new fusion gene TPM3-ALK in anaplastic large cell lymphoma created by a (1;2)(q25;p23) translocation. Blood 1999;93:3088–3095.
153. Siebert R, Gesk S, Harder L, et al: Complex variant translocation t(1;2) with TPM3-ALK fusion due to cryptic ALK gene rearrangement in anaplastic large-cell lymphoma. Blood 1999;94:3614–3617.
154. Touriol C, Greenland C, Lamant L, et al: Further demonstration of the diversity of chromosomal changes involving 2p23 in ALK-positive lymphoma: 2 cases expressing ALK kinase fused to CLTCL (clathrin chain polypeptide-like). Blood 2000;95:3204–3207.
155. Knezevich SR, Garnett MJ, Pysher TJ, Beckwith JB, Grundy PE, Sorensen PH: ETV6-NTRK3 gene fusion and trisomy 11 established a histogenetic link between mesoblastic nephroma and congenital fibrosarcoma. Cancer Res 1998;58:5046–5048.
156. Rubin BP, Chen CJ, Morgan TW, et al: Congenital mesoblastic nephroma t(12;15) is associated with ETV6-NTRK3 gene fusion: Cytogenetic and molecular relationship to congenital (infantile) fibrosarcoma. Am J Pathol 1998;153:1451–1458.
157. Wai DH, Knezevich SR, Lucas T, Jansen B, Kay RJ, Sorensen PH: The ETV6-NTRK3 gene fusion encodes a chimeric protein tyrosine kinase that transforms NIH3T3 cells. Oncogene 2000;19:906–915.
158. Tognon C, Garnett M, Kenward E, Kay R, Morrison K, Sorensen PH: The chimeric protein tyrosine kinase ETV6-NTRK3 requires both Ras-Erk1/2 and PI3-kinase-Akt signaling for fibroblast transformation. Cancer Res 2001;61:8909–8916.
159. Eguchi M, Eguchi-Ishimae M, Tojo A, et al: Fusion of ETV6 to neurotrophin-3 receptor TRKC in acute myeloid leukemia with t(12;15)(p13;q25). Blood 1999; 93:1355–1363.

ASPL-TFE3 Gene Fusion in ASPS and Renal Tumors

160. Joyama S, Ueda T, Shimizu K, et al: Chromosome rearrangement at 17q25 and Xp11.2 in alveolar soft-part sarcoma: A case reported and review of the literature. Cancer 1999;86:1246–1250.
161. Ladanyi M, Lui MY, Antonescu CR, Krause-Boehm A, Meindl A, Argani P: The der(17)t(X;17)(p11;q25) of human alveolar soft part sarcoma fuses the TFE3 transcription factor gene to ASPL, a novel gene at 17q25. Oncogene 2001;20:48–57.
162. Sidhar SK, Clark J, Gill S, et al: The t(X;1)(p11.2;q21.2) translocation in papillary renal cell carcinoma fuses a novel gene PRCC to the TFE3 transcription factor gene. Hum Mol Genet 1996;5:1333–1338.
163. Clark J, Lu YJ, Sidhar SK, et al: Fusion of splicing factor genes PSF and NonO (p54nrb) to the TFE3 gene in papillary renal cell carcinoma. Oncogene 1997;15: 2233–2239.
164. Heimann P, el Housni H, Ogur G, Weterman MAJ, Petty EM, Vassart G: Fusion of a novel gene, RCC17, to the TFE3 gene in t(X;17)(p11.2;q25.3)-bearing papillary renal cell carcinomas. Cancer Res 2001;61:4130–4135.
165. Argani P, Antonescu CR, Illei PB, et al: Primary renal neoplasms with the ASPL-TFE3 gene fusion of alveolar soft part sarcoma: A distinctive tumor entity previously included among renal cell carcinomas of children and adolescents. Am J Pathol 2001;159:179–192.

Translocations and Other Rearrangements Involving *HMGIC* Gene

166. Ashar HR, Schoenberg Fejzo M, Tkachenko A, et al: Disruption of the architectural factor HMGI-C: DNA-binding AT hook motifs fused in lipomas to distinct transcriptional regulatory domains. Cell 1995;82: 57–65.
167. Schoenmakers EF, Wanschura S, Mols R, Bullerdiek J, Van den Berghe H, Van de Ven WJ: Recurrent rearrangements in the high mobility group protein gene, HMGI-C, in benign mesenchymal tumours. Nat Genet 1995;10:436–444.
168. Kazimierczak B, Rosigkeit J, Wanschura S, et al: HMGI-C rearrangements as the molecular basis for the majority of pulmonary chondroid hamartomas: A survey of 30 tumors. Oncogene 1996;12:515–521.
169. Manfioletti G, Giancotti V, Bandiera A, et al: cDNA cloning of the HMGI-C phosphoprotein, a nuclear protein associated with neoplastic and undifferentiated phenotypes. Nucleic Acids Res 1991;19:6793–6797.
170. Johnson KR, Lehn DA, Reeves R: Alternative processing of mRNAs encoding mammalian chromosomal high-mobility-group proteins HMG-I and HMG-Y. Mol Cell Biol 1989;9:2114–2133.
171. Fedele M, Battista S, Manfioletti G, Croce CM, Giancotti V, Fusco A: Role of the high mobility group A proteins in human lipomas. Carcinogenesis 2001;22:1583–1591.
172. Petit MM, Mols R, Schoenmakers EF, Mandahl N, Van de Ven WJM: LPP, the preferred fusion partner gene of HMGIC in lipomas, is a novel member of the LIM protein family. Genomics 1996;36:118–129.
173. Rogalla P, Kazimierczak B, Meyer-Bolte K, Tran KH, Bullerdiek J: The t(3;12)(q27;q14-q15) with underlying HMGIC-LPP fusion is not determining an adipocytic phenotype. Genes Chromosomes Cancer 1998;22: 100–104.
174. Petit MM, Schoenmakers EF, Huysmans C, Geurts JM, Mandahl N, Van de Ven WJ: LHFP, a novel translocation partner gene of HMGIC in a lipoma, is a member of a new family of LHFP-like genes. Genomics 1999;57:438–441.
175. Kazimierczak B, Wanschura S, Rosigkeit J, et al: Molecular characterization of 12q14-15 rearrangements in three pulmonary chondroid hamartomas. Cancer Res 1995;55:2497–2499.

176. Kools PF, Van de Ven WJ: Amplification of the rearranged form of the high mobility group protein gene HMGIC in OsA-CI osteosarcoma cells. Cancer Genet Cytogenet 1996;91:1–7.
177. Hauke S, Rippe V, Bullerdiek J: Chromosomal rearrangements leading to abnormal splicing within intron 4 of HMGIC? Genes Chromosome Cancer 2001;30:302–304.
178. Berner JM, Meza-Zepeda LA, Kools PF, et al: HMGIC, the gene for an architectural transcription factor, is amplified and rearranged in a subset of human sarcomas. Oncogene 1997;14:2935–2941.
179. Meza-Zepeda LA, Berner JM, Henriksen J, South AP, et al: Ectopic sequences from truncated HMGIC in liposarcomas are derived from various amplified chromosomal regions. Genes Chromosomes Cancer 2001;31:264–273.
180. Fedele M, Berlingieri MT, Scala S, et al: A truncated and chimeric HMGI-C gene induces neoplastic transformation of NIH3T3 murine fibroblasts. Oncogene 1998;17:413–418.
181. Battista S, Fidanza V, Fedele M, et al: The expression of a truncated HMGI-C gene induces gigantism associated with lipomatosis. Cancer Res 1999;59:4793–4797.
182. Arlotta P, Tai AK-F, Manfioletti G, Clifford C, Jay G, Ono SJ: Transgenic mice expressing a truncated form of the high mobility group I-C protein develop adiposity and an abnormally high prevalence of lipomas. J Biol Chem 2000;275:14394–14400.
183. Zhou X, Benson KF, Ashar HR, Chada K: Mutation responsible for the mouse pygmy phenotype in the developmentally regulated factor HMGI-C. Nature 1995;376:771–774.
184. Kazimierczak B, Dal Cin P, Wanschura S, et al: HMGIY is the target of 6p21.3 rearrangements in various benign mesenchymal tumors. Genes Chromosomes Cancer 1998;23:279–285.
185. Xiao S, Lux ML, Reeves R, Hudson TJ, Fletcher JA: HMGI(Y) activation by chromosome 6p21 rearrangements in multilineage mesenchymal cells from pulmonary hamartoma. Am J Pathol 1997;150:901–910.
186. Williams AJ, Powell WL, Collins T, Morton CC: HMGI(Y) expression in human uterine leiomyomata. Involvement of another high-mobility group architectural factor in a benign neoplasm. Am J Pathol 1997;150:911–918.
187. Tkachenko A, Ashar HR, Meloni AM, Sandberg AA, Chada KK: Misexpression of disrupted HMGI architectural factors activates alternative pathways of tumorigenesis. Cancer Res 1997;57:2276–2280.
188. Melillo RM, Pierantoni G, Scala S, et al: Critical role of the HMGI (Y) proteins in adipocytic cell growth and differentiation. Mol Cell Biol 2001;21:2485–2495.

Detection of Translocations and Gene Fusion Products

189. Stark B, Zoubek A, Hattinger C, et al: Metastatic extraosseous Ewing tumor. Association of the additional translocation der(16)t(1;16) with the variant EWS/ERG rearrangement in a case of cytogenetically inconspicuous chromosome 22. Cancer Genet Cytogenet 1996;87:161–166.
190. Åström AK, Voz ML, Kas K, et al: Conserved mechanism of PLAG1 activation in salivary gland tumors with and without chromosome 8q12 abnormalities: Identification of SII as a new fusion partner gene. Cancer Res 1999;59:918–923.
191. Geurts van Kessel A, de Bruijn D, Hermsen L, et al: Masked t(X;18)(p11;q11) in a biphasic synovial sarcoma revealed by FISH and RT-PCR. Genes Chromosomes Cancer 1998;23:198–201.
192. Kaneko Y, Kobayashi H, Hanada M, Satake N, Maseki N: EWS-ERG fusion transcript produced by chromosomal insertion in a Ewing sarcoma. Genes Chromosomes Cancer 1997;18:228–231.
193. Trumper L, Pfreundschuh M, Bonin FV, Daus H: Detection of the t(2;5)-associated NPM/ALK fusion cDNA in peripheral blood cells of healthy individuals. Br J Haematol 1998;103:1138–1144.
194. Ji W, Qu G, Ye P, Zhang X-Y, Halabi S, Erlich M: Frequent detection of bcl-2/J_H translocations in human blood and organ samples by a quantitative polymerase chain reaction assay. Cancer Res 1995;55: 2876–2882.
195. Biernaux C, Loos M, Sels A, Huez G, Stryckmans P: Detection of major bcr-able gene expression at a very low level in blood cells of some healthy individuals. Blood 1995;86:3118–3122.

DNA Amplification in STTs

196. Schwab M: Oncogene amplification in solid tumors. Semin Cancer Biol 1999;9:319–325.
197. Collins S, Groudine M: Amplification of endogenous myc-related sequences in a human myeloid leukaemia cell line. Nature 1982;298:679–681.
198. Dalla-Favera R, Wong-Staal F, Gallo RC: Oncogene amplification in promyelocytic leukaemia cell line HL-60 and primary leukaemic cells of the same patient. Nature 1982;299:61–63.
199. Yokota J, Tsunetsugu-Yokota Y, Battifora H, Le Fevre C, Cline MJ: Alterations of myc, myb, and ras(Ha) proto-oncogenes in cancers are frequent and show clinical correlation. Science 1986;231:261–265.
200. Barrios C, Castresana JS, Ruiz J, Kreicbergs A: Amplification of the c-myc proto-oncogene in soft tissue sarcomas. Oncology 1994;51:13–17.
201. Kohl NE, Kanda N, Schreck RR, et al: Transposition and amplification of oncogene-related sequences in human neuroblastomas. Cell 1983;35:359–367.
202. Schwab M, Varmus HE, Bishop JM, et al: Chromosome localization in normal human cells and neuroblastomas of a gene related to c-myc. Nature 1984; 308:288–291.
203. Brodeur GM, Seeger RC, Schwab M, Varmus HE, Bishop JM: Amplification of N-myc in untreated human neuroblastomas correlates with advanced disease stage. Science 1984;224:1121–1124.
204. Seeger RC, Brodeur GM, Sather H, et al: Association of multiple copies of the N-myc oncogene with rapid

progression of neuroblastomas. N Engl J Med 1985; 313:1111–1116.
205. Brodeur GM, Azar C, Brother M, et al: Neuroblastoma: Effect of genetic factors on prognosis and treatment. Cancer 1992;70:1685–1694.
206. Wolf M, Aaltonen LA, Szymanska J, et al: Complexity of 12q13-22 amplicon in liposarcoma: Microsatellite repeat analysis. Genes Chromosomes Cancer 1997;18: 66–70.
207. Berner JM, Forus A, Elkahloun A, Meltzer PS, Fodstad O, Myklebost O: Separate amplified regions encompassing CDK4 and MDM2 in human sarcomas. Genes Chromosome Cancer 1996;17:254–259.
208. Elkahloun AG, Bittner M, Hoskins K, Gemmill R, Meltzer PS: Molecular cytogenetic characterization and physical mapping of 12q13-15 amplification in human cancer. Genes Chromosomes Cancer 1996;17: 205–214.
209. Reifenberger G, Ichimura K, Reinferberger G, Elkahloun AG, Meltzer PS, Collins VP: Refined mapping of 12q13-15 amplicons in human malignant gliomas suggests CDK4/SAS and MDM2 as independent amplification targets. Cancer Res 1996;56: 5141–5145.
210. Fakharzadeh SS, Trusko SP, George DL: Tumorigenic potential associated with enhanced expression of a gene that is amplified in a mouse tumor cell line. EMBO J 1991;10:1565–1569.
211. Kussie P, Gorina S, Marechal V, et al: Structure of the MDM2 oncoprotein bound to the p53 tumor suppressor transactivation domain. Science 1996;274: 921–922.
212. Buschmann T, Fuchs SY, Lee CG, Pan ZQ, Ronai Z: SUMO-1 modification of Mdm2 prevents its self-ubiquitination and increases Mdm2 ability to ubiquitinate p53. Cell 2000;101:753–762.
213. Xiao ZX, Chen J, Levine AJ, et al: Interaction between the retinoblastoma protein and the oncoprotein MDM2. Nature 1995;375:694–698.
214. Kanoe H, Nakayama T, Murakami H, et al: Amplification of the CDK4 gene in sarcomas: Tumor specificity and relationship with the RB gene mutation. Anticancer Res 1998;18:2317–2321.
215. Nakayama T, Toguchida J, Wadayama B, Kanoe H, Kotoura Y, Sasaki MS: MDM2 gene amplification in bone and soft tissue tumors: Association with tumor progression in differentiated adipose tissue tumors. Int J Cancer 1995;64:342–346.
216. Pedeutour F, Forus A, Coindre JM, et al: Structure of the supernumerary ring and giant rod chromosomes in adipose tissue tumors. Genes Chromosomes Cancer 1999;24:30–41.
217. Suijkerbuijk RF, Olde Weghuis DE, Van den Berg M, et al: Comparative genomic hybridization as a tool to define two distinct chromosome 12-derived amplification units in well differentiated liposarcomas. Genes Chromosomes Cancer 1994;9:292–295.
218. Szymanska J, Virolainen M, Tarkkanen M, et al: Overrepresentation of 1q21-23 and 12q13021 in lipoma-like liposarcomas but not in benign lipomas: A comparative genomic hybridization study. Cancer Genet Cytogenet 1997;99:14–18.
219. Pilotti S, Della Torre G, Lavarino C, et al: Distinct mdm2/p53 expression patterns in liposarcoma subgroups: Implication for different pathogenetic mechanisms. J Pathol 1997;181:14–24.

Tumor Suppressor Genes

Retinoblastoma Gene *(RB1)*

220. Knudson AJ: Mutation and cancer: Statistical study of retinoblastoma. Proc Natl Acad Sci USA 1971;68: 820–823.
221. Knudson AJ, Hethocte HW, Brown BW: Mutation and childhood cancer: A probabilistic model for the incidence of retinoblastoma. Proc Natl Acad Sci USA 1975; 72:5116–5120.
222. Friend SH, Bernards R, Rogelj S, et al: A human DNA segment with properties of the gene that predispose to retinoblastoma and osteosarcoma. Nature 1986;323: 643–646.
223. Fung Y-KT, Murphree AL, T'Ang A, Qian J, Hinrichs SH, Benedict WF: Structural evidence for the authenticity of the human retinoblastoma gene. Science 1987;236:1657–1661.
224. Hong FD, Huang H-JS, To H, et al: Structure of the human retinoblastoma gene. Proc Natl Acad Sci USA 1989;86:5502–5506.
225. Horowitz JM, Yandell DW, Park S-H, et al: Point mutational inactivation of the retinoblastoma antioncogene. Science 1989;243:937–940.
226. Lohmann DR: RB1 mutations in retinoblastoma. Hum Mutat 1999;14:283–288.
227. Dei Tos AP, Maestro R, Doglioni C, et al: Tumor suppressor genes and related molecules in leiomyosarcoma. Am J Pathol 1996;148:1037–1045.
228. Cohen JA, Geradts J: Loss of RB and MTS1/CDKN2 (p16) expression in human sarcomas. Hum Pathol 1997;28:893–898.
229. Stratton MR, Williams S, Fisher C, et al: Structural alterations of the RB1 gene in human soft tissue tumours. Br J Cancer 1989;60:202–205.
230. Wunder JS, Czitrom AA, Kandel R, Andrulis IL: Analysis of alterations in the retinoblastoma gene and tumor grade in bone and soft-tissue sarcomas. J Natl Cancer Inst 1991;83:194–200.
231. Cordon-Cardo C: Mutation of cell cycle regulators. Biological and clinical implications for human neoplasia. Am J Pathol 1995;147:545–560.
232. Sherr CJ: Cancer cell cycles. Science 1996;274: 1672–1677.
233. Huang H-JS, Yee J-K, Shew J-Y, et al: Suppression of the neoplastic phenotype by replacement of the RB gene in human cancer cells. Science 1988;242: 1563–1566.
234. Takahashi R, Hashimoto T, Xu H-J, et al: The retinoblastoma gene functions as a growth and tumor suppressor in human bladder carcinoma cells. Proc Natl Acad Sci USA 1991;88:5257–5261.

Tumor Protein p53 Gene *(TP53)*

235. Lane DP, Crawford LV: T antigen is bound to a host protein in SV40-transformed cells. Nature 1979;278: 261–263.
236. Linzer DI, Levine AJ: Characterization of a 54K dalton cellular SV40 tumor antigen present in SV40-transformed cells and uninfected embryonal carcinoma cells. Cell 1979;17:43–52.
237. Eliyahu D, Raz A, Gruss P, Givol D, Oren M: Participation of p53 cellular tumor antigen in transformation of normal embryonic cells. Nature 1984;312:646–649.
238. Parada LF, Land H, Weinberg RA, Wolf D, Rotter V: Cooperation between gene encoding p53 tumour antigen and ras in cellular transformation. Nature 1984; 312:649–651.
239. Finlay CA, Hinds PW, Levine AJ: The p53 proto-oncogene can act as a suppressor of transformation. Cell 1989;57:1083–1093.
240. Eliyahu D, Michalovitz D, Eliyahu S, Pinhasi-Kimhi O, Oren M: Wild-type p53 can inhibit oncogene-mediated focus formation. Proc Natl Acad Sci USA 1989; 86:8763–8767.
241. Lee JM, Bernstein A: p53 mutations increase resistance to ionizing radiation. Proc Nat Acad Sci USA 1993;90:5742–5746.
242. Levine AJ: p53, the cellular gatekeeper for growth and division. Cell 1997;88:323–331.
243. Oren M: Regulation of the p53 tumor suppressor protein. J Biol Chem 1999;274:36031–36034.
244. Vogelstein B, Kinzler KW: p53 function and dysfunction. Cell 1992;70:523–526.
245. McBride OW, Merry D, Givol D: The gene for human p53 cellular tumor antigen is located on chromosome 17 short arm (17p13). Proc Nat Acad Sci USA 1989;83: 130–134.
246. Isobe M, Emanuel BS, Givol D, Oren M, Croce CM: Localization of gene for human p53 antigen to band 17p13. Nature 1986;320:84–85.
247. Baker SJ, Fearon ER, Nigro JM, et al: Chromosome 17 deletions and p53 gene mutations in colorectal carcinomas. Science 1989;244:217–221.
248. Nigro JM, Baker SJ, Preisinger AC, et al: Mutations in the p53 gene occur in diverse human tumour types. Nature 1989;342:705–708.
249. Hollstein M, Shomer B, Greenblatt M, et al: Somatic point mutations in the p53 gene of human tumors and cell lines: Updated compilation. Nucleic Acids Res 1996;24:141–146.
250. Lavigueur A, Maltby V, Mock D, Rossant J, Pawson T, Bernstein A: High incidence of lung, bone, and lymphoid tumors in transgenic mice overexpressing mutant alleles of the p53 oncogene. Mol Cell Biol 1989;9:3982–3991.
251. Donehower LA, Harvey M, Slagle BL, et al: Mice deficient for p53 are developmentally normal but susceptible to spontaneous tumours. Nature 1992;356: 215–221.
252. Harvey M, McArthur MJ, Montgomery CA Jr, Butel JS, Bradley A, Donehower LA: Spontaneous and carcinogen-induced tumorigenesis in p53-deficiant mice. Nat Genet 1993;5:225–229.
253. Jacks T, Remington L, Williams BO, et al: Tumor spectrum analysis in p53-deficient mice. Curr Biol 1994;4: 1–7.
254. Li FP, Fraumeni JF: Rhabdomyosarcoma in children: Epidemiologic study and identification of a cancer family syndrome. J Natl Cancer Inst 1969;43: 1365–1373.
255. Li FP, Fraumeni JF: Soft tissue sarcomas, breast cancer and other neoplasms: A familial syndrome? Ann Intern Med 1969;71:747–752.
256. Malkin D, Li FP, Strong LC, Fraumeni JF, et al: Germ line p53 mutations in a familial syndrome of breast cancer, sarcomas, and other neoplasms. Science 1990; 250:1233–1238.
257. Varley JM, Evans DGR, Birch JM: Li-Fraumeni syndrome—A molecular and clinical review. Br J Cancer 1997;76:1–14.
258. Varley JM, Thorncroft M, McGown G, et al: A detailed study of loss of heterozygosity on chromosome 17 in tumours from Li-Fraumeni patients carrying a mutation to the TP53 gene. Oncogene 1997;14:865–871.

Checkpoint Kinase 2 Gene *(CHK2)*

259. Matsuoka S, Huang M, Elledge SJ: Linkage of ATM to cell cycle regulation by the Chk2 protein kinase. Science 1998;282:1893–1897.
260. Blasina A, de Weyer IV, Laus MC, Luyten WH, Parker AE, McGowan CH: A human homologue of the checkpoint kinase Cds1 directly inhibits Cdc25 phosphatase. Curr Biol 1999;14:1–10.
261. Chaturvedi P, Eng WK, Zhu Y, et al: Mammalian Chk2 is a downstream effector of the ATM-dependent DNA damage checkpoint pathway. Oncogene 1999;18:4047–4054.
262. Brown AL, Lee C-H, Schwarz JK, Mitiku N, Piwnica-Worms H, Chung JH: A human Cda1-related kinase that functions downstream of ATM protein in the cellular response to DNA damage. Proc Nat Acad Sci USA 1999;96:3745–3750.
263. Chehab NH, Malikzay A, Appel M, Halazonetis TD: Chk2/hCds1 functions as a DNA damage checkpoint in G-1 by stabilizing p53. Genes Dev 2000;14: 278–288.
264. Bell DW, Varley JM, Szydlo TE, et al: Heterozygous germ line hCHK2 mutations in Li-Fraumeni syndrome. Science 1999;286:2528–2531.
265. Vahteristo P, Tamminen A, Karvinen P, et al: p53, CHK2 and CHK1 genes in Finnish families with Li-Fraumeni syndrome: Further evidence of CHK2 in inherited cancer predisposition. Cancer Res 2001;61: 5718–5722.

Cyclin-Dependent Kinase Inhibitor 2A Gene *(CDKN2A)*

266. Kamb A, Gruis NA, Weaver-Feldhaus J, et al: A cell cycle regulator potentially involved in genesis of many tumor types. Science 1994;264:436–440.

267. Nabori T, Miura K, Wu DJ, Lois A, Takabayashi K, Carson DA: Deletions of the cyclin-dependent kinase-4 inhibitor gene in multiple human cancers. Nature 1994; 368:753–756.
268. Serrano H, Hannon GJ, Beach D: A new regulatory motif in cell-cycle control causing specific inhibition of cyclin D/CDK4. Nature 1993;366:704–707.
269. Roussel MF: The family of cell cycle inhibitors in cancer. Oncogene 1999;18:5311–5317.
270. Ruas M, Peters G: The p16INK4a/CDKN2A tumor suppressor and its relatives. Biochim Biophys Acta 1998;1378:F115–177.
271. Orlow I, Drobnjak M, Zhang ZF, et al: Alterations of INK4A and INK4B genes in adult soft tissue sarcomas: Effect on survival. J Natl Cancer Inst 1999;91: 73–79.
272. Hussussian CJ, Struewing JP, Goldstein AM, et al: Germline p16 mutations in familial melanoma. Nat Genet 1994;8:15–21.
273. Green MH: The genetics of hereditary melanoma and nevi. 1998 update. Cancer 1999;86:2464–2477.
274. Merlo A, Herman JG, Mao L, et al: 5-prime CpG island methylation is associated with transcriptional silencing of the tumour suppressor p16/CDKN2/MTS1 in human cancers. Nature Med 1995;1: 686–692.
275. Hannon GJ, Beach D: p15(INK4B) is a potential effector of TGF-beta-induced cell cycle arrest. Nature 1994; 371:257–261.
276. Okuda T, Shurtleff SA, Valentine MB, et al: Frequent deletion of p16(INK4a)/MTS1 and p15(INK4b)/MTS2 in pediatric acute lymphoblastic leukemia. Blood 1995; 85:2321–2330.
277. Serrano M, Lee H, Chin L, Cordon-Cardo C, Beach D, DePinho RA: Role of the INK4a locus in tumor suppression and cell mortality. Cell 1996;85:27–37.
278. Kamijo T, Zindy F, Roussel MF, et al: Tumor suppression at the mouse INK4a locus mediated by the alternative reading frame product p19ARF. Cell 1997;91: 649–659.

Wilms Tumor Gene *(WT1)*

279. Fitzgerald HL, Hardin HC Jr: Bilateral Wilms' tumor family: Case report. J Urol 1955;73:468–474.
280. Knudson AG Jr, Strong LC: Mutation and cancer: A model for Wilms' tumor of the kidney. J Nat Cancer Inst 1972;48:313–324.
281. Fearon ER, Vogelstein B, Feinberg AP: Somatic deletion and duplication of genes on chromosome 11 in Wilms' tumours. Nature 1984;309:176–178.
282. Koufos A, Hansen MF, Lampkin BC, et al: Loss of alleles at loci on human chromosome 11 during genesis of Wilms' tumour. Nature 1984;309:170–172.
283. Orkin SH, Goldman DS, Sallan SE: Development of homozygosity for chromosome 11p markers in Wilms' tumour. Nature 1984;309:172–174.
284. Reeve AE, Housiaux PJ, Gardner RJM, Chewings WE, Grindley RM, Millow LJ: Loss of Harvey ras allele in sporadic Wilms' tumour. Nature 1984;309:174–176.
285. Weissman BE, Saxon PJ, Pasquale SR, Jones GR, Geiser AG, Stanbridge EJ: Introduction of normal human chromosome into Wilms' tumor cell line controls its tumorigenic expression. Science 1987;236:175–180.
286. Call KM, Glaser T, Ito CY, et al: Isolation and characterization of a zinc finger polypeptide gene at the human chromosome 11 Wilms' tumor locus. Cell 1990;60:509–520.
287. Rose EA, Glaser T, Jones C, et al: Complete physical map of the WAGR region of 11p13 localizes a candidate Wilms tumor gene. Cell 1990;60:495–508.
288. Haber DA, Park S, Maheswaran S, et al: WT1-mediated growth suppression of Wilms tumor cells expressing a WT1 splicing variant. Science 1993;262:2057–2059.
289. Haber DA, Timmers HT, Pelletier J, Sharp PA, Housman DE: A dominant mutation in the Wilms tumor gene WT1 cooperates with the viral oncogene E1A in transformation of primary kidney cells. Proc Natl Acad Sci USA 1992;89:6010–6014.
290. Rauscher FJ III, Morris JF, Tournay OE, Cook DM, Curran T: Binding of the Wilms' tumor locus zinc finger protein to the EGR-1 consensus sequence. Science 1990;250:1259–1262.
291. Bickmore WA, Oghene K, Little MH, Seawright A, van Heyningen V, Hastie ND: Modulation of DNA binding specificity by alternative splicing of the Wilms' tumor wt1 gene transcript. Science 1992;257:235–237.
292. Reddy J, Licht JD: The WT1 Wilms' tumor suppressor gene: How much do we really know? Biochim Biophys Acta 1996;1287:1–28.
293. Davies RC, Calvio C, Bratt E, Larsson SH, Lamond AI, Hastie ND: WT1 interacts with the splicing factor U2AF65 in an isoform-dependent manner and can be incorporated into spliceosomes. Genes Dev 1998;12: 3217–3225.
294. Barbaux S, Niaudet P, Gubler MC, et al: Donor splice-site mutations in WT1 are responsible for Frasier syndrome. Nat Genet 1997;17:467–470.
295. Pelletier J, Bruening W, Kashtan CE, et al: Germinal mutations in the Wilms' tumor suppressor gene are associated with abnormal urogenital development in Denys-Drash syndrome. Cell 1991;67:437–447.
296. van Heyningen V, Bickmore WA, Seawright A, et al: Role for the Wilms tumor gene in genital development? Proc Nat Acad Sci USA 1990;87:5383–5386.
297. Kreidberg JA, Sariola H, Loring JM, et al: WT-1 is required for early kidney development. Cell 1993;74: 679–691.
298. Armstrong JF, Pritchard-Jones K, Bickmore WA, Hastie ND, Bard JB: The expression of the Wilms' tumour gene, WT1, in the developing mammalian embryo. Mech Dev 1993;40:85–97.
299. Moore AW, McInnes L, Kreidberg J, Hastie ND, Schedl A: YAC complementation shows a requirement for Wt1 in the development of epicardium, adrenal gland and throughout nephrogenesis. Development 1999;126:1845–1857.
300. Rackley RR, Flenniken AM, Kuriyan NP, Kessler PM, Stoler MH, Williams BR: Expression of the Wilms'

tumor suppressor gene WT1 during mouse embryogenesis. Cell Growth Differ 1993;4:1023–1031.
301. Kumar-Singh S, Segers K, Rodeck U, et al: WT1 mutations in malignant mesothelioma and WT1 immunoreactivity in relation to p53 and growth factor receptor expression, cell-type transition and prognosis. J Pathol 1997;181:67–74.
302. Park S, Schalling M, Bernard A, et al: The Wilms tumor gene WT1 is expressed in murine mesoderm-derived tissues and mutated in a human mesothelioma. Nat Genet 1993;4:415–420.
303. King-Underwood L, Renshaw J, Pritchard-Jones K: Mutations in the Wilms' tumor gene WT1 in leukemias. Blood 1996;87:2171–2179.
304. Dennis SL, Manji SS, Carrington DP, et al: Expression and mutation analysis of the Wilms' tumor 1 gene in human neural tumors. Int J Cancer 2002;97:713–715.
305. Kim J, Lee K, Pelletier J: The desmoplastic small round cell tumor t(11;22) translocation produces EWS/WT1 isoforms with differing oncogenic properties. Oncogene 1998;16:1973–1979.

SMARCB1

306. Beckwith JB, Palmer NF: Histopathology and prognosis of Wilms tumors: Results from the First National Wilms' Tumor Study. Cancer 1978;41:1937–1948.
307. Parham DM, Weeks DA, Beckwith JB: The clinicopathologic spectrum of putative extrarenal rhabdoid tumors: An analysis of 42 cases studied with immunohistochemistry or electron microscopy. Am J Surg Pathol 1994;18:1010–1029.
308. Biegel JA, Rorke LB, Packer RJ, Emanuel BS: Monosomy 22 in rhabdoid or atypical tumors of the brain. J Neurosurg 1990;73:710–714.
309. Biegel JA, Burk CD, Parmiter AH, Emanuel BS: Molecular analysis of partial deletion of 22q in a central nervous system rhabdoid tumor. Genes Chromosomes Cancer 1992;5:104–108.
310. Biegel JA, Allen CS, Kawasaki K, Shimizu N, Budarf ML, Bell CJ: Narrowing the critical region for the rhabdoid tumor locus in 22q11. Genes Chromosomes Cancer 1996;16:94–105.
311. Versteege I, Sevenet N, Lange J, et al: Truncating mutations of hSNF5/INI1 in aggressive paediatric cancer. Nature 1998;394:203–206.
312. Sevenet N, Lellouch-Tubiana A, Schofield D, et al: Spectrum of hSNF5/INI1 somatic mutations in human cancer and genotype-phenotype correlations. Hum Mol Genet 1999;8:2359–2368.
313. Sevenet N, Sheridan E, Amram D, Schneider P, Handgretinger R, Delattre O: Constitutional mutations of the hSNF5/INI1 gene predispose to a variety of cancers. Am J Hum Genet 1999;65:1342–1348.
314. Taylor MD, Gokgoz N, Andrulis IL, Mainprize TG, Drake JM, Rutka JT: Familial posterior fossa brain tumors of infancy secondary to germline mutation of the hSNF5 gene. Am J Hum Genet 2000;66: 1403–1406.

Neurofibromatosis Type 1 Gene *(NF1)*

315. Rasmussen SA, Friedman JM: NF1 gene and neurofibromatosis 1. Am J Epidemiol 2000;151:33–40.
316. Cichowski K, Jacks T: NF1 tumor suppressor gene function: Narrowing the GAP. Cell 2001;104: 593–604.
317. Cawthon RM, Weiss R, Xu GF, et al: A major segment of the neurofibromatosis type 1 gene: cDNA sequence, genomic structure, and point mutations. Cell 1990;62: 193–201
318. Wallace MR, Marchuk DA, Anderson LB, et al: Type 1 neurofibromatosis gene: Identification of a large transcript disrupted in three NF1 patients. Science 1990; 249:181–186.
319. Xu GF, Lin B, Tanaka K, et al: The catalytic domain of the neurofibromatosis type 1 gene product stimulates ras GTPase and complements ira mutants of *S. cerevisiae.* Cell 1990,63:835–841.
320. McCormick F: Ras signaling and NF1. Curr Opin Genet Dev 1995,5:51–55.
321. Skuse GR, Kosciolek BA, Rowley PT: Molecular genetic analysis of tumors in von Recklinghausen neurofibromatosis: Loss of heterozygosity for chromosome 17. Genes Chromosomes Cancer 1989;1:36–41.
322. Xu W, Mulligan LM, Ponder MA, et al: Loss of NF1 alleles in phaeochromocytomas from patients with type I neurofibromatosis. Genes Chromosomes Cancer 1992;4:337–342.
323. Legius E, Marchuk DA, Collins FS, Glover TW: Somatic deletion of the neurofibromatosis type 1 gene in neurofibrosarcoma supports a tumour suppressor gene hypothesis. Nat Genet 1993;3:122–126.
324. Shannon KM, O'Connell P, Martin GA, et al: Loss of normal NF1 allele from the bone marrow of children with type 1 neurofibromatosis and malignant myeloid disorders. N Engl J Med 1994;330:597–601.
325. Colman SD, Williams CA, Wallace RW: Benign neurofibromas in type 1 neurofibromatosis (NF1) show somatic deletions of the NF1 gene. Nat Genet 1995;11: 90–92.
326. Lothe RA, Slettan A, Saeter G, Brøgger A, Børresen A-L, Nesland JM: Alterations at chromosome 17 loci in peripheral nerve sheath tumors. J Neuropathol Exp Neurol 1995;54:65–73.
327. Serra E, Puig S, Otero D, et al: Conformation of a double-hit model for the NF1 gene in benign neurofibromas. Am J Hum Genet 1997;61:512–519.
328. Däschner K, Assum G, Eisenbarth I, et al: Clonal origin of tumor cells in a plexiform neurofibroma with LOH in NF1 intron 38 and in dermal neurofibromas without LOH of the NF1 gene. Biochem Biophys Res Commun 1997;234:346–350.
329. Kluwe L, Friedrich RE, Mautner VF: Allelic loss of the NF1 gene in NF1-associated plexiform neurofibromas. Cancer Genet Cytogenet 1999;113:65–69.
330. Eisenbarth I, Beyer K, Krone W, Assum G: Toward a survey of somatic mutation of the NF1 gene in benign neurofibromas of patients with neurofibromatosis type 1. Am J Hum Genet 2000;66:393–401.

331. John AM, Ruggieri M, Ferner R, Upadhyaya M: A search for evidence of somatic mutations in the NF1 gene. J Med Genet 2000;37:44–49.
332. Rasmussen SA, Overman J, Thomson SAM, et al: Chromosome 17 loss-of-heterozygosity studies in benign and malignant tumors in neurofibromatosis type I. Genes Chromosomes Cancer 2000;28:425–431.
333. Gutzmer R, Herbst RA, Mommert S, et al: Allelic loss at the neurofibromatosis type 1 (NF1) gene locus is frequent in desmoplastic neurotropic melanoma. Hum Genet 2000;107:357–361.
334. Perry A, Roth KA, Banerjee R, Fuller CE, Gutmann DH: NF1 deletions in S-100 protein-positive and negative cells of sporadic and neurofibromatosis 1 (NF1)-associated plexiform neurofibromas and malignant peripheral nerve sheath tumors. Am J Pathol 2001;159:57–61.
335. Kluwe L, Hagel C, Tatagiba M, et al: Loss of NF1 alleles distinguish sporadic from NF1-associated pilocytic astrocytomas. J Neuropathol Exp Neurol 2001; 60:917–920.
336. Viskochil DH: In Uphadhyaya M, Cooper DN (eds): Neurofibromatosis Type 1: From Genotype to Phenotype. Oxford, England: BIOS Scientific Publishers, 1998, pp 39–56.
337. Jacks T, Shih TS, Schmitt EM, Bronson RT, Bernards A, Weinberg RA: Tumor predisposition in mice heterozygous for a targeted mutation in Nf1. Nat Genet 1994;7:353–361.
338. Cichowski J, Shih TS, Schmitt E, et al: Mouse models of tumor development in neurofibromatosis type 1. Science 1999;286:2172–2176.

Neurofibromatosis Type 2 Gene *(NF2)*

339. Gutmann DH: Molecular insights into neurofibromatosis 2. Neurobiol Dis 1997;3:247–261.
340. Rouleau GA, Merel P, Lutchman M, et al: Alteration ina new gene encoding a putative membrane-organizing protein causes neurofibromatosis type 2. Nature 1993;363:515–521.
341. Trofatter JA, MacCollin MM, Rutter JL, et al: A novel moesin-, ezrin-, radixin-like gene is a candidate for the neurofibromatosis 2 tumor suppressor. Cell 1993;75:826.
342. Merel P, Hoang-Xuan K, Sanson M, et al: Screening for germ-line mutations in the NF2 gene. Genes Chromosomes Cancer 1995;12:117–127.
343. Ruttledge MH, Andermann AA, Phelan CM, et al: Type of mutation in the neurofibromatosis type 2 gene (NF2) frequently determines severity of disease. Am J Hum Genet 1996;59:331–342.
344. Zucman-Rossi J, Legoix P, Der Sarkissian H, et al: NF2 gene in neurofibromatosis type 2 patients. Hum Mol Genet 1998;7:2095–2101.
345. Bianchi AB, Mitsunaga SI, Cheng JQ, et al: High frequency of inactivating mutations in the neurofibromatosis type 2 gene (NF2) in primary malignant mesotheliomas. Proc Natl Acad Sci USA 1995;92: 10854–10858.
346. Cheng JQ, Lee WC, Klein MA, Cheng GZ, Jhanwar SC, Testa JR: Frequent mutations of NF2 and allelic loss from chromosome band 22q12 in malignant mesothelioma: Evidence for a two-hit mechanism of NF2 inactivation. Genes Chromosomes Cancer 1999;24:238–242.
347. Bijlsma EK, Merel P, Bosch DA, et al: Analysis of mutations in the SCH gene in schwannomas. Genes Chromosomes Cancer 1994;11:7–14.
348. Twist EC, Ruttledge MH, Rousseau M, et al: The neurofibromatosis type 2 gene is inactivated in schwannomas. Hum Mol Genet 1994;3:147–151.
349. Jacoby LB, MacCollin M, Barone R, Ramesh V, Gusella JF: Frequency and distribution of NF2 mutations in schwannomas. Genes Chromosomes Cancer 1996;17:45–55.
350. Lasota J, Fetsch JF, Wozniak A, Wasag B, Sciot R, Miettinen M: The neurofibromatosis type 2 gene is mutated in perineural cell tumors. A molecular genetic study of eight cases. Am J Pathol 2001;158:1223–1229.
351. Stemmer-Rachamimov AO, Xu L, Gonzalez-Agosti C, et al: Universal absence of merlin, but not other ERM family members, in schwannomas. Am J Pathol 1997; 151:1649–1654.
352. Gutmann DH, Giordano MJ, Fishback AS, Guha A: Loss of merlin expression in sporadic meningiomas, ependymomas and schwannomas. Neurology 1997;49: 267–270.
353. Lee JH, Sundaram V, Stein DJ, Kinney SE, Stacey DW, Golubic M: Reduced expression of schwannomin/merlin in human sporadic meningiomas. Neurosurgery 1997;40:578–587.
354. Kimura Y, Koga H, Araki N, et al: The involvement of calpain-dependent proteolysis of the tumor suppressor NF2 (merlin) in schwannomas and meningiomas. Nat Med 1998;4:915–922.

Adenomatous Polyposis Coli Gene *(APC)* and β-Catenin *(CTNNB1)* Genes

355. Kinzler KW, Nilbert MC, Su L-K, et al: Identification of FAP locus genes from chromosome 5q21. Science 1991;253:661–665.
356. Nishisho I, Nakamura Y, Miyoshi Y, et al: Mutations of chromosome 5q21 genes in FAP and colorectal cancer patients. Science 1991;253:665–669.
357. Groden J, Thliveris A, Samowitz W, et al: Identification and characterization of the familial adenomatous polyposis coli gene. Cell 1991;66:589–600.
358. Joslyn G, Carlson M, Thliveris A, et al: Identification of deletion mutation and three new genes at the familial polyposis locus. Cell 1991;66:601–613.
359. Klemmer S, Pascoe L, DeCosse J: Occurrence of desmoids in patients with familial adenomatous polyposis of the colon. Am J Med Genet 1987;28:385–392.
360. Clark SK, Neale KF, Landgrebe JC, Phillips RKS: Desmoid tumours complicating familial adenomatous polyposis. Br J Surg 1999;86:1185–1189.
361. Sen-Gupta S, van der Luijt R, Bowles LV, Meera Khan P, Delhanty JDA: Somatic mutation of APC gene in desmoid tumour in familial adenomatous polyposis. Lancet 1993;342:552–553.

362. Eccles DM, van der Luijt R, Breukel C, et al: Hereditary desmoid disease due to a frameshift mutation at codon 1924 of the APC gene. Am J Hum Genet 1996;59:1193–1201.
363. Scott RJ, Froggatt NJ, Trembath RC, Evans DG, Hodgson SV, Maher ER: Familial infiltrative fibromatosis (desmoid tumours) (MIM135290) caused by a recurrent 3′ APC gene mutation. Hum Mol Genet 1996;5:1921–1924.
364. Alman BA, Li C, Pajerski ME, Diaz-Cano S, Wolfe HJ: Increased beta-catenin protein and somatic APC mutations in sporadic aggressive fibromatoses (desmoid tumors). Am J Pathol 1997;151:329–334.
365. Couture J, Mitri A, Lagace R, et al: A germline mutation at the extreme 3′ end of the APC gene results in a severe desmoid phenotype and is associated with overexpression of beta-catenin in the desmoid tumor. Clin Genet 2000;57:205–212.
366. Miyoshi Y, Iwao K, Nawa G, Yoshikawa H, Ochi T, Nakamura Y: Frequent mutations in the beta-catenin gene in desmoid tumors from patients without familial adenomatous polyposis. Oncol Res 1998;10:591–594.
367. Gottardi CJ, Gumbiner BM: Adhesion signaling: How beta-catenin interacts with its partners. Curr Biol 2001;11:R792–794.
368. Laken SJ, Papadopoulos N, Petersen GM, et al: Analysis of masked mutations in familial adenomatous polyposis. Proc Natl Acad Sci USA 1999;96:2322–2326.
369. Yan H, Dobbie Z, Gruber SB, et al: Small changes in expression affect predisposition to tumorigenesis. Nat Genet 2002;30:25–36.
370. Lamlum H, Ilyas M, Rowan A, et al: The type of somatic mutation at APC in familial adenomatous polyposis is determined by the site of the germline mutation: A new facet to Knudson's 'two-hit' hypothesis. Nat Med 1999;5:1071–1075.

Detection of Minimal Residual Disease

371. Peter M, Magdelenat H, Michon J, et al: Sensitive detection of occult Ewing's cells by the reverse transcriptase-polymerase chain reaction. Br J Cancer 1995;72:96–100.
372. Zoubek A, Pfleiderer C, Ambros PF, et al: Minimal metastatic and minimal residual disease in patients with Ewing tumors. Klin Padiatr 1995;207:242–247.
373. Kelly KM, Womer RB, Barr FG: Minimal disease detection in patients with alveolar rhabdomyosarcoma using a reverse transcriptase-polymerase chain reaction method. Cancer 1996;78:1320–1327.
374. West DC, Grier HE, Swallow MM, Demetri GD, Granowetter L, Sklar J: Detection of circulating cells in patients with Ewing's sarcoma and peripheral primitive neuroectodermal tumor. J Clin Oncol 1997;15:583–588.
375. de Alava E, Lozano MD, Patino A, Sierrasesumaga L, Pardo-Mindan FJ: Ewing family tumors: Potential prognostic value of reverse-transcriptase polymerase chain reaction detection of minimal residual disease in peripheral blood samples. Diagn Mol Pathol 1998;7:152–157.
376. Fagnou C, Michon J, Peter M, et al: Presence of tumor cells in bone marrow but not in blood is associated with adverse prognosis in patients with Ewing's tumor. J Clin Oncol 1998;16:1707–1711.
377. Willeke F, Ridder R, Mechtersheimer G, et al: Analysis of FUS-CHOP fusion transcripts in different types of soft tissue liposarcoma and their diagnostic implications. Clin Cancer Res 1998;4:1779–1784.
378. Willeke F, Mechtersheimer G, Schwarzbach M, et al: Detection of SYT-SSX1/2 fusion transcripts by reverse transcriptase-polymerase chain reaction (RT-PCR) is a valuable diagnostic tool in synovial sarcoma. Eur J Cancer 1998;34:2087–2093.
379. Zoubek A, Ladenstein R, Windhager R, et al: Predictive potential of testing for bone marrow involvement in Ewing tumor patients by RT-PCR: A preliminary evaluation. Int J Cancer 1998;79:56–60.
380. Athale UH, Shurtleff SA, Jenkins JJ, et al: Use of reverse transcriptase polymerase chain reaction for diagnosis and staging of alveolar rhabdomyosarcoma, Ewing sarcoma family of tumors, and desmoplastic small round cell tumor. J Pediatr Hematol Oncol 2001;23:99–104.
381. Panagopoulos I, Åman P, Mertens F, et al: Genomic PCR detects tumor cells in peripheral blood from patients with myxoid liposarcoma. Genes Chromosomes Cancer 1996;17:102–107.
382. Montanaro L, Pession A, Trere D, et al: Detection of EWS chimeric transcripts by nested RT-PCR to allow reinfusion of uncontaminated peripheral blood stem cells in high-risk Ewing's tumor in childhood. Haematologica 1999;84:1012–1015.
383. Thomson B, Hawkins D, Felgenhauer J, Radich J: RT-PCR evaluation of peripheral blood, bone marrow and peripheral blood stem cells in children and adolescents undergoing VACIME chemotherapy for Ewing's sarcoma and alveolar rhabdomyosarcoma. Bone Marrow Transplant 1999;24:527–533.
384. Chen XQ, Stroun M, Magnenat JL, et al: Microsatellite alterations in plasma DNA of small cell lung cancer patients. Nat Med 1996;2:1033–1035.
385. Nawroz H, Koch W, Anker P, Stroun M, Sidransky D: Microsatellite alterations in serum DNA of head and neck cancer patients. Nat Med 1996;2:1035–1037.
386. Goessl C, Heicappell R, Munker R, et al: Microsatellite analysis of plasma DNA from patients with clear cell renal carcinoma. Cancer Res 1998;58:4728–4732.
387. Hibi K, Robinson CR, Booker S, et al: Molecular detection of genetic alterations in the serum of colorectal cancer patients. Cancer Res 1998;58:1205–1207.
388. Chen X, Bonnefoi H, Diebold-Berger S, et al: Detecting tumor-related alterations in plasma or serum DNA of patients diagnosed with breast cancer. Clin Cancer Res 1999;5:2297–2303.
389. Hickey KP, Boyle KP, Jepps HM, Andrew AC, Buxton EJ, Burns PA: Molecular detection of tumour DNA in serum and peritoneal fluid from ovarian cancer patients. Br J Cancer 1999;80:1803–1808.

390. Chen XQ, Bonnefoi H, Pelte MF, et al: Telomerase RNA as a detection marker in the serum of breast cancer patients. Clin Cancer Res 2000;6:3823–3826.
391. Hibi K, Nakayama H, Yamazaki T, et al: Detection of mitochondrial DNA alterations in primary tumors and corresponding serum of colorectal cancer patients. Int J Cancer 2001;94:429–431.
392. Frascella E, Rosolen A: Detection of the MyoD1 transcript in rhabdomyosarcoma cell lines and tumor samples by reverse transcription polymerase chain reaction. Am J Pathol 1998;152:577–583.
393. Gattenloehner S, Vincent A, Leuschner I, et al: The fetal form of the acetylcholine receptor distinguishes rhabdomyosarcomas from other childhood tumors. Am J Pathol 1998;152:437–444.
394. Gattenloehner S, Dockhorn-Dworniczak B, Leuschner I, Vincent A, Müller-Hermelink HK, Marx A: A comparison of MyoD1 and fetal acetylcholine receptor expression in childhood tumors and normal tissues: Implications for the molecular diagnosis of minimal disease in rhabdomyosarcomas. J Mol Diagn 1999;1: 23–31.

Assessment of Clonality Using Chromosome X Inactivation Assays

395. Lyon MF: Gene action in the X-chromosome of the mouse (Mus musculus L). Nature 1961;190:372–373.
396. Lyon MF: The William Allan Memorial Award address: X-chromosome inactivation and the location and expression of X-linked genes. Am J Hum Genet 1988;42:8–16.
397. Beutler E, Yeh M, Fairbanks VF: Normal human female as a mosaic of X-chromosome activity: Studies using the gene for G6PD deficiency as a marker. Proc Natl Acad Sci USA 1962;48:9–16.
398. Fialkow PJ: Clonal origin of human tumors. Biochem Biophys Acta 1976;458:283–321.
399. Beutler E, Collins Z, Irwin LE: Value of genetic variants of glucose-6-phosphate dehydrogenase in tracing the orgin of malignant tumors. N Engl J Med 1967; 271:389–391.
400. Boyd Y, Fraser NJ: Methylation patterns at the hypervariable X-chromosome locus DXS255 (M27β): Correlation with X-inactivation status. Genomics 1990;7: 182–187.
401. Keith DH, Singer-Sam J, Riggs AD: Active X chromosome DNA is unmethylated at eight CCGG sites clustered in a guanine-plus-cytosine-rich island at the 5′ end of the gene for phosphoglycerate kinase. Mol Cell Biol 1986;6:4122–4125.
402. Vogelstein B, Fearon ER, Hamilton SR, Feinberg AP: Use of restriction fragment length polymorphisms to determine the clonal origin of human tumors. Science 1985;227:642–645.
403. Vogelstein B, Fearon ER, Hamilton SR, et al: Clonal analysis using recombinant DNA probes from X-chromosome. Cancer Res 1987;47:4806–4813.
404. Fey MF, Liechti-Gallati S, von Rohr A, et al: Clonality and X-inactivation patterns in hematopoietic cell populations detected by the highly informative M27β DNA probe. Blood 1994;83:931-938.
405. Allen RC, Zoghbi HY, Moseley AB, Rosenblatt HM, Belmont JW: Methylation of HpaII and HhaI sites near the polymorphic CAG repeat in the human androgen-receptor gene correlates with X chromosome inactivation. Am J Hum Genet 1992;51:1229–1239.
406. Busque L, Gilliland DG: Clonal evolution in acute myeloid leukemia. Blood 1993;82:337–342.
407. Diaz-Cano SJ: Designing a molecular analysis of clonality in tumors. J Pathol 2000;191:343–344.
408. Busque L, Zhu J, DeHart D, et al: An expression based clonality assay at the human androgen receptor locus (HUMARA) on chromosome X. Nucleic Acids Res 1994;22:697–698.
409. Chen TC, Kuo T, Chan HL: Dermatofibroma is a clonal proliferative disease. J Cutan Pathol 2000;27:36–39.
410. Li M, Cordon-Cardo C, Gerald WL, Rosai J: Desmoid fibromatosis is a clonal process. Hum Pathol 1996;27: 939–943.
411. Lucas DR, Schroyer KR, McCarthy PJ, Markham NE, Fujita M, Enomoto TE: Desmoid tumor is a clonal cellular proliferation: PCR-amplification of HUMARA for analysis of patterns of X-chromosome inactivation. Am J Surg Pathol 1997;21:306–311.
412. Paradis V, Laurendeau I, Viellefond A, et al: Clonal analysis of renal sporadic angiomyolipomas. Hum Pathol 1998;29:1063–1067.
413. Saxena A, Alport EC, Cuastead S, Skinnider LF: Molecular analysis of clonality of sporadic angiomyolipoma. J Pathol 1999;189:79–84.

Genetic Instability

414. Cahill DP, Lengauert C, Yu J, et al: Mutation of mitotic checkpoint genes in cancer. Nature 1998;392: 300–303.
415. Lengauer C, Kinzler KW, Vogelstein B: Genetic instabilities in human cancers. Nature 1998;396: 643–649.
416. Cahill DP, da Costa LT, Carson-Walter EB, Kinzler KW, Vogelstein B, Lengauert C: Characterization of MAD2B and other mitotic spindle checkpoint genes. Genomics 1999;58:181–187.
417. Ionov Y, Peinado MA, Malkhosyan S, Shibata D, Perucho M: Ubiquitous somatic mutations in simple repeated sequences reveal a new mechanism for colonic carcinogenesis. Nature 1993;363:558–561.
418. Thibodeau SN, Bren G, Schaid D: Microsatellite instability in cancer of the proximal colon. Science 1993;260:816–819.
419. Leach FS, Nicolaides NC, Papadopoulos N, et al: Mutations of a MutS homolog in hereditary nonpolyposis colorectal cancer. Cell 1993;75:1215–1225.
420. Papadopoulos N, Nicolaides NC, Wei YF, et al: Mutation of a mutL homolog in hereditary colon cancer. Science 1994;263:1625–1629.
421. Arzimanoglou II, Gilbert F, Barber HR: Microsatellite instability in human solid tumors. Cancer 1998;82: 1808–1820.

422. Ottini L, Esposito DL, Richetta A, et al: Alterations of microsatellites in neurofibromas of von Recklinghausen's disease. Cancer Res 1995;55:5677–5688.
423. Sourvinos G, Parissis J, Sotsiou F, Arvanitis DL, Spandidos DA: Detection of microsatellite instability in sporadic cardiac myxomas. Cardiovasc Res 1999;42: 728–732.
424. Berg PE, Liu J, Yin J, Rhyu MG, Frantz CN, Meltzer SJ: Microsatellite instability is infrequent in neuroblastoma. Cancer Epidemiol Biomarkers Prev 1995;4: 907–909.
425. Hogarty MD, White PS, Sulman EP, Brodeur GM: Mononucleotide repeat instability is infrequent in neuroblastoma. Cancer Genet Cytogenet 1998;106:140–143.
426. Tajiri T, Suita S, Shono K, et al: A microsatellite instability in neuroblastoma based on a high resolution fluorescent microsatellite analysis. Cancer Lett 1998; 124:59–63.
427. Aue G, Hedges LK, Schwartz HS, Bridge JA, Neff JR, Butler MG: Clear cell sarcoma or malignant melanoma of soft parts: Molecular analysis of microsatellite instability with clinical correlation. Cancer Genet Cytogenet 1998;105:24–28.
428. Schneider-Stock R, Szibor R, Walter H, Plate I, Roessner A: No microsatellite instability, but frequent LOH in liposarcomas. Int J Oncol 1999;14:721–726.
429. Suwa K, Ohmori M, Miki H: Microsatellite alterations in various sarcomas in Japanese patients. J Orthop Sci 1999;4:223–230.
430. Martin SS, Hurt WG, Hedges LK, Butler MG, Schwartz HS: Microsatellite instability in sarcomas. Ann Surg Oncol 1998;5:356–360.

Techniques for Genetic Analysis

431. Caspersson T, Zech L, Johansson C: Differential binding of alkylating fluorochromes in human chromosomes. Exp Cell Res 1970;60:315–319.
432. Comings DE: Methods and mechanisms of chromosome banding. Methods Cell Biol 1978;17:115–132.
433. Mitelman F: ISCN: An International System for Human Cytogenetic Nomenclature. Basel, Karger, 1995.
434. Cremer T, Lichter P, Borden J, Ward DC, Manuelidis L: Detection of chromosome aberrations in metaphase and interphase tumor cells by in situ hybridization using chromosome-specific library probes. Hum Genet 1988;80:235–246.
435. Pinkel D, Straume T, Gray JW: Cytogenetic analysis using quantitative, high-sensitivity, fluorescence hybridization. Proc Natl Acad Sci USA 1986;83:2934–2938.
436. Speicher MR, Ballard SG, Ward BD: Karyotyping human chromosomes by combinatorial multi-fluor FISH. Nat Genet 1996;12:368–375
437. Busam KJ, Fletcher CD: The clinical role of molecular genetics in soft tissue tumor pathology. Cancer Metastasis Rev 1997;16:207–227.
438. Veldman T, Vignon C, Schrock E, Rowley JD, Ried T: Hidden chromosome abnormalities in haematological malignancies detected by multicolour spectral karyotyping. Nat Genet 1997;15:406–410.
439. Liyanage M, Coleman A, du Manoir S, et al: Multicolour spectral karyotyping of mouse chromosomes. Nat Genet 1996;14:312–315.
440. Cohen N, Betts DR, Trakhtenbrot L, et al: Detection of unidentified chromosome abnormalities in human neuroblastoma by spectral karyotyping (SKY). Genes Chromosomes Cancer 2001;31:201–208.
441. Mrozek K, Iliszko M, Rys J, et al: Spectral karyotyping reveals 17;22 fusions in a cytogenetically atypical dermatofibrosarcoma protuberans with a large marker chromosome as a sole abnormality. Genes Chromosomes Cancer 2001;31:182–186.
442. Kallioniemi A, Kallioniemi O-P, Sudar D, et al: Comparative genomic hybridization for molecular cytogenetic analysis of solid tumors. Science 1992;258: 818–821.
443. Kallioniemi O-P, Kallioniemi A, Piper J, et al: Optimizing comparative genomic hybridization for analysis of DNA sequence copy number changes in solid tumors. Gene Chromosome Cancer 1994;10: 231–243.
444. du Manoir S, Speicher MR, Joos S, et al: Detection of complete and partial chromosome gains and losses by comparative genomic in situ hybridization. Hum Genet 1993;90:590–610.
445. Knuutila S, Autio K, Aalto Y: On line access to CGH data of DNA sequence copy number changes. Am J Pathol 2000;157:689–690.
446. El-Rifai W, Sarlomo-Rikala M, Andersson LC, Knuutila S, Miettinen M: DNA sequence copy number changes in gastrointestinal stromal tumors: Tumor progression and prognostic significance. Cancer Res 2000;60:3899–3903.
447. Southern EM: Detection of specific sequences among DNA fragments separated by gel electrophoresis. J Mol Biol 1975;98:503–517.
448. Mullis KB, Faloona F: Specific synthesis of DNA in vitro via a polymerase-catalyzed chain reaction. Methods Enzymol 1987;155:335–350.
449. Saiki R, Scharf S, Faloona F, et al: Enzymatic amplification of beta-globin genomic sequences and restriction site analysis for diagnosis of sickle cell anemia. Science 1985;230:1350–1354.
450. Saiki RK, Bugawan TL, Horn GT, Mullis KB, Erlich HA: Analysis of enzymatic amplificatically amplified beta-globin and HLA-DQ alpha DNA with allele-specific oligonucleotide probes. Nature 1986;324: 163–166.
451. Embury SH, Scharf SJ, Saiki RK, et al: Rapid prenatal diagnosis of sickle cell anemia by a new method of DNA analysis. N Engl J Med 1987;316:656–661.
452. Barnes WM: PCR amplification of up to 35-kb DNA with high fidelity and high yield from λ bacteriophage templates. Proc Natl Acad Sci USA 1994;91:2216–2220.
453. Akasaka T, Muramatsu M, Ohno H, et al: Application of long-distance polymerase chain reaction to detection of junctional sequences created by chromosomal translocation in mature B-cell neoplasms. Blood 1996;88:985–994.
454. Willis TG, Jadayel DM, Coignet LJA, et al: Rapid molecular cloning of rearrangements of the IgH J

locus using long-distance inverse polymerase chain reaction. Blood 1997;90:2456–2464.
455. Vaandrager JW, Schuuring E, Zwikstra E, et al: Direct visualization of dispersed 11q13 chromosomal translocations in mantel cell lymphoma by multicolor fiber fluorescence in situ hybridization. Blood 1996;88: 1177–1182.
456. Downing JR, Khandekar A, Shurtleff SA, et al: Multiplex RT-PCR assay for the differential diagnosis of alveolar rhabdomyosarcoma and Ewing's sarcoma. Am J Pathol 1995;46:626–634.
457. Meier VS, Kuhne T, Jundt G, Gudat F: Molecular diagnosis of Ewing tumors: Improved detection of EWS-FLI-1 and EWS-ERG chimeric transcripts and rapid determination of exon combinations. Diagn Mol Pathol 1998;7:29–35.
458. Lasota J, Miettinen M. Absence of Kaposi's sarcoma-associated virus (human herpesvirus-8) sequences in angiosarcoma. Virchows Arch 1999;434:51–56.
459. Lasota J, Jasinski M, Debiec-Rychter M, Szadowska A, Limon J, Miettinen M: Detection of the SYT-SSX fusion transcripts in formaldehyde-fixed, paraffin-embedded tissue: A reverse transcription polymerase chain reaction amplification assay useful in the diagnosis of synovial sarcoma. Mod Pathol 1998;11:626–633.
460. Cotton RGH: Slowly but surely towards better scanning for mutations. Trends Genet 1997;13:43–46.
461. Fischer SG, Lerman LS: DNA fragments differing by single base-pair substitutions are separated in denaturing gradient gels: Correspondence with melting theory. Proc Natl Acad Sci USA 1983;80:1579–1583.
462. Fodde R, Losekoot M: Mutation detection by denaturing gradient gel electrophoresis (DGGE). Hum Mutat 1994;3:83–94.
463. Orita M, Iwahana H, Kanazawa H, Hayashi K, Sekiya T: Detection of polymorphism of human DNA by gel electrophoresis as single-strand conformation polymorphisms. Proc Natl Acad Sci USA 1989;86: 2766–2770.
464. Hayashi K: PCR-SSCP: A method for detection of mutations. GATA 1992;9:73–79.
465. Oefner PJ, Underhill PA: Comparative DNA sequencing by denaturing high-performance liquid chromatography (DHPLC). Am J Hum Genet 1995;57: A266.
466. Liu W, Smith DI, Rechtzigel KJ, Thibodeau SN, James CD: Denaturing high performance liquid chromatography (DHPLC) used in the detection of germline and somatic mutations. Nucleic Acids Res 1998;26: 1396–1400.
467. Han SS, Cooper DN, Upadhyaya MN: Evaluation of denaturing high performance liquid chromatography (DHPLC) for the mutational analysis of the neurofibromatosis type 1 (NF1) gene. Hum Genet 2001;109: 487–497.
468. Mies C: Molecular biology analysis of paraffin-embedded tissues. Hum Pathol 1994;25:555–560.
469. Lewis F, Maughan NJ, Smith V, Hillan KJ, Quirke P: Unlocking the archive—Gene expression in paraffin-embedded tissue. J Pathol 2001;195:66–71.
470. Jackson DP, Lewis FA, Taylor GR, Boylston AW, Quirke P: Tissue extraction of DNA and RNA and analysis by the polymerase chain reaction. J Clin Pathol 1990;43:499–504.
471. Greer CE, Peterson SL, Kiviat NB, Manos MM: PCR amplification from paraffin-embedded tissues. Effects of fixative and fixation time. Am J Clin Pathol 1991; 95:117–124.
472. Shibata D: The polymerase chain reaction and the molecular genetic analysis of tissue biopsies. In Herrington CS, McGee JOD (eds): Diagnostic Molecular Pathology: A Practical Approach, vol II. Oxford, England: IRL Press, 1992, pp 85–111.
473. Williams C, Ponten F, Moberg C, et al: A high frequency of sequence alterations is due to formalin fixation of archival specimens. Am J Pathol 1999;155: 1467–1471.
474. Sieben NL, ter Haar NT, Cornelisse CJ, Fleuren GJ, Cleton-Jansen AM: PCR artifacts in LOH and MSI analysis of microdissected tumor cells. Hum Pathol 2000;31:1414–1419.
475. Livak KJ, Flood SJ, Marmaro J, Giusti W, Deetz K: Oligonucleotides with fluorescent dyes at opposite ends provide a quenched probe system useful for detecting PCR product and nucleic acid hybridization. PCR Methods Appl 1995;4:357–362.
476. Peter M, Gilbert E, Delattre O: A multiplex real-time PCR assay for the detection of gene fusions observed in solid tumors. Lab Invest 2001;81:905–912.
477. Bijwaard KE, Fetsch JF, Przygodzki R, Taubenberger JK, Lichy JH: Detection of SYT-SSX fusion transcripts in archival synovial sarcomas by real time reverse transcriptase-polymerase chain reaction. J Mol Diagn 2002;4:59–64.
478. Pongers-Willemse MJ, Verhagen OJ, Tibbe GJ, et al: Real-time PCR for the detection of minimal residual disease in acute lymphoblastic leukemia using junctional region specific TaqMan probes. Leukemia 1998;12:2006–2014.
479. Preudhomme C, Revillion F, Merlat A, et al: Detection of BCR-ABL transcripts in chronic myeloid leukemia (CML) using a 'real time' quantitative RT-PCR assay. Leukemia 1999;13:957–964.
480. Duggan DJ, Bittner M, Yidong C, Meltzer P, Trent JM: Expression profiling using cDNA microarrays. Nat Genet 1999;21:10–14.
481. Lockhard DJ, Winzeler EA: Genomics, gene expression and DNA arrays. Nature 2000;405:827–836.
482. Golub TR, Slonim DK, Tamayo P, et al: Molecular classification of cancer: Class discovery and class prediction by gene expression monitoring. Science 1999; 286:531–536.
483. Khan J, Simon R, Bittner M, et al: Gene expression profiling of alveolar rhabdomyosarcoma with cDNA microarrays. Cancer Res 1998;58:5009–5013.

Gene Nomenclature

484. Genome International Sequencing Consortium: Initial sequencing and analysis of the human genome. Nature 2001;409:860–921.
485. Ventner JC, Adams MD, Myers EW, et al: The human genome. Science 2001;291:1304–1352.

Additional References

486. Nucci MR, Weremowicz S, Neskey DM, et al: Chromosomal translocation t(8;12) induces aberrant HMGIC expression in aggressive angiomyxoma of the vulva. Genes Chromosomes Cancer 2001;32:172–176.
487. Koontz JI, Soreng AL, Nucci M, et al: Frequent fusion of the JAZF1 and JJAZ1 genes in endometrial stromal tumors. Proc Nat Acad Sci USA 2001;98:6348–6353.
488. Mendlick M, Nelson M, Pickering D, et al: Translocation t(1;3)(p36.3q25) is a nonrandom aberration in epithelioid hemangioendothelioma. Am J Surg Pathol 2001;25:684–687.
489. Henn W, Wullich B, Thonnes M, Steudel WI, Feiden W, Zang KD: Recurrent t(12;19)(q13;q13.3) in intracranial and extracranial hemangiopericytoma. Cancer Genet Cytogenet 1993;71:151–154.
490. Schoenmakers EF, Huysmans C, van de Ven WJ: Allelic knockout of novel splice variants of human recombination repair gene RAD51B in t(12;14) uterine leiomyomas. Cancer Res 1999;59:19–23.
491. Douglass EC, Rowe ST, Valentine M, Parham DM, Meyer WH, Thompson EI: A second nonrandom translocation, der(16)t(1;16)(q21;q13), in Ewing sarcoma and peripheral neuroectodermal tumor. Cytogenet Cell Genet 1990;53:87–90.
492. Astrom A, D'Amore ES, Sainati L, et al: Evidence of involvement of the PLAG1 gene in lipoblastomas. Int J Oncol 2000;16:1107–1110.
493. Hibbard MK, Kozakewich HP, Dal Cin P, et al: PLAG1 fusion oncogenes in lipoblastoma. Cancer Res 2000;60:4869–4872.
494. Gisselsson D, Hibbard MK, Dal Cin P, et al: PLAG1 alterations in lipoblastoma: Involvement in varied mesenchymal cell types and evidence for alternative oncogenic mechanisms. Am J Pathol 2001;159: 955–962.
495. Panagopoulos I, Mencinger M, Dietrich CU, et al: Fusion of the RBP56 and CHN genes in extraskeletal myxoid chondrosarcomas with translocation t(9;17) (q22;q11). Oncogene 1999;18:7594–7598.

Benign Fibroblastic and Myofibroblastic Proliferations

CHAPTER 5

Introduction

Benign fibroblastic tumors and tumor-like lesions form a large and heterogeneous group of nonneoplastic and neoplastic tumor entities. Some of these are specific for or predominantly occur in children, and some occur in adults only. The benign fibroblastic proliferations are here arbitrarily divided into three groups: (1) putative reactive lesions (including fasciitis and related lesions), (2) benign fibrous neoplasms (fibromas and related tumors), and (3) potentially locally aggressive fibrous lesions (fibromatoses, solitary fibrous tumor). The classification has been summarized in Table 5–1. The fibrous proliferations in children are discussed in Chapter 6.

Common to all lesions included in this chapter is their inability to metastasize (except rare examples of malignant solitary fibrous tumor). Fibromatoses, especially the ones of desmoid type, have a significant tendency to local recurrence.

Although many fibrous lesions are generally believed to be reactive, lack of hard evidence makes it difficult to clearly separate reactive and neoplastic conditions in many instances. Likewise, some lesions, believed to be neoplasms, may actually be reactive. In some cases, the commonly used designations are actually misleading in regard to the true nature of the lesion; for example, nuchal fibroma, penile fibromatosis, and fibromatosis colli all are probably reactive processes.

Dermatofibrosarcoma, fibrosarcoma, and related tumors have metastatic potential or the capability of progression unless completely excised. Malignant fibrous histiocytoma is also included among malignant fibroblastic neoplasms. These tumors are discussed in Chapter 7.

Biology of Fibroblasts

Fibroblasts are collagen-producing mesenchymal cells that form the collagenous matrix of dense connective tissue composed of fibrillary collagens, mainly of collagen type I. Fibroblasts are also present in the dispersed loose connective tissue in fibrous septa adjacent to muscles, blood vessels, and other structures. Fibrocyte is the designation historically used for an "inactive" form of fibroblast.

The proliferation and differentiation of fibroblasts is regulated by interaction of several fibroblast growth factors and their receptors and other growth factors, such as proteins of the transforming growth factor beta (TGF-β) family. Interaction with the extracellular matrix also regulates fibroblast behavior.[1,2]

In nonneoplastic conditions, the fibroblastic proliferation may be activated by inflammation (through growth factors/cytokines) or by another type of tissue injury. The molecular mechanisms of fibroblastic neoplasia are still incompletely understood. However, pathologic activation of signal transduction pathways is being revealed in some tumor types, for example, in intramuscular myxoma.

Table 5–1. Classification of Benign Fibrous Lesions

Putative Reactive Lesions
Nodular fasciitis
Cranial fasciitis
Proliferative fasciitis
Proliferative myositis
Ischemic fasciitis
Elastofibroma
Nuchal type fibroma
Nuchal fibrocartilaginous pseudotumor
Idiopathic retroperitoneal fibrosis (Ormond disease)
Penile fibromatosis (Peyronie disease)
Keloid
Benign Fibroblastic Neoplasms with Limited Growth Potential
Collagenous fibroma
Fibroma of tendon sheath
Sclerotic fibroma of skin (circumscribed storiform collagenoma)
Pleomorphic fibroma of skin
Palisaded myofibroblastoma
Myofibroblastoma of breast
Benign fibrous histiocytoma and its variants
Intramuscular myxoma
Juxta-articular myxoma
Superficial angiomyxoma
Superficial acral fibromyxoma
Fibroblastic Tumors with Proliferative Capacity
Palmar fibromatosis
Plantar fibromatosis
Desmoid type fibromatosis
Solitary fibrous tumor*

*Rare malignant variants occur with metastatic capability.

Under certain conditions, fibroblasts are capable of secreting abundant proteoglycan or glycoprotein matrix. Such secretory activity of fibroblasts contributes to the histogenesis of myxoid neoplasms, which are essentially fibroblastic tumors, based on evidence of the fibroblastic and myofibroblastic nature of such tumors.

Subsets of Fibroblasts

Two specific subsets of fibroblasts can be identified based on morphology and antigen expression: myofibroblasts and the $CD34^+$ fibroblasts.

Most reactive fibroblastic lesions, stroma of malignant tumors, and most fibroblastic neoplasms contain myofibroblasts. Originally, Gabbiani and Majno identified these derivatives of fibroblasts ultrastructurally as cells with features intermediate between fibroblasts and smooth muscle cells and functionally as the cells responsible for scar contraction.[3] Like fibroblasts, myofibroblasts contain an ultrastructurally prominent rough endoplasmic reticulum, and they have some cytoplasmic bundles of actin microfilaments and membrane-attached actin filaments (attachment plaques), but less than seen in true smooth muscle cells. Unlike smooth muscle cells, they have an incomplete, only focally developed basement membrane. Immunohistochemically myofibroblasts have a broad spectrum including subsets that are positive for vimentin only, vimentin and actin, or vimentin, actin, and desmin.[4]

Another distinctive cell type that contributes to the histogenesis of many mesenchymal tumors is the $CD34^+$ fibroblast. This cell type was originally described by Nickoloff around skin adnexa and blood vessels.[5] The possible relationship of these cells with the $CD34^+$ bone marrow stem cells was originally suspected, but has not been convincingly demonstrated. The $CD34^+$ fibroblasts are present perivascularly and in connective tissue septa throughout the body. These cells are candidates for the histogenetic origin of some $CD34^+$ fibroblastic tumors, such as solitary fibrous tumor and dermatofibrosarcoma protuberans.

Putative Reactive Lesions

Nodular Fasciitis

Clinical Features

Nodular fasciitis is the designation for a presumably reactive, sometimes pseudosarcomatous spindle cell proliferation. It occurs predominantly in young adults in the third to fifth decades, occasionally in children, and sometimes in older adults. The lesion most commonly presents in the subcutis of forearm, arm, thigh, and distal upper extremity. Occurrence in the head and neck, trunk, and genital area is also possible. The lesion is often attached to fascia, and usually measures 2 to 3 cm in diameter, and occasionally reaches the size of 10 cm. The main mass is usually subcutaneous, but extension to dermis is not rare. Some involve skeletal muscle, and purely intramuscular location is possible. Only some patients elicit a history of trauma, although nodular fasciitis is believed to be a reactive process.[6–9] Local excision is considered adequate treatment.

Pathology

Grossly nodular fasciitis is typically well circumscribed and surrounded by a dense collagenous band, but it is not encapsulated. Some variants, especially the granulation tissue-like highly vascular lesions, commonly have an infiltrative, spiculated border to the subcutaneous fat. On sectioning, the lesion varies from mucoid to firm. It is tan and often discolored with focal hemorrhage. Older lesions may have multiple microcysts or sometimes a larger central cyst.

The histologic features of nodular fasciitis vary according to the age of the lesion. It has been suggested that the lesion evolves from a myxoid early stage to a cellular phase and later to a fibrous phase with progressive cystic change. The excised lesions are often usually slightly myxoid, moderately cellular spindle cell proliferations with pale staining streaks of evolving collagenous matrix. They are composed of randomly oriented, uniform myofibroblasts with the appearance of tissue culture, separated by varying numbers of collagen fibers that often increase toward the periphery and on maturation of the lesion (Fig. 5–1). Sprinkled extravasated erythrocytes, lymphocytes, and scattered osteoclast-like giant cells, which can be more numerous, often give the lesions a heterogeneous appearance.

Cytologically, the myofibroblasts often have a "tissue culture appearance" with large hypochromatic nucleus with a delicate nucleolus and angulated cytoplasmic processes. Numerous mitoses may be present, especially in the highly cellular variants. Some examples are highly vascular with a granulation tissue-like appearance, and these examples typically infiltrate in fat as multiple spicules.

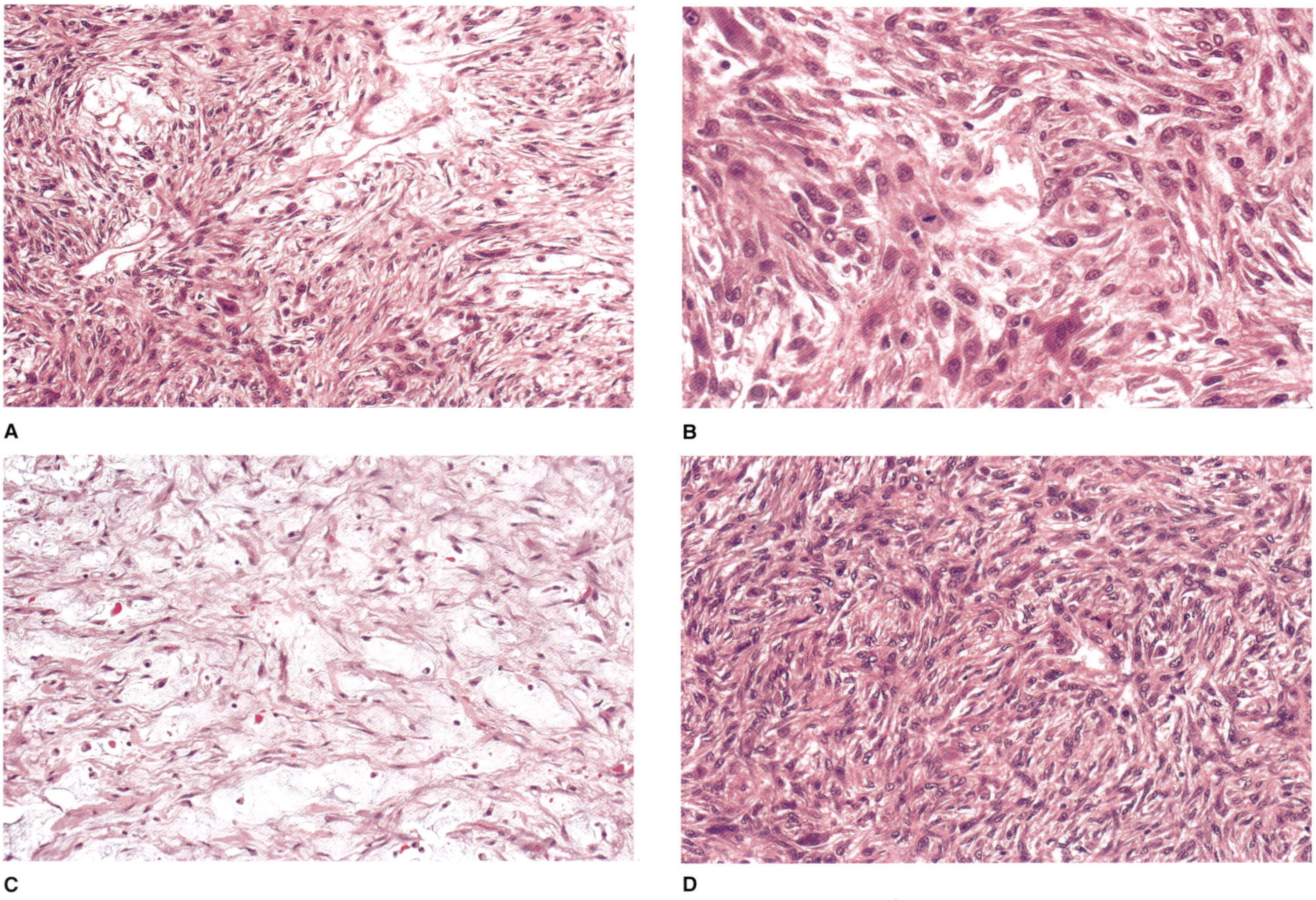

Figure 5–1. Different appearances of nodular fasciitis. *A,* Cellular myofibroblastic spindle cell proliferation with alternating myxoid areas. *B,* High magnification of a highly cellular example with mitotic activity. *C,* Myxoid lesion with a lower cellularity. *D,* A lesion with numerous osteoclast giant cells.

Intravascular Fasciitis and Penile "Myointimoma"

Those cases of nodular fasciitis with a dominant intravascular component are termed intravascular fasciitis.[10] These lesions involve the lumina of small vessels (Fig. 5–2). The clinical course is indolent and cellular composition is similar to that of nodular fasciitis. The designation of parosteal fasciitis is used of those lesions that are apposed to a bone. Their cellular composition is similar to that of classical variants.

Fetsch et al.[11] recently reported myofibroblastic intravascular proliferations in the glans penis of males of various ages, including three young children. These lesions were small nodules (<1 cm) that were mostly treated by excisional biopsy and were benign in clinical follow-up. Histologically, the intravascular proliferation resembled the myofibroblastic component of myofibroma, but a relationship with intravascular fasciitis could not be ruled out.

Immunohistochemistry of Nodular Fasciitis and Related Lesions

Immunohistochemically, the lesional cells are positive for vimentin, muscle actins, and smooth muscle actin (SMA); prominent actin positivity should not result in misclassification as a smooth muscle tumor. There may be a significant CD68$^+$ histiocytic component although this marker may also react with some nonhistiocytic cells.[12] The lesional cells are negative for desmin, S-100 protein, CD34, and bcl-2. Electron microscopic studies have shown a major myofibroblastic component.[13]

Differential Diagnosis

Some carcinomas, notably a variant thyroid papillary carcinoma, may contain nodular fasciitis-like stroma; therefore, thorough sampling is required to rule out the presence of carcinoma components before nodular fasciitis is diagnosed in parenchymal locations, such as the thyroid.[14]

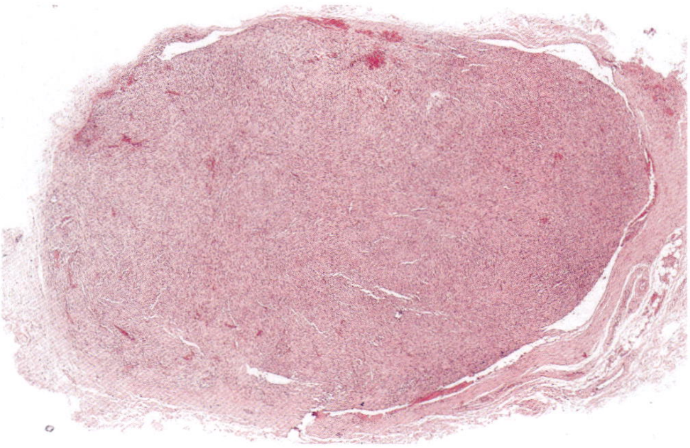

Figure 5–2. Intravascular fasciitis grows inside a small vein.

Desmoid and low-grade fibrosarcomas/myofibroblastic sarcomas may contain areas resembling nodular fasciitis, and definitive differential diagnosis may therefore be impossible with limited material, such as a needle biopsy. Areas of myofibroblastic proliferation with relative uniformity and prominent blood vessels are typical of desmoid, and the presence of enlarged nuclei with atypia should alert one to the possibility of low-grade sarcoma. Such atypia should be sought for, especially in the case of large lesions and those occuring in older people.

Genetics

Clonal gene rearrangements at 3q21 have been reported, representing a reciprocal translocation of t(13;15) in one case.[15,16] Such findings raise the question whether some cases of nodular fasciitis could be true neoplasms.

Cranial Fasciitis

Cranial fasciitis[17,18] is analogous to nodular fasciitis, and it occurs as a deep scalp mass in infants (see Chapter 6).

Proliferative Fasciitis

Clinical Features

This is a reactive fibroblastic/myofibroblastic proliferation probably related to nodular fasciitis. It is distinctive by its content of ganglion cell-like fibroblasts. Proliferative fasciitis is much less common than nodular fasciitis. In contrast to the latter, proliferative fasciitis occurs predominantly in adults with a mild male predominance; 70% of patients are between 31 and 70 years of age (Armed Forces Institute of Pathology unpublished data). Rare occurrence in children (7% of all cases) has been documented. The most common sites of presentation are subcutis of the thigh, forearm, arm, back, shoulder, chest wall, and buttock. About one third of patients have a history of recent local trauma. The lesion grows rapidly and is often tender. Local excision is sufficient, and there is no tendency for recurrence.[19–21]

Pathology

Proliferative fasciitis forms a poorly circumscribed, infiltrative, subcutaneous mass of 1 to 4 cm that is sometimes attached to fascia. Grossly, the tumor is yellowish gray to tan, and it often has a ragged or spiculated margin.

Histologically, the lesion is composed of a nodular fasciitis-like cellular spindle cell proliferation with admixed clusters and streaks of ganglion cell-like fibroblasts with abundant amphophilic or basophilic cytoplasm and large nuclei often with a prominent eosinophilic nucleolus (Fig. 5–3*A*). Moderate mitotic activity may be present. The lesion often infiltrates in the fat. In children it can be alarmingly cellular and when predominantly composed of ganglion-like cells, it can be confused with rhabdomyosarcoma (Fig. 5–3*B*). Immunohistochemically the lesional spindle cells are negative for CD34 and desmin, but they may be positive for muscle actins and SMA; the ganglion-like cells are typically negative for actins.[19–22]

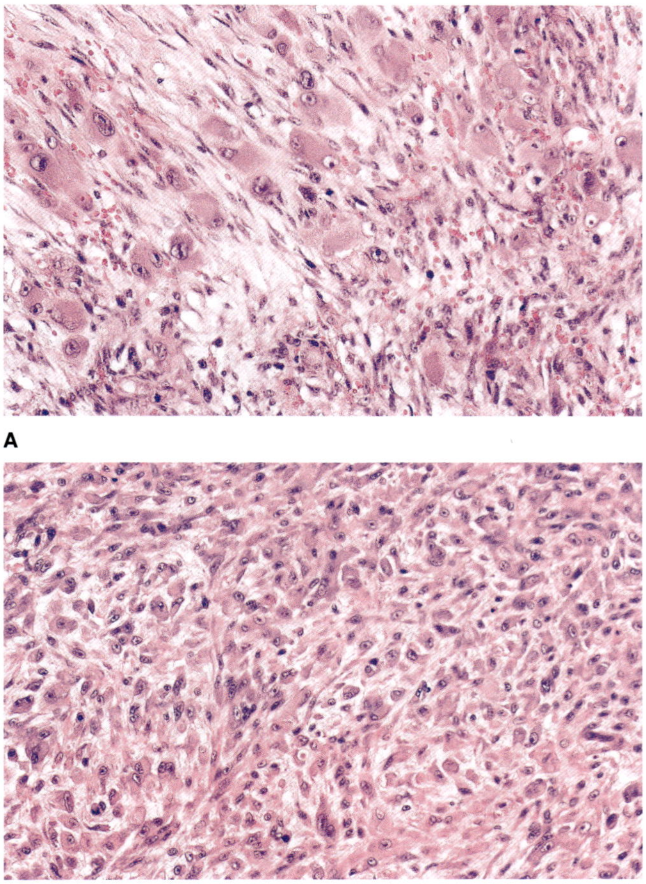

Figure 5–3. *A,* Proliferative fasciitis typically contains clusters of large ganglion cell-like fibroblasts in a stroma resembling nodular fasciitis. *B,* Proliferative fasciitis lesions in children may be composed entirely of the ganglion cell-like fibroblasts. These tumors can be separated from rhabdomyosarcoma by the uniform cellular appearance and lack of desmin positivity.

Proliferative Myositis

Clinical Features

Proliferative myositis is the designation for an intramuscular lesion that shows histologic features similar to proliferative fasciitis. The lesion probably represents a reparative process of unknown origin; it is benign and self-limited.

Similar to proliferative fasciitis, proliferative myositis occurs predominantly in middle-aged adults and has a mild male predominance. The most common sites of presentation are the muscles of the neck, shoulder, and upper trunk. The lesion presents as a rapidly growing painless mass. Local excision is sufficient, and there is no tendency to recur.[23,24]

Pathology

Grossly, the lesions are typically small, poorly delineated pale, fibrous foci involving the skeletal muscle tissue and surrounding muscle fibers and fascia. Histologically, the lesion typically expands the space between the muscle fibers and widens the connective tissue septa. In evolving lesions, foci of muscle cell degeneration and lymphoid and histiocytic infiltration are present. The more cellular, early phase shows essentially similar components as proliferative fasciitis with spindle cells and large cytoplasmic ganglion-like cells (Fig. 5–4); the latter have been shown to be modified fibroblasts by electron microscopy.[22,25]

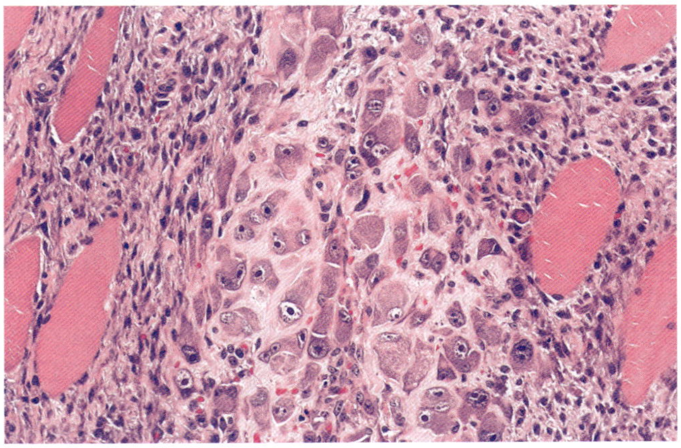

Figure 5–4. Proliferative myositis lesion contains numerous ganglion cell-like fibroblasts and infiltrates in the skeletal muscle.

Mitoses are inconspicuous. Foci of metaplastic bone may be present. A resolved lesion may develop into paucicellular, diagnostically nonspecific scar.

Differential Diagnosis

The histologically unusual, large ganglion-like cells and cellular spindle cell component should not be confused with sarcoma; in fact, the gross appearance does not resemble a tumor. However, skeletal muscle infiltration of low-grade sarcomas may resemble the histologic pattern of proliferative myositis in a biopsy specimen. In the differential diagnosis, attention should be paid to cellular atypia and radiologic or surgical evidence of a dominant tumor mass (almost always seen with true sarcomas).

Focal myositis is the designation for a nonspecific fibroinflammatory lesion of skeletal muscle. This condition may represent a reparative phase of a muscle rupture. Histologically, there is a mixture of evolving fibrosis with lymphoid infiltration and degenerative skeletal muscle fibers. No ganglion-like cells are present, in contrast to proliferative myositis.

Ischemic Fasciitis (Atypical Decubital Fibroplasia)

Clinical Features

This is a reactive, pseudoneoplastic fibroblastic proliferation in soft tissues on top of bony prominences; it typically occurs in old or chronically bedridden patients. This condition probably represents a faulty reparative fibrovascular process in an ischemic environment.

The lesions typically occur as tumor-like bulges in the scapular, trochanteric, or shoulder in older adults, usually between the 8th and 10th decades. However, it may occur in very old patients without an underlying condition, suggesting that this lesion may be an age-specific histologic reaction. The lesion is subcutis based but may extend to the periosteum.

Pathology

The lesion bulges underneath an overlying hyperemic skin, but the skin is rarely ulcerated. It typically ranges from 1 to 8 cm in diameter, and larger examples are often centrally cystic. Histologically, the lesions contain scattered atypical, bipolar spindled, or epithelioid reactive fibroblasts with an abundant basophilic cytoplasm and smudged nuclei with prominent nucleoli. These cells are embedded in a myxoid matrix with foci or lakes of fibrin.

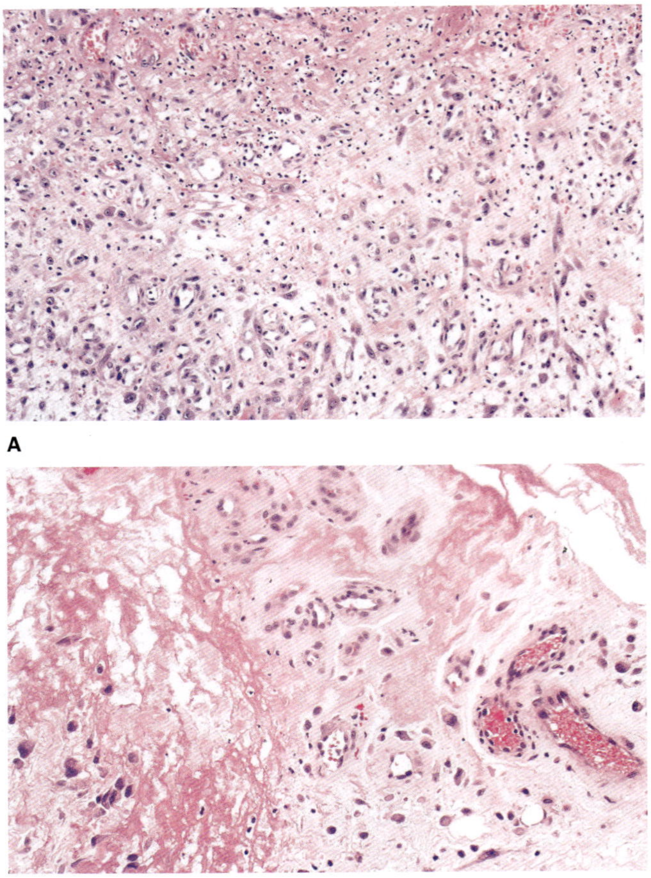

A

B

Figure 5-5. *A,* Ischemic fasciitis lesion is highly vascular with florid capillary proliferation bordering necrosis. *B,* The lesion contains scattered plump fibroblasts and capillaries dilated by fibrin deposition.

Prominent hemangioma-like clusters and zones of newly formed capillaries bordering necrosis are typical of this condition and probably reflect the fact that tissue ischemia is one of the most powerful angiogenic stimuli (Fig. 5–5).

Although nonneoplastic, these lesions may show alarming histologic features and can be confused with neoplasms such as myxoid malignant fibrous histiocytoma (MFH). The presence of fibrin, zones of capillary proliferation, and clinical setting help this distinction.[26,27]

The lesional cells may be positive for CD34 and muscle actins, but they are negative for desmin.

Other Conditions Named "Fasciitis"

Eosinophilic fasciitis is an inflammatory autoimmune condition seen together with scleroderma; it does not form a discrete mass. Necrotizing fasciitis refers to bacterial soft tissue infection involving deep soft tissues, which can form a localized inflammatory mass. This condition may arise as a complication of surgery.

Elastofibroma

Clinical Features

Originally described by Järvi et al.,[28] elastofibroma is a clinicopathologically distinctive fibrous proliferation rich in thick, convoluted elastic fibers. It occurs in middle-aged and older adults almost exclusively underneath the scapula in the posterior chest wall. Autopsy and radiologic studies have suggested that incidental, microscopic elastofibromas are quite common (10–20%).[29] Reactive origin, possibly caused by chronic minor trauma, has been suggested. Behavior is benign, and recurrences do not develop. Histologically, similar lesions designated as elastofibroma or elastofibromatous nodules have been reported in the plantar foot and in the gastric wall with peptic ulcer.[30–32]

Pathology

Elastofibroma typically forms an ill-defined subscapular mass of 3 to 10 cm in diameter. It is firm and rubbery, and on sectioning often shows yellow and gray stripes corresponding to alternating fatty and fibrous tissue. The appearance varies according to the proportions of the yellow fatty and gray fibrous components.

Microscopically, elastofibroma shows a major fibrous and a minor fatty component. It typically shows a low cellularity with regular fibroblasts in a densely collagenous matrix containing thick, convoluted elastic fibers that are fragmented and appear beaded in the section plane and are highlighted in elastin staining (Fig. 5–6). The lesional cells have been found positive for collagen type II, which is normally found only in hyaline cartilage and fibrocartilage.[33]

Elastofibroma is so characteristic for its presentation and histologic appearance that it can hardly be confused with other tumors. However, desmoid and sarcomas (MFH) may occur in the same location and can be distinguished by their much greater cellularity.

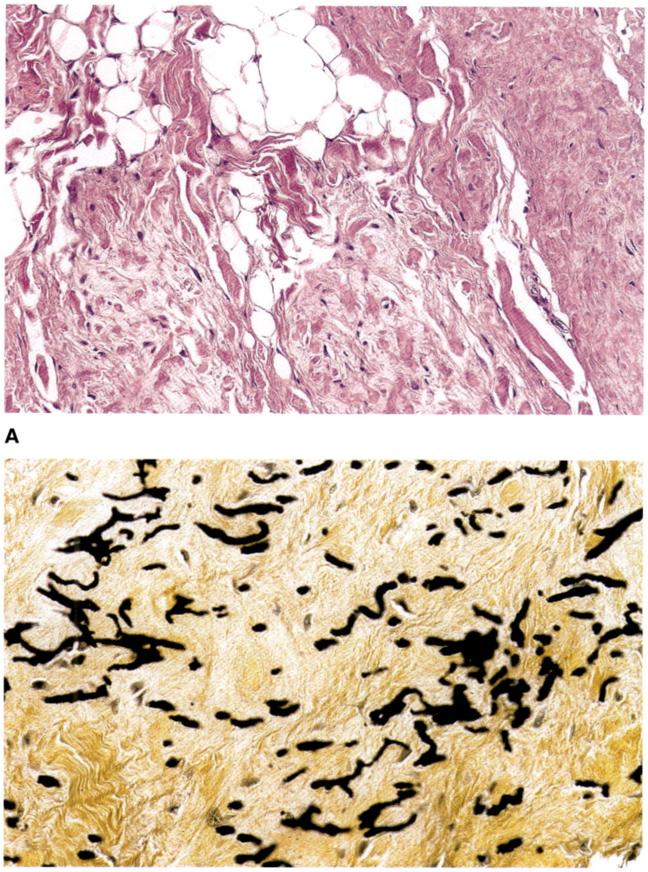

A

B

Figure 5–6. Histologically, elastofibroma shows the typical thick pale staining elastic fibers in a collagenous background *(A)*. Elastin stain highlights fragmented thick elastic fibers *(B)*.

Nuchal-Type Fibroma

Clinical Features

This designation refers to paucicellular dermal and subcutaneous accumulation of collagen, predominantly presenting in the posterior neck.[34,35] Because similar lesions may present in extranuchal sites, the designation of nuchal-type fibroma has been proposed.[36]

According to our series of 50 patients, nuchal-type fibroma presents in a wide age range but the frequency peaks at the sixth decade. There is a strong male predominance. Over 70% of the lesions present in the posterior neck, but similar lesions may also occur in the back, shoulder, and face and occasionally elsewhere. The etiology is unknown, but there is an association with diabetes, and coexistence with Gardner syndrome in some cases.[36–38] A recent report also verified the connection between diabetic scleredema, a cutaneous swelling that occurs in diabetes, and nuchal type fibroma.[39] Occasional lesions have recurred following simple excision, but it is not sure whether this is a true recurrence or persistency of the triggering factors. The lesion probably represents a reactive condition to unknown stimulus. There is currently no evidence that this condition is neoplastic.

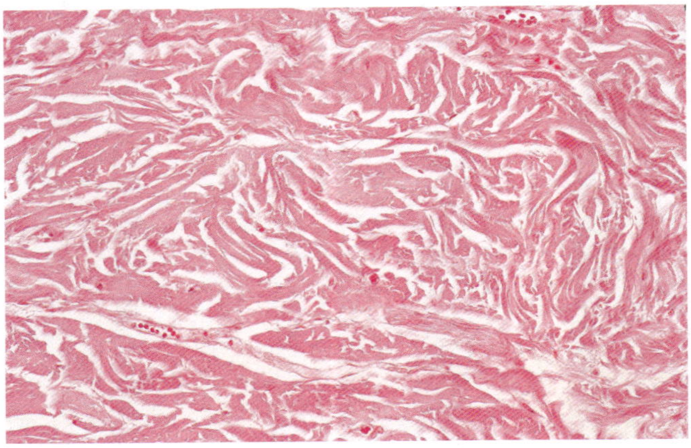

A

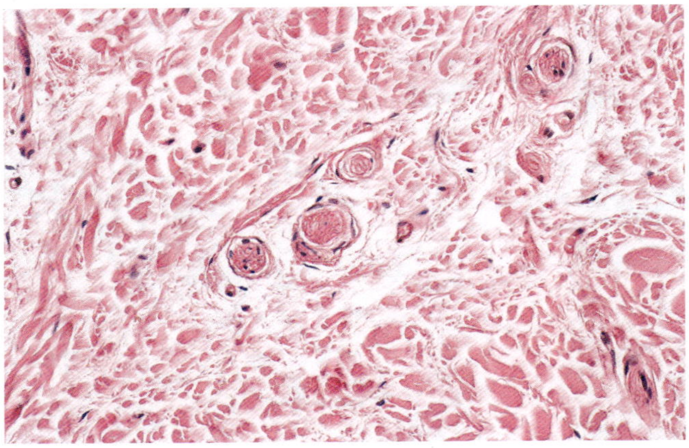

B

Figure 5–7. *A*, Nuchal fibroma is paucicellular and contains dense lobules of coarse collagen. *B*, Neuroma-like clusters of small nerves are often present.

Pathology

Nuchal-type fibroma appears as a firm tumor-like mass that measures 1 to 6 cm in diameter (mean, 3 cm). Histologically, it is composed of paucicellular accumulation of lobulated bundles of collagen often containing entrapped islands of fat. The lesional fibroblasts are few and inconspicuous. Small, apparently proliferating nerve twigs resembling traumatic neuroma are often present (Fig. 5–7). The lesion may extend to skeletal muscle.

Nuchal Fibrocartilaginous Pseudotumor

Clinical Features

This designation refers to an uncommon, acquired fibrocartilaginous metaplasia of the nuchal ligament. The lesion presents in adult life, predominantly in young adults and early middle age. The median age of 11 reported patients is 39 years. Seven of the reported cases have been in women and four in men. The lesion may be tender and is located in the posterior neck overlying the posterior aspect of the lower cervical vertebrae. Some patients have elicited a history of past cervical trauma suggesting posttraumatic etiology. Follow-up studies have shown no recurrences.[40,41]

Pathology

The lesions measure 1 to 3 cm in diameter and are located in the deep soft tissue above the cervical vertebrae involving the nuchal ligament. Microscopically, it is a poorly delineated nodular fibrocartilaginous proliferation with linear arrays of chondrocytes within a fibrocartilage-type of dense matrix, surrounded by dense fibrosis (Fig. 5–8).

Idiopathic Retroperitoneal Fibrosis (Ormond Disease) and Related Disorders

Clinical Features

This reactive fibrous proliferation of retroperitoneum is often clinically distinctive by causing ureteral obstruction. The process is believed to begin as a plaquelike inflammatory cuffing around the aorta. Later it draws the ureters toward the midline, ultimately encasing them with a potential to cause obstructive renal damage. By comparison, retroperitoneal tumors often displace the ureters laterally. This condition usually occurs in middle-aged and older individuals, and it has a male predominance.[42–44] *Idiopathic mediastinal fibrosis* probably represents a similar disease in thoracic location and may cause superior vena cava obstruction. It may occur in younger patients.[45]

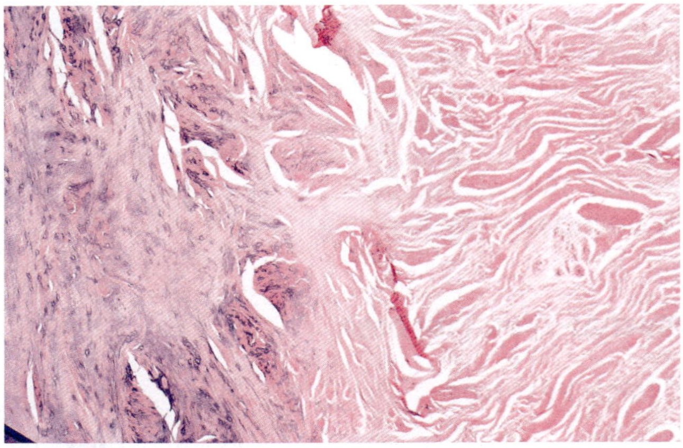

Figure 5–8. Nuchal fibrocartilaginous pseudotumor is composed of focus of cartilage and paucicellular fibrous proliferation.

Inflammatory aneurysm of the aorta and *perianeurysmal retroperitoneal fibrosis* are believed to be part of the same disease process, and immunologic reaction to atherosclerotic aortic lesions could have an etiologic role in some cases. Lesions associated with etiologic factors such as drugs (methysergide used for migraine treatment, practolol, a β-receptor blocker) and tumors (carcinoid) may be histologically and clinically somewhat similar, but they do not qualify under the rubric "idiopathic."

Systemic symptoms, such as fever and weight loss, and elevated erythrocyte sedimentation rate, are common. Surgical relief of ureteral obstruction, corticosteroids, and aortic aneurysm repair in some cases are the most important treatment modalities.

Pathology

The lesion presents as ill-defined tumor-like plaques and nodules typically located in the midline adjacent to the aorta and around the ureters. The lesional tissue is typically excised as single or multiple plaque-like strips or nodules, which appear grossly as gray-white and firm. Histologically, the lesional tissue shows dense, sclerosing fibrosis with plasma cells, histiocytes, and clusters of lymphocytes, often with focal germinal center formation. The fibrous component contains fibroblasts and myofibroblasts, but the fibrous tissue is usually less cellular than that seen in the desmoplastic stroma of carcinomas (Fig. 5–9).

Imunohistochemically, the lymphoid component contains B cells, T cells, and polyclonal plasma cells.

Differential Diagnosis

Caution is needed in interpretation of small biopsies because the diagnosis requires exclusion of specific infections and sclerosing neoplasms, and clinical or radiologic correlation is necessary. Sclerosing (follicular) lymphoma, mesothelioma, or metastatic carcinoma (prostatic, sclerosing carcinoid) have to be ruled out. Lack of a dominant mass and heterogeneous cellular composition help to separate this condition from fibromatosis, sclerosing liposarcoma with an inflammatory fibrous component, and inflammatory myofibroblastic tumor, which it may histologically resemble.

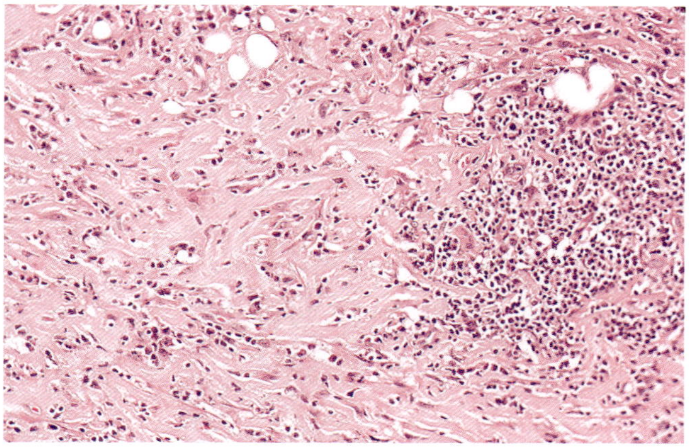

Figure 5–9. Retroperitoneal fibrosis lesion typically contains streaks of mildly cellular fibroblastic proliferation sprinkled with lymphoplasmacytic infiltration.

Penile Fibromatosis

Penile fibromatosis (Peyronie disease, plastic induration of the penis) is a reactive, sclerosing fibrous proliferation that involves the inner thin part of the penile fascia (tunica albuginea) around the corpora cavernosa. The plaquelike fibrous proliferation of penile fibromatosis may cause pain or penile curvature on erection. Histologically, the lesion is composed of dense fibrous tissue, often with focal perivascular lymphoid infiltration, and sometimes with osseous metaplasia.[46]

Caution is necessary to rule out sclerosing carcinoma and epithelioid sarcoma; the presence of atypical epithelial cells is diagnostic and is aided by keratin immunohistochemistry.

Keloid

Clinical Features

Keloid is a reactive, hyperplastic fibrous overgrowth typically presenting in surgical and other scars and sites of recent trauma, such as in body piercing sites. It can be considered a pathologic wound-healing process. Keloids predominantly occur in young adults and are more common in blacks. Chronic inflammation is believed to be etiologically significant, probably via local excess of fibrosis-promoting cytokines such as TGF-β. Recurrence following excision is common. It probably reflects the persistence of the causative stimulus.[47,48]

Pathology

Grossly keloid specimens are firm and resilient to rubbery on sectioning, sometimes with trabeculated or whorled surface. Histologically, keloid is composed of thick, deeply eosinophilic "waxy" collagen fibers surrounded by scattered hyperplastic fibroblasts or myofibroblasts (Fig. 5–10); this component separates keloid from a hypertrophic scar. The vascular pattern may be prominent with focal perivascular lymphoplasmacytic infiltration, but inflammation may be absent.

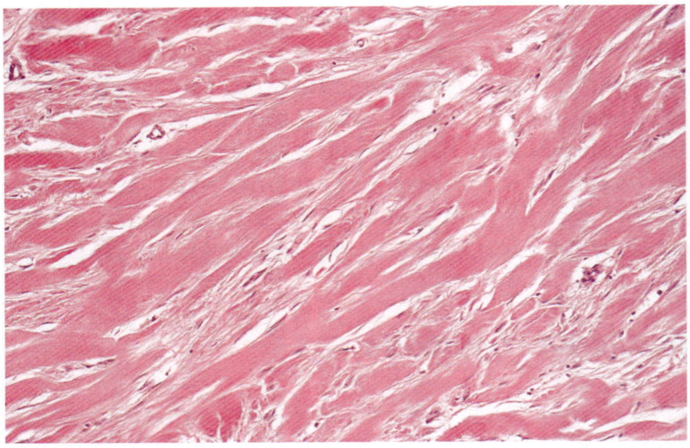

Figure 5–10. Keloid is composed of thick fibers of collagen and inconspicuous fibroblasts.

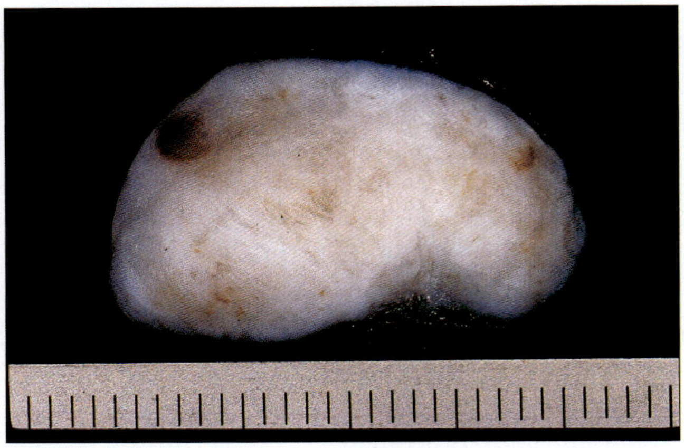

Figure 5–11. Collagenous fibroma lesion is a sharply circumscribed-appearing pearl-gray nodule.

Benign Fibroblastic Tumors with Limited Growth Potential

Collagenous Fibroma (Desmoplastic Fibroblastoma)

Clinical Features

Collagenous fibroma is a grossly and microscopically distinctive benign fibrous tumor that predominantly occurs in older men. The tumor occurs chiefly between the fifth and seventh decades (70%), and rarely in adolescents. It has a strong male predominance (3:1) and occurs in a wide variety of body sites usually the subcutis, but may also be purely intramuscular. The most common locations are arm (24%), shoulder (19%), back, upper extremity, and feet. The behavior is benign, and none of the published series have had documented recurrences.[49–52]

Pathology

The tumor usually measures 1 to 4 cm in greatest dimension, but examples over 10 cm and as large as 20 cm have occurred. Grossly, it appears well circumscribed and oval, elongated, or disk-shaped; it may be lobulated. On sectioning the tissue is firm, pearl-gray, homogeneous, and sometimes feels cartilage-like (Fig. 5–11).

Microscopically, collagenous fibroma is composed of scattered spindled or stellate-shaped fibroblasts and myofibroblasts in a dense, mainly amorphous collagenous matrix (Fig. 5–12). Myxoid stroma is seen in some cases. Despite the apparent circumscription, the lesion microscopically infiltrates in the subcutaneous fat in 70% of cases and extends into the skeletal muscle in 25% of cases; even in these cases, the lesion appears grossly circumscribed. The vessels are usually inconspicuous and have thin walls. Lower cellularity, predominance of amorphous collagenous matrix, and inconspicuous vasculature separate it from desmoid tumor.

Immunohistochemically, the lesional cells are variably positive for smooth muscle actin and occasionally for keratins. They are negative for desmin, endothelial membrane antigen (EMA), S-100 protein, and CD34.[52]

Differential Diagnosis

Intramuscular examples of this tumor are often suspected as desmoids. Collagenous fibroma is more collagenous and less cellular than desmoid, and its

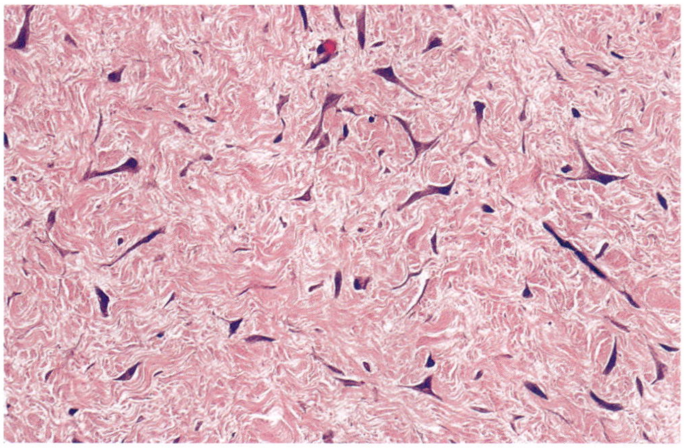

Figure 5–12. Microscopically, collagenous fibroma lesion is composed of stellate-shaped fibroblasts in a densely collagenous background.

vascular pattern is inconspicuously lacking prominent muscle cells or endothelia. The fibroblasts are stellate-shaped in collagenous fibroma, whereas they are more spindled and fascicularly arranged in desmoid.

Genetics

Cytogenetic studies have been reported in two cases. Both showed involvement of 11q12, similar to that previously observed in fibroma of tendon sheath, suggesting a possible genetic relationship of these entities.[53]

Fibroma of Tendon Sheath

Clinical Features

This tumor occurs predominantly in young and middle-aged adults with a strong male predominance. Examples in children have also been reported. The lesion typically occurs as a small painless mass in the subcutis of fingers and hands closely associated with tendon sheaths, but location in the knee region and feet has also been reported. Simple, conservative excision is curative, and the tumor does not recur.[54–61]

Pathology

The lesion is usually small, 1 to 2 cm in diameter, and appears well circumscribed and sometimes lobulated. Histologically, it is composed of uniform spindled fibroblasts and myofibroblasts in a variably myxoid to densely fibrous, often highly vascular stroma. Slitlike blood vessels are typically present (Fig. 5–13).

Differential Diagnosis

This entity may sometimes be difficult to histologically distinguish from nodular fasciitis and collagenous fibroma. The former has a more heterogeneous composition, and the latter has stellate-shaped fibroblasts. Although fibroma of tendon sheath has been suggested as a hyalinized variant of tenosynovial giant cell tumor,[62] there is no general consensus of such a relationship.

Ultrastructural studies have revealed a significant myofibroblastic component, and immunohistochemical studies have shown muscle actin positivity.

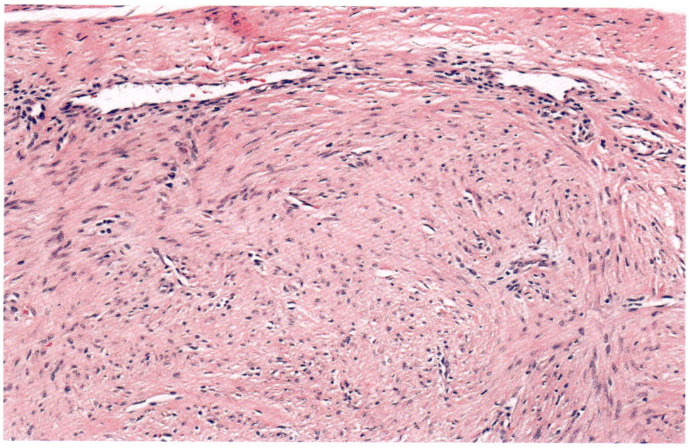

A

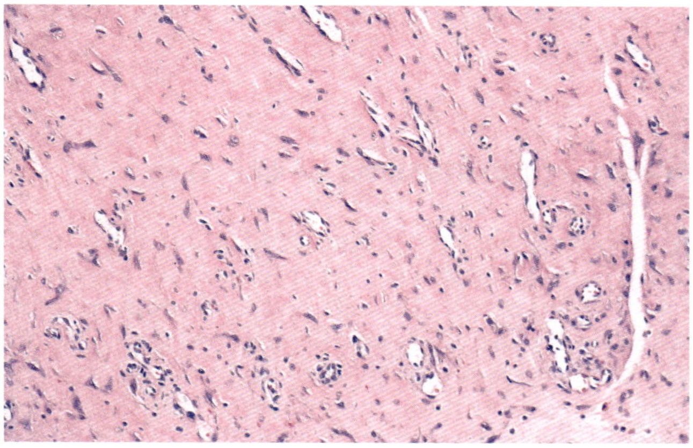

B

Figure 5–13. Fibroma of tendon sheath is sharply circumscribed and often contains slitlike vascular spaces in the periphery *(A)*. The tumor is highly vascular but relatively paucicellular *(B)*.

Genetics

Cytogenetic analysis has revealed translocation t(2;11) in one patient.[63]

Sclerotic Fibroma of Skin

Sclerotic fibroma (circumscribed storiform collagenoma) is a designation for a skin tumor that forms a small, solitary spherical dermal nodule usually measuring less than 1 cm. It occurs in adults with no site predilection and is sometimes seen in connection with Cowden disease (multiple hamartoma syndrome). Local excision is curative.[64–66]

Histologically, the nodule is paucicellular and is composed of inconspicuous fibroblasts in a dense collagenous background with a storiform organization and pericellular cleavages (Fig. 5–14).

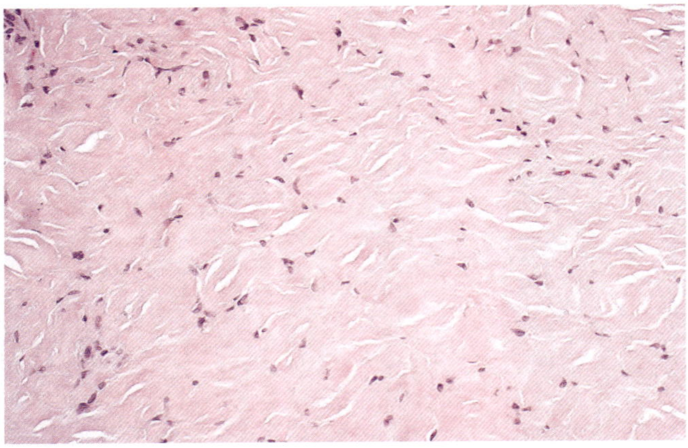

Figure 5–14. Sclerotic fibroma is composed of dense collagen with narrow cleavage spaces and inconspicuous fibroblasts.

Pleomorphic Fibroma of the Skin

Pleomorphic fibroma is the designation for a relatively rare skin tumor that presents as polypoid, small (4–16 mm), dome-shaped cutaneous fibrous lesion in young and middle-aged adults. Clinical course has been benign in all cases.[67]

Histologically, these tumors are paucicellular but contain distinctive, atypical fibroblasts with large, irregularly shaped and variably hyperchromatic nuclei in a dense collagenous background (Fig. 5–15). The lesional cells have been found to be positive for CD34 and negative for S-100 protein. Positivity for CD34 differentiates this fibroma from benign fibrous histiocytoma with giant (monster) cells.[68]

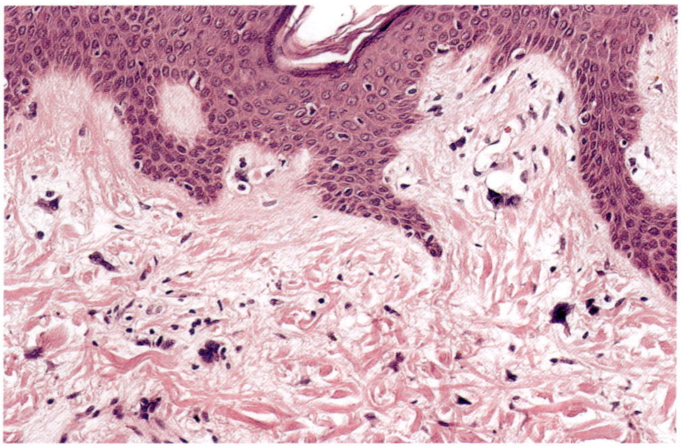

Figure 5–15. Pleomorphic fibroma forms a dermal nodule containing scattered fibroblasts with nuclear atypia in a dense collagenous background.

Palisaded Myofibroblastoma

Clinical Features

This rare condition, also described as "hemorrhagic spindle cell tumor with amianthoid fibers" involves lymph nodes, usually the inguinal ones, where it forms a painless mass; few similar lesions in submandibular location have been reported.[66] The tumor occurs mainly in middle-aged adults, and largest series showed 2:1 male predominance.[69–74] Although the condition is benign, recurrence has been reported at least in one instance.[75]

Pathology

Grossly, the tumor is a sharply demarcated, firm gray-white mass within a lymph node. Histologically, it is highly distinctive with large collections of amorphous "amianthoid" collagen fibers often radiating to the periphery of the clusters (Fig. 5–16).

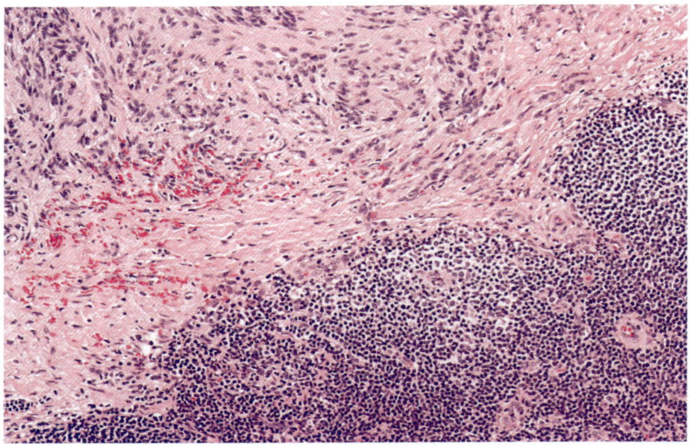

A

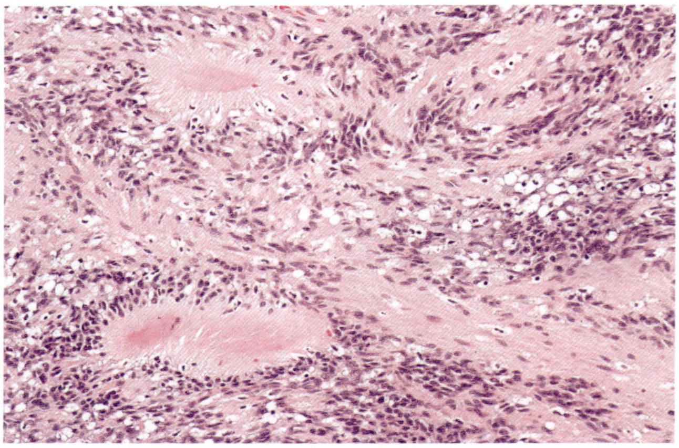

B

Figure 5–16. Palisaded myofibroblastoma forms a sharply circumscribed nodule located in a lymph node *(A)*. A higher magnification shows crystalloid collagen deposits surrounded by spindled myofibroblasts *(B)*.

Focal hemorrhage and solid cellular areas are often present. The bland, spindled lesional fibroblasts and myofibroblasts often have a focal palisading nuclear pattern simulating that of schwannoma. Cytoplasmic eosinophilic globules, resembling those seen in digital fibroma, may also be present. A rim of lymphoid tissue is identified in all thoroughly sampled lesions.

Immunohistochemically, the lesional cells are positive for muscle actins and vimentin and negative for desmin and S-100 protein.[69,70] According to one study, the crystalloid "amianthoid" collagen fibers may not truly be "amianthoid," that is, abnormally thick collagen fibers, but are rather composed of multiple coalesced fibers consisting of collagen types I and III.[73]

Differential Diagnosis

Although the intranodal location and hemorrhagic spindle cell appearance has some resemblance to Kaposi sarcoma, the thick collagen fibers are unique to this lesion; palisaded myofibroblastoma is a myofibroblastic, not endothelial process. Negative immunostaining for S-100 protein separates this tumor from schwannoma, as which these tumors often were historically diagnosed.

Myofibroblastoma of the Breast

Clinical Features

This tumor, originally described by Wargotz et al.,[76] predominantly occurs in the breasts of older men and occasionally in women. The median age in the largest series was 64 years (range, 40–85 years). The tumor forms a firm, circumscribed and relatively small nodule. Follow-up information indicates that this tumor neither recurs nor metastasizes and is therefore amenable to a simple excision.[76-79]

Pathology

Grossly, this tumor is typically well circumscribed, rubbery gray-tan, and 1 to 4 cm in size, with a mean diameter of 2.3 cm in the largest series.[76]

Histologically, the tumor is quite cellular and has a pushing, noninfiltrative border. It is composed of plump, uniform, spindled or sometimes oval to slightly epithelioid myofibroblasts separated by broad streaks of collagen (Fig. 5–17). Nuclear grooves are often seen, but there is no pleomorphism. Mitotic activity is low. Immunohistochemically the tumor cells are positive for actin and CD34, focally for desmin, and negative for S-100 protein and keratins.[76-80] Positivity for

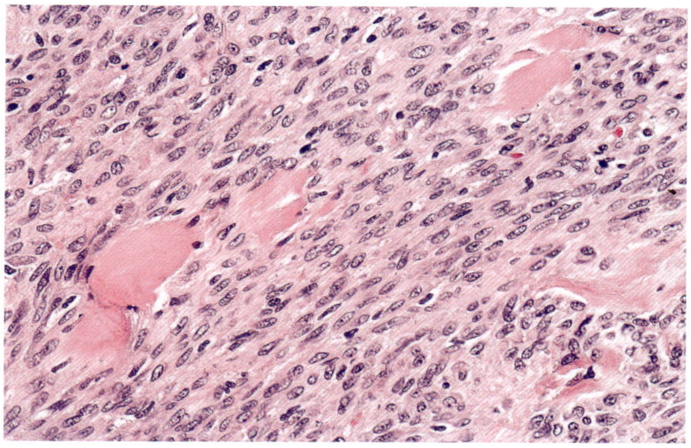

Figure 5–17. Myofibroblastoma of the breast is composed of uniform ovoid myofibroblasts and broad bands of collagen.

estrogen and progesterone receptors has been reported, whereas androgen-receptor positivity appears rare.[81]

The presence of lipomatous component in some tumors and cytogenetic studies showing losses in 16q, similar to those found in spindle cell lipoma, suggest a relationship between these tumors.[82] There may also be a continuum between myofibroblastoma and solitary fibrous tumor that may represent a less myofibroblastic CD34$^+$ stromal tumor. Sharp circumscription and intermixed foci of collagen, as opposed to infiltrative margin with finger-like tumor extensions and solid sheets of fibroblasts and myofibroblasts, separate this tumor from fibromatosis of breast.

The occurrence of tumors with features intermediate between myofibroblastoma and spindle cell lipoma also suggests that these entities may be related.

Benign Fibrous Histiocytoma (Dermatofibroma)

Clinical Features

Benign fibrous histiocytoma (BFH, dermatofibroma, previously also called histiocytoma) is among the most common benign soft tissue neoplasms. This designation refers to tumors that mainly occur in the dermis, but sometimes also in the subcutis and in deeper soft tissues. BFH occurs in wide age range and skin sites. It is most common in the extremities, especially the leg and thigh.[73-85]

The small lesions of the typical variant most commonly present as slightly elevated pigmented nodules. Larger tumors may form sessile polypoid or hemispherical cutaneous elevations and sometimes extend to subcutis.

The tumor may recur unless completely excised. However, the cellular variant has a much higher recurrence rate. Extremely rare pulmonary metastases of cellular BFH have been reported.[86] In these cases it was not possible to histologically predict the metastatic behavior.

Pathology

The lesions vary in gross appearance. The most common variants are small hyperpigmented nodules or plaques, the latter often showing a central depression. Larger tumors may be sessile polypoid masses. The cut surface is often yellow to brown by extensive lipid and hemosiderin content.

The typical variant forms a small lesion composed of fibroblasts, xanthoma cell-like foamy histiocytes, focal hemosiderin pigment, and wide streaks of entrapped collagen. Most lesions are highly vascular and often show perivascular hyalinization. Some tumors are storiform, and many contain mild lymphohistiocytic infiltration. The lesional periphery is typically ragged and infiltrative, but the margin to the subcutis may be of pushing quality. The cellularity varies in a wide range.

Several histologic variants have been identified, some of them clinically distinctive. The most important are (1) dermatomyofibroma, (2) lipidized, (3) aneurysmal, (4) epithelioid, (5) granular cell, (6) cellular, and (7) atypical fibrous histiocytoma (with "monster cells").[85–98]

Dermatomyofibroma is the designation for the 1- to 2-cm plaquelike lesion that typically occurs in young adults in the arm and shoulder region.[87] Histologically, it is composed of uniform, horizontally oriented spindled myofibroblasts and fibroblasts admixed with thin collagen fibers resembling superficial variants of fibromatosis (Fig. 5–18*A*). Foamy histiocytes and giant cells are not present, and inflammatory cells are scant. These lesions are positive for muscle actins but negative for desmin.

The aneurysmal variant occurs in a wide age range with an apparent predilection to proximal parts of extremities and some tendency to recurrence. The tumor usually measures less than 2 cm and has a blue or dark surface and cystic consistency. Histologically, it contains blood-filled spaces and extravasated erythrocytes, in addition to a highly cellular pattern of BFH (Fig. 5–18*B*). The presence of xanthoma cells and blood pools help to distinguish it from Kaposi sarcoma.[88,89]

The lipidized variant occurs especially in the lower extremity in the ankles and legs.[85] It contains abundant lipid-laden histiocytes, and often has a rich vascular pattern with hyalinized vessel walls (Fig. 5–18*C*).

The epithelioid variant typically forms a small dome-shaped or polypoid lesion 1 to 2 cm in diameter, most commonly in the lower extremity. It occurs in a wide age range, with the median age 40 to 42 years in the largest series.[90–92] Histologically, it is composed of uniform polygonal cells with abundant cytoplasm and distinct borders giving the cells an epithelioid appearance (Fig. 5–18*D*). This tumor should not be confused with Spitz nevus, which usually shows nevoid type clusters in the periphery and often has a spindle cell component.

The granular cell variant is rare. It occurs especially in the skin of the shoulder area in middle-aged adults. The tumor contains cells with abundant granular cytoplasm quite similar to granular cell tumors, but the cells are negative for S-100 protein, in contrast to typical granular cell tumor.[93]

Cellular fibrous histiocytoma is the designation for densely cellular benign fibrous histiocytoma composed of compact sheets of spindle cells without significant atypia.[94] These tumors occur predominantly in young adults in similar locations as other fibrous histiocytomas. The lesions usually measure 0.5 to 2.5 cm in maximum diameter, have higher mitotic rate than typical fibrous histiocytomas, occasional necrosis, and often extend to the subcutis (Fig. 5–18*E*). Recurrence has been noted in 25% of patients. Immunohistochemically, the tumors do not differ from other fibrous histiocytomas and are negative for CD34, in contrast to dermatofibrosarcoma protuberans (DFSP).

Atypical fibrous histiocytoma, pseudosarcomatous fibrous histiocytoma, or dermatofibroma with monster cells are the designations used for BFHs with marked focal cytologic atypia.[95–98] These tumors are clinically similar to other variants and occur in a wide age range with a predilection to extremities. The scattered atypical cells have large nuclei, and some also have abundant cytoplasm, but mitotic activity is very low (Fig. 5–18*F*). Although such lesions have had a benign behavior, complete excision is advisable to avoid recurrence.

Differential Diagnosis and Immunohistochemistry

When infiltrating the subcutis, BFH has a pushing margin or infiltrates fibrous septa, in contrast to the diffuse fat infiltration typically seen in DFSP. The lesional cells in BFH are typically negative for CD34, in contrast to DFSP.[99,100] Focal myofibroblastic differentiation and actin positivity are possible, but the lesional cells are negative for S-100 protein and histiocytic markers (factor XIIIa, lysozyme); the latter are seen in the rich histiocytic "passenger cell" infiltration in these tumors.[101] The coexpression of

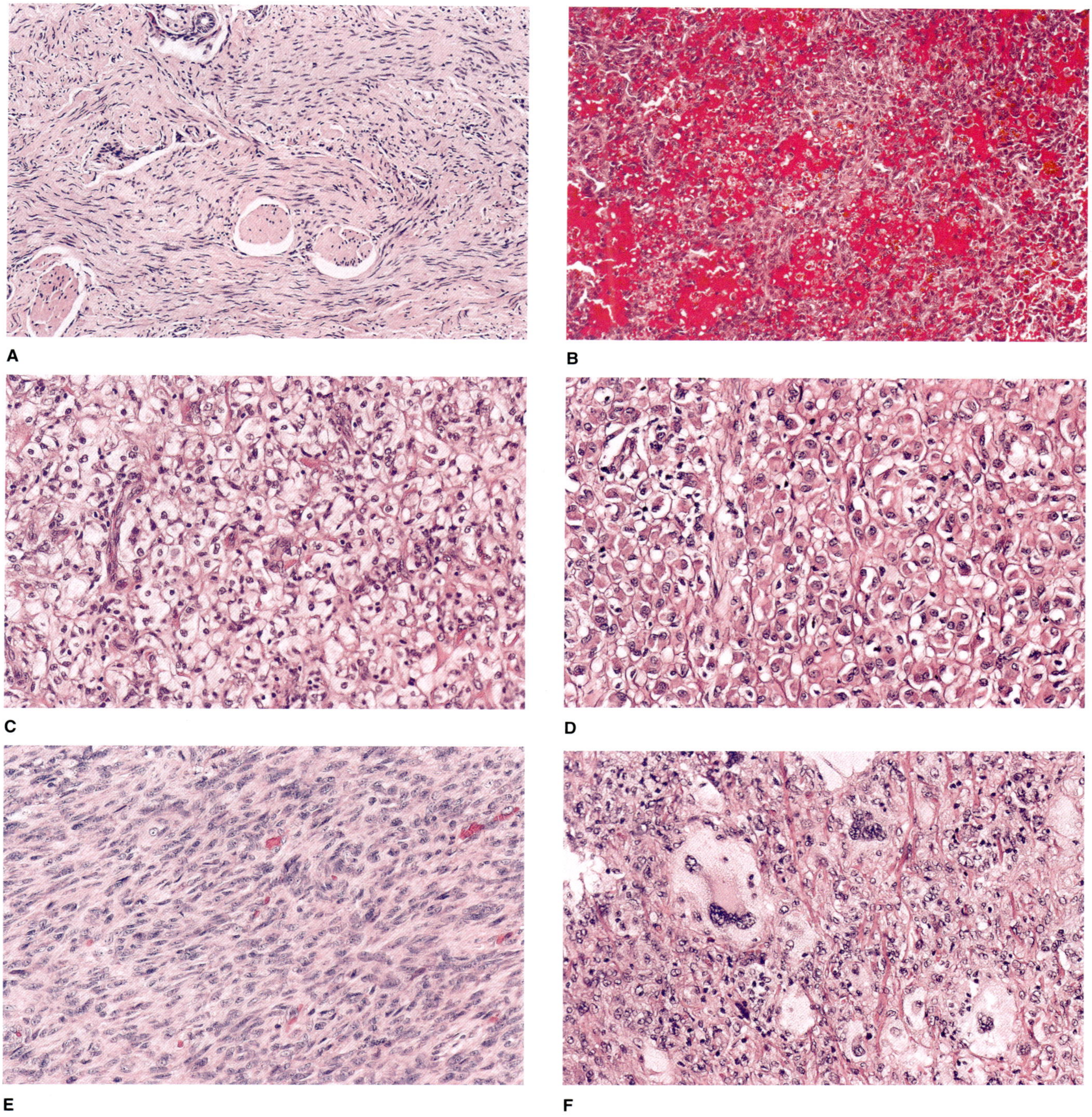

Figure 5-18. Variants of benign fibrous histiocytoma. *A,* Dermatomyofibroma is composed of uniform spindled cells with limited atypia. *B,* Aneurysmal variant with bloody cyst. *C,* Lipidized fibrous histiocytoma with hyalinized blood vessels. *D,* Epithelioid variant composed of cells with sharp demarcation and abundant cytoplasm. *E,* Cellular fibrous histiocytoma. *F,* Atypical fibrous histiocytoma contains scattered atypical large cells.

proliferative markers preferentially seen in the lesional fibroblasts but not histiocytes indicates that the fibroblasts are the proliferative compartment.

Atypical fibrous histiocytoma differs conceptually from atypical fibroxanthoma (AFX) by the presence of widespread cytologic atypia in the latter.

Plexiform fibrohistiocytic tumor is a distinctive multinodular childhood lesion. It has a rare potential for metastasis, and is discussed in Chapter 6.

Juvenile xanthogranuloma is a true histiocytic lesion typically seen in children and young adults (see Chapter 21).

Genetics

The BFHs have been proven monoclonal by HUMARA analysis.[102] Cytogenetic data on 14 cases also revealed clonal chromosomal changes in 38% of cases, more commonly in the cellular fibrous histiocytomas.[103]

Intramuscular Myxoma

Clinical Features

This tumor typically presents in middle-aged adults with a female predominance. The most common locations are the thigh, buttock, arm, and forearm. The tumors vary from small nodule to a sizable mass up to 10 cm; the ones located in the lower extremity tend to be larger. The tumor does not recur after simple excision. Specific preoperative diagnosis by radiologic studies or biopsy allow for conservative surgery. Fewer than 10% of the patients have multiple intramuscular myxomas together with fibrous dysplasia of adjacent bone. This is part of McCune-Albright syndrome.[104–111] Minor, other radiologic bony abnormalities may also be present.[107]

Pathology

Grossly, the tumor often appears sharply demarcated, although microscopically the tumor commonly infiltrates between the skeletal muscle fibers (Fig. 5–19*A*). On sectioning the tumor is gelatinous, gray-white, and glistening. Central cysts may be present, especially in larger tumors.

Microscopically, the tumor is paucicellular and hypovascular, but often contains edematous fibrous streaks (Fig. 5–19*B*). The inconspicuous fibroblasts and myofibroblasts are embedded in a myxoid matrix containing acid mucopolysaccharides, including hyaluronic acid. The lesional cells may be oval or stellate-shaped and have small, dense nuclei and sometimes have a vacuolated cytoplasm. Variants with higher cellularity have been reported; these do not seem to have an increased risk for recurrence.[110] In some cases, the apparently higher cellularity is contributed by histiocytic infiltration. The tumor cells are negative for S-100 protein and desmin.

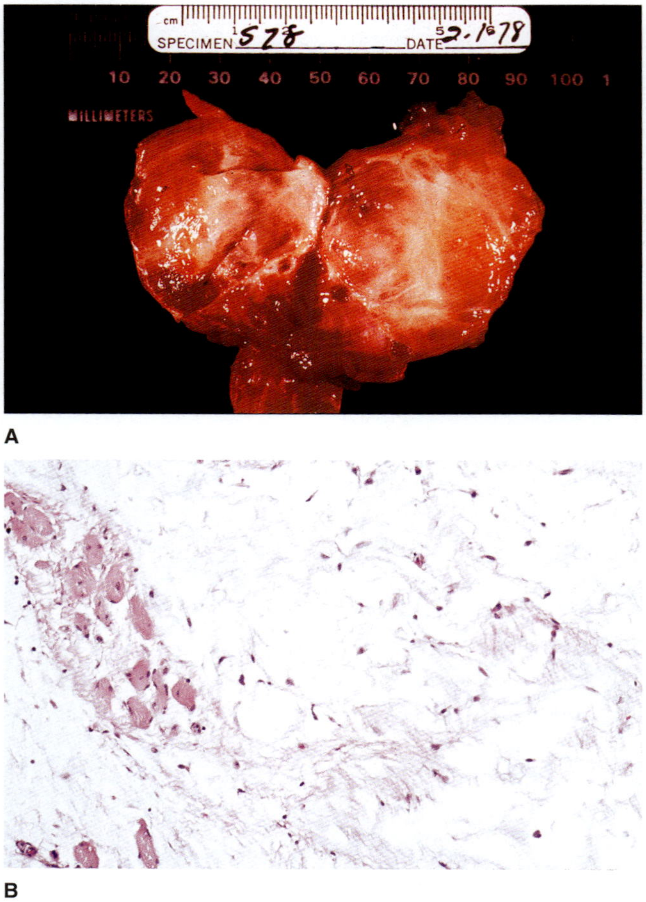

Figure 5–19. *A,* A small intramuscular myxoma appears grossly well circumscribed and has a mucoid, glistening grayish surface. *B,* Histologically, intramuscular myxoma is paucicellular and hypovascular and infiltrates the skeletal muscle.

Genetics

Activating mutations in the *GNAS1* gene encoding a signal transduction protein that regulates the cellular cyclic adenosine monophosphate level have been recently demonstrated in intramuscular myxomas. These mutations have been seen in tumors with and without fibrous dysplasia,[111] and they are similar to the mutations previously reported in fibrous dysplasia of bone,[112,113] indicating that these diverse pathologic processes may have the same molecular pathogenesis.

Juxta-articular Myxoma

Clinical Features

This form of myxoma typically occurs adjacent to joint spaces and ligamentous tissue. It occurs almost at any age except early childhood, and the median age in the

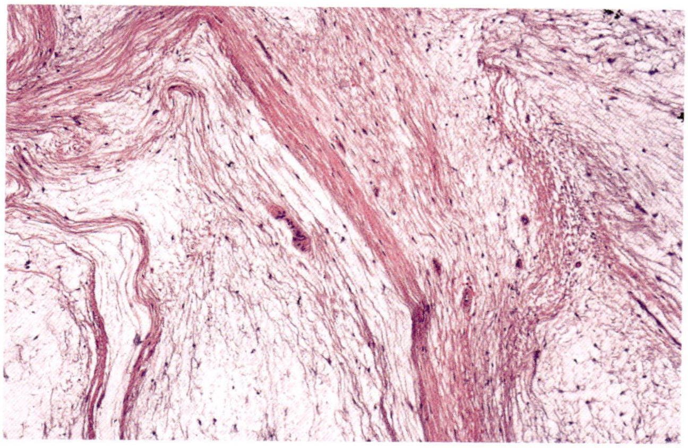

Figure 5–20. Juxta-articular myxoma contains large cells in a fibromyxoid background.

large series by Meis and Enzinger was 43 years with nearly a 3:1 male predominance. The most common location was the knee region, and the majority of lesions were small (<5 cm), manifested by swelling or pain, or occasionally were incidentally detected. Recurrence seems to be relatively common and was seen in 34% of cases in the largest published series.[114]

Pathology

Grossly, the lesion is gelatinous and gray-white to pale tan. Microscopically, it is paucicellular with fine alternating streaks of collagen and myxoid areas; it commonly has ganglion-like cysts with a collagenous, acellular lining. This type of myxoma trends to have a better developed vascular pattern and higher cellularity than intramuscular myxoma (Fig. 5–20). Some tumors have hypercellular areas containing multinucleated histiocytoid cells; these features separate juxta-articular myxoma from intramuscular myxoma.

Genetics

Several chromosomal changes were reported in one case of juxta-articular myxoma. They involved an inversion in chromosome 2, a translocation t(8;22)(q11-12;q12-13), and trisomy of chromosome 7.[115]

Superficial Angiomyxoma (Cutaneous Myxoma)

Clinical Features

Originally cutaneous myxoma was described as one lesion of the familial myxoma syndrome (Carney complex), together with spotty pigmentation of skin, Cushing syndrome, and cardiac myxoma in some patients.[116] Patient series with similar tumors, reported as superficial angiomyxomas, have not had associated lesions, suggesting that the syndrome association of superficial angiomyxoma is weak.[117–120] However, the presence of multiple superficial angiomyxomas in a young patient should raise a suspicion of Carney complex.[116]

The tumor has predilection to young adults between 20 and 40 years equally in men and women, but it may occur at any age. The most common locations are the trunk, thigh, and head and neck. One series reported tumors in female external genitalia.[119] Although the tumor is benign, it may recur locally in 30% of patients, sometimes multiple times.

Pathology

The lesion usually measures between 1 and 5 cm, but may occasionally reach the size of over 10 cm. Grossly, the tumor is soft and has a gray-white, gelatinous surface on sectioning. Microscopically, it usually involves both dermis and subcutis. It is typically composed of multiple lobules separated by collagenous septa. The tumor is paucicellular with a myxoid background and prominent capillary pattern commonly sprinkled with perivascular lymphocytes. Cytologically, there is a mixture of small inconspicuous cells and larger irregularly shaped, mildly atypical cells, but mitoses are scant (Fig. 5–21). Cystic skin adnexal or squamous elements are present within some lesions.

Immunohistochemically, the tumor cells are typically positive for muscle actins, CD34, and, occasionally and focally, for S-100 protein and are negative for AE1/AE3 keratin cocktail.[119]

Differential Diagnosis

Digital mucous cyst is a small, cystic myxoid lesion in the fingers and toes. It has limited cellularity and lacks the prominent vascular component seen in superficial angiomyxoma. Superficial acral fibromyxoma is a distinctive lesion often seen in the nailbed area. This tumor is less myxoid and more cellular than superficial angiomyxoma and lacks lobulation typical of the latter.

Genetics

The familial myxoma syndrome (Carney complex) has been linked to loci on 2p16 and 17q22-24.[121] In the latter, the *PRKAR1A* gene encoding type I regulatory subunit of protein kinase A (PKA) has been implicated. This gene acts as a tumor suppressor gene, and

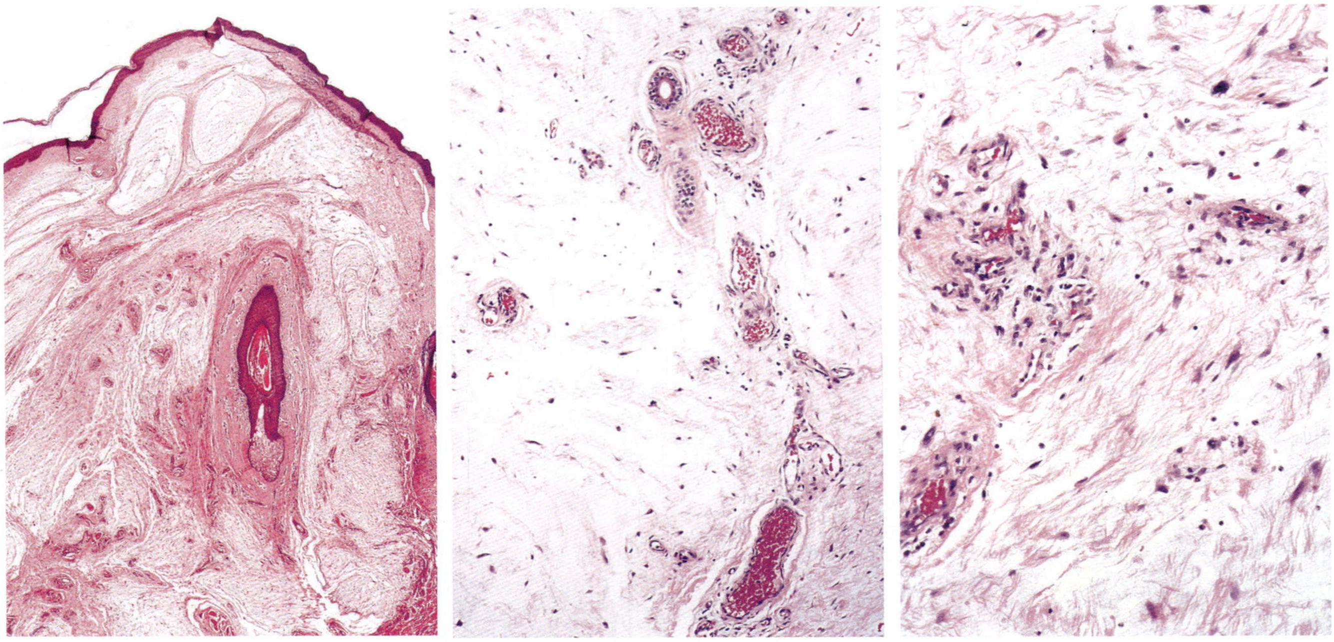

A B C

Figure 5-21. Superficial angiomyxoma is composed of coalescent myxoid lobules. Entrapped skin adnexa are present in this lesion *(A)*. Higher magnification shows focal nuclear atypia *(B)* and perivascular lymphocytes *(C)*.

nonsense mutations resulting in stop codons have been identified in the lesions from some patients.[122,123]

Superficial Acral Fibromyxoma

Clinical Features

This designation refers to a fibromyxoid neoplasm that typically occurs in the distal extremities, often in the nail bed area. The reported 37 tumors occurred in a wide age range with median age of 43 and male predominance 2:1. Most tumors were relatively small, and a long history of local lesion is common. Benign behavior was documented with a low (<10%) frequency of recurrences.[124]

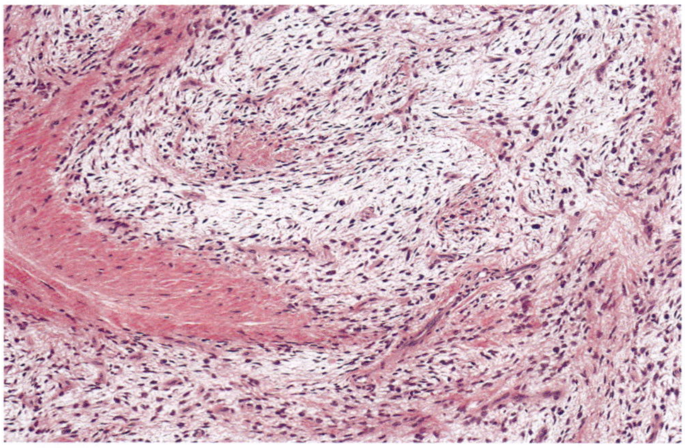

Figure 5-22. Superficial acral fibromyxoma is composed of alternating myxoid and fibrous areas.

Pathology

Grossly superficial acral fibromyxoma is soft to firm and on sectioning has a gray-white, sometimes slightly gelatinous surface. Histologically, it is composed of hypervascular, myxoid spindle cell proliferation often with alternating fibrous areas (Fig. 5–22). Scattered mast cells are often present. Nuclear atypia and mitotic activity are exceptional, but rare atypical variants have been identified as part of the spectrum. No instances of malignant behavior have been documented.

The tumor cells are usually (>90% of cases) positive for CD34 and often for EMA. They are negative for actins, desmin, keratins, and S-100 protein.[124] There are no data on genetics.

Benign Fibroblastic Tumors with Proliferative Capacity

The designation fibromatosis refers to locally recurring and potentially aggressive but nonmetastasizing fibroblastic and myofibroblastic tumors. They include superficial variants of palmar and plantar fibromatosis. Digital fibroma(tosis) is a childhood tumor (see Chapter 6). The terms "deep musculoaponeurotic fibromatosis" and "aggressive fibromatosis" are synonymous with desmoid tumor. All fibromatoses are composed of fibroblasts with a substantial myofibroblastic component.

Palmar Fibromatosis (Dupuytren Contracture)

Clinical Features

This common condition involving the superficial palmar fascia usually occurs in men over the age of 60, and it is believed to occur preferentially in men of northern or eastern European descent. Rarely, similar lesions occur in younger persons, including children and young adults. Autosomal dominant inheritance has been suggested in familial cases. An association with smoking, alcoholism, diabetes, and seizure disorders has been suggested, but its nature is unclear. Although the pathogenetic mechanism is unknown, microvascular changes have been suggested to have a role. The condition manifests as multiple discontinuous nodules along the palmar fascia on the volar surface of hand and fingers, and flexion contractures of fingers may develop over time.[125-128]

Pathology

Grossly, the lesions of palmar fibromatosis are firm, white nodules that are resilient on sectioning. Histologically, they are composed of variably cellular small nodules surrounded by dense collagenous tissue (Fig. 5–23). The cellular nodules contain spindle-shaped fibroblasts and myofibroblasts. Based on the cellularity and amount of collagen, the lesions are sometimes divided into proliferative, involutional, and residual phases. The cellular areas may have prominent neovascularization. Slight mitotic activity may be present, but cytologic atypia is not a feature of this lesion.[127,128]

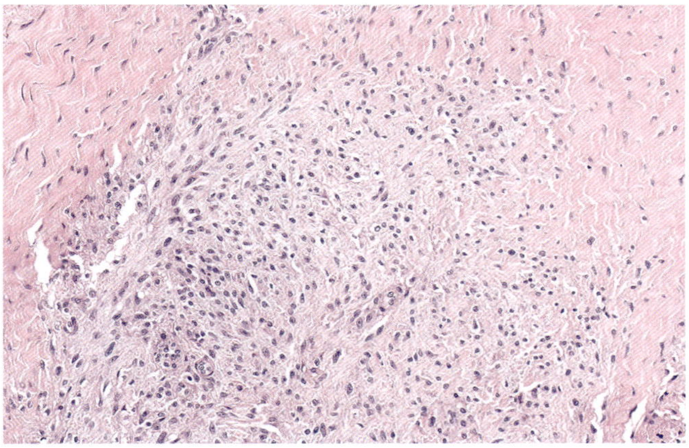

Figure 5–23. Palmar fibromatosis lesion is focally quite cellular and composed of myofibroblasts with no atypia.

Genetics

Cytogenetic studies have shown multiple clonal chromosomal changes; one study suggested recurrent trisomies of chromosomes 7 and 8.[129,130] The HUMARA test, however, has suggested polyclonal nature of the proliferation.[131] The divergent results on the clonal nature of palmar fibromatosis have left open the question whether this process is a reactive hyperplasia or a clonal neoplasm.

Plantar Fibromatosis

Clinical Features

This condition manifests as single or multiple nodules in the plantar fascia of the foot. In contrast to palmar fibromatosis, the plantar fibromatosis occurs often in young adults and has a less prominent male predominance. Some patients have synchronous lesions of plantar and palmar fibromatosis. The lesions have a high rate of recurrence unless completely excised.[132] Familial occurrence has been rarely reported.[133]

Pathology

Grossly, the lesions measure 1.5 to 2 cm in diameter and are firm, gray-white, often with a visible fascial association. Histologically, they are generally similar to those of palmar fibromatosis, but the cellular areas are often larger. They consist of single or multiple cellular nodules surrounded by dense fascial connective tissue. The nodules are composed of uniform often parallel-oriented spindled fibroblasts and myofibroblasts in a dense, collagenous background. When cut cross-sectionally, the lesional cells may have a round appearance with pericellular halos (Fig. 5–24). Profiles of blood vessels with prominent endothelia and smooth muscle layer are present inside and around the nodules. Moderate mitotic activity may be present. Scattered mast cells are often seen.

Differential Diagnosis

Synovial sarcoma may present in the plantar area and the hand. It is typically more homogenous and more highly cellular than the fibromatoses. It lacks the homogenous collagenous background, although it may

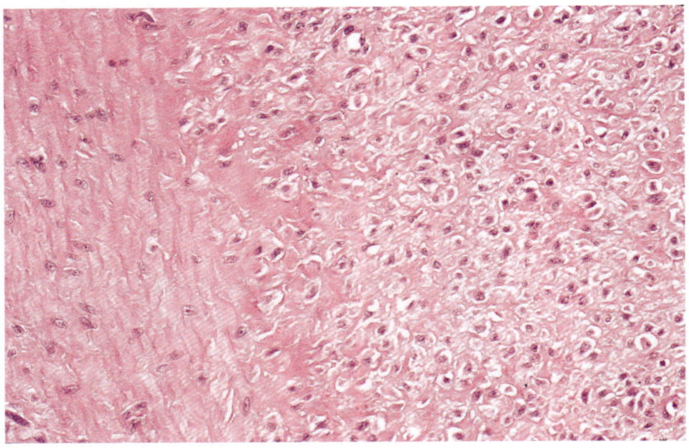

A

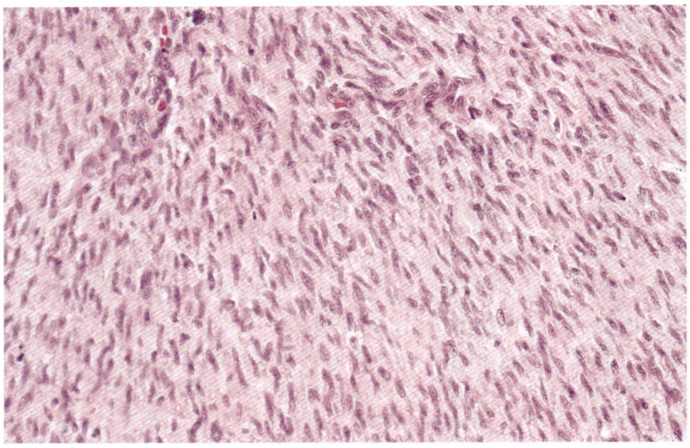

B

Figure 5-24. Plantar fibromatosis nodule is composed of densely cellular fibroblasts arranged in well-circumscribed nodules. *A*, Epithelioid pattern. *B*, Spindle cell pattern.

have collagenous areas. Immunohistochemical demonstration of epithelial markers is helpful in problem cases. Fibrous histiocytomas are skin-based lesions and rarely involve the fascia.

Genetics

Trisomies of chromosomes 8 and 14 have been reported in plantar fibromatosis.[134]

Desmoid-Type Fibromatosis (Aggressive Fibromatosis)

Desmoid is subclassified by location into abdominal wall (often referred to as "abdominal desmoid"), extra-abdominal, and mesenteric forms. They are essentially similar grossly and histologically but their potential for recurrence seems to vary.[135–142] Desmoid tumors are typically located in deep soft tissues intramuscularly or intra-abdominally in the mesentery. Fibromatosis of the breast has histologic similarities with desmoid, but may present unassociated with skeletal muscle.

Clinical Features

Abdominal (wall) and pelvic desmoids comprise 30% to 40% of all desmoids.[137,138] They usually present in young women between ages 20 and 35 years and occasionally in men. Location inside the rectus muscle sheath is most common. Some abdominal desmoids develop in scars, for example, those after a cesarean section. Because of their location, abdominal wall desmoids are easily amenable to curative surgery, and probably therefore have a lower recurrence rate and uniformly favorable course.

Extra-abdominal desmoids (over 50% of all desmoids) typically occur in young adults with a female predominance, and 80% of them are diagnosed in patients younger than 40 years.[135,136] These tumors may also occur in small children and represent part of what has been called "infantile fibromatosis" and "juvenile fibromatosis." According to our experience, desmoid is the most common type of fibromatosis in children.

Extra-abdominal desmoids most commonly appear in the shoulder girdle, chest wall, arm, and the musculatures of the thigh. Occurrence in hands and feet is rare. Extra-abdominal desmoids, especially the larger ones in the shoulder girdle, may be clinically troublesome by extensive infiltration near the neurovascular bundles necessitating extensive reconstructions or sometimes even an amputation. Repeated recurrences may occur following incomplete excision, but long-term follow-up studies have not revealed distant metastases. The slow growth rate of the recurrent tumor may justify a conservative approach in some instances. Antiestrogens, nonsteroidal anti-inflammatory drugs, and even conventional tumor chemotherapies have been used to inhibit tumor growth as an alternative to surgery.

Mesenteric desmoids (10–15%) usually occur in the small bowel mesentery, and approximately 10% of them are associated with Gardner syndrome with intestinal adenomatosis, skull osteomas, and epidermal cysts. Mesenteric desmoids vary from relatively small nodules to complex tumors that may encase multiple loops of small bowel and stomach. Despite a grossly ominous appearance, these tumors have a rather good prognosis. Patients who have Gardner syndrome have a higher risk of recurrence and complications including some tumor-related mortality, mainly due to intestinal obstruction or postsurgical short bowel syndrome. Patients with Gardner syndrome may also develop gastrointestinal carcinomas related to the adenomatosis. Nevertheless, many patients, even with unresectable mesenteric desmoid, do well, and therefore radical surgery is not always mandatory.[140–142]

Multiple desmoids may occur synchronously or metachronously. Sometimes the lesions occur in different regions, and in some cases in different parts of the same extremity. In the latter case, the multiplicity probably represents regional recurrences of the original tumor, a phenomenon sometimes referred to as "tumor migration." In a large study of extra-abdominal desmoids, 10% of the cases were multicentric, and 20% demonstrated such tumor migration.[136] Familial occurrence of multicentric desmoid has also been reported unassociated with Gardner syndrome.[139]

Pathology

Grossly, desmoids vary greatly in size from a small nodule to bulky tumor, but they usually measure 3 to 20 cm in diameter. They are typically located inside the muscle and attached to fascia sometimes with a grossly spiculated periphery due to infiltrative intramuscular growth. On sectioning, the tissue is white and firm and has a whorled or trabeculated surface (Fig. 5–25). Some lesions show focal blood color on sectioning reflecting the well-vascularized nature of the lesions.

Microscopically, desmoids show longitudinally oriented fascicles of spindled fibroblasts and myofibroblasts in a prominently collagenous background. The cell borders are not well defined and merge with the abundant extracellular collagen.

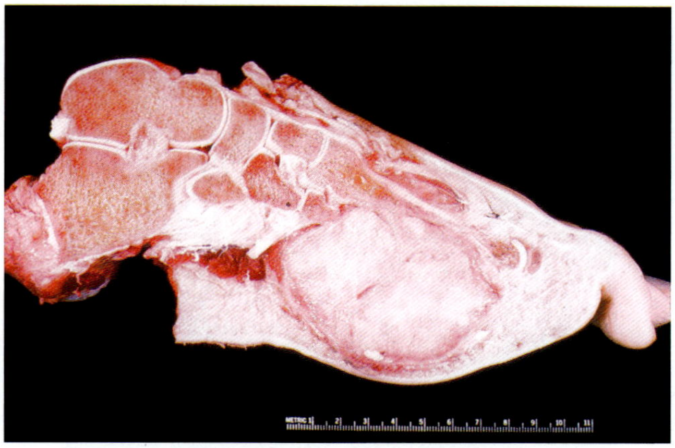

Figure 5–25. Grossly, desmoid tumor appears sharply demarcated, and the cross section reveals trabeculation. (Courtesy of Dr. John F. Fetsch, MD.)

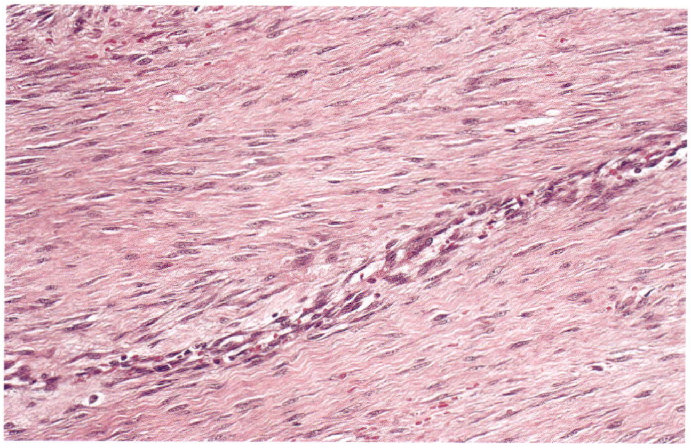

A

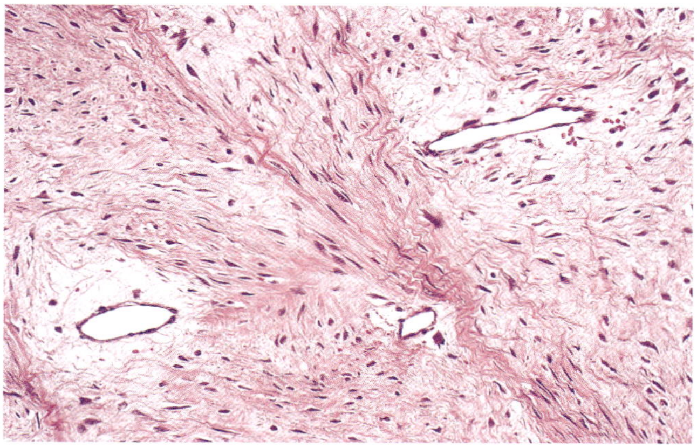

B

Figure 5–26. Variants of desmoid fibromatosis, *A*, Moderately cellular, with mildly gaping vessels. *B*, Example with myxoid features.

The nuclei are oval, are of moderate size, and have one or more delicate nucleoli. The collagenous matrix may contain thick keloid-like collagen fibers. The lesions have a prominent, evenly spaced vascular pattern composed of mildly gaping vessels which often have prominent endothelia and hypercellular smooth muscle (Fig. 5–26). Mitotic activity is typically low. Focal myxoid change may occur, especially in the mesenteric tumors. Atrophic skeletal muscle fibers are often entrapped in the periphery of intramuscular lesions.

Immunohistochemically, desmoid tumors may be focally positive for α-smooth muscle actin and desmin, but they are negative for CD34 and S-100 protein.

Differential Diagnosis

Small biopsies of desmoid may sometimes be difficult to distinguish from nodular fasciitis. A more homogeneous appearance, desmoid-type gaping vessels, and lack of scattered lymphohistiocytic infiltrate support the diagnosis of desmoid. Highly cellular desmoids, especially with mitotic activity, have to be separated from fibrosarcoma. Uniform cytologic features, lack of atypia, and a high amount of extracellular collagen support the diagnosis of desmoid. Solitary fibrous tumors demonstrate higher cellularity, hemangiopericytoma-like vessels, and CD34 immunoreactivity.

Genetics

The demonstration of cytogenetic abnormalities and clonal X-chromosome inactivation patterns in HUMARA analysis has proven desmoid as a monoclonal and neoplastic process.[143,144] Recurrent cytogenetic anomalies reported in desmoid include trisomies of chromosomes 8 and 20.[145,146] Two independent studies have shown the former as a risk factor for recurrence.[146,147]

Desmoid tumors, especially those associated with Gardner syndrome, may have mutations in the adenomatous polyposis *(APC)* gene at 5q, but at least some studies have failed to show such changes in sporadic desmoids.[148,149] *APC* gene mutations lead to overexpression of β-catenin gene *(CTNNB1)*, encoding for a cytoskeleton associated protein. Mutations of *CTNNB1* gene are another pathogenetic pathway, especially in desmoids unassociated with Gardner syndrome.[150,151] Recently, comparative genomic hybridization has shown a common gain in 1q32, but no specific gene involvement is known yet in this region.[152]

Solitary Fibrous Tumor

History

Originally known as a neoplasm of the pleura[153,154] and mediastinum,[155] this tumor was historically designated as (benign or malignant) fibrous mesothelioma in the pleura. Its proven nonepithelial and nonmesothelial nature prompted its renaming as localized fibrous tumor, or more commonly as solitary fibrous tumor of the pleura. The designation has been used for analogous extrapleural tumors that were first described on peritoneal serous surfaces[156,157] and later in a wide variety of anatomic sites, including peripheral soft tissues.[158–174]

Clinical Features

The solitary fibrous tumors present in adults of all ages, but most tumors occur in adults over age 30 years, often in the sixth and seventh decade. Rare occurrence in children has been reported. Some series show a significant female predominance (up to 1.5:1).

Extraserosal solitary fibrous tumors have been reported in a variety of locations, including the orbit,[158,159] upper respiratory tract,[160,161] and peripheral soft tissues.[162–167] A small number of cases have been reported in skin,[168] salivary gland,[169] thyroid, breast, lung (intraparenchymal), liver,[170] kidney, lower urogenital tract including bladder and prostate,[171,172] oral cavity and meninges.[173] Although most tumors have behaved in a benign fashion, some have recurred locally, and others have behaved as soft tissue sarcomas indicating that this tumor has a clinical spectrum from benign to fully malignant.

A peculiar clinical feature of some large solitary fibrous tumors is tumor-induced hypoglycemia, which resolves following tumor removal. The hypoglycemia has been attributed to secretion of insulin-like growth factors I and II by the tumor cells.[175,176] Quite likely, historical reports on fibrosarcomas with hypoglycemia have dealt with solitary fibrous tumors. The pleural lesions may also be associated with clubbing of fingernails.

Pathology

The lesions vary greatly in size from 1 to over 10 cm, but tumors larger than 20 cm may occur in the serous cavities. Grossly, solitary fibrous tumor is well circumscribed but unencapsulated. The pleural and peritoneal tumors are often attached with a narrow pedicle to outer surfaces of lung, liver, or intestines. The tissue is homogeneously firm and gray-white or pale tan on sectioning (Fig. 5–27). Malignant examples appear softer on sectioning and may show areas of necrosis; sometimes one tumor has both benign and malignant areas.

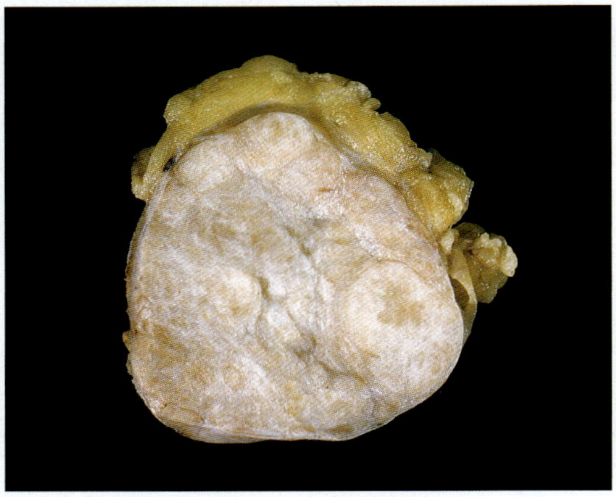

Figure 5–27. Grossly solitary fibrous tumor is a gray-white, apparently sharply circumscribed tumor.

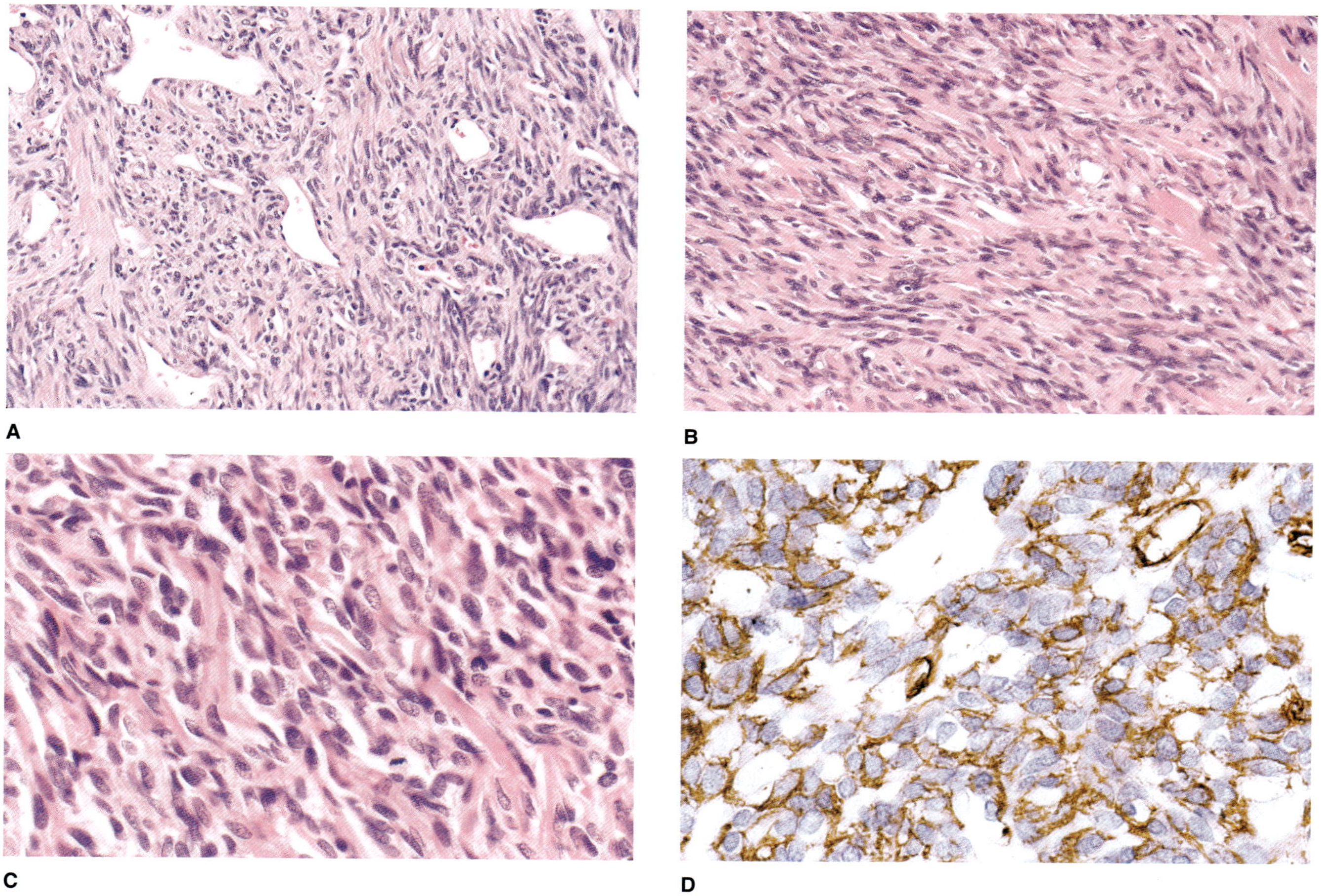

Figure 5–28. Histologic spectrum of solitary fibrous tumor. *A,* A solitary fibrous tumor with a hemangiopericytoma-like vascular pattern. *B,* A moderately cellular tumor with weak palisading of the tumor cells. *C,* Malignant transformation with high cellularity and mitotic activity. *D,* Solitary fibrous tumor is strongly positive for CD34.

Microscopically, alternating collagenous, cellular, and myxoid areas are typical. A hemangiopericytoma-like vascular pattern is seen at least focally in most cases (Fig. 5–28*A*). Cytologically these tumors have relatively uniform spindle cell population often separated by wide bands of collagen (Fig. 5–28*B*). The tumor cells have indistinct cytoplasm and oval nuclei usually with inconspicuous nucleoli. Mitotic activity is low (<2 mitoses/10 high-power field [HPF]) in most cases, but some tumors show overtly sarcomatous features with a high mitotic activity (Fig. 5–28*C*).

Immunohistochemistry

Solitary fibrous tumor cells are typically uniformly positive for vimentin, CD34 (Fig. 5–28*D*) and bcl-2.[159,169,174,177–180] Focal reactivity for muscle actins (and myofibroblastic features) has been reported, but these tumors are uniformly negative for desmin, S-100 protein, and EMA. Although most tumors are negative for keratins, malignant examples have been reported occasionally as focally positive for keratins.[169]

Tumor Behavior

Features correlating with risk of malignant behavior and metastasis include overtly sarcomatous features with high cellularity, mitotic rate over 4/10 HPF, and tumor necrosis. Similar criteria seem to apply to pleural and extrapleural tumors. In one series, 5 of 10 of such tumors metastasized to liver, lung, or bones and 4 of 10 developed a local recurrence.[165] However, some series reporting histologically malignant tumors had neither recurrences nor metastases, although the follow-up was relatively brief.[164,166] Long-term follow-up studies of histologically benign and malignant tumors are needed to fully define the potential of these tumors, especially in extrapleural sites. Any tumor with atypia or mitotic activity should be approached with caution, and such lesions should be considered having an at least uncertain (if not definite) malignant potential until more precise criteria to define tumor behavior become available.

Differential Diagnosis

The separation of solitary fibrous tumor from a hemangiopericytoma is often arbitrary. Tumor with a more well-developed staghorn-type vascular pattern and oval or round versus spindle cell cytology are classified as hemangiopericytomas, and spindle cell tumors and those with fibrous background are classified as solitary fibrous tumors. Lack of S-100 protein reactivity separates this tumor from nerve sheath tumors. Many examples of these tumors were earlier classified as deep fibrous histiocytomas or fibrosarcomas of soft tissues.

Giant cell angiofibroma of orbit and peripheral soft tissues is a variant of solitary fibrous tumor; both are $CD34^+$ fibroblastic tumors (see following).

Genetics

Heterogeneous results have been obtained on cytogenetic analysis of isolated cases. One tumor showed trisomy 21,[181] one had a translocation t(6;17) and a rearrangement of 12q13-15,[182] and a third had translocation t(9;22).[183] Comparative genomic hybridization studies have shown no changes in small tumors, whereas the larger and malignant ones have shown gain of chromosome 8, like many other soft tissue sarcomas on tumor progression.[180]

Giant Cell Angiofibroma

This tumor was originally reported in the orbit,[185] but has been more recently documented in other soft tissue locations (head and neck, back, retroperitoneum, hip, vulva), and convincing arguments have been presented for its belonging to the spectrum of solitary fibrous tumor.[180]

The reported tumors have occurred in adult patients with a wide age range, with some predilection to young adults (median age, 45 years). The aggregate data show equal gender distribution. The reported orbital tumors were small (1–3 cm), whereas the ones in peripheral soft tissues varied from 1 to 11 cm. The tumor has a benign behavior, although one orbital tumor was reported to have recurred.[185]

Histologically, the tumor is highly vascular, often with a hemangiopericytoma-like vascular pattern with hyalinized vessel walls. The main tumor cell population is composed of uniform oval or spindled cells in a collagenous stroma with little or no mitotic activity. Distinctive is the presence of scattered multinucleated giant cells, which often line pseudovascular spaces and have peripheral nuclei.

The tumor cells are strongly positive for CD34 and negative for desmin, similar to solitary fibrous tumor and hemangiopericytoma. Although the original report found the tumor negative for SMA and S-100 protein, a later series reports some cases as positive for these markers.[180]

REFERENCES

Introduction—Biology of Fibroblasts

1. McKeehan WL, Wang F, Kan M: The heparan sulfate-fibroblast growth factor family: Diversity of structure and function. Prog Nucleic Acid Res Mol Biol 1998; 59:135–176.
2. Eckes B, Kessler D, Aumailley M, Krieg T: Interactions of fibroblasts with the extracellular matrix: Implications for the understanding of fibrosis. Springer Semin Immunopathol 1999;21:415–429.
3. Schurch W, Seemayer TA, Gabbiani G: The myofibroblast: A quarter century after its discovery. Am J Surg Pathol 1998;22:141–147.
4. Skalli O, Schurch W, Seemayer T, et al: Myofibroblasts from diverse pathologic settings are heterogeneous in their content of actin isoforms and intermediate filament proteins. Lab Invest 1989;60:275–285.
5. Nickoloff BJ: CD34. The human progenitor cell antigen (CD34) is localized on endothelial cells, dermal dendritic cells, and perifollicular cells in formalin-fixed normal skin, and on proliferating endothelial cells and stromal spindle-shaped cells in Kaposi's sarcoma. Arch Dermatol 1991;127:523–529.

Putative Reactive Lesions

Nodular Fasciitis

6. Allen PW: Nodular fasciitis. Pathology 1972;4:9–26.
7. Dahl I, Jarlstedt J: Nodular fasciitis in the head and neck. A clinicopathological study on 18 cases. Acta Otolaryngol 1980;90:152–159.
8. Bernstein KE, Lattes R: Nodular (pseudosarcomatous) fasciitis, a nonrecurrent lesion: Clinicopathologic study of 134 cases. Cancer 1982;49:1668–1678.
9. Shimizu S, Hashimoto H, Enjoji M: Nodular fasciitis: An analysis of 250 patients. Pathology 1984;16:161–166.
10. Patchefsky AS, Enzinger FM: Intravascular fasciitis: A report of 17 cases. Am J Surg Pathol 1981;5:29–36.
11. Fetsch JF, Brinsko RW, Davis CJ, Mostofi FK, Sesterhenn IA: A distinctive myointimal proliferation ("myointimoma") involving the corpus spongiosum of the glans penis. A clinico-pathologic and immunohistochemical analysis of 10 cases. Am J Surg Pathol 2000; 24:1524–1530.

12. Montgomery EA, Meis JM: Nodular fasciitis. Its morphologic spectrum and immunohistochemical profile. Am J Surg Pathol 1991;15:942–948.
13. Wirman JA: Nodular fasciitis, a lesion of myofibroblasts: An ultrastructural study. Cancer 1976;38: 2378–2389.
14. Chan JK, Carcangiu ML, Rosai J: Papillary carcinoma of thyroid with exuberant nodular fasciitis-like stroma. Report of three cases. Am J Clin Pathol 1991;95:309–314.
15. Sawyer JR, Sammartino G, Baker GF, Bell JM: Clonal chromosome aberrations in a case of nodular fasciitis. Cancer Genet Cytogenet 1994;76:154–156.
16. Weibolt VM, Buresh CJ, Roberts CA, et al: Involvement of 3q21 in nodular fasciitis. Cancer Genet Cytogenet 1998;106:177–179.

Cranial Fasciitis

17. Lauer DH, Enzinger FM: Cranial fasciitis in childhood. Cancer 1980;45:401–406.
18. Sarangarajan R, Dehner LP: Cranial and extracranial fasciitis of childhood: A clinicopathologic and immunohistochemical study. Hum Pathol 1999;30:87–92.

Proliferative Fasciitis and Proliferative Myositis

19. Chung EM, Enzinger FM: Proliferative fasciitis. Cancer 1975:36:1450–1458.
20. Kitano M, Iwasaki H, Enjoji M: Proliferative fasciitis. A variant of nodular fasciitis. Acta Pathol Jpn 1977;27: 485–493.
21. Meis JM, Enzinger FM: Proliferative fasciitis and myositis in childhood. Am J Surg Pathol 1992;16: 364–372.
22. Lundgren L, Kindblom LG, Willems J, Falkmer U, Angervall L: Proliferative myositis and fasciitis. A light and electron microscopic, cytologic, DNA-cytometric and immunohistochemical study. APMIS 1992; 100:437–448.
23. Kern WH: Proliferative myositis: A pseudosarcomatous reaction to injury. Arch Pathol 1960;69:209.
24. Enzinger FM, Dulcey F: Proliferative myositis: Report of 33 cases. Cancer 1967;20:2213–2223.
25. Rose AG: An electron microscopic study of the giant cells in proliferative myositis. Cancer 1974;33:1543–1547.

Ischemic Fasciitis (Atypical Decubital Fibroplasia)

26. Montgomery EA, Meis JM, Mitchell MS, Enzinger FM: Atypical decubital fibroplasia. A distinctive fibroblastic pseudotumor occurring in debilitated patients. Am J Surg Pathol 1992;16:708–715.
27. Perosio PM, Weiss SW: Ischemic fasciitis: A juxtaskeletal fibroblastic proliferation with a predilection for elderly patients. Mod Pathol 1993;6:69–72.

Elastofibroma

28. Järvi OH, Saxén EA, Hopsu-Havu VK, Vartiovaara JJ, Vaissalo VT: Elastofibroma—A degenerative pseudotumor. Cancer 1969;23:42–63.
29. Järvi OH, Länsimies PH: Subclinical elastofibromas in the scapular region in an autopsy series. Acta Pathol Microbiol Scand A 1975;83:87–108.
30. Nagamine N, Nohary Y, Ito E: Elastofibromas in Okinawa: A clinicopathologic study of 170 cases. Cancer 1982;50:1794–1805.
31. Cross DL, Mills SE, Kulund DN: Elastofibroma arising in the foot. South Med J 1984;77:1194–1196.
32. Enjoji M, Sumiyoshi K, Sueyoshi K: Elastofibromatous lesion of the stomach in a patient with elastofibroma dorsi. Am J Surg Pathol 1985;9:233–237.
33. Madri JA, Dise CA, LiVolsi VA, Merino MJ, Bibro MC: Elastofibroma dorsi: An immunohistochemical study of collagen content. Hum Pathol 1981;12: 186–190.

Nuchal-Type Fibroma

34. Balachandran K, Allen PW, MacCormac LB: Nuchal fibroma. A clinicopathologic study of nine cases. Am J Surg Pathol 1995;19:313–317.
35. Abraham Z, Rosenbaum M, Rosner I, Nashitz Y, Boss Y, Rosenmann E: Nuchal fibroma. J Dermatol 1997; 24:262–265.
36. Michal M, Fetsch JF, Hes O, Miettinen M: Nuchal-type fibroma. A clinicopathologic study of 52 cases. Cancer 1999;85:156–163.
37. Diwan AH, Graves ED, King JA, Horenstein MG: Nuchal-type fibroma in two related patients with Gardner's syndrome. Am J Surg Pathol 2000; 24:1563–1567.
38. Dawes CL, LaHei ER, Tobias V, Kern I, Stening W: Nuchal fibroma should be recognized as a new extracolonic manifestation of Gardner-variant familial adenomatous polyposis. Aust N Z J Surg 2000; 70:824–826.
39. Banney LA, Weedon D, Muir JB: Nuchal fibroma associated with scleredema, diabetes mellitus and organic solvent exposure. Australas J Dermatol 2000; 41:39–41.

Nuchal Fibrocartilaginous Pseudotumor

40. O'Connell JX, Janzen DL, Hughes TR: Nuchal fibrocartilaginous pseudotumor: A distinctive soft tissue lesion associated with prior neck injury. Am J Surg Pathol 1997;21:836–840.
41. Laskin WB, Fetsch JF, Miettinen M: Nuchal fibrocartilaginous pseudotumor: A clinicopathologic study of five cases and review of the literature. Mod Pathol 1999;12:663–668.

Idiopathic Retroperitoneal Fibrosis and Related Disorders

42. Mitchinson MJ: Retroperitoneal fibrosis revisited. Arch Pathol Lab Med 1986;110:784–786.
43. Gilkeson GL, Allen NB: Retroperitoneal fibrosis. A true connective tissue disease. Rheum Dis Clin North Am 1996;22:23–38.
44. Dehner LP, Coffin CM: Idiopathic fibrosclerotic disorders and other inflammatory pseudotumors. Semin Diagn Pathol 1998;15:161–173.

45. Flieder DB, Suster S, Moran CA: Idiopathic fibroinflammatory (fibrosing/sclerosing) lesions of the medistinum: A study of 30 cases with emphasis on morphologic heterogeneity. Mod Pathol 1999;12:257–264.

Penile Fibromatosis (Peyronie Disease)

46. Davis CJ: The microscopic pathology of Peyronie's disease. J Urol 1997;157:282–284.

Keloid

47. Niessen FB, Spauwen PH, Shalkwijk J, Kon M: On the nature of hypertrophic scars and keloids: A review. Plast Reconstr Surg 1999;104:1435–1458.
48. Tuan TL, Nichter LS: The molecular basis of keloid and hypertrophic scar formation. Mol Med Today 1998;4:19–24.

Benign Fibroblastic Tumors with Limited Growth Potential

Collagenous Fibroma (Desmoplastic Fibroblastoma)

49. Evans HL. Desmoplastic fibroblastoma. A report of seven cases. Am J Surg Pathol 1995;19:1077–1081.
50. Nielsen GP, O'Connell JX, Dickersin GR, Rosenberg AE: Collagenous fibroma (Desmoplastic fibroblastoma): A report of seven cases. Mod Pathol 1996;9: 781–785.
51. Hasegawa T, Shimoda T, Hirohashi S, Hizawa K, Sano T: Collagenous fibroma (desmoplastic fibroblastoma): Report of four cases and review of the literature. Arch Pathol Lab Med 1998;122:455–460.
52. Miettinen M, Fetsch JF: Collagenous fibroma (desmoplastic fibroblastoma). A lesion with stellate-shaped fibroblasts. Hum Pathol 1998;28:1504–1510.
53. Sciot R, Samson I, van den Berghe H, van Damme B, Dal Cin P: Collagenous fibroma (desmoplastic fibroblastoma): Genetic link with fibroma of tendon sheath? Mod Pathol 1999;12:565–568.

Fibroma of Tendon Sheath

54. Chung EB, Enzinger FM: Fibroma of tendon sheath. Cancer 1979;44:1945–1954.
55. Smith PS, Pieterse AS, McClure J: Fibroma of tendon sheath. J Clin Pathol 1992;35:842–848.
56. Azzopardi JG, Tanda F, Salm R: Tenosynovial fibroma. Diagn Histopathol 1983;6:69–76.
57. Lundgren LG, Kindblom LG: Fibroma of tendon sheath. A light and electron microscopic study of 6 cases. Acta Pathol Microbiol Immunol Scand [A]. 1984;92:401–409.
58. Hashimoto H, Tseneyoshi M, Daimaru Y, Ushijama M, Enjoji M: Fibroma of tendon sheath: A tumor of myofibroblasts. A clinocopathologic study of 18 cases. Acta Pathol Jpn 1985;35:1099–1107.
59. Humphreys S, McKee PH, Fletcher CD: Fibroma of tendon sheath: A clinicopathologic study. J Cutan Pathol 1986;13:331–338.
60. Pulitzer DR, Martin PC, Reed RJ: Fibroma of tendon sheath. A clinicopathologic study of 32 cases. Am J Surg Pathol 1989;13:472–479.
61. Millon SJ, Bush DC, Garbes AD: Fibroma of tendon sheath in the hand. J Hand Surg (Am) 1994;19:788–793.
62. Satti MB: Tendon sheath tumors: A pathological study of the relationship between giant cell tumor of tendon sheath and fibroma of tendon sheath. Histopathology 1992;20:213–220.
63. Dal Cin P, Sciot R, Se Smet L, Van den Berghe H: Translocation 2;11 in a fibroma of tendon sheath. Histopathology 1988;32:433–435.

Sclerotic Fibroma of Skin

64. Rapini RP, Golitz LS: Sclerotic fibromas of the skin. Am J Acad Dermatol 1989;20:266–271.
65. Lo WL, Wong CK: Solitary sclerotic fibroma. J Cutan Pathol 1990;17:269–273.
66. Metcalf JS, Maize JC, le Boit PW: Circumscribed storiform collagenoma (sclerosing fibroma). Am J Dermatopathol 1991;13:122–129.

Pleomorphic Fibroma of the Skin

67. Kamino H, Lee JY, Berke A: Pleomorphic fibroma of the skin: A benign neoplasm with cytologic atypia. Am J Surg Pathol 1989;13:107–113.
68. Rudolph P, Schubert C, Zelger BG, Parwaresch R: Differential expression of CD34 and Ki-M1p in pleomorphic fibroma and dermatofibroma with monster cells. Am J Dermatopathol 1999;21:414–419.

Palisaded Myofibroblastoma

69. Weiss SW, Gnepp DR, Bratthauer GL: Palisaded myofibroblastoma: A benign mesenchymal tumor of lymph node. Am J Surg Pathol 1989;13:341–346.
70. Suster S, Rosai J: Intranodal hemorrhagic spindle cell tumor with amianthoid fibers. Report of six cases of a distinctive mesenchymal neoplasm of the inguinal region that simulates Kaposi's sarcoma. Am J Surg Pathol 1989;13:347–357.
71. Fletcher CD, Stirling RW: Intranodal myofibroblastoma presenting in the submandibular region: Evidence of a broader clinical and histological spectrum. Histopathology 1990;16:287–293.
72. Michal M, Chlumska A, Povysilova V: Intranodal "amianthoid" myofibroblastoma. Report of six cases: Immunohistochemical and electron microscopical study. Pathol Res Pract 1992;188:199–204.
73. Skalova A, Michal M, Chlumska A, Leivo I: Collagen composition and ultrastructure of the so-called amianthoid fibres in palisaded myofibroblastoma. Ultrastructural and immunohistochemical study. J Pathol 1992;167:335–340.
74. Hisaoka M, Hashimoto H, Daimaru Y: Intranodal palisaded myofibroblastoma with so-called amianthoid fibers: A report of two cases with a review of the literature. Pathol Int 1998;48:307–312.

75. Creager AJ, Garwacki CP: Recurrent intranodal palisaded myofibroblastoma with metaplastic bone formation. Arch Pathol Lab Med 1999;123:433–436.

Myofibroblastoma of the Breast

76. Wargotz ES, Weiss SW, Norris HJ: Myofibroblastoma of the breast. Sixteen cases of a distinctive benign mesenchymal tumor. Am J Surg Pathol 1987;11:493–502.
77. Lee AH, Sworn MJ, Theaker JM, Fletcher CD: Myofibroblastoma of breast: An immunohistochemical study. Histopathology 1993;22:75–78.
78. Damiani S, Miettinen M, Peterse JL, Eusebi V: Solitary fibrous tumour (myofibroblastoma) of the breast. Virchows Arch 1994;425:89–92.
79. Lazaro-Santander R, Garcia-Prats MD, Nieto S, et al: Myofibroblastoma of the breast with diverse histological features. Virchows Arch 1999;434:547–550.
80. Eyden BP, Shanks JH, Ioachim E, Ali HH, Christensen L, Howat AJ: Myofibroblastoma of breast: Evidence favoring smooth-muscle rather than myofibroblastic differentiation. Ultrastruct Pathol 1999;23:249–257.
81. Magro G, Bisceglia M, Michal M: Expression of steroid hormone receptors, their regulated proteins, and bel-2 protein in myofibroblastoma of the breast. Histopathology 2000;36:515–521.
82. Pauwels P, Sciot R, Croiset F, Rutten H, Van Den Berghe H, Dal Cin P: Myofibroblastoma of the breast: Genetic link with spindle cell lipoma. J Pathol 2000;191:282–285.

Benign Fibrous Histiocytoma

83. Gonzalez S. Duatte I: Benign fibrous histiocytoma of the skin. A morphologic study of 290 cases. Path Res Pract 1982;174:379–391.
84. Requena L, Farina MC, Fuente C, et al: Giant dermatofibroma. A little known clinical variant of dermatofibroma. J Am Acad Dermatol 1994;30:714–718.
85. Calonje E, Fletcher CDM: Cutaneous fibrohistiocytic tumors: An update. Adv Anat Pathol 1994:1:2–15.
86. Colome-Grimmer MI, Evans HL: Metastasizing cellular dermatofibroma: A report of two cases. Am J Surg Pathol 1996;20:1361–1367.
87. Kamino H, Reddy VB, Gero M, Greco MA: Dermatomyofibroma. A benign, cutaneous, plaque-like proliferation of fibroblasts and myofibroblasts in young adults. J Cutan Pathol 1992;19:85–93.
88. Santa-Cruz DJ, Kyriakos M: Aneurysmal ("angiomatoid") fibrous histiocytoma of the skin. Cancer 1981;47:2053–2061.
89. Calonje E, Fletcher CDM: Aneurysmal benign fibrous histiocytoma: Clinicopathological analysis of 40 cases of a tumour frequently misdiagnosed as a vascular neoplasm. Histopathology 1995;26:323–331.
90. Wilson Jones E, Cerio R, Smith NP: Epithelioid fibrous histiocytoma: A new entity. Br J Dermatol 1989;120:185–195.
91. Mehregan AH, Mehregan DR, Broecker A: Epithelioid cell histiocytoma. J Am Acad Dermatol 1992;26:243–246.
92. Singh Gomez C, Calonje E, Fletcher CDM: Epithelioid benign fibrous histiocytoma of skin: Clinico-pathological analysis of 20 cases of a poorly known variant. Histopathology 1994;24:123–129.
93. Val-Bernal JF, Mira C: Dermatofibroma with granular cells. J Cutan Pathol 1996;23:562–565.
94. Calonje E, Mentzel T, Fletcher CD: Cellular benign fibrous histiocytoma. Clinicopathologic analysis of 74 cases of a distinctive variant of cutaneous fibrous histiocytoma. Am J Surg Pathol 1994;18:668–676.
95. Fukamizu H, Oku T, Inoue K, Matsumoto K, Okayama H, Tagami H: Atypical pseudosarcomarous cutaneous fibrous histiocytoma. J Cutan Pathol 1983; 10:327–333.
96. Levya WH, Santa Cruz DJ: Atypical cutaneous fibrous histiocytoma. Am J Dermatopathol 1986;8:467–471.
97. Tamada S, Ackerman AB: Dermatofibroma with monster cells. Am J Dermatopathol 1987;9:380–387.
98. Beham A, Fletcher CDM: Atypical "pseudosarcomatous" variant of cutaneous benign fibrous histiocytoma: Report of eight cases. Histopathology 1990;17: 167–169.
99. Abenoza P, Lillemoe T: CD34 and factor XIIIa in the differential diagnosis of dermatofibroma and dermatofibrosarcoma protuberans. Am J Dermatopathol 1993;15:429–434.
100. Prieto VG, Reed JA, Shea CR: Immunohistochemistry of dermatofibromas and benign fibrous histiocytomas. J Cutan Pathol 1995;22:336–341.
101. Li DF, Iwasaki H, Kikuchi M, Ichiki M, Ogata K: Dermatofibroma: Superficial fibrous proliferation with reactive histiocytes. A multiple immunostaining analysis. Cancer 1994;74:66–73.
102. Chen TC, Kuo T, Chan HL: Dermatofibroma is a clonal proliferative disease. J Cutan Pathol 2000;27:36–39.
103. Vanni R, Fletcher CD, Sciot R, et al: Cytogenetic evidence of clonality in cutaneous benign fibrous histiocytomas: A report of the CHAMP study group. Histopathology 2000;37:212–217.

Intramuscular Myxoma

104. Enzinger FM: Intramuscular myxoma. Am J Clin Pathol 1965;43:104–110.
105. Wirth WA, Leavitt D, Enzinger FM: Multiple intramuscular myxomas. Another extraskeletal manifestation of fibrous dysplasia. Cancer 1971;27:1167–1173.
106. Kindblom LG, Stener B, Angervall L: Intramuscular myxoma. Cancer 1974;34:1737–1744.
107. Miettinen M, Hockerstedt K, Reitamo J, Totterman S: Intramuscular myxoma. A clinicopathological study of 23 cases. Am J Clin Pathol 1985;84:265–272.
108. Hashimoto H, Tsuneyoshi M, Daimaru Y, Enjoji M, Shinohara N: Intramuscular myxoma. A clinicopathologic, immunohistochemical, and electron microscopic study. Cancer 1986;58:740–747.
109. Szendroi M, Rahoty P, Antal I, Kiss J: Fibrous dysplasia associated with intramuscular myxoma (Mazabraud's syndrome): A long term follow-up of three cases. J Cancer Res Clin Oncol 1998;124:401–406.
110. Nielsen GP, O'Connell JX, Rosenberg AE: Intramuscular myxoma: A clinicopathologic study of 51 cases

with emphasis on hypercellular and hypervascular variants. Am J Surg Pathol 1998;22:1222–1227.

111. Okamoto S, Hisaoka M, Ushijima M, Nakahara S, Toyoshima S, Hashimoto H: Activating Gs α mutation in intramuscular myxomas with and without fibrous dysplasia of bone. Virchows Arch 2000;437:133–137.
112. Malchoff CD, Reardon G, Macgillivray DC, Yamase H, Rogol AD, Malchoff DM: An unusual presentation of McCune-Albright syndrome confirmed by an activating mutation of the Gs alpha-subunit from a bone lesion. J Clin Endocr Metab 1994;78:803–806.
113. Shenker A, Weinstein LS, Sweet DE, Spiegel AM: An activating Gs alpha mutation is present in fibrous dysplasia of bone in the McCune-Albright syndrome. J Clin Endocrinol Metab 1994;79:750–755.

Juxta-articular Myxoma

114. Meis JM, Enzinger FM: Juxta-articular myxoma: A clinical and pathologic study of 65 cases. Hum Pathol 1992;23:639–646.
115. Sciot R, DalCin P, Samson I, van den Berghe H, van Damme B: Clonal chromosomal changes in juxta-articular myxoma. Virchows Arch 1999;434:177–180.

Superficial Angiomyxoma (Cutaneous Myxoma)—Clinicopathologic

116. Carney JA, Headington JT, Su WP: Cutaneous myxomas. A major component of myxomas, spotty pigmentation, and endocrine overactivity. Arch Dermatol 1986;122:790–798.
117. Carney JA: Carney complex: The complex of myxomas, spotty pigmentation, endocrine overactivity, and schwannomas. Semin Dermatol 1995;14:90–98.
118. Allen PW, Dymock RB, MacCormac LB: Superficial angiomyxomas with and without epithelial components. Report of 30 tumors in 28 patients. Am J Surg Pathol 1988;12:519–530.
119. Fetsch JF, Laskin WB, Tavassoli FA: Superficial angiomyxoma (cutaneous myxoma): A clinicopathologic study of 17 cases arising in the genital region. Int J Gynecol Pathol 1997;16:325–334.
120. Calonje E, Guerin D, McCormick D, Fletcher CD: Superficial angiomyxoma: Clinicopathologic analysis of a series of a distinctive but poorly recognized cutaneous tumors with tendency for recurrence. Am J Surg Pathol 1999;23:910–917.

Superficial Angiomyxoma (Cutaneous Myxoma)—Genetics

121. Goldstein MM, Casey M, Carney JA, Basson CT: Molecular genetic diagnosis of the familial myxoma syndrome (Carney complex). Am J Med Genet 1999;86:62–65.
122. Kirschner LS, Carney JA, Pack SD, et al: Mutations of the gene encoding the protein kinase A type I-alpha regulatory subunit in patients with the Carney complex. Nat Genet 2000;26:89–92.
123. Kirschner LS, Sandrini F, Monbo J, Lin JP, Carney JA, Stratakis CA: Genetic heterogeneity and spectrum of mutations of the PRKAR1A gene in patients with the Carney complex. Hum Mol Genet 2000;12:3037–3046.

Superficial Acral Fibromyxoma

124. Fetsch JF, Laskin WB, Miettinen M: Superficial acral fibromyxoma: A clinicopathologic and immunohistochemical analysis of 37 cases of a distinctive soft tissue tumor with a predilection for the fingers and toes. Hum Pathol 2001;32:704–714.

Benign Fibroblastic Tumors with Proliferative Capacity

Palmar Fibromatosis

125. Ross DC: Epidemiology of Dupuytren's disease. Hand Clin 1999;15:53–62.
126. Benson LS, Williams CS, Kahle M: Dupuytren's contracture. J Am Acad Orthop Surg 1998;6:24–35.
127. Ushijima M, Tsuneyoshi M, Enjoji M: Dupuytren type fibromatoses. A clinicopathologic study of 62 cases. Acta Pathol Jpn 1984;34:991–1001.
128. Casalone R, Mazzola D, Meroni E, et al: Cytogenetic and interphase cytogenetic analyses reveal chromosome instability but no clonal trisomy 8 in Dupuytren contracture. Cancer Genet Cytogenet 1997;99:73–76.
129. Dal Cin P, De Smet L, Sciot R, van Damme B, Van den Berghe H: Trisomy 7 and trisomy 8 in dividing and non-dividing tumor cells in Dupuytren's disease. Cancer Genet Cytogenet 1999;108:137–140.
130. Chansky HA, Trumble TE, Conrad EU, Wolff JF, Murray LW, Raskind WH: Evidence for a polyclonal etiology of palmar fibromatosis. J Hand Surg 1999;24: 339–344.
131. Allen PW: The fibromatoses: A clinicopathologic classification based on 140 cases. Am J Surg Pathol 1977;1:255–270.

Plantar Fibromatosis

132. Aluisio FV, Mair SD, Hall RL: Plantar fibromatosis: Treatment of primary and recurrent lesions and factors associated with recurrence. Foot Ankle Int 1996; 17:672–678.
133. Chen KT, van Dyne TA: Familial plantar fibromatosis. J Surg Oncol 1985;29:240–241.
134. Brainer JA, Nelson M, Bredthauer BD, Neff JR, Bridge JA: Trisomy 8 and trisomy 14 in plantar fibromatosis. Cancer Genet Cytogenet 1999;108:176–177.

Desmoid Fibromatosis—Clinicopathologic

135. Enzinger FM, Shiraki M: Musculo-aponeurotic fibromatosis of the shoulder girdle (extra-abdominal desmoid): Analysis of 30 cases followed-up for 10 or more years. Cancer 1967;20:1131–1140.
136. Rock MG, Pritchard DJ, Reiman HM, Soule EH, Brewster AR: Extra-abdominal desmoid tumors. J Bone Joint Surg Am 1984;66:1369–1374.
137. Reitamo JJ, Häyry P, Nykyri E, Saxén E: The desmoid tumor I. Incidence, sex, age and anatomical distribu-

tion in the Finnish population. Am J Clin Pathol 1982;77:665–673.
138. Häyry P, Reitamo JJ, Totterman S, Hopfner-Hallikainen D, Sivula A: The desmoid tumor II. Analysis of factors possibly contributing to the etiology and growth behavior. Am J Clin Pathol 1982;77: 674–680.
139. Zayid I, Dihmis C: Familial multicentric fibromatosis—desmoids. Cancer 1969;24:786–795.
140. Burke AP, Sobin LH, Shekitka KM, Federspiel BH, Helwig EB: Intra-abdominal fibromatosis. A pathologic analysis of 130 tumors with comparison of clinical subgroups. Am J Surg Pathol 1990;14:335–341.
141. Burke AP, Sobin LH, Shekitka KM: Mesenteric fibromatosis. A follow-up study. Arch Pathol Lab Med 1990;114:832–835.
142. Heiskanen I, Järvinen H: Occurrence of desmoid tumours in familial adenomatous polyposis and results of treatment. Int J Colorectal Dis 1996;11:157–162.

Desmoid Fibromatosis—Molecular Genetics

143. Li M, Cordon-Cardo C, Gerald WL, Rosai J: Desmoid fibromatosis is a clonal process. Hum Pathol 1996;27: 939–943.
144. Lucas DR, Schroyer KR, McCarthy PJ, Markham NE, Fujita M, Enomoto TE: Desmoid tumor is a clonal cellular proliferation: PCR-amplification of HUMARA for analysis of patterns of X-chromosome inactivation. Am J Surg Pathol 1997;21:306–311.
145. Fletcher JA, Naeem R, Xiao S, Corson JM: Chromosome aberrations in desmoid tumors. Trisomy 8 may be a predictor of recurrence. Cancer Genet Cytogenet 1995;79:139–143.
146. Mertens F, Willen H, Rydholm A, et al: Tri-some 20 is a primary chromosome aberration in desmoid tumors. Int J Cancer 1995;63:527–529.
147. Kouho H, Aoki T, Hisaoka M, Hashimoto H: Clinicopathological and interphase cytogenetic analysis of desmoid tumors. Histopathology 1997;31:336–341.
148. Miyaki M, Konishi M, Kikuchi-Yanoshita R, et al: Coexistence of somatic and germ-line mutations in APC gene in desmoid tumors from patients with familial adenomatous polyposis. Cancer Res 1993;53:5079–5082.
149. Alman BA, Li C, Pajerski ME, Diaz-Cano S, Wolfe HJ: Increased beta-catenin protein and somatic APC mutations in sporadic aggressive fibromatosis. Am J Pathol 1997;151:329–334.
150. Miyoshi Y, Iwao K, Nawa G, Ochi T, Nakamura Y: Frequent mutations in the beta-catenin gene in desmoid tumors from patients without familial adenomatous polyposis. Oncol Res 1998;10:591–594.
151. Tejpar S, Nollet F, Li C, et al: Predominance of beta-catenin mutations and beta-catenin dysregulation in sporadic aggressive fibromatosis (desmoid tumor). Oncogene 1999;18:6615–6620.
152. Larramendy ML, Virolainen M, Tukiainen E, Elomaa I, Knuutila S: Chromosome band 1q21 is recurrently gained in desmoid tumors. Genes Chromosomes Cancer 1998;23:183–186.

Solitary Fibrous Tumor—Clinicopathologic

153. England DM, Hochholzer L, McCarthy MJ: Localized benign and malignant fibrous tumors of the pleura. A clinicopathologic review of 223 cases. Am J Surg Pathol 1989;13:640–658.
154. Briselli M, Mark EJ, Dickersin GR: Solitary fibrous tumors of the pleura: Eight new cases and review of 360 cases in the literature. Cancer 1981;47: 2678–2689.
155. Witkin GB, Rosai J: Solitary fibrous tumor of the mediastinum. A report of 14 cases. Am J Surg Pathol 1989;13:547–557.
156. el-Naggar AK, Ro JY, Ayala AG, Ward R, Ordonez NG: Localized fibrous tumor of the serosal cavities. Immunohistochemical, electron-microscopic, and flow-cytometric DNA study. Am J Clin Pathol 1989;92:561–565.
157. Young RH, Clement PB, McCaughey WT: Solitary fibrous tumors ("fibrous mesotheliomas") of the peritoneum. A report on three cases and a review of literature. Arch Pathol Lab Med 1990;114:493–495.
158. Dorfman DM, To K, Dickersin GR, Rosenberg AE, Pilch BZ: Solitary fibrous tumor of the orbit. Am J Surg Pathol 1994;18:281–287.
159. Westra WH, Gerald WL, Rosai J: Solitary fibrous tumor. Consistent CD34 immunoreactivity and occurrence in the orbit. Am J Surg Pathol 1994;18:992–998.
160. Zukerberg LR, Rosenberg AE, Randolph G, Pilch BZ, Goodman ML: Solitary fibrous tumor of the nasal cavity and paranasal sinuses. Am J Surg Pathol 1991;15:126–130.
161. Witkin GB, Rosai J: Solitary fibrous tumor of the upper respiratory tract. A report of six cases. Am J Surg Pathol 1991;15:842–848.
162. Suster S, Nascimento AG, Miettinen M, Sickel JZ, Moran CA: Solitary fibrous tumor of soft tissue. A clinicopathologic and immunohistochemical study of 12 cases. Am J Surg Pathol 1995;19:1257–1266.
163. Fukunaga M, Naganuma H, Nikaido T, Harada T, Ushigome S: Extrapleural solitary fibrous tumor: A report of seven cases. Mod Pathol 1997;10:443–450.
164. Nielsen GP, O'Connell JX, Dickersin GR, Rosenberg AE: Solitary fibrous tumor of soft tissue: A report of 15 cases, including 5 malignant examples with light microscopic, immunohistochemical and ultrastructural data. Mod Pathol 1997;10:1028–1037.
165. Vallat-Decouvelaere AV, Dry SM, Fletcher CD: Atypical and malignant solitary fibrous tumors in extrathoracic locations: Evidence of their comparability to intra-thoracic tumors. Am J Surg Pathol 1998;22: 1501–1511.
166. Brunnemann RB, Ro JY, Ordonez NG, Mooney J, El-Naggar AK, Ayala AG: Extrapleural solitary fibrous tumor: A clinicopathologic study of 24 cases. Mod Pathol 1999;12:1034–1042.
167. Hasegawa T, Matsuno Y, Shimoda T, Hasegawa F, Sano T, Hirohashi S: Extrathoracic solitary fibrous tumors: Their histological variability and potentially aggressive behavior. Hum Pathol 1999;30:1464–1473.
168. Cowper SE, Kilpatrick T, Proper S, Morgan MB: Solitary fibrous tumor of the skin. Am J Dermatopathol 1999;21:213–219.

169. Hanau CA, Miettinen M: Solitary fibrous tumor: Histological and immunohistochemical spectrum of benign and malignant variants presenting at different sites. Hum Pathol 1995;26:440–449.
170. Moran CA, Ishak KG, Goodman ZD: Solitary fibrous tumor of the liver: A clinicopathologic and immunohistochemical study of nine cases. Ann Diagn Pathol 1998;2:19–24.
171. Bainbridge TC, Singh RR, Mentzel T, Katenkamp D: Solitary fibrous tumor of urinary bladder: Report of two cases. Hum Pathol 1997;28:1204–1206.
172. Westra WH, Grenko RT, Epstein J: Solitary fibrous tumor of the lower urogenital tract: A report of five cases involving the seminal vesicles, urinary bladder, and prostate. Hum Pathol 2000;31:63–68.
173. Carneiro SS, Scheithauer BW, Nascimento AG, Hirose T, Davis DH: Solitary fibrous tumor of the meninges: A lesion distinctive from fibrous meningioma. A clinicopathologic and immunohistochemical study. Am J Clin Pathol 1996;106:217–224.
174. Nascimento AG: Solitary fibrous tumor: A ubiquitous neoplasm of mesenchymal differentiation. Adv Anat Pathol 1006;3:388–395.
175. Strom EH, Skjorten F, Aarseth LB, Haug E: Solitary fibrous tumor of the pleura. An immunohistochemical, electron microscopic and tissue culture study of a tumor producing insulin-like growth factor I in a patient with hypoglycemia. Pathol Res Pract 1991;187: 109–113.
176. Fukasawa Y, Takada A, Tateno M, et al: Solitary fibrous tumor of the pleura causing recurrent hypoglycemia by secretion of insulin-like growth factor II. Pathol Int 1998;48:47–52.
177. van de Rijn M, Lombard CM, Rouse RV: Expression of CD34 by solitary fibrous tumors of the pleura, mediastinum, and lung. Am J Surg Pathol 1994;18: 814–820.
178. Flint A, Weiss SW: CD-34 and keratin expression distinguishes solitary fibrous tumor (fibrous mesothelioma) of pleura from desmoplastic mesothelioma. Hum Pathol 1995;26:428–431.
179. Chilosi M, Facchetti F, DeiTos AP, et al: bcl-2 expression in pleural and extrapleural solitary fibrous tumours. J Pathol 1997;181:362–367.
180. Guillou L, Gebhard S, Coindre JM: Orbital and extraorbital giant cell angiofibroma: A giant cell-rich variant of solitary fibrous tumor? Clinicopathologic and immunohistochemical analysis of a series in favor of a unifying concept. Am J Surg Pathol 2000;24:971–979.

Solitary Fibrous Tumor—Genetics

181. Dal Cin P, Sciot R, Fletcher CD, et al: Trisomy 21 in solitary fibrous tumor. Cancer Genet Cytogenet 1996; 86:58–60.
182. Donner LR, Silva MT, Dobin SM: Solitary fibrous tumor of the pleura: A cytogenetic study. Cancer Genet Cytogenet 1999;111:169–171.
183. Havlik DM, Farnath DA, Bocklage T: Solitary fibrous tumor of the orbit with a t(9;22)(q31;p13). Arch Pathol Lab Med 2000;124:756–758.
184. Miettinen MM, el-Rifai W, Sarlomo-Rikala M, Anderson LC, Knuutila S: Tumor size-related DNA copy number changes occur in solitary fibrous tumors but not in hemangiopericytomas. Mod Pathol 1997;10:1194–1200.

Giant Cell Angiofibroma

185. Dei Tos A, Seregard S, Calonje E, Chan JKC, Fletcher CDM: Giant cell angiofibroma. A distinctive orbital tumor in adults. Am J Surg Pathol 1995;19:1286–1293.

Fibroblastic Proliferations in Children

CHAPTER 6

A number of benign and few malignant fibroblastic proliferations are typical of children. Other fibroblastic proliferations also may occur in children, in addition to their more common presentation in adults. Among them, fibromatoses (desmoid) are discussed in Chapter 5 and low-grade fibromyxoid sarcoma in Chapter 7. On the other hand, many of the lesions included here occur in adults as well, especially in young age groups.

All childhood fibroblastic proliferations are relatively rare. They cover a wide clinicopathologic spectrum from reactive lesions to benign, borderline malignant, and malignant tumors (Table 6–1). Nevertheless, only few of these tumors are truly malignant and clinically aggressive, although histologically some are clearly malignant appearing. For example, infantile fibrosarcoma has an excellent prognosis and rarely metastasizes.

Understanding of molecular genetics of some childhood tumors has markedly increased, and tumor-specific translocations resulting in specific gene fusions have been described in infantile fibrosarcoma and inflammatory myofibroblastic tumor. This has not only given new tools for diagnosis, but may also help to devise pathogenesis-oriented treatments in the future.

Cranial Fasciitis

Clinical Features

Cranial fasciitis is the designation of a rare nodular fasciitis-like fibroblastic proliferation that presents as a rapidly growing scalp mass in infants and young children, usually before the age of 2 years. The lesions often erode the outer table of skull and occasionally extend to the underlying bone and dura. Conservative treatment is considered sufficient.

Pathology

The lesions are generally similar to nodular fasciitis, often with a more myxoid appearance. They also coexpress vimentin and muscle actins.[1,2]

Cranial fasciitis should be differentiated from a desmoid tumor, which may occur in the cranium in small children. These tumors are more highly cellular and typically have a prominent vascular pattern. Myofibroma contains pale myofibroblastic clusters and an immature hemangiopericytoma-like vascular component; this tumor is usually subcutaneous.

Table 6–1. Benign Fibrous Tumors and Tumor-like Lesions in Children

Probable Nonneoplastic Conditions
Cranial fasciitis
Fibromatosis colli
Calcifying fibrous pseudotumor
Juvenile hyaline fibromatosis
Benign Neoplasms
Fibrous hamartoma of infancy
Infantile digital fibroma
Nasopharyngeal angiofibroma
Myofibromatosis and myofibroma
Calcifying aponeurotic fibroma
Juvenile diffuse fibromatosis
Lipofibromatosis
Borderline Malignant or Malignant Tumors
Plexiform fibrohistiocytic tumor
Inflammatory myofibroblastic tumor*
Infantile fibrosarcoma

*Tumors with malignant variants

Fibromatosis Colli (Congenital Torticollis)

Clinical Features

This reactive, reparative condition in newborns is probably caused by perinatal trauma to sternocleidomastoid muscle. The lesion develops during the first 2 months of life, and appears as a 2- to 3-cm mass in any part of the sternocleidomastoid muscle, more often in its lower portion.[3] Because of general awareness of the harmless nature of these lesions, surgery is avoided, and fine-needle aspiration biopsy has been advocated for the confirmation of the diagnosis and to rule out a true tumor.[4] The condition termed congenital or acquired muscular fibrosis is probably a similar reactive process that can occur in muscles of other regions.

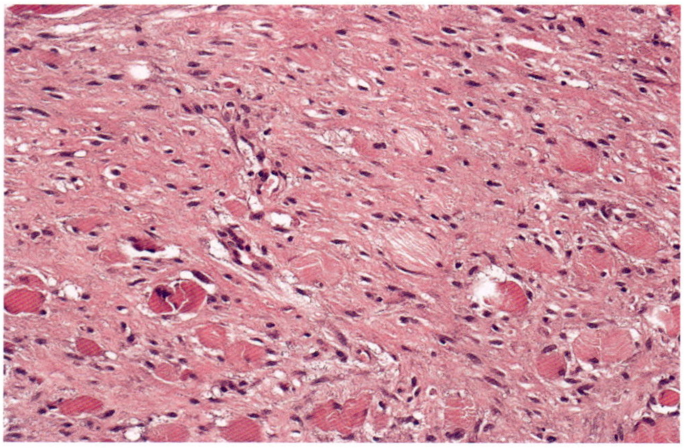

Figure 6–1. Fibromatosis colli lesion contains degenerating skeletal muscle fibers and intervening scarlike fibrous proliferation.

Pathology

The needle aspirates typically show fibroblasts and fragments of degenerated skeletal muscle cells. Histologically the lesions shows cellular, collagenous scarlike tissue, which separates muscle to single fibers or clusters of them. Both degenerating and regenerating muscle fibers are present (Fig. 6–1). Compared to desmoid fibromatosis, the cytologic composition is more heterogeneous with fewer spindle cells and lack of confluent areas of lesional cells.

Calcifying Fibrous Pseudotumor

Clinical Features

This histologically distinctive fibrous tumor occurs practically only in children and young adults; sex distribution is equal. The tumor presents in a wide variety of sites, and the reported examples have varied in size from 2.5 to 15 cm in diameter. The tumor may involve both the subcutis and deep soft tissues, and occurrence in the pleura has been reported. Intra-abdominal location is also possible, and such lesions may be bigger and composed of multiple nodules. Recurrence was reported in one case.[5–8]

Pathology

Grossly, the tumor is white and firm and appears without texture on sectioning, except for possible calcifications. Histologically, it is composed of thick, partly amorphous collagen fibers and scattered psammomatous calcifications, mild diffuse lymphoplasmacytic infiltrate, and lymphoid foci (Fig. 6–2). In one case, the coexistence of calcifying fibrous pseudotumor and inflammatory myofibroblastic tumor with transitional features was suggested to indicate the relationship of these entities.[8] However, we have not been able to document such a connection. Many features of this process suggest reactive nature.

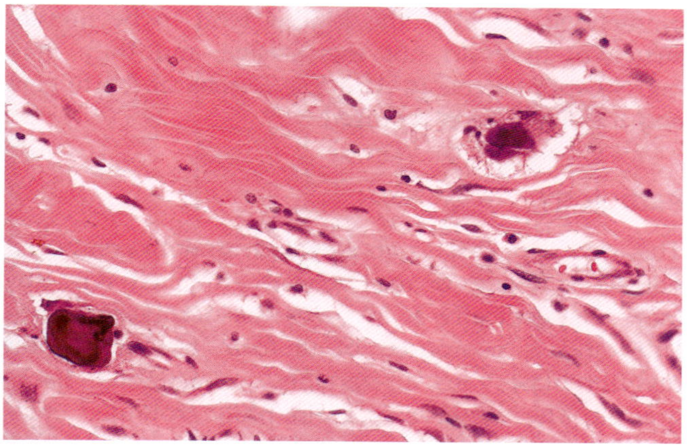

Figure 6-2. Calcifying fibrous pseudotumor has a low cellularity and contains psammomatous calcification and focal lymphoid infiltration.

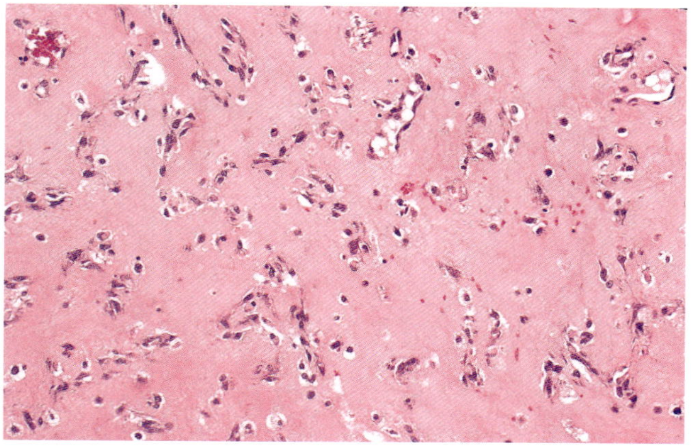

Figure 6-3. Juvenile hyaline fibromatosis contains amorphous material between fibroblasts in a vascular background.

Calcifying fibrous pseudotumor is much less cellular than inflammatory myofibroblastic tumor; the latter does not usually feature psammomatous calcifications.

Juvenile Hyaline Fibromatosis

Clinical Features

This rare hereditary syndrome (also called fibromatosis hyalinica multiplex) is transmitted in an autosomal recessive manner, and sometimes affects children of consanguineous parents. It manifests in young children with slowly growing multiple fibrous tumors in the head and neck, back, or extremities. Associated manifestations include fibrous gingival hyperplasia, flexion contractures of joints, and osteolytic lesions.[9-13] The fibrous tumors involve the skin and subcutis, and when located in the scalp and face can reach disfiguring proportions. When multiple skin tumors develop, this syndrome can be clinically misinterpreted as neurofibromatosis, especially if the other manifestations are not prominent. Infantile systemic hyalinosis is probably a variant of the same syndrome that presents in early childhood.

Pathology

Histologically, the nodules are composed of bland fibroblasts separated by abundant hyaline-myxoid eosinophilic, collagenous matrix (Fig. 6–3). It is felt that the key change is accumulation of extracellular mucopolysaccharide material in the connective tissue due to a yet unidentified inborn error of metabolism.

Although clinically this lesion may have resemblance to neurofibromatosis 1 because of multiplicity of lesions, histologic features of fibroblasts in myxohyaline matrix differ from neurofibroma.

Fibrous Hamartoma of Infancy

Clinical Features

This histologically distinctive lesion typically presents in the trunk of small children, more often in boys by a 2:1 margin. It usually occurs in children younger than 2 years old and may be congenital. The lesion commonly reaches the size of 3 to 4 cm. It is subcutaneous and most commonly located in the axilla or chest wall. Rarely, it presents in the proximal extremities, but never in hands, fingers, and toes.[14-19] Simple excision is almost always curative.

Pathology

A typical fibrous hamartoma of infancy is grossly poorly circumscribed merging with the surrounding fat and usually measuring 1 to 5 cm. Histologically, the lesion consists of mature adipose tissue interspersed with curving streaks of variably cellular fibroblasts in collagenous background. Distinctive and unique to this lesion are rounded clusters of oval fibroblasts, which are often seen at the interface of fat and fibrous tissue (Fig. 6–4*A*). This constellation of components is virtually diagnostic for fibrous hamartoma of infancy. Sometimes (our estimate, 20%) the lesion is entirely composed of cellular fibrous elements with wavy collagen, and such lesions may resemble a neurofibroma (Fig. 6–4*B*). However, true Schwann cell elements are absent, and the lesion is negative for S-100 protein.

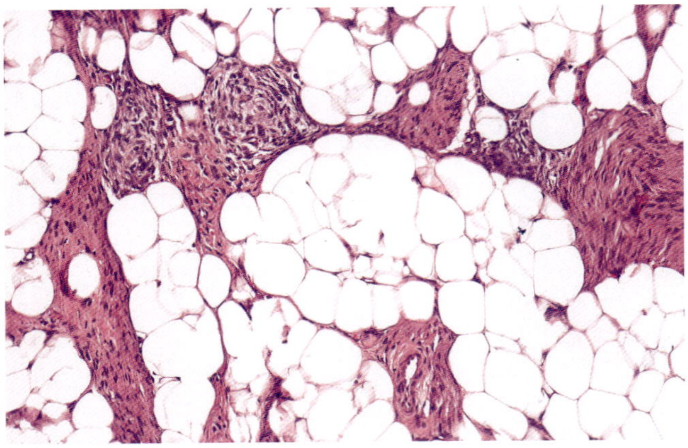

A

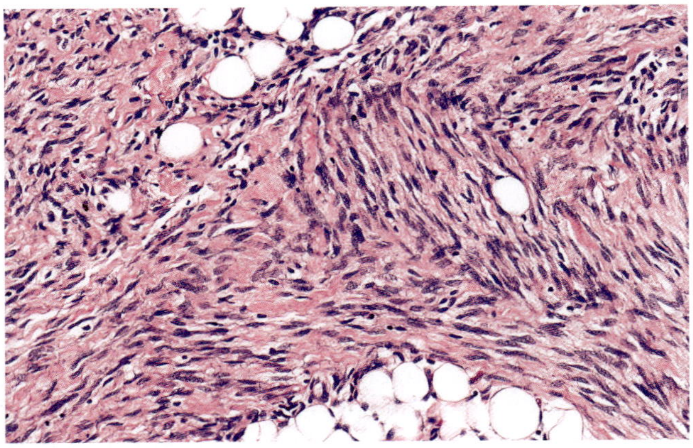

B

Figure 6–4. *A,* Typical fibrous hamartoma of infancy contains a fatty component, narrow streaks of fibrous tissue, and small clusters of oval more primitive cells. *B,* Some fibrous hamartoma lesions are more cellular, and their wavy collagen resembles that of neurofibroma.

Somewhat similar tumors in distal parts of extremities lack the clusters of oval fibroblasts and have been classified as lipofibromatosis (see pp. 180 and 181).

Infantile Digital Fibroma

Clinical Features

This rare tumor (infantile digital fibromatosis, inclusion body fibromatosis), previously also known as recurrent digital fibroma, typically occurs in infants and small children on the extensor surfaces of the second to fifth fingers and toes; the lesion appears to spare the thumb and great toe. Some of these tumors are congenital, and some may be multiple. Pathogenesis of this tumor is unknown, and attempts to isolate viruses have been unsuccessful. Although local recurrence is common, aggressive surgery is not recommended; because the lesions tend to be nondestructive, they do not metastasize and they may regress spontaneously. Multiple lesions in the fingers and toes have been reported.[20–26]

Pathology

The lesion appears as an elevated, smooth contoured nodule in fingers or toes beneath stretched skin surface. Histologically, it involves the dermis and subcutis and is composed of uniform fibroblasts and myofibroblasts in a variably collagenous background. The presence of eosinophilic, rounded cytoplasmic perinuclear inclusions is typical of this tumor, but the number of inclusions varies in a wide range (Fig. 6–5). The inclusions have been shown to contain actin microfilaments, as demonstrated by immunohistochemistry and heavy meromyosin binding.[27–30] Ultrastructural studies have also revealed a filamentous nature of the inclusion and shown myofibroblastic cellular features.

Fibrous tumors with cytoplasmic inclusions similar to those of infantile digital fibromatosis have been sporadically reported in adults in nondigital sites. These include occurrence in fibroma of the arm, phyllodes tumor, and other fibroepithelial tumors of the breast, and in the peculiar scleroderma-like fibrous lesions that developed in conjunction with the epidemic toxic oil syndrome, especially reported from Spain.[31–35]

Differential Diagnosis

Although the lesion may resemble fibromatosis (desmoid) at first glance, the superficial location, distinctive eosinophilic cytoplasmic globules, and lack of prominent vessels are differentiating features.

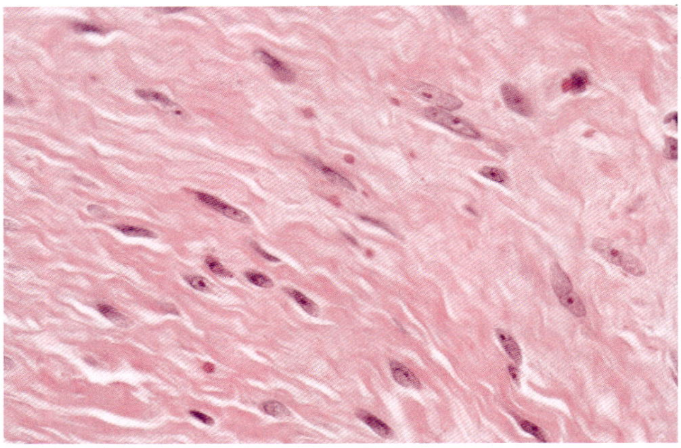

Figure 6–5. Infantile digital fibroma contains perinuclear eosinophilic inclusions. The fibroblasts in this lesion are quite bland.

Nasopharyngeal Angiofibroma

Clinical Features

This histologically distinctive tumor occurs in the nasopharynx almost exclusively in young boys between 10 and 15 years old,[36] and therefore the prefix "juvenile" was previously attached to this diagnosis. Occurrence in older adult men and women has been reported on occasion.

The tumor usually presents a nasal mass or by repeated episodes of epistaxis. Because of the striking male predilection, androgen receptors have been evaluated and demonstrated by some investigators.[37] The tumor often recurs after a simple excision, sometimes after a long interval. Based on the abnormal vascular structure, as revealed by electron microscopy and immunohistochemistry, some authors have suggested that nasopharyngeal angiofibroma is a vascular malformation rather than a true neoplasm.[38] Malignant transformation has been reported in isolated cases but has been considered most likely related to radiation treatment.[39]

Pathology

Grossly, the tumor is solid and rubbery and measures on average 3 to 5 cm. Histologically, it is distinctive by the presence of gaping vessels with flaccid contours, lined by a thin endothelial layer, and surrounded by a variably dense fibrous stroma containing scattered plump fibroblasts with mild nuclear pleomorphism (Fig. 6–6). The degree of cellularity varies, but mitotic activity is rare.

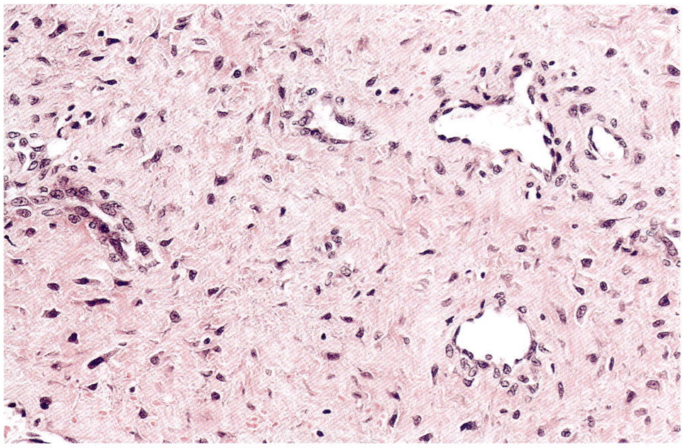

Figure 6–6. Nasopharyngeal angiofibroma is composed of gaping vessels and plump fibroblasts in a dense collagenous background.

Differential Diagnosis

Sinonasal hemangiopericytoma and solitary fibrous tumor are more highly cellular, with more densely packed spindled or round tumor cells. Choanal polyps have an edematous stroma, often with inflammatory cells, and the blood vessels are dilated thin-walled capillaries.

Myofibromatosis and Myofibroma

Clinical Features

Originally reported in infants and children,[40,41] the clinicopathologic spectrum of this tumor has expanded to cover similar lesions in adults of all ages.[42–44] The designation of myofibromatosis is applied to multiple lesions, which were historically sometimes referred to as congenital generalized fibromatosis or fibrosarcoma. The multiple infantile lesions are more common in girls. Presentation as a solitary nodule is more common and is referred to as myofibroma or solitary myofibroma. Rare familial occurrence in an autosomal dominant pattern has been reported,[45] and some cases have occurred in siblings of different generations of one family.[40,44] According to one clinical review, myofibroma is the most common fibrous tumor of infancy.[46]

The tumor may occur in a wide variety of peripheral soft tissue locations, and the multiple lesions, seen in 20% of infantile cases, may widely involve the superficial soft tissues, internal organs, bone, and bone marrow. More common is the occurrence in proximal than distal parts of the extremities, and occurrence in the head and neck and trunk is not rare. The peripheral lesions usually involve dermis or subcutis or they may be intramuscular.[40,44] A large series reported occurrence in the oral region, most commonly in the mandible, lips, cheeks, and tongue, where the tumor often presents as a polypoid intraoral projection.[44]

The behavior of tumors in peripheral soft tissue locations is benign. Some lesions in small children are multifocal and involve internal organs. In rare cases, the tumor has caused the death of a newborn by internal organ compromise, with 20% mortality for the multicentric disease in the original series.[40] Two other fatal cases were also reported with widely disseminated lesions involving heart, lungs, and liver.[47] Recurrence rate in the largest series has been 7% to 13%, with all recurrences having been cured by a local excision. In many cases the tumor undergoes spontaneous regression. This has been attributed to tendency of lesional cells for apoptosis.[48] Many older patients have a long history of a stable lesion before the excision.

Pathology

The tumor usually measures 1 to 5 cm and is sharply demarcated but unencapsulated, often with a histologically infiltrative margin. Grossly, the nodules may be lobulated, and on sectioning they are firm or gritty and vary from white to gray-pink/tan, often with hemorrhagic discoloration.

Microscopically, typically two components are seen: a central highly vascular and cellular hemangiopericytoma-like component with plump, oval intervascular cells, and peripheral bundles of spindled, pale-staining bland myofibroblasts, with the bundles crossing at random angles (Fig. 6–7). When the latter component is not present in the biopsy, the diagnosis may be difficult; tumors lacking the former component can be more easily recognized. In many cases the central immature part of the lesion has extensive coagulative necrosis, calcification, hyalinization, or cystic change. The more differentiated, eosinophilic myofibroblastic component often forms distinctive, histologically paler and more paucicellular foci and swirling nests of spindle cells often separated by collagen fibers. In some cases, this component is seen as the only preserved component in extensively centrally necrotic lesions, and in others it may comprise most of the lesion. This component may also show intimal vascular involvement, often outside of the confines of the main lesion; this has no further clinical significance.

The solitary cutaneous lesions and tumors in adults are generally similar to those in children, except they often have a more prominent myofibroblastic component and a less prominent vascular hemangiopericytoma-like component. The more cellular areas may have mitotic rate as high as 8/10 high power fields (HPF),[40] although usually less than 5/10 HPF.

Immunohistochemically, the differentiated myofibroblastic component is positive for α-smooth muscle actin and negative for desmin and S-100 protein.

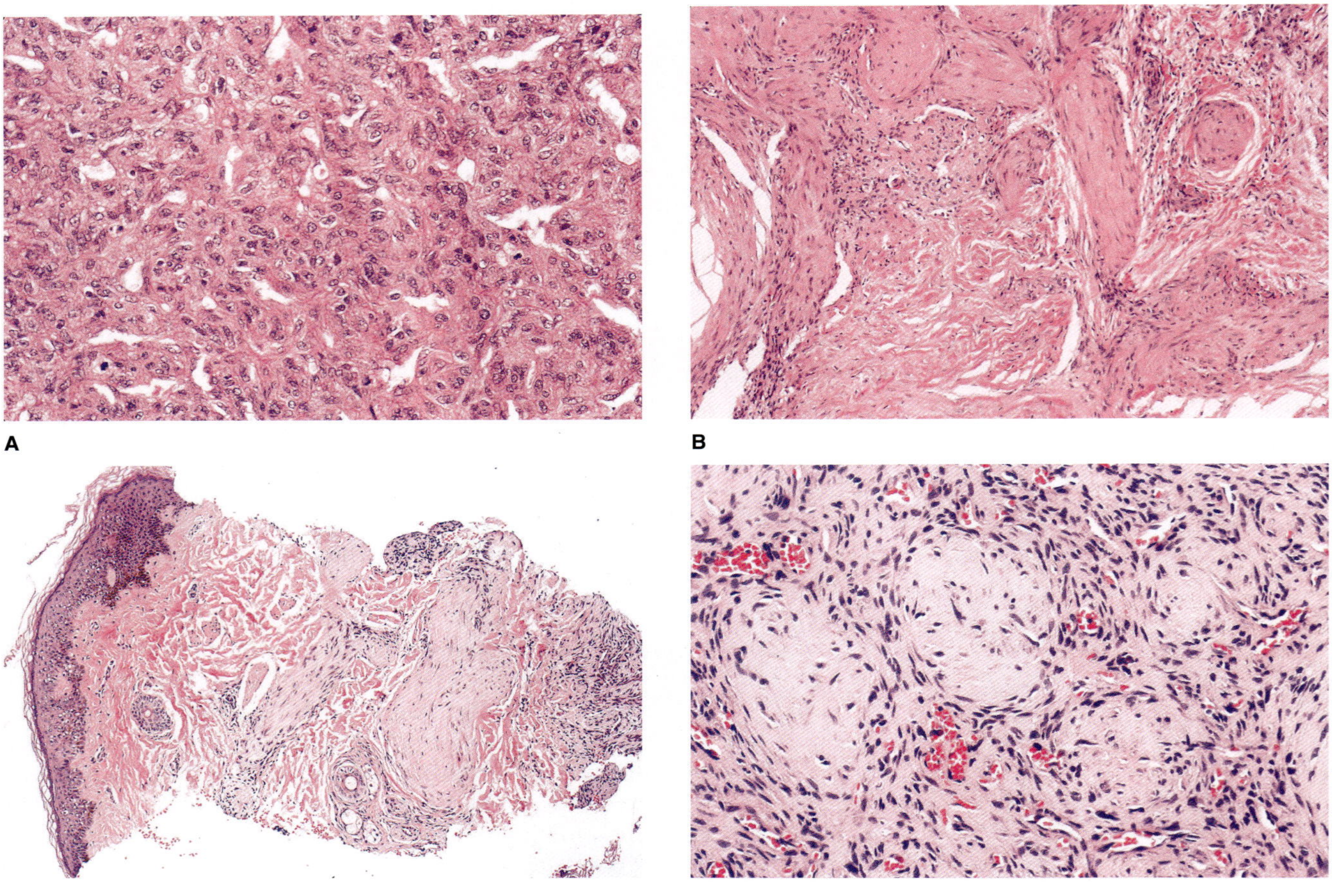

A B C D

Figure 6–7. Histologic spectrum of myofibroma. Infantile myofibroma contains two types of areas: A highly vascular component with a pericytoma-like pattern *(A)* and a more differentiated sharply demarcated myofibroblastic foci *(B)*. *C*, Cutaneous solitary myofibroma in an adult patient is predominantly composed of streaks of smooth muscle-like myofibroblasts. *D*, This solitary myofibroma contains a vascular component and round clusters of myofibroblasts.

Genetic data are scant, but an interstitial deletion of 6q12q15 has been reported in one case.[49]

Differential Diagnosis

Cellular variants of myofibromas may resemble vascular tumors or even sarcomas, but differ from them by the biphasic composition by vascular and myofibroblastic components. Myofibromas were historically classified as fibromatosis (e.g., under the designation congenital fibromatosis), from which they differ by lack of a uniform fibroblastic proliferation with collagen formation. Many tumors classified earlier as hemangiopericytomas in infants represent this entity, because careful search often reveals myofibroblastic foci typical of myofibroma.[50]

Calcifying (Juvenile) Aponeurotic Fibroma

Clinical Features

Calcifying aponeurotic fibroma is a very rare, distinctive fibrous lesion of childhood, previously designated as juvenile aponeurotic fibroma or aponeurotic fibroma.[51–53] This tumor occurs almost exclusively in children and young adults, nearly half in the first decade with the median age of 11 years in the Armed Forces Institutes of Pathology material.[54] Occasional cases are seen in older individuals. There is a 2:1 male predominance. Eighty percent of the lesions occur in the distal extremities, especially in the palmar side of hand and fingers, and 20% occur in the proximal parts of extremities and trunk. The lesions have a significant tendency to recur locally, and in some cases the recurrences have occurred in the span of over 20 years. Malignant transformation does not occur. Because the recurrences are not destructive, and lesional maturation or regression may occur over time, a complete but function-preserving excision is considered optimal.

Pathology

Grossly, the lesion has irregular contours and is usually relatively small with median size of 2 to 3 cm and size, rarely exceeding 4 to 5 cm. It has a rubbery consistency and may have visibly calcified foci. Histologically, these tumors have a spindle cell fibroblastic component that often extends to subcutaneous fat and may resemble the appearance of fibromatosis or even fibrosarcoma, but mitotic activity is low (<2/10 HPF). Most cases also contain distinctive round or oval fibrocartilaginous foci, often with central calcification. Nodular foci of epithelioid

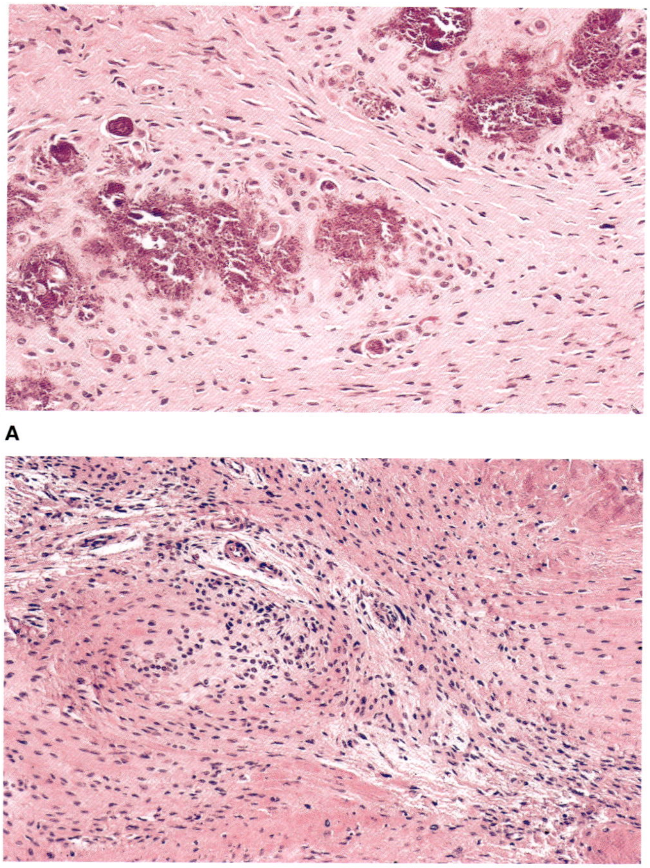

Figure 6–8. *A*, Calcifying aponeurotic fibroma contains a fibromatosis-like spindle cell component and rounded clusters of focal cartilaginous differentiation with an epithelioid pattern and central calcification. *B*, A lesion with predominantly fibromatosis-like elements.

fibroblasts may precede the formation of such cartilaginous foci (Fig. 6–8*A*). Some lesions have a prominent fibromatosis-like component (Fig. 6–8*B*). In such cases, the presence of epithelioid foci with calcification elsewhere in the tumor establishes the diagnosis. The predominance of the fibrous component in lesions of small children and cartilaginous components in older individuals suggests that the cartilaginous component increases during the evolution of the lesion. Genetic data have not been reported.

Juvenile Diffuse Fibromatosis

This is a heterogeneous and poorly understood group of tumors. It includes probably as the largest group conventional desmoids that may present in early childhood. Perhaps the most distinctive rare variant of this category is the diffuse form of

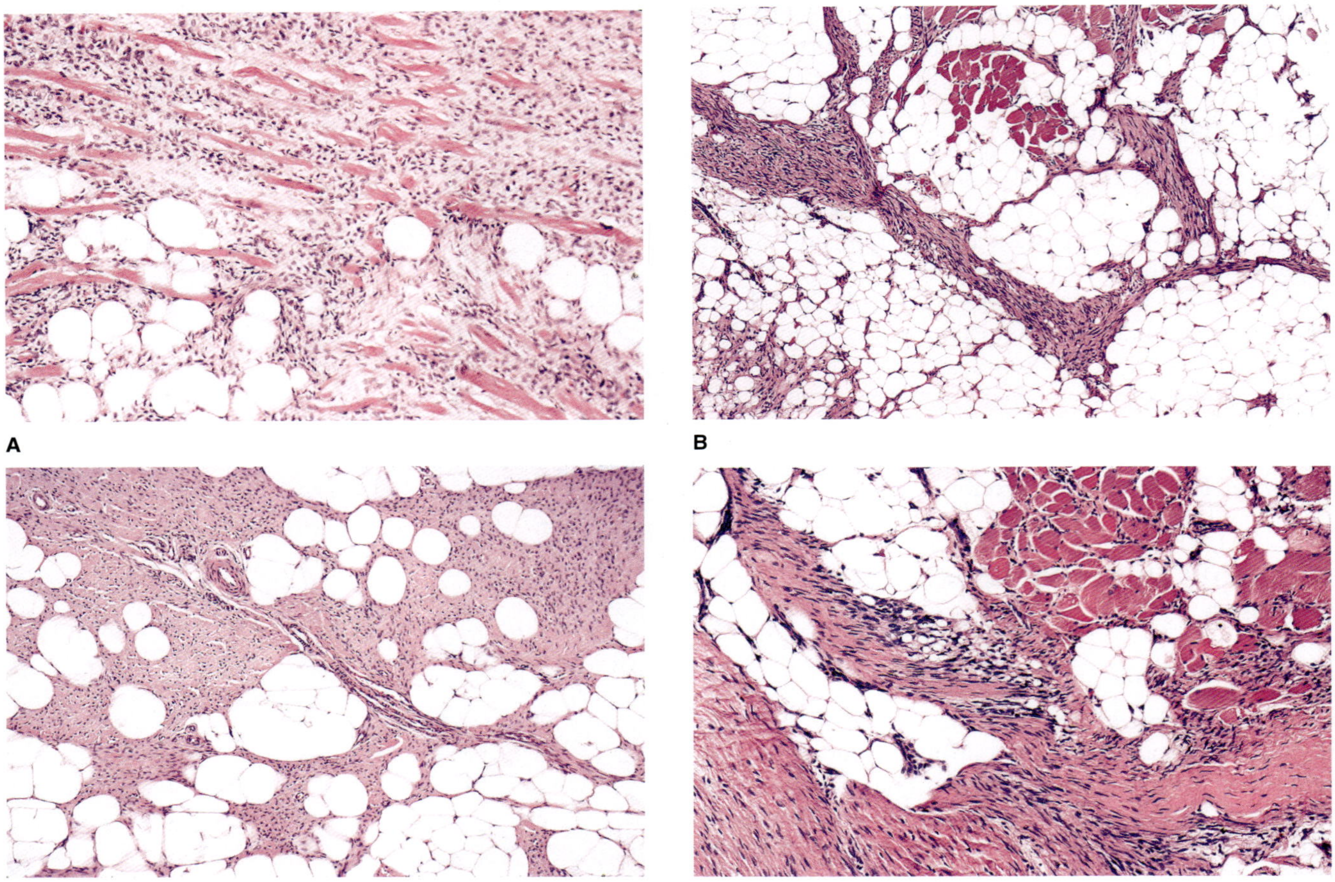

A B C D

Figure 6–9. Juvenile fibromatosis. *A,* Juvenile diffuse fibromatosis contains round cells diffusely infiltrating in the skeletal muscle and subcutaneous fat. *B* and *C,* Lipofibromatosis lesions contain streaks of moderately cellular fibroblastic foci and intervening fat somewhat resembling fibrous hamartoma of infancy. *D,* The lesion typically infiltrates in skeletal muscle and may have lipoblast-like foci.

juvenile fibromatosis. These lesions chiefly occur in small children in deep soft tissues at a wide variety of body sites in the extremities, trunk, and head and neck. Local recurrence is common.[55]

Histologically, the lesions are composed of oval to round fibroblast-like cells that diffusely infiltrate in fat and skeletal muscle (Fig. 6–9*A*). There is no nuclear atypia, and mitotic activity is inconspicuous.

Lipofibromatosis

Clinical Features

This pediatric tumor was recently reported by Fetsch et al.[56] It typically occurs in hands and feet in children aged 5 to 15. The tumor has a high tendency for local recurrence, but it does not metastasize. Previously, lesions of this type were called juvenile fibromatosis or examples of fibrous hamartoma of infancy in distal extremities.

Pathology

Grossly, the lesion is fibrolipomatous, having an integral fatty component with visible fibrous streaks. Microscopically, the fatty and maturing fibrous components resemble those of fibrous hamartoma of infancy, except that there is no primitive round cell component. The lesions differ from other forms of fibromatosis by the architectural preservation of fat and lack of solid fibrous growth. The lesion is typically composed of mature adipose tissue element with streaks of cellular fibrous tissue involving the septa of fat and skeletal muscle (Fig. 6–9*B* to *D*). Mitotic activity is low and atypia is absent. Focal lipoblast-like cells, probably representing evolving fat, are sometimes present in the interphase of the fatty and fibrous components.[56]

Characteristic combination of streaks of fibrous tissue and islands of fat distinguish this tumor from lipoblastoma, which is typically composed of well-organized lobules of highly vascular, often myxoid, embryonal type fat.

Plexiform Fibrohistiocytic Tumor

This histologically distinctive multinodular skin tumor typical of children and young adults was described by Enzinger and Zhang.[57] Smaller series have been reported since then.[58-60]

Clinical Features

Over half of the cases have been reported in children, and two thirds occur in children under the age of 20 years. There is a significant female predominance. The tumor most commonly occurs in the superficial soft tissues of the upper extremity (shoulder, forearm) and less commonly in the lower extremity, trunk, and head and neck.

The original series reported local recurrences in 37.5% and lymph node metastases in 6% of cases, but there were no distant metastases. Subsequent reports show occasional pulmonary metastasis, but fatalities have been exceedingly rare.[60]

Pathology

The lesion is typically centered in the lower dermis, but often extends into the entire dermis and often subcutis, where a minority of lesions are centered. The tumor is typically poorly circumscribed and usually measures 1 to 3 cm in diameter, and rarely over 5 cm.

Histologically, a multinodular "plexiform" growth pattern is typical (Fig. 6–10). The nodules and streaks of tumor may be confluent or separated by dermal collagen or subcutaneous fat. Some nodules are surrounded by a dense band of fibrosis.

The tumor foci are composed of spindle cells with scattered osteoclastic giant cells, sometimes seen in the center of the nodules, sometimes evenly dispersed. Some elements of tumor may be composed of spindle cells only, whereas others may be rich in osteoclastic giant cells. The nodules often contain foci of hemosiderin and focal lymphocytic infiltration. Many tumors have streaks of spindle cells in a collagenous background resembling fibromatosis. Focal cytologic atypia may be present, but mitotic activity is usually low not exceeding 3 mitoses/10 HPF.

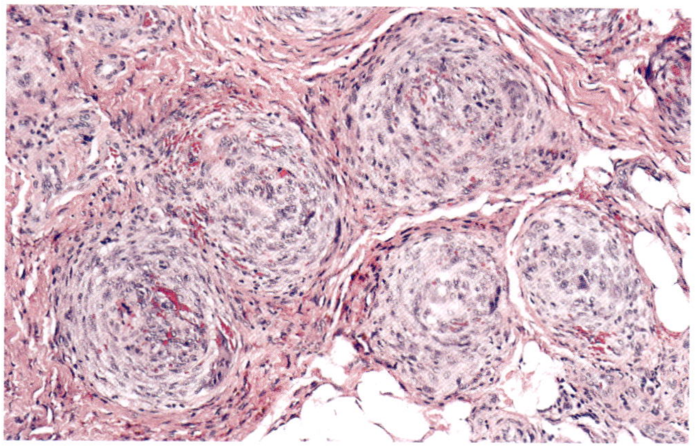

Figure 6–10. Plexiform fibrohistiocytic tumor is composed of multiple nodules of oval histiocytes, multinucleated giant cells, and fibroblasts.

Genetics

Two cytogenetic studies show different changes. One study[61] showed a simple karyotype with a translocation t(4;15)(q21;q15). Another study[62] reported complex changes, including deletion of 4q25q31, suggesting that a gene in 4q21-q25 could be pathogenetically important.

Inflammatory Myofibroblastic Tumor

Inflammatory myofibroblastic tumor (IMT) is a peculiar spindle cell tumor that combines ample cytoplasmic spindle cells and an inflammatory background. IMT usually occurs in children and young adults in the lung, abdominal cavity, and urinary bladder. The presence of clonal chromosomal changes suggests neoplastic nature.[63-65]

The term inflammatory pseudotumor has been used for IMT lesions at different sites, but this designation has also been used in a generic sense of any inflammatory tumefactions whether infectious (mycobacterial pseudotumor) or noninfectious.[66] Whether IMTs ultimately represent a single biologic entity is unknown. Especially not sure is whether the peripheral soft tissue tumors designated as IMT are fully comparable to the abdominal ones. Heterogeneous terminology and controversy over whether some cases should be designated as sarcomas also surround this entity. There is at least one report on progression into sarcoma after repeated recurrences.[67]

A variety of designations have been used for IMTs at various sites. In the lung IMT has been designated as plasma cell granuloma, postinflammatory tumor, xanthomatous pseudotumor, and inflammatory myofibrohistiocytic tumor. In the bladder the designations have been inflammatory myofibroblastic pseudotumor, inflammatory pseudosarcomatous myofibroblastic tumor, pseudosarcomatous fibromyxoid tumor, and pseudosarcomatous myofibroblastic tumor. Quite likely, at least some postoperative spindle cell nodules also represent IMTs.[68]

The term inflammatory fibrosarcoma has been used mainly for the highly cellular abdominal lesions of children,[69,70] but most authors currently designate all lesions as IMT, because of lack of clear distinguishing criteria and the expressed uncertainty whether true metastases occur. Some of these tumors have been designated as leiomyosarcomas in the past, especially when located in the gastrointestinal tract.

Clinical Features

The most common site of presentation is the lung. Other common sites for IMT are omentum and mesenteries, stomach and intestines, peripheral soft tissues, upper respiratory tract, mediastinum, pelvis, and retroperitoneum. The specific clinical features of the pulmonary[71] and urinary bladder tumors[72–74] will not be discussed here in detail, but their histologic and immunohistochemical features are in many aspects similar to IMTs presenting in soft tissue sites.

Lesions designated as inflammatory myofibroblastic tumors of the liver and spleen include dendritic reticulum cell sarcomas.[66] Inflammatory pseudotumors of lymph node[75] and spleen differ from IMT in several respects and probably represent a different entity.

The IMTs of soft tissue, similar to those in the lungs and bladder, have mainly been reported in children and young adults. The median and mean ages of the largest series have been 9 to 12 years. These tumors have been reported in infants and in late adulthood as well. Two series reported IMTs of soft tissues and larynx, respectively, in adults with median ages of 55 to 59 years (range, 19–83), but it is not clear whether all these tumors represent the same entity as IMT in childhood.[76,77] No clear sex predilection has emerged.

The peripheral and larger abdominal tumors may present as mass lesions, and tumors involving the intestines may cause obstruction. Multiple lesions are seen in some intra-abdominal cases. The intra-abdominal tumors are commonly large, over 10 cm.

A minority of patients (15–30%) have constitutional symptoms that disappear after tumor removal and may reappear with tumor recurrence. They include fever, malaise, and weight loss. Some children have experienced growth retardation. Pathologic laboratory findings include anemia (normochromic or hypochromic, microcytic), leukocytosis, thrombocytosis, elevated erythrocyte sedimentation rate, and polyclonal hypergammaglobulinemia. Rarely reported cultured pathogens may be coincidental rather than etiologic. Studies based on polymerase chain reactions on abdominal lesions have been negative for Epstein-Barr virus and cytomegalovirus DNA.[70]

Pathology

Grossly, the lesions have a wide size range of 1 to 20 cm. The mesenteric and other intra-abdominal lesions (including those reported as inflammatory fibrosarcoma) are typically larger, often exceeding 10 cm. Multiple tumor nodules are common with lobular, multinodular, and sometimes with whorled texture on sectioning. The tumor tissue is gray-white on tan-pink. The cut surface is usually rubbery, but may be myxoid in some areas.

Histologically, IMT is composed of a mixture of spindle or polygonal cells, plasma cells, and lymphocytes in varying proportions (Fig. 6–11A.) Some lesions contain eosinophils and neutrophils. The spindle cells may show a dense storiform or fascicular arrangement with relatively few inflammatory cells in between, or there may be extensive inflammatory infiltration. The pulmonary lesions are often rich in xanthomatous histiocytes. Myxoid, paucicellular areas with a rich network of delicate capillaries or foci with dense fibrosis are seen in some cases. Focal calcifications may also occur.

Cytologically, the spindle cells have typically oval to elongated nuclei, often resembling smooth muscle cells. The cytoplasm is amphophilic and often abundant. A histologic spectrum includes relatively bland lesions in one end and more highly cellular and atypical lesions in the other end (Fig. 6–11*B*). Some cases show cells with abundant cytoplasm and epithelioid or ganglion-like features, typically mixed with less cytoplasmic spindle cells. These cells typically show prominent, eosinophilic nucleoli. Some elongated large cells with ample cytoplasm may resemble rhabdomyoblasts. Mitotic frequency varies, but is generally low, and necrosis is rare. It has been suggested that tumors with a high content of large ganglion-like cells behave more aggressively. Vascular invasion may occur, but this has no adverse prognostic significance. It has been suggested that tumor aneuploidy correlates with a higher risk for recurrence.[78]

Immunohistochemistry

The lesional cells show myofibroblastic features. They are often positive for anaplastic lymphoma kinase (ALK) (Fig. 6–11*C*). They are also positive for vimentin, muscle actin (HHF-35), α-smooth muscle actin, and occasionally and focally for desmin.

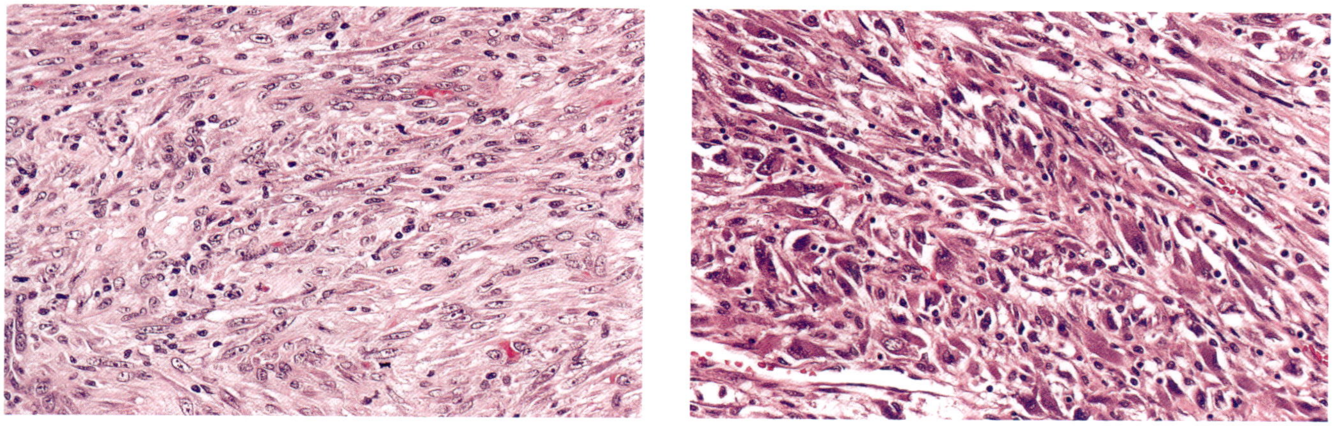

A B

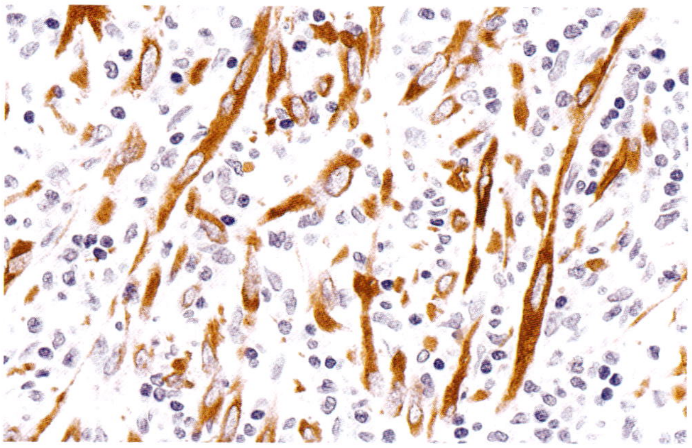

C

Figure 6–11. *A,* Inflammatory myofibroblastic tumor is composed of plump myofibroblasts and moderate lymphoplasmacytic infiltration. *B,* The tumor cells often have an epithelioid appearance with abundant, amphophilic cytoplasm. *C,* Immunohistochemically, the tumor cells show strong cytoplasmic positivity for anaplastic lymphoma kinase (ALK).

Keratin positivity with AE1/AE3 cocktail and CAM5.2 antibodies has been often reported in abdominal and bladder tumors, but not in pulmonary lesions. The lesional cells are always negative for myoglobin and S-100 protein.[64,70]

Differential Diagnosis

The childhood lesions may both clinically and histologically resemble embryonal rhabdomyosarcoma (RMS), especially when located in the bladder. However, the extensive inflammatory background differs from RMS; also the IMT occurs in older children. The large cytoplasmic cells are always negative for myoglobin, and IMT usually shows extensive smooth muscle actin reactivity not seen in RMS; the latter is usually positive for skeletal muscle-specific transcriptional regulators (MyoD1, myogenin).

The IMTs should be also separated as specific and nonspecific inflammatory pseudotumors and from malignant fibrous histiocytoma.

Leiomyosarcomas typically have eosinophilic, fibrillary cytoplasm not seen in IMT. Compared to IMT, gastrointestinal stromal tumors (GISTs) have a more homogeneous cellular composition and almost exclusively present in adults over 40 years of age. Apparently some childhood tumors reported as GISTs are IMTs. In contrast to GISTs, IMTs are negative for KIT.

Tumor Behavior and Treatment

The biologic potential of these lesions is difficult to predict with certainty. Local recurrences have been observed in 15% in a series of extrapulmonary IMT[63] and in 37% among the mainly abdominal-mesenteric tumors diagnosed as inflammatory fibrosarcomas.[70]

Malignant behavior has been reported in three contexts: malignant transformation of IMT, metastatic disease, and patient death due to nonmetastatic complications. One tumor that was primary in the forearm underwent malignant transformation after five local recurrences and led to subsequent pulmonary metastasis and death.[67] No metastases were reported in a large series of extrapulmonary IMT,[63] whereas three patients (11%) diagnosed with inflammatory fibrosarcoma[69] developed metastasis (two in lung, one in brain). Additionally, 18% of patients diagnosed with abdominal inflammatory fibrosarcoma died from locally aggressive disease, including exsanguination by tumor infiltration in one case.[69] In view of the clinical unpredictability and potential for low-grade malignant behavior, complete excision of the tumor and satellite nodules and metastases and close clinical follow-up are advisable.

Genetics

Several reports describe clonal chromosomal changes supporting neoplastic nature of these tumors.[79] Common to all specific gene rearrangements found in IMT has been involvement of the *ALK* gene at 2p23; overexpression of *ALK* by immunohistochemistry has also been shown.[80,81] Recently, a chromosomal translocation resulting in fusion of the tropomyosin 3 *(TPM3)* or tropomyosin 4 *(TPM4)* and *ALK* genes was reported.[82] A similar translocation has also been found in anaplastic large cell lymphoma, which more often has the t(2;5) translocation with *ALK-NPM* fusion.[83]

Immunohistochemical evaluation of ALK expression may have a role in the differential diagnosis, because other inflammatory pseudotumors are typically negative for ALK.[84] Correlative molecular genetic and immunohistochemical studies and extensive evaluation of ALK expression in different tumors are necessary to understand its practical diagnosis.

Infantile (Congenital) Fibrosarcoma

This tumor has recently proved to be a specific molecular entity with a typical gene fusion; the clinical features are also characteristic.

Clinical Features

This rare tumor usually arises during the first year of life, and half of the tumors are congenital; occurrence beyond 5 years of age is exceptional. The tumor has a 6:4 male predominance and affects mainly the distal parts of the upper and lower extremities: hands, forearm, ankle, and feet. It is typically rapidly growing and poorly circumscribed and may infiltrate both superficial and deep soft tissues and reach a considerable size. Because this tumor has a relatively good prognosis despite the ominous clinical features, conservative primary treatment is now advocated, although complete excision should be performed.[85–91] Chemotherapy may obviate amputations in some cases in which amputation would otherwise be required for complete excision.[92] The tumor is prone to local recurrences, but lung metastases are rare. The series of Chung and Enzinger showed a 5-year survival of 84%,[86] with a few fatalities caused by lung or brain metastases. Subsequent series have shown similar good survival results. Compared with fibrosarcomas of older children, the prognosis is more favorable.[87]

Pathology

Grossly, infantile fibrosarcoma varies from a small nodule to a bulky tumor, with the mean size 4 cm in the largest series.[86] On sectioning the tumor is pale tan or fleshy, and varies from firm to soft. Larger tumors often have areas of hemorrhage and necrosis.

Histologically, infantile fibrosarcoma varies from a well-differentiated collagen-forming fibrosarcomatous pattern to a highly cellular noncollagenous spindle cell tumor arranged in fascicles or diffuse sheets (Fig. 6–12). Mitotic activity is often high. Malignant fibrous histiocytoma-like pleomorphic transformation may occur and has been shown to carry a poor prognosis.[93]

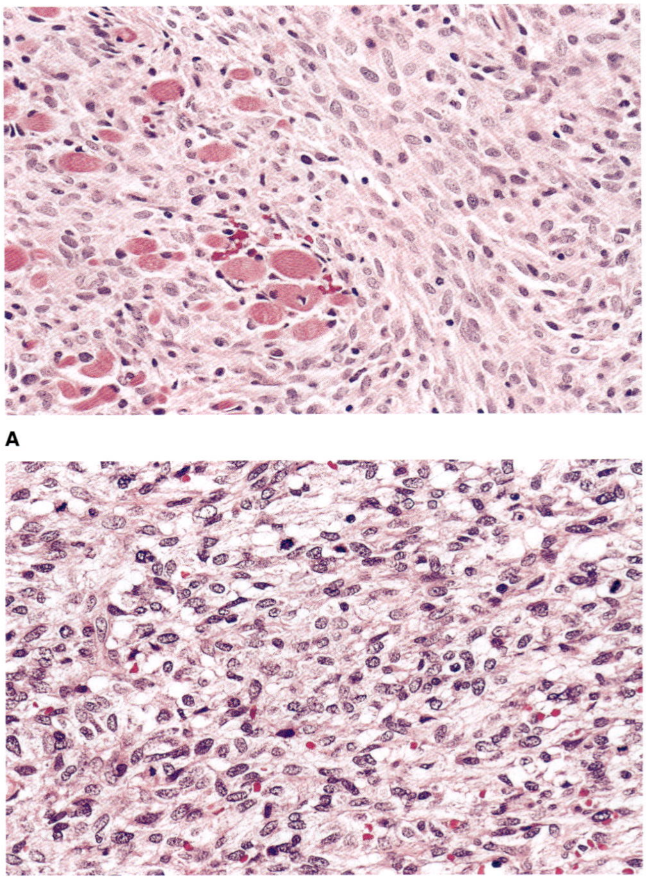

A

B

Figure 6–12. *A* and *B,* Infantile fibrosarcoma infiltrates in the skeletal muscle and is composed of uniform plump spindle cells.

Differential Diagnosis

The diagnoses of spindle cell and poorly differentiated embryonal rhabdomyosarcoma have to be ruled out, especially in the case of tumors in the genital region and pelvis. Immunohistochemistry is required for this in every case, and a wide panel of markers, including desmin and skeletal muscle transcriptional regulators (MyoD1, myogenin), should be evaluated. Intratumoral hemorrhage seen in some cases should not be mistaken for a vascular tumor.

Genetics

Trisomy of chromosome 11 along with variable trisomies of chromosomes 17 and 20 and occasionally of 8 and 10 occur as nonrandom cytogenetic changes with possible differential diagnostic value.[94–97]

A reciprocal translocation t(12;15)(p13;q25) resulting in the fusion of *ETV6* and *NTRK3* genes has been found in most cases.[98] The same translocation occurs in the cellular (but not the typical) variant of mesoblastic nephroma indicating virtual genetic identity of these tumors.[99–101] The translocation can be evaluated by reverse transcription-polymerase chain reaction using frozen or formalin-fixed and paraffin-embedded tissue.[102,103] This gene fusion has not been detected in other spindle cell tumors of childhood.

The *NTRK3* gene encodes for a tyrosine kinase receptor C. According to two studies, this protein is similarly present in infantile fibrosarcoma and in other spindle cell tumors of childhood, indicating that this protein is not a tumor-specific immunohistochemical marker.[103,104]

REFERENCES

Cranial Fasciitis

1. Lauer DH, Enzinger FM: Cranial fasciitis in childhood. Cancer 1980;45:401–406.
2. Sarangarajan R, Dehner LP: Cranial and extracranial fasciitis of childhood: A clinicopathologic and immunohistochemical study. Hum Pathol 1999;30:87–92.

Fibromatosis Colli

3. MacDonald D: Sternomastoid tumor and muscular torticollis. J Bone Joint Surg [Br] 1969;51:432–443.
4. Sauer F, Sehner L, Freng A: Cytologic features of fibromatosis colli of infancy. Acta Cytol 1997;41:633–635.

Calcifying Fibrous Pseudotumor

5. Rosenthal NS, Abdul-Karim FW: Childhood fibrous tumor with psammoma bodies. Clinicopathologic features in two cases. Arch Pathol Lab Med 1988; 112:798–800.
6. Fetsch JF, Montgomery EA, Meis JM: Calcifying fibrous pseudotumor. Am J Surg Pathol 1993;17:502–508.
7. Pinkard NB, Wilson RW, Lawless N, et al: Calcifying fibrous pseudotumor of pleura. A report of three cases of a newly described entity involving the pleura. Am J Clin Pathol 1996;105:189–194.
8. Van Dorpe J, Ectors N, Geboes K, D'Hoore A, Sciot R: Is calcifying fibrous pseudotumor a late sclerosing stage of inflammatory myofibroblastic tumor? Am J Surg Pathol 1999;23:329–335.

Juvenile Hyaline Fibromatosis

9. Remberger K, Krieg T, Kunze D, Weinmann HM, Hubner G: Fibromatosis hyalinica multiplex (juvenile hyalin fibromatosis). Light microscopic, electron microscopic, immunohistochemical, and biochemical findings. Cancer 1985;56:614–624.
10. Fayad MN, Yacoub A, Salman S, Khudr A, Der Kaloustian VM: Juvenile hyaline fibromatosis: Two new patients and review of the literature. Am J Med Genet 1987;26:123–131.
11. Mancini GM, Stojanov L, Willemsen R, et al: Juvenile hyaline fibromatosis: Clinical heterogeneity in three patients. Dermatology 1999;198:18–25.
12. Senzaki H, Kiyozuka Y, Uemura Y, Shikata N, Ueda S, Tsubura A: Juvenile hyaline fibromatosis: A report of two unrelated adult sibling cases and a literature review. Pathol Int 1998;48:230–236.
13. Allen PW: Selected case from the Arkadi M. Rywlin International Pathology slide Seminar: Hyaline fibromatosis. Adv Anat Pathol 2001;8:173–178.

Fibrous Hamartoma of Infancy

14. Enzinger FM: Fibrous hamartoma of infancy. Cancer 1965;18:241–248.
15. Michal M, Mukensnabl P, Chlumska A, Kodet R: Fibrous hamartoma of infancy. A study of eight cases with immunohistochemical and electron microscopic findings. Pathol Res Pract 1992;188:1049–1053.
16. Efem SE, Ekpo MD: Clinicopathological features of untreated fibrous hamartoma of infancy. J Clin Pathol 1993;46:522–524.
17. Popek EJ, Montgomery EA, Fourcroy JL: Fibrous hamartoma of infancy in the genital region: Findings in 15 cases. J Urol 1994;151:990–993.
18. Sotelo-Avila C, Bale PM: Subdermal fibrous hamartoma of infancy: Pathology of 40 cases and differential diagnosis. Pediatr Pathol 1994;14:39–52.
19. Dickey GE, Sotelo-Avila C: Fibrous hamartoma of infancy. Current review. Pediatr Dev Pathol 1999;2: 236–243.

Infantile Digital Fibroma(tosis)

20. Reye RDK: Recurring digital fibrous tumor of childhood. Arch Pathol 1965;80:228–223.
21. Allen PW: Recurring digital fibrous tumor of childhood. Pathology 1972;4:215–223.
22. Beckett JH, Jacobs AH: Recurring digital fibrous tumor of childhood: A review. Pediatrics 1977;59:401–406.
23. Santa-Cruz DJ, Reiner CB: Recurrent digital fibroma of childhood. J Cutan Pathol 1978;5:339–346.
24. Bhawan J, Bacchetta C, Joris I, Majno G: A myofibroblastic tumor. Infantile digital fibroma (recurrent digital fibrous tumor of childhood). Am J Pathol 1979;94:19–36.
25. Ishii N, Matsui K, Ichiyama S, Takahashi Y, Nakajima H: A case of infantile digital fibromatosis showing spontaneous regression. Br J Dermatol 1989;121:129–133.
26. Rimareix F, Bardot J, Anmdrac L, Vasse D, Galinier P, Magalon G: Infantile digital fibroma—Report on eleven cases. Eur J Pediatr Surg 1997;7:345–348.
27. Iwasaki H, Kikuchi M, Ohtsuki I, Enjoji M, Suenaga N, Mori R: Infantile digital fibromatosis. Identification of actin filaments in cytoplasmic inclusions by heavy meromyosin binding. Cancer 1983;52:1653–1661.
28. Fringer B, Thais H, Bohm N, Altmannsberger M, Osborn M: Identification of actin microfilaments in the intracytoplasmic inclusions present in recurring infantile digital fibromatosis (Reye tumor). Pediatr Pathol 1986;6:311–324.
29. Mukai M, Torikata C, Iri H, Hata J, Naito M, Shimoda T: Immunohistochemical identification of aggregated actin filaments in formalin-fixed, paraffin embedded sections I. A study of infantile digital fibromatosis by a new pretreatment. Am J Surg Pathol 1992;16:110–115.
30. Hyashi T, Tsuda N, Chowdhury PR, et al: Infantile digital fibromatosis: A study of the development and regression of cytoplasmic inclusion bodies. Mod Pathol 1995;8:548–552.
31. Sarma DP, Hoffmann EO: Infantile digital fibroma-like tumor in an adult. Arch Dermatol 1980;116:578–579.
32. Viale G, Doglioni C, Iuzzolino P, et al: Infantile digital fibromatosis-like tumour (inclusion body fibromatosis) of adulthood: Report of two cases with ultrastructural and immunocytochemical findings. Histopathology 1988;12:415–424.
33. Bittesini L, DeiTos AP, Doglioni C, DellaLibera D, Laurino L, Fletcher CD: Fibro-epithelial tumor of the breast with digital fibroma-like inclusions in the stromal component. Case report with immunocytochemical and ultrastructural analysis. Am J Surg Pathol 1994;18:296–301.
34. Hiraoka N, Mukai M, Hosoda Y, Hata J: Phyllodes tumor of the breast containing the intracytoplasmic inclusion bodies identical with infantile digital fibromatosis. Am J Surg Pathol 1994;18:506–511.
35. Navas-Palacios JJ, Conde-Zurita JM: Inclusion body myofibroblasts other than those seen in recurrent digital fibroma of childhood. Ultrastruct Pathol 1984;7:109–121.

Nasopharyngeal Angiofibroma

36. Neel HB, Whicker JH, Devine KD, Weiland JH: Juvenile angiofibroma: Review of 120 cases. Am J Surg 1973;126:547–556.
37. Hwang HC, Mills SE, Patterson K, Gown AM: Expression of androgen receptors in nasopharyngeal angiofibroma: An immunohistochemical study of 24 cases. Mod Pathol 1998;11:1122–1126.
38. Beham A, Beham-Schmid C, Regauer S, Aubock L, Stammberger H: Nasopharyngeal angiofibroma: True neoplasm or vascular malformation. Adv Anat Pathol 2000;7:36–46.
39. Makek MS, Andrews JC, Fisch U: Malignant transformation of a nasopharyngeal angiofibroma. Laryngoscope 1990;100:791–792.

Myofibromatosis and Myofibroma

40. Chung EB, Enzinger FM: Infantile myofibromatosis. A review of 59 cases with localized and generalized involvement. Cancer 1981;48:1807–1818.
41. Briselli MF, Soule EH, Gilchrist GS: Congenital fibromatosis. Report of 18 cases of solitary and 4 cases of multiple tumors. Mayo Clin Proc 1980;55:554–562.
42. Daimaru Y, Hashimoto H, Enjoji M: Myofibromatosis in adults (adult counterpart of infantile myofibromatosis). Am J Surg Pathol 1989;13:859–865.
43. Smith KJ, Skelton HG, Barrett TL, Lupton GP, Graham JH: Cutaneous myofibroma. Mod Pathol 1989;2:603–609.
44. Foss RD, Ellis GL: Myofibromas and myofibromatosis of the oral region: A clinicopathologic analysis of 79 cases. Oral Surg Oral Med Oral Pathol Oral Radiol Endod 2000;89:57–65.
45. Jennings T, Duray PH, Collins FS, et al: Infantile myofibromatosis. Evidence for an autosomal-dominant disorder. Am J Surg Pathol 1984;8:529–538.
46. Wiswell TE, Davis J, Cunningham BE, Solenberger L, Thomas PJ: Infantile myofibromatosis: The most common fibrous tumor of infancy. J Pediatr Surg 1988;23:315–318.
47. Coffin CM, Neilson KA, Ingels S, Frank-Gerszberg R, Dehner LP: Congenital generalized fibromatosis: A disseminated angiocentric myofibromatosis. Pediatr Pathol Lab Med 1995;15:571–587.
48. Fukasawa Y, Ishikura H, Takada A, et al: Massive apoptosis in infantile myofibromatosis. A putative mechanism for tumor regression. Am J Pathol 1995;144:480–485.
49. Stenman G, Nadal N, Persson S, Gunterberg B, Angervall L: del(6)(q12q15) as the sole cytogenetic abnormality in a case of solitary infantile myofibromatosis. Oncol Rep 1999;6:1101–1104.

50. Mentzel T, Calonje E, Nascimento AG, Fletcher CDM: Infantile hemangiopericytoma versus infantile myofibromatosis. Study of a series suggesting a continuous spectrum of infantile myofibroblastic lesions. Am J Surg Pathol 1994;18:922–930.

Calcifying Aponeurotic Fibroma

51. Keasbey LE: Juvenile aponeurotic fibroma (calcifying fibroma): A distinctive tumor arising in the palms and soles of young children. Calcifying aponeurotic fibroma. Cancer 1953;6:338–346.
52. Goldman RL: The cartilage analogy of fibromatosis (aponeurotic fibroma): Further observations based on seven new cases. Cancer 1970;26:1325–1331.
53. Allen PW, Enzinger FM: Juvenile aponeurotic fibroma. Cancer 1970;26:857–867.
54. Fetsch JF, Miettinen M: Calcifying aponeurotic fibroma: A clinicopathologic study on 22 cases arising in uncommon sites. Hum Pathol 1998;29:1504–1510.

Juvenile Diffuse Fibromatosis and Lipofibromatosis

55. Enzinger FM: Fibrous tumors of infancy. In: Tumors of Bone and Soft Tissue. Chicago, Year Book Medical Publishers, 1965, pp. 231–268.
56. Fetsch JF, Miettinen M, Laskin WB, Michal M, Enzinger FM: A clinicopathologic study of 45 pediatric soft tissue tumors with an admixture of adipose tissue and fibroblastic elements, and a proposal for classification as lipofibromatosis. Am J Surg Pathol 2000;24:1491–1500.

Plexiform Fibrohistiocytic Tumor

57. Enzinger FM, Zhang R: Plexiform fibrohistiocytic tumor presenting in children and young adults. An analysis of 65 cases. Am J Surg Pathol 1988;12:818–826.
58. Hollowood K, Holley MP, Fletcher CDM: Plexiform fibrohistiocytic tumour: Clinicopathological, immunohistochemical and ultrastructural analysis in favour of a myofibroblastic lesion. Histopathology 1991;19:503–513.
59. Zelger B, Weinlich G, Steiner H, Zelger BG, Egarter-Vigl E: Dermal and sub-cutaneous variants of plexiform fibrohistiocytic tumor. Am J Surg Pathol 1997;21:235–241.
60. Remstein ED, Arndt CAS, Nascimento AG: Plexiform fibrohistiocytic tumor: Clinicopathologic analysis of 22 cases. Am J Surg Pathol 1999;23:662–670.
61. Redlich GC, Montgomery KD, Allgood GA, Joste NE: Plexiform fibrohistiocytic tumor with a clonal cytogenetic anomaly. Cancer Genet Cytogenet 1999;108:141–143.
62. Smith S, Fletcher CD, Smith MA, Gusterson BA: Cytogenetic analysis of a plexiform fibrohistiocytic tumor. Cancer Genet Cytogenet 1990;48:31–34.

Inflammatory Myofibroblastic Tumor—Clinicopathologic

63. Coffin CM, Watterson J, Priest JR, Dehner LP: Extrapulmonary inflammatory myofibroblastic tumor (inflammatory pseudotumor). A clinicopathologic and immunohistochemical study of 84 cases. Am J Surg Pathol 1995;19:859–872.
64. Coffin CM, Dehner LP, Meis-Kindblom JM: Inflammatory myofibroblastic tumor, inflammatory fibrosarcoma, and related lesions: An historical review with differential diagnostic considerations. Semin Diagn Pathol 1998;15:102–110.
65. Coffin CM, Humphrey PA, Dehner LP: Extrapulmonary inflammatory myofibroblastic tumor: A clinical and pathological survey. Semin Diagn Pathol 1998;15:85–101.
66. Chan JKC: Inflammatory pseudotumor—A family of lesions of diverse nature and etiologies. Adv Anat Pathol 1996;3:156–171.
67. Donner LR, Trompler RA, White RR: Progression of inflammatory myofibroblastic tumor (inflammatory pseudotumor) of soft tissue into sarcoma after several recurrences. Hum Pathol 1996;27:1095–1098.
68. Proppe KH, Scully RE, Rosai J: Postoperative spindle cell nodules of genitourinary tract resembling sarcomas. Am J Surg Pathol 1984;8:101–108.
69. Meis JM, Enzinger FM: Inflammatory fibrosarcoma of the mesentery and retroperitoneum. A tumor closely simulating inflammatory pseudotumor. Am J Surg Pathol 1991;15:1146–1156.
70. Meis-Kindblom JM, Kjellström C, Kindblom LG: Inflammatory fibrosarcoma: Update, reappraisal, and perspective on its place in the spectrum of inflammatory myofibroblastic tumors. Semin Diagn Pathol 1998;15:133–143.
71. Pettinato G, Manivel JC, De Rosa N, Dehner LP: Inflammatory myofibroblastic tumor (plasma cell granuloma): Clinicopathologic study of 20 cases with immunohistochemical and ultrastructural observations. Am J Clin Pathol 1990;94:538–546.
72. Albores-Saavedra J, Manivel JC, Essenfeld H, et al: Pseudosarcomatous myofibroblastic proliferations in the urinary bladder of children. Cancer 1990;66:1234–1241.
73. Ro JY, el-Naggar AK, Amin MB, Sahin AA, Ordonez NG, Ayala AG: Pseudosarcomatous fibromyxoid tumor of the urinary bladder and prostate: Immunohistochemical, ultrastructural and DNA flow cytometric analyses of nine cases. Hum Pathol 1993;24:1203–1210.
74. Hojo H, Newton WA Jr, Hamoudi AB, et al: Pseudosarcomatous myofibroblastic tumor of the urinary bladder in children: A study of 11 cases with review of the literature. An intergroup rhabdomyosarcoma study. Am J Surg Pathol 1995;19:1224–1236.
75. Perrone T, De Wolf-Peeters C, Frizzera G: Inflammatory pseudotumor of lymph nodes. A distinctive pattern of nodal reaction. Am J Surg Pathol 1988;12:351–361.

76. Ramachandra S, Hollowood K, Bisceglia M, Fletcher CDM: Inflammatory pseudotumor of soft tissues: A clinicopathological and immunohistochemical analysis of 18 cases. Histopathology 1995;27:313–323.
77. Wenig BM, Devaney K, Bisceglia M: Inflammatory myofibroblastic tumor of the larynx. A clinicopathologic study of eight cases simulating a malignant spindle cell neoplasm. Cancer 1995;76:2217–2229.
78. Hussong JW, Brown M, Perkins SL, Dehner LP, Coffin CM: Comparison of DNA ploidy, histologic and immunohistochemical findings with clinical outcome in inflammatory myofibroblastic tumors. Mod Pathol 1999;12:279–286.

Inflammatory Myofibroblastic Tumor—Genetics

79. Snyder CS, Dell-Aquila M, Haghighi P, Baergen RN, Suh YK, Yi ES: Clonal changes in inflammatory pseudotumor of the lung. Cancer 1995;76:1545–1549.
80. Su LD, Atayde-Perez A, Sheldon S, Fletcher JA, Weiss SW: Inflammatory myofibro-blastic tumor: Cytogenetic evidence supporting clonal origin. Mod Pathol 1998; 11:364–368.
81. Griffin CA, Hawkins AL, Dvorak C, Henkle C, Ellingham T, Perlman EJ: Recurrent involvement of 2p23 in inflammatory myofibroblastic tumors. Cancer Res 1999; 59:2776–2780.
82. Lawrence B, Perez-Atayde A, Hibbard MK, et al: TPM3-ALK and TPM4-ALK oncogenes in inflammatory myofibroblastic tumors. Am J Pathol 2000;157: 377–384.
83. Siebert R, Gesk S, Harder L, et al: Complex variant translocation t(1;2) with TPM3-ALK fusion due to cryptic ALK gene rearrangement in anaplastic large-cell lymphoma. Blood 1999;94:3614–3617.
84. Chan JKC, Cheuk W, Shimizu M: Anaplastic lymphoma kinase expression in inflammatory pseudotumors. Am J Surg Pathol 2001;25:761–768.

Infantile (Congenital) Fibrosarcoma—Pathology

85. Balsaver AM, Butler JJ, Martin RG: Congenital fibrosarcoma. Cancer 1967;20:1607–1616.
86. Chung EB, Enzinger FM: Infantile fibrosarcoma. Cancer 1976;38:729–739.
87. Soule EH, Pritchard DJ: Fibrosarcoma in infants and children: A review of 110 cases. Cancer 1977;40: 1711–1721.
88. Iwasaki H, Enjoji M: Infantile and adult fibrosarcomas of the soft tissues. Acta Pathol Jpn 1979;29: 377–388.
89. Coffin CM, Jaszcz W, O'Shea PA, Dehner LP: So-called congenital-infantile fibrosarcoma—Does it exist and what is it? Pediatr Pathol 1994;14:133–150.
90. Kodet R, Stejskal J, Pilat D, Kocourkova M, Smelhaus V, Eckschlager T: Congenital-infantile fibrosarcoma: A clinicopathological study of five patients entered on the Prague Children's Tumor Registry. Pathol Res Pract 1996;192:845–853.
91. Cofer BR, Vescio PJ, Wiener ES: Infantile fibrosarcoma: Complete excision is the appropriate treatment. Ann Surg Oncol 1996;3:159–161.
92. Kynaston JA, Malcolm AJ, Craft AW, et al: Chemotherapy in the management of infantile fibrosarcoma. Med Pediatr Oncol 1993:21:488–493.
93. Salloum E, Caillaud JM, Flamant F, Landman J, Lemerle J: Poor prognosis infantile fibrosarcoma with pathologic features of malignant fibrous histiocytoma after local recurrence. Med Pediatr Oncol 1990;18: 295–298.

Infantile Fibrosarcoma—Genetics

94. Adam LR, Davison EV, Malcolm AJ, Pearson AD, Craft AW: Cytogenetic analysis of a congenital fibrosarcoma. Cancer Genet Cytogenet 1991;52:37–41.
95. Dal Cin P, Brock P, Casteels-Van Daele M, De Wever I, Van Damme B, Van den Berghe H: Cytogenetic characterization of congenital or infantile fibrosarcoma. Eur J Pediatr 1991;150:579–581.
96. Sankary S, Dickman PS, Wiener E, et al: Consistent numerical chromosome aberrations in congenital fibrosarcoma. Cancer Genet Cytogenet 1993;65: 152–156.
97. Bernstein R, Zeltzer PM, Lin F, Carpenter PM: Trisomy 11 and other nonrandom trisomies in congenital fibrosarcoma. Cancer Genet Cytogenet 1994;78:82–86.
98. Knezevich SR, Mcfadden DE, Tao W, Lim JF, Sorensen PH: A novel ETV6-NTRK3 gene fusion in congenital fibrosarcoma. Nat Genet 1998;18:184–187.
99. Knezevich SR, Garnett MJ, Pysher TJ, Beckwith JB, Grundy PE, Sorensen PH: ETV6-NTRK3 gene fusions and trisomy 11 establish a histogenetic link between mesoblastic nephroma and congenital fibrosarcoma. Cancer Res 1998;58:5046–5048.
100. Rubin BP, Chen CJ, Morgan TW, et al: Congenital mesoblastic nephroma t(12;15) is associated with ETV6-NTRK3 gene fusion: Cytogenetic and molecular relationship to congenital (infantile) fibrosarcoma. Am J Pathol 1998;153:1451–1458.
101. Argani P, Fritsch M, Kadkol SS, Schuster A, Beckwith JB, Perlman EJ: Detection of the ETV6-NTRK3 chimeric RNA of infantile fibrosarcoma/cellular congenital mesoblastic nephroma in paraffin-embedded tissue: Application to challenging pediatric renal stromal tumors. Mod Pathol 2000:13:29–36.
102. Bourgeois JM, Knezevich SR, Mathers JA, Sorensen PH: Molecular detection of the ETV6-NTRK3 gene fusion differentiates congenital fibrosarcoma from other childhood spindle cell tumors. Am J Surg Pathol 2000;24:937–946.
103. Dubus P, Coindre JM, Groppi A, et al: The detection of the Tel-TrkC chimeric transcripts is more specific than TrkC immunoreactivity for the diagnosis of congenital fibrosarcoma. J Pathol 2001;193:88–94.
104. Sheng WQ, Hisaoka M, Okamoto S, et al: Congenital-infantile fibrosarcoma. A clinicopathologic study of 10 cases and molecular detection of the ETV6-NTRK3 fusion transcripts using paraffin-embedded tissues. Am J Clin Pathol 2001;115:348–355.

Malignant and Potentially Malignant Fibroblastic and Myofibroblastic Tumors

CHAPTER 7

This group includes tumors that have a significant potential for recurrence and some metastatic potential, although metastatic potential varies and is low for many tumors discussed here.

Dermatofibrosarcoma protuberans (DFSP) and its pigmented variant (Bednar tumor) are clinicopathologically distinctive $CD34^+$ fibroblastic tumors. Although they typically behave indolently if completely excised, they are capable of transformation to a more aggressive form and may metastasize. Giant cell fibroblastoma is the juvenile variant of DFSP with a lower biologic potential.

Low-grade fibromyxoid sarcoma is a histologically distinctive tumor, which despite its bland histologic appearance, may metastasize. Like the typical DFSP, this tumor may also progress to a more aggressive form.

Infantile (congenital) fibrosarcoma is a clinically, pathologically, and genetically distinct tumor entity with a specific chromosomal translocation and gene fusion. This was discussed in Chapter 6.

Adult fibrosarcoma is a designation for a nonpleomorphic malignant fibroblastic tumor and is a diagnosis made by exclusion. It is a rarely diagnosed tumor, and tumors historically classified as fibrosarcomas included monophasic synovial sarcomas, low-grade fibromyxoid tumors, desmoids, solitary fibrous tumors, and even fasciitis and related lesions.

Recently, some tumors have been classified as myofibrosarcomas based on their prominent myofibroblastic differentiation. The term myxofibrosarcoma is synonymous with myxoid malignant fibrous histiocytoma (MFH).

Sclerosing epithelioid fibrosarcoma is the designation for a clinically heterogeneous group of tumors with histologically distinctive features.

Acral myxoinflammatory fibroblastic sarcoma (inflammatory myxohyaline tumor) is a newly described fibroblastic lesion of low malignant potential. Although this tumor commonly recurs, metastases are exceptional if they occur.

Malignant fibrous histiocytoma is now understood to be a fibroblastic and myofibroblastic tumor diagnosed by exclusion, except the angiomatoid variant, which is a separate entity with a very low malignant potential; it will be discussed separately (Chapter 20).

The pleomorphic-storiform, myxoid, and giant cell variants of MFH are discussed here, along with a group of low malignant potential or borderline giant cell tumors of soft tissue. In those giant cell-rich tumors, the fibroblastic spindle cell component probably is the only neoplastic component. Plexiform fibrohistiocytic tumor is a giant cell-rich childhood tumor (see Chapter 6).

Dermatofibrosarcoma Protuberans and Bednar Tumor

Dermatofibrosarcoma protuberans is a relatively common superficial low-grade sarcoma and Bednar tumor is its rare pigmented variant. Giant cell fibroblastoma is the juvenile variant of DFSP, as supported by their occasional coexistence and genetic similarity. These clinically and histologically distinctive tumors present in the dermis or subcutis. Their immunohistochemical positivity for CD34 and a specific t(17;22) translocation with *COL1A-PDGFB* (collagen type I–platelet-derived growth factor β) gene fusion are important diagnostic features and help to distinguish DFSP from benign fibrous histiocytoma (BFH) and from other sarcomas.

Clinical Features

The tumor occurs in a wide age range but is particularly common in young and middle-aged adults with a male predominance. It may also present in children, as well as in old age. Most commonly DSFP is located in the trunk, especially the chest or abdominal wall, and sometimes around the external genitalia.[1–4] DFSP occurs less commonly in the proximal parts of extremities and very rarely in distal extremities. Occurrence in the head and neck, especially the scalp, is not uncommon.

An early lesion may present as a plaquelike cutaneous induration clinically resembling localized scleroderma or as an apparently sharply demarcated cutaneous and subcutaneous nodule. Some tumors present as multiple nodules protruding to the skin surface, and an advanced tumor may form a fungating mass with surface ulceration. The lesions are slowly growing, and they often have been observed for a long time before the excision.

The tumor behaves as a low-grade sarcoma and typically recurs unless completely excised. However, the prognosis is excellent if the tumor is completely excised. This generally requires a wide excision with a clear margin of 1 to 2 cm, because the lesion often infiltrates beyond its grossly visible margins. Mohs microsurgery with incremental excision until normal tissue, as documented by repeated frozen sections, has been advocated to avoid unnecessarily wide excision. Typical DFSP rarely develops lymph node metastases, and distant metastases are very rare, unless fibrosarcomatous transformation has occurred.

Fibrosarcomatous transformation may occur over time or at first presentation. It more commonly occurs in older patients. This condition may increase the likelihood of metastasis.[5–11] Although some reports have shown a metastatic rate as high as 5% to 15%, a recent series found no risk of metastasis, provided that adequate wide excision was performed.[10]

Pathology of Typical DFSP

Grossly, DFSP may form a dense dermal fibrous plaquelike lesion or a solitary circumscribed-appearing cutaneous-subcutaneous nodule, multiple nodules, or a polypoid lesion, which is gray-white on sectioning. Pure subcutaneous location without a dermal component is possible.[11]

Histologically, the tumor typically diffusely infiltrates the subcutaneous fat and between the adnexal structures. Some tumors (approximately 10%) are histologically well circumscribed and may even appear encapsulated. The tumor may infiltrate the whole thickness of dermis, but often leaves a hypocellular zone just below the epidermis. Epidermal hyperplasia, usually seen in BFH, is not present. DFSP is typically composed of uniform, mildly atypical, oval fibroblasts often arranged in a storiform, cartwheel-like pattern (Fig. 7–1). However, sometimes the whorled pattern is very inconspicuous and the cells are more longitudinally oriented.

Superficial portions of the tumor and the plaquelike lesions are often less cellular and more collagenous and may have a deceptively benign appearance on biopsy. Significant myxoid matrix is seen in some cases, and some tumors are myxoid throughout.[12] Peculiar myointimal vascular proliferation occurs in some tumors; this component, although originally believed to indicate myoid differentiation of the tumor, is nonneoplastic.[13–15] This component has a low mitotic activity and is probably analogous to the myofibroblastic component in myofibroma.

Pathology of Fibrosarcomatous Transformation

Fibrosarcomatous transformation of DFSP (DFSP-FS) is the designation for DFSP that has attained a fascicular (no longer storiform), more highly cellular fibrosarcoma-like histologic pattern, often with a "herringbone pattern," with the fascicles crossing at 45-degree angles. It often has a higher mitotic activity than typical DFSP. The fibrosarcomatous component is sometimes sharply demarcated from the area of typical DFSP. The studies assessing the significance of DFSP-FS have used different cutoff values (10–30% of tumor area) versus 1 cm of minimum area.[5–10] Occasionally, a pleomorphic, MFH-like pattern develops in DFSP.[16] Both the DFSP-FS and the MFH-like

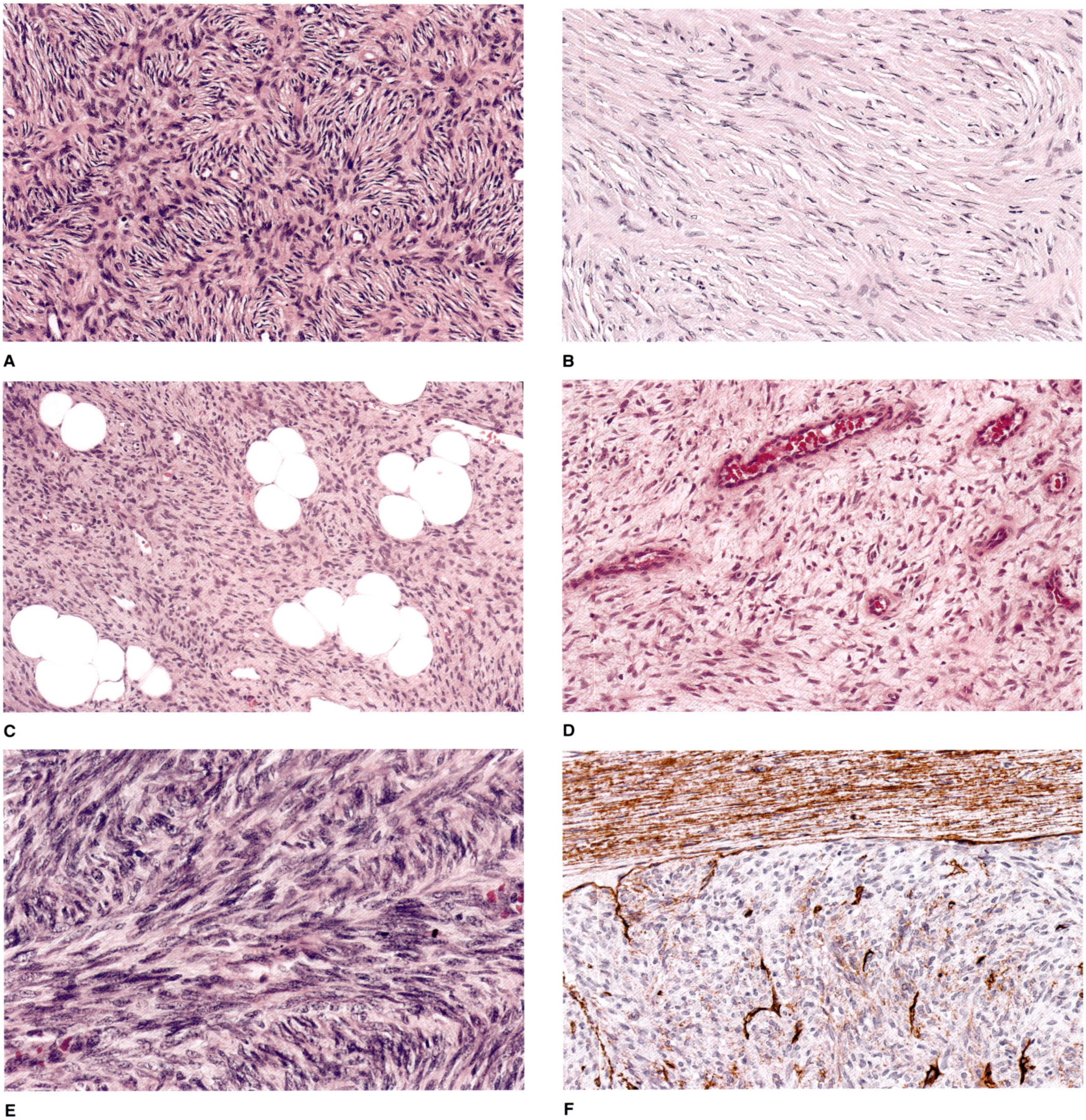

Figure 7–1. Histologic spectrum of dermatofibrosarcoma protuberans. *A,* A homogenous cartwheel pattern. *B,* Parallel arrangement of spindle cells in fibrous background. *C,* Subcutaneous fat infiltration. *D,* Myxoid variant with a prominent vascular pattern. *E,* Fibrosarcomatous transformation with a highly cellular fascicular pattern. *F,* The typical DFSP component is strongly positive for CD34, whereas the sharply demarcated fibrosarcomatous component is only weakly positive.

pleomorphic pattern may occur at the first presentation or in the recurrent tumor.

Specific Histologic Variant: Bednar Tumor

Pigmented DFSP (Bednar tumor) refers to the rare variant that contains scattered melanin-pigmented slender spindle cells with melanocytic differentiation, and was originally described as pigmented neurofibroma (Fig. 7–2*A*). This tumor does not clinically differ from the ordinary DFSP, and like ordinary DFSP, it may recur locally unless completely excised.[17–19] Fibrosarcomatous transformation is very rare.

Specific Histologic Variant: Giant Cell Fibroblastoma

Giant cell fibroblastoma (GCF) is the juvenile variant of DFSP; the typical DFSP may also occur in children. GCF usually occurs in the first decade, predominantly in the trunk or proximal lower extremity. Similar to typical DFSP, it has a male predominance. Its relationship with DFSP is supported by the common coexistence of these lesions and the similar *COL1A-PDGF* gene fusion. The tumor may recur, but fibrosarcomatous transformation has not been reported.[20–23]

The tumor forms a painless mass of usually less than 5 cm. Histologically distinctive is the presence of large, hyperchromatic mononucleated or multinucleated tumor cells often lining slitlike pseudovascular spaces in a collagenous background. The cellular density is only moderate and lower than in typical DFSP, and the collagen content is often higher giving the lesion a fibrosing appearance (Fig. 7–2*B*). Mitotic activity is scant. Areas typical of DFSP are present in some tumors, and coexistence with Bednar tumor has also been reported. Immunohistochemically, this tumor is similar to the typical DFSP and is positive for CD34.

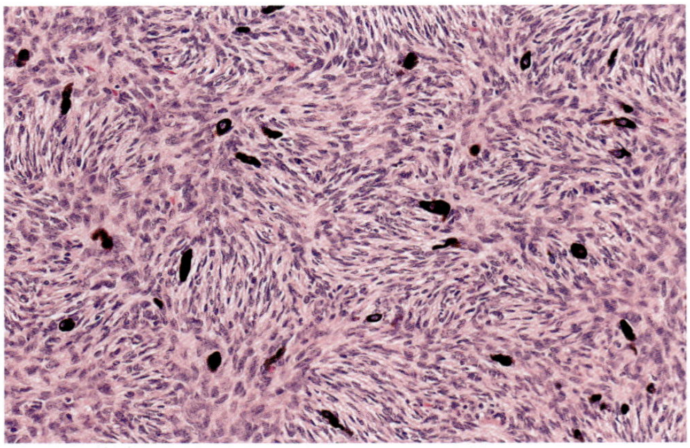

A

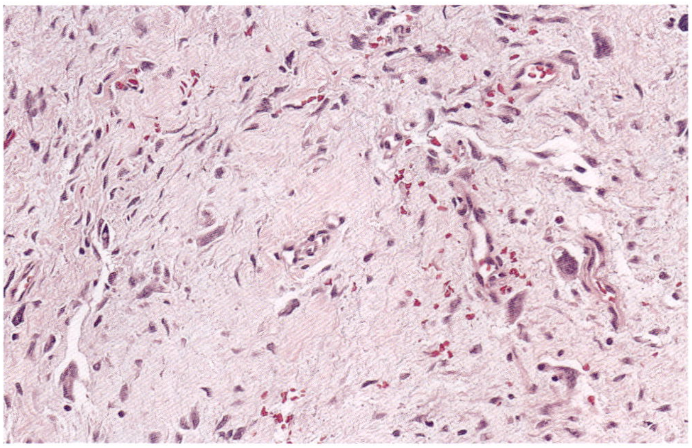

B

Figure 7–2. Rare variants of dermatofibrosarcoma protuberans (DFSP). *A,* The pigmented variant (Bednar tumor) contains scattered heavily melanin-laden cells but otherwise has a typical appearance of DFSP. *B,* Giant cell fibroblastoma has only moderate cellularity, and it contains nonvascular spaces lined by multinucleated tumor giant cells.

Immunohistochemistry of DFSP

The DFSP cells in typical and variant tumors are positive for vimentin and CD34.[24–27] The tumor cells are negative for S-100 protein, actins, desmin, keratins, and epithelial membrane antigen (EMA). Therefore, the tumor cell differentiation resembles that of $CD34^{+}$ dermal periadnexal fibroblasts that are the most significant candidate for its origin. Although earlier ultrastructural studies suggested nerve sheath differentiation, the markers do not support this. The fibrosarcomatous transformation differs from the ordinary DFSP by its less consistent positivity for CD34 (see Fig. 7–1*F*); this probably represents antigen loss on tumor progression.[27,28] Another marker typically seen in DFSP but not in BFH is low affinity nerve growth factor receptor, p75.[29] In contrast to BFH, DFSP does not have a tenascin-positive dermoepidermal zone.[30]

The pigmented cells in Bednar tumor have melanocytic differentiation and are positive for S-100 protein, tyrosinase and melan A.[31] One study suggested that p53 overexpression indentifies a more aggressive subset of DFSP.[32]

Differential Diagnosis

The lack of epidermal hyperplasia and a more homogeneous and less collagenous appearance separate DFSP from benign and cellular fibrous histiocytoma (BFH, dermatofibroma). The border is also different; its is typically diffusely infiltrative in DFSP as opposed to pushing border or septal infiltration in BFH. Also helpful is the fact DFSP is CD34$^+$; BFHs are negative or have only a focally positive spindle cell component. DFSP and diffuse neurofibroma share diffuse subcutis infiltration; the latter is distinctly positive for S-100 protein, often with Meissner-like tactile corpuscles.

True pigmented neurofibroma usually shows distinct foci of cells with melanocytic differentiation, and the tumor is positive for S-100 protein.

Genetics

Ring chromosomes containing low level amplifications of material from chromosomes 17 and 22 were shown as a typical cytogenetic change in DFSP.[33–35] The translocation t(17;22)(q22;q13) creating a fusion of the *COL1A* gene in chromosome 17q and *PDGFB* in chromosome 22q has been shown a consistent event in DFSP and GCF.[36] The fusion transcript has a transforming effect in vitro and is likely a key pathogenetic event.[37,38] Demonstration of the *COL1A-PDGFB* fusion transcript by reverse transcription-polymerase chain reaction or fluorescein in situ hybridization will probably become the ultimate diagnostic test for problem cases.[39]

Low-Grade Fibromyxoid Sarcoma

Clinical Features

This histologically distinctive low-grade sarcoma was initially described by Evans in 1987 and definitively in 1993 with a larger series.[40] The tumor occurs predominantly in young and middle-aged adults, aged 25 to 45, and sometimes in children. Male predominance has been shown in one series.[41] The tumor is usually located intramuscularly, and the most common sites of presentation are the thigh and buttocks, inguinal area, shoulder region, and chest wall. Tumors have been reported in the retroperitoneum and mesentery. The tumor has an extremely slow course. Local recurrences may occur during a long time span (up to 50 years). Lung metastases occurred in two early series in 7 of 12 and 1 of 11 cases, often after a long period of repeated local recurrences.[40,41] A larger, later series found a much lower frequency of pulmonary metastases. The tumor nevertheless shows an undeniable metastatic capability, which may be lower than initially reported but underestimated in a recent series with a relatively short follow-up.[42] We have seen cases in which pulmonary metastases have occurred before a detection of a large, occult apparently primary soft tissue tumor.

Pathology

Grossly, the tumor is firm and rubbery and it may have mucoid foci. Although it appears sharply circumscribed, it often infiltrates in skeletal muscle (Fig. 7–3). Histologically, the tumor typically shows alternating densely fibrous and myxoid areas. The vascularity is often well developed, and more cellular foci may be seen perivascularly. In many areas, the tumor shows a swirling or storiform appearance. The tumor cells show mild to moderate nuclear atypia, but mitotic activity is low (Fig. 7–4*A* and *B*). In some cases, the tumor may undergo transformation to a higher histologic grade with sheets of ovoid cells (Fig. 7–4*C*). Such a pattern can be seen in pulmonary metastases or sometimes in the primary tumor.

A histologic variant of low-grade fibromyxoid sarcoma was described as hyalinizing spindle cell tumor with giant rosettes.[42,43] The reported cases predominantly occurred in young adults (mean age, 38 years) intramuscularly in the proximal extremities showing similar clinicopathologic features as the main variant. This tumor contains peculiar giant rosettes formed by epithelioid fibroblasts with a core of dense, hyalinized collagen (Fig. 7–4*D*). Otherwise the histologic features are similar to those of low-grade fibromyxoid sarcoma.

Differential Diagnosis

Low-grade myxofibrosarcoma (low-grade myxoid MFH) differs from low-grade fibromyxoid sarcoma by a more developed vascular pattern, more myxoid matrix, presence of greater nuclear atypia, and

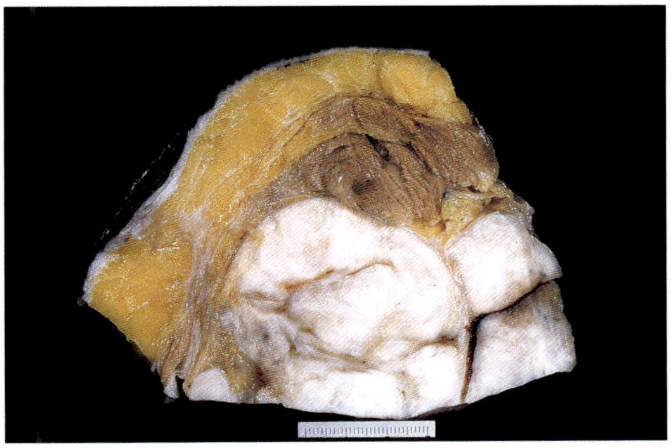

Figure 7–3. Low-grade fibromyxoid sarcoma forms of a deep intramuscular mass with vague lobulation.

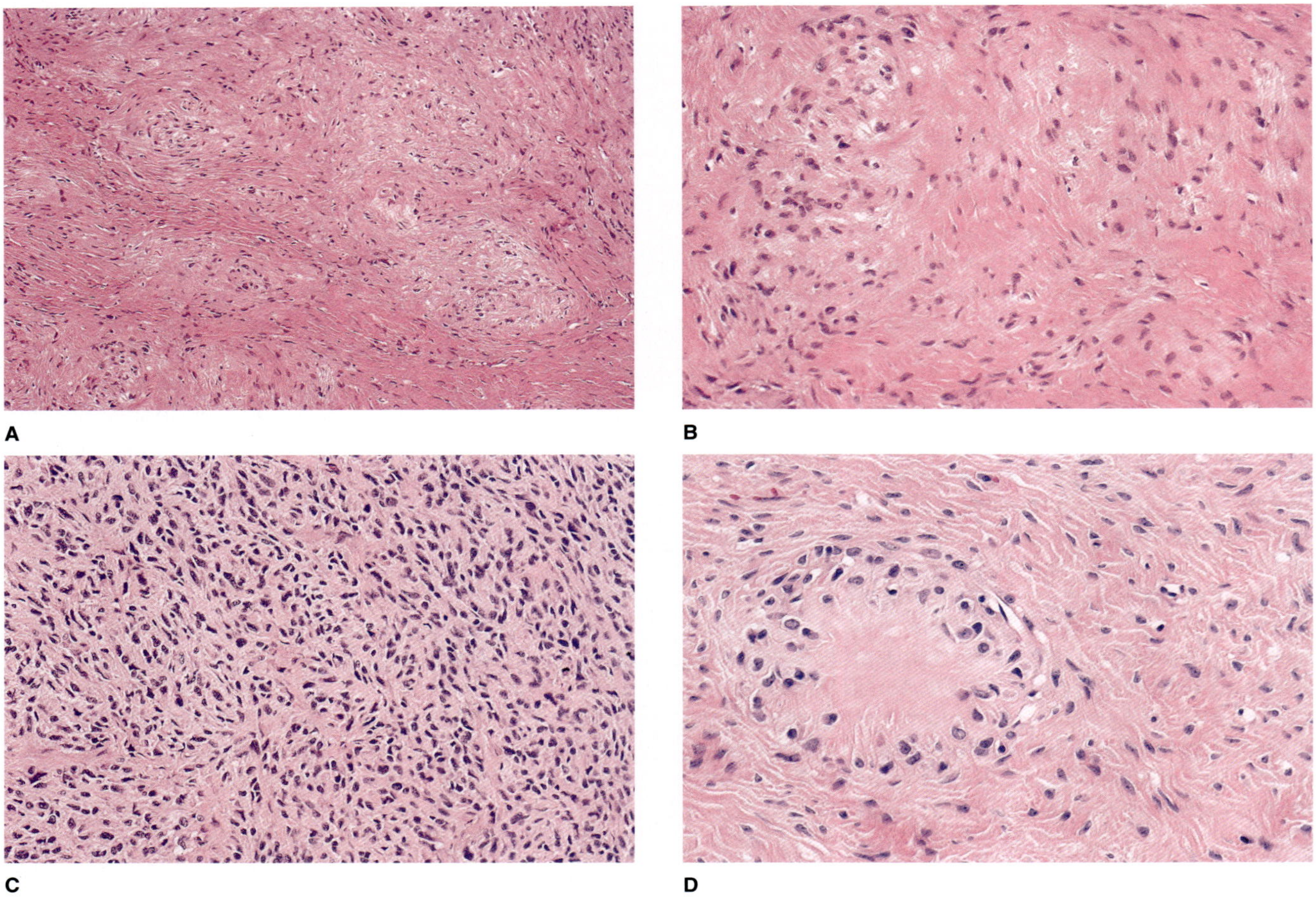

Figure 7-4. Histologic spectrum of low-grade fibromyxoid sarcoma and its variants. *A,* Low magnification reveals alternating cellular and myxoid areas. *B,* Higher magnification shows focal cellular atypia. *C,* A more cellular example that metastasized to the lungs. *D,* A variant with giant hyaline rosettes shows a collagen core in the rosette, which is surrounded by epithelioid fibroblasts.

tendency for perivascular hypercellular zones. This distinction is important, because low-grade fibromyxoid sarcoma may have a greater metastatic potential. Desmoid is less cellular and shows spindled cells with less atypia.

Immunohistochemistry

Low-grade fibromyxoid sarcoma is vimentin-positive and shows no specific differentiation markers. In some cases, the tumor cells have been focally positive for smooth muscle actin, but they are negative for desmin, S-100 protein, CD34, EMA, and keratins.

Genetics

Comparative genomic hybridization showed losses in 13q as the most common recurrent change, observed in 4 of 12 cases (Kiuru-Kuhlefelt et al., unpublished observations).

Adult Fibrosarcoma

Adult fibrosarcoma is a collagen-forming nonpleomorphic spindle cell sarcoma that cannot be classified into any other category (i.e., malignant peripheral nerve sheath tumor, synovial sarcoma, solitary fibrous tumor, low-grade fibromyxoid sarcoma, cellular desmoid, dermatofibrosarcoma protuberans with fibrosarcomatous transformation). It is rare and is diagnosed by exclusion. Most such tumors occur in deep soft tissues of the extremities or trunk.[44] The fibrosarcomas most commonly occur in middle age, but presentation in any age after the first decade is possible. A recent study showed that some superficial fibrosarcomas represent DFSP-based fibrosarcomas, based on demonstration of the typical fusion transcript.[45]

Because of the changed diagnostic practice, the old series of fibrosarcomas are difficult to compare in modern terms. The older series undoubtedly

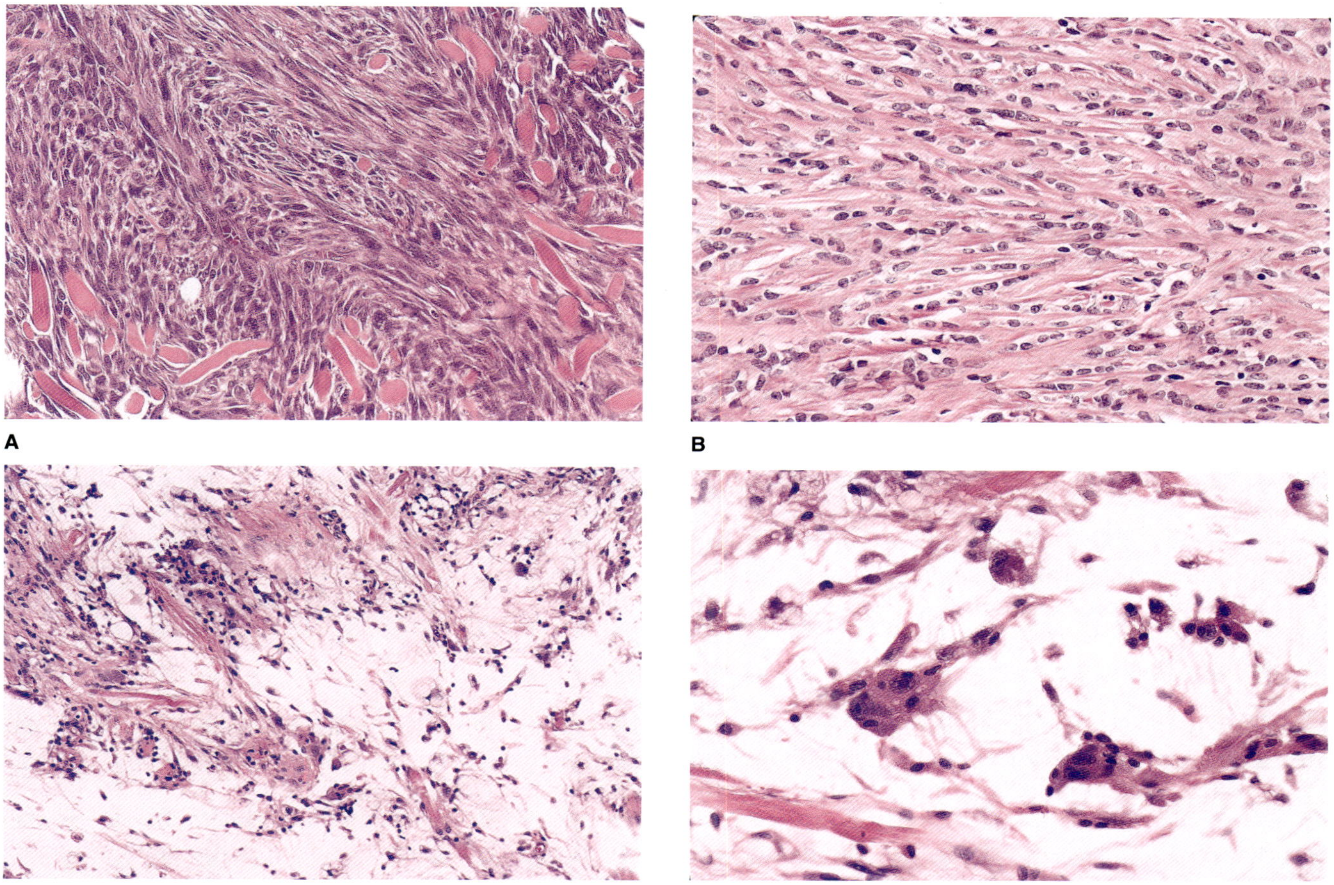

A B C D

Figure 7–5. Adult fibrosarcomas and related tumors. *A,* Adult fibrosarcoma with myofibroblastic features and keloid-like collagen. *B,* Sclerosing epithelioid fibrosarcoma has a trabecular pattern of cells in densely collagenous background. *C,* Low-power magnification of acral fibrosarcoma. *D,* High magnification reveals several Reed-Sternberg-like cells with large nuclei and prominent nucleoli.

include tumors now classified as the previously mentioned tumor entities.

Adult fibrosarcoma is now rarely diagnosed, because most fibroblastic tumors have at least some pleomorphic features, and consequently are preferentially classified as MFHs. However, some authors designate myxoid MFH, especially the low-grade variants, as myxofibrosarcomas. These tumors will be discussed with MFHs.

Myofibrosarcoma is a designation given to fibrosarcoma with myofibroblastic differentiation, usually detected by electron microscopy (Fig. 7–5*A*). Tumors reported under this name have mostly been low-grade sarcomas in adult patients presenting in a wide variety of locations.[46,47]

Inflammatory fibrosarcoma[48] belongs to the category of inflammatory myofibroblastic tumor and is discussed among fibroblastic tumors of children (see Chapter 6). Sclerosing epithelioid fibrosarcoma, a recently described fibrosarcoma variant, is discussed in the following section.

Sclerosing Epithelioid Fibrosarcoma

This histologic variant of fibrosarcoma was reported by Meis-Kindblom et al.[49] and subsequently by others.[50,51] Further studies are needed to determine whether this a homogeneous biologic entity, and how it is related to other fibrosarcomas.

Clinical Features

Based on the three published series, the tumor occurs in a wide age range (14–87 years), with a mean age between 40 and 45 years and no sex predilection. The tumors have been located in a wide variety of sites, mostly in deep soft tissues of the proximal parts of the extremities, trunk, and head and neck region. Nearly half the tumors have been 10 cm or larger.

The tumors have behaved as fully malignant sarcomas causing death in over half the patients. The most common metastatic sites are the lungs and bones. In some patients, the metastases have developed in less than 2 years, whereas in others they have developed 10 or more years after resection of the primary lesion.

Pathology

Grossly, sclerosing epithelioid fibrosarcoma forms a large oval or discoid mass measuring 2 to 15 cm. It has a fleshy to hard consistency on sectioning, often with necrosis.

A microscopically distinctive feature is the presence of oval to epithelioid cells with a clear cytoplasm, in a dense collagenous matrix (Fig. 7–5*B*). Mitotic activity can vary from 0 to 15 mitoses per 10 high-power field (HPF). The tumor may have areas of conventional fascicular fibrosarcoma, and one series[51] reported the coexistence with low-grade fibromyxoid sarcoma-like elements, suggesting the possibility that some examples of this entity may represent high-grade transformation from low-grade fibromyxoid sarcoma.

Immunohistochemically, the tumor cells do not generally display specific differentiation, and they are usually negative for muscle actins, desmin, CD34, S-100 protein, and keratins.[51] Weak positivity for EMA occurs in some cases, and the initial series reported two tumors positive for keratins with AE1/AE3 and CAM5.2 antibodies.[49]

Differential Diagnosis

Sclerosing carcinoma and synovial sarcoma have to be ruled out. Solitary fibrous tumor may have a somewhat similar histologic pattern, but this tumor is $CD34^+$.

Genetics

Amplification of 12q13 and 12q15 sequences has been reported in one case.[52]

Acral Myxoinflammatory Fibroblastic Sarcoma (Inflammatory Myxohyaline Tumor)

Clinical Features

Two series of this tumor of low malignant potential were recently described under different names.[53,54] The reports collectively detailed similar clinical and histologic distinctive features of 95 examples. This tumor was formerly variably classified as exuberant reactive processes or low-grade myxoid MFH.

The tumor occurs at all ages with the median age varying from 44 to 53 years with an equal sex distribution. The tumors had a strong predilection for distal extremities: fingers and hands, 56%; toes and feet, 17%; ankles/lower legs, 14%; and wrists/forearms, 11%. Some patients had a long history of mass, and the median duration of symptoms was 1 year in one series.[53]

Although the follow-up was not long in all cases, recurrences, sometimes multiple, were documented. One of the series documented pulmonary metastasis in one patient and lymph node metastasis in another;[53] the other series had only local recurrences.[54]

Based on definitive potential for recurrence and possible metastatic potential, we believe that this tumor can be classified as low-grade malignant. The tumor should probably be treated with a complete excision, which at times can lead to amputation of a finger.

Pathology

The tumor typically measures 1 to 8 cm with the median size in the two series 3 to 3.4 cm. Grossly, the tumor is white and multinodular, often poorly circumscribed, and sometimes gelatinous. It primarily involves the subcutis, and sometimes also dermis, skeletal muscle or tendons, and aponeuroses.

Histologically, the tumor is distinctive for a multinodular pattern. There is variably prominent mixed inflammatory infiltrate composed of lymphocytes, plasma cells, neutrophils, and eosinophils in a variably myxoid and collagenous background (Fig. 7–5*C*). The neoplastic cells vary from spindled to rounded. A distinctive feature is the presence of scattered large atypical ganglion-like cells with prominent, eosinophilic nucleoli that may resemble Hodgkin cells or viral inclusion cells, although they typically have more cytoplasm than Hodgkin cells (Fig. 7–5*D*). Multivacuolated polygonal fibroblasts with intracellular mucins may resemble lipoblasts. Studies for CD30 and cytomegalovirus and Epstein-Barr virus have been negative. The pathogenesis of this tumor most likely includes cytokine-stimulated lymphohistiocytic infiltration in a fibroblastic neoplasm.

Differential Diagnosis

This tumor can be confused with proliferative synovitis because of prominent inflammatory infiltration, and potentially with epithelioid sarcoma because of occurrence in the distal extremities; occasionally reported keratin-positive cells could also lead to such a confusion.

Malignant Fibrous Histiocytoma

Pleomorphic sarcomas not belonging to previously recognized types were increasingly recognized in the 1970s and named fibroxanthosarcoma and malignant fibrous histiocytoma. This designation currently refers to a group of essentially fibroblastic sarcomas that may also have myofibroblastic features. The name could be substituted with the designation of pleomorphic fibrosarcoma. Although the concept of histiocytic origin has proven incorrect, these tumors have a significant reactive histiocytic component, which originally led to the ultrastructural interpretation of histiocytic features.[55-60]

The diagnosis is made by exclusion and requires that other pleomorphic sarcomas, carcinomas, melanoma, and lymphomas are ruled out. According to our experience, MFH remains the single most common sarcoma in adults, even after careful exclusion of other specific diagnoses. MFH is the most common type of postirradiation sarcoma.

The pleomorphic-storiform variant is the most common. The myxoid variant has been synonymously called myxofibrosarcoma. Giant cell and inflammatory MFH are rare. Angiomatoid malignant fibrous histiocytoma (now preferably angiomatoid fibrous histiocytoma) is an unrelated tumor predominantly occurring in children and will be discussed separately in the section of tumors of unknown histogenesis (Chapter 20).

Clinical Features of Pleomorphic and Myxoid MFH

A population-based study from Sweden determined the annual incidence of MFH as 0.42/100,000.[61] The tumor typically occurs in older adults in the deep soft tissues of the proximal parts of the extremities, such as muscles of the thigh and arm. A minority of tumors occurs in the trunk wall and in the retroperitoneum. The median age of patients in large series has been between 60 and 70 years, and occurrence before the age of 40 is rare. Male predominance has been noted in some series. Pleomorphic storiform variants are usually high-grade tumors, with development of pulmonary metastases in up to 50% of cases. Several clinicopathologic series have demonstrated that tumors under 5 cm have a better prognosis, especially if not high grade.[55-66]

The myxoid subtype usually presents in the extremities, often in a subcutaneous location.[67-70] Its prognosis is better than that of the pleomorphic type. In particular, grade 1 tumors with no pleomorphism were found to never metastasize based on the largest published study.[69] Survival is also grade dependent, the 5-year survival varying from over 90% in grade 1 tumors to 60% in grade 4 tumors.[69]

Pathology

The pleomorphic-storiform MFH is often a large tumor commonly measuring 10 to 15 cm in diameter, and it often involves both the muscles and the subcutis and may ulcerate overlying skin. A majority of tumors appear grossly well circumscribed, although histologically they typically infiltrate in the periphery (Fig. 7–6). On sectioning, MFH is often multilobulated and relatively soft; larger tumors tend to have central necrosis. The color varies from gray-white to tan on sectioning.

Histologically, the storiform-pleomorphic variant of MFH is composed of a mixture of spindled, pleomorphic, and occasionally polygonal epithelioid cells. Multinucleated tumor giant cells may be present. A collagenous background is variably present. Mitotic

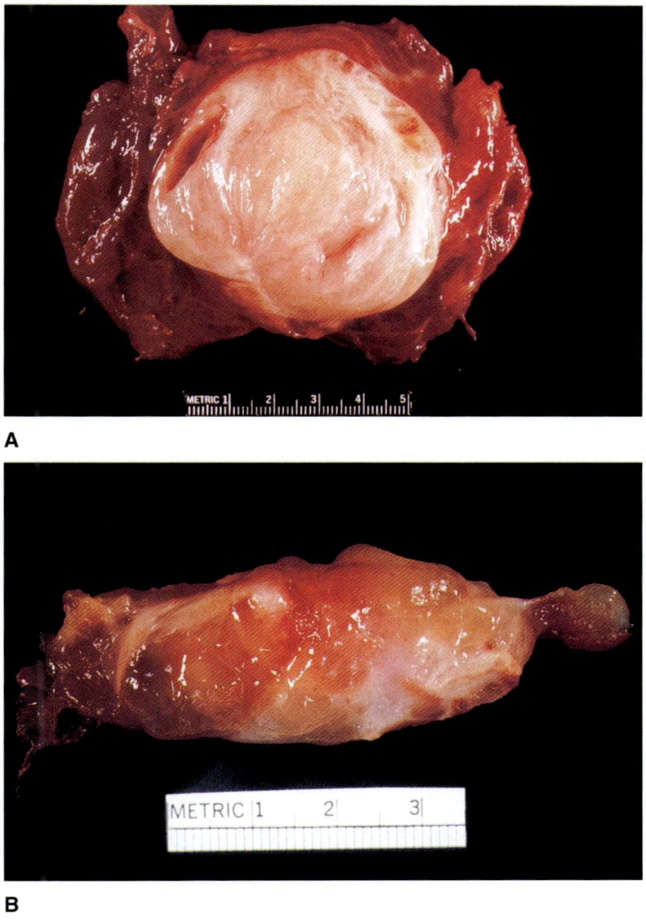

Figure 7–6. Gross appearances of typical variants of malignant fibrous histiocytoma. *A,* An intramuscular pleomorphic storiform variant. *B,* A subcutaneous myxoid variant. (Courtesy of Dr. John Fetsch, Washington, DC.)

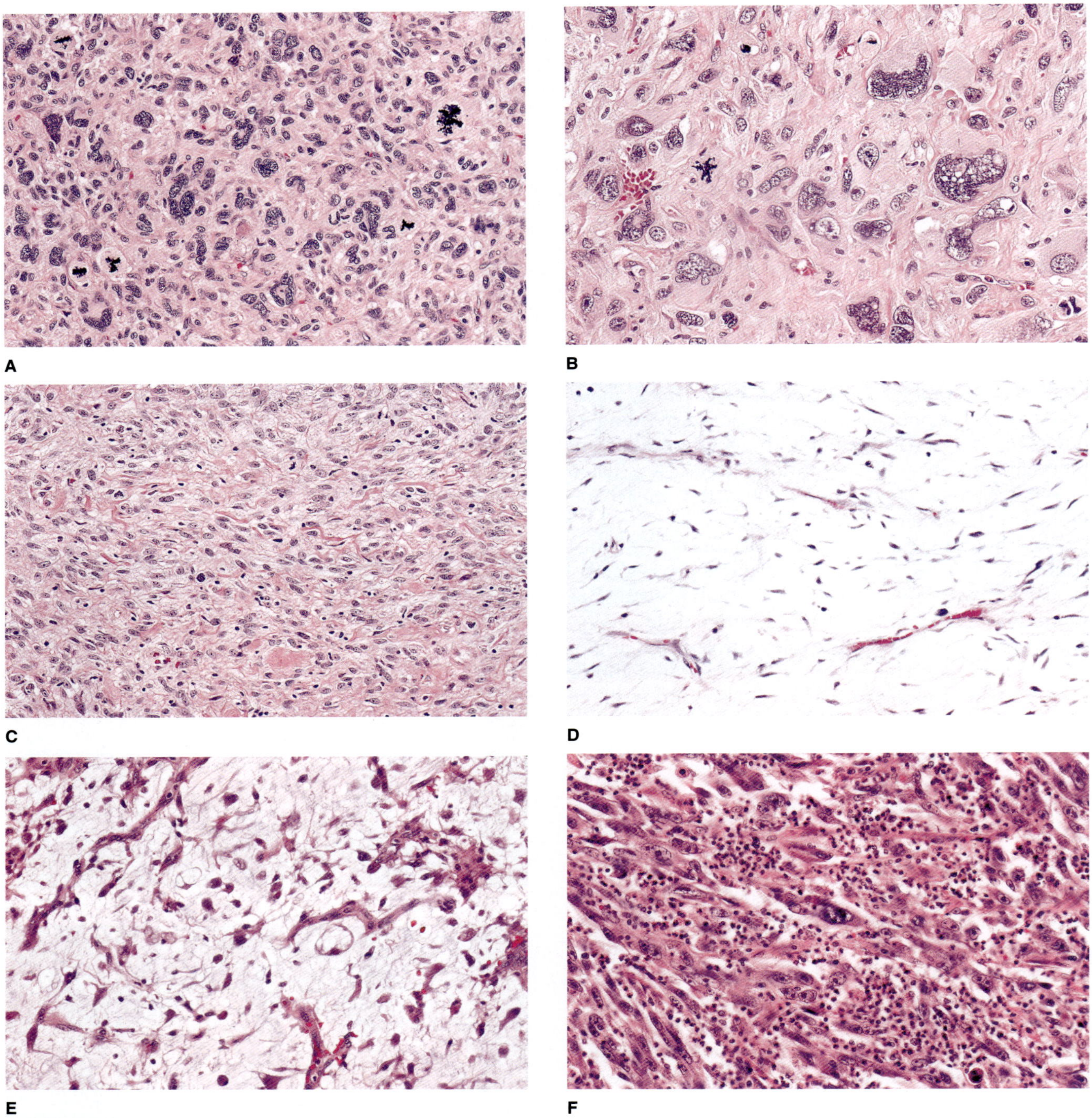

Figure 7–7. Histologic spectrum of malignant fibrous histiocytoma. *A* and *B*, Storiform pleomorphic variant with marked nuclear pleomorphism and atypical mitoses. *C*, A more collagenous variant. *D*, A low-grade myxoid variant (myxofibrosarcoma). Note a coarse vascular pattern and atypical cells around the vessels. *E*, A more cellular example of myxoid MFH. Several vacuolated "pseudolipoblasts" are present. *F*, Inflammatory MFH with scattered atypical spindle cells in an inflammatory background.

activity is usually easily identified, and atypical mitoses are common (Fig. 7–7*A* to *C*). The tumor may be storiform, but this pattern is not present in all tumors, and it is not required for diagnosis.

The myxoid variant (myxofibrosarcoma) has been generally defined as a MFH with a myxoid component rich in acid mucopolysaccharides in at least 50% of the tumor area, but tumors with 10% myxoid stroma were classified as such in one series.[70] Tumors of the myxoid subtype often appear mucoid (see Fig. 7–6).

Histologically, the myxoid type[67–70] is often low grade, but it may be intermediate or rarely high grade based on the presence of degree of cellularity, mitosis, and necrosis. Low-grade variants are only mildly hypercellular, but have a prominent plexiform vascular pattern. The presence of thin collagen fibers and more coarse and thick-walled capillaries with perivascular fibrosis separate this variant from myxoid liposarcoma. Cellular pleomorphism occurs in all except grade 1 tumors. More highly cellular intermediate-grade tumors have higher cellularity around the prominent thick-walled capillaries and higher numbers of large atypical cells. Some tumors have a trabecular pattern mimicking chordoma, and the tumor cells often contain vacuoles filled with acid mucopolysaccharides. Such cells are sometimes called pseudolipoblasts (Fig. 7–7*D* and *E*).

The rare inflammatory variant (Fig. 7–7*F*) contains large atypical cells typical of MFH in a background rich in xanthoma cells and often neutrophils. Clinicopathologically, these tumors were found to be highly aggressive with all seven patients dead of disease, although 4 survived longer than 5 years.[71]

Biology and Immunohistochemistry

The diagnosis of MFH is one of exclusion, and currently no specific markers are available to document this diagnosis. The MFH-like transformation described from many types of sarcomas (liposarcoma, chondrosarcoma, chordoma) suggests that MFH itself may represent a heterogeneous group of sarcomas that have developed by transformation from differentiated tumors, as hypothesized by Brooks.[72]

Several studies have agreed that the tumor cells are not of histiomonocytic origin, but more related to fibroblasts. They are negative for true histiocytic markers, such as lysozyme and histiocyte-specific leukocyte antigens, such as CD45 and CD14,[73,74] but instead have enzyme histochemical profile closer to that of fibroblasts.[74] However, MFH cells are commonly positive for the serin protease inhibitors α_1-antitrypsin and α_1-antichymotrypsin. Although these findings were previously considered diagnostically helpful and indicating a histiocytic differentiation, more recent studies have shown widespread distribution of these antigens (in melanomas, carcinomas, lymphomas), therefore limiting their diagnostic value and their support for histiocytic differentiation.[75–78] Similarly CD68 antibodies (KP1) may label MFH cells, but this marker, reacting with a lysosomal constituent, also lacks histiocytic specificity.

The cytokine production of MFH cells has been demonstrated in some cases and could explain the high content of intratumoral histiocytes, the morphologic pattern of the inflammatory MFH, and the constitutional symptoms observed in some patients. Indeed, leukemoid reaction detected in some patients has been attributed to cytokines, such as interleukin 6, secreted by MFH cells,[79–80] and production of multiple hematopoietic growth factors-cytokines, such as granulocyte-monocyte colony-stimulating factor (GM-CSF) and monocyte colony-stimulating factor (M-CSF), has been verified in MFH cell cultures.[81]

No specific diagnostic markers for MFH are available. A monoclonal antibody study concluded that MFH shared phenotypic features with perivascular fibroblast-like mesenchymal cells.[82] In various relatively small series, and in our experience, MFHs have shown heterogeneous features. All tumors have been consistently positive for vimentin, like most other sarcomas. The tumor cells may be positive for muscle actins and α-smooth muscle actin, but they are generally negative for desmin and S-100 protein; the latter is present in the interdigitating reticulum cells and Langerhans cells infiltrating in the tumor. Keratin positivity (usually focal) may occur, and it is probably comparable to the phenotype of transformed fibroblasts.[82–84]

Electron Microscopy

More recent studies emphasize fibroblastic and myofibroblastic features in the tumor cells. These typically have prominent rough endoplasmic reticulum, often with dilated profiles, and may have scattered bundles of actin filaments.[85,86] Cells with truly histiocytic differentiation are believed to be tumor infiltrating histiocytes.

Genetics

Complex cytogenetic changes are typical.[87–89] Some recurrent changes and possible candidate genes have been identified in the classical cytogenetic and comparative genomic hybridization (CGH) studies. However, various studies highlight different genetic changes, and the CGH results are not very comparable, perhaps because of heterogeneity of the tumor material.

Cytogenetic observations have shown that 19p13 aberration with addition of new material from unknown source correlates with an unfavorable outcome.[90] In one series, comparative genomic hybridization identified gains in 7q32 as a possible prognostically adverse sign,[91] and another series found, among others, amplifications of 12q12-15, similar to those seen in many liposarcomas.[92] Yet another study identified common loss of chromosome 13 as the most common chromosomalimbalance.[93] A gene, named as *MASL1* (MFH-amplified sequences with leucine-rich tandem repeats) was identified in the amplification region of 8p23.[94] A multimethod study using classic cytogenetics, CGH, and Southern blot analysis found losses in 9p, including p16 (INK4).[95] Losses in 13q14-q21 were found in nearly 80% of tumors in another study, and *RB1* gene was included in the area with losses.[96] Amplification of the *MDM2* gene[97,98] and mutations in the β-catenin gene[99] have also been reported.

Differential Diagnosis

Malignant fibrous histiocytoma is a diagnosis of exclusion, and the possibility of other sarcomas, sarcomatoid carcinoma, melanoma, and lymphoma needs to be ruled out. If a pleomorphic sarcoma of the extremities or trunk has no evidence for differentiation, except for fibroblastic and myofibroblastic, MFH is the likely diagnosis. The specific sarcomas that have to be ruled out are pleomorphic liposarcoma (if lipoblasts are present), leiomyosarcoma (evidence for smooth muscle differentiation, not merely smooth muscle actin positivity), and pleomorphic rhabdomyosarcoma. The latter is extremely rare and can be verified by immunohistochemical positivity for desmin and skeletal muscle-specific transcriptional regulators, such as MyoD1 and myogenin. In the gastrointestinal tract, the KIT^+ gastrointestinal stromal tumors can be pleomorphic and sometimes simulate MFH.

It has been suggested that most MFHs can be reclassified as other tumors, especially as specific sarcomas, if studied carefully.[100] Although thorough sampling may reveal specific mesenchymal differentiation in some cases, extensive reclassification of MFHs, for example as smooth muscle tumors, has to rely on relaxed criteria for smooth muscle differentiation, which will "contaminate" the data on differentiated smooth muscle tumors.

Although MFH has been reported at almost any site, this diagnosis should be made with caution in parenchymal organs (e.g., in the kidney), where sarcomatoid carcinomas can have a pleomorphic, MFH-like appearance. Extensive sampling is recommended in these situations.

Malignant melanoma (either primary or metastatic) needs to be ruled out, because these tumors can be quite pleomorphic. Metastatic subcutaneous and mucosal melanomas or those at other unusual sites are more likely to be confused with MFH.

Lymphomas that may simulate MFH include rare variants of large cell anaplastic lymphoma[101] and sarcomatoid variants of Hodgkin disease. The diagnosis of the latter is facilitated by immunohistochemistry for leukocyte antigens CD15 and CD30, which are absent in the potentially lymphoma-like inflammatory variant of MFH.[102]

Atypical Fibroxanthoma

Clinical Features

This designation refers to a superficial analog to MFH. The lesion typically occurs in the sun-exposed skin of elderly individuals, especially in the head and neck area, particularly the face and scalp. It may form an elevated cutaneous nodule or ulcerated plaque. Despite high-grade malignant histologic appearance, the behavior is indolent if the tumor is adequately excised.[103,104] Occasional lymph node metastases have been reported, but if this tumor is defined appropriately (and narrowly), the rate of metastasis is extremely low.

Pathology

By definition, atypical fibroxanthoma is limited to skin or shows minimal subcutaneous involvement, typically with a pushing margin. The lesional size is usually less than 1 cm, and almost never exceeds 2 cm. Lesions that show significant (more than minimal) subcutaneous involvement are more appropriately diagnosed as MFH. The diagnosis can be usually made only based on excision specimen where the extent of the lesion is clearly visible.

The histologic spectrum varies from conspicuous cellular pleomorphism similar to MFH, and atypical mitoses are common. Variants composed of nonpleomorphic spindle cells[105] and containing osteoclast-like giant cells have been described.[106]

Differential Diagnosis

Similar to MFH, the diagnosis of atypical fibroxanthoma is made by exclusion. Important differential diagnoses that almost always require immunohistochemical evaluation are melanoma (positive for S-100 protein and variably for other melanoma markers) and pleomorphic carcinoma, which often shows more clearly epithelial component and epithelial markers (keratins and EMA). Large cell anaplastic lymphoma may have pleomorphism, but usually shows a more uniform cellular population that is always $CD30^+$ and usually $CD45^+$. Pleomorphic leiomyosarcomas are distinguished by presence of more typical areas and expression of muscle actin, desmin, or both.[107–109]

Giant Cell Tumor of Soft Parts and Giant Cell MFH

The giant cell tumors of soft tissue and giant cell type of MFH are a spectrum of giant cell-rich tumors of probably fibroblastic or myofibroblastic origin. The benign and low malignant potential tumors are now generally classified as giant cell tumors of soft parts, whereas the designation of giant cell MFH is reserved for high-grade sarcomas.

Plexiform fibrohistiocytic tumor is an architecturally distinctive giant cell-rich soft tissue tumor, which is separate from the preceding tumors. It is a childhood tumor and is discussed in Chapter 6.

The tenosynovial giant cell tumor (giant cell tumor of tendon sheath) is a clinically and pathologically distinctive tumor that should be separated from this group. Tenosynovial giant cell tumors are almost always benign (Chapter 21).

Giant Cell Tumors of Soft Parts

Salm and Sissons described tumors that were histologically analogous to giant cell tumors of bone and lack an atypical mononuclear cell component.[110] Recently, three series reported similar tumors and emphasized that they should be separated from giant cell MFH because of their limited malignant potential. Opinions vary whether these tumors should be considered nearly benign or should be classified among tumors of uncertain malignant potential.[111-113]

Clinical Features

The tumor occurs in a wide age range, including children. The collective data from the four series suggest a mild male predominance. The majority of tumors occur in the proximal parts of the extremities, some in the trunk, and a few are reported from intra-abdominal sites. Arm, thigh, knee, and leg are among the most common locations, and examples have also been reported from the hands and feet. Approximately 60% of the tumors are subcutaneous or dermal, and 40% are deep to the superficial fascia. By definition, origin from bone has to be ruled out.

Provided that tumors with an atypical mononuclear cell population are excluded, the prognosis seems excellent, with some potential for local recurrence after an incomplete excision. However, none of the series have extensive long-term follow-up, and further studies are needed to confirm the potential of these lesions. This especially applies to large and deep tumors.

Pathology

The tumor typically presents as a circumscribed nodule or larger mass measuring 1 to 10 cm. The median sizes in the four published series have been 2 to 4 cm. Grossly, the cut surface appears reddish or gray and varies from fleshy to rubbery.

Histologically typical is a multinodular pattern with fibrous septa dividing the tumor into cellular lobules. Many tumors contain a peripheral rim of metaplastic bone. The cellular areas are conspicuously rich in osteoclast-like giant cells, which are evenly spaced throughout the cellular areas (Fig. 7–8*A*). There is a mononuclear component,

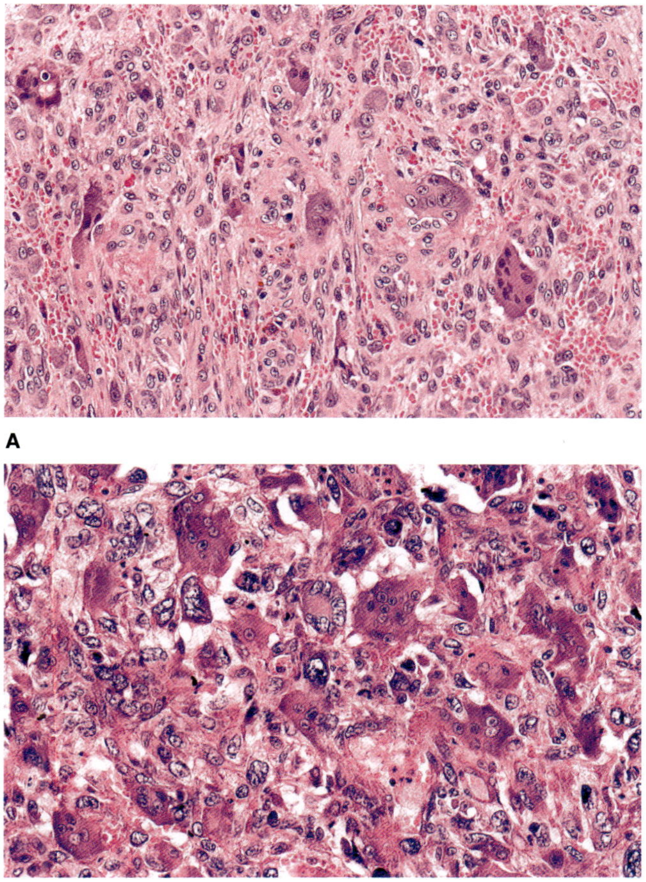

A

B

Figure 7–8. *A,* The cellular nodules of giant cell tumor of soft parts are composed numerous osteoclasts and a mononuclear population with oval of spindle cells with limited atypia. *B,* A giant cell MFH, in comparison, shows highly atypical mononuclear cells in the background of osteoclasts.

which may be composed or round, oval, or spindled cells. Atypia is limited in this component, and bizarre giant cells do not occur. The mitotic rate varies in a wide range, being on average 3/10 HPF, but counts as high as more than 30 mitoses/10 HPF have been included under this definition. Necrosis is uncommon.

The opinions vary whether these tumors should be classified as benign or potentially malignant; some segregate a malignant group that seems to be comparable with giant cell MFH.

Giant Cell MFH

This designation should be reserved for high-grade malignant tumors with osteoclast-like giant cells in a highly atypical pleomorphic or spindle cell component. The need to rule out specific differentiation also applies to this variant. Other sarcomas (leiomyosarcoma) and carcinomas (e.g., pancreatic) with osteoclastic giant cells should not be confused with this entity.

Clinicopathologic Features

The tumor typically occurs in older adults in deep soft tissues of extremities and often reaches a large size. Metastatic rate is high.[114,115]

Grossly, the tumor is typically divided into multiple lobules by collagenous septa. On sectioning the tumor is red-brown, and often contains areas with hemorrhage and necrosis. Histologically, the giant cell MFH is composed of multiple cellular nodules separated by paucicellular fibrous septa. The nodules contain markedly atypical mononuclear cells mixed with osteoclast-like cells (Fig. 7–8*B*). Mitotic activity may be considerable, and atypical mitoses are often present. Larger nodules often have necrosis.

Pleomorphic Hyalinizing Angiectactic Tumor

This designation refers to a histologically distinctive tumor that shows the combination of pleomorphic MFH-like cells with low if any mitotic activity and prominent vasculature with degenerative changes resembling the vascular changes seen in schwannoma (Fig. 7–9). Perivascular hyalinization is often prominent, and many tumors have foci of hemosiderin. The tumor differs from MFH by lack of mitotic activity. Nuclear pseudoinclusions are another histologically distinctive feature.[116,117]

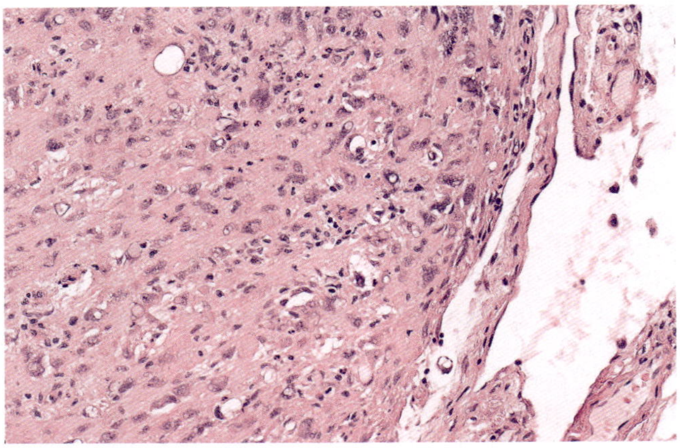

Figure 7–9. Pleomorphic hyaline angiectatic tumor shows large cells with pleomorphic nuclei but little mitotic activity. Dilated vascular channels are also present.

The series describing these tumors showed a wide age distribution with equal sex incidence. Most tumors were subcutaneous and measured 2 to 8 cm. Local recurrences were seen in half the patients with follow-up, but there were no metastases.

The tumor cells are characteristically positive for CD34, and in contrast to schwannoma, they are negative for S-100 protein.

REFERENCES

Dermatofibrosarcoma Protuberans—Clinicopathologic Studies

1. Taylor HB, Helwig EB: Dermatofibrosarcoma protuberans: A study of 115 cases. Cancer 1962;15:717–725.
2. McPeak CJ, Cruz T, Nicastri AD: Dermatofibrosarcoma protuberans: An analysis of 86 cases—Five with metastasis. Ann Surg 1968;166:803–816.
3. Pappo AS, Rao BN, Cain A, Bodner S, Pratt CB: Dermatofibrosarcoma protuberans: The pediatric experience at St. Jude Children's Research Hospital. Pediatr Hematol Oncol 1997;14:563–568.
4. Ghorbani RP, Malpica A, Ayala A: Dermatofibrosarcoma protuberans of the vulva: A clinicopathologic and immunohistochemical analysis of four cases, one with fibro-sarcomatous change, and review of the literature. Int J Gynecol Pathol 1999;18:366–373.
5. Wrotnowski U, Cooper PH, Shmookler BM: Fibrosarcomatous change in dermatofibrosarcoma protuberans. Am J Surg Pathol 1988;12:287–293.
6. Ding J, Hashimoto H, Enjoji M: Dermatofibrosarcoma protuberans with fibrosarcomatous areas. A clinicopathologic study of nine cases and comparison with allied tumors. Cancer 1989;64:721–729.
7. Connelly JH, Evans HL: Dermatofibrosarcoma protuberans. A clinicopathologic review with emphasis on

fibrosarcomatous areas. Am J Surg Pathol 1992;16: 921–925.
8. Eisen RN, Tallini G: Metastatic dermatofibrosarcoma protuberans with fibrosarcomatous change in the absence of local recurrence. A case report of simultaneous occurrence with a malignant giant cell tumor of soft parts. Cancer 1993;72:462–468.
9. Mentzel T, Beham A, Katenkamp D, Dei Tos AP, Fletcher CDM: Fibrosarcomatous ("high-grade") dermatofibrosarcoma protuberans: Clinicopathologic and immunohistochemical study of a series of 41 cases with emphasis on prognostic significance. Am J Surg Pathol 1998;22:576–587.
10. Goldblum JR, Reith JD, Weiss SW: Sarcomas arising in dermatofibrosarcoma protuberans. A reappraisal of biologic behavior in eighteen cases treated by wide local excision with extended clinical follow-up. Am J Surg Pathol 2000;24:1125–1130.
11. Diaz-Cascajo C, Weyers W, Rey-Lopez A, Borghi S: Deep dermatofibrosarcoma protuberans: A subcutaneous variant. Histopathology 1998;32:552–555.
12. Frierson HF, Cooper PH: Myxoid variant of dermatofibrosarcoma protuberans. Am J Surg Pathol 1983; 7:445–450.
13. Calonje E, Fletcher CDM: Myoid differentiation in dermatofibrosarcoma protuberans and its fibrosarcomatous variant: Clinicopathologic analysis of 5 cases. J Cutan Pathol 1996;23:30–36.
14. Morimitsu Y, Hisaoka M, Okamoto S, Hashimoto H, Ushijima M: Dermatofibro-sarcoma protuberans and its fibrosarcomatous variant with areas of myoid differentiation: A report of three cases. Histopathology 1998; 32:547–551.
15. Sanz-Trelles A, Ayala-Carbonero A, Rodrigo-Fernandez I, Weil-Lara B: Leiomyomatous nodules and bundles of vascular origin in the fibrosarcomatous variant of dermatofibrosarcoma protuberans. J Cutan Pathol 1998;25:44–49.
16. O'Dowd J, Laidler P: Progression of dermatofibrosarcoma protuberans to malignant fibrous histiocytoma: Report of a case with implications for tumor histogenesis. Hum Pathol 1988;19:368–370.

Dermatofibrosarcoma Protuberans Variants—Bednar Tumor and Giant Cell Fibroblastoma

17. Dupree WB, Langloss JM, Weiss SW: Pigmented dermatofibrosarcoma protuberans (Bednar tumor). A pathologic, ultrastructural, and immunohistochemical study. Am J Surg Pathol 1985;9:630–639.
18. Fletcher CD, Theaker JM, Flanagan A, Krausz T: Pigmented dermatofibrosarcoma protuberans (Bednar tumour): Melanocytic colonization or neuroectodermal differentiation? A clinicopathologic and immunohistochemical study. Histopathology 1988;13: 631–643.
19. Ding JA, Hashimoto H, Sugimoto T, Tsuneyoshi M, Enjoji M: Bednar tumor (pigmented dermatofibrosarcoma protuberans). An analysis of six cases. Acta Pathol Jpn 1990;40:744–754.
20. Abdul-Karim FV, Evans HL, Silva EG: Giant cell fibroblastoma. A report of three cases. Am J Clin Pathol 1985;83:165–170.
21. Dymock RB, Allen PW, Stirling JW, Gilbert EF, Thornbery JM: Giant cell fibroblastoma. A distinctive, recurrent tumor of childhood. Am J Surg Pathol 1987;11: 263–271.
22. Shmookler BM, Enzinger FM, Weiss SW: Giant cell fibroblastoma. A juvenile form of dermatofibrosarcoma protuberans. Cancer 1989;64:2154–2161.
23. De Chadarevian JP, Coppola D, Billmire DF: Bednar tumor pattern in recurring giant cell fibroblastoma. Am J Clin Pathol 1993;100:164–166.

Dermatofibrosarcoma Protuberans—Immunohistochemistry

24. Aiba S, Tabata N, Ishii H, Ootani H, Tagami H: Dermatofibrosarcoma protuberans is a unique fibrohistiocytic tumour expressing CD34. Br J Dermatol 1992; 127:79–84.
25. Altman DA, Nickoloff BJ, Fivenson DP: Differential expression of factor XIIIa and CD34 in cutaneous mesenchymal tumors. J Cutan Pathol 1993;20:154–158.
26. Kutzner H: Expression of the human progenitor cell antigen (CD34, HPCA1) distinguishes dermatofibrosarcoma protuberans from fibrous histiocytoma in formalin-fixed, paraffin embedded tissue. J Am Acad Dermatol 1993;28:613–617.
27. Sato N, Kimura K, Tomita Y: Recurrent dermatofibrosarcoma protuberans with myxoid and fibrosarcomatous changes paralleled by loss of CD34 expression. J Dermatol 1995;22:665–627.
28. Goldblum JR, Tuthill RJ: CD34 and Factor XIIIa immunoreactivity in dermato-fibrosarcoma protuberans and dermatofibroma. Am J Dermatopathol 1997; 19:147–153.
29. Fanburg-Smith JC, Miettinen M: Low-affinity nerve growth factor in dermatofibrosarcoma protuberans and schwannian and neural tumors. A study of 1130 tumors. Hum Pathol 2001;32:976–983.
30. Kahn HJ, Fekete E, From L: Tenascin differentiates dermatofibroma from dermatofibrosarcoma protuberans: Comparison with CD34 and factor XIIIa. Hum Pathol 2001;32:50–56.
31. Fetsch JF, Michal M, Miettinen M: Pigmented (melanotic) neurofibroma. A clinicopathologic and immunohistochemical analysis of 19 lesions from 17 patients. Am J Surg Pathol 2000;24:331–343.
32. Sasaki M, Ishida T, Horiuchi H, Machinami R: Dermatofibrosarcoma protuberans: An analysis of proliferative activity, DNA flow cytometry and p53 overexpression with emphasis on its progression. Pathol Int 1999;49:799–806.

Dermatofibrosarcoma Protuberans—Genetics

33. Naeem R, Lux ML, Huang SF, Naber SP, Corson JM, Fletcher JA: Ring chromosomes in dermatofibrosarcoma protuberans are composed of interspersed

sequences from chromosomes 17 and 22. Am J Pathol 1995;147:1553–1558.

34. Pedeutour F, Simon MP, Minoletti F, et al: Ring 22 chromosomes in dermatofibrosarcoma protuberans are low-level amplifiers of chromosome 17 and 22 sequences. Cancer Res 1995;55:2400–2403.
35. Mandahl N, Limon J, Mertens F, Arheden K, Mitelman F: Ring marker containing 17q and chromosome 22 in a case of dermatofibrosarcoma protuberans. Cancer Genet Cytogenet 1996;89:88–91.
36. Simon MP, Pedeutour F, Sirvent N, et al: Deregulation of the platelet derived growth factor B-chain via fusion with collagen gene COL1A1 in dermatofibrosarcoma protuberans and giant cell fibroblastoma. Nat Genet 1997;15:95–98.
37. Greco A, Fusetti L, Villa R, et al: Transforming activity of the chimeric sequence formed by the fusion of collagen gene COL1A1 and the platelet growth factor b-chain gene in dermatofibrosarcoma protuberans. Oncogene 1998;17:1313–1319.
38. Shimizu A, O'Brien KP, Sjoblom T, et al: The dermatofibrosarcoma protuberans-associated collagen type Ialpha1/platelet-derived growth factor (PDGF) β-chain fusion gene generates a transforming protein that is processed to functional PDGF-BB. Cancer Res 1999;59: 3719–3723.
39. Wang J, Hisaoka M, Shimajiri S, Morimitsu Y, Hashimoto H: Detection of COL1A1-PDGFB fusion transcripts in dermatofibrosarcoma protuberans by reverse transcription-polymerase chain reaction using archival formalin-fixed, paraffin-embedded tissues. Diagn Mol Pathol 1999;8:113–119.

Low-Grade Fibromyxoid Sarcoma

40. Evans HL: Low-grade fibromyxoid sarcoma. A report of 12 cases. Am J Surg Pathol 1993;17:595–600.
41. Goodlad JR, Mentzel T, Fletcher CD: Low-grade fibromyxoid sarcoma: Clinico-pathological analysis of eleven new cases in support of a distinct entity. Histopathology 1995;26:229–237.
42. Folpe AL, Lane KL, Paull G, Weiss SW: Low-grade fibromyxoid sarcoma and hyalinizing spindle cell tumor with giant rosettes. A clinicopathologic study of 73 cases supporting their identity and assessing the impact of high-grade areas. Am J Surg Pathol 2000; 24:1353–1360.
43. Lane KL, Shannon RJ, Weiss SW: Hyalinizing spindle cell tumor with giant rosettes: A distinctive tumor closely resembling low-grade fibromyxoid sarcoma. Am J Surg Pathol 1997;21:1481–1488.

Other Fibrosarcomas

44. Scott SM, Reiman HM, Pritchard DJ, Ilstrup DM: Soft tissue fibrosarcoma: A clincopathologic study of 132 cases. Cancer 1989;64:925–931.
45. Shen WQ, Hashimoto H, Okamoto S, et al: Expression of COLIAI-PDGFB fusion transcripts in superficial adult fibrosarcoma suggests close relationship to dermatofibrosarcoma protuberans. J Pathol 2001;194: 88–94.
46. Mentzel T, Dry S, Katenkamp D, Fletcher CDM: Low-grade myofibroblastic sarcoma: Analysis of 18 cases in the spectrum of myofibroblastic tumors. Am J Surg Pathol 1998;22:1228–1238.
47. Montgomery EA, Goldblum JR, Fisher C: Myofibrosarcoma. A clinicopathologic study. Am J Surg Pathol 2001;25:219–228.
48. Meis JM, Enzinger FM: Inflammatory fibrosarcoma of the mesentery and retroperitoneum: A tumor closely simulating inflammatory pseudotumor. Am J Surg Pathol 1991;15:1146–1156.
49. Meis-Kindblom JM, Kindblom LG, Enzinger FM: Sclerosing epithelioid fibrosarcoma. A variant of fibrosarcoma simulating carcinoma. Am J Surg Pathol 1995; 19:979–993.
50. Eyden BP, Manson C, Banerjee SS, Roberts IS, Harris M: Sclerosing epithelioid fibrosarcoma: A study of five cases emphasizing diagnostic criteria. Histopathology 1998;33:354–360.
51. Antonescu C, Rosenblum MK, Pereira P, Nascimento AG, Woodruff JM: Sclerosing epithelioid fibrosarcoma. A study of 16 cases and confirmation of a clinicopathologic entity. Am J Surg Pathol 2001;25:699–709.
52. Gisselsson D, Andreasson P, Meis-Kindblom JM, Kindblom LG, Mertens F, Mandahl N: Amplification of 12q13 and 12q15 sequences in a sclerosing epithelioid fibrosarcoma. Cancer Genet Cytogenet 1998;107: 102–106.
53. Meis-Kindblom JM, Kindblom LG: Acral myxoinflammatory fibroblastic sarcoma. A low grade tumor of the hands and feet. Am J Surg Pathol 1998;22:911–924.
54. Montgomery EA, Devaney KO, Giordano TJ, Weiss SW: Inflammatory myxohyaline tumor of distal extremities with virocyte or Reed-Sternberg-like cells: A distinctive lesion with features simulating inflammatory conditions, Hodgkin's disease, and various sarcomas. Mod Pathol 1998;11:384–391.

Malignant Fibrous Histiocytoma—Clinicopathologic Studies

55. Kempson RL, Kyriakos M: Fibroxanthosarcoma of the soft tissues: A type of malignant fibrous histiocytoma. Cancer 1972;29:961–976.
56. Weiss SW, Enzinger FM: Malignant fibrous histiocytoma: An analysis of 200 cases. Cancer 1978;41: 2250–2266.
57. Enjoji M, Hashimoto H, Tsuneyoshi M, Iwasaki H: Malignant fibrous histiocytoma: A clinicopathologic study of 130 cases. Acta Pathol Jpn 1980;30:727–741.
58. Lattes R: Malignant fibrous histiocytoma: A review article. Am J Surg Pathol 1982;6:761–771.
59. Weiss SW: Malignant fibrous histiocytoma—A reaffirmation. Am J Surg Pathol 1982;6:773–784.
60. Enzinger FM: Malignant fibrous histiocytoma 30 years after Stout. Am J Surg Pathol [Suppl] 1986;10:S43–S53.
61. Bertoni F, Capanna R, Biagini R, et al: Malignant fibrous histiocytoma of soft tissue: An analysis of 78

cases located and deeply seated in the extremities. Cancer 1985;56:356–367.
62. Rydholm A, Syk I: Malignant fibrous histiocytoma of soft tissue. Correlation between clinical variables and histologic malignancy grade. Cancer 1986;57: 2323–2324.
63. Rööser B, Willen H, Gustafson P, Alvegård TA, Rydholm A: Malignant fibrous histiocytoma of soft tissue: A population-based epidemiologic and prognostic study of 137 patients. Cancer 1991;67: 499–505.
64. Pezzi CM, Rawlings MS, Esgro JJ, Pollock RE, Romsdahl MM: Prognostic factors in 227 patients with malignant fibrous histiocytoma. Cancer 1992;69: 2098–2103.
65. LeDoussal V, Coindre JM, Leroux A, et al. Prognostic factors for patients with localized primary malignant fibrous histiocytoma: A multicenter study of 216 patients with multivariate analysis. Cancer 1996;77: 1823–1830.
66. Salo JC, Lewis JJ, Woodruff JM, Leung DH, Brennan MF: Malignant fibrous histiocytoma of the extremity. Cancer 1999;85:1765–1772.
67. Weiss SW, Enzinger FM: Myxoid variant of malignant fibrous histiocytoma. Cancer 1977;39:1672–1685.
68. Angervall L, Kindblom LG, Merck C: Myxofibrosarcoma. A study of 30 cases. Acta Pathol Microbiol Scand 1977;85:127–140.
69. Merck C, Angervall L, Kindblom LG, Oden A: Myxofibrosarcoma. A malignant soft tissue tumor of fibroblastic-histiocytic origin. A clinicopathologic and prognostic study of 110 cases using a multivariate analysis. APMIS 1983;91(Suppl 282):1–40.
70. Mentzel T, Calonje E, Wadden C, et al: Myxofibrosarcoma. Clinicopathologic analysis of 75 cases with emphasis on the low-grade variant. Am J Surg Pathol 1996;20:391–405.
71. Kyriakos M, Kempson RL: Inflammatory fibrous histiocytoma. An aggressive and lethal lesion. Cancer 1976; 37:1584–1606.

Malignant Fibrous Histiocytoma—Biology and Immunohistochemistry

72. Brooks JJ: The significance of double phenotypic patterns and markers in human sarcomas. A new model of mesenchymal differentiation. Am J Pathol 1986;125: 113–123.
73. Roholl PJ, Kleyne J, Van Unnik JAM: Characterization of tumor cells in malignant fibrous histiocytomas and other soft tissue tumours, in comparison with malignant histiocytes. II: Immunoperoxidase study on cryostat sections. Am J Pathol 1985;121: 269–274.
74. Wood GS, Beckstead JH, Turner RR, Hendrickson MR, Kempson RL, Warnke RA: Malignant fibrous histiocytoma tumor cells resemble fibroblasts. Am J Surg Pathol 1986;10:323–335.
75. Leader M, Patel J, Collins M, Henry K: Anti-alpha 1-antichymotrypsin staining of 194 sarcomas, 38 carcinomas, and 17 malignant melanomas. Its lack of specificity as a tumour marker. Am J Surg Pathol 1987;11:133–139.
76. Soini Y, Miettinen M: Widespread immunoreactivity for alpha-1-antichymotrypsin in different types of tumors. Am J Clin Pathol 1988;90:131–136.
77. Soini Y, Miettinen M: Alpha-1-antitrypsin and lysozyme. Their limited significance in fibrohistiocytic tumors. Am J Clin Pathol 1989;91:515–521.
78. Iwasaki H, Isayama T, Johzaki H, Kikuchi M: Malignant fibrous histiocytoma. Evidence of perivascular mesenchymal cell origin. Immunocytochemical studies with monoclonal anti-MFH antibodies. Am J Pathol 1987;128:528–537.
79. Melhem MF, Meisler AI, Saito R, Finley CG, Hockman HR, Koski RA: Cytokines in inflammatory malignant fibrous histiocytoma presenting with leukemoid reaction. Blood 1993;82:2038–2044.
80. Hamada T, Komiya S, Hiraoka K, Zenmyo M, Morimatsu M, Inoue A: IL-6 in a pleomorphic type of malignant fibrous histiocytoma presenting high fever. Hum Pathol 1998;29:758–761.
81. Reinecke P, Moll R, Hildebrandt B, et al: A novel human malignant fibrous histiocytoma cell line of heart (MFH-H) with secretion of hematopoietic growth factors. Anticancer Res 1999;19:1901–1907.
82. Miettinen M, Soini Y: Malignant fibrous histiocytoma Heterogeneous patterns of intermediate filament proteins by immunohistochemistry. Arch Pathol Lab Med 1989;113:1363–1366.
83. Litzky LA, Brooks JJ: Cytokeratin immunoreactivity in malignant fibrous histiocytoma and spindle cell tumors: Comparison between frozen and paraffin-embedded tissues. Mod Pathol 1992;5:30–34.
84. Rosenberg AE, O'Connell JX, Dickersin GR, Bhan AK: Expression of epithelial markers in malignant fibrous histiocytoma of the musculoskeletal system: An immunohistochemical and electron microscopic study. Hum Pathol 1993;23:284–293.
85. Antonescu CR, Erlandson RA, Huvos AG: Primary fibrosarcoma and malignant fibrous histiocytoma of bone—a comparative ultrastructural study: Evidence of a spectrum of fibroblastic differentiation. Ultrastruct Pathol 2000;24:83–91.
86. Suh CH, Ordonez NG, Mackay B: Malignant fibrous histiocytoma: An ultrastructural perspective. Ultrastruct Pathol 2000;24:243–250.

Malignant Fibrous Histiocytoma—Genetics

87. Mandahl N, Heim S, Willen H, et al: Characteristic karyotypic anomalies identify subtypes of malignant fibrous histiocytoma. Genes Chromosomes Cancer 1989;1:9–14.
88. Szymanska J, Tarkkanen M, Wiklund T, et al: A cytogenetic study of malignant fibrous histiocytoma. Cancer Genet Cytogenet 1995;85:91–96.
89. Schmidt H, Korber S, Hinze R, et al: Cytogenetic characterization of ten malignant fibrous histiocytomas. Cancer Genet Cytogenet 1998;100:134–142.

90. Choong PF, Mandahl N, Mertens F, et al: 19p+ marker chromosome correlates with relapse in malignant fibrous histiocytoma. Genes Chromosomes Cancer 1996;16:88–93.
91. Larramendy ML, Tarkkanen M, Blomqvist C, et al: Comparative genomic hybridization of malignant fibrous histiocytoma reveals a novel prognostic marker. Am J Pathol 1997;151:1153–1161.
92. Hinze R, Schagdarsurengin U, Taubert H, et al: Assessment of genomic imbalances in malignant fibrous histiocytomas by comparative genomic hybridization. Int J Mol Med 1999;3:75–79.
93. Mairal A, Terrier P, Chibon F, Sastre X, Lecesne A, Aurias A: Loss of chromosome 13 is the most frequent genomic imbalance in malignant fibrous histiocytomas. A comparative genomic hybridization analysis of a series of 30 cases. Cancer Genet Cytogenet 1999; 111:134–138.
94. Sakabe T, Shinomiya T, Mori T, et al: Identification of a novel gene, MASL1, within an amplicon at 8p23.1 detected in malignant fibrous histiocytomas by comparative genomic hybridization. Cancer Res 1999;59: 511–515.
95. Simons A, Schepens M, Jeuken J, et al: Frequent loss of 9p21 (p16(INK4A)) and other genomic imbalances in human malignant fibrous histiocytoma. Cancer Genet Cytogenet 2000;118:89–98.
96. Chibon F, Mairal A, Freneaux P, et al: The RB1 gene is the target of chromosome 13 deletions in malignant fibrous histiocytoma. Cancer Res 2000;60:6339–6345.
97. Reid AH, Tsai MM, Venzon DJ, Wright CF, Lack EE, O'Leary TJ: MDM2 amplification, P53 mutation, and accumulation of the P53 gene product in malignant fibrous histiocytoma. Diagn Mol Pathol 1996;5: 65–73.
98. Molina P, Pellin A, Navarro S, Boix J, Carda C, Llombart-Bosch A: Analysis of p53 and mdm2 proteins in malignant fibrous histiocytoma in absence of gene alteration: Prognostic significance. Virchows Arch 1999;435:596–605.
99. Iwao K, Miyoshi Y, Nawa G, Yoshikawa H, Ochi T, Nakamura Y: Frequent beta-catenin abnormalities in bone and soft tissue tumors. Jpn J Cancer Res 1999; 90:205–209.

Malignant Fibrous Histiocytoma—Differential Diagnosis

100. Fletcher CDM: Malignant fibrous histiocytoma: Fact or fiction? A critical reappraisal based on 159 tumors diagnosed as a pleomorphic sarcoma. Am J Surg Pathol 1992;16:213–228.
101. Chan JK, Buchanan R, Fletcher CD: Sarcomatoid variant of anaplastic large cell Ki-1 lymphoma. Am J Surg Pathol 1990;14:983–988.
102. Khalidi HS, Singleton TP, Weiss SW: Inflammatory malignant fibrous histiocytoma: Distinction from Hodgkin's disease and non-Hodgkin's lymphoma by a panel of leukocyte markers. Mod Pathol 1997;10: 438–442.

Atypical Fibroxanthoma

103. Fretzin DF, Helwig EB: Atypical fibroxanthoma of the skin. A clinicopathologic study of 140 cases. Cancer 1973;31:1541–1552.
104. Dahl I: Atypical fibroxanthoma of the skin. A clinicopathological study of 57 cases. Acta Pathol Microbiol Scand A 1976;84:183–197.
105. Calonje E, Wadden C, Wilson-Jones E, Fletcher CD: Spindle-cell non-pleomorphic atypical fibroxanthoma: Analysis of a series and delineation of a distinctive variant. Histopathology. 1993;22:247–254.
106. Tomaszewski MM, Lupton GP: Atypical fibroxanthoma. An unusual variant with osteoclast-like giant cells. Am J Surg Pathol 1997;21:213–218.
107. Longacre TA, Smoller BR, Rouse RV: Atypical fibroxanthoma. Multiple immunohistologic profiles. Am J Surg Pathol 1993;17:1199–1209.
108. Wick MR, Fitzgibbon J, Swanson PE: Cutaneous sarcomas and sarcomatoid neoplasms of the skin. Semin Diagn Pathol. 1993;10:148–558.
109. Kamino H, Salcedo E: Histopathologic and immunohistochemical diagnosis of benign and malignant fibrous and fibrohistiocytic tumors of the skin. Dermatol Clin 1999;17:487–505.

Giant Cell Tumor of Soft Parts and Giant Cell MFH

110. Salm R, Sissons HA: Giant cell tumours of soft tissues. J Pathol 1972;107:27–39.
111. Folpe AL, Morris RJ, Weiss SW: Soft tissue giant cell tumor of low malignant potential: A proposal for the reclassification of malignant giant cell tumor of soft parts. Mod Pathol 1999;12:894–902.
112. Oliveira AM, Dei Tos AP, Fletcher CDM, Nascimento AG: Primary giant cell tumor of soft tissues. A study of 22 cases. Am J Surg Pathol 2000;24:248–256.
113. O'Connell JX, Wehrli BM, Nielsen GP, Rosenberg AE: Giant cell tumors of soft tissue: A clinicopathologic study of 18 benign and malignant tumors. Am J Surg Pathol 2000;24:386–395.
114. Guccion JG, Enzinger FM: Malignant giant cell tumor of soft parts. An analysis of 32 cases. Cancer 1972; 29:1518–1529.
115. Angervall L, Hagmar B, Kindblom LG, Merck C: Malignant giant cell tumor of soft tissues: A clinicopathologic, cytologic, ultrastructural, angiographic and microangiographic study. Cancer 1981;47:736–747.

Pleomorphic Hyaline Angiectatic Tumor

116. Smith MEF, Fisher C, Weiss SW: Pleomorphic hyalinizing angiectatic tumor of soft parts. A low-grade neoplasm resembling neurilemoma. Am J Surg Pathol 1996;20:21–29.
117. Groisman GM, Bejar J, Amar M, Ben-Izhak O: Pleomorphic hyalinizing angiectatic tumor of soft parts: Immunohistochemical study including the expression of vascular endothelial growth factor. Arch Pathol Lab 2000;124:423–426.

Benign Fatty Tumors

CHAPTER 8

Lipomas and their variants comprise more than half of all benign soft tissue tumors. They greatly outnumber liposarcomas, their malignant counterparts, by a margin of over 100:1. Lipomas mainly occur in adults; lipoblastoma is the corresponding tumor in children. Most lipomas present in superficial soft tissues, but some occur intramuscularly or intermuscularly, and rarely in body cavities. Recent genetic findings support the neoplastic versus hyperplastic nature of most lipomas and the separation of several lipoma types as specific disease entities (Table 8–1). A group of diffuse fat lesions, termed lipomatosis, and nonneoplastic conditions simulating fatty tumors, are also reviewed in this chapter.

Lipoma

Clinical Features

Lipomas are the most common benign soft tissue tumors in adults and were estimated to comprise almost half of all benign soft tissue tumors in a large series.[1] They usually occur in adults over age 40 years, with a male predominance. Lipomas present in a wide variety of body sites, most commonly in the upper body, especially the back, shoulder, arm, forearm, and other extremity sites, usually proximally.

A wide variety of other locations may be involved, including the intracranial space, orbit, interventricular septum of the heart, and submucosa of the respiratory and gastrointestinal tracts (especially colon). The diagnosis of mediastinal and intraabdominal lipoma should be made with great caution because most fatty neoplasms in these locations are well-differentiated liposarcomas.

Some lesions named as lipomas, especially the synovial lipoma with villous pattern (lipoma arborescens), lipoma of the hernia sac, and some lesions designated as lipomas of the foot and heel may be actually reactive hyperplasias rather than true neoplasms.

The majority of lipomas are subcutaneous, circumscribed, mobile tumors. According to a large series, 80% of them are smaller than 5 cm.[2] Multiple lipomas occur in some patients, sometimes on hereditary basis.[3] A minority of lipomas are intramuscular or located in intermuscular septa. Simple excision is the recommended treatment, but recurrence is possible. The diffuse intramuscular lipomas have a much higher local recurrence rate.[4,5]

Whether malignant transformation of ordinary lipoma occurs at all is questionable; it is quite possible that cases believed to represent such an occurrence were lipoma-like liposarcomas already at inception.

Gross Findings

Grossly and histologically lipomas resemble mature white adipose tissue. Although typically less than 5 cm, they may reach a size of over 20 cm. Lipomas often appear to be surrounded by a thin capsule-like

Table 8–1. Classification and Key Features of Benign Fatty Tumors

Tumor Type	Comment/Additional Elements/Difference from Ordinary Lipoma	Regions with Genetic Changes
Lipoma (ordinary lipoma)	Composed of mature adipose tissue	12q, 6p
Intra/intermuscular lipoma	Lipomas with deep locations	
Fibrolipoma	Prominent fibrous septa	
Myxoid lipoma (myxolipoma)	Myxoid matrix	
Lipomas with heterologous elements		
Myolipoma	Foci of mature smooth muscle	
Chondrolipoma	Islands of mature cartilage	
Osteolipoma	Foci of metaplastic bone	
Angiolipoma	Capillaries with fibrin microthrombi, usually in young adults	None found
Angiomyolipoma	Immature, HMB45^{+} smooth muscle cells, in kidney or retroperitoneum	12q, 16p13
Chondroid lipoma	Epithelioid cartilage-like differentiation	11q13, 16p12-13
Myelolipoma	Fatty and hematopoietic marrow elements, in adrenal or retroperitoneum	
Spindle cell and pleomorphic lipoma	Lipoma with spindle cells or giant cells, posterior neck of older men. CD34^{+}	16q
Hibernoma	Benign tumor with features of brown fat	11q13
Lipoblastoma	A childhood fatty tumor. Lobulated, myxoid composed of immature fat	8q
Atypical lipoma (atypical lipomatous tumor)	Lipoma with significant nuclear atypia	12q15

membrane and are sometimes lobulated. Intramuscular lipomas may be circumscribed or diffuse and tend to be larger than subcutaneous lipomas (Fig. 8–1). Fibrolipomas are firmer and may show grayish streaks of fibrous tissue. Some lipomas are mucoid (myxoid lipoma); this change is more common in spindle cell lipoma.

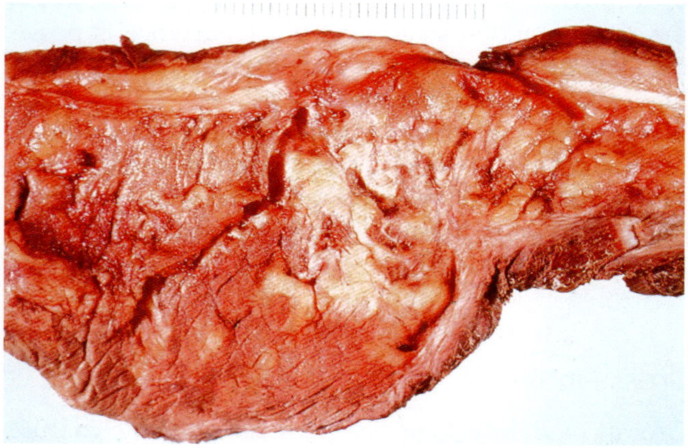

Figure 8–1. This intramuscular lipoma appears grossly as poorly demarcated yellow streaks in the middle of brown skeletal muscle tissue.

Microscopic Findings

Histologically, typical lipomas are composed of mature adipocytes indistinguishable from normal adipose tissue. Minor to moderate variation in adipocyte size may occur. Nuclei in lipomas are typically small and peripherally located. Tumors with significant nuclear atypia are classified as atypical lipomas when subcutaneous, or as well-differentiated, lipoma-like liposarcomas when intramuscular or located in deep soft tissues.

Intramuscular lipomas often involve skeletal muscle in a checkerboard pattern with alternating fat and skeletal muscle cells (Fig. 8–2), but they may also be well-demarcated similar to subcutaneous lipomas.

The variants showing prominent fibrous septa are referred to as fibrolipomas (Fig. 8–3). Those lipomas

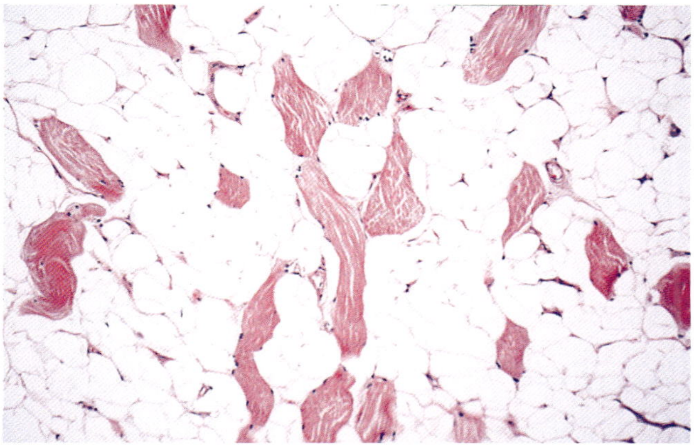

Figure 8-2. Histologically, many intramuscular lipomas grow between the muscle fibers in a checkerboard pattern.

that have a myxoid stroma—myxoid lipoma (Fig. 8-4) and myxoid spindle cell lipoma—should not be confused with myxoid liposarcoma. Lack of a prominent plexiform capillary pattern and lipoblasts separate them from the latter. Also, myxoid liposarcomas are almost always intramuscular.

Differential Diagnosis

Large lipomas, especially the deep and intra-abdominal ones, should be sampled adequately (ideally one section per each centimeter of tumor diameter) to not miss atypia. Significant atypia in deep tumors confers the diagnosis of well-differentiated liposarcoma, whereas the subcutaneous tumors may be designated as atypical lipomas because of their lower potential. Because well-differential retroperitoneal liposarcomas may have areas indistinguishable from lipomas, small needle biopsies are of limited value to definitively diagnose lipoma and rule out well-differentiated liposarcoma.

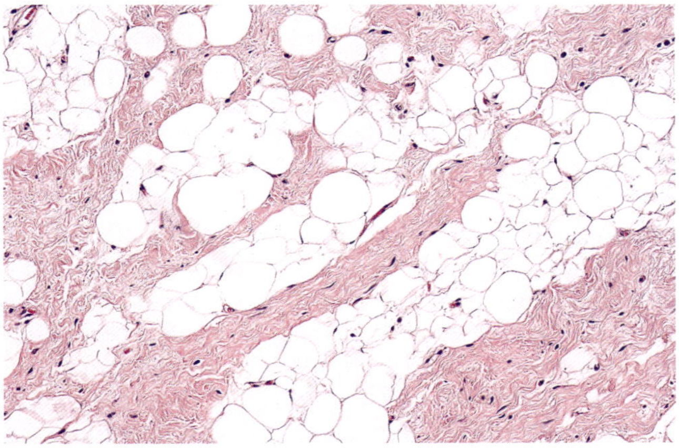

Figure 8-3. Fibrolipoma is the designation used for lipomas with prominent fibrous septa.

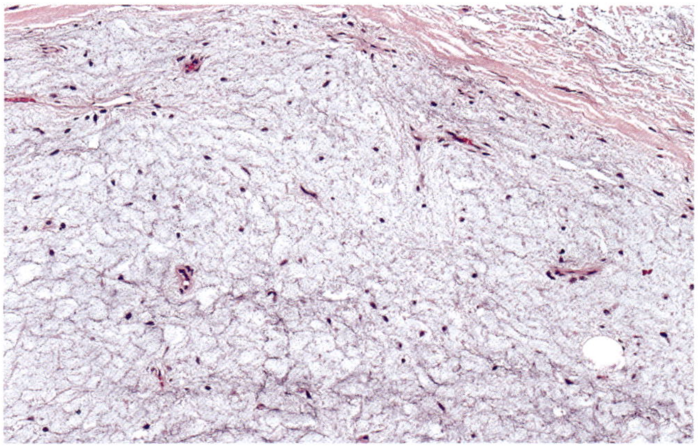

Figure 8-4. Myxoid lipoma shows abundant myxoid matrix and moderate vascularity. Only a single adipocyte is seen in this field.

In some instances it may be difficult to determine whether well-differentiated fat represents lipoma or normal fat. Muscular dystrophy may cause massive fatty replacement in the involved muscles, histologically simulating a lipomatous process. Also intramuscular hemangiomas can have a significant lipomatous component; in this tumor the presence of the hemangiomatous component overweighs the presence of fat (although historically the designation of infiltrative angiolipoma has been used of these fatty hemangiomas).

Genetics

The chromosomal regions most commonly involved in different types of lipomas, and the specific genes involved are listed in Table 8-2. Several balanced translocations and other gene rearrangements involving different chromosomal areas, especially 12q15, have been described in ordinary lipomas.[6] The presence of such genetic changes supports the neoplastic versus hyperplastic nature of lipomas. A large series found karyotypic abnormalities in 78% of lipomas, and such abnormalities were more common in older patients.[7] Among the most common recurrent changes were rearrangements of 12q13-15, 6p, 13q, and 8q11-13. The described translocations include, for example, t(12;14)(q14-15;q24).

The gene involved in lipoma gene rearrangements involving 12q15 encodes for a nuclear nonhistone protein, named high-mobility group protein IC *(HMGIC)* based on its high mobility in polyacrylamide gel electrophoresis. This DNA-binding protein participates in the transcriptional regulation as a cofactor (architectural transcription factor, regulating

Table 8–2. The Chromosomal Regions and Genes Involved in Different Types of Benign Fatty Tumors

Tumor	Chromosomal Region Type of Involvement		Gene and Encoded Protein
Lipoma	12q15 rearrangements including translocations	*HMGC1*	High-mobility group protein, overexpression Transcriptional regulator
	13q rearrangements	*LHFP*	Lipoma *HMGC1* fusion partner Function unknown
	6p, 8q rearrangements including translocations	Not known	
Angiolipoma	None		
Angiomyolipoma	16p13 deletions	*TSC2*	Tuberous sclerosis 2 tumor suppressor Loss of hamartin expression
Chondroid lipoma	t(11;16)(q13;p12-13)	Not known	
Spindle cell lipoma	16q deletions 13q rearrangements	Not known	
Hibernoma	11q13 rearrangements	Not known	
Lipoblastoma(tosis)	8q11-13 rearrangements	*PLAG1*	Overexpression
Atypical lipoma	12q13-15 rearrangements	*HMGC1*	Overexpression

Note that different tumors may have the same chromosomal regions involved. It is not known in all of these instances whether the same or different genes are involved.

DNA configuration) and is commonly rearranged and overexpressed in different types of tumors, among them benign tumors such as lipomas and uterine leiomyomas.[8]

The lipoma HMGIC fusion partner *(LHFP)* is a gene in 13q that was found to participate in a t(12;13) translocation in lipoma.[9]

Lipomas with Heterologous Elements: Myolipoma, Chondrolipoma, and Osteolipoma

Several types of well-differentiated nonlipomatous elements may rarely occur within benign lipoma. Designations "myolipoma," "chondrolipoma," and "osteolipoma" refer to lipomas that have focal elements of mature smooth muscle, cartilage, or metaplastic bone, respectively. These tumors have a benign behavior similar to ordinary lipoma, and their recognition is only significant in the sense that they should not be confused with variants of liposarcoma.

Myolipomas present in adult patients with female predominance.[10] They are often large tumors, located in superficial or deep peripheral soft tissues or in the retroperitoneum. Grossly, the periphery of the tumor is fatty. The smooth muscle component can be seen as a grossly recognizable element or sometimes as microscopic foci. Histologically, myolipomas contain mature fatty elements admixed with foci of mature smooth muscle cells. Tumors that have predominant smooth muscle elements with focal fat are designated as lipoleiomyomas.

Chondrolipoma is the designation for lipoma that has small islands of well-differentiated hyaline cartilage in the middle of the mature fatty component. These tumors usually occur in peripheral soft tissues, but examples have also been reported in the subcutis of breast and in the larynx.[11,12] Chondrolipoma should not be confused with chondroid lipoma, which is histologically quite different and shows ill-defined epithelioid chondroid-like areas intermixed with fatty elements without demarcation. This tumor does not have well-differentiated islands of hyaline cartilage. Osteolipoma is a designation for mature lipoma that contains spicules of mature bone. We have seen such lesions especially in the hand. This designation has also been used for a lipoma that contains a central inclusion from an underlying bony osteochondroma.[13]

Genetics

There is no specific genetic information on these variants of lipoma.

Angiolipoma

Clinical Features

Angiolipomas are common tumors that present as circumscribed, small, subcutaneous nodules, typically in young adults with a male predominance. The lesions are often painful. Multiple lesions commonly occur, and some patients may have up to several hundred angiolipomas. Typical locations include forearm, arm, trunk, and breast; in the latter location they are typically superficial and not intraparenchymal.[14] Behavior is benign.

Pathology

Grossly, angiolipomas are small, ovoid, circumscribed nodules usually measuring 1 to 2 cm in greatest diameter. They may appear firmer than ordinary lipomas. Histologically, angiolipomas show the combination of mature white fat with clusters of thick-walled capillaries, often located in the periphery of the tumors and extending as streaks into the center. The vessels are typically filled with erythrocytes and often contain eosinophilic fibrin microthrombi, a typical feature of this entity (Fig. 8–5).

Cellular angiolipoma is the designation for angiolipoma with an extensive vascular component and scattered fat cells or a narrow rim of them (Fig. 8–6). These tumors may simulate a spindle cell vascular neoplasm, especially Kaposi sarcoma or spindle cell angiosarcoma. Although cellular angiolipomas can have mitotic activity, sharp demarcation, packeting of the vessels as lobules, slitlike vascular spaces, lack of piling up of endothelial cells and presence of fibrin thrombi help to separate them from hemangiomas and malignant vascular tumors.[15]

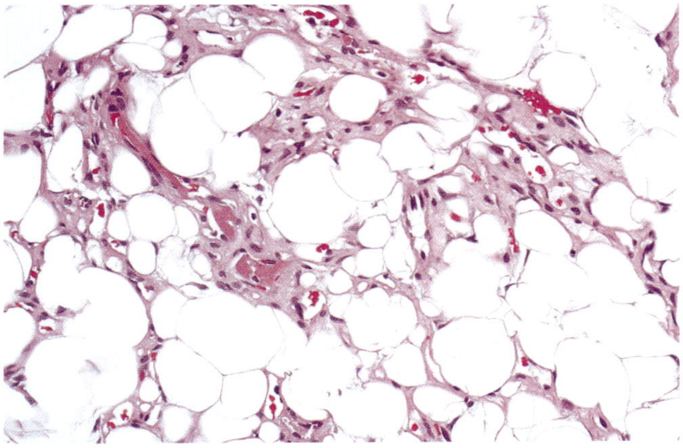

Figure 8-5. Angiolipoma typically contains peripheral streaks of thick-walled capillaries filled with erythrocytes and often fibrin microthrombi.

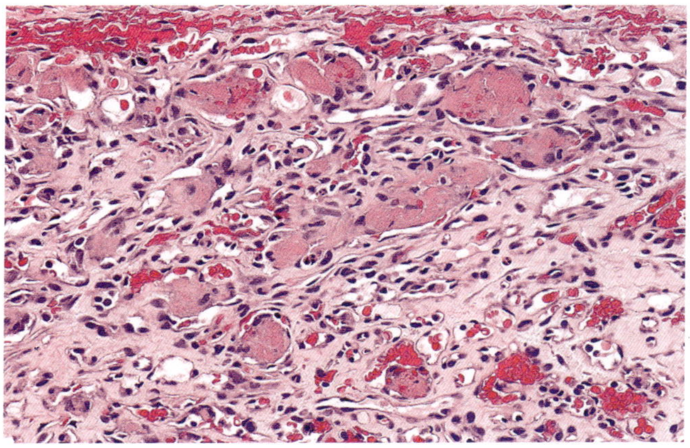

Figure 8-6. Cellular angiolipoma shows a dominant vascular component, and prominent fibrin thrombosis is present.

The term angiolipoma, especially in the form of "infiltrative angiolipoma," has also been used for an unrelated lesion, intramuscular hemangioma, which often combines vascular and lipomatous elements.[16]

Genetics

No cytogenetic alterations were reported in a study of 20 angiolipomas, suggesting a genetic difference from ordinary lipomas.[17] The apparent lack of genetic changes suggests that either these tumors have subtle, undetectable genetic changes or, if they have no changes, that they may be reactive rather than neoplastic.

Angiomyolipoma and Related Tumors

Angiomyolipoma (AML) is a relatively rare mesenchymal tumor that primarily occurs in the kidney. It contains mature lipomatous, vascular, and peculiar smooth muscle cell components; the latter is usually positive for smooth muscle markers and the melanoma marker HMB45, showing a unique "myomelanocytic" differentiation. The term myomelanocytic tumor or perivascular epithelioid cell tumor also includes clear cell (sugar) tumor of the lung, similar tumors rarely described in pancreas and intestines, and lymphangiomyoma(tosis) of the lung or retroperitoneum.[18–20] The latter tumors will be discussed in Chapter 10.

Clinical Features

Although most commonly presenting in the kidney, AMLs may also occur primarily in the retroperitoneum, liver, and other abdominal and extra-abdominal sites. AMLs usually occur in adults and sporadically in children. Most series show a significant female predominance (3:1 or more).

In the kidney and liver, AMLs range from minute, incidental small nodules to large tumors over 10 to 20 cm. Larger tumors in the kidney may cause hematuria or pain and in the liver present as space-occupying lesions. Some angiomyolipomas present as retroperitoneal masses. Rupture of a lesional vessel can cause abdominal hemorrhage of AMLs at any location. Some patients, especially those with the tuberous sclerosis complex, have multiple and bilateral renal AMLs. In clinicopathologic series, approximately 20% of renal and 10% of hepatic AMLs have this association.[21–29]

Because most renal AMLs are indolent tumors, there is a tendency toward their specific preoperative diagnosis by combined radiologic and cytologic or histologic methods. This allows for conservative management, either by follow-up only, by conservative kidney-sparing resection, or sometimes by selective embolization in the case of larger tumors. Rare fatal cases (especially of epithelioid variants) with metastatic spread have been described, and sarcomatous transformation has been described on rare occasions.[18]

Pathology

The gross appearance varies according to the proportions of the components. Predominantly fatty tumors are pale yellow, whereas the tumors with an extensive smooth muscle component are brownish (Fig. 8–7).

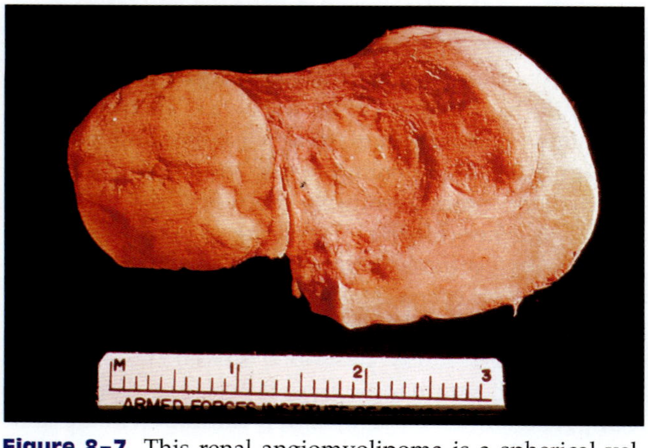

Figure 8–7. This renal angiomyolipoma is a spherical yellowish mass in the periphery of the kidney *(left)*.

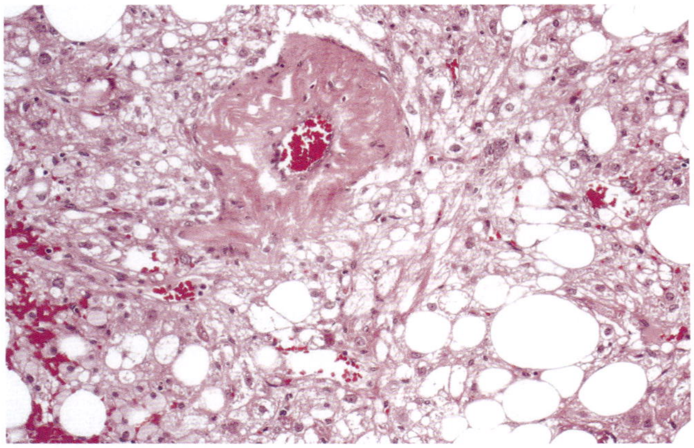

Figure 8–8. Typical angiomyolipoma with thick-walled blood vessels, a clear cytoplasmic smooth muscle component, and a mature fatty component.

Histologically, the mature adipose tissue, smooth muscle, and vascular components occur in various proportions (Fig. 8–8). Some AMLs are predominantly composed of mature fat that lacks atypia (Fig. 8–9*A*) and only show inconspicuous clusters of immature smooth muscle cells, but adipocyte size may vary greatly. The smooth muscle component is typically composed of hollow-appearing, glycogen-rich, spindled or polygonal smooth muscle cells that may be present in clusters around the blood vessels or form inconspicuous foci within the fatty component.[30]

In some cases the smooth muscle component is predominant,[31] presenting either as a spindled component resembling lymphangiomyoma, or sometimes an epithelioid component that can resemble renal carcinoma.[25–27] The epithelioid component may be pleomorphic and may have alarming nuclear atypia, but mitoses are extremely rare. With eccentric nuclei, such a component may resemble ganglion cells (Fig. 8–9*B*).

The vascular component is composed of blood vessels that often have a thick smooth muscle layer. Massive intratumoral hemorrhage may disrupt the architecture and make the diagnosis more difficult.

Lymph node involvement may occur and does not indicate malignant behavior; it has been suggested to indicate multifocality rather than true metastasis. Vascular invasion into the renal vein or vena cava has been rarely noted and has no adverse prognostic significance either.

Immunohistochemistry

The smooth muscle components of AML are positive for smooth muscle actin, usually for desmin, although some series report less consistent positivity for both markers. Subsets of smooth muscle component almost always show granular cytoplasmic

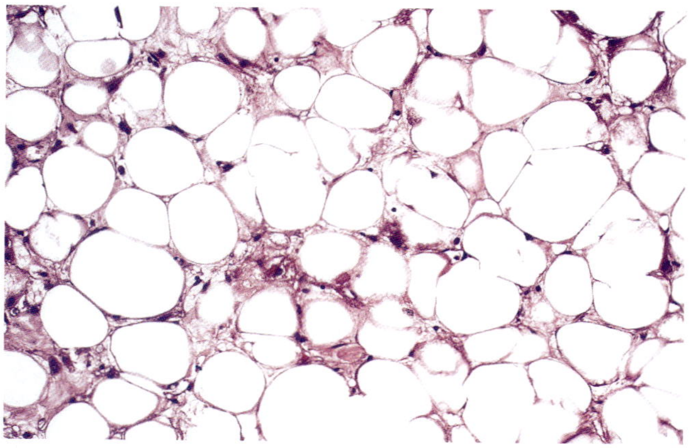

A

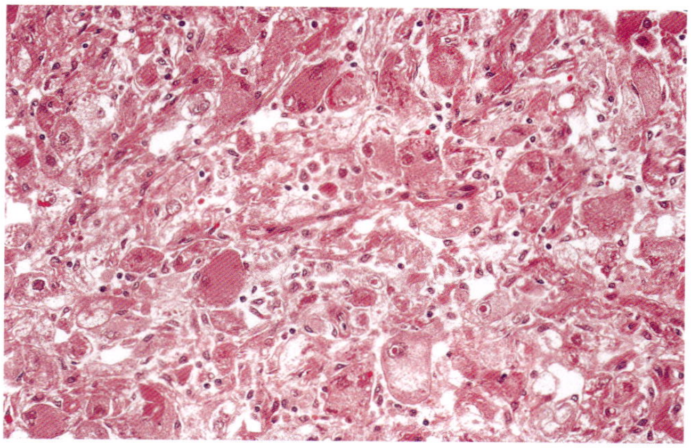

B

Figure 8-9. Histologic variants of angiomyolipoma include *(A)* tumors dominated by fat with small streaks of smooth muscle, and *(B)* rare variants primarily composed of epithelioid cells with eosinophilic cytoplasm.

immunostaining for melanoma markers HMB45 (Fig. 8–10) and MelanA in varying numbers of tumor cells.[32–34] A minority of tumors show focal nuclear and cytoplasmic S-100 protein positivity, but they are CD34^{-}. Estrogen and progesterone receptor immunoreactivity has been reported and could indicate hormonal dependence and explain the female predominance. HMB45 positivity in some renal capsular leiomyomas suggests that they may be related to AML.[35]

Differential Diagnosis

Retroperitoneal AML has to be differentiated from well-differentiated lipoma-like liposarcoma.[30] Lack of adipocytic atypia and the presence of HMB45 and Melan A-positive smooth muscle elements are diagnostic. The epithelioid variants should not be confused with renal cell carcinoma.[25–27] Some nasal and cutaneous tumors diagnosed as AMLs that were HMB45^{-} represent vascular leiomyomas with a lipomatous component rather than AMLs.

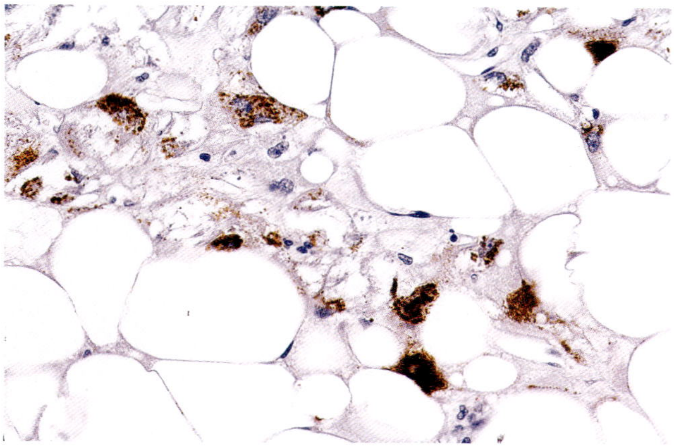

Figure 8-10. Angiomyolipoma contains varying numbers of HMB45^{+} epithelioid smooth muscle cells.

Genetics

The involvement of the tuberous sclerosis 2 *(TSC2)* tumor suppressor locus of chromosome band 16p13 is a candidate for the underlying genetic change in AML. Allelic losses at 16p13 have been found in both sporadic AMLs and those associated with tuberous sclerosis complex.[36,37] Also, lack of *TSC2* gene product (hamartin) expression has been reported, consistent with the possibility that AML development may be caused by lack of *TSC2* gene function.[38] Recurrent cytogenetic findings include trisomy 7, and there are sporadic reports on trisomy 8 and chromosomal rearrangements in 12q13-15 in a region also involved in liposarcomas.[39–41] Comparative genomic hybridization studies have shown recurrent losses in 5q33-q34, suggesting the possible involvement of a tumor suppressor gene in this region.[42] Clonality of this tumor is supported by HUMARA analysis (Chapter 4).[43,44]

Chondroid Lipoma

Clinical Features

This uncommon lesion, described by Meis and Enzinger,[45] is a peculiar, benign lipomatous tumor that combines diffuse cartilage-like, myxoid, and lipomatous elements. The tumor chiefly presents in young adults with a female predominance (80%). The most common locations are shoulder, arm, and thigh. The tumors may be subcutaneous or intramuscular. The reported lesions have measured 1.5 to 11 cm in diameter (average 3–4 cm). The behavior is benign, but we have seen local recurrences.

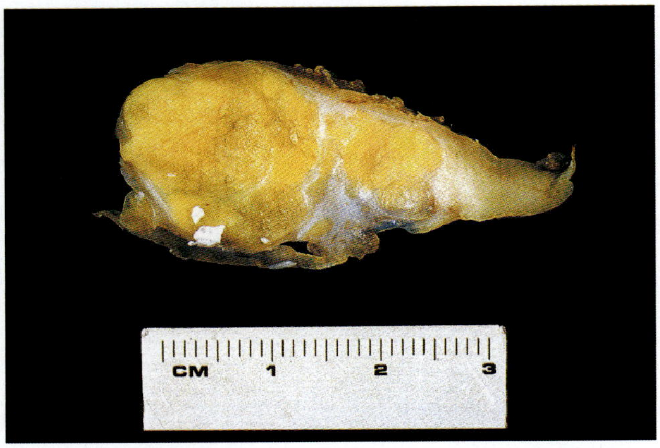

Figure 8–11. Chondroid lipoma is grossly composed of lobules of fatty tissue. This tumor is a recurrence.

Pathology

Grossly, the tumors are yellow and slightly firmer than lipomas, and lobulation may be visible (Fig. 8–11). Microscopically, the lesions are lobulated and consist of alternating ordinary white fat cells, epithelioid-appearing tumor cells with well-demarcated cell borders and variably vacuolated bubbly cytoplasm, and clearly chondroid cells with eosinophilic cytoplasm and myxoid matrix (Fig. 8–12*A*). A corded pattern in some lesions may resemble extraskeletal myxoid chondrosarcoma (Fig. 12*B*).

Immunohistochemically, the lesional cells are typically positive for S-100 protein with variable CD68 positivity, and they may also be positive for keratins. Collagen IV immunoreactivity around tumor cells reflects the presence of basement membranes.

Electron microscopic findings typically include prominent pinocytic vesicles and numerous cytoplasmic lipid vacuoles, interpreted to support white fat differentiation.[46]

Lipomas with true cartilaginous differentiation do not belong to this category but are rather classified as lipomas with chondroid foci (chondrolipoma).

Genetics

Balanced translocation t(11;16)(q13;p12-13) has been described in one case. The breakpoint in chromosome 11 is similar to that of hibernoma, whereas the breakpoint in chromosome 16 is different from that of myxoid liposarcoma.[47]

Myelolipoma

Myelolipoma is a rare tumor-like process resembling the components of bone marrow with fatty and hematopoietic components. It usually involves the adrenal cortex but occasionally presents in the extra-adrenal soft tissues in retroperitoneum, especially in the pelvis. It is usually incidentally detected in radiologic studies for cancer staging or at surgery for another condition, but larger tumors or those that have ruptured may be symptomatic. Myelolipoma occurs in older adults and has no connection with hematologic disease. However, it is associated with obesity and hypercortisolism, either endogenous or iatrogenic.[48–52]

Pathology

Grossly, myelolipoma shows lipoma-like features and soft blood-colored material corresponding to hematopoietic bone marrow. Histologically, it is composed of areas of mature fat and cellular hematopoietic bone marrow, especially with maturing erythroid cells and megakaryocytes (Fig. 8–13). It is not known whether myelolipoma is a peculiar tumor-like hyperplasia or

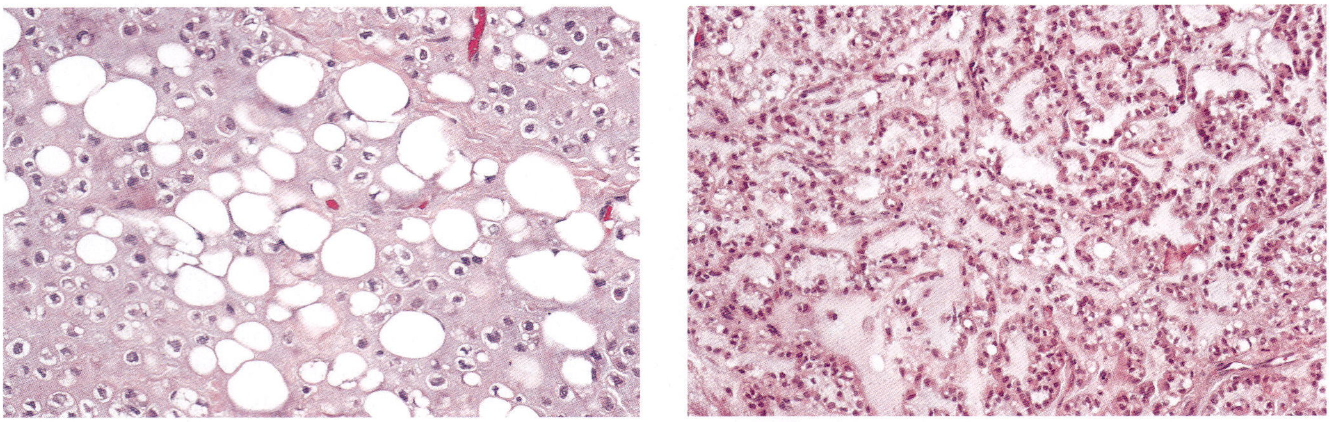

A B

Figure 8–12. *A,* Typical chondroid lipoma contains epithelioid chondroid cells and a mature lipomatous component. *B,* Chondroid lipomas may have a trabecular or alveolar pattern resembling extraskeletal myxoid chondrosarcoma.

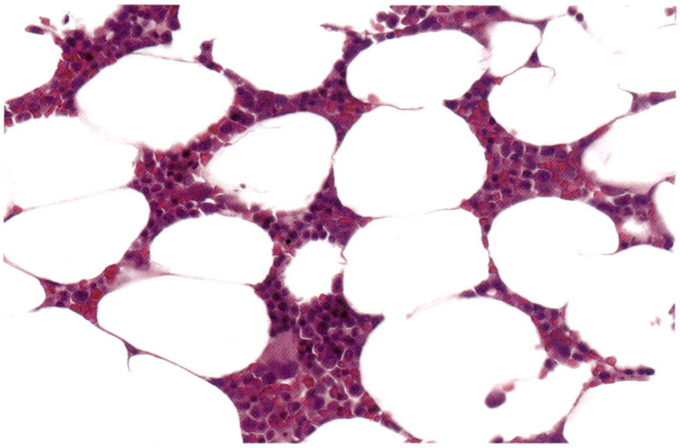

Figure 8-13. Myelolipoma simulates bone marrow with fatty and hematopoietic elements.

a true neoplasm. It should be separated from extramedullary myeloid tumors that have abnormal hematopoietic cell components, tend to be multifocal, and are often associated with splenomegaly.

Spindle Cell Lipoma and Pleomorphic Lipoma

Clinical Features

Spindle cell lipoma, first described by Enzinger and Harvey in 1975,[53] is a relatively rare benign lipomatous tumor that shows a variably prominent, nonlipogenic, spindle cell component. Pleomorphic lipoma, described by Shmookler and Enzinger in 1981 is its histologic variant with floret-like adipocytes with some nuclear pleomorphism.[54] Both spindle cell and pleomorphic lipomas typically present in older men (85–90%) with a median age of over 55 years.[53–58] The lesions have often a long history and occur chiefly in the subcutis of the posterior neck, back, and shoulder area (over 80%). On occasion, spindle cell and pleomorphic lipomas present elsewhere in the trunk or in the extremities, orofacial region, orbit, and skin,[59] but very rarely if ever in deep soft tissues. These tumors, although usually relatively small, may reach a size over 10 cm. Some patients have multiple lesions, and familial occurrence has been reported, mostly in men.[58] Spindle cell and pleomorphic lipomas have a benign behavior and conservative local excision is considered sufficient.

Pathology

Grossly, spindle cell lipoma forms an oval or discoid yellowish to grayish white mass depending on the relative extent of the fatty and spindle cell components. The tumor has a firmer texture than ordinary lipoma.

Histologically, spindle cell lipoma is composed of mature fat and bland spindled mesenchymal cells that may present as small clusters between the fat cells or dominate the tumor.[53–57] The spectrum of spindle cell lipomas varies from tumors that resemble ordinary lipomas but have narrow streaks of spindle cells to tumors that are mostly composed of spindle cells with just a few fat cells (Fig. 8–14*A*). Large numbers of mast cells are often seen in between the spindle cells, and lymphocytes and plasma cells may occur, especially in the pleomorphic lipoma. Coarse collagen bands often occur between the spindle cells. Some spindle cell lipomas show myxoid stromal change, which may be a dominant feature (Fig. 8–14*B*). Mitoses are exceptional. Some spindle cell lipomas contain slitlike cleavage spaces resembling vascular slits; this has been termed as "pseudoangiomatoid variant."[60]

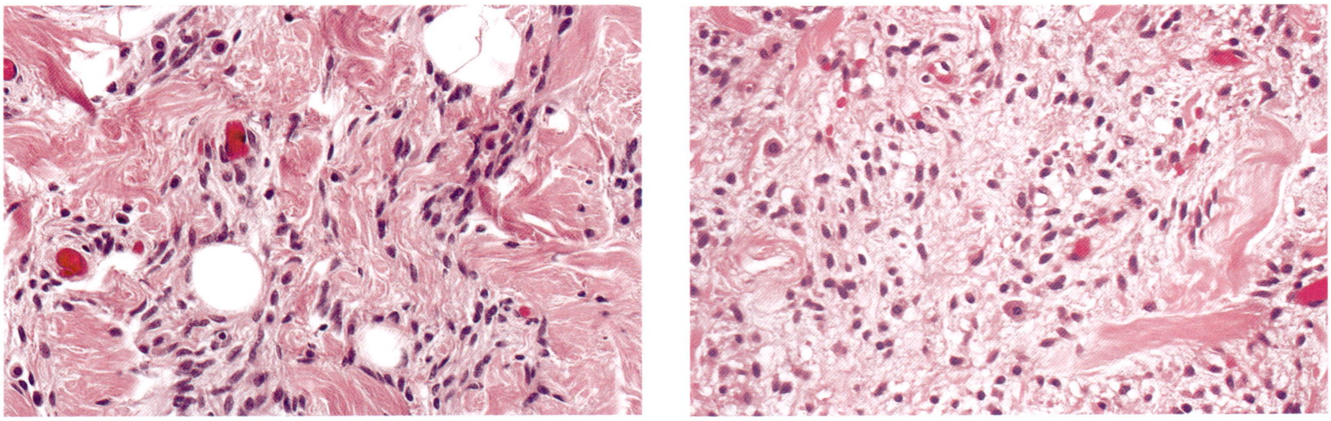

A **B**

Figure 8-14. Spindle cell lipomas with different appearances. *A,* Spindle cell component in a coarse collagenous background. *B,* Cellular spindle cell pattern in a myxoid background.

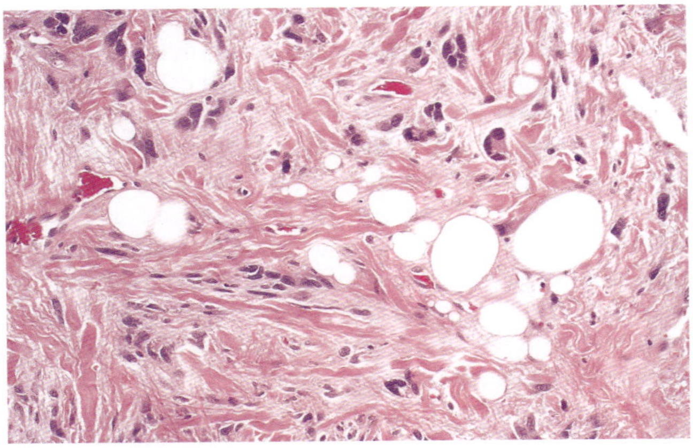

Figure 8–15. Pleomorphic lipoma resembles spindle cell lipoma but has floret-like giant cells.

Pleomorphic lipoma is a variant of spindle cell lipoma. In addition to the above features, this tumor contains multinucleated floret-like giant cells with radially arranged nuclei, like petals of flowers (Fig. 8–15). Some of these tumors have prominent nuclear atypia with hyperchromasia and even occasional atypical mitoses. In such instances the border between pleomorphic lipoma and atypical lipoma is arbitrary. Clinical features and behavior are similar to spindle cell lipoma.

Immunohistochemically, the spindle cells in both spindle cell and pleomorphic lipomas are strongly CD34$^+$ (Fig. 8–16) and usually negative for S-100 protein, desmin, and smooth muscle actin.[61–63]

Differential Diagnosis

Uniformity of spindle cells, mature collagen fibers, and absence of lipoblasts separate spindle cell and pleomorphic lipoma from liposarcoma. The subcutaneous location also differs from liposarcoma.

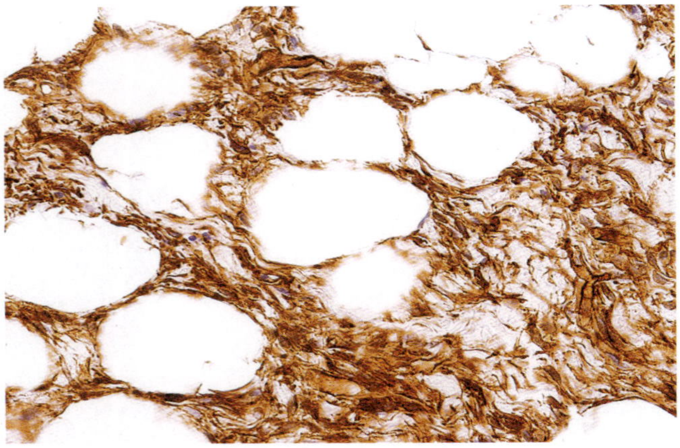

Figure 8–16. Spindle cell lipoma cells are strongly positive for CD34.

Genetics

The 16q losses with partial monosomy are typical of spindle cell and pleomorphic lipoma and differ from the changes seen in other lipomas. The involved genes have not been specifically identified. Recurrent involvement of chromosome 13q has also been reported.[64,65] Hypertetraploid cell populations have been reported in pleomorphic lipomas, probably corresponding to the cells with bizarre, hyperchromatic nuclei.

Hibernoma

Hibernoma is a rare tumor that mimics the differentiation of brown fat, which is involved in metabolic thermogenesis in hibernating animals by regulated uncoupling of mitochondrial oxidative phosphorylation. Brown fat is normally seen in the posterior neck and axilla, and may be seen for example, around cervical and axillary lymph nodes.[66–68]

Clinical Features

Based on data from 170 cases published from the Armed Forces Institute of Pathology, hibernoma occurs predominantly in young adults (61% in the third and fourth decades). The youngest patients have been children aged 2 to 15 years (5%); rarely hibernomas are seen in persons over age 60 (7%). The tumor occurs most commonly in the thigh (29%), shoulder and back (22%), neck, chest, arm, and abdomen. A minority are intramuscular. Behavior does not differ from that of ordinary lipoma.[68]

Pathology

Grossly, the hibernomas that show brown fat cells amidst white fat are not recognizable from ordinary lipomas. Those tumors that have extensive brown fat differentiation are yellow brown to brown. Otherwise they resemble lipomas, usually measure between 3 and 10 cm in diameter, and appear well-demarcated (Fig. 8–17).

Histologically, hibernomas show a mixture of brown fatlike multivacuolar adipocytes and brown fat cells with granular, eosinophilic cytoplasm and univacuolar white fat cells in various proportions. The nuclei of brown fat cells are small and centrally placed, and some have prominent nucleoli. Mitoses are very rare. The cytoplasm of multivacuolar hiber-

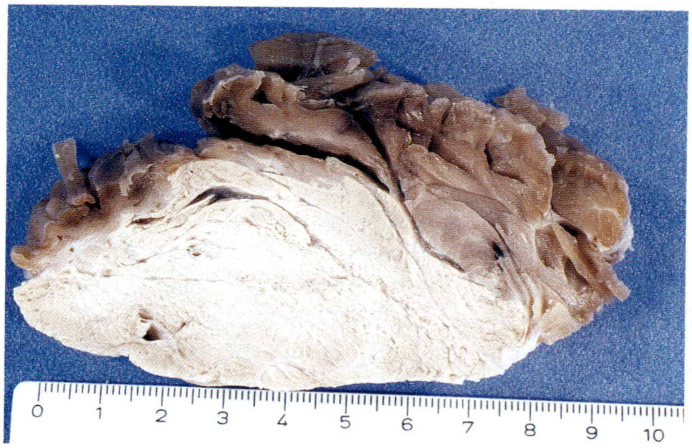

Figure 8-17. Hibernoma containing high numbers of brown fat cells is grossly brown. Note the sharp demarcation of this intramuscular tumor.

noma cells varies from pale staining to eosinophilic and granular (Fig. 8–18). Rare myxoid and spindle cell variants do occur. Immunohistochemically, they are often strongly positive for S-100 protein. Hibernomas have to be distinguished from myxoid liposarcomas that may have hibernoma-like cytoplasmic features. Recently, expression of uncoupling protein, typical of brown fat, was shown in hibernoma cells by immunohistochemistry.[69]

Genetics

Rearrangements of 11q13, sometimes involved in complex translocations involving multiple chromosomes, appear to be a recurrent cytogenetic change.[70–72] Homozygous deletion of multiple endocrine neoplasia I *(MEN1)* gene in this region was also observed.[73] Breakpoints have also been repeatedly found in 12q13-15 and 6p.[71]

Lipoblastoma and Lipoblastomatosis

Clinical Features

Lipoblastoma is a designation for specific, rare, grossly well-defined benign fatty tumors occurring in young children, and lipoblastomatosis is the designation of similar lesions that have diffuse borders. These tumors typically present in the subcutis of the extremities or less commonly trunk, but they may also be intramuscular. Occasional retroperitoneal intra-abdominal examples have been reported. Most patients are under 3 years of age, and there is a 2:1 male predominance. The tumor is benign, but may recur, especially if diffuse. Therefore, complete but conservative excision is advisable.[74–79]

Pathology

Grossly, lipoblastoma is yellow or yellowish gray, often lobulated, and may show extensive myxoid change (Fig. 8–19). The majority of lesions measure less than 5 cm, but lipoblastomas as large than 20 cm have been reported in the retroperitoneum.

Histologically, lipoblastoma and lipoblastomatosis are typically clearly lobulated by connective tissue septa, as seen at low magnification (Fig. 8–20*A*). The lobules are composed of highly vascular fat with variably myxoid stroma, with resemblance to embryonic white fat (Fig. 8–20*B*). Foci of multivacuolated lipoblasts may occur. Some lipoblastomas are composed predominantly of immature spindle cells (Fig. 8–20*C*) and others of lobulated mature white fat, and as such may resemble fibrolipoma (Fig. 8–20*D*). Lipoma-like features have also been reported in recurrent lipoblastoma suggesting that the lesions may undergo maturation over time.

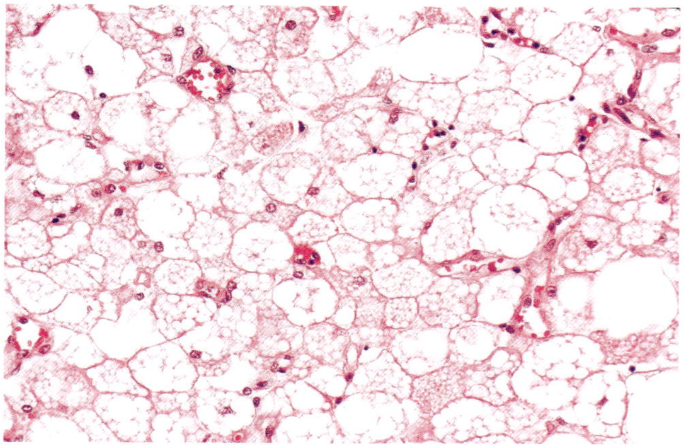

A

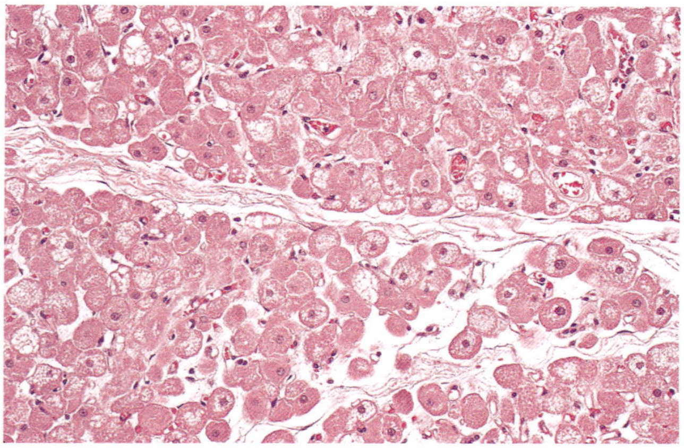

B

Figure 8-18. Histologically hibernoma cells vary from pale cytoplasmic, multivacuolated *(A)* to eosinophilic cells with granular cytoplasm *(B)*.

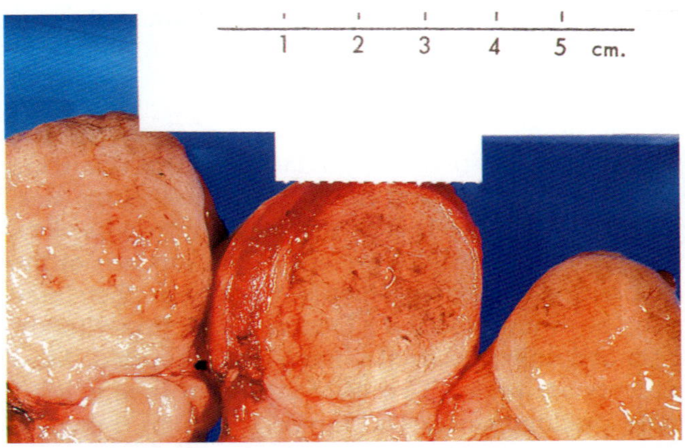

Figure 8-19. Lipoblastoma shows multiple lobules of myxoid fatty tissue. Note the sharp circumscription of this tumor.

Differential diagnosis from fibrolipoma is based on prominent lobulation of lipoblastoma; fibrolipomas do not generally occur in children. distinction from myxoid liposarcoma is aided by the lobular and more organized nature and more commonly subcutaneous location of lipoblastoma. Molecular genetic studies may be useful in problem cases.

Genetics

Genetic changes described in lipoblastoma typically include structural rearrangements, especially translocations and inversions involving chromosome 8q11-13 region.[80-83] Recently, overexpression of the *PLAG1* gene in this region was reported, suggesting that this gene may be the target in the 8q changes in lipoblastoma.[84]

Atypical Lipoma (Atypical Lipomatous Tumor)

This designation is used for those well-differentiated lipomatous tumors that show significant nuclear atypia, detectable by low magnification (4–10× objective), and are located in subcutaneous tissue. However, similar tumors in intramuscular and retroperitoneal locations are by convention designated as well-differentiated liposarcomas because of

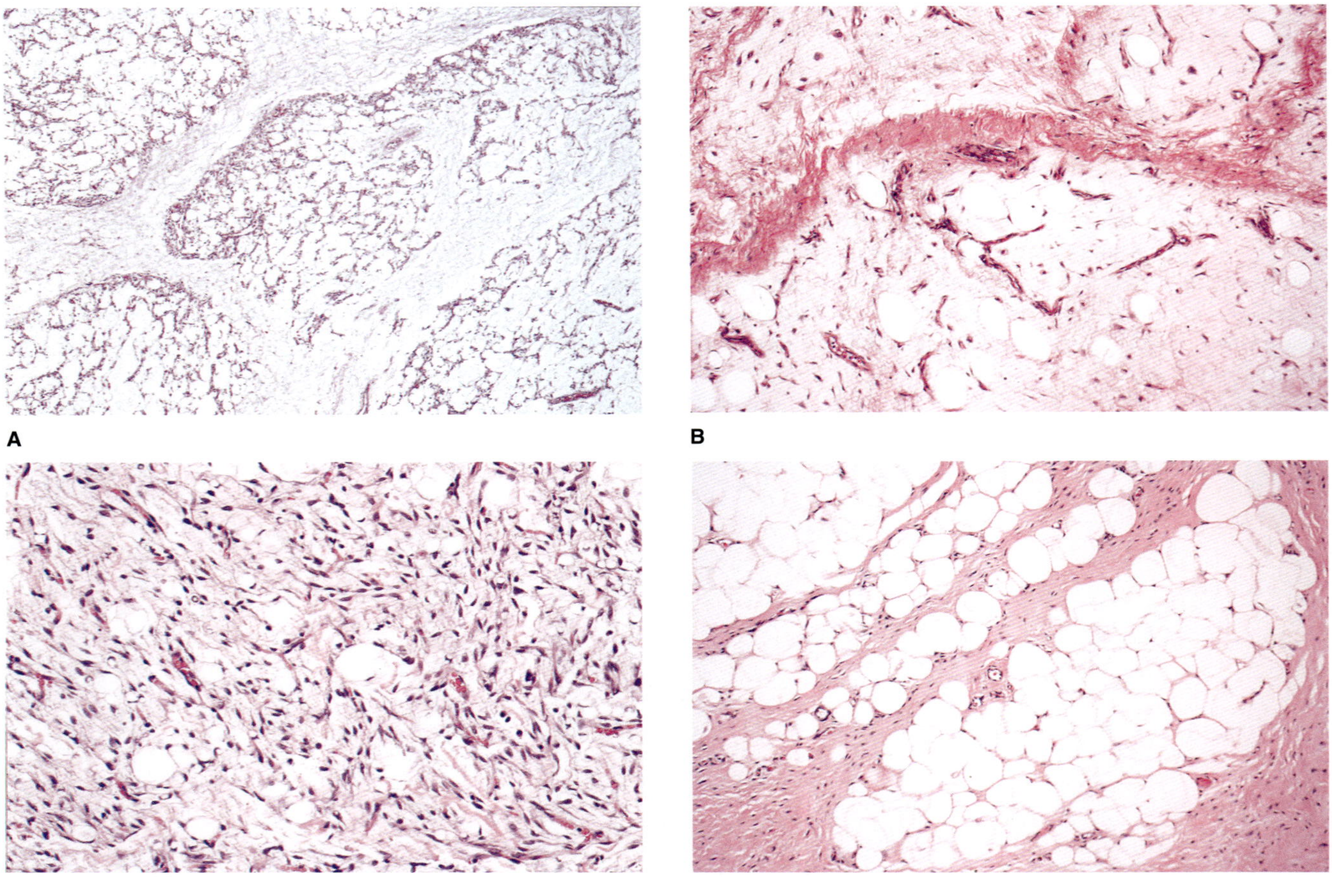

A B C D

Figure 8-20. Histologically lipoblastomas typically have microlobulation *(A),* and vary in maturation. *B,* Immature lipoblastoma with myxoid features and high vascularity. *C,* Lipoblastoma with spindle cell features. *D,* Mature lipoma-like lipoblastoma lobulated by fibrous septa.

their much greater tendency to undergo high-grade transformation (dedifferentiation).[85,86] Also, tumors whose cellularity and atypia are equal to that of pleomorphic liposarcoma are classified as such regardless of location. Pathology of these tumors is discussed with liposarcomas.

Atypical lipoma and well-differentiated liposarcoma are histologically identical, and they also show similar genetic changes consistent with their close relationship.[85,86] A subset of spindle cell and pleomorphic lipomas with pronounced atypia can also be classified into this group. Lipomas showing less significant atypia are sometimes designated as lipoma with focal or mild atypia; the specific significance of this finding is not known.

Clinical Features

The atypical lipomas predominantly occur in older age groups from the fifth to sixth decade on. They may present in a wide variety of subcutaneous locations, most commonly in the shoulder area, back, arm, and buttock. These tumors may recur locally, but transformation to high-grade sarcoma (dedifferentiation) and subsequent metastasis are very rare.

Pathology

The atypical nuclei are seen at the low magnification (4–10× objective) and show a wide variety of appearances, described with well-differentiated liposarcoma. Mitoses are not usually found. The occurrence of multinucleated histiocytes in focal fat necrosis should not be confused with atypia, although this feature often coexists with atypia. In some cases, the border between pleomorphic lipoma with marked atypia and atypical lipoma becomes arbitrary, and it will be safer to classify such tumors as the latter. These lesions are further discussed and illustrated in Chapter 9.

Genetics

Similar chromosomal rearrangements in 12q involving the gene encoding HMGIC have been found in atypical lipoma as seen in lipoma and in well-differentiated liposarcoma.[87,88]

Lipomatosis

Clinical Features

Table 8–3 summarizes the lipomatosis syndromes. This designation is used for a heterogeneous group of conditions all of which manifest as a diffuse regional collection of adipose tissue without a well-defined tumor mass.[89–95] Some lipomatoses are part of syndromes that may be hereditary, at least in some cases (diffuse symmetric lipomatosis, Madelung disease), and others may be based on acquired metabolic changes (e.g., steroid lipomatosis, by added corticosteroid stimulation).

Table 8–3. Summary of the Most Important Clinical Lipomatosis Syndromes[88–94]

Condition	Description
Diffuse lipomatosis	Lipomatous growth involving an entire region, such as an extremity
	Involves different tissue planes (subcutis, muscle), analogous to angiomatosis
Symmetrical lipomatosis (Madelung disease, Launois-Bensaude) syndrome)	Prominent fat collection symmetrically in the neck, upper trunk, arm. Some cases are hereditary, also reported in association with alcoholism
	Plastic surgery for debulking to prevent neurovascular and respiratory compromise
Pelvic lipomatosis	Pelvic fat collection. May cause urinary tract or colorectal obstruction. Predilection to blacks.
Encephalocraniocutaneous lipomatosis	Congenital hamartomatous condition with skin lesions, lipomas, and ipsilateral oculocerebral malformations. Reported in connection with neurofibromatosis type I.
Spinal epidural lipomatosis	May be associated with corticosteroid use or be idiopathic. Spinal decompression may be needed.
Steroid lipomatosis	Designation of lipomatous masses caused by excessive corticosteroid stimulation. May be endogenous (Cushing syndrome) or iatrogenic. A variety of sites can be affected.

Patients with diffuse symmetric lipomatosis (Madelung disease) have a diffuse fat collection in the anterior neck, shoulders, and upper body.[89–91] Pelvic lipomatosis presents often in black men, and the lipomatous masses may compromise urinary tract or colorectum.[92]

Pathology

Although these conditions are clinically distinctive, they are rarely seen as surgical specimens. Extensive regional disease in the extremity may clinically simulate a tumor, such as liposarcoma, and often has to be biopsied. Histologically, the fat does not differ from normal adipose tissue.

Genetics

Point mutations in codon 8344 in mitochondrial DNA encoding the transfer RNA gene for lysine have been detected in some patients with multiple symmetric lipomatosis.[96] Experimental truncation of the *HMGC1* gene in mouse was found to lead to abdominal and pelvic lipomatosis.[97] *HMCGC1* gene is known to be also involved in typical and atypical lipomas and in well-differentiated liposarcomas. If human pelvic lipomatosis shows similar changes, it raises the question whether some forms of lipomatosis may actually be lipomatous neoplasms.

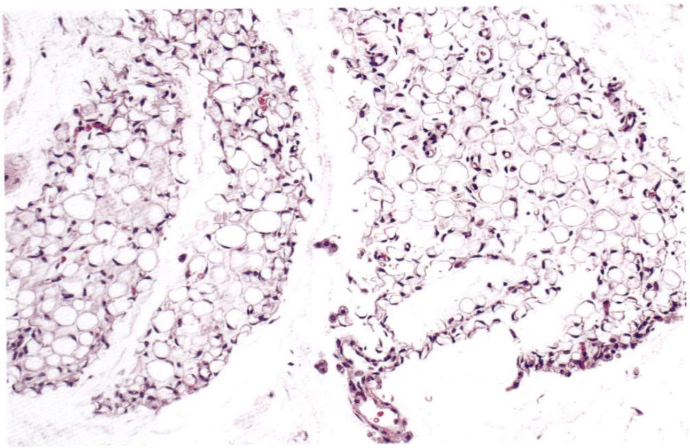

Figure 8–21. Fat atrophy shows distinct but shrunken lobules of well-differentiated fat.

Fatty or Fatlike Changes That Can Simulate Lipomatous Tumors

Fat Atrophy

Focal fat atrophy causes an area of skin depression and does not grossly look like a tumor. However, histologically it has a hypercellular appearance, because it shows shrunken fatty lobules partially or totally depleted of fat containing a prominent capillary pattern. There is no adipocytic atypia (Fig. 8–21).

Fat Necrosis

The response of adipose tissue to mechanical trauma or inflammation is fat necrosis with histiocyte infiltration. It is commonly seen at surgical sites and sometimes as small subcutaneous nodules. By added cellularity and mild pleomorphism seen in benign histiocytes, this condition may simulate liposarcoma. The infiltrating histiocytes often have larger nuclei than the fat cells and may include slightly atypical and multinucleated forms (Fig. 8–22). The appearance of the background adipocytes needs to be evaluated, because lipomatous neoplasms may also have fat necrosis.

Sclerosing Lipogranuloma

This is a reaction to lipid substance, which may be exogenous and related to paraffin oil injection for the cosmetic purposes of body part augmentation, or it may be of endogenous origin. The lesions usually occur in the external genitalia. The lipid material is found in extracellular spaces surrounded by sclerotic collagen, and there may be fat necrosis and lympho-

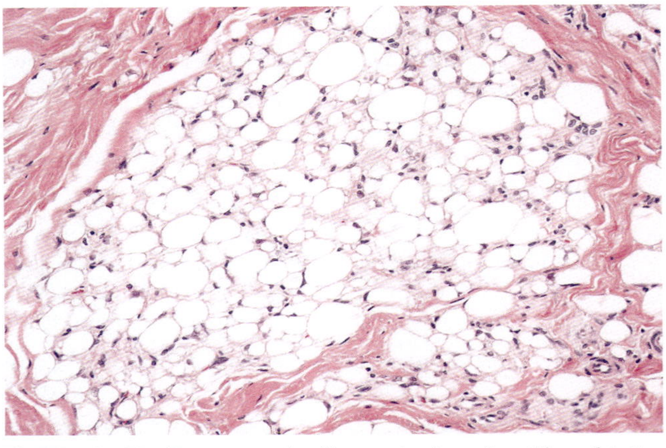

Figure 8–22. Fat necrosis (lipogranuloma) with a histiocytic reaction.

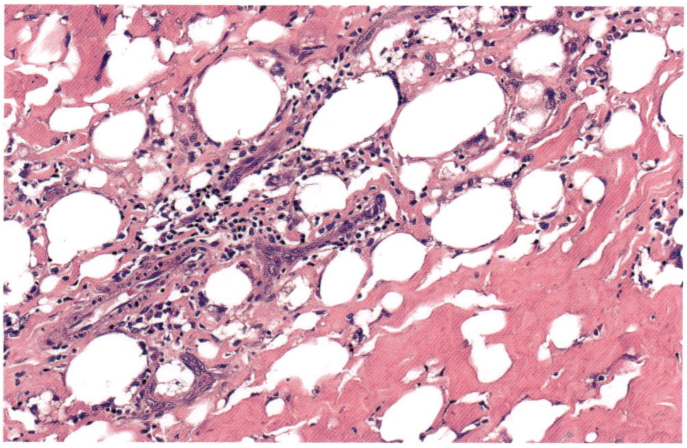

Figure 8–23. Sclerosing lipogranuloma shows empty fatty spaces surrounded by a sclerosing collagenous background with focal lymphoplasmacytoid reaction.

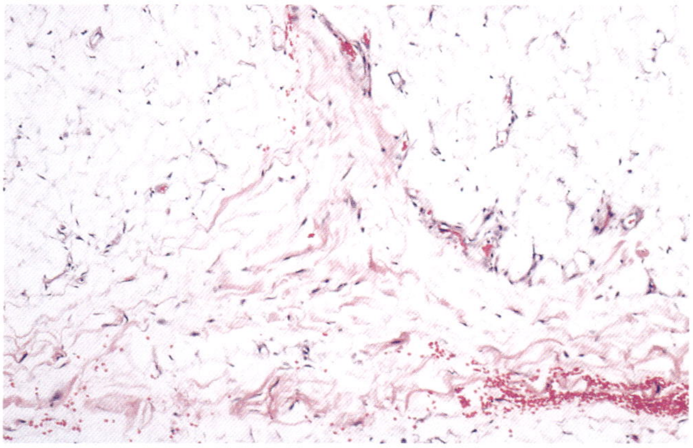

Figure 8–24. Lymphedema in obese patients shows adipose tissue with reactive changes, including enhanced edematous fibrous septa and periseptal vascular proliferation. The latter feature is not seen in liposarcoma.

plasmacytic reaction (Fig. 8–23). Systemic and tissue eosinophilia may accompany the endogenous lipogranulomas.[98,99]

Silicone Granuloma

Silicone seepage from tissue implants may resemble fat, but the deposition is in histiocytes usually around the fibrous capsule-like surrounding of the implant, such as silicone breast implants or less commonly silicone joint implants. The silicone material from breast implants may also reach the axillary lymph nodes.

Histologically, the extracellular silicone material becomes easily visible as birefringent when lowering the microscope condenser, but it is less easy to verify when in histiocytes. Histiocytic giant cells are present in some cases. Silicone often elicits a prominent fibrous reaction around breast implants. If specific verification is desired, silicone can be detected by x-ray microanalysis or laser-Raman microprobe analysis from lesional cells or tissue sections.[100–102]

Massive Localized Lymphedema in the Obese

This condition described by Farshid and Weiss usually involves the subcutis of medial thigh or less commonly proximal arm, where a large, pendulous tumor-like fatty prominence develops.[103] This lesion typically occurs in middle-aged patients who weigh more than 150 to 200 kg and may be precipitated by lymphadenectomy for carcinoma, varicose vein stripping, or local trauma. The lesions commonly weigh 5 to 10 kg and measure 20 to 30 cm. However, there is no distinct mass radiologically or clinically. The histologic findings may simulate well-differentiated liposarcoma by edematous, expanded, moderately cellular fibrous septa and interstitial fibrosis disturbing the normal lobular architecture of fat. The adipose elements also show interstitial expansion by fibroblastic proliferation and lymphoid infiltration. The presence of zones of neovascular capillaries bordering the fat and fibrous tissue and lack of adipocytic atypia separate this condition from liposarcoma (Fig. 8–24). Reactive inflammatory changes may also involve the overlying skin.

Neural Fibrolipoma (Fibrolipomatous Hamartoma of Nerves)

This rare condition occurs predominantly in children and young adults. It presents with an ill-defined, sometimes painful tumor-like lesion developing on the volar aspects of fingers and hands, usually around the median nerve. In many cases, the lesions are congenital, and there may be concomitant deformities in fingers and hands. Neural fibrolipoma is a nonneoplastic tumor-like condition and should not be treated by radical excision to avoid unnecessary nerve sacrifice; rather it should be diagnosed by biopsy and treated by nerve decompression when necessary.[104–106]

Grossly, the lesion represents a fibrofatty fusiform enlargement around a nerve, usually the median nerve. Histologically, it shows fibrofatty tissue containing nerves with surrounding fibrosis and sometimes mild perineurial cell proliferation (Fig. 8–25).

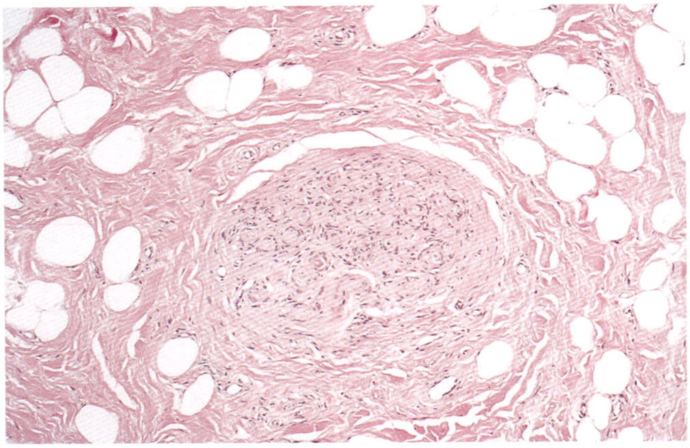

Figure 8-25. Neural fibrolipoma typically contains nerve branches with perineurial fibrosis in a fibrolipoma-like background.

Hemosiderotic Fibrohistiocytic Lipomatous Lesion

This condition, occurring mainly in middle-aged women in the foot and ankle, probably is a benign neoplasm with accompanying reactive changes. Grossly, it resembles lipoma with yellow-brown pigment. It is characterized by a well-delineated mass of homogeneously sized adipocytes with a quiltlike periseptal, periadipocytic, and perivascular proliferation of spindle cells, histiocytes, mast cells, and coarsely granulated iron pigment (Fig. 8-26). The spindled cells resemble those of spindle cell lipoma and are $CD34^+$. The lesion may reach a large size and locally recur.[107]

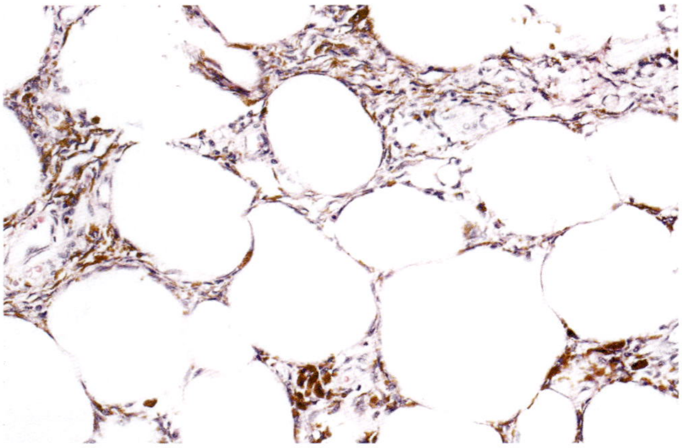

Figure 8-26. Hemosiderotic fibrohistiocytic lipomatous lesion contains a major mature fatty component, streaks of spindle cells, and hemosiderin.

REFERENCES

Lipoma

1. Myhre-Jensen O: A consecutive 7-year series of 1331 benign soft tissue tumours. Clinicopathologic data. Comparison with sarcomas. Acta Orthop Scand 1981; 52:287–293.
2. Rydholm A, Berg NO: Size, site and clinical incidence of lipoma. Factors in the differential diagnosis of lipoma and sarcoma. Acta Orthop Scand 1983;54:929–934.
3. Chalk CH, Mills KR, Jacobs JM, Donaghy M: Familial multiple symmetric lipomatosis with peripheral neuropathy. Neurology 1990;40:1246–1250.
4. Bjerregaard P, Hagen K, Daugaard S, Kofoed H: Intramuscular lipoma of the lower limb. Long-term follow-up after local resection. J Bone Joint Surg [Br] 1989;71:812–815.
5. Fletcher CD, Martin-Bates E: Intramuscular and intermuscular lipoma: Neglected diagnoses. Histopathology 1988;12:275–287.
6. Mrozek K, Karakousis CP, Bloomfield CD: Chromosome 12 breakpoints are cytogenetically different in benign and malignant lipogenic tumors: Localization of breakpoints in lipoma to 12q15 and in myxoid liposarcoma to 12q13.3. Cancer Res 1993;53:1670–1675.
7. Willen H, Akerman M, Dal Cin P, et al: Comparison of chromosomal patterns with clinical features in 165 lipomas: A report of the CHAMP study group. Cancer Genet Cytogenet 1998;102:46–49.
8. Petit MM, Schoenmakers EF, Hyusmans C, Geurts JM, Mandahl N, van de Ven WJ: LHFP, a novel translocation partner gene of HMGIC in a lipoma, is a member of a new family of LHFP-like genes. Genomics 1999;57:438–441.
9. Tallini G, Dal Cin P: HMGI(Y) and HMGI-C dysregulation: A common occurrence in human tumors. Adv Anat Pathol 1999;6:237–246.

Myolipoma, Chondrolipoma, and Osteolipoma

10. Meis JM, Enzinger FM: Myolipoma of soft tissue. Am J Surg Pathol 1991;15:121–125.
11. Marsh WL, Lucas JG, Olsen J: Chondrolipoma of breast. Arch Pathol Lab Med 1989;113:369–371.
12. Nwaorgy OK, Akang EE, Ahmad BM, Nwachokor FN, Olu-Eddo AN: Pharyngeal lipoma with cartilaginous metaplasia (chondrolipoma): A case report and literature review. J Laryngol Otol 1997;111:656–658.
13. Hopkins JDF, Rayan GM: Osteolipoma of the hand: A case report. J Okla State Med Assoc 1999;92:535–537.

Angiolipoma

14. Howard WR, Helwig EB: Angiolipoma. Arch Dermatol 1960;82:924–931.
15. Hunt SJ, Santa-Cruz DJ, Barr RJ: Cellular angiolipoma. Am J Surg Pathol 1990;14:75–81.
16. Pribyl C, Burke SW, Roberts JM, Mackenzie F, Johnston CE: Infiltrating angiolipoma or intramuscular heman-

gioma? A report of five cases. J Pediatr Orthop 1986; 6:172–176.
17. Sciot R, Akerman M, Dal Cin P, et al: Cytogenetic analysis of subcutaneous angiolipoma: Further evidence supporting its difference from ordinary pure lipomas: A report of the CHAMP study group. Am J Surg Pathol 1997;21:441–444.

Angiomyolipoma

18. Eble JN: Angiomyolipoma of the kidney. Semin Diagn Pathol 1998;15:21–40.
19. Bonetti F, Pea M, Martignoni G, et al: Clear cell "sugar" tumor of the lung is a lesion strictly related to angiomyolipoma: The concept of a family of lesions characterized by the presence of perivascular epitheloid cell (PEC). Pathology 1994;26:230–236.
20. Zamboni G, Pea M, Martignoni G, et al: Clear cell "sugar" tumor of the pancreas. A novel member of the family of lesions characterized by the presence of perivascular epithelioid cells. Am J Surg Pathol 1996; 20:722–730.
21. Tong YC, Chieng PU, Tsai TC, Lin SN: Renal angiomyolipoma: Report of 24 cases. Br J Urol 1990; 66: 585–589.
22. Kennelly MJ, Grossman HB, Cho KJ: Outcome analysis of 42 cases of renal angiomyolipoma. J Urol 1994; 152:1998–1991.
23. Chen SS, Lin AT, Chen KK, Chang LS: Renal angiomyolipoma—Experience of 20 years in Taiwan. Eur Urol 1997;32:175–178.
24. L'Hostis H, Deminiere C, Ferriere JM, Coindre JM: Renal angiomyolipoma: A clinicopathologic, immunohistochemical, and follow-up study of 46 cases. Am J Surg Pathol 1999;23:1011–1020.
25. Eble JN, Amin MB, Young RH: Epithelioid angiomyolipoma of the kidney: A report of five cases with a prominent and diagnostically confusing epithelioid smooth muscle component. Am J Surg Pathol 1997; 21:1123–1130.
26. Martignoni G, Pea M, Bonetti F, et al: Carcinomalike monotypic epithelioid angiomyolipoma in patients without evidence of tuberous sclerosis: A clinicopathologic and genetic study. Am J Surg Pathol 1998;22: 663–672.
27. Delgado R, de Leon Bojorge B, Albores-Saavedra J: Atypical angiomyolipoma of the kidney: A distinct morphologic variant that is easily confused with a variety of malignant neoplasms. Cancer 1998;83:1581–1592.
28. Goodman ZD, Ishak KG: Angiomyolipomas of the liver. Am J Surg Pathol 1984;8:745–750.
29. Tsui WM, Colombari R, Portmann BC, et al: Hepatic angiomyolipoma: A clinicopathologic study of 30 cases and delineation of unusual morphologic variants. Am J Surg Pathol 1999;23:34–48.
30. Nonomura A, Minato H, Kurumaya H: Angiomyolipoma predominantly composed of smooth muscle cells: Problems in histological diagnosis. Histopathology 1998;33:20–27.
31. Hruban RH, Bhagavan BS, Epstein JH: Massive retroperitoneal angiomyolipoma. A lesion that may be confused with well-differentiated liposarcoma. Am J Clin Pathol 1989;92:805–808.
32. Pea M, Bonetti F, Zamboni G, Martignoni G, et al: Melanocyte-marker HMB-45 is regularly expressed in angiomyolipoma of the kidney. Pathology 1991; 23:185–188.
33. Chan JK, Tsang WY, Pau MY, Tang MC, Pang SW, Fletcher CD: Lymphangio-myomatosis and angiomyolipoma: Closely related entities characterized by hamartomatous proliferation of HMB-45-positive smooth muscle cells. Histopathology 1993;22:445–455.
34. Fetsch PA, Fetsch JF, Marincola FM, Travis W, Batts KP, Abati A: Comparison of melanoma antigen recognized by T-cell (MART-1) to HMB-45: Additional evidence to support a common lineage for angiomyolipoma, lymphangiomyomatosis and clear cell sugar tumor. Mod Pathol 1998;11:699–703.
35. Bonsib SM: HMB-45 reactivity in renal leiomyomas and leiomyosarcomas. Mod Pathol 1996;9:664–669.
36. Green AJ, Smith M, Yater RRW: Loss of heterozygosity on chromosome 16p13.3 in hamartomas from tuberous sclerosis patients. Nat Genet 1994;6: 193–196.
37. Henske EP, Neumann HP, Scheithauer BW, Herbst EW, Short MP, Kwiatkowski DJ: Loss of heterozygosity in the tuberous sclerosis (TSC2) region of chromosome band 16p13 occurs in sporadic as well as TSC-associated angiomyolipomas. Genes Chromosom Cancer 1995;13:295–298.
38. Plank TL, Loggindou H, Klein-Szanto A, Henske EP: The expression of hamartin, the product of the TSC1 gene, in normal human tissues and in TSC1- and TSC2-linked angiomyolipomas. Mod Pathol 1999;12: 539–545.
39. Dal Cin P, Sciot R, Van Poppel H, Baert L, Van Damme B, Van den Berghe H: Chromosome analysis in angiomyolipoma. Cancer Genet Cytogenet 1997; 99:132–134.
40. De Jong B, Castedo SM, Oosterhuis JW, Dam A: Trisomy 7 in a case of angiomyolipoma. Cancer Genet Cytogenet 1998;34:219–222.
41. Debiec-Rychter M, Saryusz-Wolska H, Salagierski M: Cytogenetic analysis of renal angiomyolipoma. Genes Chromosom Cancer 1992;4:101–103.
42. Kattar MM, Grignon DJ, Eble JN, et al: Chromosomal analysis of renal angiomyolipoma by comparative genomic hybridization: Evidence for clonal origin. Hum Pathol 1999;30:295–299.
43. Paradis V, Laurendeau I, Viellefond A, et al: Clonal analysis of renal sporadic angiomyolipomas. Hum Pathol 1998;29:1063–1067.
44. Saxena A, Alport EC, Cuastead S, Skinnider LF: Molecular analysis of clonality of sporadic angiomyolipoma. J Pathol 1999;189:79–84.

Chondroid Lipoma

45. Meis JM, Enzinger FM: Chondroid lipoma. A unique tumor simulating liposarcoma and myxoid chondrosarcoma. Am J Surg Pathol 1993;17:1103–1112.

46. Nielsen GP, O'Connell JX, Dickersin GR, Rosenberg AE: Chondroid lipoma. Am J Surg Pathol 1995; 19:1272–1276.
47. Thomson TA, Horsman D, Bainbridge TC: Cytogenetic and cytologic features of chondroid lipoma of soft tissue. Mod Pathol 1999;12:88–91.

Myelolipoma

48. Noble MJ, Montague DK, Levin HS: Myelolipoma: An unusual surgical lesion of the adrenal gland. Cancer 1982;49:952–958.
49. Fowler MR, Williams RM, Alba JM, Burd CR: Extraadrenal myelolipomas compared with extramedullary hematopoietic tumors: A case of presacral myelolipoma. Am J Surg Pathol 1983;6:363–374.
50. Hunter SB, Schemankewitz EH, Patterson C, Varma VA: Extraadrenal myelolipoma. A report of two cases. Am J Clin Pathol 1992;97:402–404.
51. Sanders R, Bissada N, Cutty N, Gordon B: Clinical spectrum of adrenal myelolipoma: Analysis of 8 tumors in 7 patients. J Urol 1995;153:1791–1793.
52. Shapiro JL, Goldblum JR, Bobrow DA, Ratliff NB: Giant bilateral extraadrenal myelolipoma. Arch Pathol Lab Med 1995;119:283–285.

Spindle Cell and Pleomorphic Lipoma

53. Enzinger FM, Harvey DA: Spindle cell lipoma. Cancer 1975;36:1852–1859.
54. Shmookler BM, Enzinger FM: Pleomorphic lipoma: A benign tumor simulating liposarcoma. A clinicopathologic analysis of 48 cases. Cancer 1981;47:126–133.
55. Angervall L, Dahl I, Kindblom LG, Save-Soderbergh J: Spindle cell lipoma. Acta Pathol Microbiol Scand [A] 1976;84:477–487.
56. Fletcher CD, Martin-Bates E: Spindle cell lipoma: A clinicopathologic study with some original observations. Histopathology 1987;11:803–817.
57. Azzopardi JG, Iocco J, Salm R: Pleomorphic lipoma: A tumor simulating liposarcoma. Histopathology 1983;7:511–523.
58. Fanburg-Smith JF, Miettinen M, Weiss SW: Multiple spindle cell lipomas. Am J Surg Pathol 1998;22:40–48.
59. Zelger BW, Zelger BG, Plorer A, Steiner H, Fritsch PO: Dermal spindle cell lipoma: Plexiform and nodular variants. Histopathology 1995;27:533–540.
60. Hawley ICV, Krausz T, Evans DJ, Fletcher CD: Spindle cell lipoma—A pseudoangiomatous variant. Histopathology 1994;24:565–569.
61. Suster S, Fisher C: CD34 in lipomatous tumors. Am J Surg Pathol 1997;21:195–200.
62. Templeton SF, Solomon AR: Spindle cell lipoma is strongly CD34 positive. An immunohistochemical study. J Cutan Pathol 1996;23:546–550.
63. Beham A, Schmid C, Hodl S, Fletcher CD: Spindle cell and pleomorphic lipoma: An immunohistochemical study and histogenetic analysis. J Pathol 1989;158: 219–222.
64. Mandahl N, Mertens F, Willen H, Rydholm A, Brosjo O, Mitelman F: A new cytogenetic subgroup in lipomas: Loss of chromosome 16 material in spindle cell and pleomorphic lipomas. J Cancer Res Clin Oncol 1994;120:707–711.
65. Dal Cin P, Sciot R, Polito P, et al: Lesions of 13q may occur independently of deletion of 16q in spindle cell/pleomorphic lipomas. Histopathology 1997; 31:222–225.

Hibernoma

66. Kindblom LG, Angervall L, Stener B, Wickbom I: Intramuscular and intermuscular lipomas and hibernomas. A clinical roentgenologic, histologic and prognostic study of 46 cases. Cancer 1974;33:754–762.
67. Gaffney EF, Hargreaves HK, Semple E, Vellios F: Hibernoma: Distinctive light and electron microscopic features and relationship to brown adipose tissue. Hum Pathol 1983;14:677–687.
68. Furlong MA, Fanburg-Smith JC, Miettinen M: The morphologic spectrum of hibernoma: A clinicopathologic study of 170 cases. Am J Surg Pathol 2001;25: 809–814.
69. Zancanaro C, Pelosi G, Accordini C, Balercia G, Sbabo L, Cinti S: Immunohistochemical identification of the uncoupling protein in human hibernoma. Biol Cell 1994;80:75–78.
70. Meloni AM, Spanier SS, Bush CH, Stone JF, Sandberg AA: Involvement of 10q22 and 11q13 in hibernoma. Cancer Genet Cytogenet 1994;72:59–64.
71. Mertens F, Rydholm A, Brosjo O, Willen H, Mitelman F, Mandahl N: Hibernomas are characterized by rearrangements of chromosome bands 11q13-21. Int J Cancer 1994;58:503–505.
72. Mrozek K, Karakousis CP, Bloomfield CD: Band 11q13 is nonrandomly rearranged in hibernomas. Genes Chromosomes Cancer 1994;9:145–147.
73. Gisselson D, Hoglund M, Mertens F, Dal Cin P, Mandahl N: Hibernomas are characterized by homozygous deletions in the multiple endocrine neoplasia type I region. Metaphase fluorescence in situ hybridization reveals complex rearrangements not detected by conventional cytogenetics. Am J Pathol 1999;155:61–66.

Lipoblastoma

74. Chung EB, Enzinger FM: Benign lipoblastomatosis. An analysis of 35 cases. Cancer 1973;32:482–492.
75. Mahour GH, Bryan BJ, Isaacs H: Lipoblastoma and lipoblastomatosis—A report of six cases. Surgery 1988;104:577–579.
76. Mentzel T, Calonje E, Fletcher CD: Lipoblastoma and lipoblastomatosis: A clinicopathological study of 14 cases. Histopathology 1993;23:527–533.
77. Coffin CM: Lipoblastoma: An embryonal tumor of soft tissue related to organogenesis. Semin Diagn Pathol 1994;11:98–103.
78. Collins MH, Chatten J: Lipoblastoma/lipoblastomatosis: A clinicopathologic study of 25 tumors. Am J Surg Pathol 1997;21:1131–1137.
79. Miller GC, Yanchar NL, Magee JF, Blair GK: Lipoblastoma and liposarcoma in children: An analysis of

9 cases and review of the literature. Can J Surg 1998; 41:455–458.
80. Ohjimi Y, Iwasaki H, Kaneko Y, Ishiguro M, Ohgami A, Kikuchi M: A case of lipoblastoma with t(3;8) (q12;q11.2). Cancer Genet Cytogenet 1992;62: 103–105.
81. Fletcher JA, Kozakewich HP, Schoenberg ML, Morton CC: Cytogenetic findings in pediatric adipose tissue tumors: Consistent rearrangement of chromosome 8 in lipoblastoma. Genes Chromosomes Cancer 1993; 6:24–29.
82. Dal Cin P, Sciot R, DeWever I, van Damme B, van den Berghe H: New discriminative chromosomal marker in adipose tissue tumors. The chromosome 8q11-q13 region in lipoblastoma. Cancer Genet Cytogenet 1994;78:232–235.
83. Sawyer JR, Parsons EA, Crowson ML, Smith S, Erickson S, Bell JM: Potential diagnostic implications of breakpoints in the long arm of chromosome 8 in lipoblastoma. Cancer Genet Cytogenet 1994;76:39–42.
84. Astrom A, D'Amore ES, Sainati L, et al: Evidence of involvement of the PLAG1 gene in lipoblastomas. Int J Oncol 2000;16:1107–1110.

Atypical Lipoma

85. Evans HL, Soule EH, Winkelmann RK: Atypical lipoma, atypical intramuscular lipoma, and well-differentiated retroperitoneal liposarcoma: A reappraisal of 30 cases formerly classified as well-differentiated liposarcoma. Cancer 1979;43:574–584.
86. Weiss SW, Rao VK: Well-differentiated liposarcoma (atypical lipoma) of deep soft tissue of the extremities, retroperitoneum and miscellaneous sites. A follow-up study of 92 cases with analysis of the incidence of "dedifferentiation." Am J Surg Pathol 1992; 167:1051–1058.
87. Tallini G, Dal Cin P, Rhoden KJ, et al: Expression of HMGI-C and HMGI(Y) in ordinary lipoma and atypical lipomatous tumors: Immunohistochemical reactivity correlates with karyotypic alterations. Am J Pathol 1997;151:37–43.
88. Szymanska J, Virolainen M, Tarkkanen M, et al: Overrepresentation of 1q21-23 and 12q13-21 in lipoma-like liposarcomas but not in benign lipomas: A comparative genomic hybridization study. Cancer Genet Cytogenet 1997;99:14–18.

Lipomatosis

89. Enzi G: Multiple symmetric lipomatosis: Updated clinical report. Medicine 1984;63:56–64.
90. Plotnicov NA, Babayev TA, Lamberg MA, Aaltonen M, Syrjänen SM: Madelung's disease (benign symmetric lipomatosis). Oral Surg Oral Med Oral Pathol 1988; 66:171–175.
91. Smith PD, Stedelmann WK, Wassermann RJ, Kearney RE: Benign symmetric lipomatosis (Madelung's disease). Ann Plast Surg 1998;41:671–673.
92. Klein FA, Smith MJ, Kasenetz I: Pelvic lipomatosis: 35-year experience. J Urol 1988;139:998–1001.
93. Stern JD, Quint DJ, Swaesey TA, Hoff JT: Spinal epidural lipomatosis: Two new idiopathic cases and a review of the literature. J Spinal Disord 1994;7: 343–349.
94. Legius E, Wu R, Eyssen M, Marynen P, Fryns JP, Cassiman JJ: Encephalocraniocutaneous lipomatosis with a mutation in the NF1 gene. J Med Genet 1995; 32:316–319.
95. Carlsen A, Thomsen M: Different clinical types of lipomatosis. A case report. Scand J Plast Reconstr Surg 1978;12:75–79.
96. Battista S, Fidanza V, Fedele M, et al: The expression of truncated HMGI-C gene induces giantism associated with lipomatosis. Cancer Res 1999;59:4793–4797.
97. Munoz-Malaga A, Bautista J, Salazar JA, et al: Lipomatosis, proximal myopathy, and the mitochondrial 8344 mutation. A lipid storage myopathy? Muscle Nerve 2000;23:538–542.

Reactive Conditions Simulating Fatty Neoplasms

98. Oertel YC, Johnson FB: Sclerosing lipogranuloma of male genitalia. Review of 23 cases. Arch Pathol Lab Med 1977;101:321–326.
99. Matsuda T, Shichiri Y, Hida S, et al: Eosinophilic sclerosing lipogranuloma of the male genitalia not caused by exogenous lipids. J Urol 1988;140:1021–1024.
100. Greene WB, Raso DS, Walsh LG, Harley RA, Silver RM: Electron probe microanalysis of silicon and the role of macrophage in proximal (capsule) and distant sites in augmentation mammoplasty patients. Plastic Reconstr Surg 1995;95:513–519.
101. Luke JL, Kalasinsky VF, Turnicky RP, Centeno JA, Johnson FB, Mullick FG: Pathological and biophysical findings associated with silicone breast implants: A study of capsular tissues from 86 cases. Plastic Reconstr Surg 1997;100:1558–1565.
102. Centeno JA, Mullick FG, Panos RG, Miller FW, Valenzuela-Espinoza A: Laser-Raman microprobe identification of inclusions in capsules associated with silicone gel breast implants. Mod Pathol 1999;12: 714–721.
103. Farshid G, Weiss SW: Massive localized lymphedema in the morbidly obese: A histologically distinct reactive lesion simulating liposarcoma. Am J Surg Pathol 1998;22:1277–1283.
104. Haverbush TJ, Kendrick JI, Nelson CL: Intraneural lipoma of the median nerve: Report of two cases. Cleveland Clin Q 1970;37:145–149.
105. Silverman TA, Enzinger FM: Fibrolipomatous hamartoma of the nerve: A clinicopathologic analysis of 26 cases. Am J Surg Pathol 1985;9:7–14.
106. Brodwater BK, Major NM, Goldner RD, Layfield LJ: Macrodystrophia lipomatosa with associated fibrolipomatous hamartoma of the median nerve. Pediatr Surg Int 2000;16:216–218.
107. Marshall-Taylor C, Fanburg-Smith JC: Hemosiderotic fibrohistiocytic lesion: 10 cases of a previously undescribed fatty lesion of the foot/ankle. Mod Pathol 2000;3:1192–1199.

Liposarcoma

CHAPTER 9

Liposarcoma is the designation for a group of histologically and genetically distinct sarcomas with fatty differentiation. Together these tumors are among the most common sarcomas (25–35%). The two histologically and genetically distinct main types are well-differentiated and myxoid-round cell liposarcoma. Round cell liposarcoma, originally considered a type of its own, is now considered a high grade variant of myxoid liposarcoma. Dedifferentiated liposarcoma is a transformed variant usually developing from well-differentiated liposarcoma and represents its histologic disease progression. A third type, pleomorphic liposarcoma, is histologically well defined but is genetically less understood; its possible genetic and histogenetic relationship with the other types is open. All these types[1,2] represent clinicopathologic entities and are therefore considered here separately. Table 9–1 shows an overview of liposarcoma types and their clinicopathologic features.

The different types of liposarcomas present in different ages and sites. The well-differentiated type occurs primarily in middle-aged and older persons in the extremities and retroperitoneum, myxoid-round cell type in the extremities of young adults, and pleomorphic liposarcomas in the extremities and retroperitoneum of older patients. Well-documented liposarcomas, especially the myxoid ones, are sometimes seen in children in the second decade and very rarely in small children.[3–5]

Most liposarcomas occur in deep soft tissues, whereas lipomas are usually subcutaneous. No significant etiologic clues are available. However, liposarcomas seem to be distinctly uncommon among postirradiation sarcomas. Genetic studies on liposarcomas have led to discovery of many genes important in the transcriptional regulation and metabolism of fatty tissue, and a molecular genetic test is available to test for the fusion transcripts for myxoid liposarcoma translocation.

Promising results were recently reported from experimental treatment of patients with liposarcoma with a peroxisome proliferator, troglitazone, previously used for the treatment of diabetes.[6]

The diagnosis of liposarcoma is based on recognition of the typical histologic pattern of any specific type of liposarcoma. Adipocytic atypia is present by definition. Although multivacuolated lipoblasts are often found in all types of liposarcoma, they are not required for diagnosis and are uncommon in well-differentiated tumors. Fat stains are not very useful, because fat is present in other tumors, for example, in malignant fibrous histiocytoma (MFH; undifferentiated sarcoma) and in renal carcinoma.

Well-Differentiated Liposarcoma

Clinical Features

Well-differentiated liposarcoma (WDLS) is the most common variant of liposarcoma, accounting for up to 50% of the cases. It occurs virtually exclusively in adults and generally presents in the fifth to eighth decades. Among liposarcomas, WDLS shows the

Table 9–1. Overview of Liposarcoma Types and Their Clinicopathologic Features

Type	Estimated Frequency	Age at Presentation	Typical Sites	Behavior	Genetics
Well-differentiated	>50%	Middle-aged to old	Extremities Retroperitoneum	Local recurrence and risk of dedifferentiation	12q amplification
Dedifferentiated	5%	Middle-aged to old	Extremities Retroperitoneum	Risk for metastasis	
Myxoid-round cell	30–40%	Rarely in children Adults, often below the age of 40 yr	Extremities, especially the thigh	Recurrence if not widely excised. Metastases low in myxoid, high in round cell variants	t(12;16)
Pleomorphic	<5%	Old age	Extremities Retroperitoneum	High risk for recurrence and metastasis	Complex, poorly known

greatest resemblance to normal adipose tissue. This tumor is most common in the deep soft tissues of the extremities, including buttocks and shoulder area (60–70%), followed by retroperitoneum, inguinal region, and paratesticular location in the scrotum (together 30–40%). Occurrence in distal extremities is rare. Rare sites for WDLS include larynx and mediastinum.[7–12]

By definition, the subcutaneous well-differentiated adipose tissue tumors are preferentially classified as atypical lipomatous tumors because of their low overall potential and nonexistent metastatic potential. Although these tumors are histologically and genetically identical with WDLS, they are classified in the borderline group because of their low biologic potential and very low risk for progression into dedifferentiated liposarcoma.

Well-differentiated liposarcoma in any location has a high tendency to recur locally unless the tumor is completely excised. WDLS of the extremities has a very low disease-related mortality, but we have seen patients who died of pulmonary metastasis following dedifferentiation, a relatively rare event with the extremity-based tumors. WDLS of the retroperitoneum has a greater tendency to develop multiple recurrences, sometimes over 10 to 15 years. These tumors may be ultimately fatal due to locally uncontrollable disease or following dedifferentiation and metastasis, which is much more common in retroperitoneal tumors. However, some patients with dedifferentiated tumors may live years with the tumor, even after lung metastases. Two published series both found 14% mortality of WDLS, one of them only related to retroperitoneal disease.[9,10] However, this figure probably underestimates the mortality of retroperitoneal liposarcoma in long-term follow-up.

Wide excision is the preferred treatment in the case of extremity tumors. It is often impossible to perform wide excision for a retroperitoneal liposarcoma, and therefore tumors of this location are prone to relentless recurrences and subsequent transformation (dedifferentiation).

Gross Pathology

Grossly, WDLSs are often large tumors. Their maximum diameter in the thigh often exceeds 10 cm and in the retroperitoneum 20 cm and several kilograms in weight. WDLS of the extremities may be homogeneous tumors with a lipomatous appearance (Fig. 9–1), but they may also contain

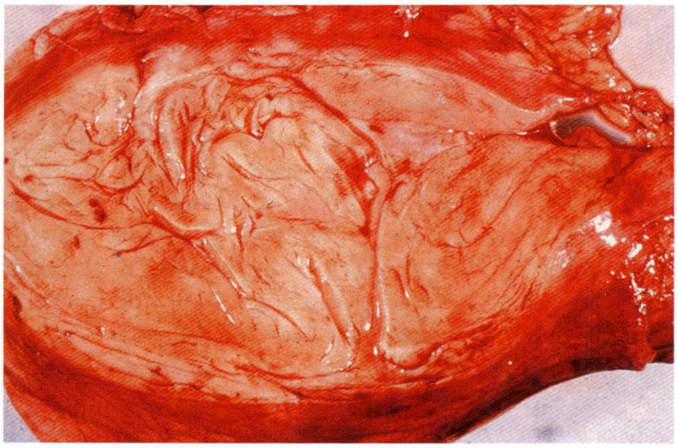

Figure 9–1. Well-differentiated intramuscular lipoma-like liposarcoma is a yellow tumor. Narrow streaks of fibrosis are present.

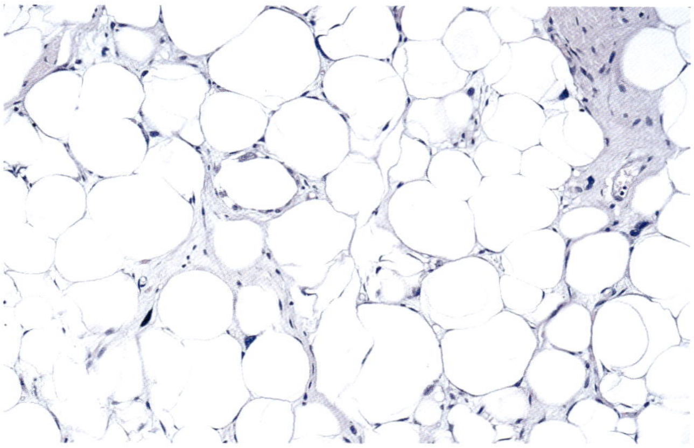

Figure 9-2. WDLS has significant nuclear atypia and widened fibrous septa at low magnification.

firm, white areas. The fatlike areas often have a paler yellow color than mature lipomas. Increased fibrous septa often give the tumors a slightly firmer consistency than observed in lipomas. The retroperitoneal WDLS often show significant macroscopic heterogeneity including yellow lipoma-like, gray myxoid to rubbery and firm, gray, sclerosing components.

Histologic Features

Five main histologic patterns are recognized for WDLS: lipoma-like, sclerosing, myxoid, inflammatory (lymphocyte-rich), and spindle cell; the last, if nonlipogenic, may represent dedifferentiation. The patterns overlap and often coexist in the same tumor, especially in the larger retroperitoneal liposarcomas.

Histologically, the lipoma-like areas may closely simulate lipoma and may be impossible to diagnose as liposarcoma if taken out of context or in a small biopsy. However, widened fibrous septa with hypercellularity and convincing cytologic atypia (diagnosable at low magnification with 4–10 × objective) are always present at least focally (Fig. 9–2). In such cells the atypical, crescent-shaped or pleomorphic, multilobated nucleus is seen in the cell periphery (Fig. 9–3*A* and *B*). Multivacuolated lipoblasts may

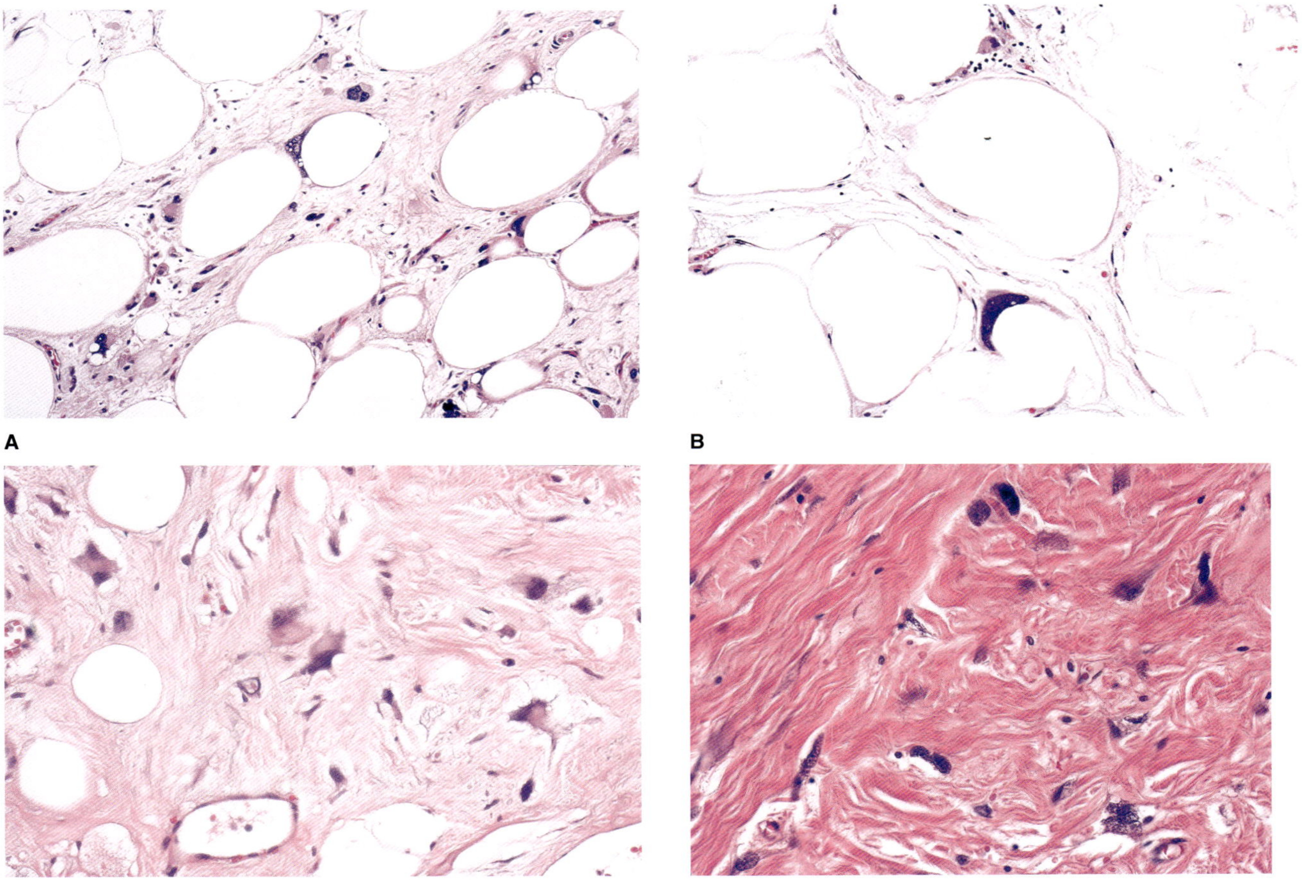

A B C D

Figure 9-3. Different appearances of WDLS, all with significant fat cell atypia. *A* and *B*, Lipoma-like. *C* and *D*, Sclerosing.

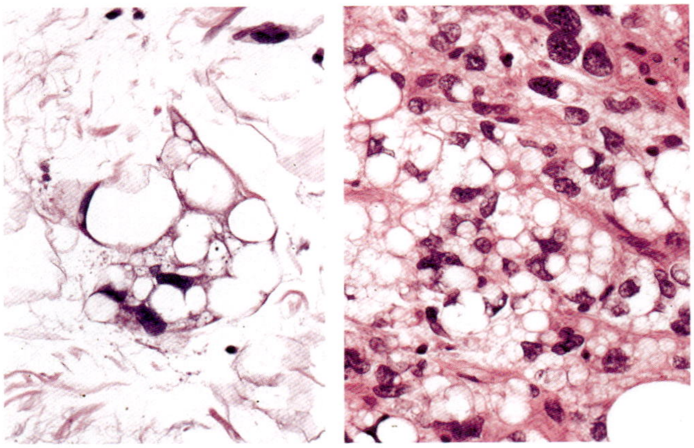

Figure 9-4. Atypical, multivacuolated lipoblasts are often seen in WDLS, but they are not required for diagnosis *(left)*. Lipoblasts are more numerous in pleomorphic liposarcomas *(right)*.

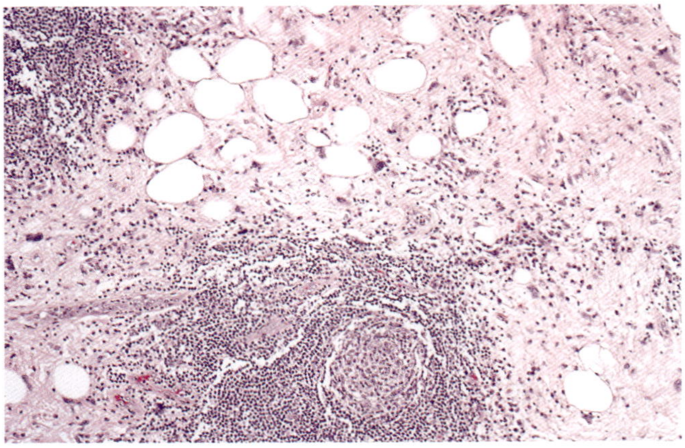

Figure 9-6. Inflammatory well-differentiated liposarcoma contains lymphoplasmacytoid infiltration around the atypical lipomatous component.

be present but their presence is not required for the diagnosis (Fig. 9–4).

Other features often seen in WDLS more often than lipoma are focal lymphoid infiltration, adipocyte cell size variation, and single-cell fat necrosis. However, to some degree these features may also occur in ordinary lipoma. Mitotic activity is very low and is not required for diagnosis.

The sclerosing WDLS seen as the only pattern or a component of WDLS contains atypical cells embedded in a dense collagenous or variably myxoid matrix; some of these cells show fatty differentiation. Prominent nuclear pleomorphism with mild mitotic activity may be present (Fig. 9–3*C* and *D*). Nevertheless, the pleomorphism in the context of a fibrous matrix-rich liposarcoma should not be considered pleomorphic liposarcoma, which is a densely cellular, high-grade liposarcoma. A peculiar change often seen in well-differentiated liposarcoma is vascular smooth muscle proliferation with mild atypia in medium-sized tumoral vessels (Fig. 9–5).

The inflammatory variant of WDLS shows scattered and clustered lymphoid cells, sometimes with germinal center formation. The tumor may have a myxoid-sclerosing stroma and be confused with inflammatory pseudotumor.[13,14] Lipomatous atypia, presence of lipoblasts, or both allow for the identification of this as a WDLS (Fig. 9–6).

Spindle cell areas may be seen in WDLS, especially in retroperitoneal tumors, but similar features may also be seen in peripheral WDLS (Fig. 9–7). With increasing cellularity and pleomorphism the border between well-differentiated and pleomorphic liposarcoma may become arbitrary.

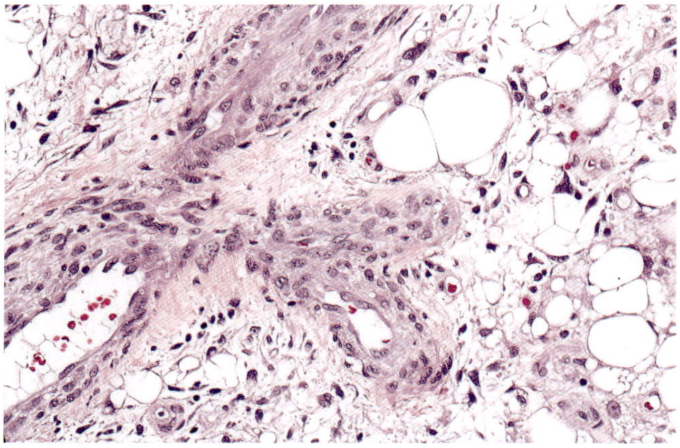

Figure 9-5. WDLS showing blood vessels with smooth muscle proliferation with mild atypia.

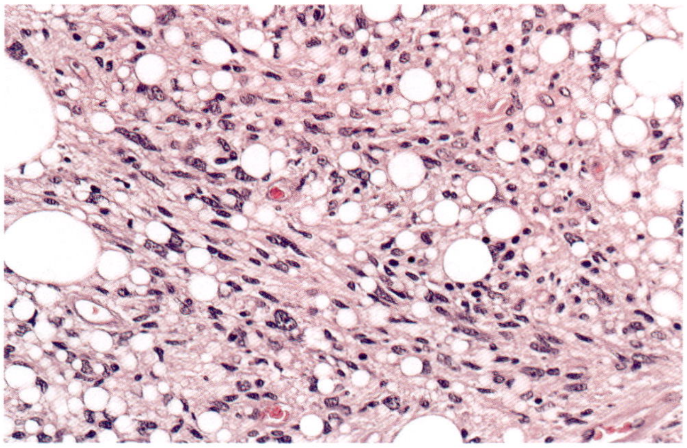

Figure 9-7. An unusual cellular spindle cell pattern in WDLS. This is not dedifferentiation because fatty differentiation is present.

Immunohistochemistry

Immunohistochemistry is currently of limited value in the diagnosis of liposarcoma, but if antibodies to transcriptional regulators or another proteins specific for adipose tissue become available they would be of great interest. Although normal fat cells are positive for S-100 protein, neoplastic adipocytes react inconsistently. CD34 positivity is common in the spindle cells and fat cells in WDLSs. Desmin and keratin positivity may also occur, in our experience.

Differential Diagnosis

Conditions that may simulate WDLS include fat necrosis, reactive fatty changes in extremely obese persons, and categories of benign lipoma, especially spindle cell, pleomorphic, and chondroid lipoma. Lipogranuloma and silicone deposition may superficially resemble WDLS. Sclerosing extramedullary myeloid tumor with atypical megakaryocytes in a fibrosclerotic background may also simulate liposarcoma; these tumors occur in connection with chronic myeloproliferative disorders.[15] This distinction is aided by documentation of the large atypical cells as megakaryocytes (Factor-VIII-related antigen [FVIIIRAg], $CD61^{+}$), and observation of other immature hematopoietic components, especially eosinophilic myelocytes (Fig. 9–8).

Deep lipomatous tumors with limited atypia (especially those in retroperitoneum) are often problematic. They should be sampled extensively. If in doubt, they should be diagnosed as well-differentiated lipomatous tumors, with the statement added that the possibility of WDLS cannot be ruled out.

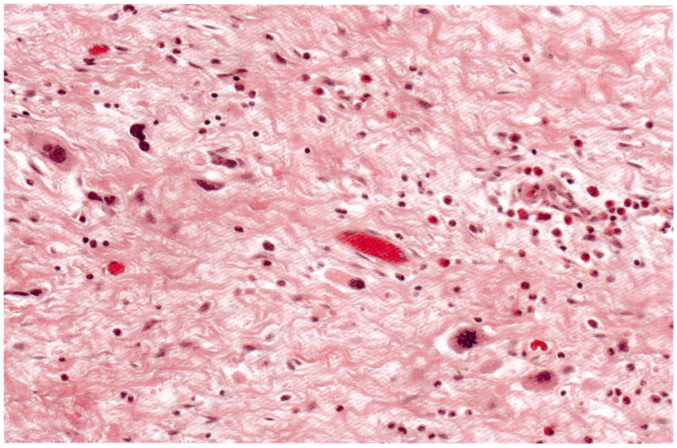

Figure 9–8. Sclerosing extramedullary myeloid tumor may simulate well-differentiated sclerosing liposarcoma. The large, atypical cells are megakaryocytes. Note also scattered eosinophilic myelocytes.

Genetics

The genetic changes described in WDLS include most importantly gene rearrangements of 12q.[16–18] The giant marker chromosomes and ring chromosomes seen in cytogenetic studies are derived from the amplified sequences of the 12q. Comparative genomic hybridization and fluorescent in situ hybridization (FISH) studies have also shown gains or amplifications in this area. Genes that are located in this area and may be involved include *SAS* (sarcoma amplified sequence), *MDM2* (murine double minute chromosome), and *CDK4* (cyclin-dependent kinase 4).[19]

Dedifferentiated Liposarcoma

Clinical Features

This term refers to the presence of solid sheets (not only small foci) of undifferentiated, nonlipogenic areas in WDLS. According to suggested definition of Hendricks and colleagues,[20] the nonlipogenic solid area has to be grossly visible and measure at least 1 cm in diameter.

The dedifferentiated components may present in the primary tumor or in a recurrence. Most commonly dedifferentiation occurs in retroperitoneal WDLSs, but it may also occur in the deep extremity-based WDLSs, and rarely in subcutaneous tumors often designated as atypical lipomas.[20–24] Low-grade dedifferentiation has a more favorable course than high-grade dedifferentiation; the latter carries a significant risk for distant metastasis.

Pathology

Grossly, the dedifferentiated components are often distinctive. Foci of high-grade dedifferentiation may appear as sharply demarcated soft, white nodules (Fig. 9–9). Lower grade components may be firm, white to tan.

Histologically, the dedifferentiated components often have an abrupt transition from the well-differentiated areas (Fig. 9–10*A*). They may have a spindle pattern resembling hypercellular fibromatosis or fibrosarcoma (low grade) or be storiform and resemble low-grade MFH (Fig. 9–10*B*), or they may be high-grade pleomorphic with the features of high-grade fibrosarcoma (Fig. 9–10*C*) or MFH (Fig. 9–10*D*). The high-grade dedifferentiation indicates significant

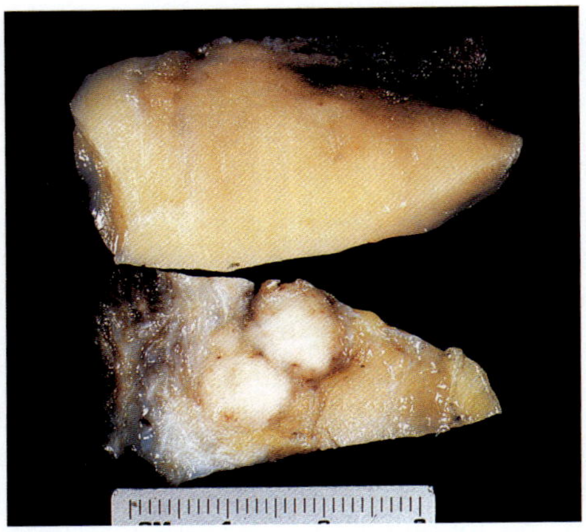

Figure 9–9. Dedifferentiated liposarcoma appears grossly as white nodules in the middle of yellow adipose tissue. The other section shows only the lipoma-like component.

risk for distant (lung) metastasis. However, such tumors have an unpredictable behavior. In several instances, we have seen retroperitoneal sarcomas originally interpreted as high-grade MFH recur as lipoma-like liposarcoma; in these cases the primary tumor evidently was a dedifferentiated liposarcoma.

A rare variant of dedifferentiated liposarcoma contains meningothelial-like whorls that form concentric perivascular proliferations (Fig. 9–11) These changes may include spicules of metaplastic bone.[25,26] In the earlier literature, such changes have been referred to as "malignant mesenchymoma." Such tumors usually occur in the retroperitoneum, and they have a variable prognosis with potential for lung metastases.

Heterologous elements are occasionally seen in dedifferentiated liposarcomas. Usually they are high-grade components representing extraskeletal osteosarcoma, chondrosarcoma, leiomyosarcoma, or rhabdomyosarcoma (Fig. 9–12), often with extensive rhabdomyoblastic differentiation.[27,28] Previously, tumors

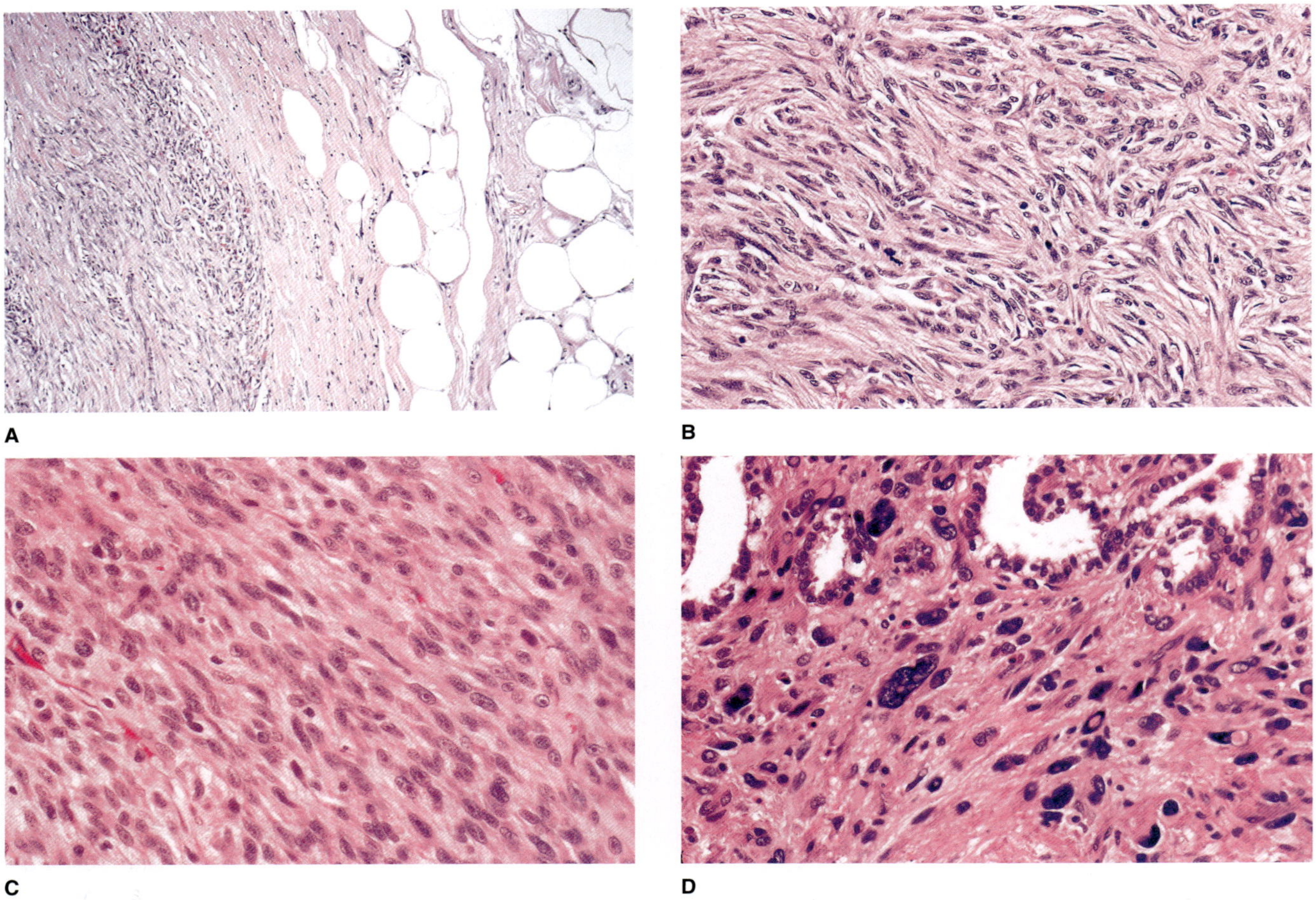

Figure 9–10. Different histologic appearances of dedifferentiated liposarcoma. *A,* Low-power micrograph showing sharp demarcation of the components. *B,* Low-grade dedifferentiation with a storiform pattern. *C,* High-grade dedifferentiation with fibrosarcoma-like pattern. *D,* Lung metastasis of a pleomorphic dedifferentiated liposarcoma with an MFH-like pattern.

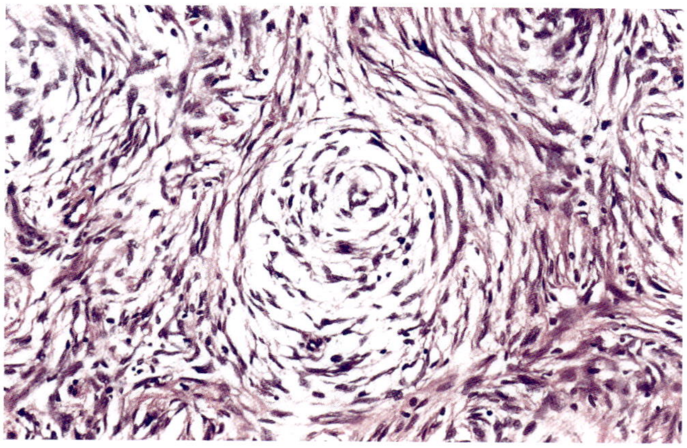

Figure 9–11. Dedifferentiated liposarcoma with meningothelial-like whorls. This is a low-grade pattern.

with such combined lipomatous and heterologous elements may also have been classified as "malignant mesenchymoma," but we support the view that they are part of the high-grade dedifferentiated liposarcoma and should be classified as liposarcomas with heterologous differentiation and specified as applicable.

Genetics

The genetic aspects of dedifferentiated liposarcoma are poorly understood.

Myxoid and Round Cell Liposarcoma

Clinical Features

Myxoid and round cell liposarcoma belong to the same genetic entity, and the latter can be considered a poorly differentiated or hypercellular variant of the former. The round cell variant is significant for its increased potential for recurrence and metastasis. Myxoid liposarcoma is customarily assigned grade 1 to 2 of 4, and round cell liposarcoma grade 3 to 4 of 4, depending on the degree of cellularity.

Myxoid liposarcoma is the second most common type after WDLS and comprises 30% to 40% of all liposarcomas. It occurs most commonly in young adults and middle-aged individuals with the median age 44 years and no sex predilection in the largest recent series.[29] It is occasionally seen in children 10 to 16 years of age,[3–5] and sometimes in elderly patients.

Myxoid liposarcoma occurs almost exclusively intramuscularly in the deep soft tissues of the extremities, most commonly in the thigh (60–70%), where the tumor often reaches a large size, over 15 cm. Other locations include popliteal fossa, leg and calf (30%), upper extremity, and rarely retroperitoneum. Most intra-abdominal liposarcomas with grossly myxoid features are not myxoid liposarcomas but well-differentiated ones with a myxoid component.[29–31]

If incompletely excised, myxoid liposarcoma is prone to recur locally. Approximately 20% to 30% of patients develop metastases. Myxoid liposarcoma often metastasizes to one or multiple soft tissue sites over years, which may pose a question of multiple primary tumors versus metastatic disease.[32] Lung and liver metastases occur in a minority of cases. One study found metastases in 35% of patients.[29] We have seen a patient who died of massive pericardial sac metastasis 2 years after the excision of myxoid liposarcoma of the thigh. Bone metastases may also occur.

Myxoid liposarcomas in children are low-grade tumors that have a favorable prognosis if complete excision can be performed.

Tumors with a round cell component show a significantly higher risk for metastasis. One study suggested a threshold of 25%,[29] and another 5% for the significance of the round cell component.[30] Patient age over 45 years and spontaneous tumor necrosis were also found to be unfavorable prognostic factors.[29] Myxoid liposarcoma with high cellularity but without a distinctive round cell component does not appear to increase the risk for metastasis. One study found infiltrative margin as a significant adverse prognostic factor.[31]

The optimal treatment is wide excision. If the tumor cannot be excised widely by its proximity to neurovascular bundles, use of postoperative radiation may prevent recurrence. Chemotherapy may also be beneficial.[33] Excision of soft tissue metastases and solitary pulmonary metastases appears beneficial because of the slow course of disease.

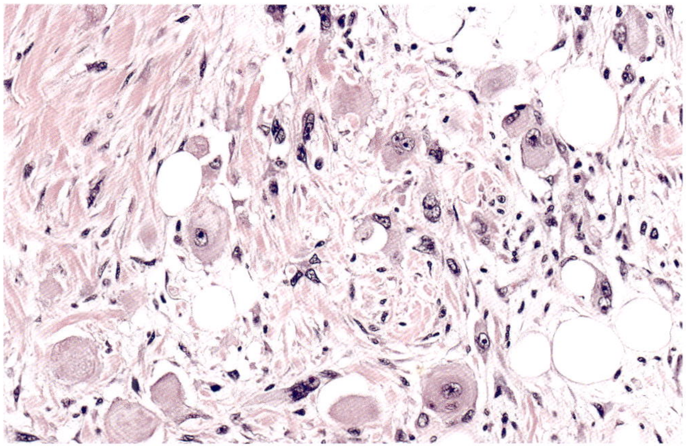

Figure 9–12. Heterologous rhabdomyoblastic differentiation in dedifferentiated retroperitoneal liposarcoma.

Gross Pathology

Grossly, myxoid liposarcoma is sometimes detected as a small tumor less than 5 cm in diameter especially when located in the upper extremity. When located in the deep thigh muscles these tumors typically reach a size of 15 cm or larger. Grossly myxoid liposarcoma is typically gelatinous, jelly-like, soft, and friable on sectioning. The cut surface is gray, often with a red tinge due to high vascularity (Fig. 9–13). Large tumors may have significant spontaneous necrosis.

Histologic Features

Histologically, myxoid liposarcoma is composed of evenly dispersed, relatively small oval or plump cells with scant cytoplasm in myxoid matrix. There is a background with prominent, arborizing thin-walled, fine capillary vessels, often seen in a "chicken-footprint" configuration (Fig. 9–14). Foci of fatty differentiation may also be present, especially in the periphery of the tumors, and this may focally resemble WDLS or even lipoma. Small numbers of signet ring cell and multivacuolated lipoblasts are usually present, but are not required for diagnosis. Some tumors contain hibernoma-like cells (Fig. 9–15*A*). Prominent cystic change reminiscent of lymphangioma is a common feature (Fig. 9–15*B*). However, the cystic spaces containing pools of mucinous material are lined by tumor cells and not endothelia. Trabecular corded patterns may be dominant in some cases (Fig. 9–15*C*). Chondroid differentiation has been described.[34] Some myxoid liposarcomas have a spindle cell pattern in some areas of the tumor (Fig. 9-15*D*).

Round cell liposarcoma may be seen focally in an otherwise typical myxoid liposarcoma, or rarely as the only pattern in a tumor (pure round cell liposarcoma). These tumors may have solid sheets of round cells with only focal evidence of adipocytic differentiation (Fig. 9–16). Round cell liposarcoma may resemble lymphoma in a small biopsy, if the fatty component is not included.

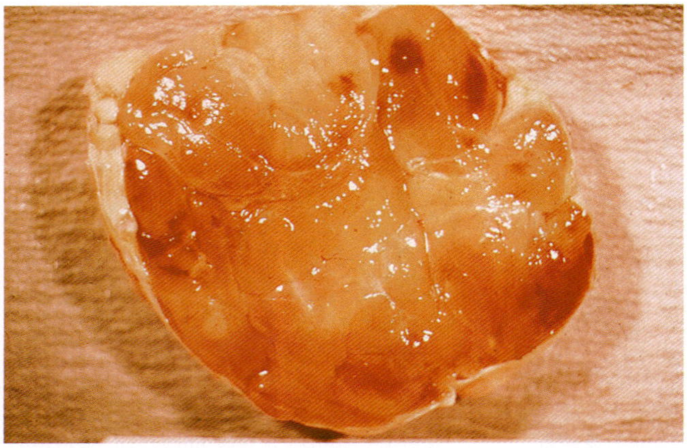

Figure 9–13. Grossly myxoid liposarcoma has a gelatinous yellowish appearance.

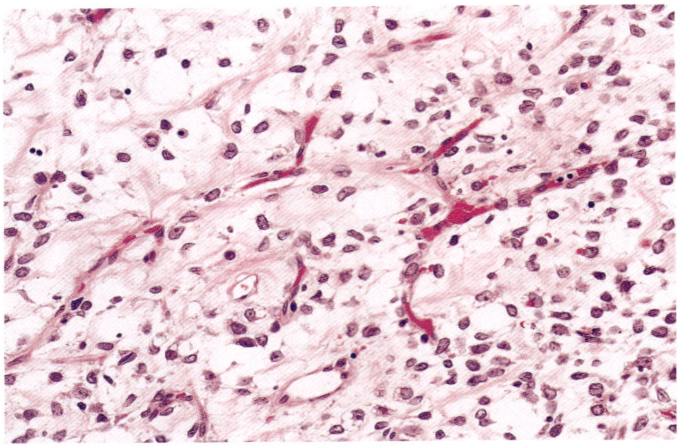

Figure 9–14. Typical myxoid liposarcoma has evenly dispersed tumor cells and prominent, branching capillary pattern.

Myxoid liposarcoma following preoperative radiation has typically a nonspecific histologic appearance as the tumor cells and the prominent vasculature are replaced by nearly acellular hyalinized with only scattered fat cells (Fig. 9–17).

Immunohistochemistry

When present, positivity for S-100 protein in round cell liposarcoma may help in the differential diagnosis. In contrast to WDLSs, myxoid and round cell variants are usually $CD34^-$, except for the endothelia.

According to one study, up-regulation of cyclin-dependent kinases CDK4 or CDK6 is very common (85%), and a third of tumors have loss of retinoblastoma locus/product. Overexpression of *MDM2* gene is also common.[35]

Differential Diagnosis

Intramuscular myxoma is a paucicellular tumor with a scant vascular pattern. Myxoid MFH and myxofibrosarcoma have a prominent vascular pattern, but the vessels are often thick-walled and coarse appearing, and the tumor tends to have focal fibrous matrix and variable cellular pleomorphism. Deep lipoblastoma shows lobulation; sometimes genetic studies are needed for the differential diagnosis from myxoid liposarcoma. Extraskeletal myxoid chondrosarcoma is similarly myxoid, but the tumor cells have a rim of eosinophilic cytoplasm arranged in cords or rounded clusters in a hypovascular background.

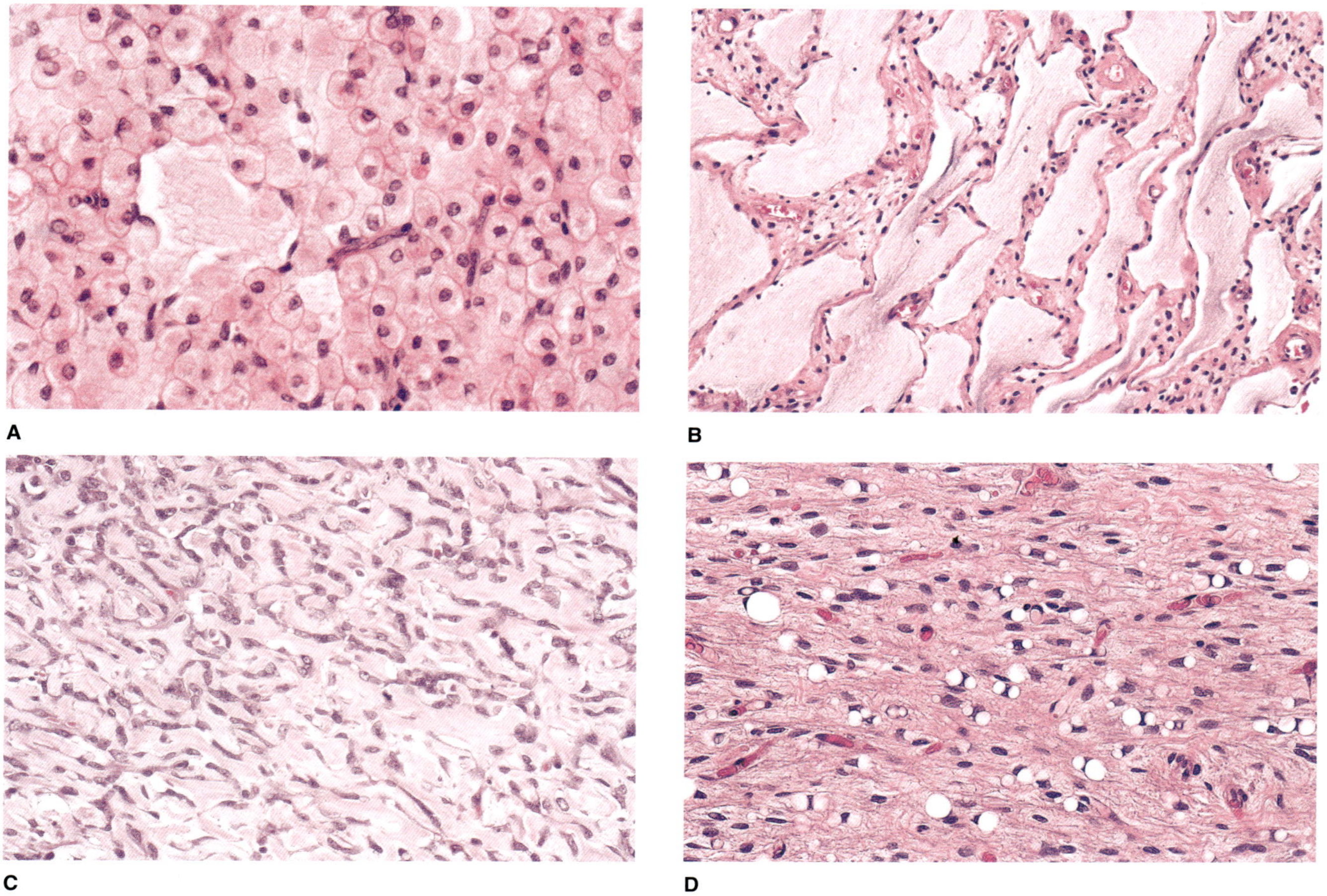

Figure 9–15. Histologic patterns of myxoid liposarcoma. *A*, Tumor with hibernoma-like cells. *B*, Lymphangioma-like pattern with spaces filled with mucoid material. *C*, Trabecular pattern. *D*, Spindle cell pattern.

Genetics

The typical, most common cytogenetic change in myxoid as well as round cell liposarcoma is the translocation t(12;16)(q13;p11) supporting the genetic identity of these histologic types.[36–40] The involved gene in the chromosome 12q13 is named as *CHOP*; this gene encodes for a DNA-binding transcriptional regulator protein. The involved gene in the short arm of chromosome 16p11 is named as *FUS* (formerly *TLS* or translocated in liposarcoma), and encodes for an RNA-binding protein. The *FUS* gene is also involved in translocations in acute myeloid leukemia.[41] Variant translocations include one involving the Ewing sarcoma gene (*EWS*) in 22q12, another gene encoding an RNA-binding protein, instead of *FUS*.[42–44] The myxoid liposarcoma translocations are listed in Chapter 4.

These translocations lead to the formation of fusion transcripts that can be detected by reverse transcription-polymerase chain reaction or FISH. However, the fusion transcript assay is complicated by the heterogeneity of the breakpoints of the t(12;16) translocation.[45] Production of FUS-CHOP oncoprotein has also been detected upon the t(12;16) translocation. The fusion protein of the translocation appears to be pathogenetically significant, and it has

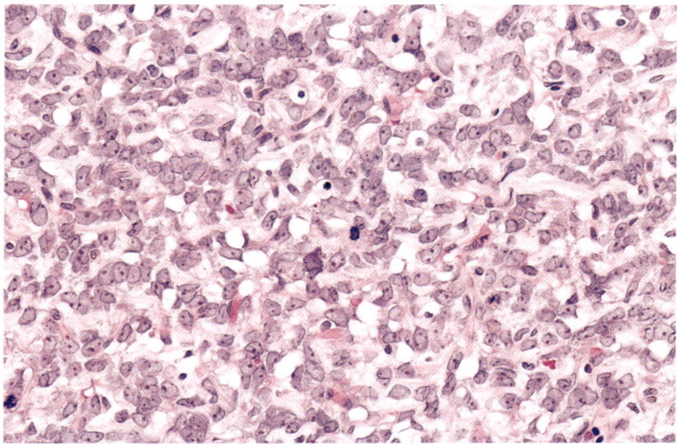

Figure 9–16. Round cell liposarcoma containing few cells with adipocytic differentiation. This tumor had also areas typical of low-grade liposarcoma. Same tumor as shown in Figure 9–14.

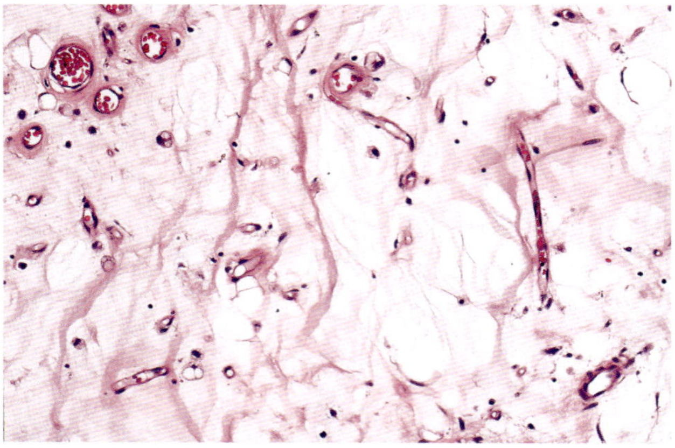

Figure 9–17. Typical myxoid liposarcoma following radiation shows hyalinized vessels and low cellularity. Pretreatment biopsy was typical, but these features are no longer diagnostic of myxoid liposarcoma.

shown to prevent normal adipocytic differentiation by abnormal expression of *DOL54* gene, normally only transiently expressed during adipocyte differentiation.[46,47]

A FUS-CHOP fusion transcript assay may be performed on fresh or fixed tissues, but the heterogeneity of the breakpoints necessitates the use of multiple primer systems.[45,48,49] One study detected the fusion transcript in the peripheral blood indicating the presence of circulating tumor cells.[50]

Pleomorphic Liposarcoma

Clinical Features

Pleomorphic liposarcoma is relatively rare, comprising less than 5% of all liposarcomas. This variant usually occurs in older individuals, predominantly in the deep muscles of the extremities and occasionally in the retroperitoneum.[1,2] Pleomorphic liposarcomas are high-grade tumors with a tendency to metastasize to lungs. Rare examples of cutaneous pleomorphic liposarcomas (along with occasional examples of cutaneous liposarcomas of other types) have been described. Contrary to other pleomorphic liposarcomas, the cutaneous examples are indolent tumors if completely excised.[51] Wide surgical excision is the standard treatment for limited tumors.

Pathology

Grossly, pleomorphic liposarcomas are often yellow, but tumors with limited fatty differentiation may be gray-white, without specific gross evidence for lipomatous differentiation. These tumors are typically large, intramuscular masses.

Histologic variants include pleomorphic MFH-like bizarre tumors, which show focal evidence of lipomatous differentiation in atypical multinucleated tumor cells (Fig. 9–18*A*). Some cases show large, bizarre lipoblasts (Fig. 9–18*B*), and the number of lipoblasts is typically higher in this variant as compared with WDLS. An epithelioid variant has also recently been described that shows solid sheets of epithelioid appearing cells with areas of obvious fatty differentiation.[52] The epithelioid variant should not be confused with metastatic carcinoma, because it may resemble adrenocortical or renal clear cell carcinoma (Fig. 9–19).

Immunohistochemically, the lipogenic tumor cells may be positive for S-100 protein, but the reaction is variable, and the lack of it does not rule out adipose tissue differentiation. Those pleomorphic liposarcomas that contain keratin-positive cells (in our experience especially keratins 7, 8, and 18), should not be confused with carcinomas.

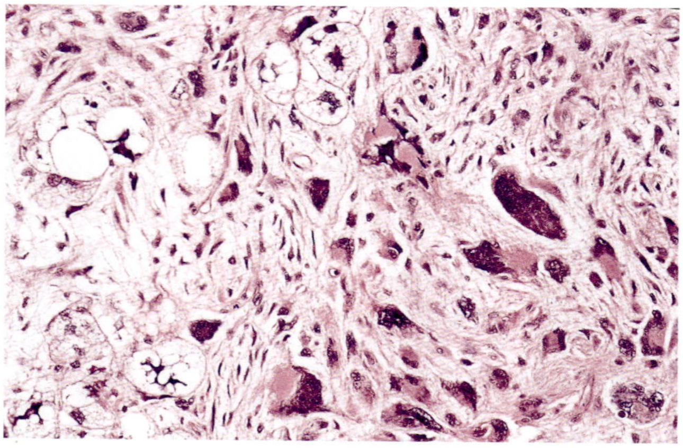

A

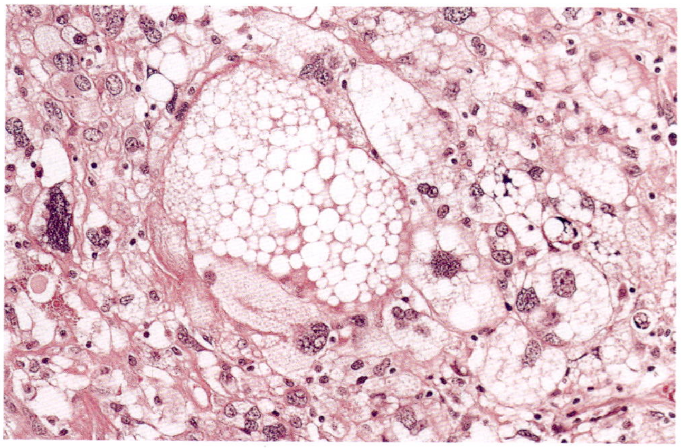

B

Figure 9–18. *A* and *B*, Two pleomorphic liposarcomas contain multivacuolated, highly atypical tumor cells and undifferentiated large cells similar to those seen in MFH.

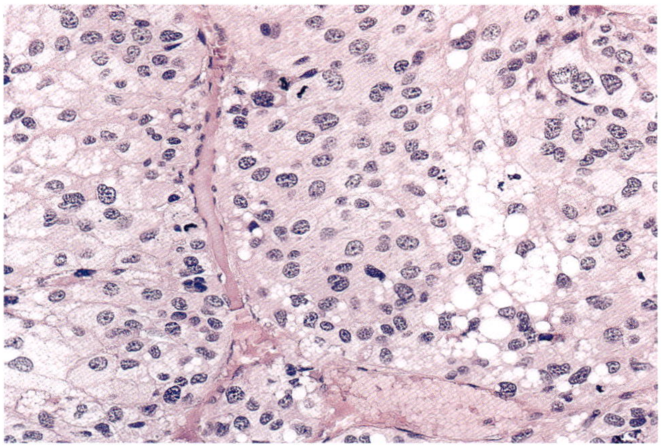

Figure 9–19. Epithelioid variant of pleomorphic liposarcoma may simulate adrenal or renal carcinoma. Focal adipocytic differentiation is diagnostic.

Genetics

The specific genetic changes of pleomorphic liposarcoma are not known. It is quite possible that many of these tumors are high-grade progression variants of WDLS because these liposarcoma types occur in the same sites in a similar patient group. The presence of t(12;16) translocation in some pleomorphic liposarcomas supports their origin from myxoid/round cell liposarcoma.[49]

REFERENCES

Liposarcoma (General)

1. Enzinger FM, Winslow DJ: Liposarcoma: A study of 103 cases. Virchows Arch Anat Pathol [A] 1962;335:367–388.
2. Kindblom LG, Angervall L, Svendsen P: Liposarcoma: A clinicopathologic, radiographic, and prognostic study. Acta Pathol Microbiol Scand 1992;253(suppl):1.
3. Shmookler BM, Enzinger FM: Liposarcomas occurring in children: An analysis of 17 cases and review of the literature. Cancer 1983;53:567–574.
4. Miller GG, Yanchar NL, Magee JF, Blair GK: Lipoblastoma and liposarcoma in children: An analysis of 9 cases and a review of the literature. Can J Surg 1998;41:455–458.
5. La Quaglia MP, Spiro SA, Ghavimi F, Hajdu SI, Meyers P, Exelby PR: Liposarcoma in patients younger than or equal to 22 years of age. Cancer 1993;72:3114–3119.
6. Demetri GD, Fletcher CD, Mueller E, et al: Induction of solid tumor differentiation by the peroxisome proliferator-activated receptor-gamma ligand troglitazone in patients with liposarcoma. Proc Natl Acad Sci USA 1999;96:3951–3956.

Well-Differentiated Liposarcoma

7. Evans HL, Soule EH, Winkelmann RK: Atypical lipoma, atypical intramuscular lipoma, and well-differentiated retroperitoneal liposarcoma: A reappraisal of 30 cases formerly classified as well-differentiated liposarcoma. Cancer 1979;43:574–584.
8. Azumi N, Curtis J, Kempson RL: Atypical and malignant neoplasms showing lipomatous differentiation. A study of 111 cases. Am J Surg Pathol 19897;11:161–183.
9. Weiss SW, Rao VK: Well-differentiated liposarcoma (atypical lipoma) of deep soft tissue of the extremities, retroperitoneum, and miscellaneous sites. A follow-up study of 92 cases with analysis of the incidence of "dedifferentiation." Am J Surg Pathol 1992;167:1051–1058.
10. Lucas DR, Nascimento AG, Sanjay BK, Rock MG: Well-differentiated liposarcoma. The Mayo clinic experience with 58 cases. Am J Clin Pathol 1994;102:677–683.
11. Klimstra DS, Moran CA, Perino G, Koss MN, Rosai J: Liposarcoma of the anterior mediastinum and thymus. A clinicopathologic study of 28 cases. Am J Surg Pathol 1995;19:782–791.
12. Wenig BM, Weiss SW, Gnepp DR: Laryngeal and hypopharyngeal liposarcoma. A clinicopathologic study of 10 cases with a comparison to soft-tissue counterparts. Am J Surg Pathol 1990;14:134–141.
13. Argani P, Facchetti F, Inghirami G, Rosai J: Lymphocyte-rich well-differentiated liposarcoma: Report of nine cases. Am J Surg Pathol 1997:21:884–895.
14. Kraus MD, Guillou L, Fletcher CD: Well-differentiated inflammatory liposarcoma: An uncommon and easily overlooked variant of a common sarcoma. Am J Surg Pathol 1997;21:518–527.
15. Remstein E, Kurtin PJ, Nascimento AG: Sclerosing extramedullary hematopoietic tumor in chronic myeloproliferative disorders. Am J Surg Pathol 2000;24:51–55.
16. Stephenson CF, Berger CS, Leong SP, Davis JR, Sandberg AA: Analysis of a giant marker chromosome in well-differentiated liposarcoma using cytogenetics and fluorescence in situ hybridization. Cancer Genet Cytogenet 1992;15:134–138.
17. Pedeutour F, Suikerbuijk RF, Forus A, et al: Complex composition and co-amplification of SAS and MDM2 in ring and giant rod marker chromosomes in well-differentiated liposarcomas. Genes Chromosomes Cancer 1994;10:85–94.
18. Szymanska J, Virolainen M, Tarkkanen M, et al: Overrepresentation of 1q21-23 and 12q13-21 in lipoma-like liposarcomas but not in benign lipomas: A comparative genomic hybridization study. Cancer Genet Cytogenet 1997;99:14–18.
19. Pilotti S, Della Torre G, Mezzelani A, et al: The expression of MDM2/CDK4 gene product in the differential diagnosis of well-differentiated liposarcoma and large deep-seated lipoma. Br J Cancer 2000;82:1271–1275.

Dedifferentiated Liposarcoma

20. Henricks W, Chu YC, Goldblum JR, Weiss SW: Dedifferentiated liposarcoma. A clinicopathological analysis of 155 cases with a proposal for an expanded definition of dedifferentiation. Am J Surg Pathol 1997;21:271–281.
21. McCormick D, Mentzel T, Beham A, Fletcher CDM: Dedifferentiated liposarcoma. Clinicopathologic analysis of 32 cases suggesting a better prognostic subgroup

among pleomorphic sarcomas. Am J Surg Pathol 1994; 18:1213–1223.
22. Elgar F, Goldblum JR: Well-differentiated liposarcoma of the retroperitoneum: A clinicopathologic analysis of 20 cases, with particular attention to the extent of low-grade dedifferentiation. Mod Pathol 1997;10:113–120.
23. Hisaoka M, Morimitsu Y, Hashimoto H, et al: Retroperitoneal liposarcoma with combined well-differentiated and myxoid malignant fibrous histiocytoma-like myxoid areas. Am J Surg Pathol 1999;23:1480–1492.
24. Hasegawa T, Seki K, Hasegawa F, et al: Dedifferentiated liposarcoma of retroperitoneum and mesentery: Varied growth patterns and histological grades: A clinicopathologic study of 32 cases. Hum Pathol 2000;31: 717–727.
25. Nascimento AG, Kurtin PJ, Guillou L, Fletcher CD: Dedifferentiated liposarcoma: A report of nine cases with a peculiar neurallike whorling pattern associated with metaplastic bone formation. Am J Surg Pathol 1998;22:945–955.
26. Fanburg-Smith J, Miettinen M: Liposarcoma with meningothelial whorls. An analysis of 17 cases of a distinctive histologic pattern associated with dedifferentiated liposarcoma. Histopathology 1998;33:414–424.
27. Tallini G, Erlandson RA, Brennan MF, Woodruff JM: Divergent myosarcomatous differentiation in retroperitoneal liposarcoma. Am J Surg Pathol 1993;17:546–556.
28. Evans HL, Khurana KK, Kemp BL, Ayala AG: Heterologous elements in the dedifferentiated component of dedifferentiated liposarcoma. Am J Surg Pathol 1994;18:1150–1157.

Myxoid and Round Cell Liposarcoma

29. Kilpatrick SE, Doyon J, Choong PF, Sim FH, Nascimento AG: The clinicopathologic spectrum of myxoid and round cell liposarcoma. A study of 95 cases. Cancer 1996;77:1450–1458.
30. Smith TA, Easley KA, Goldblum JR: Myxoid/round cell liposarcoma of the extremities. A clinocopathologic study of 29 cases with particular attention to extent of round cell liposarcoma. Am J Surg Pathol 1996;20:171–180.
31. Fukuda T, Oshiro Y, Yamamoto I, Tsuneyoshi M: Long-term follow-up of pure myxoid liposarcomas with special reference to local recurrence and progression to round cell lesions. Pathol Int 1999;49:710–715.
32. Spillane AJ, Fisher C, Thomas JM: Myxoid liposarcoma—The frequency and the natural history of nonpulmonary soft tissue metastases. Ann Surg Oncol 1999;6:389–394.
33. Patel SR, Burgess MA, Plager C, Papadopoulos NE, Linke KA, Benjamin RS: Myxoid liposarcoma. Experience with chemotherapy. Cancer 1994;74:1265–1269.
34. Siebert JD, Williams RP, Pulitzer DR: Myxoid liposarcoma with cartilaginous differentiation. Mod Pathol 1996;9:249–252.
35. DeiTos AP, Piccinin S, Doglioni C, et al: Molecular aberrations of the G1-S checkpoint in myxoid and round cell liposarcoma. Am J Pathol 1997;151:1531–1539.
36. Crozat A, Aman P, Mandahl N, Ron D: Fusion of CHOP to a novel RNA-binding protein in human myxoid liposarcoma. Nature 1993;363:640–644.
37. Panagopoulos I, Mandahl N, Ron D, et al: Characterization of the CHOP breakpoints and fusion transcripts in myxoid liposarcomas with the 12;16 translocation. Cancer Res 1994;54:6500–6503.
38. Gibas Z, Miettinen M, Limon J, et al: Cytogenetic and immunohistochemical profile of myxoid liposarcoma. Am J Clin Pathol 1995;103:20–26.
39. Knight JC, Renwick PJ, Dal Cin PD, van den Berghe H, Fletcher CD: Translocation t(12;16)(q13;p11) in myxoid liposarcoma and round cell liposarcoma: Molecular and cytogenetic analysis. Cancer Res 1995;55:24–27.
40. Tallini G, Akerman M, Dal Cin P, et al: Combined morphologic and karyotypic study of 28 myxoid liposarcomas. Implications for a revised morphological typing (a report from the CHAMP-group). Am J Surg Pathol 1996;20:1047–1055.
41. Panagopoulos I, Mandahl N, Mitelman F, Aman P: Two distinct FUS breakpoint clusters in myxoid liposarcoma and acute myeloid leukemia with the translocations t(12;16) and t(16;21). Oncogene 1995;11:1133–1137
42. Panagopoulos I, Hoglund M, Mertens F, Mandahl N, Mitelman F, Aman P: Fusion of the EWS and CHOP genes in myxoid liposarcoma. Oncogene 1996; 12:489–494.
43. Dal Cin P, Sciot R, Panagopuolos I, et al: Additional evidence of a variant translocation t(12;22) with EWS/CHOP fusion in myxoid liposarcoma: Clinicopathological features. J Pathol 1997;182:437–441.
44. Panagopoulos I, Lassen C, Isaksson M, Mitelman F, Mandahl N, Aman P: Characteristic sequence motifs at the breakpoints of the hybrid genes FUS/CHOP, EWS/CHOP and FUS/ERG in myxoid liposarcoma and acute myeloid leukemia. Oncogene 1997;15:1357–1362.
45. Kuroda M, Ishida T, Horiuchi H, et al: Chimeric TLS/FUS-CHOP gene expression and the heterogeneity of its junction in human myxoid and round cell liposarcoma. Am J Pathol 1995;147:1221–1227.
46. Kuroda M, Wang X, Sok J, et al: Induction of a secreted protein by the myxoid liposarcoma oncogene. Proc Natl Acad Sci USA 1999;96:5025–5030.
47. Adelmant G, Gilbert JD, Freytag SO: Human translocation liposarcoma-CCAAT/enhancer binding protein (C/EBP) homologous protein (TLS/CHOP) oncoprotein prevents adipocyte differentiation by directly interfering with C/EBPbeta function. J Biol Chem 1998; 273:15574–15581.
48. Hisaoka M, Tsuji S, Morimitsu Y, et al: Detection of TLS/FUS-CHOP fusion transcript in myxoid and round cell liposarcomas by nested reverse transcription-polymerase chain reaction using archival paraffin-embedded tissues. Diagn Mol Pathol 1998;7:96–101.
49. Willeke F, Ridder R, Mechtersheimer G, et al: Analysis of FUS-CHOP fusion transcripts in different types of soft tissue liposarcoma and their diagnostic implications. Clin Cancer Res 1998;4:1779–1784.
50. Panagopoulos I, Aman P, Mertens F, et al: Genomic PCR detects tumor cells in peripheral blood from

patients with myxoid liposarcoma. Genes Chromosom Cancer 1996;17:102–107.

Pleomorphic Liposarcoma

51. Dei Tos AP, Mentzel T, Fletcher CD: Primary liposarcoma of the skin: A rare neoplasm with unusual high grade features. Am J Dermatopathol 1998;20: 332–338.
52. Miettinen M, Enzinger FM: Epithelioid variant of pleomorphic liposarcoma. A study of 12 cases of a distinctive variant of high-grade liposarcoma. Mod Pathol 1999;12:722–728

Smooth Muscle Tumors

CHAPTER 10

Smooth muscle tumors generally arise from tissues with normal smooth muscle components, consistent with their origin from the replication-capable pool of the resident smooth muscle cells. The nearly ubiquitous presence of vascular smooth muscle in the body could explain the origin of smooth muscle tumors at a wide variety of sites. The most important clinicopathologic categories of smooth muscle tumors are listed in Table 10–1.

Benign smooth muscle tumors, leiomyomas and their malignant counterparts leiomyosarcomas (LMSs), are histologically separated by mitotic count and atypia, and sometimes using additional parameters, such as the presence of coagulative necrosis. In general, smooth muscle tumors of peripheral soft tissues in the extremities, trunk, and retroperitoneum should be considered at least suspicious of malignancy if mitotic activity is present. The criteria are different in the case of uterine and other female genital tumors, in which more mitotic activity is allowed. A borderline group of smooth muscle tumors of uncertain potential covers those tumors that are difficult to categorize as benign or malignant.

Leiomyomas of the soft tissues include the rare dermal ones arising from arrector pili muscles (piloleiomyomas), angioleiomyomas (vascular leiomyomas) that chiefly present in the subcutis, solitary leiomyomas in external genitalia, very rare leiomyomas of deep soft tissues, and uterine type, extrauterine, intra-abdominal leiomyomas. Organ-based benign leiomyomas may arise as small nodules in the tracheobronchial tree and upper respiratory tract. Uterine leiomyomas are probably more common than all other leiomyomas counted together. In the gastrointestinal tract, true leiomyomas are rare, and occur mainly in the esophagus and colon and rectum. They are much less common than the gastrointestinal stromal tumors (GISTs). Practically all gastrointestinal tumors previously classified as cellular leiomyomas, epithelioid leiomyomas, leiomyoblastomas, and LMSs are now reclassified as GISTs (see Chapter 11).

The LMSs are histologically relatively similar regardless of the site of origin, but their clinicopathologic features differ. A special group are the Epstein-Barr virus (EBV)-associated LMSs arising in immunosuppressed patients. LMSs at different sites and EBV-associated tumors are discussed separately, following a common pathologic description.

Congenital Smooth Muscle Hamartoma

Clinical Features

This rare lesion presents in the skin of infants, usually in the lower trunk, arm, or thigh, and has been reported more often in boys. It forms a pigmented or flesh-colored patch up to several centimeters in diameter, sometimes covered by prominent hair.

Table 10–1. Most Important Clinicopathologic Categories of Smooth Muscle Tumors

Developmental
Congenital smooth muscle hamartoma
Benign neoplasms
Pilar leiomyoma of skin
Angioleiomyoma of subcutis
Angiomyomatous hamartoma of lymph nodes
Leiomyoma of external genitalia
Retroperitoneal leiomyoma
Intravenous leiomyomatosis
Peritoneal leiomyomatosis
Esophageal leiomyoma
Colorectal leiomyoma of muscularis mucosae
Myomelanocytic: Lymphangiomyoma(tosis)
Malignant neoplasms: Leiomyosarcomas of
Skin
Subcutis and deep peripheral soft tissues
Retroperitoneum
Vascular origin
Uterus
Gastrointestinal tract
Miscellaneous other sites
Children
Immunosuppressed patients, EBV-associated

Histology

Congenital smooth muscle hamartoma is composed of bundles of well-differentiated arrector pili smooth muscle that are often periadnexally located. Some of these lesions have also been termed as a Becker nevus or melanosis.[1–3]

Pilar Leiomyoma (Piloleiomyoma)

Clinical Features

These relatively rare skin tumors, derived from the arrector pili smooth muscle, occur usually as multiple clustered or linearly arranged cutaneous papules or less commonly as single nodules that range from a few millimeters to 2 cm in diameter; the tumors presenting as single lesions tend to be larger. Pilar leiomyomas most commonly occur in young adults, usually on the extensor surfaces of legs and arms. The lesions are typically chronically painful, eliciting a burning or pinching sensation. Familial occurrence has been noted in rare cases.[4,5]

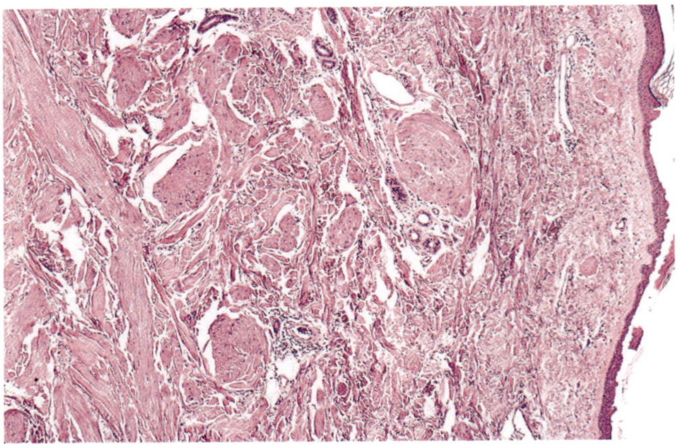

Figure 10–1. Pilar leiomyoma is composed of clusters of well-differentiated smooth muscle cells whose configuration resembles arrector pili muscles.

Pathology

Pilar leiomyomas are composed of radially or haphazardly arranged, poorly circumscribed clusters of mature smooth muscle cells that may resemble the configuration of expanded arrector pili muscles separated from each other by abundant collagenous stroma (Fig. 10–1). Small lesions may be concentrated around adnexa. A less organized architecture and presentation in adults separates this tumor from the congenital smooth muscle hamartoma.

Angioleiomyoma (Angiomyoma, Vascular Leiomyoma)

Clinical Features

According to the largest clinicopathologic series of 562 cases, the lesion appears as a small solitary subcutaneous nodule, usually in the extremities, and occurs in a wide age range.[6] Two thirds of the patients are between 30 and 50 years, and there is a significant female predominance (1.7:1).

The most common sites of involvement are the lower leg, ankle and foot, and two thirds of lesions are in the lower extremity. Upper extremity is involved in 22% of cases, hands and fingers predominantly, head occasionally, and trunk only rarely.[6–9]

Over half of the angioleiomyomas are painful, and this has been attributed to the presence of nerve fibers within the external aspect of the tumor. It has been suggested that only the painful tumors contain nerves.[10,11]

Pathology

Grossly, the lesions are sharply circumscribed, whitish rubbery nodules that usually measure 1 to 2 cm. The lesions that have calcification may appear gritty on sectioning.

Histologically, three variants have been recognized. The most common (67%) is the capillary or solid type with large numbers of narrow vascular slits surrounded by well-differentiated smooth muscle cells (Fig. 10–2*A* and *B*). The vessels are almost always small veins, but on rare occasions, arterial involvement has been noted. Foci of dystrophic calcification and fat cells may be present, and the tumors of older persons tend to be less cellular and more often calcified, perhaps as a sign of tumor regression.

The venous type (23%) has gaping venous lumina surrounded by thick smooth muscle layer that merges with adjacent vessel walls. The cavernous type (11%) has wide vascular lumina resembling cavernous hemangioma, but the septal elements are composed of smooth muscle cells (Fig. 10–2*C*). Unlike the solid variant, the cavernous one has a significant male predominance and occurs more often in the upper extremity. The venous variant has a mild male predominance.

Some angioleiomyomas have a round-cell, myopericytic component slightly resembling glomus cells (Fig. 10–2*D*). Occasionally, angioleiomyoma has cytologic atypia; tumors with such atypia without mitotic activity have a benign behavior as angioleiomyomas in general; only rare recurrences were reported in the largest series.

Genetics

Heterogeneous clonal chromosomal changes have been reported in each of the three published cytogenetic reports on angioleiomyomas.[12–14] They include interstitial deletions of 6p21-23 and 21q21, monosomy of chromosome 13, and translocation X;10 (q22;q23.2).

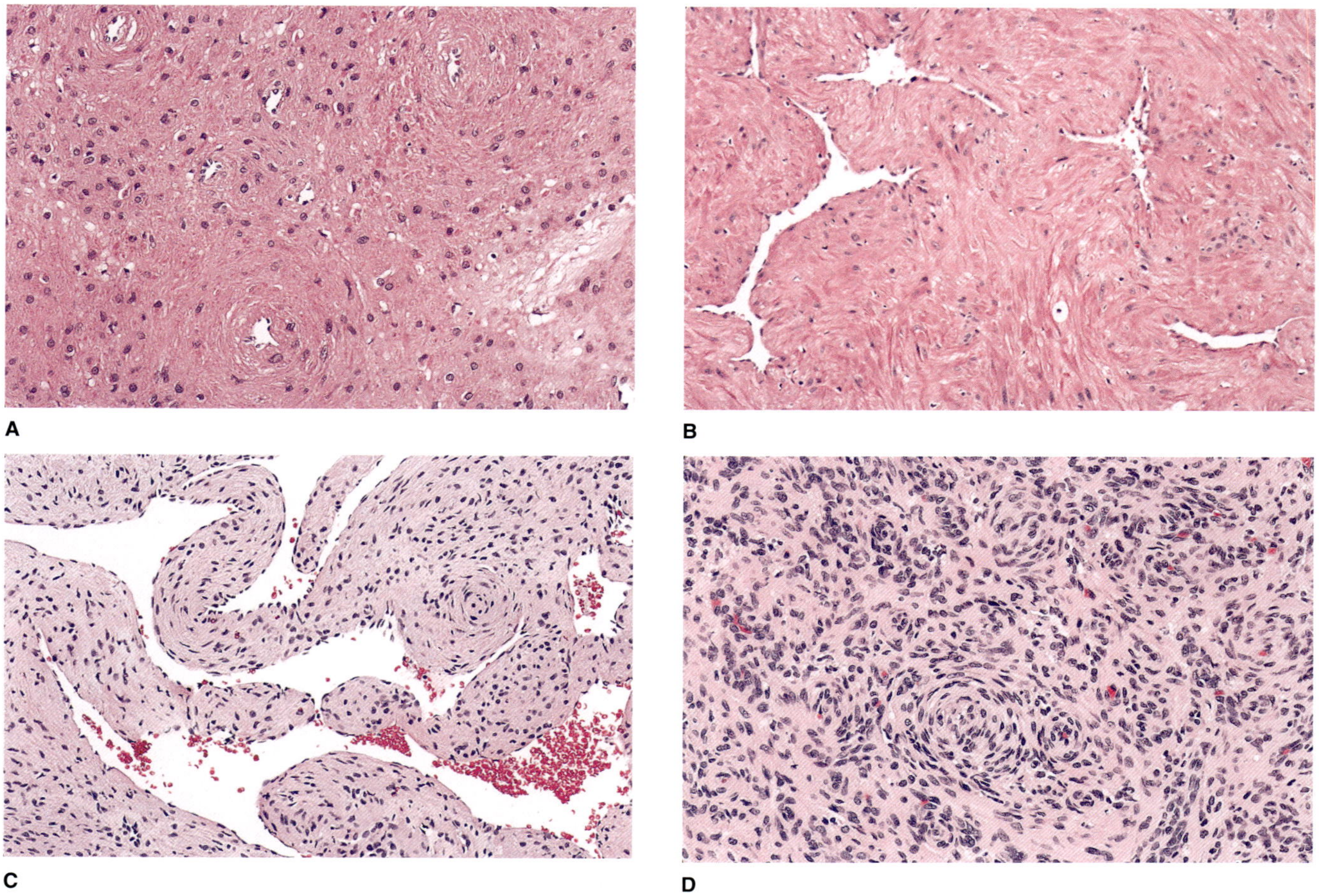

Figure 10–2. Histologic spectrum of angioleiomyoma. *A,* Solid pattern. *B,* Tumor with slitlike vascular lumina. *C,* Cavernous hemangioma-like variants. *D,* Tumor with myopericytic component.

Angiomyomatous Hamartoma of Lymph Node

Clinical Features

This designation coined by Chan and colleagues[15] refers to benign angioleiomyoma-like vascular smooth muscle proliferation involving a lymph node. The lesion forms a mass that almost always involves an inguinal lymph node, but has also been reported in a cervical lymph node.[16] It occurs in a wide age range, with an apparent strong male predominance.

Pathology

Grossly, white, firm tissue replaces much of the involved lymph node. The reported lesions have measured 1 to 3.5 cm (median, 2 cm). The tumor involves principally the hilus but may also replace the nodal cortex. Histologically, the proliferation resembles angioleiomyoma, but it has additional fibrous stroma and occasionally contains hemangioma-like elements (Fig. 10–3). There is neither smooth muscle atypia nor mitotic activity, so that the lesion is unlikely to be confused with lymph node metastasis of leiomyosarcoma (which is rare in all circumstances).

Leiomyomas of the External Genitalia

Clinical Features

Leiomyomas of the vulva and scrotal area are typically solitary, well-circumscribed nodules, and it is likely that in these locations they are related to the locally abundant, subcutaneous bandlike smooth muscle elements. In the vulva, these tumors typically arise in the labia majora, where they appear as painless small masses.[17,18] In the scrotum, the male homologue to labia majora, leiomyomas may reach a larger size.[18]

Pathology

The genital leiomyomas are usually well-circumscribed but unencapsulated masses. On sectioning they are white and rubbery. Microscopically, they are spindle cell tumors composed of well-differentiated smooth muscle cells (Fig. 10–4). Focal calcifications may be present. The criteria for malignancy developed so far is based on a limited number of cases. Invasive border and mitotic activity are features of malignancy, and the criteria for vulvar and scrotal tumors differ.

Vulvar leiomyomas, which are probably hormonally responsive tumors, are allowed some mitotic activity, up to 5/10 high-power field (HPF); in fact only 1 of 5 tumors with mitotic activity more than 5/10 HPF recurred.[17] Pregnancy associated smooth muscle tumors of external genitalia tend to have a low mitotic activity and a benign course.[17] Many epithelioid tumors formerly classified as epithelioid leiomyomas are now classified as angiomyofibroblastomas.

Nuclear atypia in scrotal leiomyomas should lead to an intense search for mitoses. Even if mitotic activity is not found, the lesions should be approached with great caution. Such lesions have been termed as "bizarre leiomyoma or symplastic leiomyoma."[19] Practically any mitotic activity in scrotal smooth muscle tumors signifies risk of malignant behavior, and therefore the designation of leiomyosarcoma would be more appropriate.

Peculiar mass-forming smooth muscle hyperplasia of the testicular adnexa can clinically simulate a tumor.[20] Such lesions were reported in middle-aged to elderly adults. The lesional size varied in a wide range (6 mm to 7 cm), and the smooth muscle hyper-

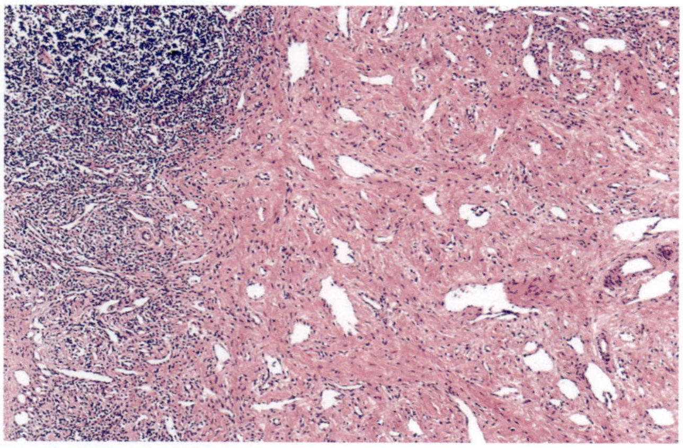

Figure 10–3. Angiomyomatous hamartoma of lymph node contains angioleiomyoma-like areas sharply demarcated from the lymphoid tissue.

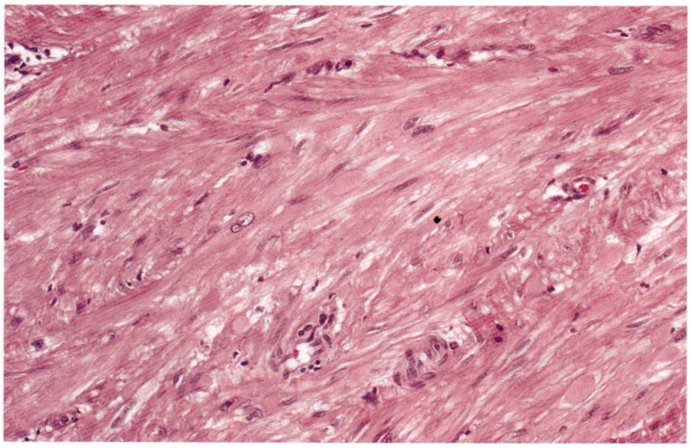

Figure 10–4. A solitary genital leiomyoma is composed of solid sheets of well-differentiated smooth muscle cells with no mitotic activity.

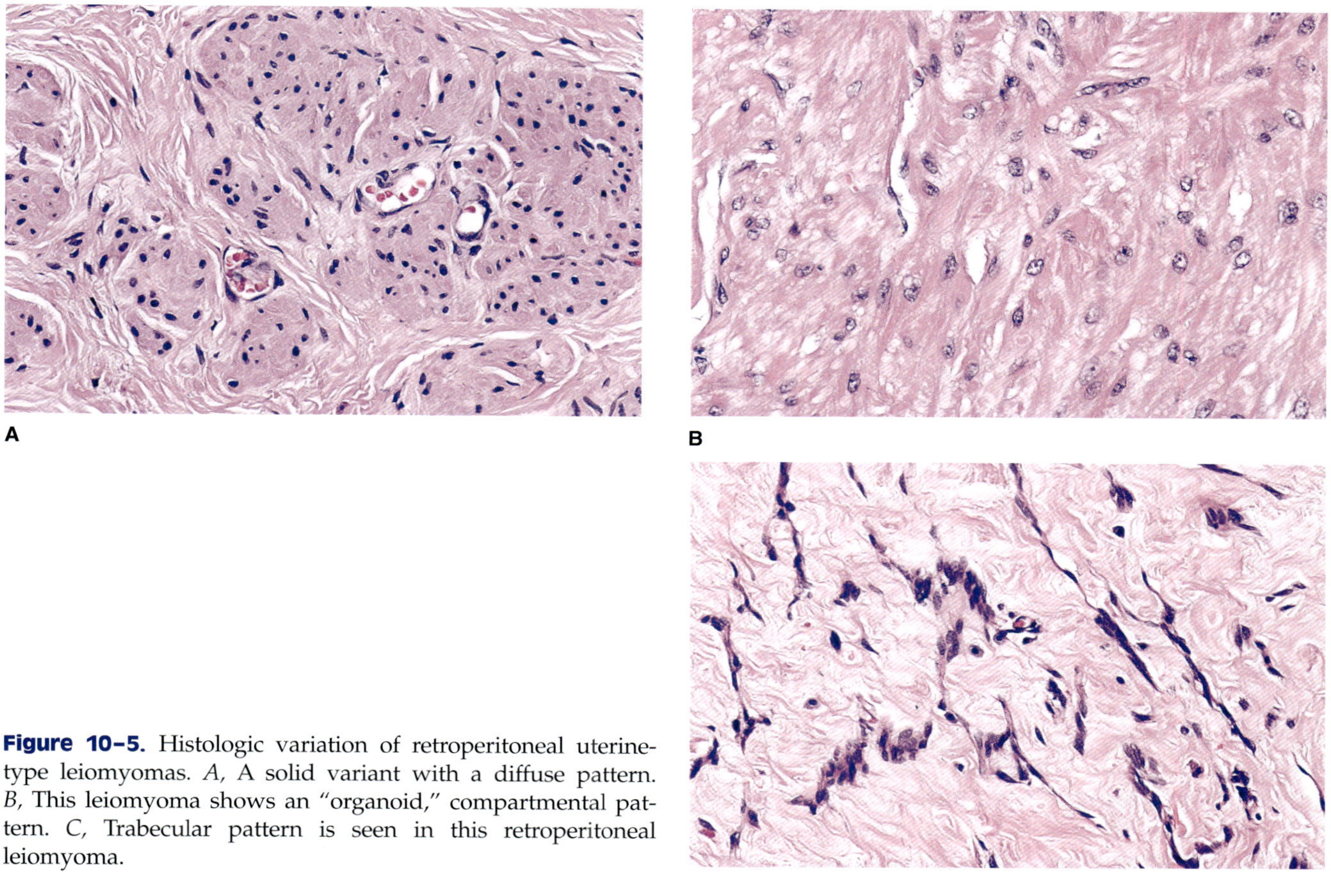

Figure 10–5. Histologic variation of retroperitoneal uterine-type leiomyomas. *A,* A solid variant with a diffuse pattern. *B,* This leiomyoma shows an "organoid," compartmental pattern. *C,* Trabecular pattern is seen in this retroperitoneal leiomyoma.

plasia was seen around the spermatic cord or associated with tunica albuginea periductally, perivascularly, or interstitially. The proliferation differed from true leiomyoma by being less compact and more orderly in nature.

Retroperitoneal Leiomyoma

Clinical Features

These tumors occur almost exclusively in women, typically in early middle age, and are histologically similar to uterine leiomyomas. In fact, they can be considered extrauterine examples of uterine leiomyomas. Retroperitoneal leiomyomas often reach a considerable size.[21]

Pathology

Retroperitoneal leiomyomas tend to be large, and they often measure 10 to 15 cm or more and can weigh more than 1 kg. They are typically paucicellular to moderately cellular and have features similar to those of their uterine counterparts. Myxoid change, hyalinization, and trabecular patterns may be seen (Fig. 10–5). As uterine leiomyomas, they are immunohistochemically positive for desmin, muscle actins, and estrogen receptor. Highly cellular examples with mitotic activity greater than 3 per 50 HPFs have to be classified as having uncertain malignant potential or as leiomyosarcomas, even if they are hormone receptor positive because there is no data on their behavior.[21]

A focal fatty component occurs in some retroperitoneal and uterine leiomyomas. These tumors are designated as lipoleiomyomas (Fig. 10–6).

Deep Peripheral Leiomyomas

Clinical Features

Benign leiomyomas occur in deep peripheral soft tissues very rarely. Such a diagnosis, especially of any larger tumor, should always be made with great caution and following extensive sampling, because some well-differentiated leiomyosarcomas may have mitotically inactive, leiomyoma-like areas. Occasionally the uterine type, hormone receptor-positive leiomyomas, occur in the inguinal canal or abdominal wall of women.

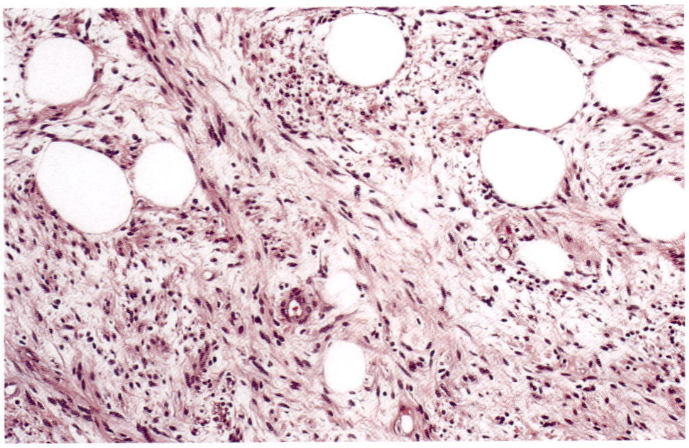

Figure 10–6. Lipoleiomyoma shows foci of mature fat amidst well-differentiated smooth muscle cells.

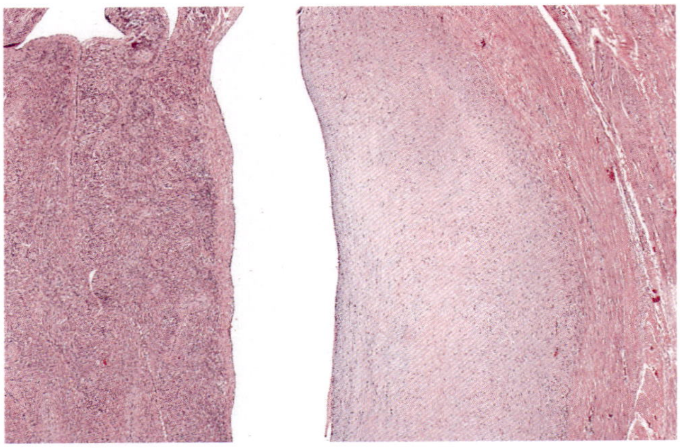

Figure 10–7. Intravenous leiomyomatosis of the uterus shows an intravenous plug of histologically benign leiomyoma. Note also vascular smooth muscle proliferation.

Intravenous Leiomyomatosis

Clinical Features

This rare condition occurs primarily in the uterus. It is defined as nodular intravascular growth of histologically benign smooth muscle cells, extending beyond a uterine leiomyoma, if coexisting with leiomyoma (i.e., an apparent intravascular smooth muscle protrusion within a uterine leiomyoma does not constitute intravenous leiomyomatosis). Intravenous leiomyomatosis usually occurs in women between the ages of 35 and 50, and occasionally at an older age.[22–24] The symptoms are similar to those seen with uterine leiomyoma. The tumor presents as a pelvic mass and usually (in 80% of cases) extends outside the uterus into pelvic veins. It extends into the vena cava in 30% of cases and may extend as an intravenous column up to the right side of heart and rarely in the pulmonary arteries. Cardiac involvement is often surgically treatable and may have a surprisingly good prognosis but has been fatal in some cases. Rarely, the cardiac involvement has been the first sign of the tumor.

The treatment consists of total abdominal hysterectomy and removal of the extrauterine intravenous extension whenever possible. Overall prognosis is good, but recurrent tumor develops in 30% of cases and may grow in the pelvic veins and to the right side of heart causing potentially fatal complications. Rare pulmonary metastases, with apparently an indolent course, have been reported. Surgery is advocated in recurrences, and tamoxifen may be useful.

Pathology

Grossly, intravenous leiomyomatosis typically forms a large uterine mass (mean size, 6–7 cm, up to 20 cm) containing convoluted, coiled, or wormlike intravenous plugs. The mass may sometimes involve the entire uterus. Intravenous extension of the tumor into pelvic veins is often noted by the surgeon.

Histologically, the intravascular plugs have varied histologic appearances in the spectrum of uterine leiomyomas, but they rarely contain mitotic activity (Fig. 10–7). The patterns include hyaline change and hydropic degeneration.[21–24] In some cases, the smooth muscle proliferation also extends to the walls of veins. Morphologic variants of uterine leiomyoma may be represented by myxoid, epithelioid, bizarre (atypia without mitoses), and clear cell changes. Lipoleiomyoma-like lesions containing mature fat have also been reported.[25] Mitotic activity is low (<1/10 HPF, occasionally up to 4/10 HPF).

Intravenous leiomyomatosis differs from LMS by lack of mitotic significant activity and it differs from endometrial stromal sarcoma by the lack of myometrial and endometrial involvement and extensive microscopic permeation of small vessels. The vascular invasion of endometrial stromal sarcoma may be grossly evident but cytologically these are round cell tumors.

Periotoneal Leiomyomatosis (Leiomyomatosis Peritonealis Disseminata)

Clinical Features

This rare condition occurs almost exclusively in fertile-age women, but occasionally it appears at postmenopausal age. Associated factors include pregnancy or exogenous estrogen intake in most cases. Innumerable small smooth muscle nodules develop on the pelvic and sometimes all peritoneal surfaces in a manner that may clinically and grossly simulate peritoneal carcinomatosis. In most cases, the condition is asymptomatic and diagnosed incidentally at cesarean section or surgery for uterine leiomyomas, which often coexist consistent with the lesion.[26–29] Treatment is usually conservative and may include antiestrogen or gonadotropin agonists. Prognosis is very good even if the lesions are not completely excised. Rare examples of malignant transformation to LMS have been reported,[30] but they may represent coincidental rather than causal association.

Pathology

Leiomyomatous nodules that usually measure from 2 to 3 mm and rarely exceed 1 cm involve the peritoneal surfaces. They are most commonly seen in the omentum and pelvic peritoneum and less commonly intestinal serosa and mesenteries. Grossly, the nodules are gray-white, firm, and rubbery. Histologically, they are composed of well-differentiated smooth muscle cells with no atypia and low mitotic activity (<2 mitoses per 10 HPF). Decidual stromal components may coexist in the lesions in pregnant patients. This condition probably represents the multipotentiality of the peritoneal mesenchyme and its capability to smooth muscle metaplasia.

This condition differs from disseminated LMS by the lack of atypia and dominant tumor seen in primary abdominal LMS.

Esophageal Leiomyoma and Leiomyomatosis

Clinical Features

Esophageal leiomyomas most commonly occur in young adults with the median age of 30 to 35 years, but they may also occur in children and in older adults. There is a strong male predominance (2:1) and predilection to the lower third of esophagus. Relatively rare esophageal leiomyomas occur in the middle portion, very few in the upper third. Dysphagia is a typical complaint, but as many as half of these tumors are asymptomatic when incidentally detected by chest x-ray as a mediastinal mass. Due to their intramural location they are not easily accessible to endoscopic biopsy, and when operated can almost always be excised extramucosally.[31,32]

Leiomyomatosis is a rare condition with an extensive longitudinal involvement of the esophagus by a smooth muscle tumor similar to leiomyoma. Most patients are young, and some are children. Esophageal leiomyomatosis may occur in connection with Alport syndrome with glomerular basement membrane disease and sensineural hearing loss, and familial occurrence has been reported.[33–37]

Pathology

Grossly, esophageal leiomyoma forms a circumscribed, white, rubbery, intramural mass that usually measures 3 to 5 cm, but it is sometimes detected as microscopic focus, and can occasionally reach a large size (>500 g) and bulge into the mediastinum. Some esophageal leiomyomas form a circumferential mass, and others may have a large longitudinal dimension and present as sausage-shaped masses along the muscle layer. Recurrence is rare after simple enucleation.

Microscopically, esophageal leiomyomas and leiomyomatosis are paucicellular and show sparsely distributed small nuclei while the cell borders are difficult to see on a hematoxylin and eosin-stained section (Fig. 10–8*A*). Focal nuclear atypia may be present in some leiomyomas, but mitotic activity is rare. There is often eosinophilic granulocyte infiltration within the tumor, and the presence of numerous mast cells is typical. Some tumors have areas of calcification. True leiomyomas can be distinguished from GISTs by their low cellular density.

Immunohistochemically, esophageal leiomyomas are positive for smooth muscle actin and desmin. They are negative for vimentin, CD34, and KIT, but numerous mast cells are KIT^+ (Fig. 10–8*B*). The immunohistochemical findings are in sharp contrast with GISTs that are always vimentin and KIT^+.

Genetics

Deletion of the genes encoding the basement membrane collagen type IV α5 and α6 has been reported in both sporadic esophageal leiomyoma and leiomyomatosis. The latter may form a complex longitudinally extending intramural mass that is often seen in connection with Alport syndrome together with renal glomerular disease and neurosensory hearing loss.[34–37] The similar genetic changes suggest that sporadic leiomyoma and leiomyomatosis are genetically related. Based on the preceding genetic findings, basement membrane collagen abnormality may be related to the pathogenesis of esophageal smooth muscle tumors. The esophageal leiomyomas commonly have gains in chromosome 5 in comparative genomic hybridization.[38]

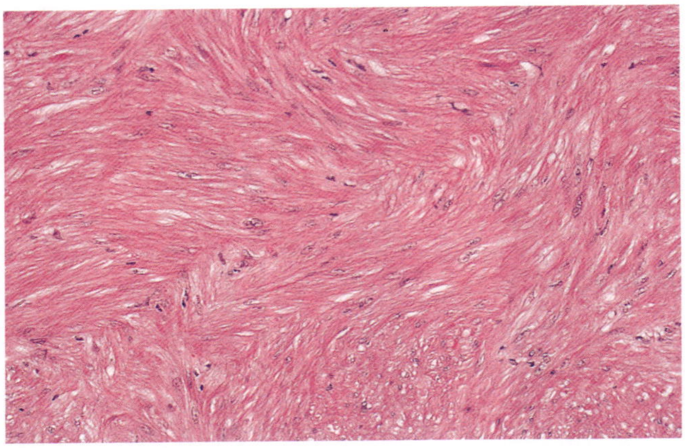

A

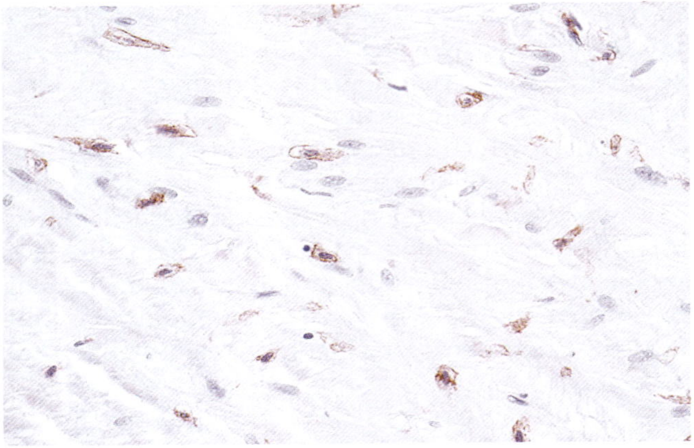

B

Figure 10–8. *A,* Esophageal leiomyoma is composed of well-differentiated smooth muscle cells. *B,* The tumor cells are KIT^-, in contrast to gastrointestinal stromal tumor, but a high number of mast cells positive for KIT are typically present.

Colorectal Leiomyoma of Muscularis Mucosae

Clinical Features

These tumors appear as small pedunculated polyps, and they are almost always incidental findings at colonoscopy. The leiomyomas of muscularis mucosae occur in adults, usually in the age range of 50 to 80 years. There is a male predilection. There is no morbidity associated with this lesion.[39,40]

Pathology

Grossly, the lesions are polyps with a clear stalk and usually measure less than 1 cm (average, 4 mm); only rarely do they reach the size of 2 cm. The lesion is firm, grayish yellow, and almost always covered by intact mucosa. Histologically, it is composed of well-differentiated smooth muscle cells similar to the muscularis mucosae, where the lesions merge and apparently arise from it (Fig. 10–9). Nuclear atypia is present on occasion.

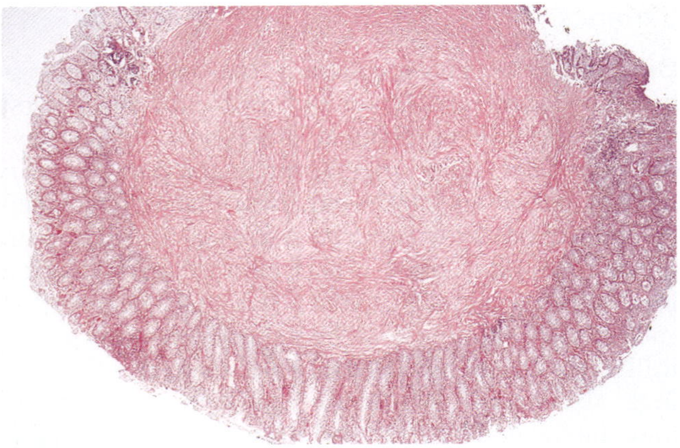

Figure 10–9. Leiomyoma of the muscularis mucosae of colon is composed of well-differentiated smooth muscle cells that merge with the muscularis mucosae.

Lymphangio(leio)myoma and Lymphangio(leio)myomatosis

Clinical Features

Lymphangiomyoma (or lymphangioleiomyoma; LAM) is a smooth muscle proliferation of the lymphatic vessels and lymph nodes related to angiomyolipoma of the kidney and retroperitoneum; 10% to 20% of the patients have also angiomyolipomas. LAM can involve the lymph nodes and thoracic duct in the retroperitoneum and mediastinum. It occurs exclusively in women, usually below the age of 50 years.[41–46]

Lymphangiomyomatosis is the designation of diffuse involvement of lungs by minute, innumerable lesions. This condition also occurs exclusively in women, usually below the age of 50 years. The changes involve the lungs diffusely and usually bilaterally. The involvement leads to complications such as pulmonary emphysema, pneumothorax, sometimes chylothorax, and ultimately loss of pulmonary function over time, but the severity of the course of disease varies. Unilateral or bilateral lung transplantation has been successfully performed on many patients, but the disease may recur in the transplants.

The condition may occur sporadically or in patients with tuberous sclerosis complex, who have a high frequency of pulmonary LAM. The coexistence

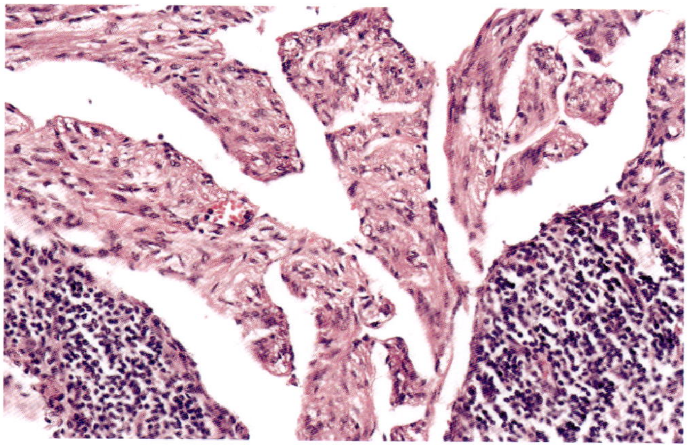

Figure 10–10. Lymphangiomyoma involves lymph nodes as trabeculae lined by endothelium. Note residual foci of lymphoid tissue.

of LAM and pulmonary sugar tumor has been observed at least in one instance.[47]

Pathology

In lymph nodes, LAM (previously called lymphangiopericytoma) forms trabecular smooth muscle proliferation separated by endothelium-lined sinusoidal spaces (Fig. 10–10).

The pulmonary involvement, when fully developed, is grossly remarkably cystic, resembling severe emphysema. In the lungs, microscopic foci of lymphangiomyoma are seen perivascularly, peribronchially, and interstitially, often associated with emphysematous cyst formation. The emphysematous change has been attributed to activation of the matrix metalloproteinase system in this disease.[47]

Histologically, the lung lesions are seen as microscopic nodules in the walls of the peripheral airways involving the interstitial lymphatics. The smooth muscle cells resemble those of angiomyolipoma, and often have a "hollow," vacuolated, clear cell appearance (Fig. 10–11). Immunohistochemically, the lesional cells are positive for smooth muscle actins and desmin, but they are unique among smooth muscle tumors with some lesional cells being positive for HMB45, similar to the related angiomyolipoma.[47]

Genetics

Mutation of the tuberous sclerosis 2 (*TSC2*) gene have recently been shown in lymphangiomyoma. This gene is also mutated in angiomyolipomas consistent with the genetic similarity between these tumors.[48]

Leiomyosarcoma

Leiomyosarcomas (LMSs) are tumors whose lesional cells resemble well-differentiated smooth muscle cells; mitotic activity over 1/10 HPF (5/50 HPF) generally establishes the diagnosis of LMS of peripheral soft tissue. A lower limit (1 mitosis per 20 HPF) may be applied to retroperitoneal smooth muscle tumors (except the uterine type leiomyomas, see following). Uterine smooth muscle tumors are classified as LMSs if they have coagulative necrosis or atypia and have mitoses over 5/10 HPF. However, cellular leiomyomas without significant atypia may have mitoses up to 15/10 HPF. Collectively, LMSs are among the most common soft tissue sarcomas.

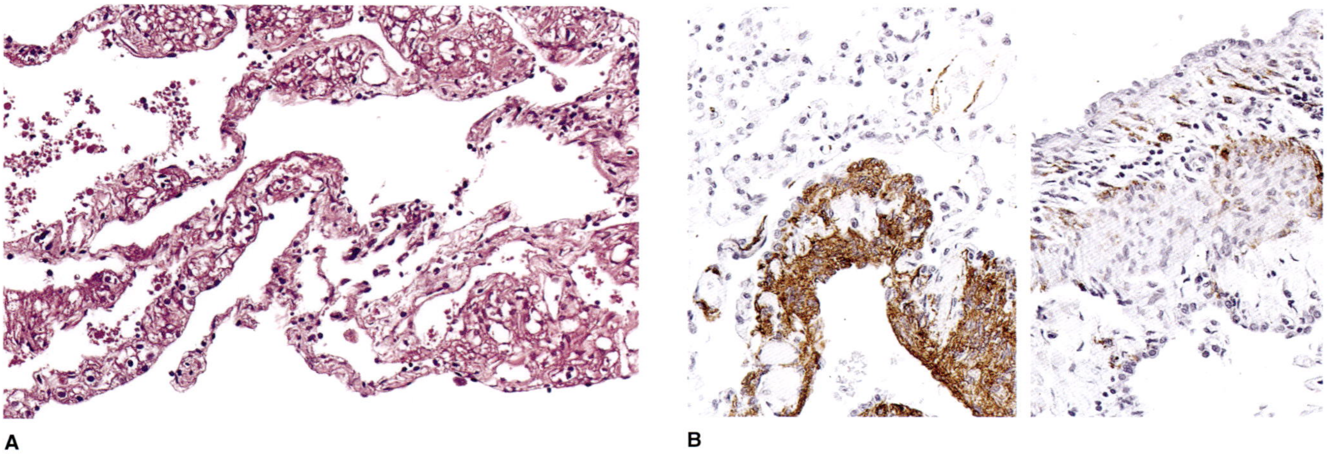

Figure 10–11. *A,* A pulmonary lymphangiomyomatosis lesion contains smooth muscle cells with a clear cytoplasm, resembling the smooth muscle component of angiomyolipoma. *B,* Immunostaining for smooth muscle actin highlights the smooth muscle proliferation of pulmonary lymphangiomyomatosis *(left)* and focal HMB45 positivity is present *(right).*

Although histologically essentially similar at different sites, the LMSs differ greatly in their clinical presentation.

There are site-related differences in the behavior, especially in that superficial cutaneous tumors behave indolently, and tumors of vascular smooth muscle origin tend to behave better than other deep tumors. Although usually tumor of adults, LMSs may occasionally occur in children. Immunosuppressed patients with acquired immunodeficiency syndrome (AIDS) and posttransplant patients may develop EBV-associated LMSs. Rare histologic variants of LMS have been described, including those with granular cell features. The genetic changes in LMSs are complex and no single typical recurrent changes have been described. Most gastrointestinal LMSs and all epithelioid smooth muscle tumors, especially the intra-abdominal ones, are now reclassified as GISTs. These tumors are discussed in Chapter 11. The clinicopathologic features of LMS of different sites are summarized in the following sections, and their pathology, common to tumors presenting at different sites, is summarized separately.

Cutaneous Leiomyosarcomas

Cutaneous LMSs occur in a wide age range (median, 50 years) with a clear male predominance. They have a strong predilection for extremities and occur more often on the extensor aspect. The most common sites are the lower extremity, especially thigh and leg (50%) and upper extremity, predominantly proximally (30%). Head and neck and trunk are less common locations. Cutaneous LMSs typically present as relatively small solitary, elevated skin nodules, some of which ulcerate. Half of them are smaller than 2 cm, and they rarely reach the size of 5 cm.[49–53] Histologically, these tumors are often poorly circumscribed. Recurrence is common if treated by enucleation only, but nevertheless purely cutaneous LMSs have an excellent prognosis, independent of histology, and they almost never metastasize, including those tumors that have a very small subcutaneous component. Wide excision is the optimal treatment.

Subcutaneous and Deep Leiomyosarcomas

Subcutaneous LMSs differ from the cutaneous ones by their significant potential to metastasize. They are similar to cutaneous LMSs in their occurrence in a wide age range, male predominance, and predilection to extremities, especially the thigh. Origin from small vessels can sometimes be demonstrated.[50,54–57] Clinically, subcutaneous LMS appears as a hemispherical mass that tends to be larger than cutaneous LMS with the median size of 4 cm. As many as one third metastasize, often following a local recurrence, which is common unless the tumor is widely excised. The possibility of metastasis from a previously diagnosed or undisclosed internal LMS (retroperitoneal, uterine) has to be considered, especially if multiple subcutaneous LMSs occur.[49]

Deep, intramuscular LMSs tend to be diagnosed as large tumors. They most commonly occur in the thigh and buttock, and they have a high metastatic rate. Many of these tumors are probably also of vascular smooth muscle origin.

Retroperitoneal Leiomyosarcoma

Retroperitoneal LMSs form one of the largest groups of malignant smooth muscle tumors of soft tissue. They have a strong female predominance (70–80%), occur in a wide age range chiefly in the older middle age, and tend to be large (>10 cm) when diagnosed. The prognosis is poor with 80% tumor-related mortality, and smooth muscle tumors with as few as 1 mitosis per 10 HPF have to be classified as LMS because they may metastasize, especially to lungs and liver and less commonly to peripheral soft tissues and bone.[58–60]

Vascular Leiomyosarcoma

Venous vascular origin is detected for some soft tissue LMSs, sometimes at surgery, and thorough gross and microscopic examination reveals vascular origin for some additional cases. Overall, the true frequency of vascular origin of LMS of soft tissues is probably underestimated. The most common vessels involved are the inferior vena cava, saphenous vein, and small peripheral veins.[61–65] Vascular LMSs have a strong female predominance, especially the tumors originating from the vena cava, and they usually occur in middle-aged and older patients. The prognosis is better than for other deep LMSs, even if the tumor has significant mitotic activity. However, recurrences and metastases may occur after a long interval.

A minority of sarcomas of the pulmonary artery and aorta are intramural LMSs, whereas the majority are intimal sarcomas with myofibroblastic, undifferentiated, or endothelial phenotypes. The prognosis of sarcomas of the great vessels is generally poor, but long-term survival has been reported of some LMSs.[66]

Uterine Leiomyosarcomas

Uterine LMSs probably outnumber all other LMSs and predominantly occur in postmenopausal women. The premenopausal patients and those whose tumors are confined to a single nodule or have a low mitotic count have a better prognosis with the overall 5-year survival rate 60% to 70%.[67–70]

Uterine LMSs are usually larger than 10 cm in diameter, although are occasionally quite small. With multiple smooth muscle tumors present, close attention should be paid to the dominant mass, because such a tumor may represent sarcoma with a greater likelihood. Uterine LMSs are often less circumscribed than leiomyomas, but some are well-defined and simulate a leiomyoma.

The defining mitotic counts for uterine smooth muscle tumors are different from other smooth muscle tumors and quite complex, taking into account several features such as presence of atypia, coagulative tumor necrosis, and special cell type (myxoid or epithelioid). However, 90% of uterine LMSs have more than 15 mitoses per 10 HPF. [71]

Tumors with no or minimal atypia are allowed 15 (possibly even more) mitoses per 10 HPF, and they are classified as cellular leiomyomas with mitotic activity. Tumors with significant atypia are classified as LMS if 10 or more mitoses per 10 HPFs are present; below that they may be classified as bizarre, symplastic leiomyomas, although such tumors usually have fewer than 2 to 3 mitoses per 10 HPF. Coagulative tumor necrosis is a warning sign and should lead to search of other signs of malignancy, such as mitotic activity and foci of atypia. The presence of coagulation necrosis has been suggested to upgrade a tumor to low-grade malignant, even if mitotic count is less than 10/10 HPF, and atypia is limited. Also the classification of myxoid and epithelioid tumors as LMS has been suggested with mitotic counts as low as 0 to 2 mitoses per 10 HPF.[71,72]

Hydropic degeneration, hemorrhagic infarction (often accompanied by reactive changes), and focal myxoid change in ordinary leiomyoma are not worrisome features.[71] Tumors that fall in-between the diagnostic criteria and present indeterminate features are best classified as smooth muscle tumors of uncertain (or low) malignant potential.

Gastrointestinal Leiomyosarcomas

The true LMS with phenotypic properties of smooth muscle cells (actin, desmin positive, KIT^-) are very rare in the gastrointestinal tract, because most tumors previously classified as gastrointestinal LMSs are now considered GISTs. Many well-documented LMSs of the gastrointestinal tract are polypoid intraluminal tumors, and such tumors in the colon might be derived from the muscularis mucosae structures. Most primary LMSs of the gastrointestinal tract are clinically and histologically highly malignant tumors, but there have been long-term survivors among patients with relatively small, polypoid intraluminal tumors. In some cases it has been difficult to determine whether a solitary gastrointestinal tumor or a synchronous soft tissue LMS is the primary tumor.[73]

Miscellaneous Leiomyosarcomas

Less common sites for LMSs of which clinicopathologic series have been reported include tumors from sinonasal tract, oral cavity, lungs, urinary bladder, and prostate.[74–78] These tumors predominantly occur in older patients. Prognosis varies, and some grade dependency of survival has been observed. Primary osseous LMS may secondarily involve the surrounding soft tissues.

Leiomyosarcomas in Children

Leiomyosarcomas very rarely occur in children; among them the most common are the LMSs in immunosuppressed patients (see following). According to the largest series, LMSs in immunocompetent children present at a variety of sites, and most are low-grade tumors with a good prognosis.[79–81] According to our experience, most tumors originally considered intra-abdominal LMSs in children are actually inflammatory myofibroblastic tumors (synonymous to inflammatory fibrosarcoma).

EBV-Associated Leiomyosarcomas in Immunosuppressed Patients

Immunosuppressed patients, usually those with AIDS, or less commonly posttransplant patients, may develop EBV-associated LMSs. The posttransplant LMSs have analogy with posttransplant lymphoproliferative disorders, which also are associated with EBV. Most of the reported AIDS-related, EBV-associated LMSs have occurred in children, predominantly in the abdomen or thorax, but intracranial occurrence has also been reported.[82–93]

In the posttransplant patients, the LMS originates either from the donor cells when in the graft or from recipient tissue when arising outside of the graft.[84,88] High numbers of EBV copies have been reported in the tumor tissue, but not in the normal tissue or control LMSs in nonimmunosuppressed patients suggesting the etiologic role of EBV in LMSs of immunosuppressed patients.[87,88] EBV-associated LMSs have also been reported in patients with congenital immunodeficiency syndromes.[91]

Many immunosuppression-associated LMSs are low-grade tumors, and antiviral therapy has been proven useful in some cases. The prognosis greatly depends on the underlying disease.

Pathology of Leiomyosarcomas

Grossly, LMSs vary according to tumor differentiation. The low-grade tumors resemble leiomyomas and tend to be hard masses with a whitish, whorled surface on sectioning. High-grade tumors resemble other high-grade sarcomas and are typically composed of homogeneous, soft gray-tan tissue. Many large high-grade LMSs show extensive central necrosis appearing as a yellowish central area with a peripheral rim of viable tumor tissue.

Microscopically, LMSs are almost always composed of spindled cells, which commonly show longitudinally oriented intersecting fascicles (Fig. 10–12*A*). Cytologically, the tumor cells typically have blunt-ended "cigar-shaped" nuclei, and the cytoplasm is variably eosinophilic, sometimes distinctly clumped. Eosinophilic cytoplasmic "contraction bands" may be visible. Some tumors have myxoid stroma, with the tumor cells arranged in a "basket-weave-pattern" (Fig. 10–12*B*) Focal pleomorphism is common (Fig. 10–12*C*), and some cases show extensive pleomorphism resembling malignant fibrous histiocytoma (Fig. 10–12*D*). In such tumors, the nature of the tumor as a poorly differentiated LMS may become apparent only after extensive sampling. These tumors occur especially in the retroperitoneum.

The LMSs arising in connection with AIDS or other immunosuppression tend to be less differentiated with a smaller amount of eosinophilic cytoplasm (Fig. 10–13).

Rare histologic variants of LMS include tumors with granular cells[94] and foci of osteoclast giant

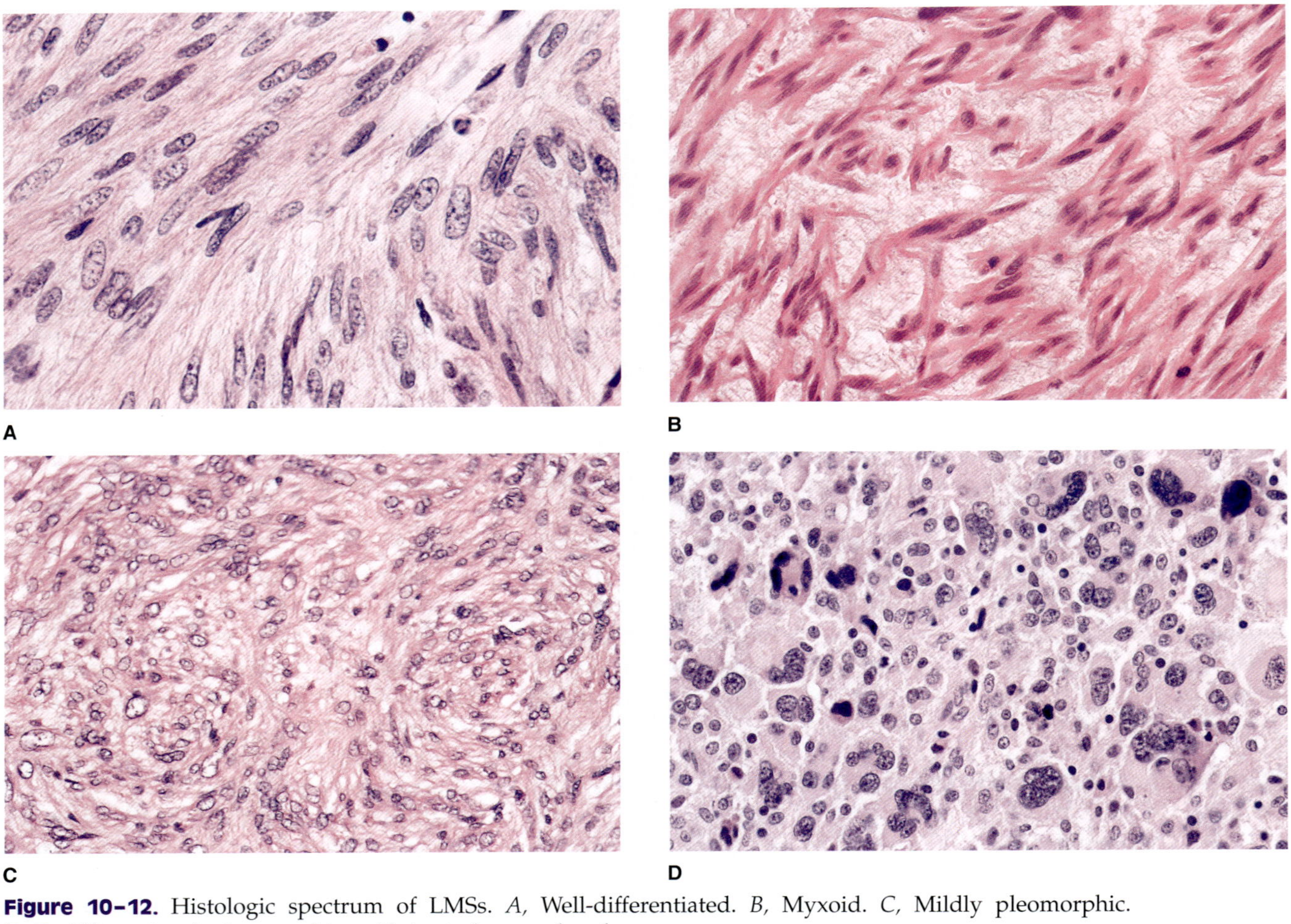

Figure 10–12. Histologic spectrum of LMSs. *A,* Well-differentiated. *B,* Myxoid. *C,* Mildly pleomorphic. *D,* Dedifferentiated, pleomorphic, with typical areas elsewhere.

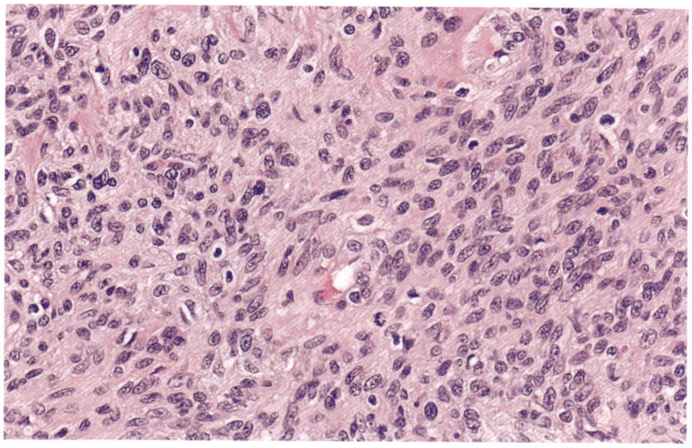

Figure 10–13. A HIV-associated leiomyosarcoma in the paraspinal soft tissues has a less differentiated appearance than typical soft tissue LMS.

cells.[71] Occasional peripheral epithelioid LMS are described in the skin;[95] these and some similar uterine tumors may be the only true epithelioid LMSs, because most gastrointestinal and other intra-abdominal tumors previously classified as epithelioid smooth muscle tumors are KIT$^+$ and are now considered epithelioid GISTs. Heterologous rhabdomyoblastic differentiation has been reported both in uterine and retroperitoneal LMS.[96]

Immunohistochemistry of Leiomyosarcomas

Immunohistochemically, LMSs are nearly always positive for α smooth muscle actin and muscle actins (HHF35), which can be considered part of the definition. Desmin positivity varies and is overall 70% to 80% with poorly differentiated tumors being less consistently, often only focally positive (Fig. 10–14).[97,98]

Smooth muscle myosin, heavy caldesmon, and calponin are other cytoskeletal components of smooth muscle cells typically present in LMS. Of these heavy caldesmon is smooth muscle specific, whereas calponin is also expressed in myofibroblasts and myofibroblastic tumors.[99,100] CD34 is expressed in as many as 30% of typical retroperitoneal LMSs; expression of this marker is by no means limited to GIST versus LMS.[101,102] Although LMSs are generally KIT$^-$ (CD117), on occasion they may have isolated cells that are strongly KIT$^+$.[102]

Epithelial markers, including keratins of simple epithelia and epithelial membrane antigen (EMA), are expressed in approximately 10% to 30% of LMSs. The expression of keratins can be especially prominent in uterine and cutaneous LMSs but are also present in some retroperitoneal and vascular leiomyosarcomas.[103,104] The keratin polypeptides expressed in leiomyosarcomas, in our experience, especially include keratins 8 and 18. Uterine leiomyosarcomas are often positive for estrogen and progesterone receptors, but extrauterine tumors are generally negative.

Ultrastructure of Leiomyosarcomas

Electron microscopic findings of typical smooth muscle tumors include abundant cytoplasmic actin filaments with dense bodies and variable intermediate filaments, actin filaments as attachment plaques at the cell membrane, pinocytic vesicles, and basement membranes surrounding the cells. These features are often incompletely developed in LMSs. The actin filaments are usually abundant, but basement membranes are often incomplete.

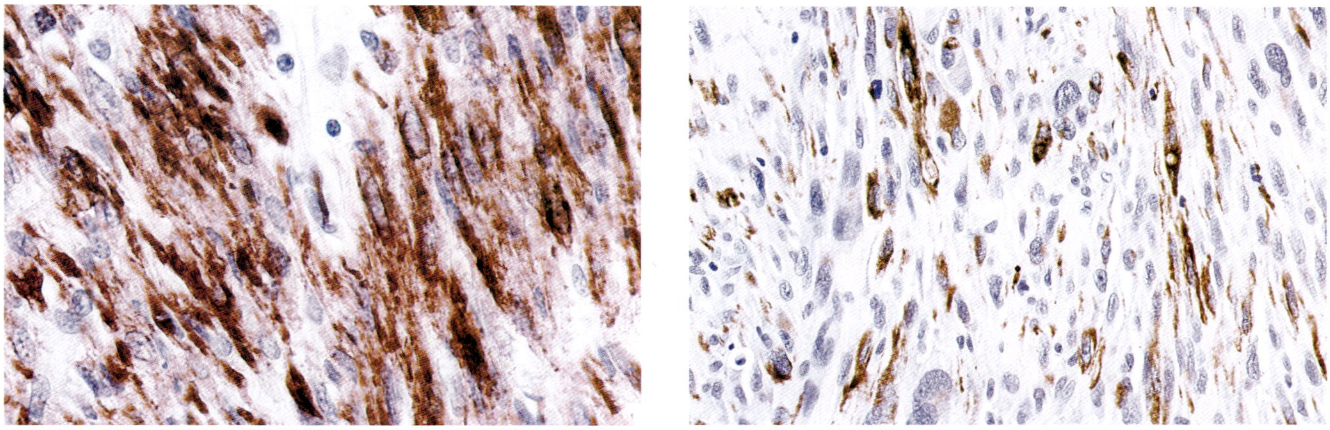

A B

Figure 10–14. Desmin positivity is usually global in well-differentiated LMSs *(A)*, but is often limited in less-differentiated tumors *(B)*.

Molecular Oncology of Leiomyosarcomas

Leiomyosarcomas have been reported to have p53 mutations with a variable frequency.[105–107] One study reported 10% to 20% frequency and showed more common loss of retinoblastoma gene protein 1 (*RB1*) and overexpression of cyclin D1, suggesting that the RB1-cyclin D1 pathway may be more important in their deranged cell cycle control.[108]

Genetics of Leiomyosarcomas

Leiomyosarcomas do not show any single typical cytogenetic changes and tend to show complex, heterogeneous changes. Comparative genomic hybridization studies have also shown multiple, complex, heterogeneous changes, suggesting a genetically advanced disease.[109–112]

REFERENCES

Congenital Smooth Muscle Hamartoma

1. Berger TG, Levin MW: Congenital smooth muscle hamartoma. J Am Acad Dermatol 1984;11:709–712.
2. Johnson MD, Jacobs AH: Congenital smooth muscle hamartoma. A report of six cases and review of the literature. Arch Dermatol 1989;125:820–822.
3. Zvulunov A, Rotem A, Merlob P, Metzker A: Congenital smooth muscle hamartoma. Prevalence, clinical findings, and follow-up in 15 patients. Am J Dis Child 1990;144:782–784.

Pilar Leiomyoma

4. Fisher WC, Helwig EB: Leiomyomas of the skin. Arch Dermatol 1963;88:78–88.
5. Raj S, Calonje E, Kraus M, Cavanagh G, Newman PL, Fletcher CD: Cutaneous pilar leiomyoma: Clinicopathologic analysis of 53 lesions in 45 patients. Am J Dermatopathol 1997;19:2–9.

Angioleiomyoma

6. Hachisuga T, Hashimoto H, Enjoji M: Angioleiomyoma. A clinicopathologic reappraisal of 562 cases. Cancer 1984;54:126–130.
7. Katenkamp D, Kohmehl H, Lengbein L: Angiomyome. Eine pathologish-anatomische Analyse von 229 Fallen. Zentralbl Allg Pathol 1988;134:423–433.
8. Calle SC, Eaton RG, Littler JW: Vascular leiomyomas in the hand. J Hand Surg [Am] 1994;19:281–286.
9. Lawson GM, Salter DM, Hooper G: Angioleiomyomas of the hand. A report of 14 cases. J Hand Surg [Br] 1995;20:479–483.
10. Fox SB, Heryet A, Khong TY: Angioleiomyomas: An immunohistochemical study. Histopathology 1990;16: 495–496.
11. Hasegawa T, Seki K, Yang P, Hirose T, Hizawa K: Mechanism of pain and cytoskeletal properties in angioleiomyomas: An immunohistochemical study. Pathol Int 1994;44:66–72.
12. Heim S, Mandahl N, Kristofferson U, et al: Structural chromosome aberrations in a case of angioleiomyoma. Cancer Genet Cytogenet 1986;20:325–330.
13. Nilbert M, Mandahl N, Heim S, Rydholm A, Willen H, Mitelman F: Cytogenetic abnormalities in angioleiomyoma. Cancer Genet Cytogenet 1989;37:61–64.
14. Sonobe H, Ohtsuki Y, Mizobuchi H, Toda M, Shimizu K: An angiomyoma with t(X;10)(q22;q23.2). Cancer Genet Cytogent 1996;90:54–56.

Angiomyomatous Hamartoma of Lymph Node

15. Chan JKC, Frizzera G, Fletcher CDM, Rosai J: Primary vascular tumors of lymph nodes other than Kaposi's sarcoma. Am J Surg Pathol 1992;16:335–350.
16. Laeng RH, Hotz MA, Borisch B: Angiomyomatous hamartoma of a cervical lymph node combined with hemangiomatosis and vascular transformation of sinuses. Histopathology 1996;29:80–84.

Leiomyoma of External Genitalia and Retroperitoneum

17. Tavassoli FA, Norris HJ: Smooth muscle tumors of the vulva. Obstet Gynecol 1979;53:213–217.
18. Newman PL, Fletcher CDM: Smooth muscle tumours of the external genitalia: Clinicopathologic analysis of a series. Histopathology 1991;18:523–529.
19. Slone S, O'Connor D: Scrotal leiomyomas with bizarre nuclei: A report of three cases. Mod Pathol 1998; 11:282–287.
20. Barton JH, Davis CJ, Sesterhenn IA, Mostofi FK: Smooth muscle hyperplasia of the testicular adnexa clinically mimicking neoplasia: Clinicopathological study of sixteen cases. Am J Surg Pathol 1999;23: 903–909.
21. Paal E, Miettinen M: Retroperitoneal leiomyomas: A clinicopathologic and immunohistochemical study of 56 cases with a comparison to retroperitoneal leiomyosarcomas. Am J Surg Pathol 2001;25:1355–1363.

Intravenous Leiomyomatosis

22. Clement PB: Intravenous leiomyomatosis of the uterus. Pathol Annu 1988;23 (part 2):153–183.
23. Norris HJ, Parley T: Mesenchymal tumors of the uterus. V. Intravenous leiomyomatosis. A clinical and pathological study of 14 cases. Cancer 1975;36:2164–217.
24. Mulvany NJ, Slavin JL, Ostor AG, Fortune DW: Intravenous leiomyomatosis of the uterus: A clinicopathologic study of 22 cases. Int J Gyn Pathol 1994;13:1–19.
25. Brescia RJ, Tazelaar HD, Hobbs HJ, Miller AW: Intravascular leiomyomatosis. A report of two cases. Hum Pathol 1989;20:252–256.

Peritoneal Leiomyomatosis (Leiomyomatosis Peritonealis Disseminata)

26. Tavassoli FA, Norris HJ: Peritoneal leiomyomatosis (Leiomyomatosis peritonealis disseminata): A clinicopathologic study of 20 cases with ultrastructural observations. Int J Gynecol Pathol 1982;1:59–74.
27. Valente PT: Leiomyomatosis peritonealis disseminata. A report of two cases and review of the literature. Arch Pathol Lab Med 1984;108:669–672.
28. Hardman WJ, Majmudar B: Leiomyomatosis peritonealis disseminata: Clinicopathologic analysis of five cases. Southern Med J 19886;89:291–294.
29. Zotalis G, Nayar R, Hicks DG: Leiomyomatosis peritonealis disseminata, endometriosis and multicystic mesothelioma: An unusual association. Int J Gynecol Pathol 1998;17:178–182.
30. Bekkers RL, Willemsen WN, Shijf CP, Massuger LF, Bulten J, Merkus JM: Leiomyomatosis peritonealis disseminata: Does malignant transformation occur? A literature review. Gynecol Oncol 1999;75:158–163.

Esophageal Leiomyoma and Leiomyomatosis

31. Seremetis MG, Lyons WS, deGuzman VC, Peabody JW: Leiomyomata of the esophagus. An analysis of 838 cases. Cancer 1976;38:2166–2177.
32. Miettinen M, Sarlomo-Rikala M, Sobin LH, Lasota J: Esophageal stromal tumors—A clinicopathologic, immunohistochemical and molecular genetic study of seventeen cases and comparison with esophageal leiomyomas and leiomyosarcomas. Am J Surg Pathol 2000;24:211–222.
33. Lonsdale RN, Roberts PF, Vaughan R, Thiru S: Familial oesophageal leiomyomatosis and nephropathy. Histopathology 1993;20:127–133.
34. Heidet L, Boye E, Cai Y: Somatic deletion of the 5′ ends of both the COL4A5 and COL4A6 genes in a sporadic leiomyoma of the esophagus. Am J Pathol 1998;152:673–678.
35. Ueki Y, Naito I, Oohashi T, et al: Topoisomerase I and II consensus sequences in a 17-kb deletion junction of the COL4A5 and COL4A6 genes and immunohistochemical analysis of esophageal leiomyomatosis associated with Alport syndrome. Am J Hum Genet 1998;62:253–261.
36. Ueki Y, Naito I, Oohashi T, et al: Topoisomerase I and II consensus sequences in a 17-kb deletion junction of the COL4A5 and COL4A6 genes and immunohistochemical analysis of esophageal leiomyomatosis associated with Alport syndrome. Am J Hum Genet 1998;62:253–261.
37. Segal Y, Peissel B, Renieri A, et al: LINE-1 elements at the sites of molecular rearrangements in Alport syndrome-diffuse leiomyomatosis. Am J Hum Genet 1999;64:62–69.
38. Sarlomo-Rikala M, El-Rifai W, Andersson L, Miettinen M, Knuutila S: Different patterns of DNA copy number changes in gastrointestinal stromal tumors, leiomyomas and schwannomas. Hum Pathol 1998;29:476–481.

Leiomyoma of Muscularis Mucosae of Colon and Rectum

39. Walsh TH, Mann CV: Smooth muscle neoplasms of the rectum and anal canal. Br J Surg 1987;71: 597–599.
40. Miettinen M, Sarlomo-Rikala M, Sobin LH: Mesenchymal tumors of muscularis mucosae of colon and rectum are benign leiomyomas that should be separated from gastrointestinal stromal tumors: A clinicopathologic and immunohistochemical study of eighty-eight cases. Mod Pathol 2001; 14:950–956.

Lymphangiomyoma(tosis)

41. Cornog JL, Enterline HT: Lymphangiomyoma, a benign lesion of chyliferous lymphatics synonymous with lymphangiopericytoma. Cancer 1966;19:1909–1930.
42. Costello LC, Hartman TE, Ryu JH: High frequency of pulmonary lymphangioleiomyomatosis in women with tuberous sclerosis complex. Mayo Clin Proc 2000; 75:591–594.
43. Corrin B, Liebow AA, Friedman PJ: Pulmonary lymphangiomyomatosis. Am J Pathol 1975;79:348–382.
44. Taylor JR, Ryu J, Colby TV, Raffin TA: Lymphangioleiomyomatosis. Clinical course in 32 patients. N Engl J Med 1990;323:1254–1260.
45. Sullivan EJ: Lymphangioleiomyomatosis. A review. Chest 1998;114:1689–1703.
46. Johnson S: Lymphangiomyomatosis: Clinical features, management and basic mechanisms. Thorax 1999; 54:254–264.
47. Travis WB, Usuki J, Horiba K, Ferrans VJ: Histopathological studies on lymphangioleiomyomatosis. In Moss J (ed): LAM and Other Diseases Characterized by Smooth Muscle Proliferation. Lung Biology in Health and Disease. New York, Marcel Dekker, 1999, pp 171–217.
48. Carsillo T, Astrinidis A, Henske EP: Mutations in the tuberous sclerosis complex gene TSC2 are a cause of sporadic pulmonary lymphangioleiomyomatosis. Proc Natl Acad Sci USA 2000;97:6085–6090.

Leiomyosarcoma

Leiomyosarcomas of Skin and Peripheral Soft Tissue

49. Dahl I, Angervall L: Cutaneous and subcutaneous leiomyosarcoma. A clinicopathologic study of 47 patients. Pathol Eur 1974;9:307–315.
50. Fields JP, Helwig EB: Leiomyosarcoma of the skin and subcutaneous tissue. Cancer 1981;47:156–169
51. Bernstein SC, Roenigk RK: Leiomyosarcoma of the sskin. Treatment of 34 cases. Dermatol Surg 1996;22: 631–635.
52. Jensen ML, Jensen OM, Michalski W, Nielsen OS, Keller J: Intradermal and subcutaneous leiomyosarcoma: A clinicopathological and immunohistochemical study of 41 cases. J Cutan Pathol 1996;23: 458–463.

53. Kaddu S, Beham A, Cerroni L, et al: Cutaneous leiomyosarcoma. Am J Surg Pathol 1997;21:979–987.
54. Wile AG, Evans HL, Romsdahl MM: Leiomyosarcoma of the soft tissue: A clinicopathologic study. Cancer 1981;48:1022–1032.
55. Hashimoto H, Daimaru Y, Tsuneyoshi M, Enjoji M: Leiomyosarcoma of the external soft tissues. A clinicopathologic, immunohistochemical and electron microscopic study. Cancer 1986;57:2077–2088.
56. Neugut AI, Sordillo PP: Leiomyosarcomas of the extremities. J Surg Oncol 1989;40:65–67.
57. Gustafson P, Willen H, Baldetrop B, Ferno M, Akerman M, Rydholm A: Soft tissue leiomyosarcoma. A population-based epidemiologic and prognostic study of 48 patients, including cellular DNA content. Cancer 1992;70:114–119.

Retroperitoneal Leiomyosarcomas

58. Shmookler BM, Lauer DH: Retroperitoneal leiomyosarcoma: A clinicopathologic analysis of 36 cases. Am J Surg Pathol 1983;7:269–280.
59. Todd CS, Michael H, Sutton G: Retroperitoneal leiomyosarcoma: Eight cases and a literature review. Gynecol Oncol 1995;59:333–337.
60. Rajani B, Smith TA, Reith JD, Goldblum JR: Retroperitoneal leiomyosarcomas unassociated with the gastrointestinal tract: A clinicopathologic analysis of 17 cases. Mod Pathol 1999;12:21–28.

Vascular Leiomyosarcomas

61. Varela-Duran J, Oliva H, Rosai J: Vascular leiomyosarcoma: the malignant counterpart of vascular leiomyoma. Cancer 1979;44:1684–1691.
62. Berlin O, Stener B, Kindblom LG, Angervall L: Leiomyosarcoma of venous origin in the extremities. A correlated clinical, roentgenologic, and morphologic study with diagnostic surgical implications. Cancer 1984;54:2147–2159.
63. Leu HJ, Makek M: Intramural venous leiomyosarcomas. Cancer 1986;57:1395–1400.
64. Mingoli A, Cavallaro A, Sapienza P, Di Marzo L, Feldhaus RJ, Cavallari N: International registry of inferior vena cava leiomyosarcoma: Analysis of a world series on 218 patients. Anticancer Res 1996;16:3201–3205.
65. Hines OJ, Nelson S, Quinones-Baldrich WJ, Eilber FR: Leiomyosarcoma of the inferior vena cava: Prognosis and comparison with leiomyosarcoma of other anatomic sites. Cancer 1999;85:1077–1083.
66. Burke AP, Virmani R: Sarcomas of the great vessels. A clinicopathologic study. Cancer 1993;71:1761–1773.

Uterine Leiomyosarcomas

67. Van Dinh T, Woodruff JD: Leiomyosarcoma of the uterus. Am J Obstet Gynecol 1982;144:817–823.
68. Larson B, Silfversward C, Nilsson B, Petterson F: Prognostic factors in uterine leiomyosarcoma. A clinical and histopathological study of 143 cases. The Radiumhemmet series 1936–1981. Acta Oncol 1990;29: 185–191.
69. Jones MW, Norris HJ: Clinicopathologic study of 28 uterine leiomyosarcomas with metastasis. Int J Gynecol Pathol 1995;14:243–249.
70. Mayerhofer K, Obermair A, Windbichler G, et al: Leiomyosarcoma of the uterus: a clinicopathologic multicenter study of 71 cases. Gynecol Oncol 1999; 74: 196–201.
71. Clement PB: The pathology of uterine smooth muscle tumors and mixed endometrial stroma-smooth muscle tumors: A selective review with emphasis on recent advances. Int J Gyn Pathol 2000;19:39–55.
72. Bell SW, Kempson RL, Hendrickson MR: Problematic uterine smooth muscle neoplasms. Am J Surg Pathol 1994;18:535–558.

Leiomyosarcomas of Rare Sites

73. Miettinen M, Sarlomo-Rikala M, Sobin H, Lasota, J: Colonic stromal tumors and leiomyosarcomas. A clinicopathologic, immunohistochemical and molecular genetic study of 44 cases. Am J Surg Pathol 2000; 24:1339–1352.
74. Kuruvilla A, Wenig BM, Humphrey DM, Heffner DK: Leiomyosarcoma of the sinonasal tract. A clinicopathologic study of nine cases. Arch Otolaryngol Head Neck Surg 1990;116:1278–1286.
75. Dry SM, Jorgensen JL, Fletcher CD: Leiomyosarcomas of the oral cavity: An unusual topographic subset easily mistaken for nonmesenchymal tumours. Histopathology 2000;36:210–220.
76. Moran CA, Suster S, Abbondanzo SL, Koss MN: Primary leiomyosarcomas of the lung: A clinicopathologic and immunohistochemical study of 18 cases. Mod Pathol 1997;10:121–128.
77. Mills SE, Bova GS, Wick MR, Young RH: Leiomyosarcoma of the urinary bladder. A clinicopathologic and immunohistochemical study of 15 cases. Am J Surg Pathol 1989;13:480–489.
78. Cheville JC, Dundore PA, Nascimento AG, et al: Leiomyosarcoma of the prostate. Report of 23 cases. Cancer 1995;76:1422–1427.

Leiomyosarcomas in Children

79. Lack EE: Leiomyosarcomas in childhood: A clinical and pathologic study of 10 cases. Pediatr Pathol 1986; 6:181–197.
80. Swanson PE, Wick MR, Dehner LP: Leiomyosarcoma of somatic soft tissues in childhood: An immunohistochemical analysis of six cases with ultrastructural correlation. Hum Pathol 1991;22:569–577.
81. de Saint Aubain Somerhausen N, Fletcher CD: Leiomyosarcoma of soft tissues in children: Clinicopathologic analysis of 20 cases. Am J Surg Pathol 1999;23:755–763.

EBV-Associated Leiomyosarcomas in Immunosuppressed Patients

82. Ross JS, Del Rosario A, Bui HX, Sonbati H, Solis O: Primary hepatic leiomyosarcoma in a child with the

acquired immunodeficiency syndrome. Hum Pathol 1992;23:69–72.

83. Orlow SJ, Kamino H, Lawrence RL: Multiple subcutaneous leiomyosarcomas in an adolescent with AIDS. Am J Pediatr Hematol Oncol 1992;14:265–268.
84. van Hoeven KH, Factor SM, Kress Y, Woodruff JM: Visceral myogenic tumors. A manifestation of HIV infection in children. Am J Surg Pathol 1993;17: 1176–1181.
85. McClain KL, Leach CT, Jenson HB, et al: Association of Epstein-Barr virus with leiomyosarcomas in children with AIDS. N Engl J Med 1995;332:12–18.
86. Timmons CF, Dawson DB, Richards CS, Andrews WS, Katz JA: Epstein-Barr virus-associated leiomyosarcomas in liver transplantation recipients. Origin from either donor or recipient tissue. Cancer 1995;76: 1481–1489.
87. Boman F, Gultekin H, Dickman PS: Latent Epstein-Barr virus infection demonstrated in low-grade leiomyosarcomas of adults with acquired immunodeficiency syndrome, but not in adjacent Kaposi's lesion or smooth muscle tumors in immunocompetent patients. Arch Pathol Lab Med 1997;121:834–838.
88. Hill MA, Araya JC, Eckert MW, Gillespie AT, Hunt JD, Levine EA: Tumor specific Epstein-Barr virus infection is not associated with leiomyosarcoma in human immunodeficiency virus negative individuals. Cancer 1997;80:204–210.
89. Litofsky NS, Pihan G, Corvi F, Smith TW: Intracranial leiomyosarcoma: A neuro-oncological consequence of acquired immunodeficiency syndrome. J Neurooncol 1998;40:179–183.
90. Somers GR, Tesoriero AA, Hartland E, et al: Multiple leiomyosarcomas of both donor and recipient origin arising in heart-lung transplant patient. Am J Surg Pathol 1998;22:1423–1428.
91. Tulbah A, Al-Dayel F, Fawaz I, Rosai J: Epstein-Barr virus-associated leiomyosarcoma of the thyroid in a child with congenital immunodeficiency: A case report. Am J Surg Pathol 1998;23:473–476.
92. Jenson HB, Moltalvo EA, McClain KL, et al: Characterization of natural Epstein-Barr virus infection and replication in smooth muscle cells from a leiomyosarcoma. J Med Virol 1999;57:36–46.
93. Rogatsch H, Bonatti H, Menet A, Larcher C, Feichtinger H, Dirnhofer S: Epstein-Barr virus-associated multicentric leiomyosarcoma in an adult patient after heart transplantation: Case report and review of the literature. Am J Surg Pathol 2000;24:614–621.

Unusual Histologic Variants of Leiomyosarcoma

94. Mentzel T, Wadden C, Fletcher CDM: Granular cell changes in smooth muscle tumours of the skin and soft tissue. Histopathology 1994;24:223–231.
95. Suster S: Epithelioid leiomyosarcoma of the skin and subcutaneous tissue. Clinicopathologic, immunohistochemical, and ultrastructural study of five cases. Am J Surg Pathol 1994;18:232–240.
96. Roncaroli F, Eusebi V: Rhabdomyoblastic differentiation in a leiomyosarcoma of the retroperitoneum. Hum Pathol 1996;27:310–313.

Immunohistochemistry of Leiomyosarcomas

97. Schürch W, Skalli O, Seemayer TA, Gabbiani G: Intermediate filament proteins and actin isoforms as markers for soft tissue tumor differentiation and origin. I. Smooth muscle tumors. Am J Pathol 1987;128:91–103.
98. Azumi N, Ben-Ezra J, Battofora H: Immunophenotypic diagnosis of leiomyosarcomas and rhabdomyosarcomas with monoclonal antibodies to muscle-specific actin and desmin in formalin-fixed tissue. Mod Pathol 1988;1: 469–474.
99. Watanabe K, Kusakabe T, Hoshi N, Saito A, Suzuki T: h-Caldesmon in leiomyosarcoma and tumors with smooth muscle cell-like differentiation: Its specific expression in the smooth muscle cell tumor. Hum Pathol 1999;30:392–396.
100. Miettinen M, Sarlomo-Rikala M, Kovatich AJ, Lasota J: Calponin and h-caldesmon in soft tissue tumors: Consistent h-caldesmon immunoreactivity in gastrointestinal stromal tumors indicates traits of smooth muscle differentiation. Mod Pathol 1999;12: 756–762.
101. Rizeq MN, van de Rijn M, Hendrickson MR, Rouse RV: A comparative immunohistochemical study of uterine smooth muscle neoplasms with emphasis on the epithelioid variant. Hum Pathol 1994;25:671–677.
102. Miettinen M, Sobin LH, Sarlomo-Rikala M: Immunohistochemical spectrum of gastrointestinal stromal tumors at different sites and their differential diagnosis with other tumors with a special reference to CD117 (KIT). Mod Pathol 2000;13:1134–1142.
103. Miettinen M: Immunoreactivity for cytokeratin and epithelial membrane antigen in leiomyosarcoma. Arch Pathol Lab Med 1988;112:637–640.
104. Iwata J, Fletcher CD: Immunohistochemical detection of cytokeratin and epithelial membrane antigen in leiomyosarcoma: A systematic study of 100 cases. Pathol Int 2000;50:7–14.

Molecular Oncology of Leiomyosarcomas

105. de Vos S, Wilczynski SP, Fleischhacker M, Koeffler P: p53 alterations in uterine leiomyosarcomas versus leiomyomas. Gynecol Oncol 1994;54:205–208.
106. Patterson H, Gill S, Fisher C, et al: Abnormalities of the p53, MDM2 and DCC genes in human leiomyosarcomas. Br J Cancer 1994;69:1052–1058.
107. Wurl P, Taubert H, Bache M, et al: Frequent occurrence of p53 mutations in rhabdomyosarcoma and leiomyosarcoma, but not in fibrosarcoma and malignant neural tumors. Int J Cancer 1996;69:317–323.
108. Dei Tos AP, Maestro R, Doglioni C, et al: Tumor suppressor genes and related molecules in leiomyosarcoma. Am J Pathol 1996;148:1037–1045.

Cytogenetic and DNA Copy Number Changes in Leiomyosarcomas

109. Sreekantaiah C, Davis JR, Sandberg AA: Chromosomal abnormalities in leiomyosarcomas. Am J Pathol 1993;142:293–305.

110. Mandahl N, Fletcher CD, Dal Cin P, et al: Comparative cytogenetic study of spindle cell and pleomorphic leiomyosarcomas of soft tissues: A report from the CHAMP study group. Cancer Genet Cytogenet 2000; 116:66–73.
111. Packenham JP, Du Manoir S, Schrock E, et al: Analysis of genetic alterations in uterine leiomyomas and leiomyosarcomas by comparative genomic hybridization. Mol Carcinog 1997;19:273–279.
112. El-Rifai W, Sarlomo-Rikala M, Knuutila S, Miettinen M: DNA copy number changes in development and progression in leiomyosarcomas of soft tissues. Am J Pathol 1998;153:985–990.

Gastrointestinal Stromal Tumors

CHAPTER 11

Gastrointestinal stromal tumor (GIST) is the term currently used for a group of specific mesenchymal tumors of the gastrointestinal (GI) tract. These tumors were designated as GI smooth muscle tumors in the earlier literature under the designations of leiomyoma, cellular leiomyoma, epithelioid leiomyoma, leiomyoblastoma, leiomyosarcoma, and epithelioid leiomyosarcoma (Table 11–1). Because most mesenchymal tumors of the stomach and intestines are GISTs, older data on gastric and small intestinal smooth muscle tumors largely apply to GISTs.[1,2]

Because of their distinctive clinical, histologic, and molecular pathogenetic features, most importantly the KIT receptor tyrosine kinase activation as a driving mechanism, GISTs are now classified separately from true smooth muscle tumors, which are rare in the GI tract, with the notable exceptions of esophageal and colorectal leiomyomas (see Chapter 10).

The GISTs occur in the entire length of the GI tract from the esophagus to the anus, and similar tumors may occur in the omentum, mesentery, and retroperitoneum adjacent to but separate from the stomach and intestines. These tumors have a wide clinical spectrum from benign, small incidentally detected nodules to massive, malignant tumors that can fill the entire abdomen. This chapter summarizes the definition, clinical, pathologic, and molecular genetic features of GISTs.

Definition of GIST

The GISTs are defined here as a cellular spindle cell, epithelioid, or occasionally pleomorphic mesenchymal tumor primary of the GI tract, omentum, or mesentery that expresses the KIT protein (CD117) in the tumor cells, as detected by immunohistochemistry.

This definition specifically excludes true smooth muscle tumors (leiomyomas and leiomyosarcomas), schwannomas, and neurofibromas; these are KIT^-. Nonepithelial tumors that are often KIT^+ but must be separated from GIST include metastatic melanoma, angiosarcoma, and Ewing sarcoma.

A new KIT tyrosine kinase inhibitor (Imatinib mesylate, Novartis), taken orally, has shown promising results in metastatic GISTs, although long-term results are not yet available.[3,4] The treatment has been effective in a great majority of metastatic GISTs, but does not seem effective in KIT^- tumors.[4] This makes defining GISTs accurately even more important.

Clinicopathologic Features

Occurrence

The incidence of GISTs has been estimated as 10–20 per million, and benign tumors outnumber malignant ones. GISTs in any location typically occur in

Table 11–1. Past and Present Diagnostic Terminology*

Past Terminology	Present Terminology and Comment
Esophageal leiomyoma	Most of these tumors are true leiomyomas, histologically and clinically separate from GISTs
Esophageal leiomyosarcoma	Most of these tumors are GISTs, and a small minority are true leiomyosarcomas
Gastric leiomyoma	Great majority are GISTs, and very few are leiomyomas similar to those more commonly seen in the esophagus
Gastric leiomyoblastoma	Corresponds to epithelioid GIST
Gastric leiomyosarcoma	Great majority are GISTs
Small intestinal leiomyoma and leiomyosarcoma	Great majority are GISTs
Colonic and rectal leiomyoma	The small tumors involving muscularis mucosae only are true leiomyomas (benign) Some tumors externally involving colon and rectum in women are uterine type leiomyomas with estrogen and progesterone receptor positivity Most intramural tumors are GISTs, and very few are true leiomyomas
Colonic and rectal leiomyosarcoma	Great majority are GISTs Small minority are true leiomyosarcomas (see Table 11–2)
Gastrointestinal autonomic nerve tumor (GANT)	This category merges with GIST, representing its ultrastructural variant
Leiomyoma/leiomyosarcoma of omentum and mesentery	A majority of these tumors are GISTs and a minority are true leiomyosarcomas
Retroperitoneal leiomyosarcoma	Includes up to one third of GISTs, primary from stomach or intestines, omentum, mesentery and retroperitoneum. Clinical and gross pathology correlation is needed to determine the primary site

*Based on our reclassification and immunohistochemical and molecular genetic studies of over 500 cases.

patients over 50 years of age and are rare in those under the age of 40 years. The median ages in the largest GIST series of different locations ranged between 55 and 65 years.[1,2,5–16] Some series show a male predominance, and others show an equal sex distribution. GISTs are very rare in children; according to our experience, many tumors earlier classified as intestinal smooth muscle tumors in children actually are inflammatory myofibroblastic tumors and not GISTs.

The GISTs are most common in the stomach (60–70%), followed by small intestine (20–30%), colon and rectum (10%), and esophagus (<5%). Occasional GISTs primary in the omentum, mesentery, and retroperitoneum have also been reported.[15,16] The primary site of a GIST diagnosed when disseminated to multiple abdominal sites may be impossible to determine.

Clinical Presentation

Small GISTs are often incidentally detected on gastric or small intestinal serosa at surgery for other conditions, for example, at gallbladder or gynecologic surgery. GISTs may also be detected at gastroscopy as submucosal nodules or occasionally as incidental radiologic findings. For example, some esophageal GISTs analyzed by us were seen in routine chest x-ray. Small rectal GISTs may be palpated at routine physical examination, in men at prostate cancer screening and in women at gynecologic examination.[14]

The symptomatic GISTs of esophagus typically present with dysphagia or occasionally as a mediastinal tumor that at surgery is found to be connected with the esophagus. Gastric GISTs usually give vague symptoms that lead to their gastroscopic detection, and those that ulcerate typically present with upper GI bleeding. Small intestinal GISTs may present with bleeding, vague abdominal symptoms, or, less commonly, mass or obstruction. Colorectal GISTs may manifest with abdominal pain, lower GI bleeding, colonic perforation, or a combination thereof. A minority of GISTs, usually malignant tumors, may be externally palpable. A preoperative specific diagnosis may be successful via endoscopic biopsy, but those GISTs that are not accessible to endoscopic biopsy may be reached via ultrasound-guided abdominal biopsy.

Tumor Behavior and Prognostic Factors

Table 11–2 summarizes suggested criteria of malignancy. Study of larger series of GISTs, defined as KIT^+ tumors, reveals that they have a spectrum of clinical behavior at all sites of their occurrence. In the stomach, the benign GISTs outnumber the malignant ones by a wide margin, whereas higher percentages of small intestinal GISTs and most esophageal and colonic GISTs are clinically malignant. The mesenteric GISTs behave more often aggressively than the omental ones.[13–16]

Table 11–2. Summary of Tumor Size and Mitotic Rate (as Guides to the Evaluation of Mailgnancy of GISTs)

Probably Benign
- Intestinal tumors
  - Maximum diameter less than 2 cm and no more than 5 mitoses per 50 HPF
- Gastric tumors
  - Maximum diameter less than 5 cm and no more than 5 mitoses per 50 HPF

Malignant
- Intestinal tumors
  - Maximum diameter greater than 5 cm or more than 5 mitoses per 50 HPF
- Gastric tumors
  - Maximum diameter greater than 10 cm or more than 5 mitoses per 50 HPF

Uncertain or Low Malignant Potential
- Intestinal tumors
  - Maximum diameter 2–5 cm and no more than 5 mitoses per 50 HPF
- Gastric tumors
  - Maximum diameter 5–10 cm and no more than 5 mitoses per 50 HPF

The small, incidental GISTs have an invariably clinical behavior, probably contributed by the fact that they are readily completely excised. Larger tumors that show low mitotic frequency (≤5 mitoses per 50 high-power field [HPF]) usually have a benign behavior. However, there is a definite percentage of low mitotic tumors that subsequently metastasize, illustrating that low mitotic count does not rule out malignant behavior.[1,6,14] Because the GISTs with low mitotic counts that have malignant behavior are usually large, combination of low mitotic rate and small size (<5 cm) may more uniformly predict a benign behavior. However, gastric tumors seem to behave less aggressively than small intestinal tumors of similar size and mitotic activity.[12] In general, low-grade tumors (<50 mitoses per 50 HPF) show a slower course of disease compared to the high-grade ones, but in long-term follow-up many low-grade tumors metastasize as well.[8]

The GISTs with mitotic count over 5/50 HPF are customarily designated as malignant, and tumors with counts above 50/50 HPF are designated as high-grade malignant. Such tumors have a high risk for diffuse intra-abdominal spread and liver metastasis, the two principal ways of the spread of malignant GISTs. Bone, lung, and subcutaneous metastases are rare.

The prognostic factors found favorable in more than one clinicopathologic series include diploidy on DNA flow cytometry, tumor size less than 5 cm, lack of coagulative tumor necrosis, and low Ki67 analog score (<10%). Intra-abdominal metastasis noted at surgery is an adverse prognostic sign.[17–27]

Gross Features

Grossly, GISTs vary according to their location and tumor size. Small GISTs present as firm, gray-white serosal nodules of the outer surface of stomach, small intestine, or colon. They may also form small, distinct submucous, intramural nodules, especially in the stomach and rectum.

Large malignant GISTs usually involve the stomach and intestines transmurally, where they can form solid or complex, internally cystic, hemorrhagic masses. Some GISTs that communicate with the lumen may simulate GI abscesses or diverticulitis, and intestinal GISTs that grow circumferentially may cause aneurysmatic dilation or constriction of the bowel. Larger GISTs may also be attached to the external aspect of the stomach and intestines and bulge outward to mask the primary GI origin.

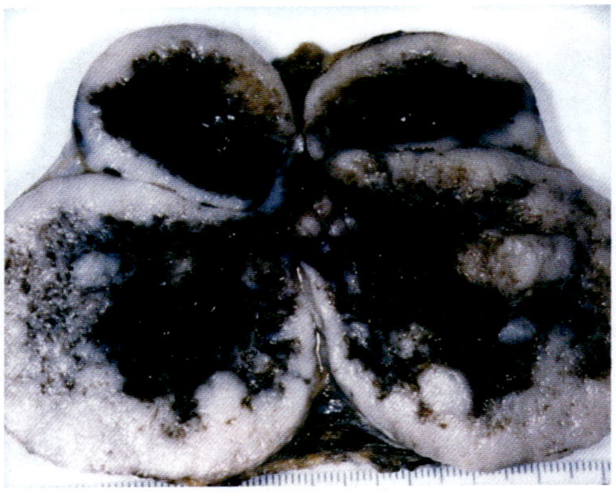

Figure 11–1. Gross appearance of an intra-abdominal metastasis of a malignant GIST. Note central hemorrhagic necrosis (fixed tissue).

Metastatic GISTs typically present as pale tan intra-abdominal nodules, often with central necrosis (Fig. 11–1).

Histologic Features

The most common histologic patterns of the gastric GISTs include cellular spindle cell tumors with moderate to slight interstitial collagen.[1,2,28] Many of these tumors have a prominent, nerve sheath tumor-like nuclear palisading pattern, whereas others show perinuclear vacuolization (Fig. 11–2).

The GISTs with epithelioid appearance correspond with the previous designation of leiomyoblastoma or epithelioid leiomyoma or leiomyosarcoma and may have either a solid or myxoid pattern (see Fig. 11–2*C*). Occasionally they have a paraganglioma

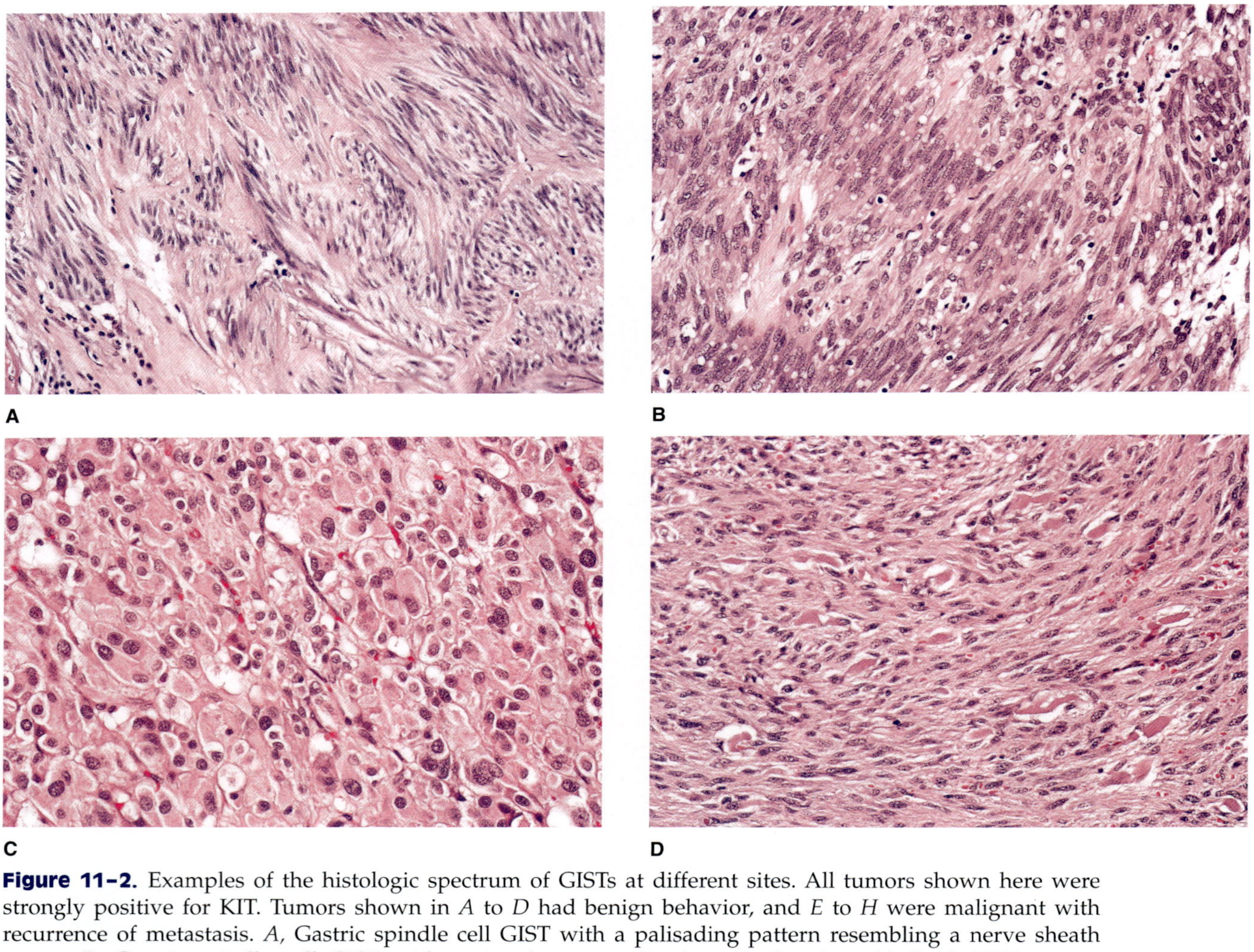

Figure 11–2. Examples of the histologic spectrum of GISTs at different sites. All tumors shown here were strongly positive for KIT. Tumors shown in *A* to *D* had benign behavior, and *E* to *H* were malignant with recurrence of metastasis. *A,* Gastric spindle cell GIST with a palisading pattern resembling a nerve sheath tumor. *B,* Gastric spindle cell GIST with perinuclear vacuolization. *C,* Gastric epithelioid GIST corresponding to the previous designation of leiomyoblastoma. *D,* Small intestinal GIST with extracellular globules of collagen.

or carcinoid-like compartmental pattern. The epithelioid tumors most commonly occur in the stomach and are rare in the intestines. They may also occur in the omentum, mesentery, or retroperitoneum. Most if not all intra-abdominal epithelioid neoplasms formerly referred to as epithelioid smooth muscle tumors are actually GISTs.

Small intestinal (benign) GISTs often contain extracellular collagen globules (skeinoid fibers) as originally ultrastructurally and histologically described by Min (see Fig. 11–2*D*).[30] GISTs of the colon and rectum are almost always spindle cell tumors, which often have a bland histology.

Malignant GISTs show various patterns including solid sheets of spindle cells, round cells, or variably epithelioid morphology. They typically have a higher cellularity and have mitotic activity, by definition 5 or more mitoses per 50 HPF. Variants with significant nuclear pleomorphism are relatively rare (see Figs. 11–2*E–H*).

Cell Differentiation of GIST

Ultrastructure

Although studies correlating KIT expression with ultrastructural features are not available, a large series by Erlandson and coworkers[30] showed complex findings. Many GISTs showed abortive smooth muscle differentiation, others showed autonomous nerve differentiation, and a number of tumors had combined features suggesting multipotential nature.

Immunohistochemistry

The GISTs are defined here as immunohistochemically KIT$^+$ tumors (Fig. 11–3). Typically such positivity is widespread in the entire tumor and appears as strong, cytoplasmic staining, often with membrane and Golgi-zone accentuation.[31–33] The KIT positivity is sometimes weaker in the epithelioid GISTs. KIT is

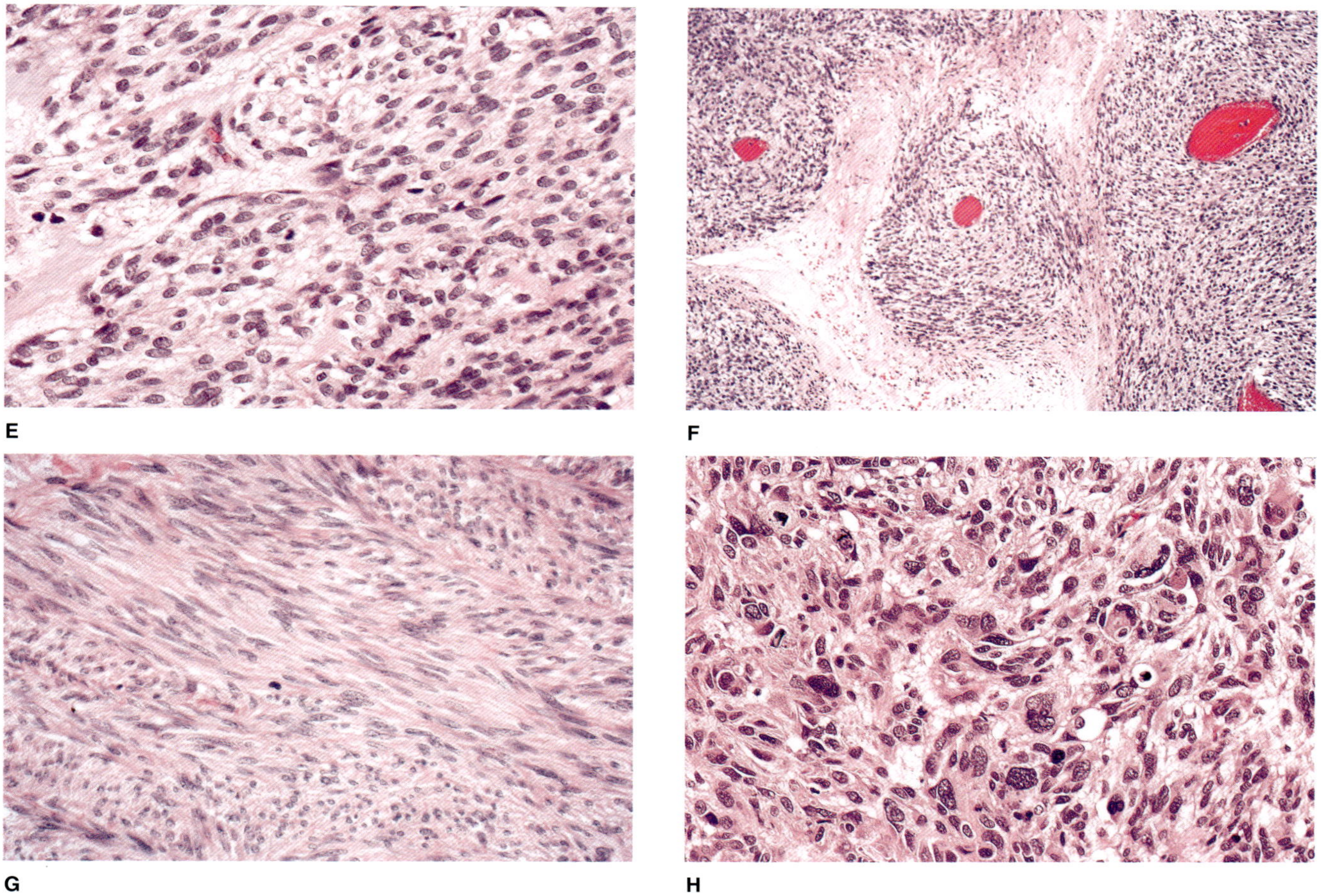

Figure 11–2 *Continued. E,* Malignant gastric GIST with a slightly epithelioid cytologic features. *F,* Malignant gastric GIST with round cells in a perivascular collar-like pattern. *G,* Spindle cell GIST of rectum with relatively bland cytology. *H,* High-grade GIST of colon with pleomorphic cytology.

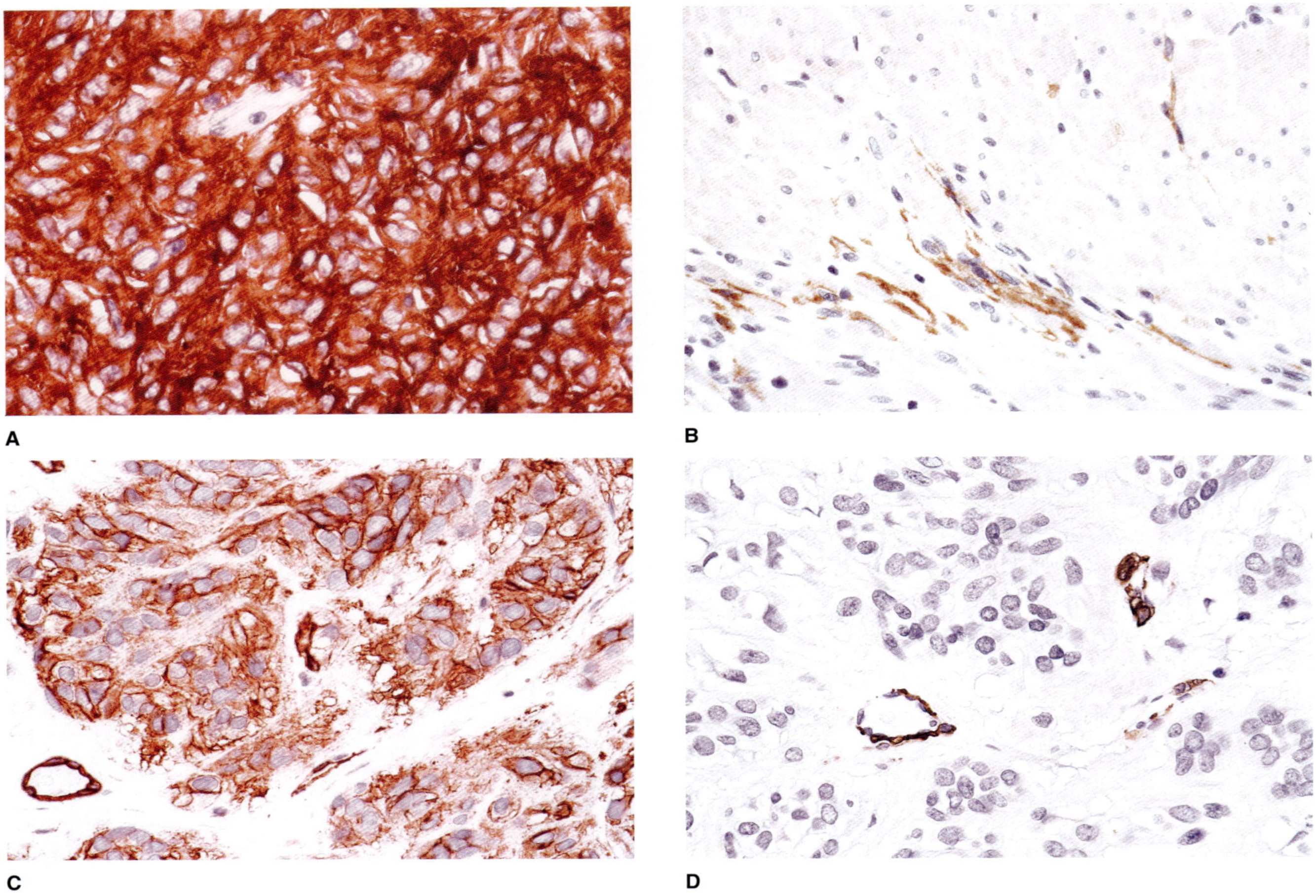

Figure 11-3. Immunohistochemical features of GIST. *A,* KIT^+ GIST with a membrane accentuation. *B,* KIT^+ Cajal cells are seen in the myenteric plexus of stomach. *C,* GISTs are typically also $CD34^+$. Note also positive endothelia. *D,* The majority of GISTs are negative for SMA; only vascular pericytes are positive.

also constitutionally expressed in mast cells and the interstitial cells of Cajal around the myenteric plexus of the GI tract; these cell types serve as excellent internal controls in KIT immunohistochemistry.

CD34 is present in approximately 60% to 70% of all GISTs with a strong apparently cytoplasmic staining sometimes showing membrane accentuation; CD34 expression was confirmed by Western blotting by van de Rijn and colleagues.[34] The esophageal and rectal GISTs have the highest frequency of CD34 positivity (>90%). Gastric benign GISTs are positive in 85% of cases, and the small intestinal ones in 50% of cases with no significant difference in expression between benign and malignant tumors.[35]

Approximately 30% of all GISTs are positive for α smooth muscle actin (SMA).[35,36] The expression may be focal or global, and interestingly is reciprocal with CD34 expression: the SMA^+ tumors are often $CD34^-$ and vice versa. Malignant GISTs are less commonly positive for SMA than the benign ones.

Desmin is only rarely expressed in GISTs. Less than 5% of GISTs contain desmin-positive tumor cells, usually focally. Desmin positivity is more common in epithelioid and esophageal GISTs. As mesenchymal tumors, GISTs are typically strongly positive for vimentin. They are negative for neurofilaments and glial fibrillary acidic protein. Expression of simple epithelial keratins is less common in GISTs than in leiomyosarcomas and occurs in our experience in 5% to 10% of cases.

Although GISTs are typically negative for S-100 protein, approximately 10% of them have cytoplasmic and nuclear S-100 protein positivity. The combination of KIT and S-100 protein positivity in GISTs separates them from schwannomas.[35]

Similar to true smooth muscle tumors (leiomyomas, leiomyosarcomas), GISTs are typically positive for heavy caldesmon (HCD), an actin-binding, cytoskeleton-associated protein.[37] Its presence in GISTs is compatible with a cell type related to smooth muscle cells.

Histogenesis

The KIT+ normal cells in the GI tract, in addition to the mast cells,[37–40] are the interstitial cells of Cajal, autonomic nerve-related GI pacemaker cells that are important for the autonomous intestinal motility. Cajal cells can be seen in the adult intestine in and around the myenteric plexus.[38,39]

Because of the morphologic and immunohistochemical similarities between Cajal cells and GISTs, histogenetic origin of GISTs from Cajal cells has been proposed.[31,33,41] Shared embryonic myosin expression in Cajal cells and GIST[40] and the coexpression of KIT and CD34 in explanted murine Cajal cells[41] was also interpreted to support the relationship of GIST and Cajal cells. Because developmental studies on birds and mice have shown origin of the Cajal cells and smooth muscle from a common precursor,[42] origin of GISTs from such precursor cells is also possible.[43,44] The reported smooth muscle conversion of Cajal cells following blockage of KIT signal transduction pathway suggests that subsets of Cajal cells may be such multipotential precursor cells.[45] This finding may reconcile the theories on GIST origin from Cajal cells versus stem cells.

Genetics of GIST

KIT Gene Mutations and Pathogenesis

Schematic drawing of the *KIT* gene and location of mutations in different diseases is shown in Figure 11–4. Hirota and coworkers first described activating mutations in the exon 11 of the c-kit gene that is an internal, juxtamembrane domain with a regulatory function.[46] The KIT protein belongs to the family of receptor tyrosine kinases of type 3 and is structurally and functionally closely related to macrophage colony-stimulating factor receptor.[47] The receptor normally becomes dimerized and its tyrosine kinase phosphorylated (activated) on the ligand binding, then enabling it to phosphorylate other proteins in the signal transduction pathway that ultimately carries the proliferation signal into the nucleus. These mutations make the KIT independent of ligand (stem cell factor or mast cell growth factor), thereby conferring the cells autonomous growth independent of the external growth factor. This scenario is common in various malignant tumors in which tyrosine kinase activation occurs and is believed to be a central pathogenetic event.

The KIT mutations in GISTs most commonly occur in exon 11. Examples of the exon 11 Kit mutations in GISTs are shown in Figure 11–5. Most often these mutations are in frame deletions of 3 to 21 base pairs in involving codon 550 to 565. Point mutations have also been shown to be activating.[46–48] Rare duplications or insertions have been reported. Several studies have confirmed the presence of exon 11 activating c-kit mutations in GISTs. Such mutations have been found in over half the malignant GISTs,[46–56] and they seem to be more common in large tumors and were suggested as an independent prognostic factor in one study.[54] Such mutations have not been found in benign GISTs; in general, esophageal leiomyomas and true leiomyosarcomas suggest different pathogenesis for these groups of tumors.[50] The KIT activation in GIST is a potential target for therapeutic intervention of GISTs.

The KIT mutation hotspots in GIST were recently discovered in exons 9 and 13. The former mutation is a two-codon duplication, and the latter a point mutation.[55] A large series recently found these mutation with combined frequency of 5%.[56] GISTs do not, at least commonly, seem to have mutations in the exon 17 of the tyrosine kinase domain, the mutation hotspot for mast cell neoplasia.[54]

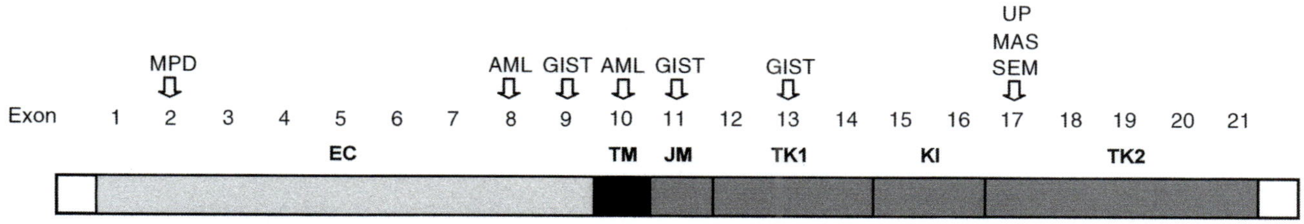

Figure 11–4. Schematic drawing of the domains of the *KIT* gene and location of KIT mutations in GISTs and other tumors. The domains from left to right: extracellular (EC), transmembrane (TM), juxtamembrane (JM), tyrosine kinase I (TK1), kinase insert (KI), tyrosine kinase 2 (TK2). The exon numbers are shown above. The location of KIT mutations in various diseases is shown above the exon numbers. AML, acute myeloid leukemia; GIST, GI stromal tumor; MAS, mastocytoma; MPD, myeloproliferative disorder; UP, urticaria pigmentosa. Note the concentration of KIT mutations of GIST in exons 9, 11, and 13. (Courtesy of Dr. Jerzy Lasota, Washington, DC.)

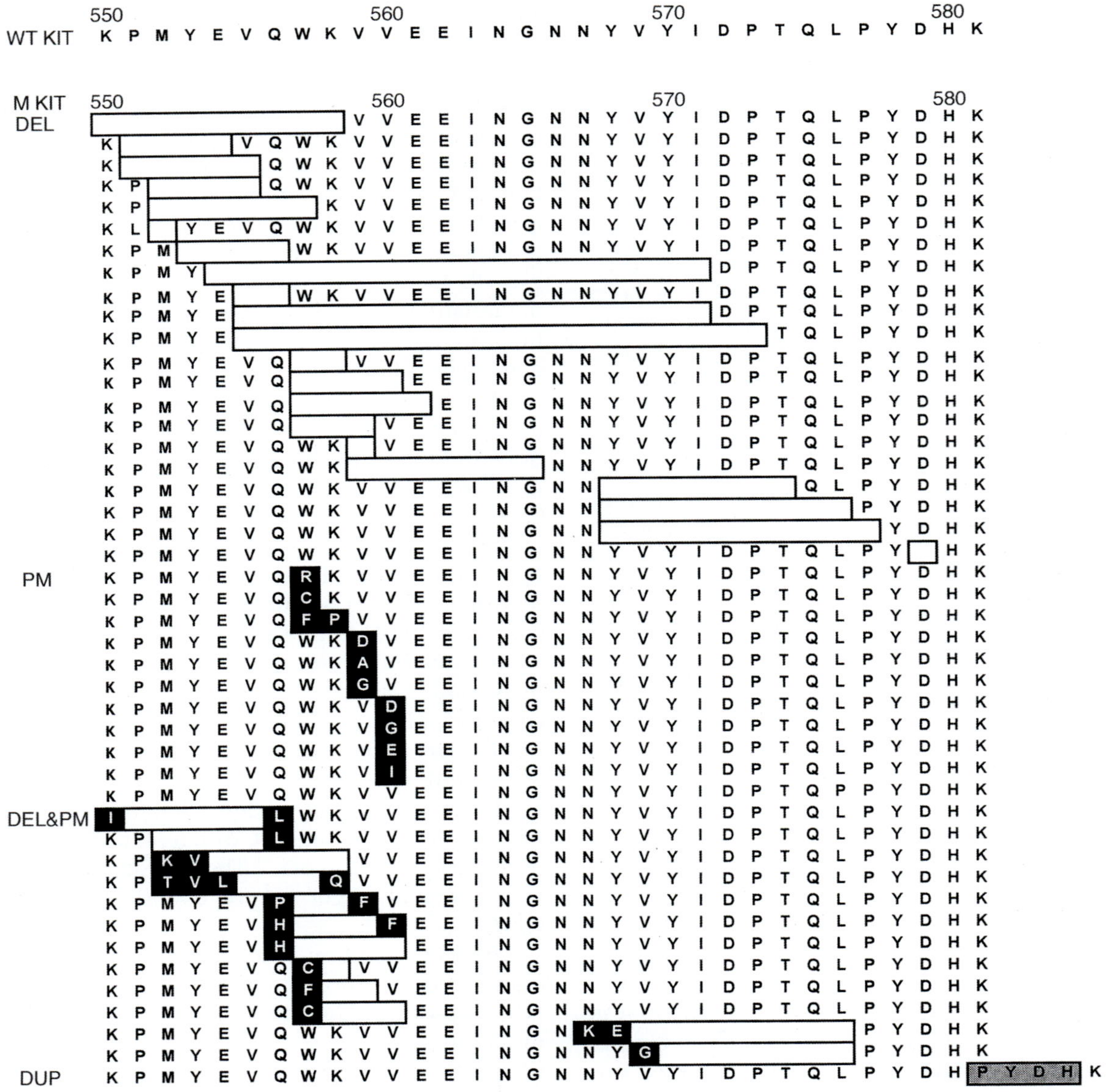

Figure 11–5. Examples of the predicted amino acid sequences of exon 11 *KIT* gene mutations in GISTs. The empty boxes show deletions, black boxes replace point mutations, and gray boxes denote insertions (duplications). Note that a number of cases have a combination of point mutations and deletions. The codon 550 to 570 are most commonly involved. (Courtesy of Dr. Jerzy Lasota, Washington, DC.)

Other Genetic Changes

The present understanding of the genetic changes in GISTs is based mainly on data based on cytogenetics and comparative genomic hybridization (CGH). Common changes include losses in 14q, 15q, and 22q.[57–62] Comparison of benign and malignant GISTs has shown that copy number gains in various loci predominantly occur in malignant GISTs suggesting the CGH evaluation could have predictive value.[62]

The GISTs have been reported in connection with neurofibromatosis 1,[63] and some patients with NF1 have multiple GISTs, although this is a very rare occurrence.

Differential Diagnosis of GIST

Table 11–3 summarizes the differential diagnoses. True leiomyomas occur in the GI tract mainly in the esophagus, colon, and rectum. They are paucicellular spindle cell tumors with histologic resemblance to normal smooth muscle. True leiomyosarcomas also resemble

Table 11-3. Differential Diagnosis of KIT^- Gastrointestinal Tumors That May Resemble GISTs Clinically or Pathologically*

Tumor Entity	Similarities and Differences from GIST
Esophageal leiomyoma	Intramural esophageal tumor composed of well-differentiated actin and desmin-positive smooth muscle cells. Much less cellular than GIST. Occurs more often in young patients than GIST
Pericolonic leiomyoma	Occurs in women; histologically similar to uterine leiomyomas. Positive for estrogen and progesterone receptors, actin and desmin
True leiomyosarcoma	A rare subset of spindle cell sarcomas (up to 10%) that show phenotypic features of well-differentiated smooth muscle cells and often mainfest as polypoid intraluminal masses, typically in older adults
Glomus tumor	Identical with glomus tumor of peripheral soft tissue. Occurs almost exclusively in the stomach in the GI-tract. Positive for smooth muscle actin; negative for desmin. May be variably $CD34^+$; only mast cells KIT^+
Inflammatory fibroid polyp	Spindle cell lesion, may be $CD34^+$. Slender spindle cells admixed with lymphoid cells and eosinophil granulocytes. Some variants are highly vascular and granulation tissue-like with a loose texture. They have a greater cellular heterogeneity than GISTs. Grossly, these lesions often represent ulcerated intraluminal polyps
Inflammatory myofibroblastic tumor (IMT)	Occurs especially in children and young adults; may form a gastric or intestinal mass simulating a GIST. More often omental or mesenteric. Many tumors reported as GISTs in children in literature are IMTs. Spindled or slightly epithelioid cells with amphophilic cytoplasm and cytoplasmic processes. Has ALK-gene expression and rearrangements. Also has been referred to as inflammatory fibrosarcoma.
Mesenteric desmoid	May have a GIST-like gastric or intestinal wall involvement. Grossly very firm and white. Fibroblasts and myofibroblasts in collagenous background. $CD34^-$
Solitary fibrous tumor	May present on the peritoneal surfaces or in the liver. Collagenous spindle cell tumor, with a focal hemangiopericytoma-like pattern. $CD34^+$
Schwannoma submucosal	Usually a small, yellow circumscribed tumor, most commonly in the stomach and secondly in the colon. Slender, often bundled S100-protein positive spindle cells, often in a microtrabecular pattern in an S100-protein-negative fibrous background. $GFAP^+$ is also common; this is almost never seen in GISTs.
Undifferentiated sarcomas	Malignant gastrointestinal tumors that do not express any specific cell-type markers and cannot currently be further defined. May grossly simulate GISTs, but histologically often show greater nuclear pleomorphism than GISTs.
Dedifferentiated liposarcoma	Mesenteric, retroperitoneal tumors that may involve intestinal walls in a GIST-like manner. May have myxoid or pleomorphic MFH- or fibrosarcoma-like features. Diagnosis is difficult if fat is not present in the sampled tissue.
Metastatic melanoma	May form a grossly GIST-like tumor with involvement of layers of the intestines or stomach. Can also be KIT^+. More often than GIST forms a polypoid intramural lesion. Positivity for melanocytic markers (tyrosinase, melanA, HMB45, in various combinations), is diagnostic.

*All types immunohistochemically tested by author.

differentiated smooth muscle cells and are positive for smooth muscle actin and desmin. Schwannomas are rare in the GI tract. They are spindle cell tumors with vague nuclear palisading and are strongly S-100 protein positive and usually positive for glial fibrillary acidic protein (GFAP) and negative for KIT. Intra-abdominal fibromatosis forms mesenteric masses that may also involve gastric and intestinal walls. These tumors are usually more collagenous and less cellular, and they are KIT^-. Inflammatory myofibroblastic tumor occurs especially in children. This tumor may form a GIST-like transmural mass in the stomach or intestines, although it is more often omental or mesenteric. The spindled tumor cells are typically admixed with lymphocytes and plasma cells and are often positive for actins but are KIT^-. Dedifferentiated retroperitoneal liposarcomas are spindle cell tumors negative for KIT. Other potentially KIT^+ neoplasms such as metastatic small cell carcinoma, melanoma, angiosarcoma, and the Ewing sarcoma family of tumors should not be confused with GIST, although these tumors are KIT^+ with a frequency of over 50%.

Gastrointestinal autonomic nerve tumors[64–66] appear to be a subset of GIST, because these tumors are KIT^+ and are histologically similar to GISTs, and have GIST-specific KIT mutations.[66]

REFERENCES

General

1. Appelman HD: Mesenchymal tumors of the gut: Histological perspectives, new approaches, new results, and does it make any difference. Monogr Pathol 1990; 31:220–246.
2. Miettinen M, Lasota J: Gastrointestinal stromal tumors—definition, clinical, histological, immunohistochemical, and molecular genetic features and differential diagnosis. Virchows Arch 2001;438:1–12.
3. Joensuu H, Roberts PJ, Sarlomo-Rikala M, et al: Effect of tyrosine kinase inhibitor ST1571 in a patient with a metastatic gastrointestinal stromal tumor. N Engl J Med 2001;344:1052–1056.
4. van Oosterom AT, Judson I, Verweij J, et al: Safety and efficacy of imatinib (ST1571) in metastatic gastrointestinal stromal tumors: A phase I study. Lancet 2001;358: 1421–1423.

Clinicopathologic Studies

5. Appelman HD, Helwig EB: Cellular leiomyomas of the stomach in 49 patients. Arch Pathol Lab Med 1977;101:373–377.
6. Ranchod M, Kempson RL: Smooth muscle tumors of the gastrointestinal tract and retroperitoneum. Cancer 1977;39:255–262.
7. DeMatteo RP, Lewis JJ, Leung D, Mudan SS, Woodruff JM, Brennan MF: Two hundred gastrointestinal stromal tumors. Recurrence patterns and prognostic factors for survival. Ann Surg 2000;231:51–58.
8. Evans HL: Smooth muscle tumors of the gastrointestinal tract. A study of 56 cases followed for a minimum of 10 years. Cancer 1985;56:2242–2250.
9. Ueyama T, Guo K-J, Hashimoto H, Daimaru Y, Enjoji M: A clinicopathologic and immunohistochemical study of gastrointestinal stromal tumors. Cancer 1992;69:947–955.
10. Lerma E, Oliva E, Tugues D, Prat J: Stromal tumours of the gastrointestinal tract: A clinicopathological and ploidy analysis of 33 cases. Virchows Arch 1994;424:19–24.
11. Rudolph P, Gloeckner K, Parvaresch R, Harms D, Schimidt D: Immunopheno-type, proliferation, DNA-ploidy, and biological behavior of gastrointestinal stromal tumors: A multivariate clinicopathologic study. Hum Pathol 1998;29:791–800.
12. Emory TS, Sobin LH, Lukes L, Lee DH, O'Leary TJ: Prognosis of gastro-intestinal smooth-muscle (stromal) tumors. Am J Surg Pathol 1999;23:82–87.
13. Miettinen M, Sarlomo-Rikala M, Sobin LH, Lasota J: Esophageal stromal tumors: A clinicopathologic, immunohistochemical and molecular genetic study of seventeen cases and comparison with esophageal leiomyomas and leiomyosarcomas. Am J Surg Pathol 2000;23:121–132.
14. Miettinen M, Furlong M, Sarlomo-Rikala M, Burke A, Sobin LH, Lasota J: Gastrointestinal stromal tumors, intramural leiomyomas, and leiomyosarcomas in the rectum and anus. A clinicopathologic, immunohistochemical and melecular genetic study of 144 cases. Am J Surg Pathol 2001;25:1121–1133.
15. Miettinen M, Monihan JM, Sarlomo-Rikala M, et al: Gastrointestinal stromal tumors/smooth muscle tumors/GISTs in the omentum and mesentery: Clinicopathologic and immunohistochemical study of 26 cases. Am J Surg Pathol 1999;22:1109–1119.
16. Reith JD, Goldblum JR, Lyles RH, Weiss SW: Extragastrointestinal (soft tissue) stromal tumors. An analysis of 48 cases with emphasis on histological predictors of outcome. Mod Pathol 2000;13:577–585.

Prognostic Factors

17. Franquemont DW: Differentiation and risk assessment of gastrointestinal stromal tumors. Am J Clin Pathol 1995;103:41–47.
18. Cooper PN, Quirke P, Hardy GJ, Dixon MF: A flow cytometric, clinical and histological study of stromal neoplasms of the gastrointestinal tract. Am J Surg Pathol 1992;16:163–170.
19. Cunningham RE, Federspiel BH, McCarthy WF, Sobin LH, O'Leary TJ: Predicting prognosis of gastrointestinal stromal smooth muscle tumors. Role of clinical and histologic evaluation, flow cytometry, and image cytometry. Am J Surg Pathol 1993;117:588–594.
20. Yu W, Fletcher CDM, Newman PL, Goodlad JR, Burton JC, Levison DA: A comparison of proliferating cell

nuclear antigen (PCNA) immunostaining, nucleolar organizing region (AgNOR) staining, and histological grading in gastrointestinal stromal tumours. J Pathol 1992;166:147–152.
21. Amin MB, Ma CK, Linden MD, Kubus JJ, Zarbo RJ: Prognostic value of proliferating cell nuclear antigen index in gastric stromal tumors. Correlation with mitotic count and clinical outcome. Am J Clin Pathol 1993;100:428–432.
22. Ray R, Tahan SR, Andrews C, Goldman H: Stromal tumors of the stomach: Prognostic value of the PCNA index. Mod Pathol 1994;7:26–30.
23. Sbaschnig RJ, Cunningham RE, Sobin LH, O'Leary TJ: Proliferating-cell nuclear antigen immunocytochemistry in the evaluation of gastrointestinal smooth-muscle tumors. Mod Pathol 1994;7:780–783.
24. Franquemont DW, Frierson HF: Proliferating cell nuclear antigen immunoreactivity and prognosis of gastrointestinal stromal tumors. Mod Pathol 1995;8:473–477.
25. Emory TS, Derringer GA, Sobin LH, O'Leary TJ: Ki-67 (MIB-1) immunohistochemistry as a prognostic factor in gastrointestinal smooth-muscle tumors. J Surg Pathol 1997;2:239–242.
26. Tsushima K, Rainwater LM, Goellner JR, Heerden JA, Lieber MM: Leiomyosarcomas and benign smooth muscle tumors of the stomach: Nuclear DNA patterns studied by flow cytometry. Mayo Clin Proc 1987;62: 275–280.
27. Kiyabu MT, Bishop PC, Parker JW, Turner RR, Fitzgibbons PL: Smooth muscle tumours of the gastrointestinal tract: Flow cytometric quantitation of DNA and nuclear antigen content and correlation with histological grade. Am J Surg Pathol 1988;12:954–960.

Histologic Spectrum and Ultrastructure

28. Suster S: Gastrointestinal stromal tumors. Semin Diagn Pathol 1996;3:297–313.
29. Min K-W: Small intestinal stromal tumors with skeinoid fibers. Clinicopathological, immunohistochemical, and ultrastructural investigations. Am J Surg Pathol 1992;16:145–155.
30. Erlandson RA, Klimstra DS, Woodruff JM: Subclassification of gastrointestinal stromal tumors based on evaluation by electron microscopy and immunohistochemistry. Ultrastruct Pathol 1996;20:373–393.

Cell Differentiation (Histogenesis)

31. Kindblom LG, Remotti HE, Aldenborg F, Meis-Kindblom JM: Gastrointestinal pacemaker cell tumor (GIPACT). Gastrointestinal stromal tumors show phenotypic characteristics of the interstitial cells of Cajal. Am J Pathol 1998;152:1259–1269.
32. Sarlomo-Rikala M, Kovatich A, Barusevicius A, Miettinen M: CD117: A sensitive marker for gastrointestinal stromal tumors that is more specific than CD34. Mod Pathol 1998;11:728–734.
33. Sircar K, Hewlett BR, Huizinga JD, Chorneyko K, Berezin I, Riddell RH. Interstitial cells of Cajal as precursors for gastrointestinal stromal tumors. Am J Surg Pathol 1999;23:377–389.
34. van de Rijn M, Hendrickson MR, Rouse RV: The CD34-expression by gastrointestinal stromal tumors. Hum Pathol 1994;25:766–771.
35. Miettinen M, Sobin LH, Sarlomo-Rikala M: Immunohistochemical spectrum of GISTs of different locations and their differential diagnosis. Mod Pathol 2000; 13:536–541.
36. Franquemont DW, Frierson HF: Muscle differentiation and clinicopathologic features of gastrointestinal stromal tumors. Am J Surg Pathol 1992;16:947–954.
37. Miettinen M, Sarlomo-Rikala M, Kovatich AJ, Lasota J: Calponin and h-caldesmon in soft tissue tumors: Consistent h-caldesmon immunoreactivity in gastrointestinal stromal tumors indicates traits of smooth muscle differentiation. Mod Pathol 1999;12:1109–1118.
38. Maeda H, Yamagata A, Nishikawa S, et al: Requirement of c-kit for development of intestinal pacemaker system. Development 1992;116:369–375.
39. Sanders KM: A case for intestinal cells as pacemakers and mediators of neurotransmission in the gastrointestinal tract. Gastroenterology 1996;111:492–515.
40. Tsuura Y, Hiraki H, Watanabe K, Igarashi S, Shimamura K, Fukuda T: Preferential localization of c-kit product in tissue mast cells, basal cells of skin, epithelial cells of breast, small cell lung carcinoma and seminoma/dysgerminoma in human: Immunohistochemical study of formalin-fixed, paraffin-embedded tissues. Virchows Arch 1994;424:135–141.
41. Sakurai S, Fukusawa T, Chong JM, Tanaka A, Fukuyama M: Embryonic form of smooth muscle myosin heavy chain (SEmb/MCH-B) in gastrointestinal stromal tumor and interstitial cells of Cajal. Am J Pathol 1999;154: 23–28.
42. Robinson TL, Sircar K, Hewlett BR, Chorneyko K, Riddell RH, Huizanga JD: Gastrointestinal stromal tumors may originate from a subset of CD34-positive interstitial cells of Cajal. Am J Pathol 2000;156:1157–1163.
43. Lecoin L, Gabella G, Le Douarin N: Origin of the c-kit positive interstitial cells in the avian bowel. Development 1996;122:725–733.
44. Young HM, Ciampoli D, Southwell BR, Newgreen DF: Origin of interstitial cells of Cajal in the mouse intestine. Dev Biol 1996;180:97–107.
45. Torihashi S, Nishi K, Tokutomi Y, Nishi T, Ward S, Sanders KM: Blockade of kit signaling induces transdifferentiation of interstitial cells of Cajal to a smooth muscle phenotype. Gastroenterology 1999;117: 140–148.

KIT Mutations

46. Hirota S, Isozaki K, Moriyama Y, et al: Gain-of-function mutations of c-kit in human gastrointestinal stromal tumors. Science 1998;279:577–580.
47. Kitamura Y, Hirota S, Nishida T: Molecular pathology of c-kit proto-oncogen and development of gastrointestinal stromal tumors. Ann Chir Gyn 1998;87: 282–286.

48. Nakahara M, Isozaki K, Hirota S, et al: A novel gain-of-function mutation of c-kit gene in gastrointestinal stromal tumors. Gastroenterology 1998;115:1090–1095.
49. Nishida T, Hirota S, Taniguchi M, et al: Familial gastrointestinal stromal tumours with germline mutation of the KIT gene. Nat Genet 1998;19:323–342.
50. Lasota J, Jasinski M, Sarlomo-Rikala M, Miettinen M: Mutations in exon 11 of c-kit occur preferentially in malignant versus benign gastrointestinal stromal tumors and do not occur in leiomyomas and leiomyosarcomas. Am J Pathol 1999;154:53–60.
51. Ernst SI, Hubbs AE, Przygodzki RM, Emory TS, Sobin LH, O'Leary TJ: KIT mutation portends poor prognosis in gastrointestinal stromal/smooth muscle tumors. Lab Invest 1998;78:1633–1636.
52. Moskaluk CR, Tian Q, Marshall CR, Rumpel CA, Franquemont DW, Frierson HF: Mutations of c-kit JM domain are found in a minority of human gastrointestinal stromal tumors. Oncogene 1999;18: 1897–1902.
53. Sakurai S, Fukasawa T, Chong JM, Tanaka A, Fukayama M: C-kit gene abnormalities in gastrointestinal stromal tumors (tumors of interstitial cells of Cajal) Jpn J Cancer Res 1999;90:1321–1328.
54. Taniguchi M, Nishida T, Hirota S, et al: Effect of c-kit mutation on prognosis of gastrointestinal stromal tumors. Cancer Res 1999;59:4297–4300.
55. Lux M, Rubin BP, Biase TL, et al: KIT extracellular and kinase domain mutations in gastrointestinal stromal tumors. Am J Pathol 2000;156:791–795.
56. Lasota J, Wozniak A, Sarlomo-Rikala M, et al: Mutations in exons 9 and 13 of KIT gene are rare events in gastrointestinal stromal tumors: A study of two hundred cases. Am J Pathol 2000;157:1091–1095.

Genetic Changes, Other Than KIT

57. Dal Cin P, Aly MS, De Wever I, van Damme B, van den Berghe H: Does chromosome investigation discriminate between benign and malignant gastrointestinal leiomyomatous tumors. Diagn Oncol 1992;2:55–59.
58. El-Rifai W, Sarlomo-Rikala M, Miettinen M, Knuutila S, Andersson LCA: DNA copy number losses in chromosome 14: An early change in gastrointestinal stromal tumors. Cancer Res 1996;56:3230–3233.
59. Sarlomo-Rikala M, El-Rifai W, Andersson L, Miettinen M, Knuutila S: Different patterns of DNA copy number changes in gastrointestinal stromal tumors, leiomyomas and schwannomas. Hum Pathol 1998;29: 476–481.
60. El-Rifai W, Sarlomo-Rikala M, Miettinen M, Knuutila S, Andersson LCA: DNA copy number losses in chromosome 14: An early change in gastrointestinal stromal tumors. Cancer Res 1996;56:3230–3233.
61. El-Rifai W, Sarlomo-Rikala M, Andersson L, Miettinen M, Knuutila S: High resolution deletion mapping of chromosome 14 in stromal tumors of the gastrointestinal tract. Genes Chrosom Cancer 2000;7:387–391.
62. El-Rifai W, Sarlomo-Rikala M, Andersson L, Knuutila S, Miettinen M: Prognostic significance of DNA copy number changes in benign and malignant GISTs. Cancer Res 2000; 60:3899–3903.
63. Schaldenbrand J, Appelman HD: Solitary solid stromal gastrointestinal tumors in von Recklinghausen's disease with minimal smooth muscle differentiation. Hum Pathol 1984;15:229–232.

Gastrointestinal Autonomic Nerve Tumors

64. Herrera GA, Cerezo L, Jones JE, et al: Gastrointestinal autonomic nerve tumors "Plexosaromas". Arch Pathol 1989;113:846.
65. Lauwers GY, Erlandson RA, Casper ES, Brennan MF, Woodruff JM: Gastrointestinal autonomic nerve tumors. A clinicopathologic, immunohistochemical, and ultrastructural study of 12 cases. Am J Surg Pathol 1993; 17:887–893.
66. Lee JR, Joshi V, Griffin JW Jr, Lasota J, Miettinen M: Gastrointestinal autonomic nerve tumor: Immunohistochemical and molecular identity with gastrointestinal stromal tumor. Am J Surg Pathol 2001;25:979–987.

Gynecologic Stromal Tumors

CHAPTER 12

Some mesenchymal tumors of the vulva, vagina, and adjacent soft tissues are specific for these sites, and common to them is origin from the hormonally responsive stromal elements, as illustrated by their estrogen and progesterone receptor positivity. Other mesenchymal tumors also occur in this region, but they are not related to the specific stromal tissues and more commonly occur elsewhere in the body; these tumors are not included in this chapter.

Tumors believed to be similar to some of the entities have also been reported in men, but their full identity with their female counterparts is open.

Some sarcomas of the uterus and adjacent genital organs, such as endometrial stromal sarcoma and carcinosarcoma (malignant mixed müllerian tumor), sometimes arise outside of the genitals in the pelvis or other abdominal locations. Also these tumors may metastasize almost anywhere in the abdominal cavity and sometimes outside it, especially to the lungs. Among such tumors is also granulosa cell tumor of the ovary, which can recur after long periods of time and sometimes simulate an intra-abdominal mesenchymal tumor. The specific recognition of genital stromal tumors is important because some of them are responsive to hormonal or antihormonal treatment.

Mesodermal Stromal Polyp (Fibroepithelial Polyp, Pseudosarcomatous Stromal Polyp)

This is a heterogeneous group of polyps usually occurring in young women, sometimes during pregnancy. Some of them have bland cytology and others are highly cellular and may be pseudosarcomatous; nevertheless all have indolent behavior.

Clinical Features

These polyps occur in the mucosa of the vagina, vulva, or rarely the cervix. They are usually diagnosed in young women (median age 35–45 years in different series) and rarely in infants and postmenopausal women. Half the patients have been asymptomatic, and the others have had local discomfort or bleeding. In some clinicopathologic series, half the patients have been pregnant, and as many as one third have had two or more polyps. The behavior was benign in published studies, and recurrence is rare.[1–7] The lesions in infants may regress warranting an extremely conservative management.[1] Because some evidence indicates that tumors with more atypical features more often recur,[6] polyps with significant atypia should be excised with normal tissue margins. Long-term follow-up studies are necessary to rule out a tumor cohort with a more adverse behavior.

Pathology

Grossly, the polyp may have a smooth surface and be pedunculated or composed of multiple finger-like polypoid protrusions potentially simulating the appearance of botryoid rhabdomyosarcoma.

Histologically, the lesions are heterogeneous. Generally they occupy the entire subepithelial zone. They can be bland and edematous, as seen in the lesions of infants, or be composed of stellate-shaped, sometimes multinucleated fibroblasts (Fig. 12–1*A*). Some lesions are highly cellular and atypical having frequent bizarre nuclei, high mitotic activity over 10/10 high-power field (HPF), and even atypical mitoses (Fig. 12–1*B*). This variant has been referred to as pseudosarcomatous stromal polyp and has histologic analogy to atypical fibroxanthoma of the skin. Such atypical polyps, in particular, are associated with pregnancy.

Immunohistochemically typical is expression of desmin and estrogen and progesterone receptors, whereas the tumor cells are generally negative for actins, S-100 protein, histiocytic markers, and keratins.[5,8]

Differential Diagnosis

The mesodermal stromal polyp should not be confused with botryoid rhabdomyosarcoma, which usually occurs in small children, is more highly cellular at the stromoepithelial interface, and contains differentiated rhabdomyoblasts at least focally. Fortunately, the rarely reported polyps in infants have been paucicellular and histologically not posing a problem with differential diagnosis.[1] Genital rhabdomyoma occurs as a polypoid lesion in adult women. These tumors show well-differentiated skeletal muscle cells without mitotic activity.

Superficial cervicovaginal myofibroblastoma forming a broad-based dome-shaped lesion has been previously included among mesodermal stromal polyps. It is now considered a separate entity, however, and is discussed in the following section.

Pedunculated fibroepithelial polyps of the skin of the labia majora represent a different entity more comparable to fibroepithelial polyps (acrochordon) of the skin.

Some mucosal melanomas and carcinomas (e.g., metastases from renal cell carcinoma), may form

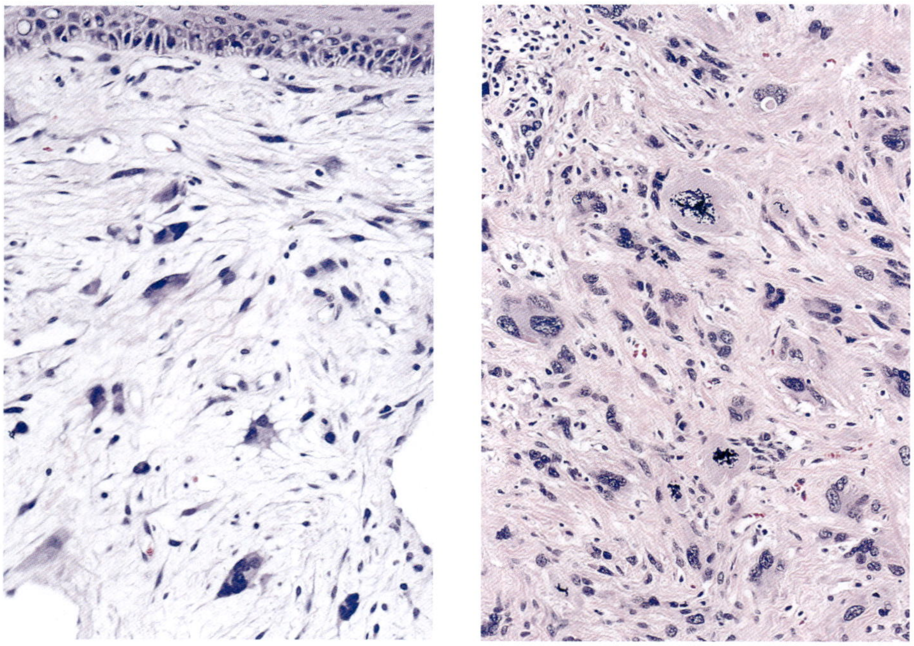

A B

Figure 12–1. Two different appearances of a mesodermal stromal polyp. *A,* Lesion with limited cellularity with numerous multinucleated giant cells. *B,* Highly cellular example with prominent mitotic activity and nuclear atypia. Note also the atypical mitoses.

polypoid lesions; exclusion of these entities and establishing the diagnosis of a pseudosarcomatous polyp may require immunohistochemical studies.

Superficial Cervicovaginal Myofibroblastoma

This lesion has clinicopathologic features distinct from the mesodermal stromal polyp, but such cases have apparently been included in previous series of the latter.

Clinical Features

The tumor occurs in patients older than those with the mesodermal stromal polyp, and 10 of 14 patients in the seminal series were over age 50. The mass is located in the vagina or less commonly in the cervix, and usually measures 1 to 2 cm, occasionally over 5 cm. Clinical behavior has been benign in all cases.[9]

Pathology

Grossly typical is a broad-based, dome-shaped elevated lesion below the mucosa, which may be hyperplastic or less commonly ulcerated. On sectioning, the tumor is glistening, mucoid, or fleshy and varies from white to pink.

Histologically, the lesion is often located beneath a zone of normal superficial stroma. It is composed of alternating cellular collagenous and myxoid areas, sometimes with a lacelike pattern with prominent capillaries (Fig. 12–2). The tumor cells are oval and uniform and have no distinct cell borders. Small amounts of eosinophilic cytoplasm may be seen as bipolar processes, especially in vimentin or desmin immunostains. The nuclei are oval with an even chromatin pattern and a small nucleolus. Mitotic activity is scant (0–2/50 HPF). Mast cells are often present.

Immunohistochemically, the tumor cells are positive for vimentin, desmin, and estrogen and progesterone receptors (Fig. 12–3). They are also variably positive for CD34, and occasionally for muscle actins, but are negative for S-100 protein, epithelial membrane antigen, and keratins.[9]

Genital (Vaginal) Rhabdomyoma

This rare, site-specific benign tumor usually occurs in the vagina. It differs from adult rhabdomyoma, which occurs in the head and neck of adults, and contains complex-shaped, typically cross-sectional profiles of skeletal muscle cells. Genital rhabdomyoma has some similarities to fetal rhabdomyoma, a highly cellular tumor usually seen in the head and neck of children and composed of less-differentiated, elongated rhabdomyoblasts (see Chapter 13).

Clinical Features

This very rare, histologically distinctive polypoid tumor typically occurs in early middle-aged women; over 20 cases have been reported.[10–13] It presents as a small broad-based mucosal polyp usually in the vagina and occasionally in the vulva or cervix. Clinical symptoms are similar to those of mesodermal stromal polyps, and behavior is benign following a simple excision.

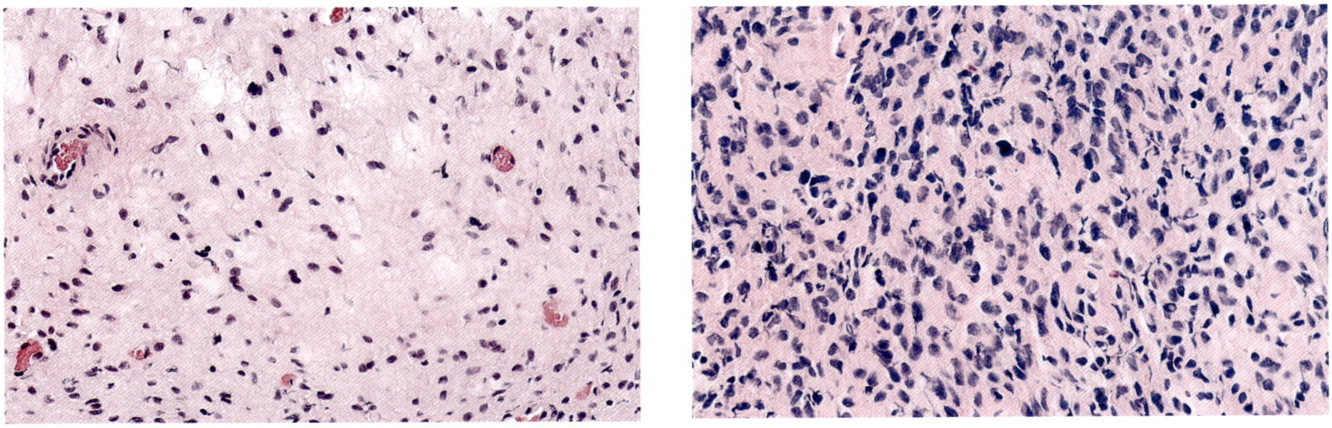

A B

Figure 12–2. Superficial cervicovaginal myofibroblastoma. *A,* Relatively low cellularity. *B,* Higher cellularity and uniform oval cells.

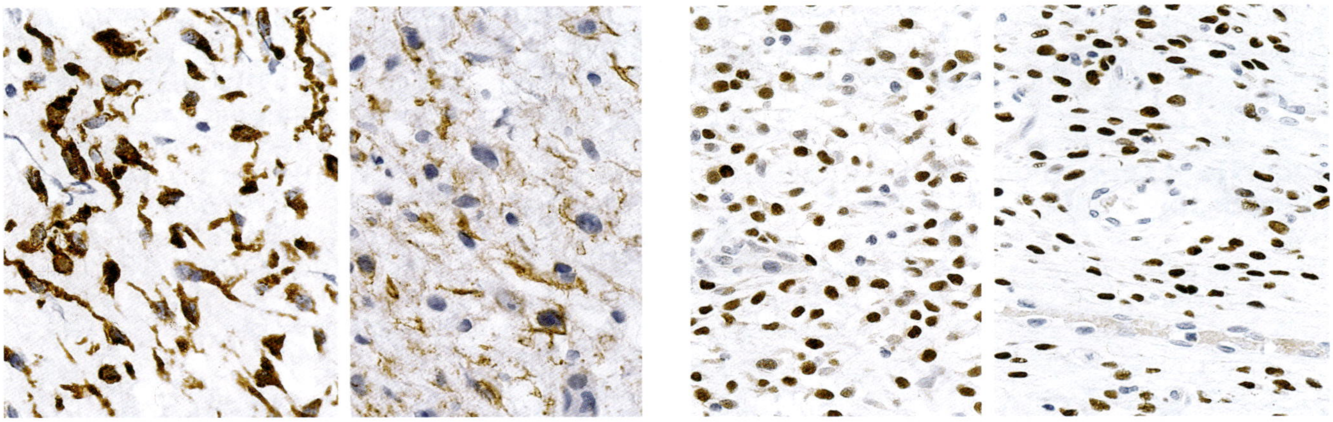

A B

Figure 12–3. *A,* Superficial cervicovaginal myofibroblastoma cells are strongly positive for desmin (*left*) and also for CD34 (*right*). *B,* The lesional cells are positive for both estrogen (*left*) and progesterone receptors (*right*).

Pathology

Grossly, genital rhabdomyoma typically forms a small lobulated polyp measuring 1 to 2 cm. Histologically, it is lined by normal or hyperplastic squamous mucosa. The stroma, especially superficially, contains lobules or random clusters of well-differentiated but immature striated muscle cells with eosinophilic cytoplasm and appearances of maturing rhabdomyoblasts in a collagenous background (Fig. 12–4). Some of these are oval, and others are elongated, probably depending on the plane of section; some have cytoplasmic cross-striations. A prominent stromal vascular pattern is often present. Mature histology and lack of atypia and mitotic activity separate this tumor from embryonal (botryoid) rhabdomyosarcoma, which in this region usually occurs in small children.

Immunohistochemically, the main lesional cells are positive for desmin and myoglobin; data on hormone receptors, MyoD1 and myogenin, are not available. Electron microscopic studies have shown features of differentiated striated muscle cells with well-aligned sarcomeres.

Angiomyofibroblastoma

Clinical Features

This histologically distinctive tumor forms a relatively small (usually <5 cm), well-circumscribed, asymptomatic mass in the vulva or labia majora clinically simulating a Bartholin cyst.[14–19] The tumor predominantly occurs in perimenopausal and postmenopausal women with the median age in the largest series being 46 years.[18] Simple excision is usually curative, and there is no tendency to recur. An exceptional case interpreted as sarcomatous transformation of a recurrent angiomyofibroblastoma was reported in an 80-year-old patient.[20]

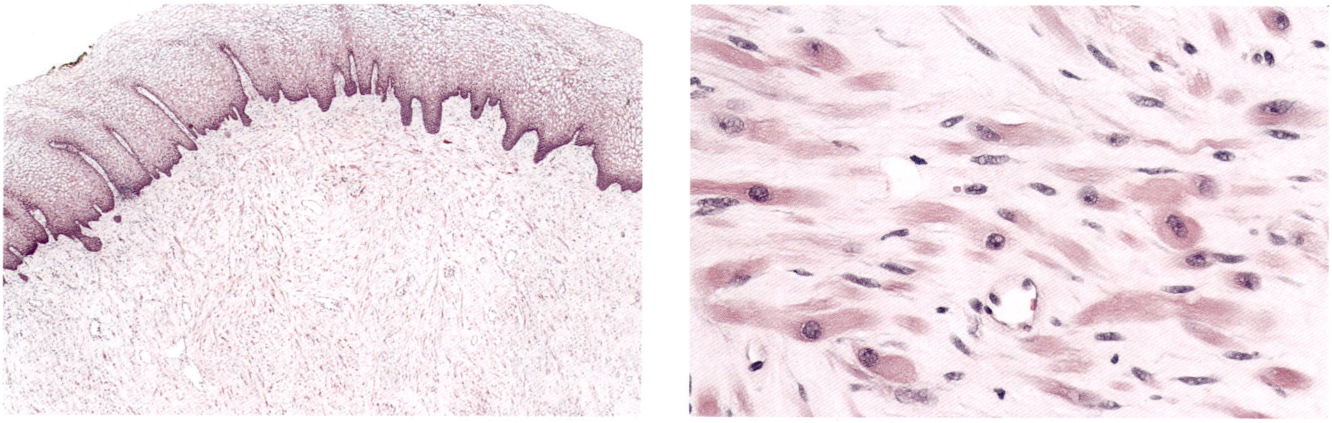

A B

Figure 12–4. *A,* Vaginal rhabdomyoma forms a broad-based vaginal polyp with moderate cellularity. *B,* The lesion contains partially aligned, well-differentiated but immature skeletal muscle cells.

Pathology

Grossly, the mass is solid and tan, and sometimes mucoid on sectioning. It is usually 1 to 5 cm in greatest diameter, but may occasionally exceed 10 cm. Histologically, the tumor is composed of alternating cellular and myxoid areas, and some lesions have an admixed mature fatty component (Fig. 12–5). The tumor cells are often grouped as trabeculae, cords, and cohesive nests around prominent, dilated thin-walled or sclerosing capillaries. The lesional cells vary from spindled to epithelioid and may form clusters (Fig. 12–5*D*). Some tumor cells have abundant cytoplasm and eccentric nucleolus imparting a plasmacytoid appearance. There is only minimal atypia and the mitotic activity is low.

Immunohistochemically, the tumor cells are positive for vimentin and usually for desmin, but rarely for smooth muscle actin. They are also positive for estrogen and progesterone receptors. The tumor cells are negative for S-100 protein, CD34, and keratins.[18–22] Ultrastructurally, the tumor cells have myofibroblastic features.

Angiomyofibroblastoma-like tumors have been recently reported in men (discussed later). These tumors are identical with those reported as cellular angiofibroma.[23,24]

Cellular Angiofibroma and Male Angiomyofibroblastoma-Like Tumors

These two designations pertain to histologically similar if not identical tumors. The former has been described in women and the latter in men in the external genital and inguinal regions. Some tumors reported as aggressive angiomyxomas in men probably belong to this category.

Clinical Features

The reported cellular angiofibromas have occurred in the vulval area of middle-aged women. These tumors are small, circumscribed nodules varying from 1 to 2.5 cm; limited follow-up has not revealed

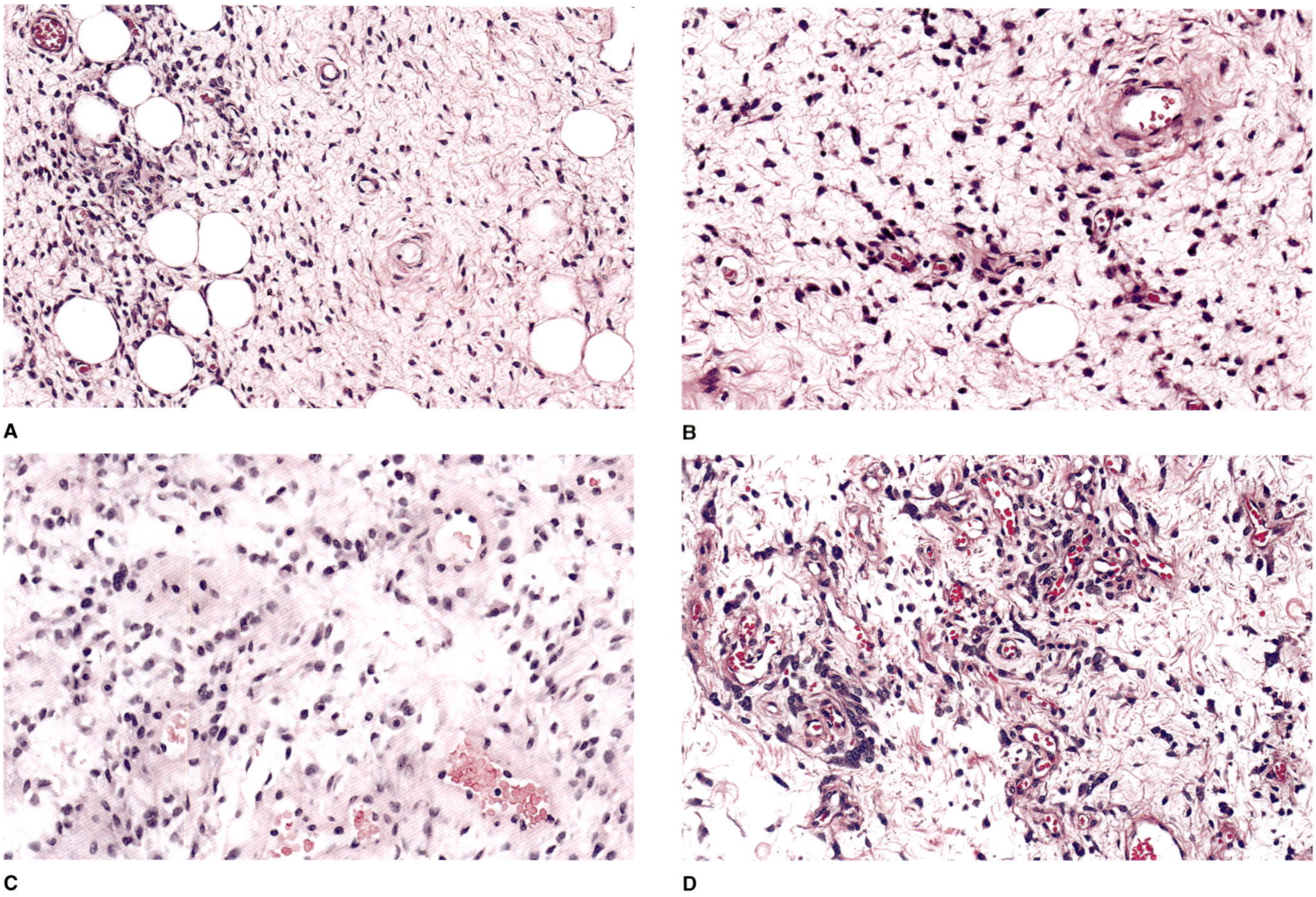

Figure 12–5. Histologic spectrum of angiomyofibroblastoma. *A,* Lesion with variable cellularity and a mature adipocytic component. *B* and *C,* Cords of epithelioid tumor cells radiating from capillary walls. *D,* Perivascular concentration of spindled and epithelioid cells with focal atypia.

recurrences.[23] The 11 tumors reported in men occurred in middle-age to old age in the scrotum or inguinal region and were larger but generally circumscribed. They varied from 2.5 to 14 cm (mean, 7.5 cm). One of the 11 tumors recurred but none metastasized.[24]

Pathology

Grossly, the tumors are circumscribed, lobulated soft to rubbery masses. Histologically, they show some resemblance to angiomyofibroblastoma, but have more prominent large vessels with perivascular hyalinization and alternating less and more cellular areas with tapered, uniform spindle cells separated by thin collagen fibers (Fig. 12–6). The tumor cells generally have a more spindled morphology than angiomyofibroblastomas with focal epithelioid change in some cases. Moderate mitotic activity was reported in some of the female tumors, whereas the male tumors were mitotically inactive. Both female and male tumors may have a fatty component suggesting the possibility of relationship with cellular spindle cell lipoma.[23,24]

Immunohistochemically, the tumor cells of female cases have been negative for desmin, muscle actins, and CD34,[23] whereas the male tumors have been variably positive for desmin, muscle actins, CD34, and estrogen and progesterone receptors.[24]

Aggressive Angiomyxoma

Clinical Features

Aggressive angiomyxoma (AAM) is a specific fibromyxoid tumor that mainly presents in adult women under the age of 50 years. The tumor occurs in the pelvis and perineum often extending to the external genital area and clinically simulating inguinal hernia or a Bartholin cyst.

The tumor is usually large, over 10 cm in diameter and sometimes much larger, filling the whole pelvic cavity. It typically has infiltrative margins and may recur, often a long time after primary surgery (in 30–40% of cases), but it does not metastasize.[25–28] Considering the problems of radical resection in a fertile-aged woman, nonsurgical treatment may be considered; tumor regression by gonadotropin- releasing hormone agonist has been observed in one patient.[29]

A small number of similar tumors in adult men have been reported.[30–32] These tumors have occurred in men between the ages of 18 and 70 years, with a median of 52 years, older than the median age of AAM. Over half of the tumors have been located in the scrotum, and others in the spermatic cord, perineum, or groin. Some of them were reportedly actin-positive but desmin-negative, differing from the typical AAM. Although some of them seem indistinguishable from AAM,[30–32] others are more consistent with tumors designated as cellular angiofibromas or male angiomyofibroblastoma-like tumors.

Pathology

Grossly, AAM is gray-tan rubbery or rubbery-myxoid with a glistening, sometimes mucoid surface (Fig. 12–7). It may appear as a circumscribed or multilobular solid mass composed of multiple finger-like projections representing tumor infiltration in soft tissues surrounding the vagina and rectum.

Microscopically, the tumor has an infiltrative margin to the surrounding fat and Bartholin glands with frequent nerve entrapment. It is paucicellular and highly vascular with dilated, often hyperemic thick-walled vessels, but recurrent tumors may be more

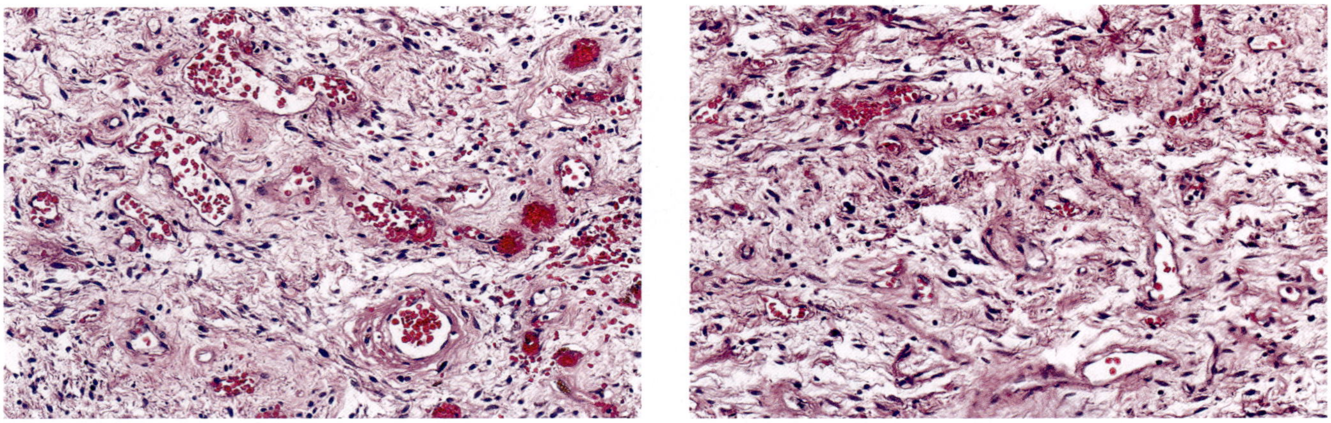

A B

Figure 12–6. *A* and *B*, Cellular angiofibroma (male angiofibromyoblastoma-like tumor) from the scrotum of an old man has prominent dilated vessels and uniform spindle cells in a collagenous stroma.

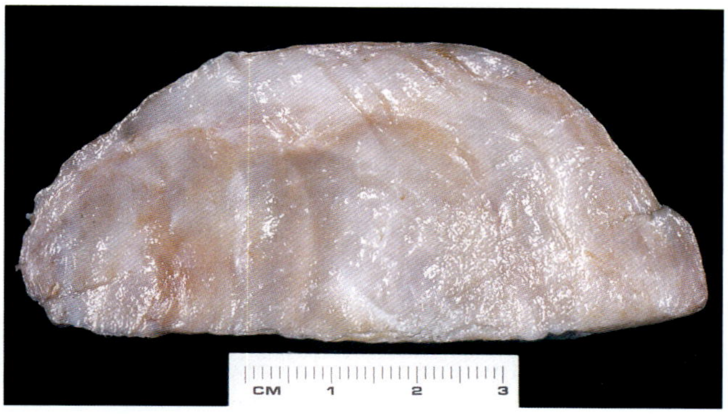

Figure 12-7. Aggressive angiomyxoma, grossly, is a rubbery mass with a glistening tan surface.

cellular. The dilated blood vessels are often surrounded by small clusters or fascicles of well-differentiated smooth muscle cells. Between tumor cells there is a background of edematous, fine collagen fibers (Fig. 12–8). The tumor cells are relatively small, uniform oval to spindled, often with bipolar cytoplasmic processes. The tumor cell nuclei are oval and uniform and have a delicate nucleolus. Mitotic activity is scant (0–4/50 HPF).

Immunohistochemically, AAM cells are typically positive for desmin and variably for muscle actins and CD34, and are negative for S-100 protein.[27,28,33] Positivity for estrogen and progesterone receptors is typical of this tumor and indicates specific gynecologic stromal cell differentiation. The portion of MIB1$^+$ proliferative cells is low, less than 1%.[27]

Ultrastructural studies have shown myofibroblastic differentiation with focal densities of actin filaments and partial basal laminas.[33]

Differential Diagnosis

Angiomyofibroblastoma is typically a well-circumscribed relatively small (<5 cm) tumor in the labial region. Histologically different from angiomyxoma

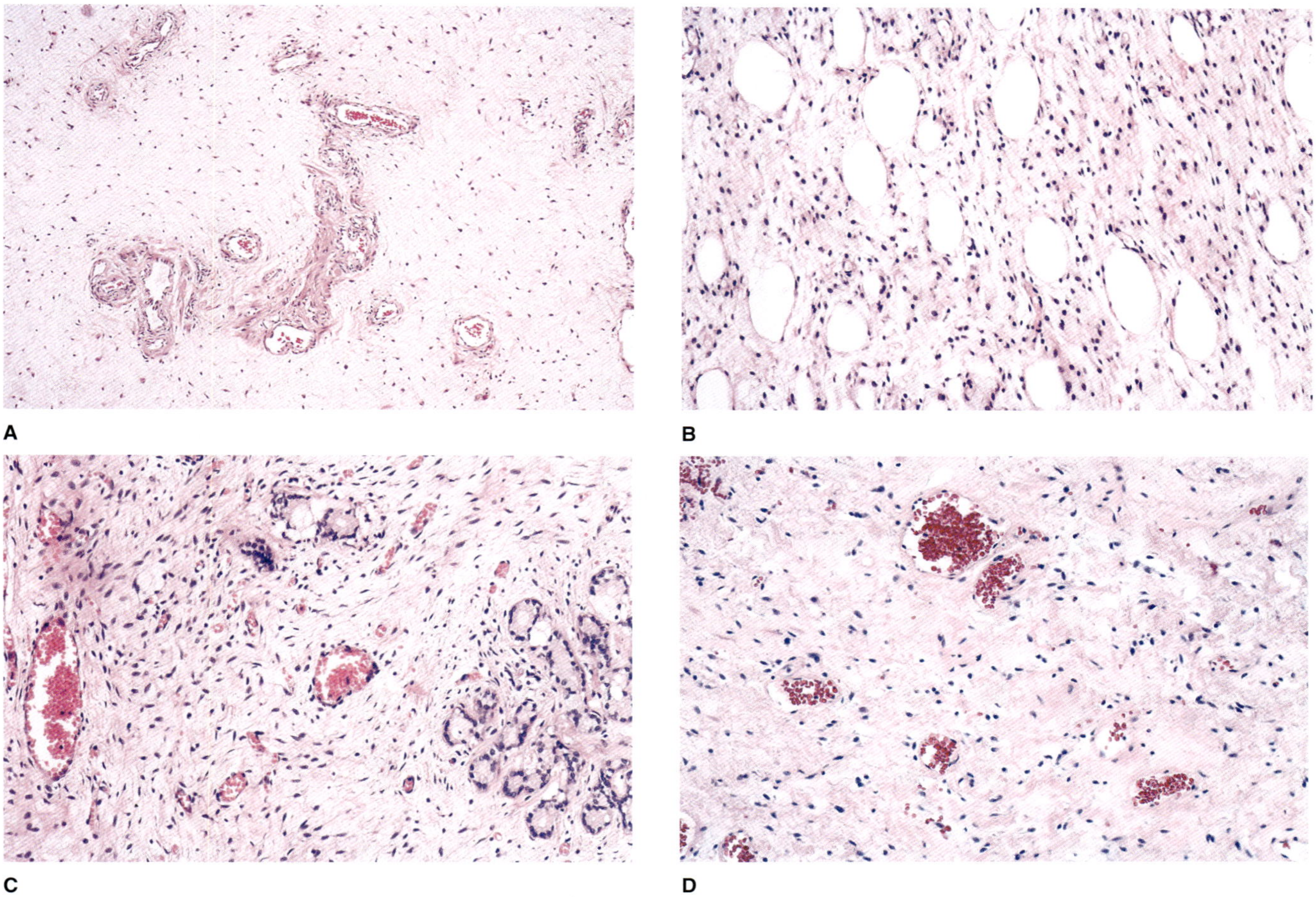

Figure 12-8. Histologic spectrum of aggressive angiomyxoma. *A,* Low magnification shows a paucicellular lesion with prominent blood vessels, often with perivascular smooth muscle proliferation. *B,* The tumor cells are uniform and evenly dispersed, and there are entrapped adipocytes. *C,* A recurrent tumor infiltrating between Bartholin glands of the vulva. *D,* A pelvic tumor of a male with a resemblance to female aggressive angiomyxoma.

are the delicate capillaries and corded perivascular pattern of tumor cells that are often epithelioid.

Superficial angiomyxoma (see Chapter 5) may present in the external genital region. It is typically a multilobulated cutaneous or subcutaneous nodule. It has a loose texture, is relatively paucicellular with abundant acid mucopolysaccharide matrix, and commonly contains perivascular lymphoid infiltration; it is estrogen and progesterone receptor negative.

Intramuscular myxoma (see Chapter 5) may occur in the buttock and inguinal region but is rarely seen in the genital region. It is a paucicellular tumor with a sparse vascularity and abundant acid mucopolysaccharides.

Myxoid liposarcoma and myxoid malignant fibrous histiocytoma contain a prominent arborizing vascular pattern; the former contains uniform evenly distributed cells with possible lipoblasts, whereas the latter typically has a pleomorphic component and perivascular zones of higher cellularity.

Myxoid leiomyomas usually have bundles of smooth muscle cells at least focally, and they are typically positive for both desmin and smooth muscle actin.

Genetics

Cytogenetic studies have shown rearrangement of 12q15 commonly involved in various translocations.[34] The *HMGIC* gene located in this region has been shown to be involved and aberrantly expressed in the tumor cells;[35] normally the expression of this DNA architectural organizer protein is restricted to fetal tissues.[36]

Low-Grade Endometrial Stromal Sarcoma (Stromatosis, Intralymphangial Stromal Myosis)

This tumor is composed of cells closely resembling those of the proliferative endometrium; it has a slow clinical course. Its older synonyms reflect the relatively indolent clinical course and commonly prominent intralymphatic invasion.

Clinical Features

The low-grade endometrial stromal sarcoma typically occurs in adult women under the age of 60 years, with the median ages in largest series being around 45 years.[37–40] Most commonly it presents with abnormal bleeding. Although most tumors are endometrial primaries and involve the uterine corpus only, some extend outside it to the cervix, parametria, and elsewhere in the abdominal cavity. Few originate in the cervix, ovaries, peritoneal cavity, or retroperitoneum.[41] Origin from the endometriosis has been postulated for some of the extrauterine tumors.

Tumors confined to the uterus have better long-term prognosis than those that have spread or originated outside of it. However, one third of patients with localized disease develop recurrences. The 10-year actuarial survival depends on the stage and varies from 75% to 90%.[39,40] The low-grade stromal sarcoma typically has a long course of disease, and late recurrences 10 to 30 years after first surgery may occur. The recurrences often occur in the pelvis, in the external aspect of the intestines, or on the peritoneal surfaces. Pulmonary metastases may also develop. Rare cardiovascular involvement of the great vessels and heart has been reported.[42] This tumor is hormonally dependent, and treatment with progesterone has been helpful in some cases.[39]

Pathology

Grossly, the low-grade stromal sarcoma is often distinctive by involvement of multiple vessels in a wormlike or complex sausage-like pattern, which can be seen both in the primary tumors and abdominal recurrences and metastases.

Histologically, the tumor is highly distinctive and generally retains the typical features in its metastases (Fig. 12–9). When involving the uterus, this tumor typically extends to the myometrium as tongues and involves lymphatics in the uterine wall; hence the previous designation "intralymphangial stromal myosis." It is composed of uniform round, oval, or sometimes spindled cells with little variation. The tumor cells are grouped around prominent, small-caliber blood vessels that may resemble the endometrial spiral arterioles or the vessels of hemangiopericytoma, if gaping vessels are present.[37,38] Some tumors have hyalinized areas, and sex cordlike or glandular epithelial differentiation has been noted on rare occasions. Endometrial-type glands may occur in these tumors whether primary in the uterus or peritoneum.[40,41] Some pulmonary metastases may have a deceptively benign appearance and histologically simulate a cystic hamartoma or cellular solitary fibrous tumor.[43] The tumor usually has a low-to-moderate mitotic activity (up to 10/10 HPF), but cases with higher mitotic counts (usually no more than 15 mitoses/10 HPF) seem to show a similar behavior, as long as they have the same cellular morphology.[38,40]

Immunohistochemically (Fig. 12–9C and *D*), the tumor cells are strongly positive for estrogen and progesterone receptors.[44] They are also positive for CD10[45] and have been described as variably positive

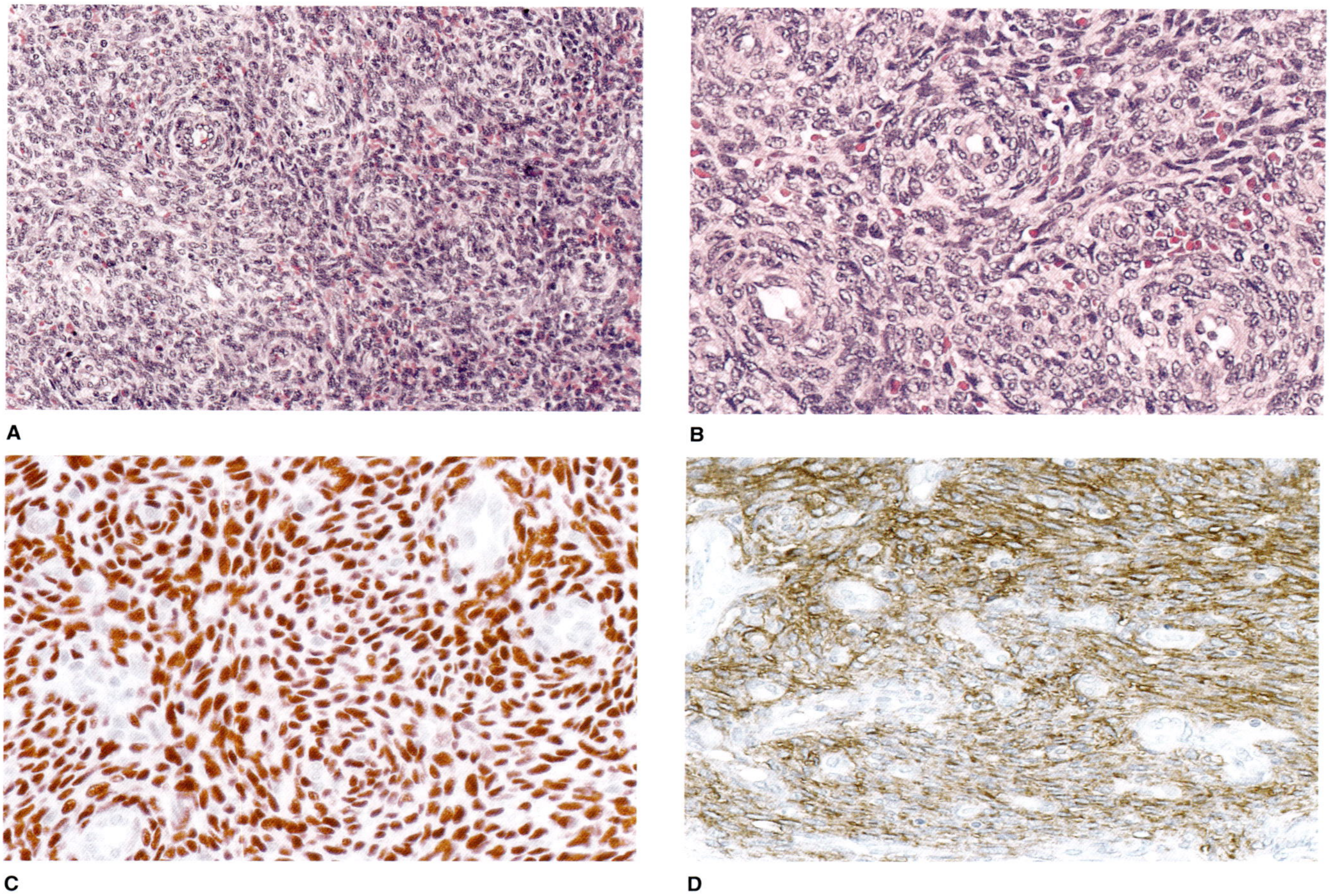

Figure 12–9. *A* and *B,* Recurrent endometrial stromal sarcoma in the abdomen shows high cellularity and prominent spiral artery-like blood vessels. Tumor cells have nuclear positivity for estrogen receptor (*C*) and cytoplasmic positivity for CD10 (*D*).

for desmin, muscle actins, and keratins, but negative for epithelial membrane antigen.[46] In contrast with smooth muscle tumors, the lesional cells are negative for h-caldesmon, which may be of differential diagnostic help in separating these tumors.[47,48]

Differential Diagnosis

Endometrial stromal nodule is a rare, histologically similar lesion that is not infiltrative with a pushing border and may occur in the myometrium or be limited to the endometrium.[37]

High-grade stromal sarcoma is a proper designation for a monomorphous sarcoma not showing endometrial stromal cell appearance; these tumors are clinically more aggressive and clinicopathologically approach carcinosarcomas.[38] They are very difficult to specifically identify outside the uterus.

Immunohistochemistry for epithelial, lymphoid, and myeloid markers may be necessary to separate low-grade stromal sarcoma from metastatic carcinoma (especially lobular carcinoma of the breast) and hematopoietic tumors, lymphoma, and extramedullary myeloid tumor.

Genetics

Recurrent translocation t (7;17)(p15;q21) seems to be the key genetic change.[49–51] It has been found to lead into the fusion of the transcription factor genes *JAZF1* at 7p15 and *JJAZ1* at 17q21, and fusion transcript has been detected in tumor cells.[52]

Carcinosarcoma (Malignant Mixed Müllerian Tumor, Malignant Mixed Mesodermal Tumor)

This tumor is now generally viewed as an endometrial carcinoma with sarcomatous differentiation, and therefore the name carcinosarcoma has been adopted.

Clinical Features

This relatively rare tumor comprising less than 5% of malignant uterine tumors usually occurs in older women between 60 and 80 years who present with postmenopausal bleeding. In some cases, the tumor has arisen in patients who had received radiation, suggesting radiation-related etiology. The tumor most commonly originates in the endometrium, but primary occurrence in the vagina, cervix, fallopian tube, ovary, and peritoneal surfaces is also possible. The primary abdominal tumors may present in the pelvic peritoneum, exterior surface of the intestines, adjacent to the liver, omentum, or retroperitoneum. Abdominal metastases can involve the same sites, and pulmonary metastases are common. Most tumors have a highly aggressive behavior, and an extended survival is rare. Exceptional, small polypoid, limited lesions may be more favorable.[53-60]

Pathology

Grossly, a uterine tumor typically forms a polypoid intracavitary mass with involvement of the uterine wall. It can reach a large size and involve large portions of the uterus and also extend outside. On sectioning, the tumor is soft, gray-tan, and often hemorrhagic and partly necrotic.

By definition, the tumor has microscopically carcinomatous and sarcomatous components (Fig. 12–10). The former typically forms sharply demarcated clusters, often with a complex cribriform pattern having endometrioid, clear-cell, serous, and often focally squamoid features. The sarcomatous component may be monomorphous and undifferentiated (homologous carcinosarcoma) or it can be composed of multiple mesenchymal components (heterologous carcinosarcoma). Cytologically, the sarcomatous component varies from round to spindle, sometimes with moderate pleomorphism. All components are typically high grade, and mitotic rate is high, especially in the epithelial component.

The heterologous sarcomatous components most commonly include an embryonal rhabdomyosarcoma-like one with varying numbers of differentiating rhabdomyoblasts (Fig. 12–10*B*). Cartilaginous, osseous, and lipomatous differentiation may also be present. Many tumors have periodic acid-Schiff–positive hyaline globules or droplets resembling those seen in some germ cell tumors.

The metastases can be composed of purely epithelial, sarcomatous, or mixed elements. The nature and extent of heterologous differentiation does not seem to have prognostic significance.

Immunohistochemical studies have shown keratin expression in both epithelial and sarcomatous components, which has been grounds for considering these tumors sarcomatoid carcinomas. Desmin and myoglobin positivity highlight heterologous skeletal muscle differentiation, and S-100 protein positivity indicates that of cartilage.[60-62] The epithelial component has been found commonly and the sarcomatous one inconsistently positive for estrogen and progesterone receptors.[63]

Genetics and Histogenesis

Complex cytogenetic changes, including inversion of 12p[64] and a translocation t(8;22)(q24;q12) have been described. However, no specific genes have been identified.[65]

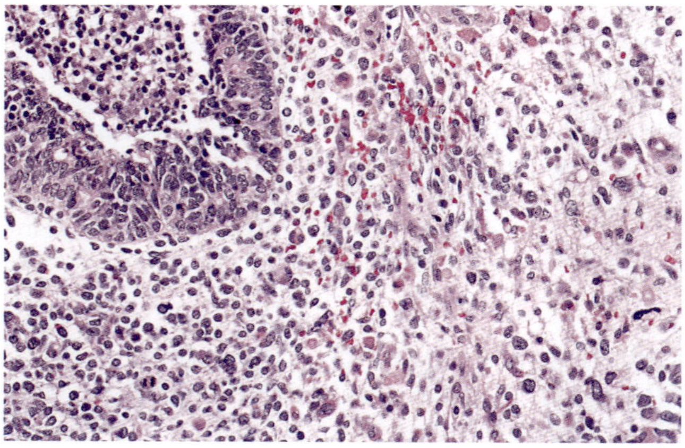

A

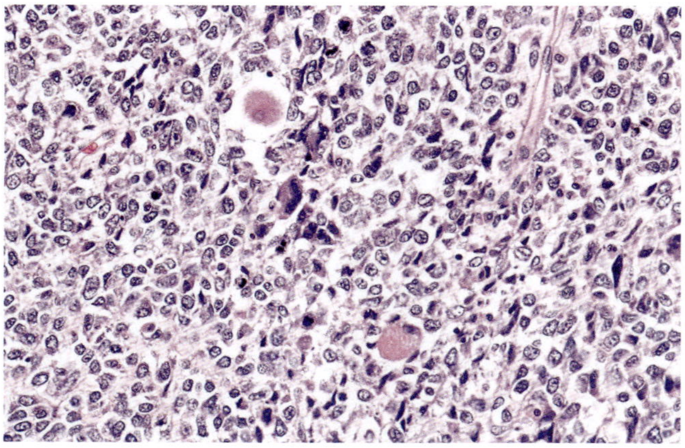

B

Figure 12–10. *A,* Carcinosarcoma is composed of atypical epithelial elements and a primitive-appearing sarcomatous component. *B,* Two large rhabdomyoblasts with abundant eosinophilic cytoplasm are present in this heterologous tumor.

Similar molecular genetic changes, namely, identical p53 mutations[66] and similar patterns of allelic losses[67] in the carcinomatous and sarcomatous components, have been found. This confirms the common clonal origin of both components and supports the concept that this tumor indeed is a metaplastic carcinoma or sarcomatoid carcinoma. This is also supported by the differentiation of carcinomatous elements into skeletal muscle in cell culture.[68]

Related Terms and Tumors

Adenosarcoma (müllerian adenosarcoma) refers to a neoplasm that typically shows a low-grade sarcomatous stroma and a benign-appearing epithelial component. It usually occurs in the endometrium or cervix, but sarcomatous components of this tumor may disseminate as intra-abdominal metastases.[53–56]

Adenofibroma has a benign-appearing epithelium and stroma and most commonly occurs in the endometrium, cervix, and ovary.[54]

Adult Granulosa Cell Tumor

The significance of this tumor in nongynecologic pathology is its common occurrence as an intra-abdominal metastasis and occasional presentation as a primary nonovarian tumor. The rare juvenile variant and granulosa cell tumors of the testis are clinicopathologically different tumors, and are not discussed here.

Clinical Features

This tumor, classified among the sex cord stromal tumors, almost always presents as an ovarian primary in middle-aged and older women, but this type rarely occurs in children. Rare examples primary in the ovary and elsewhere in the abdomen (pelvic wall) have also been reported. It often presents with postmenopausal bleeding because granulosa cell tumors typically have estrogenic activity and reactivate the endometrium; some examples have no hormonal activity, and few have androgenic activity.[69–72]

Granulosa cell tumors commonly recur in the abdominal cavity, often after a long asymptomatic period of 10 to 20 years or even more. In such a situation the history of the primary tumor is often unknown, and the diagnosis may be challenging.

Pathology

Adult granulosa cell tumors of the ovary are typically relatively large, often exceeding 10 cm. They are often grossly cystic and hemorrhagic, and the tumor tissue is typically gray-tan or yellowish. Microscopically, the histologic patterns include microfollicular and follicular ones somewhat simulating the normal graafian follicles. Many tumors have microscopic rosettes containing eosinophilic material referred to as Call-Exner bodies, and some have a trabecular pattern with or without intervening fibrous tissues. A pattern with curved trabeculae is commonly referred to as "watered silk" pattern. Some tumors have a diffuse growth with no structural differentiation (Fig. 12–11*A* and *B*). Common to all variants is dense cellularity and uniform round to oval cells with scant cytoplasm. Varying numbers of the nuclei have deep grooves imparting a "coffee-bean shape." Focal pleomorphism may rarely occur. Mitotic activity varies, but is usually less than 5 to 7/10 HPF.

The abdominal recurrences usually have a diffuse or partly trabecular pattern, but sarcomatous transformation[73] and hemangiopericytoma-like appearance[74] may occur increasing the risk for misdiagnosis (Fig. 12–11*C*).

An immunohistochemically typical and diagnostically useful feature is cytoplasmic positivity for inhibin (Fig. 12–11*D*). Inhibin positivity distinguishes granulosa cell tumors from carcinomas, which are negative, whereas fibrothecomas are also inhibin positive.[74–77] The tumor cells are also positive for vimentin and are variably but less strikingly positive for keratin-8 or keratin-18 than ovarian carcinomas in general.[78,79] They are positive for S-100 protein in 50% of the cases, but are negative for epithelial membrane antigen, in contrast to most ovarian and abdominal carcinomas.[79] Ki67 analog positivity varies in a wide range, but is higher in recurrent and mitotically highly active tumors.[80]

Genetics

Recurrent chromosomal changes, including trisomy 12,[81] trisomy 14,[82–84] and monosomy of chromosome 22 have been found in granulosa cell tumors. Translocation of t(6;16) has been described in one case.[85]

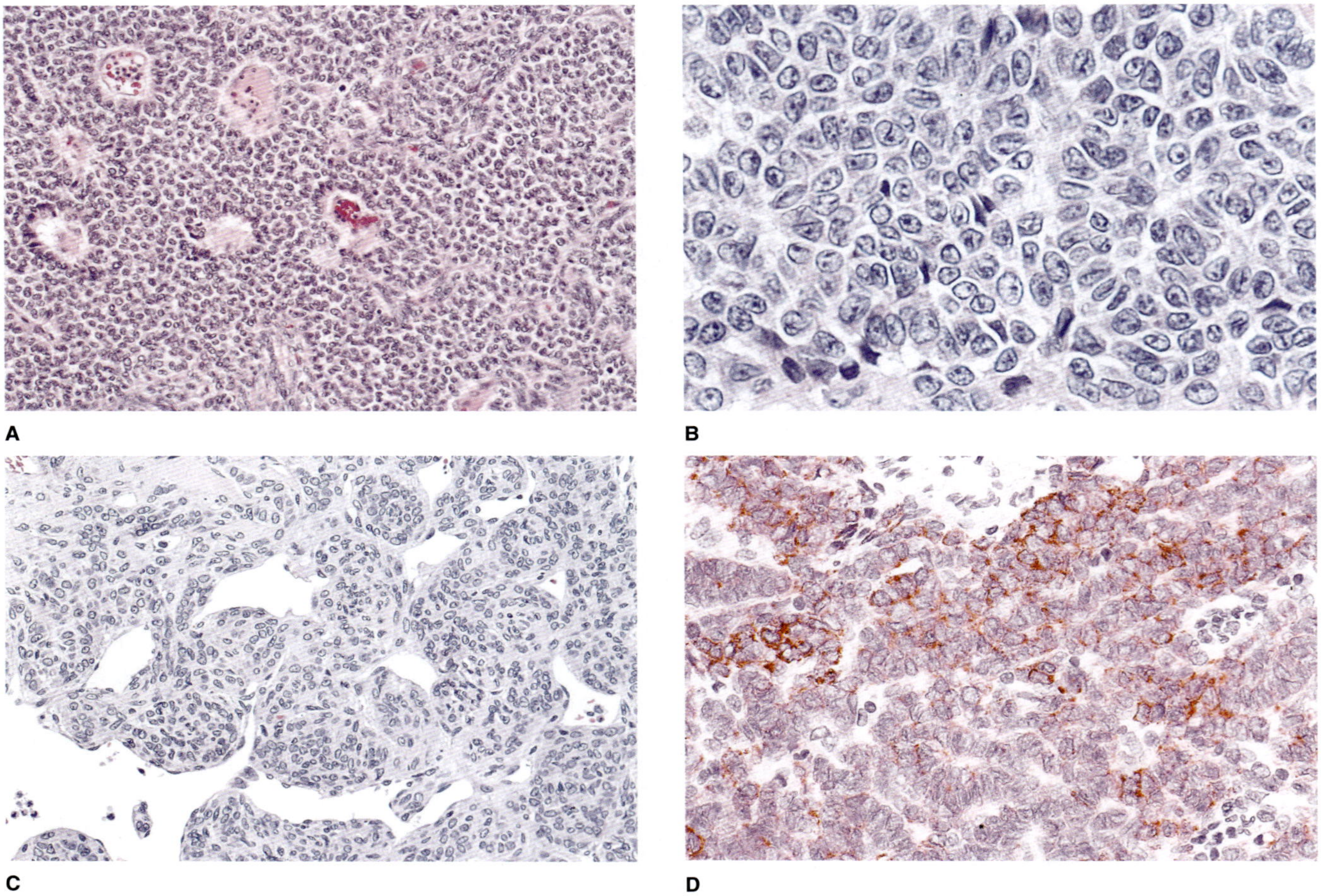

Figure 12–11. Examples of abdominal recurrences of granulosa cell tumors. *A,* Tumor with a diffuse pattern with perivascular pseudorosettes. *B,* High magnification of a diffuse pattern. *C,* A hemangiopericytoma-like pattern. *D,* The tumor cells with cytoplasmic inhibin positivity.

REFERENCES

Mesodermal Stromal Polyp and Related Lesions

1. Norris HJ, Taylor HB: Polyps of the vagina. A benign lesion resembling sarcoma botryoides. Cancer 1966; 19:227–232.
2. Chirayil SJ, Tobon H: Polyps of the vagina: A clinicopathologic study of 18 cases. Cancer 1981;47: 2904–2907.
3. Miettinen M, Wahlström T, Vesterinen E, Saksela E: Vaginal polyps with pseudosarcomatous features. A clinicopathologic study of seven cases. Cancer 1983; 51:1148–1151.
4. Östor AG, Fortune DW, Riley CB: Fibroepithelial polyps with atypical stromal cells (pseudosarcoma botryoides) of vulva and vagina. A report of 13 cases. Int J Gyn Pathol 1988;7:351–360.
5. Mucitelli DR, Charles EZ, Kraus FT: Vulvovaginal polyps. Histologic appearance, ultrastructure, immunocytochemical characteristics, and clinicopathological correlations. Int J Gyn Pathol 1990;9:20–40.
6. Nucci MR, Young RH, Fletcher CDM: Cellular pseudosarcomatous fibroepithelial stromal polyps of the lower female genital tract: An underrecognized lesion often misdiagnosed as sarcoma. Am J Surg Pathol 2000;24:231–240.
7. Rollason TP, Byrne P, Williams A: Immunohistochemical and electron microscopic findings in benign fibroepithelial vaginal polyps. J Clin Pathol 1990;43: 224–229.
8. Hartmann CA, Sperling M, Stein H: So-called fibroepithelial polyps of the vagina exhibiting an unusual but uniform antigen profile characterized by expression of desmin and steroid hormone receptors but no muscle-specific actin or macrophage markers. Am J Clin Pathol 1990;93:604–608.

Superficial Cervicovaginal Myofibroblastoma

9. Laskin WB, Fetsch JF, Tavassoli FA: Superficial cervicovaginal myofibroblastoma: Fourteen cases of a distinctive mesenchymal tumor arising from the spe-

cialized subepithelial stroma of the lower female genital tract. Hum Pathol 2001;32:715–725.

Genital Rhabdomyoma

10. Gold JH, Bossen EH: Benign vaginal rhabdomyoma. A light and electron microscopic study. Cancer 1976; 37:2283–2294.
11. Chabrel CM, Beilby JOW: Vaginal rhabdomyoma. Histopathology 1980;4:645–651.
12. Iversen UM: Two cases of benign vaginal rhabdomyoma. APMIS 1996;104:575–578.
13. Willis J, Abdul-Karim FW, di Sant'Agnese PA: Extracardiac rhabdomyomas. Semin Diagn Pathol 1994;11: 15–25.

Angiomyofibroblastoma and Related Tumors

14. Fletcher CDM, Tsang WYW, Fisher C, Lee KC, Chan JKC: Angiomyofibroblastoma of the vulva. A benign neoplasm distinct from aggressive angiomyxoma. Am J Surg Pathol 1992;16:373–382.
15. Hisaoka M, Kouho H, Aoki T, Daimaru Y, Hashimoto H: Angiomyofibroblastoma of the vulva: A clinicopathologic study of seven cases. Pathol Int 1995; 45:487–492.
16. Nielsen GP, Rosenberg AE, Young RH, Dickersin GR, Clement PB, Scully RE: Angiomyofibroblastoma of the vulva and vagina. Mod Pathol 1996;9:284–291.
17. Fukunaga M, Nomura K, Matsumoto K, Doi K, Endo Y, Ushigome S: Vulval angiomyofibroblastoma. Clinicopathologic analysis of six cases. Am J Clin Pathol 1997;107:45–51.
18. Laskin WB, Fetsch JF, Tavassoli FA: Angiomyofibroblastoma of the female genital tract: Analysis of 17 cases including a lipomatous variant. Hum Pathol 1997;28:1046–1055.
19. Ockner DM, Sayadi H, Swanson PE, Ritter JH, Wick MR: Genital angiomyofibroblastoma. Comparison with aggressive angiomyxoma and other myxoid neoplasms of skin and soft tissue. Am J Clin Pathol 1997; 107:36–44.
20. Nielsen GP, Young RH, Dickersin GR, Rosenberg AE: Angiomyofibroblastoma of the vulva with sarcomatous transformation ("angiomyofibrosarcoma"). Am J Surg Pathol 1997;21:1104–1108.
21. Vasquez MD, Ro JY, Park YW, Tornos CS, Ordonez NG, Ayala AG: Angiomyofibroblastoma. A clinicopathologic study of eight cases and review of the literature. Int J Surg Pathol 1999;7:161–169.
22. Bigotti G, Coli A, Gasbarri A, Castagnola D, Madonna V, Bartolazzi A: Angiomyofibroblastoma and aggressive angiomyxoma: Two benign mesenchymal neoplasms of the female genital tract. An immunohistochemical study. Pathol Res Pract 1999;195:39–44.
23. Nucci MR, Granter SR, Fletcher CDM: Cellular angiofibroma: A benign neoplasm distinct from angiomyofibroblastoma and spindle cell lipoma. Am J Surg Pathol 1997;21:636–644.
24. Laskin WB, Fetsch JF, Mostofi FK: Angiomyofibroblastomalike tumor of the male genital tract. Analysis of 11 cases with comparison to female angiomyofibroblastoma and spindle cell lipoma. Am J Surg Pathol 1998;22:6–16.

Aggressive Angiomyxoma

25. Steeper TA, Rosai J: Aggressive angiomyxoma of the female pelvis and perineum. Report of nine cases of a distinctive type of gynecologic soft-tissue neoplasm. Am J Surg Pathol 1983;7:463–475.
26. Begin LR, Clement PB, Kirk ME, Jothy S, McCaughey WTE, Ferenczy A: Aggressive angiomyxoma of pelvic soft parts: A clinicopathologic study of nine cases. Hum Pathol 1985;16:621–628.
27. Fetsch JF, Laskin WB, Lefkowitz M, Kindblom LG, Meis-Kindblom JM: Aggressive angiomyxoma: A clinicopathologic study of 29 female patients. Cancer 1996;78:79–90.
28. Granter SR, Nucci MR, Fletcher CDM: Aggressive angiomyxoma: Reappraisal of its relationship to angiomyofibroblastoma in a series of 16 cases. Histopathology 1997;30:3–10.
29. Fine BA, Munoz AK, Litz CE, Gershenson DM: Primary medical management of recurrent aggressive angiomyxoma with a gonadotropin-releasing hormone agonist. Gynecol Oncol 2001;81:120–122.
30. Tsang WYW, Chan JKC, Lee KC, Fisher C, Fletcher CDM: Aggressive angiomyxoma. A report of four cases occurring in men. Am J Surg Pathol 1992;16:1059–1065.
31. Clatch RJ, Drake WK, Conzalez JG: Aggressive angiomyxoma in men. A report of two cases associated with inguinal hernias. Arch Pathol Lab Med 1993;117:911–913.
32. Iezzoni JC, Fechner RE, Wong LS, Rosai J: Aggressive angiomyxoma in males. A report of four cases. Am J Clin Pathol 1995;104:391–396.
33. Skalova A, Michal M, Husek K, Zamecnik M, Leivo I: Aggressive angiomyxoma of the pelvioperineal region. Immunohistochemical and ultrastructural study of seven cases. Am J Dermatopathol 1993;15:446–451.
34. Kazmierczak B, Wanschura S, Meyer-Bolte K, et al: Cytogenetic and molecular analysis of an aggressive angiomyxoma. Am J Pathol 1995;147:580–585.
35. Nucci MR, Weremowicz S, Neskey DM, et al: Chromosomal translocation t(8;12) induces aberrant HMGIC expression in aggressive angiomyxoma of the vulva. Genes Chromosom Cancer 2001;32:172–176.
36. Hess JL: Chromosomal translocations in benign tumors. The HMGI proteins. Am J Clin Pathol 1998; 109:251–261.

Low-Grade Endometrial Stromal Sarcoma

37. Norris HJ, Taylor HB: Mesenchymal tumors of the uterus. I. A clinical and pathological study of 53 endometrial stromal tumors. Cancer 1966;19:755–766.

38. Evans HL: Endometrial stromal sarcoma and poorly differentiated endometrial sarcoma. Cancer 1982; 50:2170–2182.
39. Piver MS, Rutledge FN, Copeland L, Webster K, Bulmenson L, Suh O: Uterine endolymphatic stromal myosis: A collaborative study. Obstet Gynecol 1984; 64:173–178.
40. Chang KL, Crabtree GS, Lim-Tan SK, Kempson RL, Hendrickson MR: Primary uterine stromal neoplasms. A study of 117 cases. Am J Surg Pathol 1990; 14:415–438.
41. Chang KL, Crabtree GS, Lim-Tan SK, Kempson RL, Hendrickson MR: Primary extrauterine endometrial stromal neoplasms: A clinicopathologic study of 20 cases and a review of the literature. Int J Gynecol Pathol 1993;12:282–296.
42. Tabata T, Takeshima N, Hirai Y, Hasumi K: Low-grade endometrial stromal sarcoma with cardiovascular involvement: A report of three cases. Gynecol Oncol 1999;75:495–498.
43. Abrams J, Talcott J, Corson JM: Pulmonary metastases in patients with low-grade endometrial stromal sarcoma. Clinicopathologic findings with immunohistochemical characterization. Am J Surg Pathol 1989; 13:133–140.
44. Navarro D, Cabrera JJ, Leon L, et al: Endometrial stromal sarcoma expression of estrogen receptors, progesterone receptors and estrogen-induced srp27 (24K) suggests hormone responsiveness. J Steroid Biochem Mol Biol 1992;41:589–596.
45. Chu PG, Arber DA, Weiss LM, Chang KL: Utility of CD10 in distinguishing between endometrial stromal sarcoma and uterine smooth muscle tumors: An immunohistochemical comparison of 34 cases. Mod Pathol 2001;14:465–471.
46. Farhood AI, Abrams J: Immunohistochemistry of endometrial stromal sarcoma. Hum Pathol 1991;22: 224–230.
47. Rush DS, Tan J, Baergen RN, Soslow RA: h-Caldesmon, a novel smooth muscle-specific antibody, distinguishes between cellular leiomyoma and endometrial stromal sarcoma. Am J Surg Pathol 2001; 25:253–258.
48. Nucci MR, O'Connell JT, Huettner PC, Cviko A, Sun D, Quade BJ: h-Caldesmon expression effectively distinguishes endometrial stromal tumors from uterine smooth muscle tumors. Am J Surg Pathol 2001;25: 455–463.
49. Sreekantaiah C, Li FP, Weidner N, Sandberg AA: An endometrial stromal sarcoma with clonal cytogenetic abnormalities. Cancer Genet Cytogenet 1991;55:163–166.
50. Dal Cin P, Aly MS, De Wever I, Moerman P, Van den Berghe H: Endometrial stromal sarcoma t(7;17) (p15–21;q12–21) is a nonrandon chromosomal change. Cancer Genet Cytogenet 1992;63:43–46.
51. Hennig Y, Caselitz J, Bartnitzke S, Bullerdiek J: A third case of low-grade endometrial stromal sarcoma with a t(7;17)(p14 approximately 21;q11.2 approximately 21). Cancer Genet Cytogenet 1997;98: 84–86.
52. Koontz JI, Soreng AL, Nucci M, et al: Frequent fusion of the *JAZF1* and *JJAZ1* genes in endometrial stromal tumors. Proc Natl Acad Sci USA 2001;98: 6348–6353.

Carcinosarcoma (Malignant Mixed Müllerian Tumor)

53. Silverberg SG: Mixed mullerian tumors. Curr Top Pathol 1992;85:35–56.
54. Kempson RL, Hendrickson MR: Smooth muscle, endometrial stromal, and mixed Mullerian tumors of the uterus. Mod Pathol 2000;13:328–342.
55. Silverberg SG, Major FJ, Blessing JA, et al: Carcinosarcoma (malignant mixed mesodermal tumor) of the uterus: A gynecologic oncology group pathologic study of 203 cases. Int J Gynecol Pathol 1990;9:1–19.
56. Colombi RP: Sarcomatoid carcinomas of the female genital tract (malignant mixed mullerian tumors). Semin Diagn Pathol 1993;10:169–175.
57. Pfeiffer P, Hardt-Madsen M, Rex S, Holund B, Bertelsen K: Malignant mixed mullerian tumors of the ovary. Report of 13 cases. Acta Obstet Gynecol Scand 1991;70:79–83.
58. Garamvoelgyi E, Guillou L, Gebhard S, Salmeron M, Seematter RJ, Hadji MH: Primary malignant mixed müllerian tumor (metaplastic carcinoma) of the female peritoneum. A clinical, pathologic, and immunohistochemical study of three cases and review of the literature. Cancer 1994;74:854–863.
59. Rose PG, Rodriguez M, Abdul-Karim FW: Malignant mixed müllerian tumor of the female peritoneum: Treatment and outcome of three cases. Gynecol Oncol 1997:65:523–525.
60. Costa MJ, Khan R, Judd R: Carcinosarcoma (malignant mixed mullerian [mesodermal] tumor) of the uterus and ovary. Correlation of clinical, pathologic, and immunohistochemical features in 29 cases. Arch Pathol Lab Med 1991;115:583–590.
61. Meis JM, Lawrence WD: The immunohistochemical profile of malignant mixed mullerian tumor. Overlap with endometrial adenocarcinoma. Am J Clin Pathol 1990;94:1–7.
62. George E, Manivel JC, Dehner LP, Wick MR: Malignant mixed mullerian tumors: An immunohistochemical study of 47 cases, with histogenetic considerations and clinical correlation. Hum Pathol 1991;22:215–223.
63. Ansink AC, Cross PA, Scorer P, de Barros Lopes A, Monaghan JM: The hormonal receptor status of uterine carcinosarcomas (mixed müllerian tumours): An immunohistochemical study. J Clin Pathol 1997;50: 328–331.
64. Streekantaiah C, Rao UN, Sandberg AA: Complex karyotypic aberrations, including i(12p), in malignant mixed müllerian tumor of uterus. Cancer Genet Cytogenet 1992;60:78–81.
65. Streekantaiah C, Kwark E, Chuang LT, Ladanyi M: Cytogenetic and molecular characterization of a malignant mixed mullerian tumor of the uterus with a t(8;22)(q24.1;q12). Cancer Genet Cytogenet 1999;115: 73–76.

66. Kounelis S, Jones MW, Papadaki H, Bakker A, Swalsky P, Finkelstein SD: Carcinosarcomas (malignant mixed mullerian tumors) of the female genital tract: Comparative molecular analysis of epithelial and mesenchymal components. Hum Pathol 1998;29:82–87.
67. Abeln EC, Smit VT, Wessels JW, de Leeuw WJ, Cornelisse CJ, Fleuren GJ: Molecular genetic evidence for the conversion hypothesis of the origin of malignant mixed müllerian tumours. J Pathol 1997;183:424–431.
68. Eimoto M, Iwasaki H, Kikuchi M, Shirakawa K: Characteristics of cloned cells of mixed mullerian tumor of the human uterus: Carcinoma cells showing myogenic differentiation in vitro. Cancer 1993;71:3065–3075.

Granulosa Cell Tumor

69. Ayhan A, Tuncer ZS, Tuncer R, Mercan R, Yuce K, Ayhan A: Granulosa cell tumor of the ovary. A clinicopathological evaluation of 60 cases. Eur J Gynaecol Oncol 1994;15:320–324.
70. Miller BE, Barron BA, Wan JY, Delmore JE, Silva EG, Gershenson DM: Prognostic factors in adult granulosa cell tumor of the ovary. Cancer 1997;79:1951–1955.
71. Cronje HS, Niemand I, Bam RH, Woodruff JD: Review of the granulosa-theca cell tumors from the Emil Novak ovarian tumor registry. Am J Obstet Gynecol 1999;180:323–327.
72. Robinson JB, Im DD, Logan L, McGuire WP, Rosenshein NB: Extraovarian granulosa cell tumor. Gynecol Oncol 1999;74:123–127.
73. Susil BJ, Sumithran E: Sarcomatous change in granulosa cell tumor. Hum Pathol 1987;18:397–399.
74. Flemming P, Wellmann A, Maschek H, Lang H, Georgii A: Monoclonal antibodies against inhibin represent key markers of adult granulosa cell tumor of the ovary even in their metastases. A report of three cases with late metastases, being previously interpreted as hemangiopericytoma. Am J Surg Pathol 1995;19:927–933.
75. Rishi M, Howard LN, Bratthauer GL, Tavassoli FA: Use of monoclonal antibody against human inhibin as a marker for sex cord-stromal tumors of the ovary. Am J Surg Pathol 1997;21:583–589.
76. McCluggage WG, Maxwell P, Sloan JM: Immunohistochemical staining of ovarian granulosa cell tumors with monoclonal antibody against inhibin. Hum Pathol 1997;28:1034–1038.
77. Hildebrandt RH, Rouse RV, Longacre TA: Value of inhibin in the identification of granulosa cell tumors of the ovary. Hum Pathol 1997;28:1387–1395.
78. Otis CN, Powell JL, Barbuto D, Carcangiu ML: Intermediate filamentous proteins in adult granulosa cell tumors. An immunohistochemical study of 25 cases. Am J Surg Pathol 1992;16:962–968.
79. Costa MJ, DeRose PB, Roth LM, Brescia RJ, Zaloudek CJ, Cohen C: Immunohistochemical phenotype of ovarian granulosa cell tumors: Absence of epithelial membrane antigen has diagnostic value. Hum Pathol 1994;25:60–66.
80. Costa MJ, Walls J, Ames P, Roth LM: Transformation in recurrent ovarian granulosa cell tumors: Ki67 (MIB-1) and p53 immunohistochemistry demonstrates a possible molecular basis for the poor histopathologic prediction of clinical behavior. Hum Pathol 1996;27:274–281.
81. Fletcher JA, Gibas Z, Donovan K, et al: Ovarian granulosa-stromal cell tumors are characterized by trisomy 12. Am J Pathol 1991;138:515–520.
82. Gorski GK, McMorrow LE, Blumstein L, Faasse D, Donaldson MH: Trisomy 14 in two cases of granulosa cell tumor of the ovary. Cancer Genet Cytogenet 1992; 60:202–205.
83. Lindgren V, Waggoner S, Rotmensch J: Monosomy 22 in two ovarian granulosa cell tumors. Cancer Genet Cytogenet 1996;89:93–97.
84. Van den Berghe I, Dal Cin P, De Groef K, Michielssen P, Van der Berghe H: Monosomy 22 and trisomy 14 may be early events in the tumorigenesis of adult granulosa cell tumor. Cancer Genet Cytogenet 1999;112:46–48.
85. Verhest A, Nedoszytko B, Noel JC, Dangou JM, Simon P, Limon J: Translocation (6;16) in a case of granulosa cell tumor of the ovary. Cancer Genet Cytogenet 1992; 60:41–44.

Van H. Savell, Jr.
David M. Parham

Rhabdomyomas and Rhabdomyosarcomas

CHAPTER 13

Skeletal muscle tumors comprise a very small portion of sarcomas in adults, but are the most common soft tissue sarcomas in children. They are well studied because of multicenter studies, such as the Intergroup Rhabdomyosarcoma Study. This chapter focuses on the benign and malignant soft tissue tumors that have a principal component of skeletal muscle differentiation. A number of other tumors with heterologous skeletal muscle differentiation (Table 13–1) will be discussed in this chapter only in terms of the differential diagnosis.

Unlike tumors of adipose tissue, blood vessels, and fibrous lesions, malignant tumors with skeletal muscle differentiation are much more common than the benign ones. The reason for this is not known. According to the most widely accepted theory, an undifferentiated mesenchymal cell becomes malignant and then may differentiate along a number of tissue pathways, giving rise to sarcomas with various histologic characteristics. The appearance of rhabdomyosarcomas in the urinary bladder mucosa, a site without skeletal muscle, indeed, indicates that the pre-existing skeletal muscle is not a prerequisite for the development of rhabdomyosarcoma.

The reason rhabdomyosarcomas are overwhelmingly the most common sarcoma in childhood and the teenage years and are much rarer in adults remains a mystery. Normal myogenesis is complete by the early second fetal trimester. The association of rhabdomyosarcomas with younger age groups suggests that proliferation factors, genetic associations, and tissue differentiation processes are more likely to be involved in their pathogenesis rather than external carcinogenic factors.

Rhabdomyoma

Rhabdomyomas are benign soft tissue tumors that primarily differentiate into skeletal muscle. They are rare neoplasms, accounting for only 2% of all tumors with primary skeletal muscle differentiation in large consultation practices.[1] They can be broadly classified into cardiac and noncardiac types. Cardiac rhabdomyomas are strongly associated with tuberous sclerosis and will not be further considered in this chapter. Among the noncardiac rhabdomyomas are adult, fetal, and genital rhabdomyomas and a mixed rhabdomyomatous mesenchymal tumor that may represent a hamartoma rather than a true neoplasm.

Fetal Rhabdomyoma

Clinical Features

Fetal rhabdomyomas most commonly occur in children, usually under 3 years of age, but they may be seen in older children or young adults,[2] and even in the elderly.[3] They are more common in male patients. There is overlap in age of patients with the more common rhabdomyosarcoma; thus, distinction

Table 13–1. Tumors Other Than Rhabdomyoma and Rhabdomyosarcoma That May Contain Focal Skeletal Muscle Differentiation

Benign	Malignant
Mature teratoma	Medullomyoblastoma
Benign Triton tumor	Malignant peripheral nerve sheath tumors
Sertoli-Leydig tumor	Immature and malignant teratoma
Thymoma	Wilms tumor (nephroblastoma)
	Mixed müllerian tumor
	Carcinosarcoma
	Pleuropulmonary blastoma
	Hepatoblastoma
	Ectomesenchymoma
	Malignant mesenchymoma
	Osteosarcoma
	Dedifferentiated sarcomas: chondrosarcoma, liposarcoma
	Neuroendocrine carcinomas

between these tumors may be a source of clinical and histologic confusion. Fetal rhabdomyomas often occur in the head and neck and are outnumbered by rhabdomyosarcomas by at least 50:1.[3] Other sites of presentation are possible, although a subcutaneous rather than deep location is the rule. Fetal rhabdomyomas are cured with a local excision, although one case with progression to rhabdomyosarcoma is reported,[4] and other instances of recurrent disease are well documented.[5] Except for an association with the basal cell-nevus syndrome (Gorlin-Goltz syndrome),[3] these tumors usually occur sporadically in children without tuberous sclerosis or other genetic conditions.

Histologic Features

The usual fetal rhabdomyomas are composed of myoid tubules in a myxoid background having a component of spindle cells (Fig. 13–1). Some tumor cells may contain cross-striations. Some of these tumors have eosinophilic strap cells with little or no myxoid stroma. There should be no significant nuclear pleomorphism, and the number of mitotic

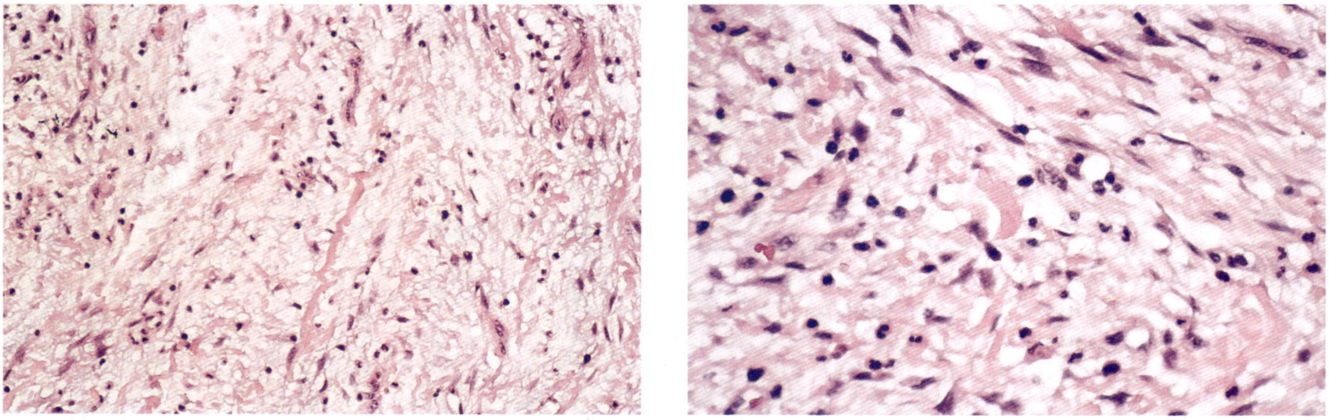

A B

Figure 13–1. *A,* Classic fetal rhabdomyoma with a myxoid background and a rare strap cell (hematoxylin & eosin [H&E], ×200). *B,* Higher power view of the same case. Note the lack of nuclear atypia or mitotic figures (H&E, ×400).

figures is small, usually 1 or less per 10 high-power (×400) magnification fields.

A histologic appearance "intermediate" between the fetal and adult rhabdomyoma and with loss of immature cells has been noted.[2,6] This tumor has also been termed a "juvenile" rhabdomyoma. The histologic differential diagnosis of a fetal rhabdomyoma includes spindle cell and embryonal rhabdomyosarcoma. The presence of a cambium layer, necrosis, significant hypercellularity, and most importantly nuclear atypia favor a malignant diagnosis. Circumscription and a low mitotic rate favor a benign diagnosis. Rhabdomyosarcomas treated with chemotherapy may also be included in the histologic differential diagnosis; however, clinical history and review of the previous material are helpful.

Ultrastructure

Fetal rhabdomyomas may contain enlarged Z-bands in addition to thick and thin filaments (myosin and actin) in more differentiated cells. Mitochondria may be abnormal.[7] The cells may be coated by an external lamina.[7] The immature cell components do not have ultrastructural evidence of cytoplasmic differentiation.[3]

Immunohistochemistry

Fetal rhabdomyomas express markers of skeletal muscle differentiation (desmin, myoglobin, and muscle-specific actin) and also may rarely express vimentin, S-100, CD57 (Leu7), glial fibrillary acidic protein, and smooth muscle actin. The tumors do not express keratin, epithelial membrane antigen, or histiocytic markers such as CD68.[2]

Genetics

No specific cytogenetic or genetic studies have been published that characterize this rare group of tumors.

Adult Rhabdomyoma

Clinical Features

Adult rhabdomyomas most commonly present in the oral cavity or superficial soft tissues of the head and neck of adults, usually in men.[8] The mean age of the affected patients is 50 years, but cases have been reported in children.[9] It has been suggested that this tumor arises from the branchial musculature (third and fourth branchial arches), due to its usual presentation in the neck; up to 20% of cases are multifocal.[1]

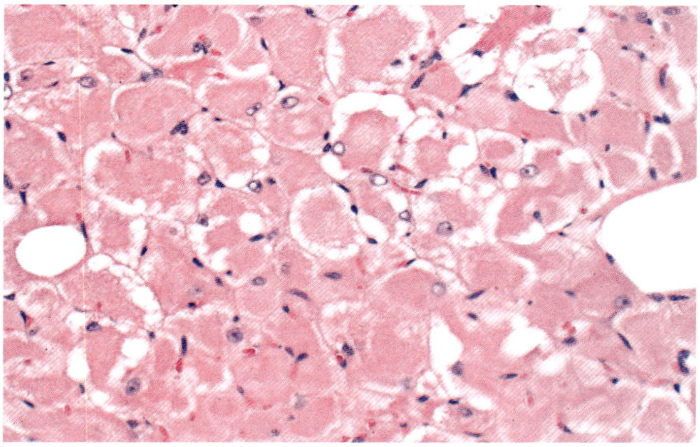

Figure 13–2. Adult rhabdomyoma with plump eosinophilic cells and focal cytoplasmic clearing (H&E). (Case courtesy of Dr. George F. Gray, Jr., Vanderbilt University and Dr. Laura W. Lamps, University of Arkansas for Medical Sciences.)

Although the tumor is benign, local recurrences occur, sometimes long after the primary surgery.

Gross and Histologic Features

Grossly, adult rhabdomyomas are brown, often lobulated masses. Histologically, they are composed of round and polygonal cells with abundant clear to eosinophilic cytoplasm (Fig. 13–2). They are strongly periodic acid-Schiff positive reflecting the high glycogen content. Cytoplasmic cross-striations can usually be identified histologically (Fig. 13–3). Due to their eosinophilic cytoplasm, the histologic differential diagnosis includes granular cell tumors and hibernomas. This differential diagnosis can easily be clarified by electron microscopy because granular cell tumors contain intracellular autophagocytic

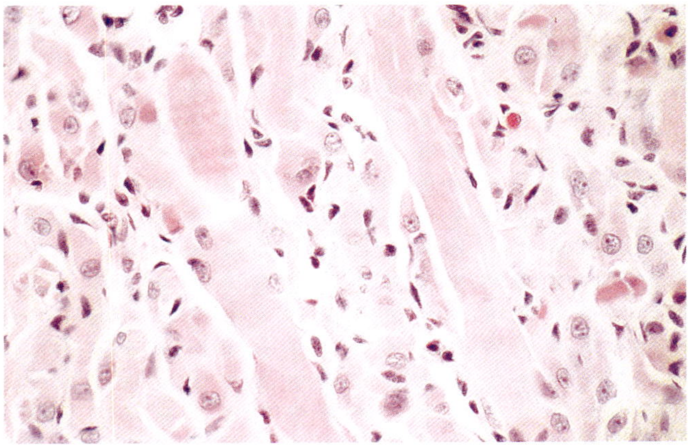

Figure 13–3. Adult rhabdomyoma with cytoplasmic cross-striations (H&E, ×400).

granules and an extracellular basal lamina, hibernomas contain lipid droplets, and rhabdomyomas contain thick and thin filaments. In general, adult rhabdomyomas are cytologically quite different from fetal rhabdomyomas, which are spindle cell tumors. However, tumors with features of both fetal and adult rhabdomyomas have been reported under various names including "juvenile rhabdomyoma" or cellular fetal rhabdomyomas.[6]

Ultrastructure

Adult rhabdomyomas have features of disorganized skeletal muscle cells. Thin and thick myofilaments are randomly dispersed with pleomorphic mitochondria, and the tumor cells are invested by a continuous basal lamina. Cytoplasmic inclusions similar to those of nemaline myopathy are present in some tumors by light microscopy and ultrastructurally correspond to hypertrophic Z-bands (Fig. 13–4).[1,7]

Immunohistochemistry

Adult rhabdomyomas are positive for α smooth muscle actin, myoglobin, desmin, and variably for vimentin[1] and smooth muscle actin. Neural markers such as S-100 and CD57 may also be positive.[3]

Genetics

Relatively little is known about the cytogenetic characteristics of adult rhabdomyoma. A recurrent parapharyngeal tumor had a reciprocal translocation of chromosomes 15 and 17 and abnormalities of the long arm of chromosome 10. The authors noted that these findings strongly supported the neoplastic nature of adult rhabdomyomas rather than a hamartomatous or reactive process.[10]

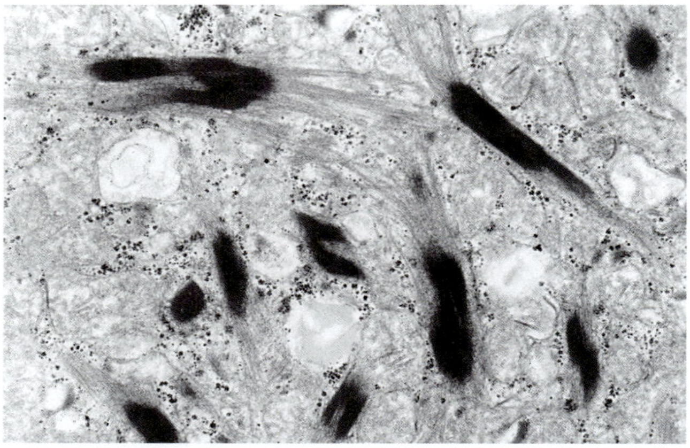

Figure 13–4. Electron microscopy shows nemaline myopathy-like inclusions in adult rhabdomyoma. (Courtesy of Dr. Markku Miettinen.)

Genital Rhabdomyomas

Clinical Features

Genital rhabdomyomas are considered by some to be a separate subtype of rhabdomyoma and are located in the vagina or cervix of postpubescent, usually reproductive-age women. Fetal rhabdomyoma has also been reported in male genitalia.[11] Histologically, however, rhabdomyomas of female genitalia are similar to fetal rhabdomyomas (Fig. 13–5) in that they also do not contain significant nuclear pleomorphism. These lesions are cured by local excision and have a benign course.

Histologic Features

Genital rhabdomyomas have many similarities with fetal rhabdomyomas (Fig. 13–6). They are usually exophytic and contain muscle cells with at least focal cross striations.[1] The extracellular matrix may be collagenous or myxoid. Some degree of pleomorphism and mitotic activity may be present, necessitating caution in the overdiagnosis of malignancy in this clinical setting.

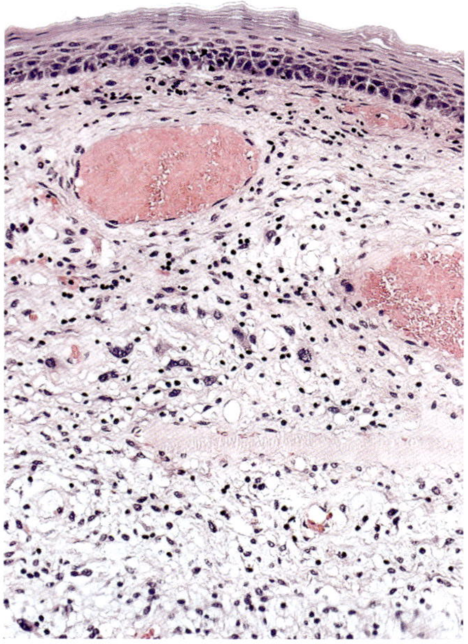

Figure 13–5. Genital rhabdomyoma with myxoid stroma in the vagina of an adolescent female following pregnancy (H&E, ×400). (From Parham DM (ed): Pediatric Neoplasia: Morphology and Biology. Philadelphia, Lippincott-Raven, 1996, with permission.)

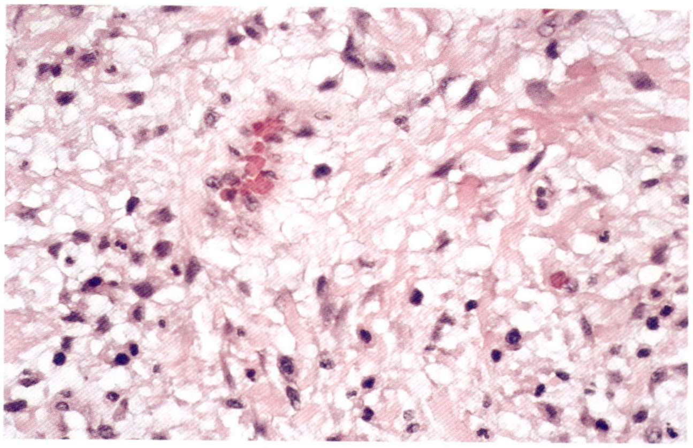

Figure 13–6. Rhabdomyoma adjacent to the labium majus in a 3-year-old girl, reportedly present since birth (H&E, ×400). (Case courtesy of Dr. Michael Kosanovich.)

Ultrastructural Features

Genital rhabdomyomas often contain myofilaments that are arranged haphazardly. They contain normal-appearing mitochondria and rarely have hypertrophied Z-bands, unlike fetal rhabdomyomas. The matrix is reportedly more prominent than that of adult or fetal rhabdomyomas.[7]

Differential Diagnosis

Hibernomas, granular cell tumors, paragangliomas, and oncocytomas enter the differential diagnosis of adult rhabdomyomas due to their eosinophilic cytoplasm. Immunohistochemistry will readily identify the skeletal muscle differentiation. Rhabdomyosarcomas should be considered in tumors containing atypical cells and mitotic activity. Chemotherapeutically treated rhabdomyosarcomas with tumor differentiation[12] may have a similar histologic appearance, although the clinical history allows for the distinction.

Miscellaneous Tumors

Rare benign tumors with skeletal muscle differentiation include the benign Triton tumor, a tumor composed of a mixture of mature neural and skeletal muscle elements,[13] and rhabdomyomatous hamartoma of the skin,[14] a tumor composed of skeletal muscle and mature adipose tissue. In our experience, another unusual phenomenon that rarely may create a mass effect on clinical examination and imaging is an accessory muscle.

Rhabdomyosarcoma

Introduction and Classification

Rhabdomyosarcomas are malignant neoplasms whose definition varies. Qualman has suggested that rhabdomyosarcomas have an exclusive component of differentiation along the line of skeletal muscle,[15] whereas Enzinger and Weiss[1] allow for other components such as cartilage. Primitive adipose tissue differentiation may be seen ultrastructurally (Fig. 13–7). Our definition is that rhabdomyosarcomas are primitive malignant mesenchymal tumors that have a strong tendency to differentiate into skeletal muscle. Whatever definition one uses to define this tumor type, its distinction as a unique entity is readily apparent. This distinction is shown by the diagnostic agreement among experts, even with different subclassification systems.[16] However, subclassification is more problematic in general practice.[15]

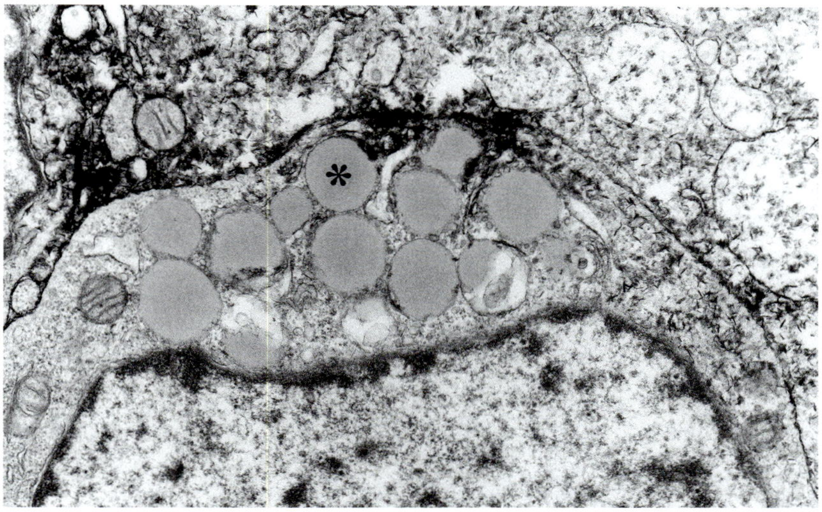

Figure 13–7. Electron microscopy of an rhabdomyosarcoma with lipid droplets (*), demonstrating focal adipose differentiation. (From Parham DM (ed): Pediatric Neoplasia: Morphology and Biology. Philadelphia, Lippincott-Raven, 1996, with permission.)

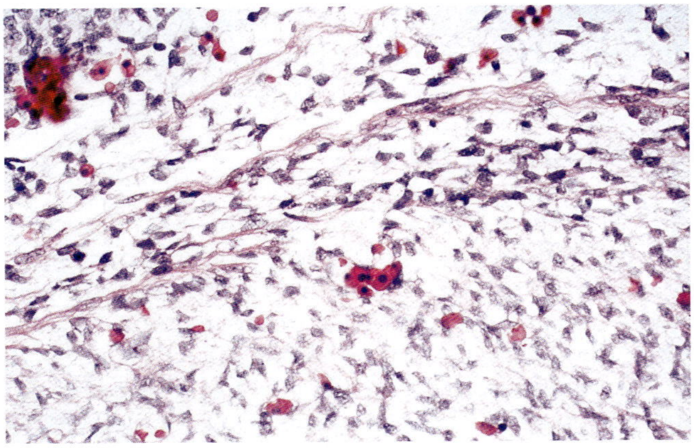

A

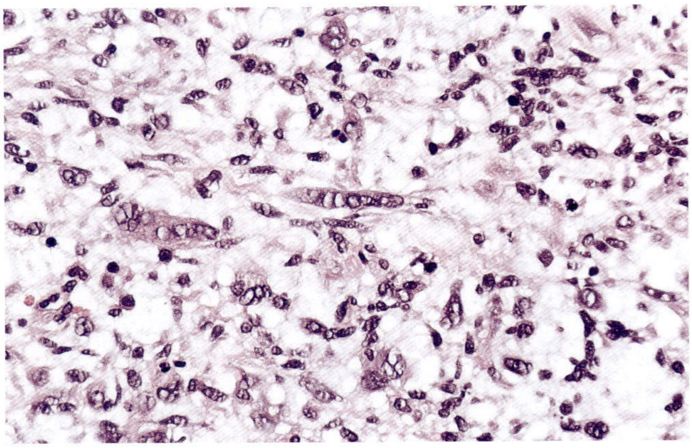

B

Figure 13–8. *A*, Fetal skeletal muscle with a myxoid matrix (H&E, ×250). *B*, Embryonal rhabdomyosarcoma showing a striking similarity to fetal skeletal muscle (H&E, ×250). (From Parham DM (ed): Pediatric Neoplasia: Morphology and Biology. Philadelphia, Lippincott-Raven, 1996, with permission.)

Rhabdomyosarcomas have histologic features similar to, yet distinct from, embryonic and very early fetal skeletal muscle. In development, immature mesenchymal cells that resemble fibroblasts develop increased amounts of cytoplasm. These cells (now called myoblasts) become mitotically active and then fuse to form myotubules. The similarity of embryonal rhabdomyosarcoma to embryonal muscle can be striking (Fig. 13–8). However, the analogy between alveolar rhabdomyosarcoma (analogous to myoblasts) and myotubules (analogous to some differentiated embryonal rhabdomyosarcomas) has, in our opinion, been somewhat overemphasized as an attempt to link embryology to neoplasia. The "alveolar" architecture is not demonstrated in embryonic development.

Subclassification of rhabdomyosarcoma is of key importance in proper diagnosis and management. The classification of rhabdomyosarcomas by the World Health Organization[17] (WHO) is shown in Table 13–2, and a similar International Classification[15,18] is shown in Table 13–3.

Table 13–2. WHO Classification of Malignant Tumors of Skeletal Muscle Differentiation[17]

Rhabdomyosarcoma with ganglionic differentiation (ectomesenchymoma)
Rhabdomyosarcoma
Embryonal
Botryoid
Spindle cell
Alveolar
Pleomorphic

Clinical Presentation

Rhabdomyosarcomas are the most common malignant soft tissue tumors in children, but they may occur in patients of all ages. The clinical presentation varies by age and histologic subtype. A male predominance and a more common occurrence in whites than in African or Asian ethnic groups has been documented.[19] A common clinical presentation for a prepubertal child is to present with a genitourinary (Fig. 13–9), retroperitoneal, or head/neck mass that on biopsy is an embryonal rhabdomyosarcoma. Occurrence in older adults has been rarely reported.

Alveolar rhabdomyosarcomas more often present in the extremity (Fig. 13–10) or head and neck region (sinonasal region, orbit) of adolescents, sometimes in small children, and very rarely in elderly

Table 13–3. International Prognostic Classification of Pediatric Rhabdomyosarcoma[18]

Superior prognosis
Botryoid embryonal rhabdomyosarcoma
Spindle cell rhabdomyosarcoma
Intermediate prognosis
Embryonal rhabdomyosarcoma
Poor prognosis
Alveolar rhabdomyosarcoma
Undifferentiated sarcoma
Rhabdomyosarcoma with diffuse anaplasia
Prognosis uncertain
Rhabdomyosarcoma with rhabdoid features

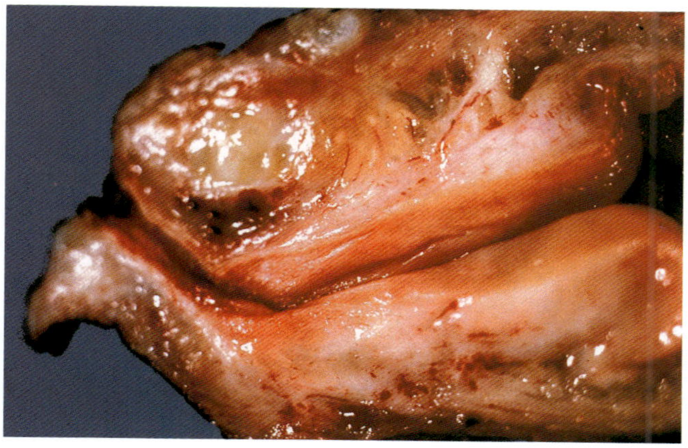

A

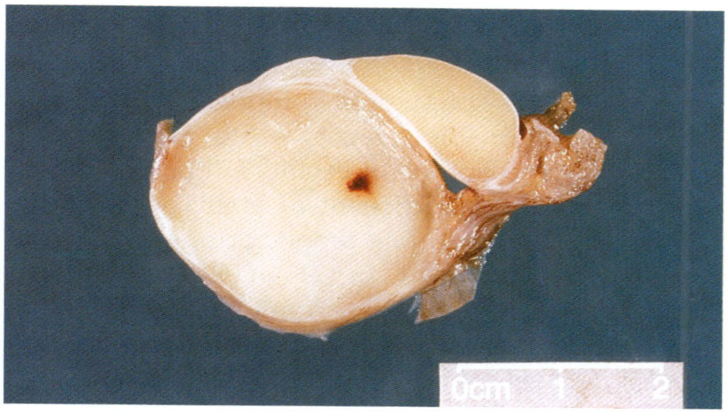

B

Figure 13–9. *A*, Gross midsagittal prostatic embryonal rhabdomyosarcoma extending into the urinary bladder. *B*, Gross of an embryonal rhabdomyosarcoma involving the testis. (*A* and *B*, Courtesy of Dr. Stephen M. Bonsib, University of Arkansas for Medical Sciences.)

adults. Spindle cell rhabdomyosarcomas have a strong predilection for the paratesticular region of children and young adults. Other sites of note for embryonal and alveolar rhabdomyosarcoma include specific regions of the head and neck (ear canal, parameningeal locations, orbit, sinuses or metastatic disease in lymph nodes), and various soft tissues, retroperitoneum, and biliary tract (Fig. 13–11). Rare cases simulate leukemia or hematopoietic neoplasms (Fig. 13–12) and may have no apparent primary site.[20–22] Currently, the vast majority of pediatric cases in industrialized nations are treated on multi-institutional protocols such as those of the Intergroup Rhabdomyosarcoma Study Group (IRSG) or Societe Internationale d' Oncologie Pediatrique.

Patients usually present with a painless mass and rarely have systemic complaints, although hypercalcemia has been reported with osteolytic lesions.[23] Symptoms may also relate to affected organs, such as urinary retention with prostatic lesions and diplopia with orbital tumors.

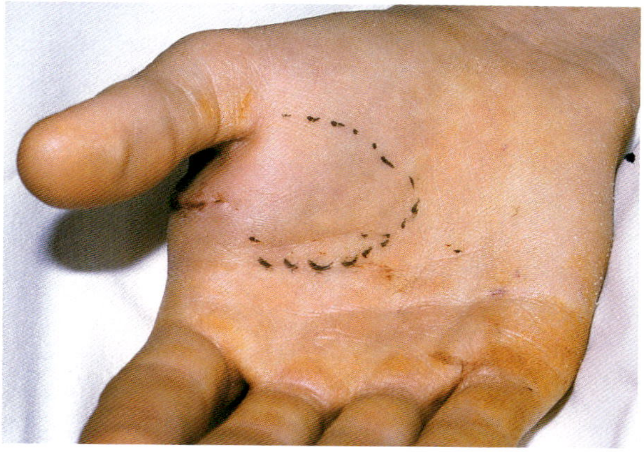

Figure 13–10. Alveolar rhabdomyosarcoma of the extremity of a teenaged male. (From Parham DM (ed): Pediatric Neoplasia: Morphology and Biology. Philadelphia, Lippincott-Raven, 1996, with permission.)

Pleomorphic rhabdomyosarcomas are rare tumors that essentially are only diagnosed in the elderly adult population, most often in the trunk and extremities. Their diagnosis is based on immunohis-

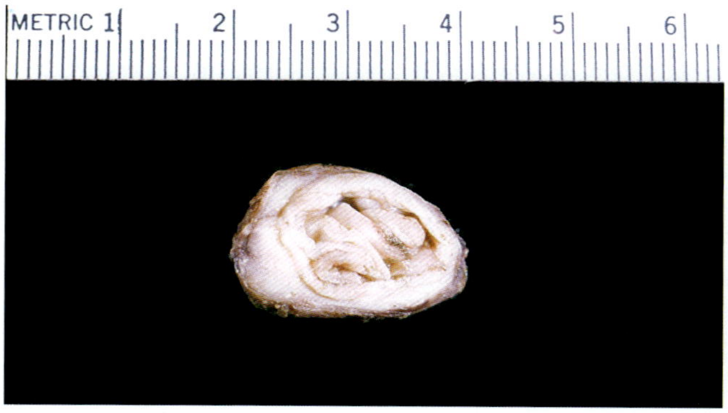

A

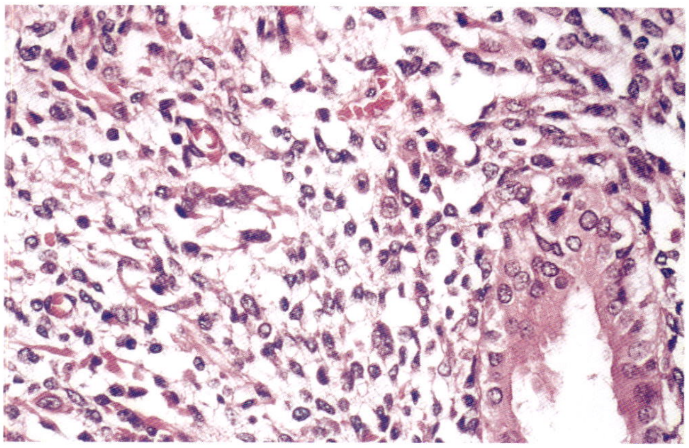

B

Figure 13–11. *A*, A cystically dilated common bile duct almost entirely filled with a polypoid mass. *B*, Microscopically an embryonal rhabdomyosarcoma is located deep to the biliary epithelium (H&E, ×400).

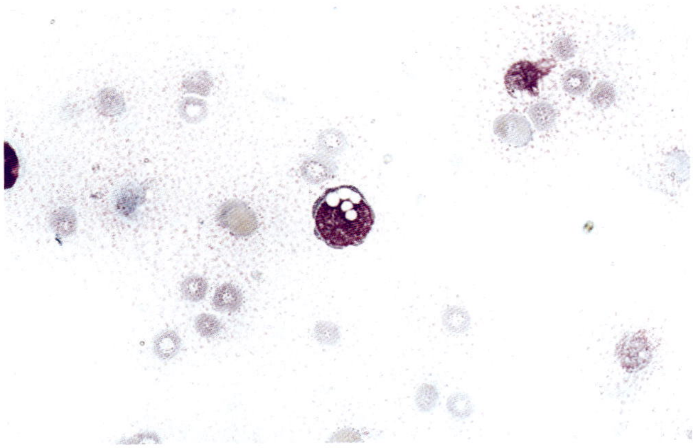

Figure 13-12. Single, discohesive rhabdomyosarcoma cells simulating a hematopoietic neoplasm (H&E, ×400).

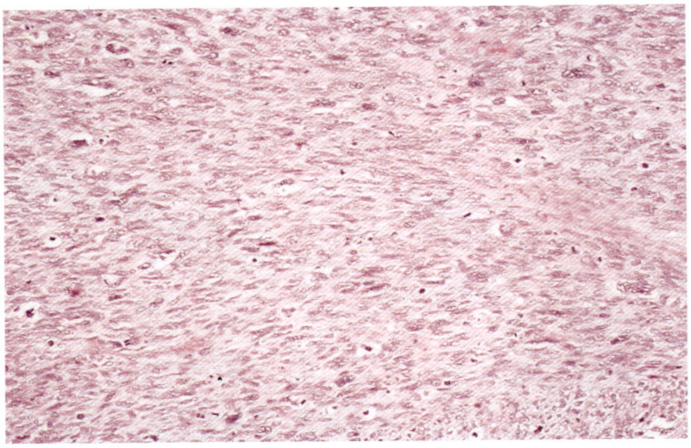

Figure 13-14. Spindle cell rhabdomyosarcoma with a fibrosarcomatous appearance (H&E, ×100).

tochemical and ultrastructural verification of skeletal muscle differentiation.

Pathology

Rhabdomyosarcomas exhibit skeletal muscle differentiation, which in primitive, poorly differentiated tumors may require documentation by immunohistochemistry or electron microscopy. Genetic findings (discussed later) may assist with undifferentiated lesion or limited samples. Grossly, the embryonal (including botryoid) tumors are often myxoid, gray-white masses, whereas the alveolar ones tend to be fleshy "lymphoma-like" tumors.

Spindle Cell Rhabdomyosarcoma

Spindle cell rhabdomyosarcomas are characterized by a large component of cells with elongate borders and a relatively dense, collagenous background stroma (Fig. 13–13). This tumor was called "type A rhabdomyosarcoma" by Palmer and colleagues.[24]

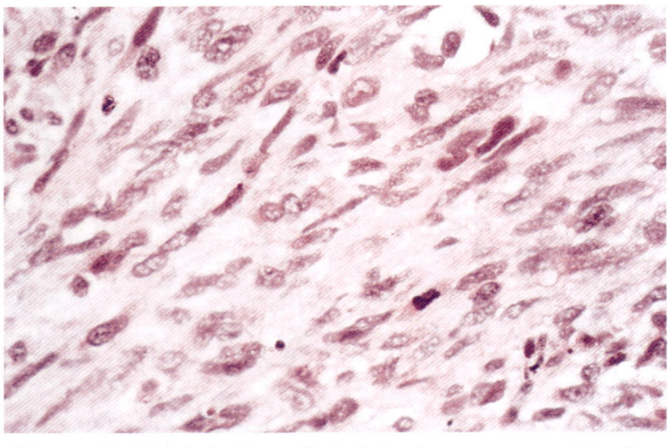

Figure 13-13. Spindle cell rhabdomyosarcoma with elongate cells and occasional cells with eosinophilic cytoplasm (H&E, ×400).

The amount of a spindle cell component required to place a tumor in this category is not well defined. Any alveolar component excludes this diagnosis, although a minor component of embryonal-appearing areas does not. In one report, cytoplasmic cross-striations were present in 21 of 21 spindle cell rhabdomyosarcomas.[25] These tumors in some areas may simulate leiomyosarcomas or fibrosarcomas (Fig. 13–14), yet they should have definitive skeletal muscle rather than smooth muscle differentiation. The spindle cell tumors may contain either abundant collagen or only scanty collagen between tumor cells.[26] Pure spindle cell tumors have the best prognosis particularly if they are located in the paratesticular region,[26] because they rarely metastasize. Eighty-eight percent of affected patients are alive at 5 years.[15] A less common location for spindle cell rhabdomyosarcomas is in the head and neck region.

Embryonal Rhabdomyosarcoma

Embryonal rhabdomyosarcomas are composed of haphazardly arranged cells, often having a myxoid stromal background (Fig. 13–15). These tumors vary from hypercellular (Fig. 13–16) to hypocellular, stroma-rich tumors (Fig. 13–17). Cellularity may be enhanced around blood vessels. The constituent cells vary from being primitive and stellate to having moderate eosinophilic cytoplasm to being very differentiated with abundant eccentric eosinophilic cytoplasm and cross-striations. Multinucleate tumor cells may recapitulate the myotube of myogenesis (Fig. 13–18). A tumor may have any combination of these stromal or cellular features. In some ways, embryonal rhabdomyosarcoma is a tumor type defined by rhabdomyoblastic differentiation and a lack of uniform features. For treatment purposes, any well-defined alveolar component establishes the diagnosis of alveolar rhabdomyosarcoma. The presence of a cambium layer or a significant spindle cell

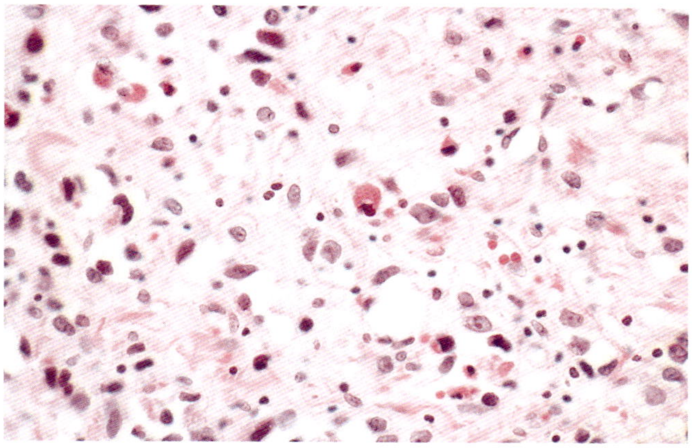

Figure 13-15. Embryonal rhabdomyosarcoma with cytologically atypical cells, some of which have eosinophilic cytoplasm consistent with myoblasts (H&E, ×200).

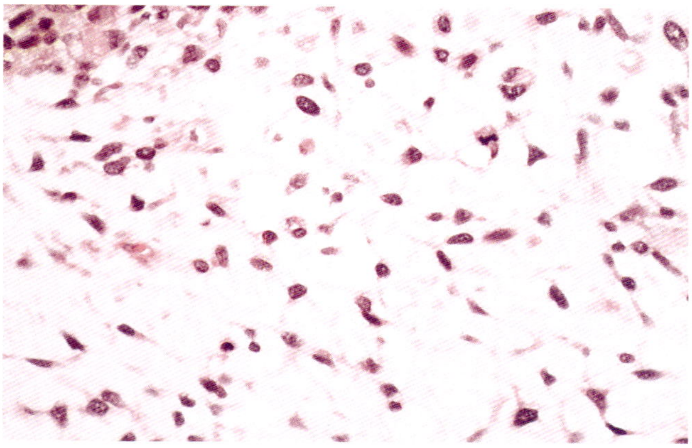

Figure 13-17. Embryonal rhabdomyosarcoma, hypocellular zone (H&E, ×200).

component distinguish botryoid and spindle cell rhabdomyosarcomas, morphologic subtypes of embryonal rhabdomyosarcomas with a superior prognosis. This designation of spindle cell or botyroid rhabdomyosarcoma, however, does not at present affect therapy. There is a danger that the term "embryonal rhabdomyosarcomas" could be used as a wastebasket category, so that we favor restricting this category to tumors with an immature stroma and features recapitulating prenatal myogenesis.

There is a strikingly wide histologic spectrum of embryonal rhabdomyosarcomas, which exhibit variable degrees of cellularity (from cellular to hypocellular examples that may lead one to question if tumor is present), matrix production (from myxoid, immature mesenchymal-appearing stroma to mature collagen), and cytoplasmic differentiation (from primitive cells to rhabdomyoblasts to myotubules or multinucleated cells to almost fully differentiated muscle cells). Cytoplasmic cross-striations similar to skeletal muscle may be seen in many cases, but their identification often requires careful searching and is no longer diagnostically essential. Embryonal rhabdomyosarcomas account for almost half of all rhabdomyosarcomas in a recent IRSG review[15] and almost 75% of cases in large consult practices.[1]

Anaplasia: Diffuse and Focal

Although alveolar rhabdomyosarcomas may have features of anaplasia, this feature is much more common in embryonal tumors.[27] Anaplasia is defined by nuclei that are three times larger than adjacent tumor nuclei at their narrowest diameter, similar to the criteria for anaplasia in Wilms tumors[27] (Fig. 13-19). Atypical mitotic figures were not required for diagnosis of anaplasia in Kodet's study,[27] but were an important histologic feature (Fig. 13-20). In Palmer's study,[24] the presence of multinucleate cells is insufficient for the

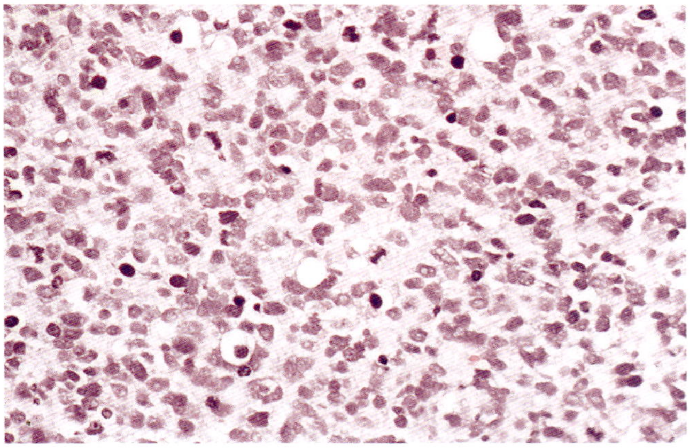

Figure 13-16. Embryonal rhabdomyosarcoma with dense cellularity (H&E, ×200).

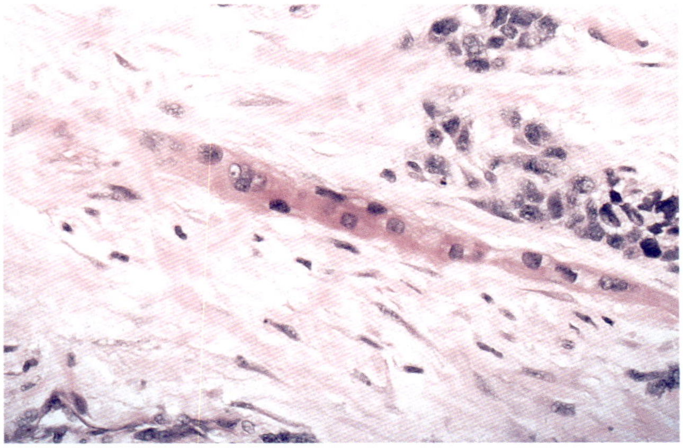

Figure 13-18. Embryonal rhabdomyosarcoma with a myotube formation (H&E, ×200).

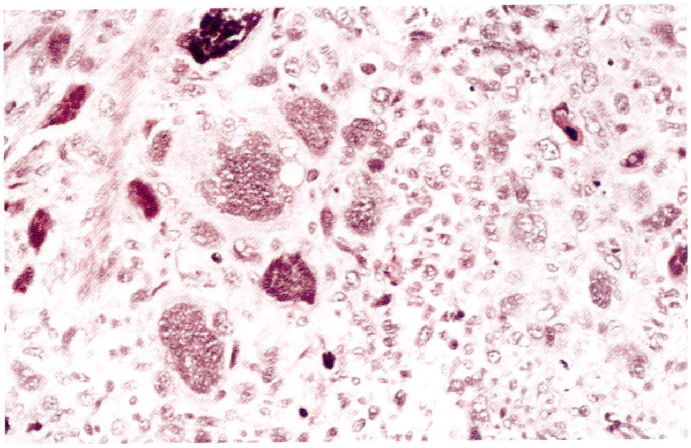

Figure 13-19. Anaplasia in an embryonal rhabdomyosarcoma with enlarged, hyperchromatic nuclei (H&E, ×400).

diagnosis of anaplasia. Anaplasia suggests a worse prognosis if it is diffuse rather than focal, the major criterion for diffuse anaplasia being sheets of anaplastic cells rather than isolated clusters.[27]

Botryoid Rhabdomyosarcoma

Botryoid rhabdomyosarcomas are embryonal rhabdomyosarcomas that occur in small children adjacent to an epithelial surface and have a condensation of neoplastic cells immediately deep to the epithelium (Fig. 13–21). This feature is called a cambium layer (similar to the cambium layer of a tree where the living cells are located subjacent to the bark). The most common locations are urinary bladder, vagina, and bile ducts. Grossly, these tumors have a polypoid configuration, similar to a bunch of grapes (Greek, "botryos"). They comprise between 5% and 10% of all rhabdomyosarcomas.[1] We believe that the cambium layer is due to tumor growth being restricted by an epithelial surface, so that instead of tumor cells infiltrating adjacent soft tissue they "pile up" against the epithelium. Botryoid rhabdomyosarcomas have an excellent prognosis with a 95% 5-year survival.[15]

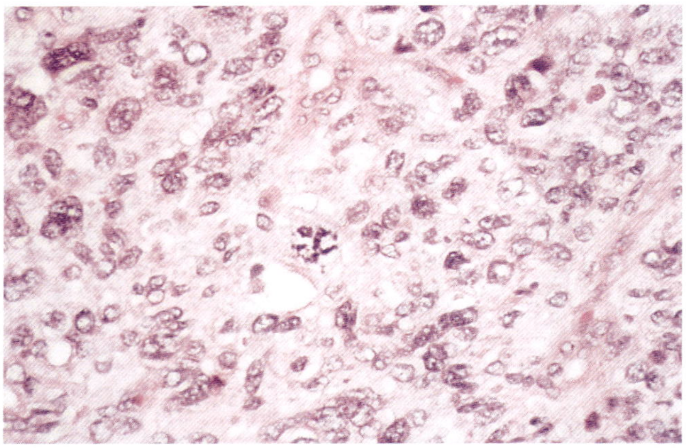

Figure 13-20. Atypical mitotic figures in an anaplastic rhabdomyosarcoma (H&E, ×400).

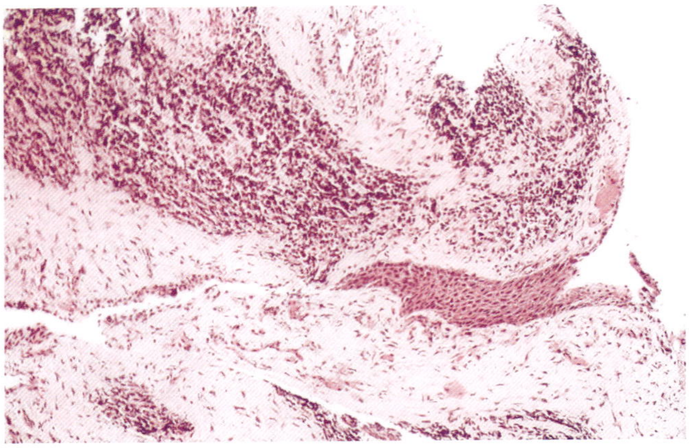

A

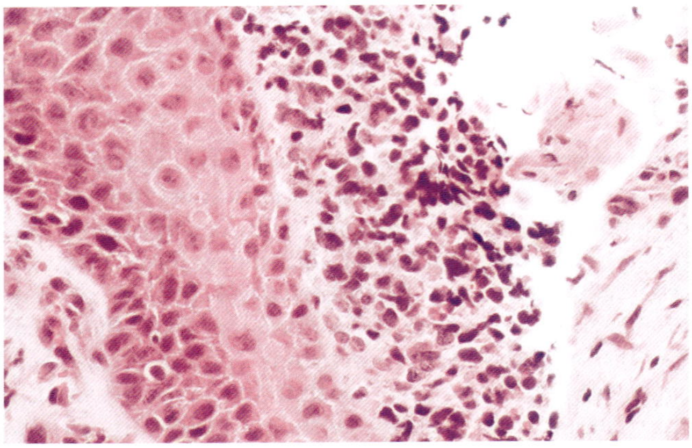

B

Figure 13-21. *A*, Low power view of a botyroid rhabdomyosarcoma (H&E, ×100). *B*, Higher power view of the same case with a distinct cambium layer deep to a mucosal surface (H&E, ×400).

Alveolar Rhabdomyosarcoma

Alveolar rhabdomyosarcoma is classically defined as a tumor composed of neoplastic cells with rhabdomyoblastic differentiation, which appear to line a hollow space. Alveolus is derived from the Latin, meaning "trough, hollow sac, or cavity." Tumors with this architecture typically have fibrous septa, lined by tumor cells that line an alveolar space. This cavity may contain discohesive tumor cells (Fig. 13–22). The presence of any alveolar pattern is adequate to place a tumor into this high-risk category. Tsokos and coworkers have expanded this category to include "solid alveolar" types (Fig. 13–23), tumors with the cytologic features of alveolar rhabdomyosaromas, but without the architectural background of septa or discohesion.[28] Cytogenetics support this designation.[29] The cytologic features of a solid alveolar rhabdomyosarcoma and typical alveolar rhabdomyosarcoma are those of a "small round cell tumor" with homogeneous, dark chromatin with or without nucleoli. Mitotic figures are often multiple. Some cases contain rhabdomyoblasts with eccentric eosinophilic

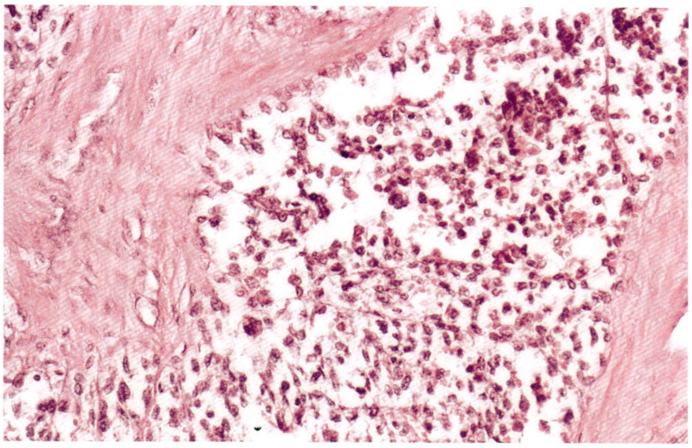

Figure 13–22. Alveolar rhabdomyosarcoma with fibrous septa and discohesive tumor cells (H&E, ×200).

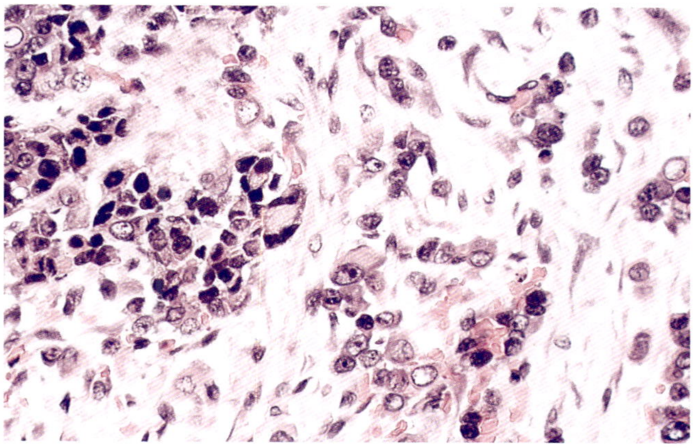

Figure 13–24. Alveolar rhabdomyosarcoma with rhabdomyoblastic differentiation (H&E, ×400).

cytoplasm (Fig. 13–24) and prominent giant cells. Rare cases may also contain areas with an epithelioid or rhabdoid appearance (Fig. 13–25). Readily identifiable rhabdomyoblasts may not be present, so that supplemental studies to document rhabdomyoblastic differentiation are required. A clear cell variant containing vacuolated cells suggestive of lipoblasts (Fig. 13–26) has been noted and in some cases has a distinct alveolar architecture.[30] Clear cell rhabdomyosarcomas contain large amounts of glycogen, similar to many other clear cell tumors.

Alveolar rhabdomyosarcoma often metastasizes into regional lymph nodes, where it maintains the same architectural pattern as seen in the primary tumors.

Pleomorphic Rhabdomyosarcoma

Pleomorphic rhabdomyosarcomas are extremely rare tumors that are felt to occur exclusively in adults. They are most common in the extremities and are composed of pleomorphic spindle cells and tumor giant cells (Fig. 13–27). The differential diagnostic considerations include liposarcoma and malignant fibrous histiocytoma. The presence of tumor cells with cytoplasmic rhabdomyoblastic differentiation is vital for diagnosis, so that a search for cross-striations seen with hematoxylin and eosin stains

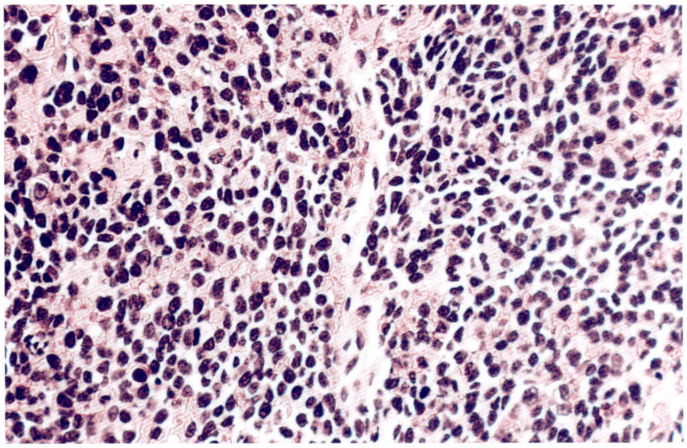

Figure 13–23. Alveolar rhabdomyosarcoma, solid pattern, with tumor cells cytologically similar to classic alveolar rhabdomyosarcomas but without the fibrous septa (H&E, ×200).

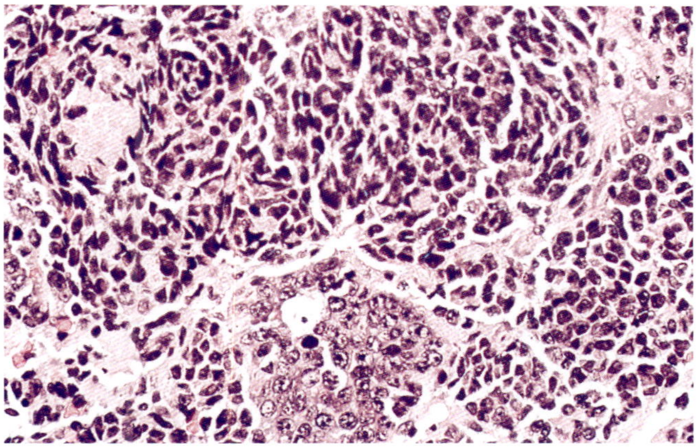

A

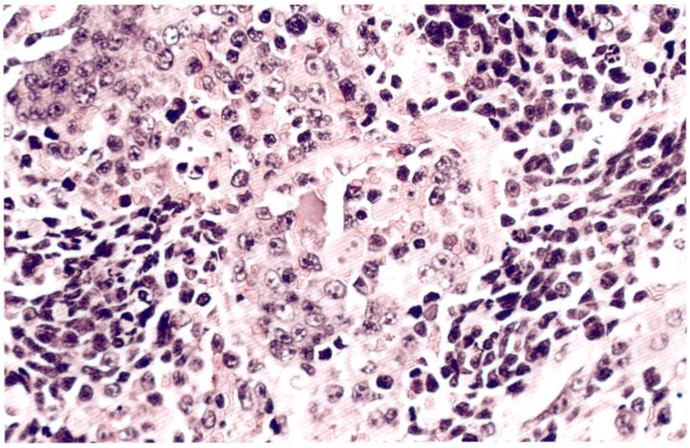

B

Figure 13–25. *A*, Low power view of a solid alveolar rhabdomyosarcoma with a focus of epithelioid cells (H&E, ×100). *B*, Higher power view with a rhabdoid phenotype (H&E, ×400).

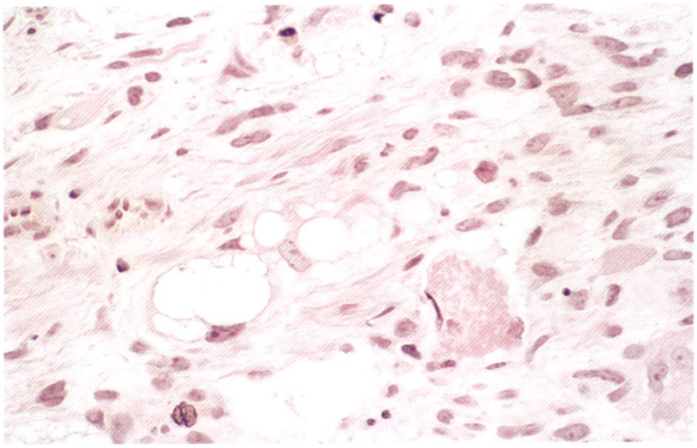

Figure 13–26. Rhabdomyosarcoma with atypical tumor cells with clear vacuoles indenting the cytoplasm similar to lipoblasts (H&E, ×400).

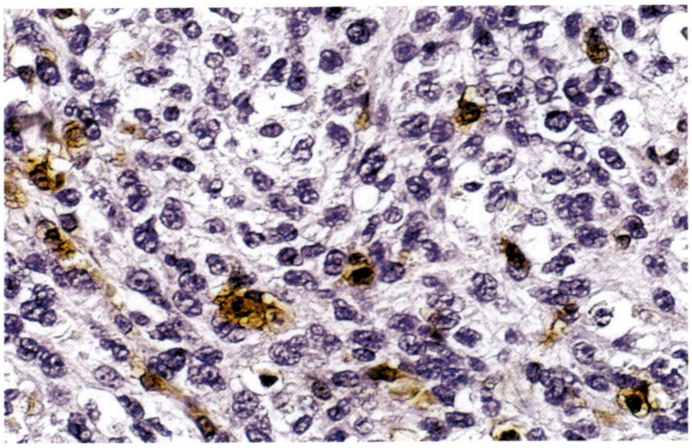

Figure 13–28. Ectomesenchymoma with immature rhabdomyoblasts and positive staining of tumor cells for S-100 (H&E, ×400).

is important. Other tumors with rhabdomyoblastic components (mixed müllerian tumors, carcinosarcomas, or malignant peripheral nerve sheath tumors, see Table 13–1) must be considered. The histologic criteria to differentiate pleomorphic rhabdomyosarcoma from anaplastic rhabdomyosarcoma have not been established, so that one might argue in some cases that these are the same tumor. However, anaplastic rhabdomyosarcomas should contain elements typical of embryonal or alveolar rhabdomyosarcoma.

Ectomesenchymoma

Ectomesenchymoma is a tumor that combines a rhabdomyosarcoma with neoplastic neuroblasts or neurons/ganglion cells. This tumor is exceedingly rare and occurs most commonly in young male patients. The lesion is often grossly well circumscribed.[31] Histologically, it may have areas that appear similar to embryonal, spindle cell, or alveolar rhabdomyosarcomas and with variable, but often scarce, neurons or neuroblasts. Immunohistochemistry documents neural differentiation in at least some portion of neoplastic cells (by definition) with positive staining for at least one of the following: neuron-specific enolase, S-100 (Fig. 13–28), synaptophysin, neurofilament, glial fibrillary acidic protein, or protein gene product 9.5. The predominant rhabdomyosarcomatous component stains similar to rhabdomyosarcomas. Rare cases stain with keratin (AE-1/AE-3).[31] Electron microscopy is another methodology to document neural and mesenchymal differentiation. Rarely a rhabdomyosarcoma will metastasize as an ectomesenchymoma.[32] Because a small neural component may be easily missed, this tumor may be underrecognized. Alternatively, this tumor can be considered a histologic variant of rhabdomyosarcoma and not a "unique" tumor type. Ectomesenchymomas are currently treated with IRSG protocols because they appear to behave similar to rhabdomyosarcomas. These tumors are also discussed in Chapter 18.

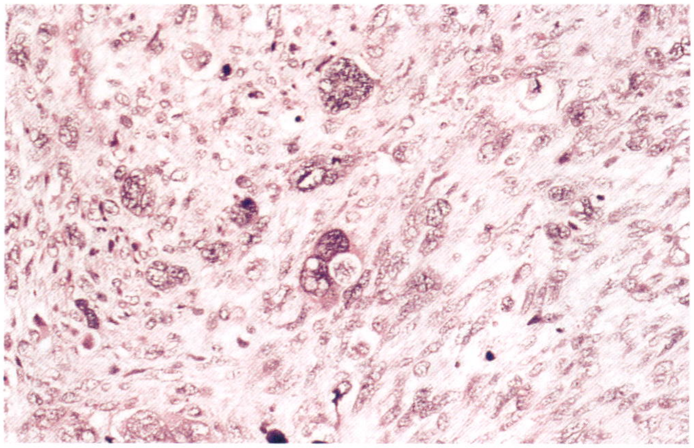

Figure 13–27. Pleomorphic rhabdomyosarcoma. Elsewhere classic areas of embryonal rhabdomyosarcoma were present (H&E, ×400).

Undifferentiated Sarcoma

Undifferentiated sarcomas are a rare group of tumors associated with a poor prognosis similar to alveolar rhabdomyosarcomas. The histologic appearance is that of a high-grade, cellular neoplasm without specific differentiation by light microscopy (Fig. 13–29), immunohistochemistry, or electron microscopy. Undifferentiated sarcomas are thus a diagnosis of exclusion.[33] These tumors express only vimentin in the majority of cases. The incidence is approximately 3% in IRSG studies.[33] Undifferentiated sarcomas that are diagnosed in the pediatric age group are included

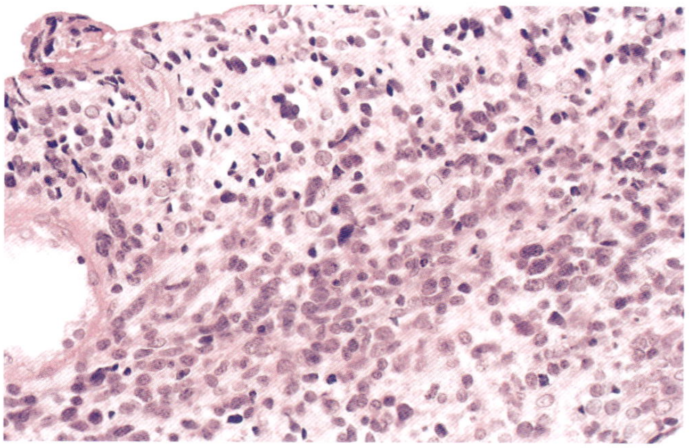

Figure 13–29. Undifferentiated rhabdomyosarcoma with an appearance similar to an embryonal rhabdomyosarcoma, except there is no light microscopic, immunohistochemical, or electron microscopic evidence of rhabdomyoblastic differentiation (H&E, ×200).

here due to some similarities with rhabdomyosarcomas and their inclusion on IRSG protocols.

Ultrastructure

In Erlandson's review of 75 cases of rhabdomyosaromas studied by electron microscopy,[7] there was no significant difference in the ultrastructural histologic appearance between various histologic types. The spectrum varies from well-differentiated rhabdomyoblasts to presumptive rhabdomyoblasts.

The most primitive cell in rhabdomyosarcoma has been termed a "presumptive rhabdomyoblast." Tumors composed entirely of this cell type are felt to be primitive embryonal rhabdomyosarcomas (also termed undifferentiated sarcomas if they only express the intermediate filament vimentin). They may have intermediate filaments and polysomes without Z-bands.

The "undifferentiated rhabdomyoblast" contains glycogen (Fig. 13–30) and may be lined by a partial basal lamina. There are 15-nm myosin filaments, large numbers of ribosomes, and occasionally "leptomeric complexes."

The "poorly differentiated" rhabdomyoblast contains one or more of the following: myosin and actin filaments (thick = 15 nm; thin = 6 nm), Z-bands, myosin-ribosome complexes, clusters of glycogen, and nuclear chromatin features. Moderately well-differentiated rhabdomyoblasts have sarcomeres that may be poorly formed (Fig. 13–31) but are still recognizable. Finally, the well-differentiated rhabdomyoblast has numerous organized sarcomeres.[31]

Immunohistochemistry

Immunohistochemical evidence for myogenic differentiation is demonstrable with markers for various actins (primarily muscle-specific), desmin, and myogenic regulatory proteins.

There are several isoforms of actin (42 kd). Rhabdomyosarcomas commonly stain for muscle-specific actin, which detects α (skeletal, smooth muscle, and cardiac) and γ smooth muscle actin.[34] Numerous other tumors are actin positive besides rhabdomyosarcomas, including fibromatosis and fibrohistiocytic

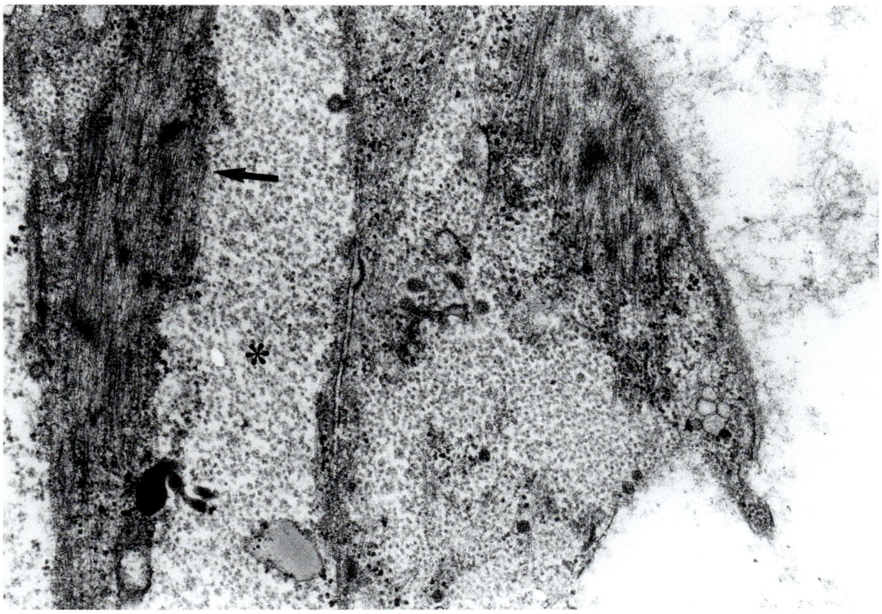

Figure 13–30. Electron microscopy of a rhabdomyosarcoma with large amounts of glycogen (*) and disorganized actin and myosin filaments *(arrow)*.

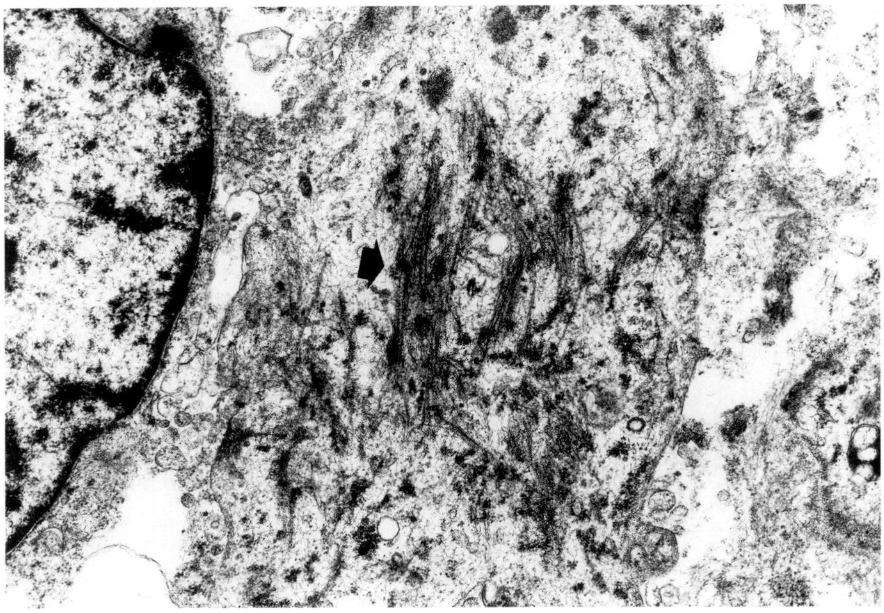

Figure 13–31. Electron microscopy of a rhabdomyosarcoma showing disorganized sarcomeres with poorly formed Z-bands *(arrow).*

lesions. Smooth muscle actin is more specific for smooth muscle tumors, but may stain rare rhabdomyosarcomas and even rhabdomyomas.[34] Positive actin staining is cytoplasmic, often in a submembranous pattern (Fig. 13–32).

Desmin is an intermediate (10-nm) filament (actin is a "thin," 7-nm filament) found in smooth and skeletal muscle tumors and nonneoplastic tissues. Early studies suggested that in formalin-fixed tissue muscle-specific actin was more sensitive than desmin.[35] At the other end of the spectrum, desmin positivity (in the absence of more specific myogenic determination protein [MyoD] positivity) has been reported in peripheral primitive neuroectodermal tumors in children.[36] Personal experience has suggested that desmin is a reliable marker of myogenic differentiation in rhabdomyosarcomas and with current methodology may be positive in tumors that are negative for actin. Like actin, desmin stains the cytoplasm (Fig. 13–33).

A specific marker of skeletal muscle (rather than smooth muscle or myofibroblastic differentiation) is myoglobin; however, it suffers greatly from the lack of sensitivity.[37] Myoglobin is the oxygen-carrying heme protein of skeletal and cardiac muscle, although it may be seen in small amounts in the thyroid and thymus.[38,39] Once a tumor shows myoglobin positivity, histologic evidence of myogenesis is usually blatantly obvious. However, myoglobin may be helpful in the evaluation of posttreatment (chemotherapy and radiotherapy) specimens with atypical cytologic features. In these cases, reactive myofibroblasts, which are positive for actin and possibly even desmin, may be suggestive of recurrent or persistent tumor. In this case, positivity for myoglobin is useful to confirm skeletal muscle differentiation, but it does not exclude regenerative skeletal muscle. Some authors suggest that radiotherapy may give misleading positivity in tumor cells,[37] but this should not be a problem in previously diagnosed rhabdomyosarcomas where the differential diagnosis is recurrent or persistent tumor versus no tumor, rather than a primary diagnosis.

At present, the most sensitive and specific markers of skeletal muscle differentiation appear to be antibodies against myogenin and MyoD1. These proteins and their relationship to rhabdomyosarcoma have been reviewed recently.[40] These two

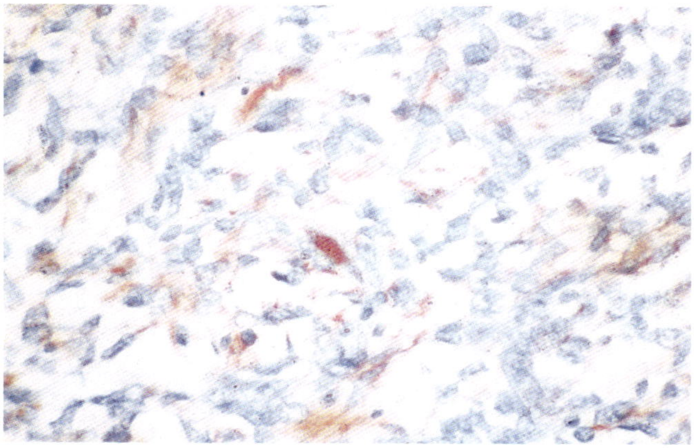

Figure 13-32. Positive cytoplasmic muscle specific actin staining in an embryonal rhabdomyosarcoma. Note the variability of staining in tumor cells (avidin-biotin complex technique with hematoxylin counterstain, ×400).

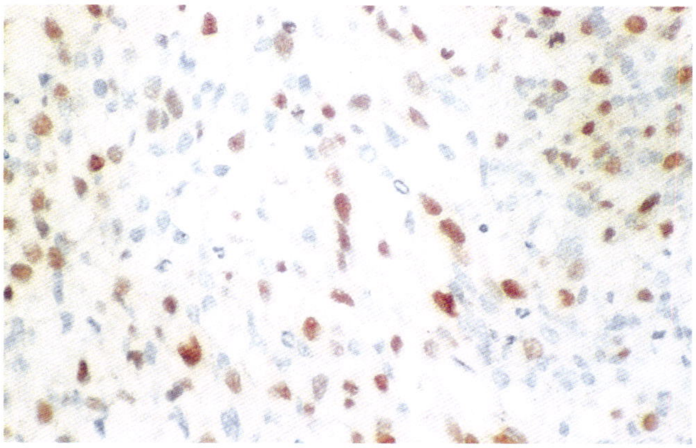

Figure 13-34. Positive nuclear staining for MyoD in an embryonal rhabdomyosarcoma (avidin-biotin complex technique with hematoxylin counterstain, ×400).

proteins are members of the MyoD family of proteins, which initiate myogenesis in tissue culture, in vivo and in vitro rhabdomyosarcoma models, and animal experimental models of myogenesis.[41] MyoD1 has been shown to be more restricted in expression than desmin.[41] Both MyoD1 and myogenin are transcriptional regulators (transcription factors) located in the nuclei (Figs. 13–34 and 13–35). They are excellent immunohistochemical markers, and nuclear staining is very specific for rhabdomyosarcoma.[42–44] One must be aware, however, that nonspecific cytoplasmic staining can occur with anti-MyoD1 and should be considered negative (Fig. 13–36).[44]

"Aberrant" immunohistochemical staining in rhabdomyosarcomas has been reported with "neural" markers, such as Leu7 and neuron-specific enolase 3 and with cytokeratin and neurofilament[45] and S-100 protein.[46] However, the strong resemblance of alveolar rhabdomyosarcoma to desmoplastic small cell tumor (see Chapter 18) leads one to question the early reports that may have preceded the recognition of desmoplastic small cell tumors, which almost uniformly express desmin. Aberrant staining has also been seen with markers of hematopoietic neoplasms (CD10, CD19, CD20) and may lead to great diagnostic difficulties.[22]

Rhabdomyosarcomas do not usually stain for CD99 (the MIC2 glycoprotein) as do the Ewing family of tumors. We have seen rare cases stain for CD99, and one study identified positive staining for CD99 with one antibody (12E7) in 4 of 14 embryonal rhabdomyosarcomas.[47]

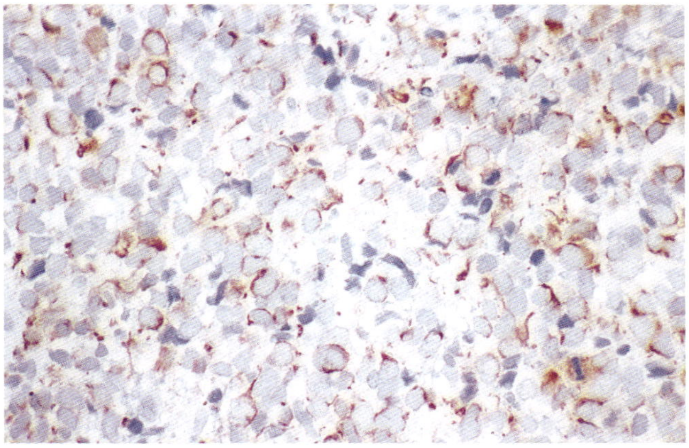

Figure 13-33. Positive cytoplasmic desmin staining in an orbital rhabdomyosarcoma without light microscopic rhabdomyoblastic differentiation (avidin-biotin complex technique with hematoxylin counterstain, ×400).

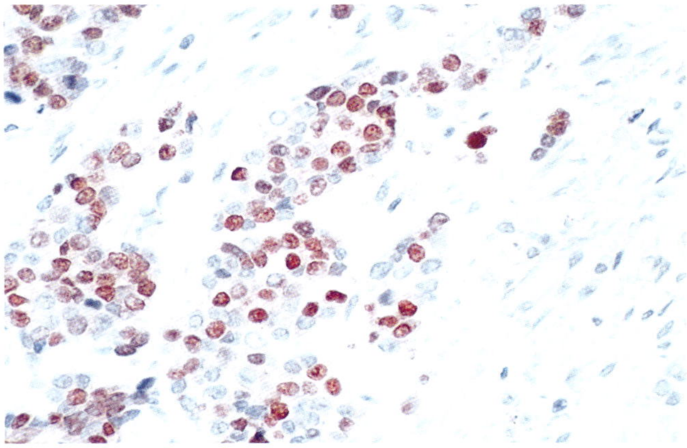

Figure 13-35. Positive nuclear staining for myogenin in an alveolar rhabdomyosarcoma (avidin-biotin complex technique with hematoxylin counterstain, ×400).

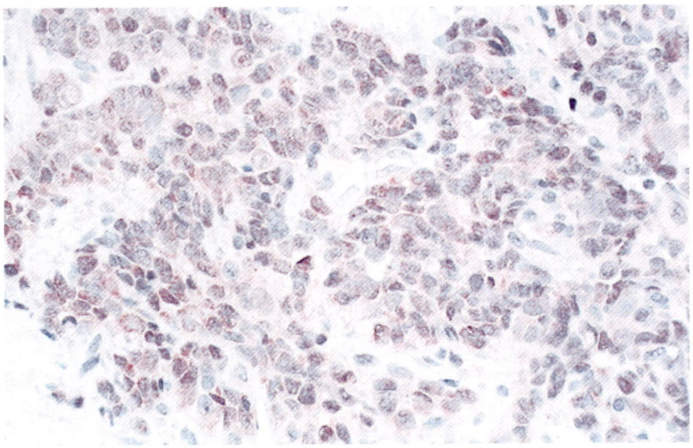

Figure 13–36. Cytoplasmic (negative) staining for MyoD1 in an alveolar rhabdomyosarcoma, the same case illustrated in Figure 13–35 (avidin-biotin complex technique with hematoxylin counterstain, ×400).

Genetic and Cytogenetic Changes

Myogenic Regulatory Proteins

Myogenic determination protein-1 (MyoD1) is one of a group of transcription factors that are expressed only in skeletal muscle. Other myogenic regulatory proteins are myogenin, myf-5, and myf-6 (MRF4). These transcription factors act on the other myogenic genes (i.e., desmin, myosin and creatine kinase), inducing their transcription and leading to skeletal muscle differentiation. MyoD family proteins may have redundant functions, but they initiate determination of a myogenesis and some degree of terminal differentiation;[48] however, they do not cause tumorigenesis. These genes are normally silent in differentiated muscle cells, but they stay active in rhabdomyosarcomas. The relationships involved in this group of transcription factors are complex,[49] but pragmatically they are specific and sensitive markers

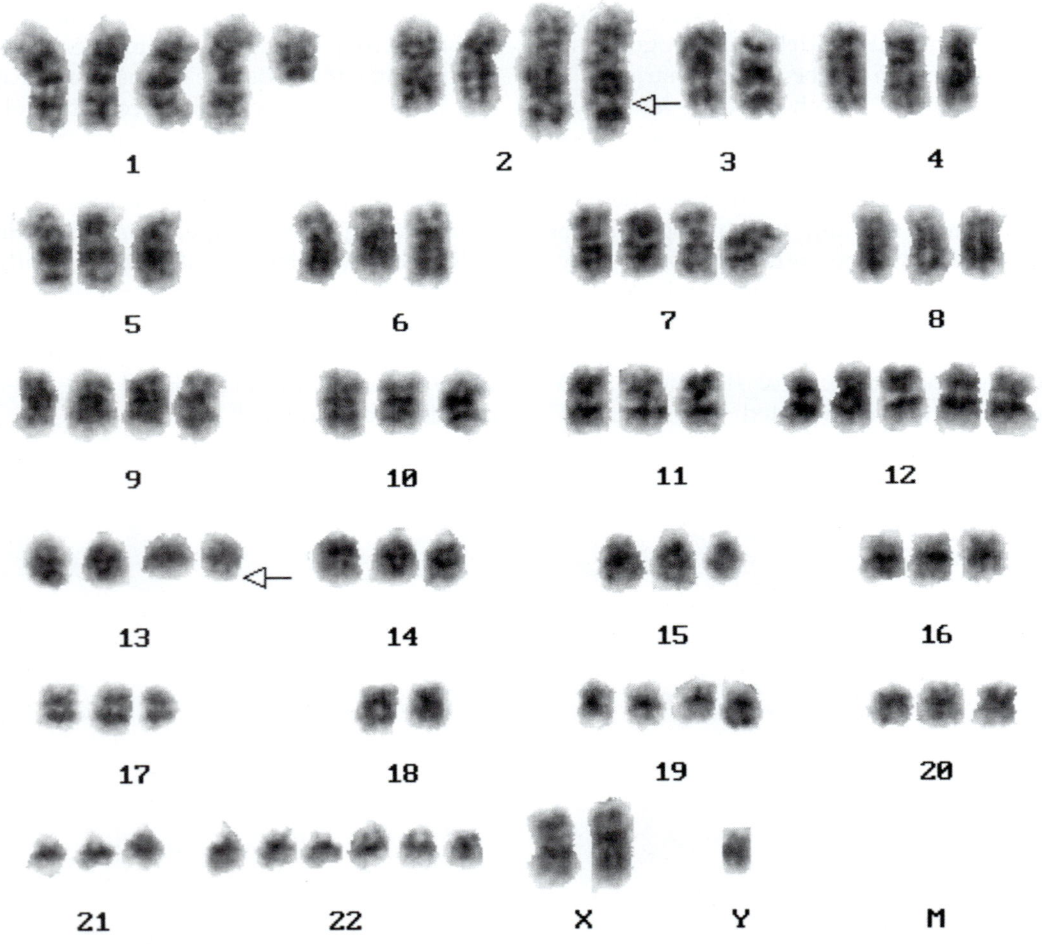

Figure 13–37. Alveolar rhabdomyosarcoma karyotype with t(2;13)(q35;q14) *(arrows)*. Note the tetraploidy, a common finding in this tumor. (Courtesy of Dr. Jeffery Sawyer and Mr. Chuck Swanson, University of Arkansas for Medical Sciences and Arkansas Children's Hospital.)

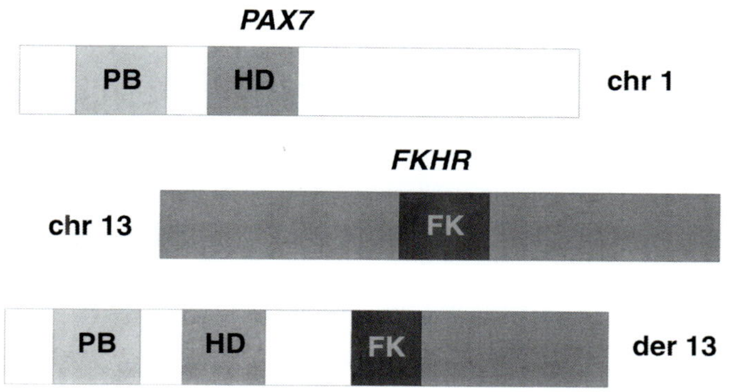

Figure 13–38. Drawing of the *PAX7-FKHR* fusion produced by the t(1;13) (p36;q14). The paired box and homeobox regions transcribe DNA-binding domains, and the FK region transcribes a locus typical of forkhead proteins. PB, paired box; HD, homeodomain; FK, forkhead.

of skeletal muscle differentiation. Transfection of complementary DNA has led to conversion of fibroblasts as well as other cell types into myoblasts.[50] Recent work has suggested that the methylation status of the gene regulatory CpG sites in the *MyoD1* gene promoter region is related to tumor type. The vast majority of alveolar rhabdomyosarcomas have unmethylated CpG sites associated with the *MyoD1* gene promoter, whereas the majority (90%) of embryonal rhabdomyosarcomas are partially methylated (similar to fetal muscle).[51] These data suggest that not only is MyoD1 expression associated with tumorigenesis, but that the degrees of expression may be related to the type of tumor produced.

Alveolar Rhabdomyosarcoma Cytogenetics

Alveolar rhabdomyosarcomas have been associated with two recurring cytogenetic translocations in over 90% of cases in one review,[40] but may be lower in the IRSG data. This has led some investigators to consider these translocations as diagnostic of the alveolar type of rhabdomyosarcoma. However, an extremely rare embryonal rhabdomyosarcoma may have this "alveolar" translocation.[52] The most common translocation is t(2;13)(q35;q14), whereas a t(1;13) (p36;q14) translocation is much less common. These translocations may be part of a complex karyotype or be partially demonstrated (Fig. 13–37). Both of these translocations fuse *FKHR* (forkhead receptor gene) on 13q14 with one of the *PAX* genes (*PAX3* on 2q35; *PAX7* on 1p36) (Figs. 13–38 and 13–39). The fusion product appears to activate aberrant DNA transcription, leading to tumorigenesis. The (2;13) and (1;13) transcripts may be identified via reverse transcriptase-polymerase chain reaction (RT-PCR) of tumor samples and cell lines (Fig. 13–40). One study,[52] however, suggests caution in the interpretation of PCR results without histologic correlation because 2 of 12 embryonal rhabdomyosarcomas had transcripts of the appropriate size. However, one possible explanation is that *PAX-FKHR*$^+$ embryonal rhabdomyosarcomas may contain alveolar foci.[53] Pending additional data,

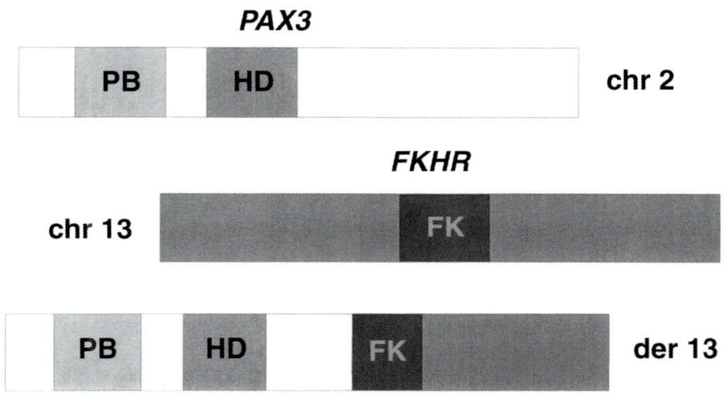

Figure 13–39. Drawing of the *PAX3-FKHR* fusion produced by the t(2;13)(q35;q14). The paired box and homeobox regions transcribe DNA-binding domains, and the FK region transcribes a locus typical of forkhead proteins. PB, paired box; HD, homeodomain; FK, forkhead.

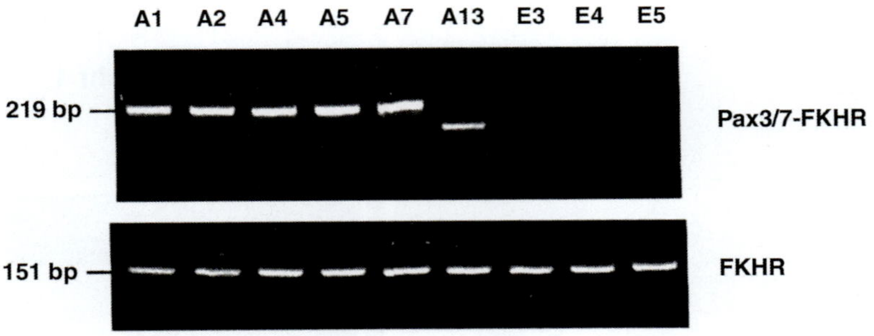

Figure 13-40. RT-PCR of the t(2;13) (lanes 1-5) and t(1;13) (lane 6) fusion products in six different alveolar rhabdomyosarcomas. There is no product in lanes 7 to 9 from embryonal rhabdomyosarcomas. The unfused forkhead receptor was amplified as a housekeeping gene in all tumors. Note the different product size in the t(1;13) (case A13, lane 6). (Courtesy of Dr. Bin Chen, University of Arkansas for Medical Sciences.)

present treatment decisions are based on histologic features. On the other side of the coin, alveolar rhabdomyosarcomas may not have cytogenetic or PCR evidence of these characteristic translocations. Tumors with the t(1;13) may predict a different clinical phenotype than the more common t(2;13).[54]

The biologic consequences of the specific translocations associated with alveolar rhabdomyosarcomas are not fully known. It is known that *PAX3* is necessary for activation of MyoD.[55] *PAX3* and possibly *PAX7* may work by maintaining cells in an undifferentiated and proliferative state in rhabdomyosarcomas.[56]

Embryonal Rhabdomyosarcoma Cytogenetics

There are no specific structural cytogenetic features of embryonal rhabdomyosarcomas, which show a variety of chromosomal gains and losses. Loss of heterozygosity does occur on chromosome 11 (11p15.5) as may occur in some Wilms tumors[57] and other small cell pediatric tumors including hepatoblastomas and neuroblastomas.[53] This region includes the insulin growth factor-2 (*IGF2*) gene, which is normally imprinted by the paternal allele. Rhabdomyosarcomas have a loss of imprinting of this region, which may lead to overexpression of oncogenic proteins such as IGF-2.[40]

Comparative genomic hybridization studies have shown gains of specific chromosomal material in embryonal rhabdomyosarcomas (especially chromosomes 2, 12, and 13) with some loss of other chromosomes.[58] The diagnostic or biologic significance of this gain in chromosomes is not yet known.

A case report of the cytogenetic findings of a spindle cell rhabdomyosarcoma has shown a hypotriploid karyotype with numerous structural translocations.[59]

Other Genetic Changes

IGF-2 has been shown to be expressed in both alveolar and embryonal rhabdomyosarcomas.[60] This overexpression may allow autocrine stimulation of tumor growth. Some tissue culture data have suggested that IGF-2 along with fused transcripts of PAX3 and FRHR may contribute to oncogenesis.[61]

Although most patients with rhabdomyosarcomas have no known underlying risk factors, some patients with Li-Fraumeni syndrome with constitutional allelic deletion of p53 are at increased risk of developing rhabdomyosarcomas. Indeed, this syndrome was first identified by the epidemiologic study of rhabdomyosarcoma patients having family members with malignancies. Germline mutations of p53 are more likely in young patients with rhabdomyosarcoma.[62] About 50% of rhabdomyosarcomas have mutations of p53.[40] p53 is a DNA binding protein involved in the cell cycle and has a short half-life. Mutant p53 appears to have a longer half-life and may disregulate the cell cycle. Wild-type p53 inhibits transcription of *IGF2*,[63] which may explain why some cases with mutant p53 overexpress this gene.

Other associations with rhabdomyosarcomas in children include the Beckwith-Wiedemann syndrome, type 1 neurofibromatosis, and basal cell-nevus syndrome.

The N-myc oncogene is sometimes amplified in alveolar rhabdomyosarcomas, but not embryonal rhabdomyosarcomas,[64] and may be associated with a worse prognosis.

Studies by flow cytometry and image analysis have suggested an association of ploidy with histologic subtype. Specifically embryonal histology correlated with hyperdiploidy, whereas alveolar histology correlated with near tetraploidy. However, no correlation with patient survival was demonstrated in one study,[65] but in another diploidy and near tetraploidy had a 5-year survival rate of approximately 30%, whereas hyperdiploidy had a survival rate of 73% at 5 years.[66]

Proliferation markers such as proliferating cell nuclear antigen (PCNA) and Ki-67 (MIB-1) have also been studied in rhabdomyosarcomas. In a study by Tokuc,[67] PCNA was shown to be associated with poor survival and relapse when the index was greater than 54%. Another study showed the lowest percentage of cells marking for Ki-67 to be found in spindle cell rhabdomyosarcomas (14%), but it did not show a significantly higher rate in alveolar rhabdomyosarcomas (23%) than in all tumors (24%).[68] It also found no relationship between Ki-67 expression and patient outcome.

Many studies have looked at p-glycoprotein, the product of the multidrug resistance gene. This protein is able to pump out chemotherapeutic agents and, thus, it confers chemoresistance to tumor cells. The importance of this protein, in addition to its biologic significance, is that it may be inhibited by some agents such as cyclosporin. A relatively large rhabdomyosarcoma study (76 patients) did not show a significant association between p-glycoprotein expression at diagnosis and clinical features or patient outcome.[69] In one study, Bcl-2 protein expression was noted in 36% of rhabdomyosarcomas, but it did not correlate with subtypes of tumor or previous treatment. Similarly, apoptosis was noted in 0.2% to 7.5% of tumor cells, but again without correlation to treatment or tumor subtype.[70] Adhesion molecule expression has also been studied in a small series of rhabdomyosarcomas; all 12 tumors stained for tenascin and thrombospondin, most were positive for fibronectin, 5 stained for laminin, and 4 stained for CD44.[71] This study found no association between the expression of these adhesion molecules and degree of tumor differentiation or presence of metastatic disease at presentation. Another small study,[72] however, has suggested that expression of CD44 in more than 60% of tumor cells is a favorable prognostic sign, compared to tumors having less than 40% of the cells expressing this adhesion molecule. Larger studies will be needed for confirmation.

Prognosis and Clinical Course

Overall 5-year survival in children with all histologic subtypes of rhabdomyosarcoma is approximately 65%. Survival depends primarily on stage, histologic subtype, and extent of resection. In general, spindle cell type has excellent prognosis, embryonal type is considered "favorable," and alveolar type "unfavorable." In adults the number of rhabdomyosarcoma cases is so small that adequate comparison with children is not possible.[73]

Staging of rhabdomyosarcomas is critically important. Two different staging systems are used: the clinicopathologic group (Table 13–4)[15] and the TNM staging system (Table 13–5).[15] Grouping is based on pathologic findings, whereas stage is based purely on clinical studies.

Diagnostic Summary and Differential Diagnosis

Modern therapy in rhabdomyosarcoma often involves an initial diagnostic biopsy followed by chemotherapy or radiotherapy or both. After systemic therapy, excision of the original mass may be performed. At this point, pathologic examination may reveal total tumor necrosis, the best outcome for the patient. Secondly, obvious viable tumor may be present, leading to continued systemic therapy or additional local

Table 13–4. Clinical Group Staging for Rhabdomyosarcoma[15]

Clinical Group	Disease Extent/Surgical Results
I	A Localized tumor, confined to site of origin, completely resected
	B Localized tumor, infiltrating beyond the site of origin, completely resected
II	A Localized tumor, gross total resection, but with microscopic residual disease
	B Locally extensive tumor (spread to regional lymph nodes), completely resected
	C Locally extensive tumor (spread to regional lymph nodes), gross total resection, but microscopic residual disease
III	A Localized or locally extensive tumor, gross residual disease after biopsy only
	B Localized or locally extensive tumor, gross residual disease after major resection (>50% debulking)
IV	Any size primary tumor with or without regional lymph node involvement, with distant metastases, without respect to surgical approach to primary tumor

Table 13-5. TNM Pretreatment (IRS-IV) Staging of Childhood Rhabdomyosarcoma[15]

Stage	Sites	T Invasiveness	T Size	Regional Nodes	Metastases
I	Orbit	T1 or T2	Any	N0, N1, or NX	M0
	Head and neck, not parameningeal	T1 or T2	Any	N0, N1, or NX	M0
	Genitourinary, not bladder and prostate	T1 or T2	Any	N0, N1, or NX	M0
II	Bladder/prostate	T1 or T2	<5 cm	N0 or NX	M0
	Extremity	T1 or T2	<5 cm	N0 or NX	M0
	Cranial parameningeal	T1 or T2	<5 cm	N0 or NX	M0
	Other	T1 or T2	<5 cm	N0 or NX	M0
III	Bladder/prostate	T1 or T2	<5 cm	N1	M0
	Extremity	T1 or T2	>5 cm	N0, N1, or NX	M0
	Cranial parameningeal	T1 or T2	>5 cm	N0, N1, or NX	M0
	Other	T1 or T2	>5 cm	N0, N1, or NX	M0
IV	All	T1 or T2	Any	N0 or N1	M1

T, tumor; T1, confined to anatomic site of origin; T2, extension beyond site of origin; M0, no distant metastasis; M1, distant metastasis present; N0, not clinically involved; N1, clinically involved; NX, clinical status unknown.

therapy. It has been observed and documented[74] that rhabdomyosarcomas undergo differentiation (Figs. 13–41 and 13–42) and have decreased mitotic activity after therapy. The degree to which this occurs and how (or if) it should affect therapy has not yet reached a point of consensus.

Differential diagnosis of rhabdomyosarcoma depends on the age of the patient and the subtype of the tumor. In alveolar rhabdomyosarcomas of children the differential may include any and all of the "small blue cell tumors," including hematopoietic malignancies (lymphoma or leukemia), the Ewing family of tumors, poorly differentiated/undifferentiated neuroblastoma, rhabdoid tumors (particularly in patients <1 year of age), and desmoplastic small cell tumor. In adults the differential diagnosis includes hematopoietic

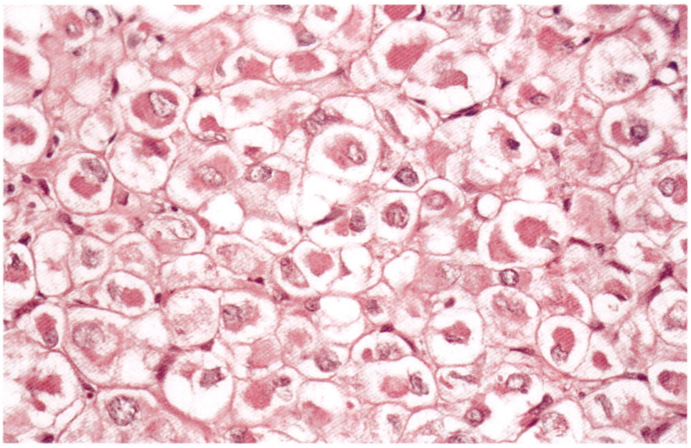

Figure 13–41. Posttreatment differentiation in a rhabdomyosarcoma with areas simulating a rhabdomyoma (H&E, ×400).

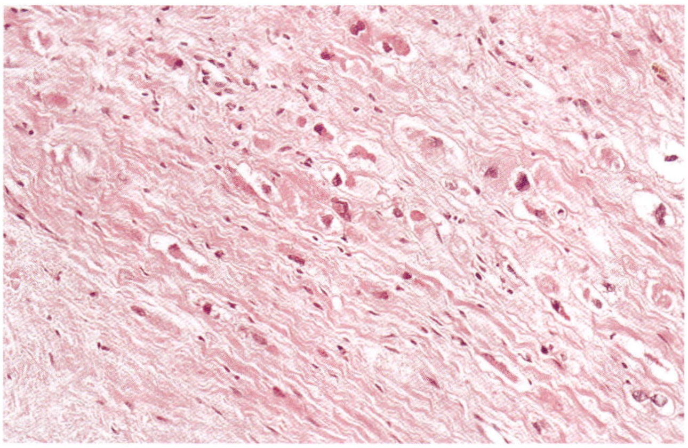

Figure 13–42. Posttreatment differentiation in a rhabdomyosarcoma with spindle cell foci, same case as in Figure 13–41 (H&E, ×400).

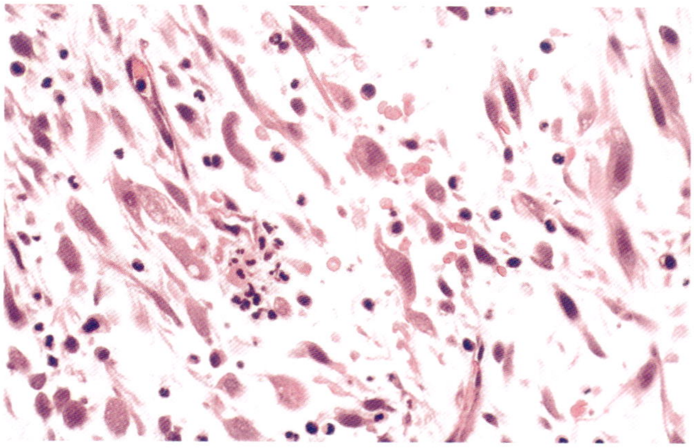

Figure 13-43. Inflammatory myofibroblastic tumor of the urinary bladder. Note the slightly basophilic rather than eosinophilic cytoplasm of the spindle cells (H&E, ×400).

neoplasms, Ewing tumors, small cell carcinomas, and desmoplastic small cell tumors. Embryonal tumors have a differential diagnosis of malignant peripheral nerve sheath tumors, myofibroblastic tumors, or other myxoid lesions. Botryoid tumors of the urinary bladder may be confused with reactive spindle cell nodules or inflammatory myofibroblastic tumors (Fig. 13–43), or rarely with inflammatory processes such as eosinophilic cystitis. Spindle cell tumors may be confused with leiomyosarcomas, fibrosarcomas, monophasic synovial sarcomas, and inflammatory (myofibroblastic) tumors.

One final difficulty in the histologic diagnosis of rhabdomyosarcomas is found in patients treated with systemic therapy. In these individuals the determination of whether differentiated tumor is present, whether it is capable of further growth and patient injury, and whether it requires further therapeutic measures can be a dilemma. Cytodifferentiation of tumor cells has been demonstrated in vivo and in vitro, with a reduction in metastatic behavior.[75] This differentiation includes increased amounts of eosinophilic cytoplasm, often with more obvious cross-striations or the formation of myotubes. Recent studies by Coffin and colleagues[12] have suggested that alveolar rhabdomyosarcomas will show differentiation less commonly than embryonal tumors and that this differentiation may relate to improved survival. They also suggest that markers of proliferation, such as MIB-1, may be useful in clinical decision-making and determining prognosis, but this is not yet clear. They also note that in some cases with differentiation, expression of the proliferative marker MIB-1 may be present. The expression of myogenin and MyoD1 is markedly decreased in posttherapy differentiated tumor cells,[46] confirming the biologic relationship between MyoD1 protein and cell cycle protein regulation.[76]

REFERENCES

Rhabdomyoma

1. Enzinger FM, Weiss SW (eds): Rhabdomyoma and rhabdomyosarcoma. In Soft Tissue Tumors, 3rd ed. St. Louis, Mosby, 1995:523, 539.
2. Kapadia SB, Meis JM, Frisman DM, et al: Fetal rhabdomyoma of the head and neck: A clinicopathologic and immunophenotypic study of 24 cases. Hum Pathol 1993;24:754.
3. O'Shea PA: Myogenic tumors of soft tissue. In Coffin CM, Dehner LP, O'Shea PA (eds): Pediatric Soft Tissue Tumors, A Clinical, Pathologic and Therapeutic Approach. Baltimore, Williams & Wilkins, 1997:214.
4. Kodet R, Fajstavr J, Kabelka Z, et al: Is fetal cellular rhabdomyosarcoma an entity or a differentiated rhabdomyosarcoma? A study of patients with rhabdomyosarcoma of the tongue and sarcoma of the tongue enrolled in the Intergroup Rhabdomyosarcoma Studies I, II, III. Cancer. 1991;67:2907.
5. Smith NM, Thorton CM: Fetal rhabdomyoma: Two instances of recurrence. Pediatr Pathol Lab Med 1996; 16:673.
6. Crotty PL, Nakhleh RE, Dehner LP: Juvenile rhabdomyoma, an intermediate form of skeletal muscle tumor in children. Arch Pathol Lab Med 1993;117:43.
7. Erlandson RA (ed): Rhabdomyoma and rhabdomyosarcoma. In Diagnostic Transmission Electron Microscopy of Tumors. New York, Raven Press, 1994:696, 700.
8. Agamanolis DP, Dasu S, Krill CE: Tumors of skeletal muscle. Hum Pathol 1986;17:778.
9. Solomon MP, Tolete-Velcek F: Lingual rhabdomyoma (adult variant) in a child. J Pediatr Surg 1979;14:91.
10. Gibas Z, Miettinen M: Recurrent parapharyngeal rhabdomyoma. Evidence of neoplastic nature of the tumor from cytogenetic study. Am J Surg Pathol 1992; 16:721.
11. Tanda F, Rocca PC, Bosincu L, et al: Rhabdomyoma of the tunica vaginalis of the testis: A histologic, immunohistochemical, and ultrastructural study. Mod Pathol 1997;10:608.

Rhabdomyosarcoma

12. Coffin CM, Rulon J, Smith L, Bruggers C, White FV: Pathologic features of rhabdomyosarcoma before and after treatment: A clinicopathologic and immunohistochemical analysis. Mod Pathol 1997;10:1175–1187.
13. Markel SF, Enzinger FM: Neuromuscular hamartoma—a benign "triton tumor" composed of mature neural and striated muscle elements. Cancer 1982; 49:140.
14. Ashfaq R, Timmons CF: Rhabdomyomatous mesenchymal hamartoma of skin. Pediatr Pathol 1992;12:731.
15. Qualman SJ, Coffin CM, Newton WA: Intergroup rhabdomyosarcoma study: Update for pathologists. Pediatr Dev Pathol 1998;1:550.
16. Asmar L, Gehan EA, Newton WA, et al: Agreement among and within groups of pathologists in the classi-

fication of rhabdomyosarcoma and related childhood sarcomas. Cancer 1994;74:2579.
17. Dehner LP: In Coffin CM, Dehner LP, O'Shea PA (eds): Pediatric Soft Tissue Tumors, A Clinical, Pathologic and Therapeutic Approach. Baltimore, Williams & Wilkins, 1997:4.
18. Newton WA, Gehan EA, Webber BL, et al: Classification of rhabdomyosarcomas and related sarcomas. Cancer 1995;76:1073.
19. Arndt CSA, Crist WM: Medical progress: Common musculoskeletal tumor of childhood and adolescence. N Engl J Med 1999;341:342.
20. Parham DM, Pinto A, Tallini G, et al: Rhabdomyosarcoma mimicking acute leukemia. Arch Pathol Lab Med 1998;122:1047.
21. Morandi S, Mana A, Sabattomo E, et al: Rhabdomyosarcoma presenting as acute leukemia. J Pediatr Hematol Oncol 1996;18:305.
22. Pinto A, Tallini G, Novak R, et al: Undifferentiated rhabdomyosarcoma with lymphoid phenotype expression. Med Pediatr Oncol 1997;28:165.
23. Locatelli F, Tonani P, Porta F, et al: Rhabdomyosarcoma with primary osteolytic lesions simulating non-Hodgkin's lymphoma. Pediatr Hematol Oncol 1991; 8:159.
24. Palmer NG, Sachs N, Foulkes M: Histopathology and prognosis in rhabdomyosarcoma [abstract]. Proc Am Soc Clin Oncol 1981;1:113.
25. Cavazzana AO, Schmidt D, Ninfo V, et al: Spindle cell rhabdomyosarcoma. A prognostically favorable variant of rhabdomyosarcoma. Am J Surg Pathol 1992;16: 229–235.
26. Leuschner I, Newton WA Jr, Schmidt D, et al: Spindle cell variants of embryonal rhabdomyosarcoma in the paratesticular region. A report of the Intergroup Rhabdomyosarcoma Study. Am J Surg Pathol 1993;17: 221–230.
27. Kodet R, Newton WA, Hamoudi AB, Asmar L, Jacobs DL, Maurer HM: Childhood rhabdomyosarcomas with anaplastic (pleomorphic) features. A report of the Intergroup Rhabdomyosarcoma Study. Am J Surg Pathol 1993;17:443–453.
28. Tsokos M, Webber BL, Parham DM, et al: Rhabdomyosarcoma: A new classification scheme related to prognosis. Arch Pathol Lab Med 1992;16:847–855.
29. Parham DM, Shapiro DN, Downing JR, et al: Solid alveolar rhabdomyosarcomas with the t(2;13). Report of two cases with diagnostic implications. Am J Surg Pathol 1994;18:474.
30. Boman F, Champigneulle J, Schmitt C, et al: Clear cell rhabdomyosarcoma. Pediatr Pathol Lab Med 1996; 16:951.
31. Mouton SC, Rosenberg HS, Cohen MC, et al: Malignant ectomesenchymoma in childhood. Pediatr Pathol Lab Med 1996;16:607.
32. Edwards V, Tse G, Doucet J, et al: Rhabdomyosarcoma metastasizing as a malignant ectomesenchymoma. Ultrastruct Pathol 1999;23:267.
33. Pawel BR, Hamoudi AB, Asmar L, et al: Undifferentiated sarcomas of children: Pathology and clinical behavior—an Intergroup Rhabdomyosarcoma study. Med Pediatr Oncol 1997;29:170.
34. Brooks JSJ: Immunohistochemistry in the differential diagnosis of soft tissue tumors. In Weiss SW, Brooks JSJ (eds): Soft Tissue Tumors, No. 38 in the USCAP Monographs in Pathology series, Baltimore, Williams & Wilkins, 1996:65.
35. Azumi N, Ben-Ezra J, Battifora H: Immunophenotypic diagnosis of leiomyosarcomas and rhabdomyosarcomas with monoclonal antibodies to muscle-specific actin and desmin in formalin-fixed tissue. Mod Pathol 1988;1:469.
36. Parham DM, Dias P, Kelly DR, et al: Desmin positivity in primitive neuroectodermal tumors of childhood. Am J Surg Pathol 1992;16:483.
37. Leader M, Patel J, Collins M, et al: Myoglobin: An evaluation of its role as a marker of rhabdomyosarcomas. Br J Cancer 1989;59:106.
38. Hayashi I: Localization of myoglobin and muscle type of creatine kinase in human skeletal muscle and thyroid. Shikoku Acta Medica (Japanese) 1981;37:15.
39. Kusaka K: The existence of myoglobin demonstrated in the human thymus and its significance. Shikoku Acta Medica (Japanese) 1980;6:637.
40. Merlino G, Helman LJ: Rhabdomyosarcoma—working out the pathways. Oncogene 1999;18:5340.
41. Dias P, Parham DM, Shapiro DN, et al: Myogenic regulatory protein (MyoD1) expression in childhood solid tumors: Diagnostic utility in rhabdomyosarcomas. Am J Pathol 1990;137:1283.
42. Cui S, Hano H, Harada T, et al: Evaluation of new monoclonal anti-MyoD1 and anti-myogenin antibodies for the diagnosis of rhabdomyosarcoma. Pathol Int 1999;49:62.
43. Engel ME, Mouton SC, Emms M: Paediatric rhabdomyosarcoma: MyoD1 demonstration in routinely processed tissue sections using wet heat pretreatment (pressure cooking) for antigen retrieval. J Clin Pathol 1997;50:37.
44. Mukunyadzi P, Dias P, Houghton PJ, et al: Comparison of MyoD1 immunostaining of pediatric tumors using frozen or paraffin-embedded sections. Appl Immunohistochem Molecul Morphol 1999;7:260.
45. Miettinen M, Rapola J: Immunohistochemical spectrum of rhabdomyosarcoma and rhabdomyosarcoma-like tumors. Am J Surg Pathol 1989;13:120-132.
46. Coindre JM, de Mascarel A, Trojani M, et al: Immunohistochemical study of rhabdomyosarcoma. Unexpected staining with S100 protein and cytokeratin. J Pathol 1988;155:127.
47. Ramani P, Rampling D, Link M: Immunocytochemical study of 12E7 in small round-cell tumours of childhood: An assessment of its sensitivity and specificity. Histopathology 1993;23:557.
48. Wang NP, Marx J, McNutt MA, Gown AM: Expression of myogenic regulatory proteins (myogenin and MyoD1) in small blue round cell tumors of childhood. Am J Pathol 1995;147:1799.
49. Dias P, Dilling M, Houghton P: The molecular basis of skeletal muscle differentiation. Semin Diagn Pathol 1994;11:3.

50. Davis RL, Weintraub H, Lassar AB: Expression of a single transfected cDNA converts fibroblasts to myoblasts. Cell 1987;51:987.
51. Chen B, Dias P, Jenkins JJ III, et al: Methylation alterations of the MyoD1 upstream region are predictive of subclassification of human rhabdomyosarcomas. Am J Pathol 1998;152:1071.
52. Downing JR, Khandekar A, Shurtleff SA, et al: Multiplex RT-PCR assay for the differential diagnosis of alveolar rhabdomyosarcoma and Ewing's sarcoma. Am J Pathol 1995;146:626.
53. Parham DM: The molecular biology of childhood rhabdomyosarcoma. Sem Diagn Pathol 1994;11:39–46.
54. Kelly KM, Womer R, Sorensen P, et al: Common and variant gene fusions predict distinct clinical phenotypes in rhabdomyosaroma. J Clin Oncol 1997; 15:1831.
55. Borycki AG, Li J, Jin F, et al: Pax3 functions in cell survival and in pax7 regulation. Development 1999; 126:1665.
56. Mansouri A: The role of Pax3 and Pax7 in development and cancer. Crit Rev Oncogen 1998;9:141.
57. Samuel DP, Tsokos M, DeBaun MR: Hemihypertrophy and a poorly differentiated embryonal rhabdomyosarcoma of the pelvis. Med Pediatric Oncol 1999;32:38.
58. Weber-Hall S, Anderson J, McManus A, et al: Gains, losses, and amplification of genomic material in rhabdomyosarcoma analyzed by comparative genomic hybridization. Cancer Res 1996;56:3220.
59. Gil-Benso R, Carda-Batalla C, Navarro-Fos S, et al: Cytogenetic study of a spindle-cell rhabdomyosarcoma of the parotid gland. Cancer Genet Cytogenet 1999; 109:150.
60. Minniti CP, Tsokos M, Newton WA Jr, et al: Specific expression of insulin-like growth factor-II in rhabdomyosarcoma tumor cells. Am J Clin Pathol 1994; 101:198.
61. Wang W, Kumar P, Wang W, et al: Insulin-like growth factor II and PAX3-FKHR cooperate in the oncogenesis of rhabdomyosarcoma. Cancer Res 1998;58:4426.
62. Diller L, Sexsmith E, Gottlieb A, et al: Germline p53 mutations are frequently detected in young children with rhabdomyosarcoma. J Clin Invest 1995;95:1606.
63. Zhang L, Zhan Q, Zhan S, et al: p53 regulates human insulin-like growth factor II gene expression through active P4 promoter in rhabdomyosarcoma cells. DNA Cell Biol 1998;17:125.
64. Hachitanda Y, Toyoshima S, Akazawa K, Tsuneyoshi M: N-myc gene amplification in rhabdomyosarcoma detected by fluorescence in situ hybridization: Its correlation with histologic features. Mod Pathol 1998;11: 1222–1227.
65. Kilpatrick SE, Teot LA, Geisinger KR, et al: Relationship of DNA ploidy to histology and prognosis in rhabdomyosarcoma. Comparison of flow cytometry and image analysis. Cancer 1994;74:3227.
66. De Zen L, Sommaggio A, d'Amore ES, et al: Clinical relevance of DNA ploidy and proliferative activity in childhood rhabdomyosarcoma: A retrospective analysis of patients enrolled onto the Italian Cooperative Rhabdomyosarcoma Study RMS88. J Clin Oncol 1997;15:1198.
67. Tokuc G, Dogan O, Ayan I, et al: Prognostic value of proliferating cell nuclear antigen immunostaining in pediatric rhabdomyosarcomas. Acta Paediatr Jpn 1998; 40:573.
68. Noguchi S, Tamiya S, Nagoshi M, et al: The prognostic importance of nuclear morphometry and the MIB-1 index in rhabdomyosarcoma. Mod Pathol 1996;9:253.
69. Kuttesch JF, Parham DM, Luo X, et al: P-glycoprotein expression at diagnosis may not be a primary mechanism of therapeutic failure in childhood rhabdomyosarcoma. J Clin Oncol 1996;14:886.
70. Boman F, Brel D, Antunes L, et al: Gene alterations and apoptosis in rhabdomyosarcoma. Pediatr Pathol Lab Med. 1997;17:233.
71. Saxon BR, Byard RW, Han P: Cellular expression of adhesion factors in childhood rhabdomyosarcoma. Pediatr Pathol Lab Med 1997;17:259.
72. Humphrey G, Hazel DL, MacLennan K, et al: Expression of CD44 by rhabdomyosarcoma: A new prognostic marker? Br J Cancer 1999;80:918.
73. Hollowood K, Fletcher CDM: Rhabdomyosarcoma in adults. Semin Diagn Pathol 1994;11:47.
74. D'Amore ESG, Tollot M, Stracca-Pansa V, et al: Therapy associated differentiation in rhabdomyosarcomas. Mod Pathol 1994;7:69.
75. Parham DM: Rhabdomyosarcomas and related tumors. In Parham, DM (ed): Pediatric Neoplasia: Morphology and Biology. Philadelphia, Lippincott-Raven, 1996:87.
76. Gu W, Schneider JW, Condorelli G, et al: Interaction of myogenic factors and the retinoblastoma protein mediates muscle cell commitment and differentiation. Cell 1993;72:309.

Vascular Tumors

CHAPTER 14

Vascular tumors include a wide variety of reactive and neoplastic proliferations composed of elements of blood vessels: endothelial cells and pericytes.[1–3] Their classification is shown in Table 14–1.

Hemangiomas are common tumors composed of units that resemble normal blood vessels, endothelial cells, pericytes, and sometimes vascular smooth muscle cells. They tend to have a lobular organization and almost invariably have limited cytologic atypia. Lymphangiomas are less common and are composed of lymphatic-type vessels. The tumors of vascular smooth muscle are discussed in Chapter 10.

Hemangioendothelioma is the designation for a group of borderline malignant vascular tumors. They may be capable of aggressive local growth, recurrence, or both but do not metastasize. However, epithelioid hemangioendothelioma refers to a low-grade angiosarcoma, and it may metastasize.

Angiosarcomas are very rare compared to hemangiomas and comprise probably around 1% of all vascular tumors and only 1% to 2% of all sarcomas. Angiosarcomas are essentially composed of malignant endothelial cells. Angiosarcomas include the low-grade variants, such as epithelioid hemangioendothelioma, and high-grade tumors. The features that aid in recognition of an angiosarcoma are disorganized and anastomosing vascular channels, permeative growth versus lobulation of the vascular units, and multilayered, atypical endothelia, often with solid areas, and general lack of pericytes of the vessel wall. Lymphangiosarcomas are not recognized separately.

Etiologically, environmental carcinogens play a known role, especially in the genesis of hepatic angiosarcomas. This is understandable because the endothelial cells are directly exposed to circulating carcinogens. However, the genetic mechanisms related to the genesis of vascular tumors are much less understood than those for many other sarcomas.

Kaposi sarcoma is etiologically related to human herpesvirus 8 (HHV8), which is probably the strongest connection between a virus and human mesenchymal neoplasia. Several clinicopathologic forms are distinguished: classic, epidemic, endemic, and transplantation associated.

Hemangiopericytoma and glomus tumor are discussed in this chapter together with the vascular tumors. Despite its name, hemangiopericytoma does not generally have phenotypic features of pericytes. This tumor overlaps with solitary fibrous tumor (see Chapter 5), but will be discussed here separately.

Glomus tumor has a significant vascular component, although the glomus cells are modified smooth muscle cells. The vascular smooth muscle tumors (vascular leiomyoma, leiomyosarcoma, and lymphangiomyoma) are discussed among smooth muscle tumors (see Chapter 10).

The following synopsis of endothelia and angiogenesis is given for biologic background information relevant for vascular tumors.

Table 14–1. Classification of Vascular Tumors

Benign, hemangioma variants
Juvenile capillary hemangioma
Lobular capillary hemangioma
Acquired tufted angioma
Microvenular hemangioma
Capillary hemangioma, not otherwise specified
Hobnail hemangioma
Cavernous hemangioma
Venous hemangioma
Spindle cell hemangioma
Benign, of lymphatic vessels
Lymphangioma
Progressive lymphangioma (lymphangioendothelioma)
Lymphangiomatosis
Borderline malignant
Kaposiform hemangioendothelioma
Papillary intralymphatic hemangioendothelioma (Dabska tumor)
Retiform hemangioendothelioma
Malignant, low grade
Epithelioid hemangioendothelioma
Malignant, generally high grade
Angiosarcoma
Site-related variants: cutaneous, breast, hepatosplenic, of serous surfaces
Morphologic variants: Epithelioid, spindled, not otherwise specified
Tumors of other vascular components (perivascular cell tumors)
Hemangiopericytoma
Glomus tumor

Biology of Endothelia and Angiogenesis

Endothelial cells are mesenchymal cells that not only form a protective epithelial-like inner lining in the lumen of the blood vessels and lymphatics, but also have several other vasoregulatory functions. These include regulation of vascular permeability and caliber, transport of nutrients and metabolites, and regulation of leukocyte adhesion, trafficking, and hemostasis. External signals from growth factors/cytokines secreted by a variety of cells modulate the differentiation, antigen expression, and functional state of endothelial cells. Hormonal activity has also been demonstrated because endothelial cells secrete vasoregulatory peptides, such as endothelin. Endothelial cells of an average human body have been estimated to line an area of 6 to 7 m^2 and weigh 1 kg in aggregate.[4,5]

The dynamic growth of endothelial cells and capillaries is important for optimal oxygen supply of tissues, inflammatory response, and wound healing, and it is one of the tissue responses to ischemia. Regulators of the endothelial proliferation include angiopoietins and several families of vascular endothelial growth factors: VEGF, VEGF-B, VEGF-C, and VEGF-D. The most widely expressed in normal tissues and cancer cells are the growth factors of the VEGF family, but growth factors of other families have also been detected in cancer cells.[6–8]

Endothelial cells have three different types of VEGF receptors. They are receptor tyrosine kinases VEGFR1, VEGFR2, and VEGFR3, which carry the external growth factor signal to the nucleus through a complex phosphorylation cascade referred to as the signal transduction pathway. Interaction with the extracellular matrix through a complex set of receptors, such as the integrins, also regulates endothelial proliferation and migration.

Angiogenesis, the formation of new blood vessels, is a requirement for any solid tumor to grow beyond the size of a few millimeters. It also occurs during wound healing, but in normal tissues only rarely, for example, in the cyclic growth of endometrium. During angiogenesis, the new capillaries arise by sprouting from the existing ones. Understanding of the molecular mechanism of angiogenesis and discovery of antiangiogenic substances such as angiostatin and endostatin has therefore been of great interest as potential cancer treatments. Thalidomide, a drug originally used for its antiemetic and sedative effects during pregnancy, is antiangiogenic. This effect is also believed to be related to its teratogenic complications, such as the truncation-type extremity malformations (phocomelia).[7,8] Promotion of angiogenesis, on the other hand, could be used to generate new blood vessels to replace the defunct ones.

Vasculogenesis is the process of formation of the blood vessels during the embryonic life. The early blood vessels come from putative mesodermal angioblasts surrounding early hematopoietic elements, but the source of the angioblasts and the process of very early vasculogenesis is not completely understood. The cardiovascular system develops further by branching out from the heart. Some evidence indicates that during a lifetime endothelia of blood vessels are replenished by circulating bone marrow stem cells. This would also explain how some endothelial neoplasms could be of stem cell origin and why some hemangiomas and angiosarcomas are multifocal.

Infection-Related Vascular Proliferations

Reactive localized vascular proliferations of infectious origin are bacillary angiomatosis and verruga peruana. In these conditions, the bacterial infection triggers a hemangioma-like local endothelial cell proliferation. Recognition of these conditions is important for specific treatment.

Bacillary Angiomatosis

Clinical Features

This rare, reactive vascular proliferation is a manifestation of an opportunistic infection caused by gram-negative, rickettsia-like bacteria of genus *Bartonella* (formerly *Rochalimae*). Two species, *B. henselae* and *B. quintana,* are equally involved, with the spectrum of clinical features somewhat different with each.[9–14] Most cases occur in patients with acquired immunodeficiency syndrome (AIDS) or individuals with other immunosuppressive conditions, and, if untreated, the infection may disseminate and be life-threatening. Because it is treatable with antibiotics (erythromycin and others), its specific recognition is important. The lesion undergoes complete regression with antibiotic therapy. Very rarely are immunocompetent persons affected, and in these circumstances the cutaneous lesion tends to be localized.

The vascular lesions occur primarily in the skin but have also been observed in deep soft tissues.[11] When disseminated the lesions may also involve lymph nodes, mucosal surfaces, liver, and spleen.

Pathology

Histologically, the cutaneous lesion resembles a florid lobular capillary hemangioma (pyogenic granuloma). It consist of lobular vascular proliferation, and the endothelia often shows epithelioid change and sometimes focal nuclear atypia. Neutrophilic microabscesses are present and should always raise a suspicion of this diagnosis when seen in a hemangioma-like process. The microabscesses and the adjacent amorphous eosinophilic extracellular material contain rodlike bacteria of 3 µm, which can be highlighted with Warthin-Starry staining (Fig. 14–1). Immunohistochemical identification may also be useful.[15]

Verruga Peruana (Acute Bartonellosis, Carrion Disease, Oroya Fever)

Clinical Features

This febrile infectious disease is geographically restricted to South America and occurs endemically in certain regions of Peru. A large epidemic occurred in the last century in the region of Oroy, and smaller epidemics have been detected since. The disease is caused by gram-negative bacteria *Bartonella bacilliformis*. The skin lesions appear during the course of the systemic disease, often as verruga-like exophytic growths.[16,17]

Pathology

The highly cellular and vascular skin lesions may resemble a vascular neoplasm because of florid endothelial proliferation and mild endothelial atypia. The organisms are seen in the cytoplasm of endothelial

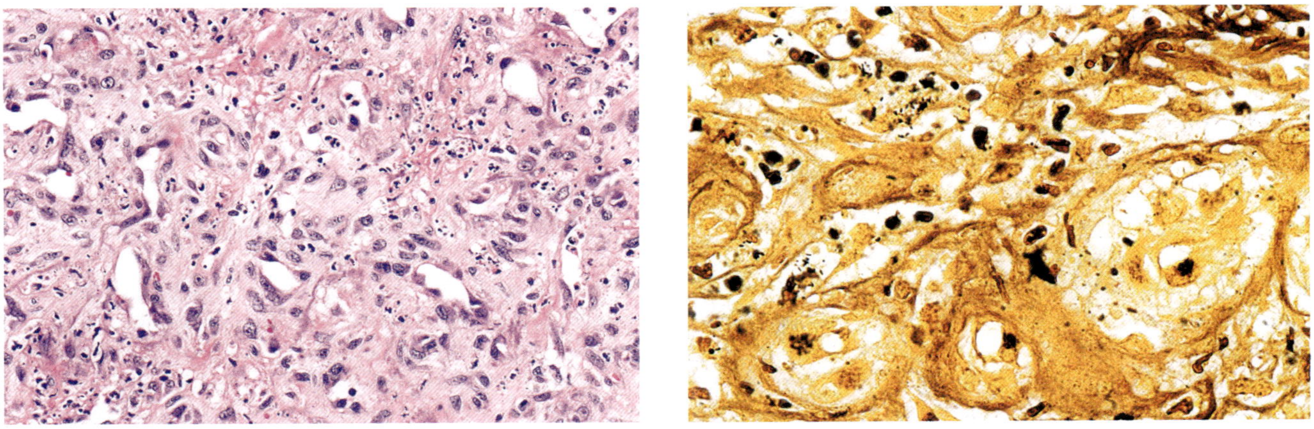

A B

Figure 14–1. *A,* Bacillary angiomatosis contains a dense capillary proliferation and distinctive interstitial microabscesses. *B,* Warthin-Starry stain shows the presence of bacteria.

cells as the so-called Rocha-Lima inclusions and can be best demonstrated with a Giemsa stain. The Bartonella bacterium has been shown to secrete angiogenic factors that are a likely source for the pathogenesis of the vascular proliferation.[18]

Other Infection-Related Reactive Vascular Proliferations

Reddish cutaneous plaques histologically representing focal reactive vascular proliferation, sometimes with papillary intraluminal endothelial hyperplasia, may occur in connection with systemic infections, such as endocarditis. Pathogenesis is likely related to angiogenic factors elicited by the infection or cytokine reaction to it.

Hemangiomas and Related Tumors

Hemangiomas are common benign tumors that form well-differentiated blood vessels with endothelia and pericytes and have a limited proliferative capacity. They occur in a wide age range, but are especially common in children. Some lesions classified among hemangiomas are closer to congenital malformations (many childhood hemangiomas), and others may be reactive (epithelioid hemangioma, glomeruloid hemangioma, lobular capillary hemangioma). Papillary endothelial hyperplasia (Masson tumor) is generally agreed to be a nonneoplastic condition related to organizing thrombi. Because their morphologic manifestations are quite similar, all hemangiomas whether hyperplasias, malformations, or true neoplasms, are discussed here together, and separated into clinicopathologic entities when pertinent.

Hemangiomas are usually classified into capillary, cavernous, and venous types according to the prevalent histologic pattern; combination tumors also occur. Capillary hemangiomas have several subtypes. Of these cellular (juvenile) capillary hemangioma, acquired tufted angioma, and targetoid hemosiderotic hemangioma will be discussed separately.

Kimura disease and epithelioid hemangioma are vascular proliferations arising in the background of inflammatory response of unknown origin. Glomeruloid hemangioma forms a skin tumor that appears as a part of multiorgan syndrome (POEMS syndrome).

Hemangiomas are associated with several clinical malformation and other syndromes.[19–24] The most important hemangioma syndromes and their key features are summarized in Table 14–2.

Capillary Hemangioma

Clinical Features

Common to all capillary hemangiomas is a composition of relatively small vessels of capillary caliber. They occur at all ages, but are particularly common in children and have a significant female predominance. Clinically, these tumors vary from small cutaneous nodules to ones that involve large areas of skin; the latter are referred to as vascular nevi under a variety of descriptive names, such as nevus flammeus, port-wine stain, and strawberry nevus. They occur especially in the head and neck area.[25–27] Subcutaneous, intramuscular, and rarely visceral involvement also occurs. Regression (gradual spontaneous disappearance of the lesion) is a common feature of capillary hemangiomas in small children. In rare cases, large hemangiomas in small children may cause significant morbidity by their disfiguring nature or high output cardiac failure.[28]

Histologically, capillary hemangiomas are composed of numerous thin-walled vascular channels. The vessels are more mature appearing with better developed vascular lumina in older children and adults, whereas the capillary hemangiomas of small children are more immature and more highly cellular; the cellular capillary hemangiomas are discussed later. In some cases it is difficult to determine whether a hemangiomatous lesion is reactive, hyperplastic, or neoplastic. For example, newly formed granulation tissue is highly vascular and has a hemangioma-like appearance. Circumscribed lobules, composed of well-formed vessels with limited nuclear atypia and presence of both endothelial cells and actin-positive pericytes, are typical features of benign hemangioma; these features help to separate hemangiomas from angiosarcoma.

Microvenular hemangioma is a rare variant presenting as a skin tumor that infiltrates as narrow vascular channels between the dermal collagen fibers.[29] This pattern should not be confused with the permeative growth of an angiosarcoma.

Cellular Capillary Hemangioma

Cellular capillary hemangiomas (juvenile hemangiomas) in small children can be alarmingly cellular and mitotically active, and therefore they were historically called "infantile hemangioendotheliomas," a term that should no longer be used because it creates a confusion with borderline malignant vascular tumors.

Grossly, cellular capillary hemangiomas are often elevated nodular lesions. The lesions grow rapidly

Table 14–2. Summary of the Most Important Syndromes That Include Hemangiomas or Related Lesions as a Component

Syndrome Genetics	Characteristics of Hemangioma	Other Tumors, Manifestations, and Complications
Blue rubber bleb nevus (Bean syndrome)	Cutaneous, gastrointestinal, pulmonary and central nervous system hemangiomas	Gastrointestinal bleeding and chronic anemia Vascular obliteration by hemangioma thrombosis
von Hippel-Lindau mutation in *VHL* gene	Retinal hemangiomas, may impair vision	Cerebellar, retinal, other hemangioblastomas Renal carcinoma
Klippel-Trenaunay-Weber autosomal dominant transmission (port-wine stains)	Cavernous or capillary hemangiomas Telangiectasias of cutaneous vessels Arteriovenous shunts When with additional arteriovenous shunt, has been referred to Parkes-Weber syndrome	Triad of systemic angiodysplasia, varicose veins and hypertrophy of soft tissue and bone of the involved leg Impaired leg function, poor durability on exercise
Osler (Osler-Rendu-Weber)	Vascular teleangiectasias in various organs	Bleeding, especially gastrointestinal
Sturge-Weber	Nevus flammeus (facial capillary hemangioma) Hemangiomas of the leptomeninges adjacent to cerebral cortex	Epilepsia
Maffucci syndrome	Multiple spindle cell hemangiomas (hemangioendotheliomas)	Multiple enchondromas, risk of chondrosarcoma
Kasabach-Merritt syndrome Acquired condition	Kaposiform hemangioendothelioma	Platelet consumption by entrapment in hemangioma

during the first postnatal weeks after which a slow phase of regression occurs.

Histologically, cellular capillary hemangiomas can be densely cellular having closely packed capillaries, which may have inconspicuous or well-defined vascular lumina (Fig. 14–2). A prominent pericytic, actin-positive component is typically present, and there is often infiltration of mast cells and factor XIII-positive histiocytes.[27] Lobulation, lack of nuclear atypia, and common circumscription help to identify them as benign tumors, despite considerable cellularity and possible mitotic activity.

Electron microscopy has revealed peculiar lamellar crystalline inclusions that measure 0.5 to 2 μm and have a periodic substructure.[30]

Immunohistochemically, only the capillary endothelia are positive for endothelial markers, and there is a substantial pericytic, smooth muscle actin positive component. The endothelial cells of juvenile capillary hemangiomas were recently reported to be selectively positive for glucose transporter type 1 (GLUT1), similar to the capillaries of placental villi.[31]

Lobular Capillary Hemangioma (Pyogenic Granuloma)

Clinical Features

This clinically distinctive form of hemangioma arises as a small purplish red, rapidly growing polypoid protrusion on the skin or mucosal surfaces, especially in the lip or gingival mucosa.[32] These tumors often occur in pregnant women (granuloma gravidarum). The surface is often ulcerated. This tumor has been thought of a superficial extension from an underlying capillary hemangioma.[33] Although some lesions of this kind may be reactive, lobular capillary hemangiomas are classified among hemangiomas.

Pathology

Microscopically, the lesion consists of proliferative capillaries arranged in lobules; mitotic activity may be present. The endothelial cells are typically enlarged (activated) and may have mild nuclear

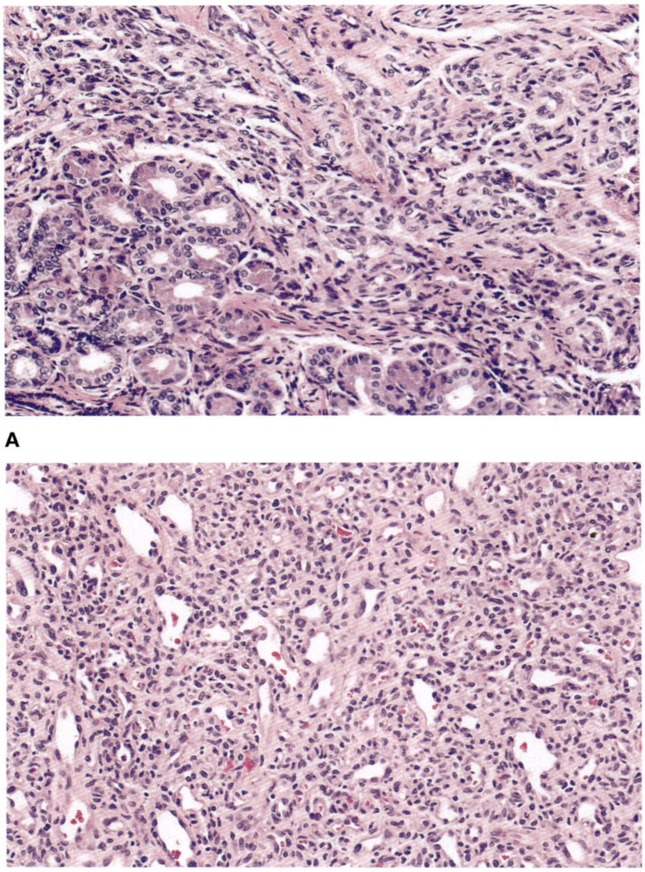

A

B

Figure 14–2. Cellular capillary hemangioma is composed of lobules of capillary-like units. They may have narrow and inconspicuous *(A)* or well-developed vascular lumina *(B).*

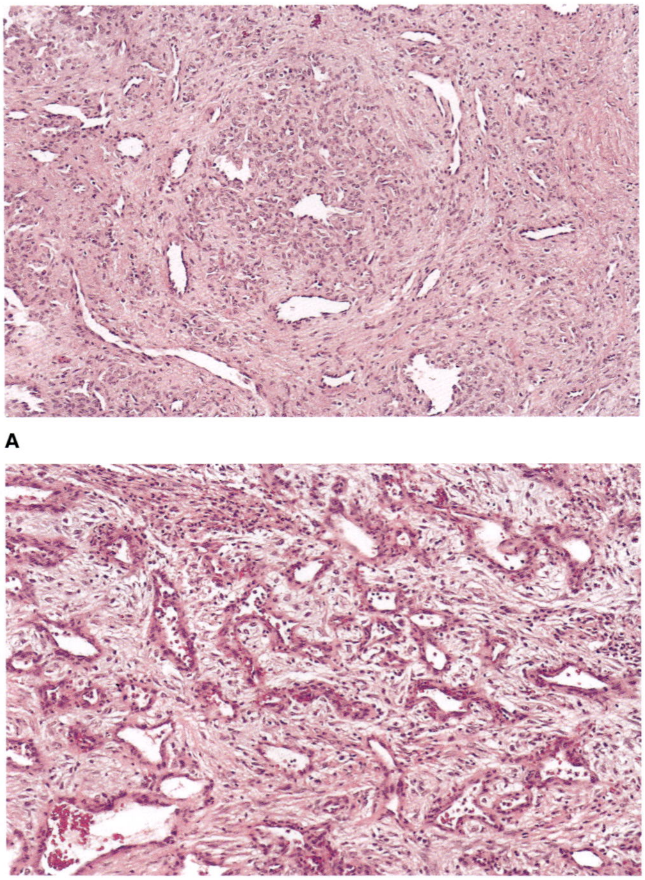

A

B

Figure 14–3. *A,* Lobular capillary hemangioma (pyogenic granuloma) is composed of lobules of proliferating capillaries. *B,* This lobular capillary hemangioma shows dilated vessels with slightly epithelioid endothelia and intervening inflammatory infiltrate.

atypia (Fig. 14–3). Cutaneous and mucosal lesions are often surrounded by a collar-like epithelial lining. Multiple satellite lesions may also occur.[34] Mild interstitial granulocytic infiltration is common, but the presence of neutrophilic microabscesses should lead to suspicion of bacillary angiomatosis, especially in immunocompromised patients.

Intravascular pyogenic granuloma refers to a histologically similar lesion that is located in a lumen of a small vein. This lesion typically occurs in the head and neck area or in the upper extremity and actually may represent an organized thrombus.[35,36]

Acquired Tufted Angioma (Progressive Angioma, Angioblastoma of Nakagawa)

This rare form of cellular capillary hemangioma occurs mainly in adults. It forms a progressively enlarging cutaneous macule and is therefore also referred to as progressive angioma. Histologically, the lesion is composed of multiple deep, sometimes bandlike dermal nodules with the appearance reminiscent of those of a cellular capillary hemangioma. The multiple, scattered, spheroidal dermal nodules are often referred to have a "cannonball pattern" (Fig. 14–4). Intravascular tufting is commonly seen. The capillaries are well formed with a single endothelial cell layer and no atypia, and pericytes are also present.[37–40]

Targetoid Hemosiderotic and Hobnail Hemangioma

This lesion was named based on the target-like clinical appearance of the early cutaneous lesion, which commonly has a darker central zone.[41] It has been later suggested that the clinical gross appearance is only part of the spectrum, and the name "hobnail hemangioma" has been suggested by the unified histologic appearance of clinically and grossly het-

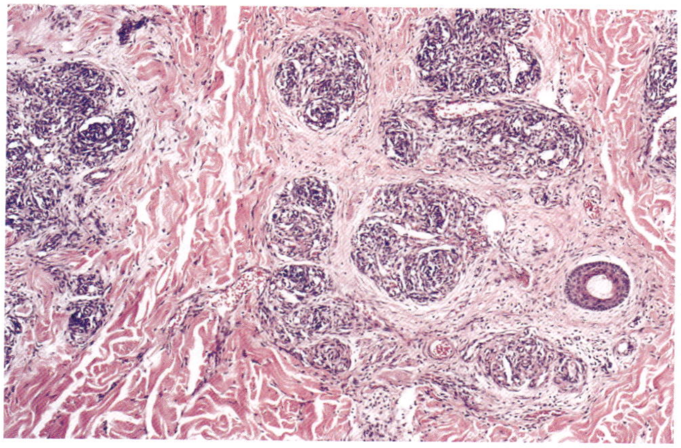

A

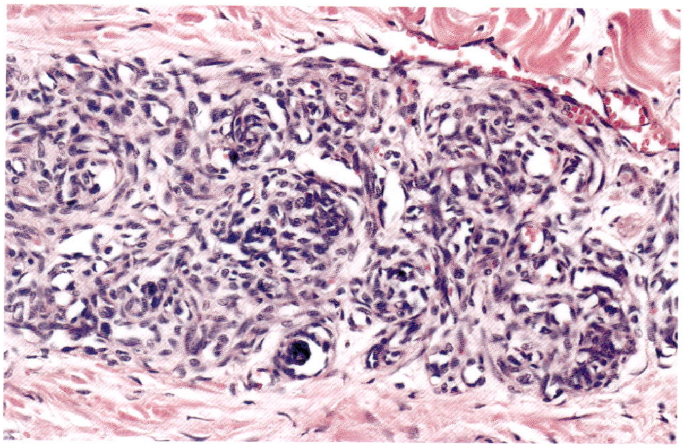

B

Figure 14-4. Acquired tufted angioma contains multiple lobules of capillary hemangioma in deep dermis *(A)*. The lobules are well demarcated and are composed of slitlike capillaries lined by spindled endothelial cells *(B)*.

erogeneous lesions of which the originally described features are only a part.[42,43]

These tumors occur predominantly in young adults without a clear sex predilection in a wide variety of locations. The lesions are typically small, usually less than 1 cm, and they have a uniformly benign behavior.

Histologically, these hemangiomas are distinctive for mildly dilated vascular channels lined by protuberant "hobnail" endothelial cells that may have mild hyperchromasia, but lack multilayered pattern and significant atypia.

Cavernous Hemangioma

These common hemangiomas occur with no age and sex predilection in a wide variety of locations, especially in the upper body. The lesions can involve skin, subcutis, deep soft tissues, and bone. A common site of presentation is the liver, where the tumor may be a small incidental nodule or a large space-occupying lesion. Cavernous hemangiomas of skin do not typically regress as the capillary ones do.

Grossly, the larger lesions have a spongy appearance because of the large vascular spaces. Histologically, the lesions are composed of a conglomerate of widely open vascular lumina lined by relatively inconspicuous endothelial cells and separated by thick nearly acellular fibrous septa (Fig. 14–5). Some tumors combine the features of cavernous and capillary hemangioma.

Sinusoidal hemangioma is the designation given to a variant of cavernous hemangioma that occurs in adults and forms sinusoidal spaces lined by delicate septa.[44]

Intramuscular Hemangioma

This rare presentation of hemangioma occurs primarily in young adults and equally in men and women. Some tumors are congenital, and the majority present before the age of 20.[45,46] The most commonly involved sites are the muscles of the thigh, followed by upper extremity and chest wall. The lesional size varies and may be large, over 10 to 15 cm. Intramuscular hemangiomas have a high recurrence rate, because complete excision may be difficult when the tumor is not well marginated.

Histologically, the intramuscular hemangiomas are composed of well-differentiated vessels and may show capillary, cavernous, or venous patterns in various combinations. Some lesions contain a fatty component, and such tumors have been earlier referred to as deep or infiltrative angiolipomas.

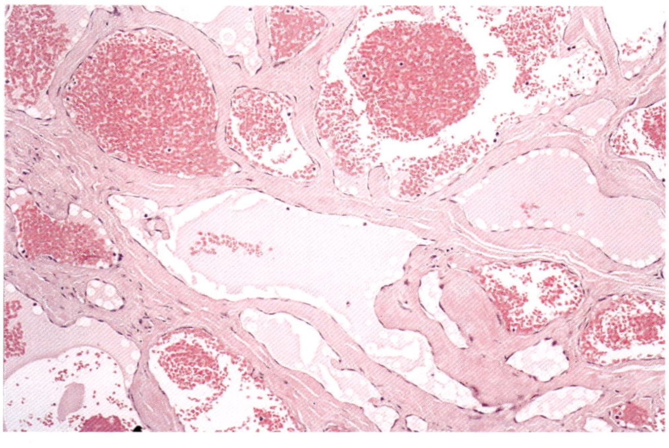

Figure 14-5. Cavernous hemangioma shows dilated vascular lumina often packed with erythrocytes. Nearly avascular vessel walls are seen between the vascular spaces.

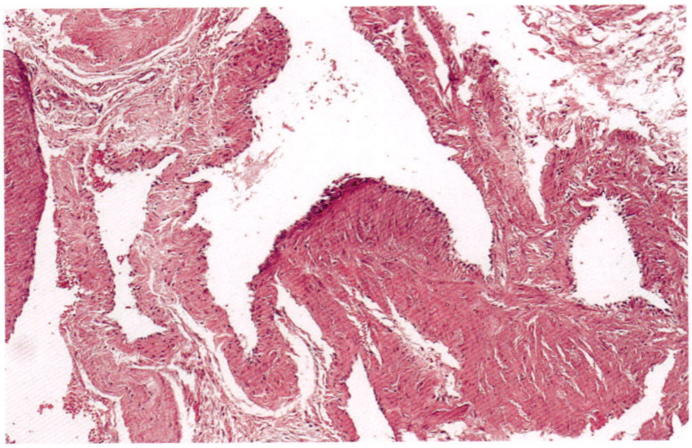

Figure 14–6. Venous hemangioma is composed of veinlike vascular units containing smooth muscle.

Venous Hemangioma

This designation refers to hemangioma that is composed of dilated veinlike vascular units with variably irregular smooth muscle walls, which distinguish it from cavernous hemangioma. The lumina are typically lined by inconspicuous endothelial cells (Fig. 14–6). The question of vascular malformation (arteriovenous hemangioma versus venous hemangioma) sometimes arises; it can be reliably resolved only with radiologic clinical correlation where arteriovenous shunting is demonstrated.

Angiomatosis

Angiomatosis has been defined as a histologically benign vascular tumor involving multiple contiguous tissue planes. These lesions are often diagnosed in early childhood, and over half of the tumors are diagnosed by the age of 20 years with a female predilection (1.5:1). The condition is often brought to attention by pain and swelling of the involved limb or region; notably skin extension appears rare. The most common region of presentation is the lower extremity with the foot, ankle, and leg being the most common sites of involvement. A number of lesions occur in the chest wall. The diagnosis is based on clinical and radiologic evidence of an extensive lesion with histologic features of a hemangioma in a biopsy. Although the lesion might recur, malignant transformation is not a feature of angiomatosis. Therefore, conservative management is possible, in view of the difficulty in complete removal without structural sacrifice.[47,48]

Histologically, the angiomatosis may show combinations of capillary, cavernous, and venous hemangioma. The presence of increased numbers of capillaries in the vein walls is also thought to be typical of this condition.

Littoral Cell Angioma of the Spleen and Other Splenic Angiomas

Falk and colleagues reported a series of 17 vascular tumors of the spleen in adult patients. They named these tumors littoral cell angiomas because they believed that these tumors originated from the splenic sinusoidal endothelia.[49]Another series of four patients was reported associated with various internal organ carcinomas.[50] Although it is possible that littoral cell angioma is specifically associated with malignancies, it is also possible that these tumors become incidentally detected during cancer staging procedures. Behavior has been benign in all cases.

The lesions vary from small, incidental nodules to massive ones that can replace much of the entire spleen. Histologically, littoral cell angioma consists of dilated and anastomosing vascular channels lined by enlarged, tall endothelial cells that do not show significant nuclear atypia or mitotic activity. Peculiar to littoral cell angioma is coexpression of von Willebrand factor and CD68, a feature believed to support sinusoidal lining cell origin.[49] Littoral cell angiomas are typically $CD34^-$ and $CD21^+$ but negative for CD8, another antigen normally present in splenic sinusoidal endothelia.[51,52]

Capillary and cavernous hemangiomas also occur in the spleen. Cellular capillary hemangiomas can be separated from angiosarcomas by their usually circumscribed nature, well-organized vascular proliferation, and lack of atypia and multilayered endothelia and anastomosing channels. Splenic capillary hemangiomas are lined by endothelia variably positive for CD34 but negative for CD8, whereas the latter marker is present in the so-called splenic hamartomas, similar to the normal splenic sinus lining cells.[52]

Kimura Disease

This rare condition is a mass-forming chronic inflammation with a vascular component. It occurs almost only in persons of Oriental descent. The tumor usually presents in the upper part of the body, especially in the head and neck, and may be multiple and accompanied by lymphadenopathy and systemic eosinophilia.[53–58]

The tumor is based in the subcutis but may involve skin, deep soft tissues, and lymph nodes. Histologically, it contains lymphoid hyperplasia with germinal centers, eosinophilic granulocytes sometimes with eosinophilic microabscesses, variably prominent dilated capillaries, and evolving fibrosis in the background. In contrast to epithelioid hemangioma, the endothelia in Kimura disease do not have a clearly epithelioid morphology.

Epithelioid Hemangioma (Angiolymphoid Hyperplasia with Eosinophilia)

Clinical Features

This condition includes a prominent capillary proliferation with at least partially epithelioid endothelial morphology. Many lesions of this kind may be rather reactive than neoplastic.[59,60] Some lesions of this type were previously designated as "histiocytoid hemangiomas."

Clinically, epithelioid hemangioma forms a cutaneous or subcutaneous lesion that often appears in the head and neck region, and multiple lesions occur in some patients. The condition is more common in middle-aged and older women. It often involves an arterial wall. In contrast to Kimura disease, systemic involvement with lymphadenopathy and peripheral blood eosinophilia is rare. Because local recurrence is possible, complete excision of the lesion is desirable. However, in some cases development of multiple lesions is felt to represent the multifocal nature of the process rather than a true recurrence. The prognosis is excellent.

Pathology

Histologically, the lesions are composed of vessels with a narrow caliber lined by epithelioid endothelial cells with abundant eosinophilic cytoplasm. Sometimes a subcutaneous artery with epithelioid transformation of endothelia is part of the tumor, suggesting that arterial trauma or other lesion may be the initiating event in some cases.[61] Endothelial proliferation may include intraluminal clustering of the epithelioid endothelia. In the background, there is inflammatory infiltration composed of eosinophils and lymphocytes, occasionally with germinal centers.[62,63] In some cases, sheets of endothelial cells in fibrous stroma may resemble an infiltrating carcinoma (Fig. 14–7).

The epithelioid morphology of the endothelial cells, lack of fibrosis, and lack of ethnic connection to an Oriental population separate this entity from Kimura disease.[54,55]

The so-called epithelioid hemangioma (histiocytoid hemangioma) of the heart is probably a mesothelial rather than endothelial proliferation.[64]

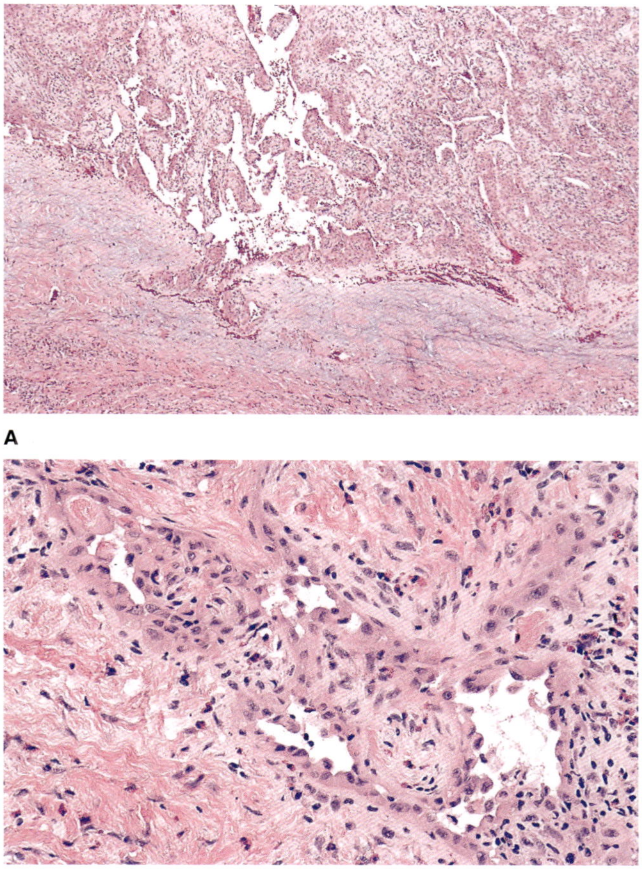

A

B

Figure 14–7. *A*, Epithelioid hemangioma lesion inside of a vessel wall. *B*, Cytologically the endothelia in this tumor show epithelioid but bland morphology. Focal solid areas are also present. Note also scattered eosinophils.

Glomeruloid Hemangioma with POEMS Syndrome

Clinical Features

This cutaneous vascular proliferation is probably reactive and is seen as part of the rare POEMS syndrome. The key pathogenetic factor is probably an underlying plasma cell neoplasia, which is seen in all patients with this syndrome. The acronym is for p = polyneuropathy, o = organomegaly, e = endocrinopathy, m = monoclonal gammopathy, s = skin lesions. The organomegaly entails hepatomegaly and splenomegaly, and the endocrinopathy includes hypothyreosis, adrenal insufficiency, and amenorrhea. The plasma cell neoplasia is the key element, and usually has λ light chain; sclerotic bone lesions are often present. The skin lesions are glomeruloid hemangiomas. Lymphadenopathy, glomerular kidney disease, and pulmonary hypertension are other common features of the syndrome.[65–67]

Pathology

The skin lesions form small red to purple papules or nodules measuring 1 to 10 mm. Histologically they consist of dilated blood vessels containing multiple profiles of tortuous capillaries, resembling the appearance of a renal glomerulus. The lymph nodes have histologic features identical with multicentric Castleman disease, where HHV8 has been detected.[68] Interestingly, this virus has been also detected in multiple myeloma. Recognition of the glomeruloid hemangioma may assist in the identification of the POEMS syndrome.[65–67]

Papillary Endothelial Hyperplasia (Masson Tumor)

Clinical Features

This benign condition is significant because it may be confused with angiosarcoma, although it represents an organizing thrombus with florid endothelial hyperplasia. It usually forms a small 1- to 2-cm, circumscribed, superficial nodule in the peripheral parts of extremities (especially fingers and hand) or head. Focal papillary endothelial hyperplasia is a relatively common finding in surgically excised hemorrhoids.[69–72]

Pathology

The intravenous location and coexistence with thrombosis point to origin from organizing vascular thrombus, although rarely, similar changes are seen outside of vessels, and rarely in organizing hematoma. Some lesions have elements of cavernous hemangioma indicating origin from a benign vascular tumor. Histologically typical are numerous intravascular papillary projections with fibrous stroma and lining of hyperplastic endothelia giving the lesion a placenta-like appearance (Fig. 14–8).

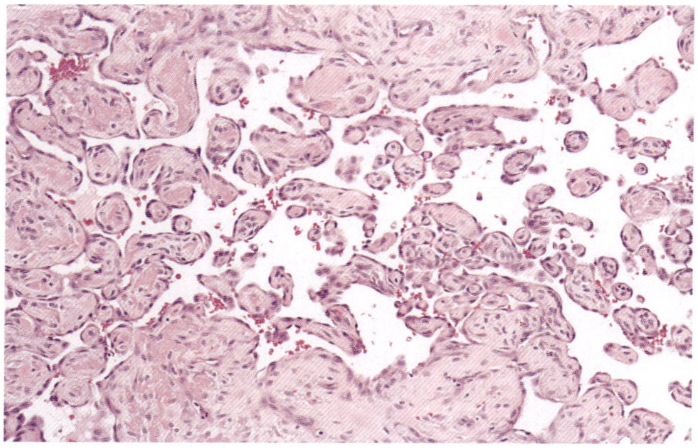

Figure 14–8. Papillary endothelial hyperplasia shows multiple papillae with fibrous cores lined by proliferative endothelial cells.

The features differing from angiosarcoma are the typical intravascular location, one-layered endothelial lining, limited atypia, lack of solid growth and necrosis, and slight if any mitotic activity.

Spindle Cell Hemangioma

Spindle cell hemangioma, formerly named spindle cell hemangioendothelioma[73] and originally believed to have a malignant potential, is now classified among hemangiomas,[74,75] and even a reactive origin has been suggested.[76]

Clinical Features

This tumor has a predilection for the distal parts of the extremities of young adults, with a male predominance. It usually develops as a slowly growing single purplish nodule or multiple lesions less than 1 cm in diameter, with cutaneous or subcutaneous involvement. A minority of lesions are intramuscular. Many patients have a long history of the lesion, and multiplicity occurs in over half the patients. Most vascular tumors in patients with Mafucci disease with enchondromas and vascular tumors are spindle cell hemangioma,[75] although they were originally believed to be cavernous hemangiomas.

Over 50% of the tumors recur locally, but they do not metastasize. New lesions often develop in the same region, but not in the exact same location, suggesting multifocality.[74–79] The rare existence of hypercellular and atypical variants may have earned this lesion its previously applied borderline designation.

Pathology

Spindle cell hemangioma resembles cavernous hemangioma with dilated vascular channels but has greater cellularity in the septa. The septa of the cavernous spaces typically contain uniform spindled cells with tapered ends in a visibly collagenous background. A significant portion of the lesions are entirely intravascular, and the cavernous spaces often contain calcified thrombi (phlebolithes). The endothelial cells often have focal epithelioid features and cytoplasmic vacuolization (Fig. 14–9). Mitotic activity and atypia are low; if present, another diagnosis such as atypical spindle cell vascular neoplasm is more appropriate in view of prognostic uncertainty.

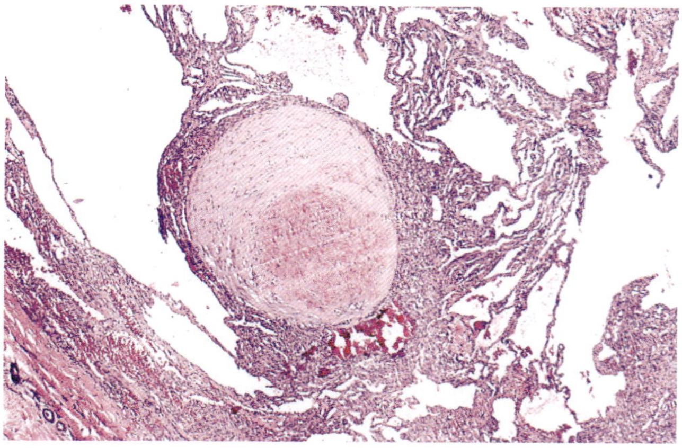

A

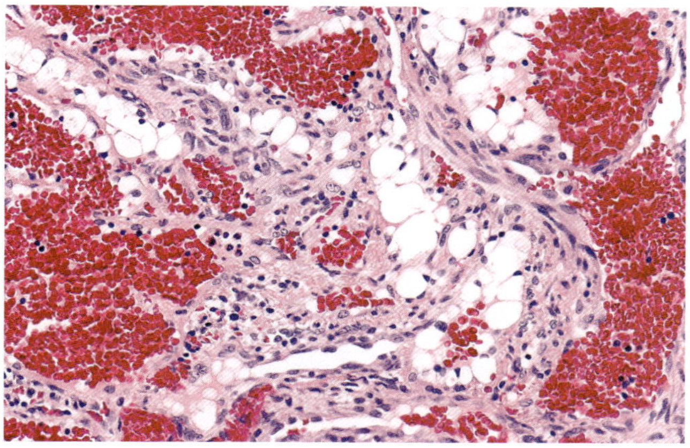

B

Figure 14-9. *A,* Low magnification of a spindle cell hemangioma with a phlebolith and multiple cavernous spaces. *B,* Spindle cell hemangioma containing multiple dilated vascular lumina with intervening spindle cells. Note focal vacuolar changes in the lining endothelia.

Immunohistochemically the slit-lining cells and the epithelioid cells have an endothelial phenotype and are positive for von Willebrand factor, UEA1, and CD31, whereas the septal spindle cells have smooth muscle or pericytic features by their positivity for smooth muscle actin and negativity for CD34. All components have been found to be negative for S-100 protein.[78]

Lymphangioma and Related Tumors

Lymphangiomas are benign tumors that are composed of lymphatic-like vessels.[80] They typically form a clinically detected tumor mass, which is often ill-defined. Most common locations are head and neck where cystic lymphangiomas (cystic hygromas) occur in newborn and older children. Such tumors have been seen with an unexpectedly high frequency in Turner syndrome.[81] Lymphangioma circumscriptum is the designation used for a localized cutaneous lymphangioma. In the gastrointestinal tract (colon) lymphangiomas have been reported as endoscopically detected polypoid masses.[82]

Grossly, the masses may appear spongy, but they are often unimpressive as tumor specimens because the lymphatic vessels often collapse after surgery. Histologically, lymphangiomas are composed of clusters of variably dilated vascular lumina filled with proteinaceous fluid. The vessels have thin walls and flaccid contours, and the endothelial cells are inconspicuous. Clusters of lymphoid tissue or more completely developed lymph nodes are often seen in the septa. Elements of smooth muscle are sometimes present in the septa. Some lymphangiomas are cystic, and in others abundant connective tissue separates the vascular units (Fig. 14–10).

Lymphangiomatosis is a designation for a lymphangioma that permeates several tissue planes, analogous to hemangiomatosis.

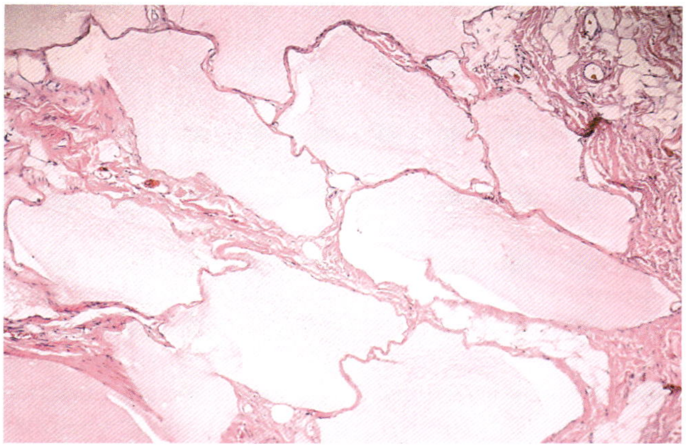

A

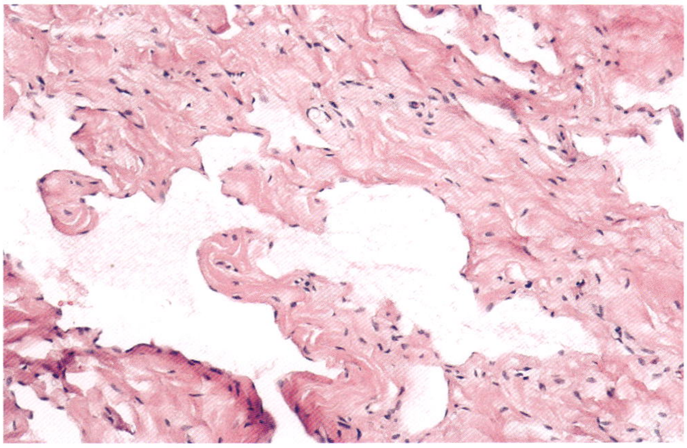

B

Figure 14-10. *A,* Cystic lymphangioma shows multiple dilated lumina with flaccid contours lined by attenuated endothelial cells. *B,* This lymphangioma shows scattered lymphatic vessels in fibrous stroma.

Lymphangioendothelioma (progressive acquired lymphangioma) is a designation for an enlarging lymphangioma that may feature anastomosing lymphatic vascular channels, but does not have the infiltrative nature typical of angiosarcoma. This feature should not lead to confusion with angiosarcoma; lymphangioendothelioma has a benign behavior, according to a series with limited follow-up.[83]

Lymphangiomyoma(tosis) is a smooth muscle proliferation related to the smooth muscle elements in the walls of lymphatics (see Chapter 10). The tumor is unique for its coexpression of HMB45, a melanoma marker, and smooth muscle markers.

Borderline Malignant Vascular Tumors

Kaposiform (Kaposi-Like) Hemangioendothelioma

Clinical Features

This tumor was originally described as Kaposi-like hemangioma,[84,85] and later as kaposiform hemangioendothelioma.[86]

This tumor predominantly occurs in young children (median age 2 years), and occasionally in young adults without a clear sex predilection. The tumor may arise in peripheral deep soft tissue and retroperitoneum, which according to one series is the most common location.[87] The tumor may cause platelet trapping and lead to potentially fatal consumption coagulopathy (Kasabach-Merritt syndrome). Although it may spread as microscopic nodules to surrounding tissues, metastases have not been detected. A retrospective study from Boston's Children's Hospital found that tumors previously diagnosed as hemangiomas with consumption coagulopathy actually were all kaposiform hemangioendotheliomas.[87]

Pathology

Grossly, the lesions are typically gray-white. Histologically, they are lobulated by fibrous septa. The lesional cells form Kaposi sarcoma-like vascular slits sometimes with microthrombosis and may be quite cellular. Pericytes are less developed than those in hemangiomas. The spindled endothelial proliferation has limited atypia and low mitotic activity (Fig. 14–11). Some tumors also have a component of lymphangiomatosis.

Papillary Intralymphatic Angioendothelioma (Dabska Tumor)

This tumor was described by Dabska in children.[88] Similar cases reported later seem to have predilection in children and young adults. The lesions occur in skin and subcutis in a wide variety of anatomic regions. Although the initial reports suggested metastatic potential, our series from the Armed Forces Institute of Pathology found favorable outcome in all cases.[89] Complete, preferably wide excision seems to be the optimal treatment.

Histologically, the tumor is composed of anastomosing, dilated vascular channels that often have papillary intravascular proliferations with radially arranged endothelial cells surrounding a fibrous core in a "match-stick pattern" (Fig. 14–12). Lymphangioma-like components with vascular lumina containing proteinaceous fluid and lymphocytes are seen in some tumors suggesting a relationship with lymphangioma. The consistent positivity of the

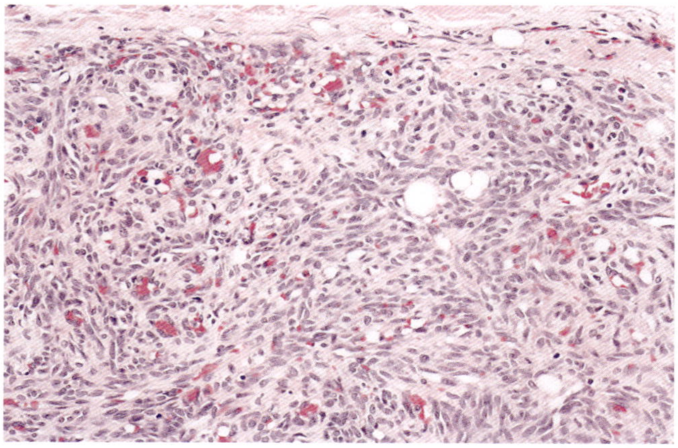

A

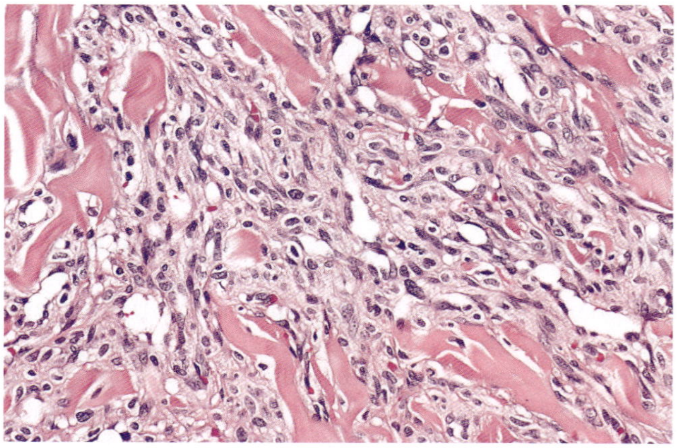

B

Figure 14–11. Kaposiform hemangioendothelioma is composed of well-demarcated lobules of spindle vascular proliferation *(A)*. The proliferation is composed of relatively uniform spindled cells *(B)*.

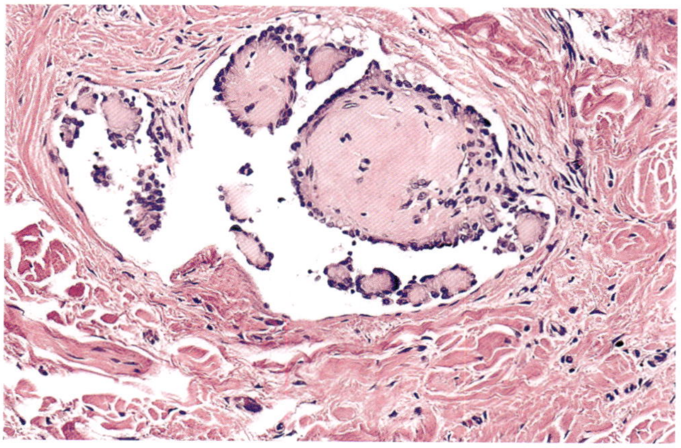

Figure 14–12. Papillary intralymphatic angioendothelioma contains papillary intravascular protrusions radially surrounded by proliferating endothelial cells with limited atypia.

lesions for vascular VEGFR3 has also been interpreted to support lymphatic vascular origin,[89] although this receptor is now known to be expressed in other vascular tumors as well.

Retiform Hemangioendothelioma

This cutaneous tumor was originally classified as a low-grade angiosarcoma,[90] but has been more recently classified among borderline malignant tumors.[3] This tumor often occurs in peripheral superficial locations, such as hands and feet, mainly in young adults of either sex. Local recurrence is common, but metastasis is exceptional and seems limited to lymph nodes. In one report, multiple synchronous tumors were described in one patient.[91]

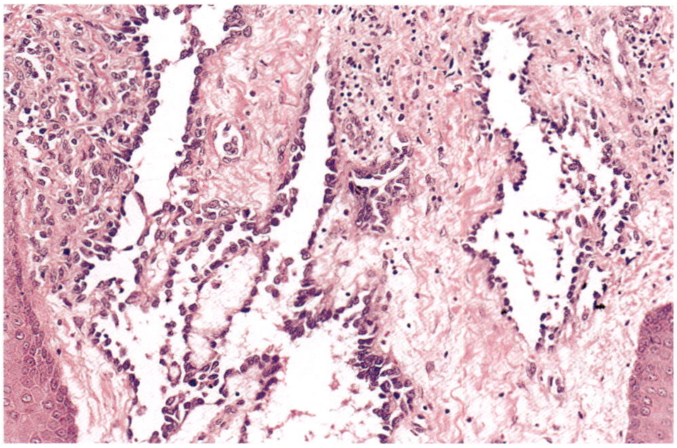

Figure 14–13. Retiform hemangioendothelioma is composed of variably dilated vascular channels with prominent, inward protruding cells.

The tumor is usually relatively small, measuring 1 to 2 cm. It is typically centered to mid-dermis, but may extend to the subcutis. Histologically typical are gaping "retiform" vessels resembling rete testis structures. The endothelium is tall, with protruding cytoplasm "hobnail cells," somewhat similar but more proliferative than that in hobnail hemangioma (Fig. 14–13). Focal solid areas are often present, but atypia and mitotic activity are limited.

Malignant Vascular Tumors

Epithelioid Hemangioendothelioma

Clinical Features

Epithelioid hemangioendothelioma (EHE) is a low-grade malignant vascular endothelial tumor, originally reported by Weiss and coworkers.[92,93] It occurs in adults of all ages, but rarely in children. In soft tissues the tumor occurs equally in males and females, but hepatic tumors have a 6:4 female predominance.[92–97]

The tumor most commonly presents in the skin, deep soft tissue, or organ-based locations, of which the most common is the liver. In the bones multifocal occurrence is common. The pulmonary EHE (previously called intravascular bronchioloalveolar tumor) typically forms multiple nodules, often bilaterally.[98] Some cases have been proven as pulmonary metastases of peripheral primary tumors.[99] Therefore, search for a primary tumor elsewhere is warranted in pulmonary lesions, especially if multifocal. The same may be true for hepatic tumors.

The tumor has an unpredictable behavior, and 20% to 30% of patients with peripheral soft tissue tumors develop metastases in liver, bones, or lungs. Regional lymph node metastases also occur. Patients diagnosed with hepatic primary tend to have multiple tumors and have a higher mortality, 43%, but liver transplantation may be curative.[96] A large series documented the 5-year survival as 43% and the 10-year survival as 25%.[97]

Pathology

Grossly, some cases of EHE are distinctive in that the mass involves a vein where a tumor thrombus can form and infiltrate surrounding tissue. The hepatic tumors have typically ill-defined, infiltrative margins.

Microscopically, EHE consists of cords of epithelioid cells in a myxoid or hyalinized matrix. The tumor cells often form primitive lumina, which may contain erythrocytes. The cellularity may vary from paucicellular, hyalinized to moderately cellular. Infiltration in the

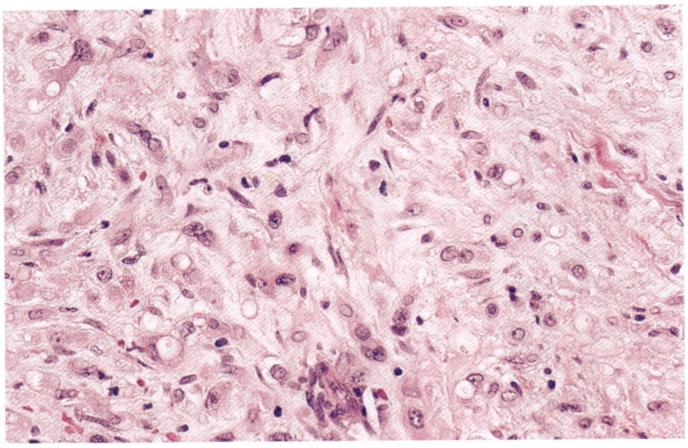

Figure 14–14. Epithelioid hemangioendothelioma is composed of streaks of epithelioid cells in a myxohyaline matrix. Note the microlumen formations.

wall of a vein is sometimes observed. In the liver, the tumor grows diffusely between focally preserved trabeculae of parenchymal cells. Cytologically, the tumor cells have small to medium-sized, pale nuclei, and mitotic activity is low (Fig. 14–14). Pronounced atypia is not a feature of this lesion, and if present, is more consistent with the diagnosis of epithelioid angiosarcoma.

Histologic features that have been found to correlate with better outcome in soft tissue tumors were low cellularity and low proliferative rate, lack of striking atypia, and low mitotic rate (2/10 high-power field [HPF] or less), whereas tumor size was not.[94] Among hepatic tumors, those with low cellularity had better behavior with 17% mortality, whereas those with high cellularity had 84% mortality. Lack of necrosis is also a favorable sign.[97]

Immunohistochemically, the lesional cells show membrane staining for CD31, cytoplasmic staining for vimentin, and usually at least focal positivity for von Willebrand factor, often in intracellular lumina. Approximately 50% of cases are positive for CD34. Keratins are commonly present. In our series, K18 was found in 100% of cases, K7 and K8 in 25% of cases, but K19 in none of the cases; antibody to the K19 or AE1 monoclonal antibody are therefore more useful in the differential diagnosis of EHE and carcinoma. Epithelial membrane antigen is rarely present, usually with weak luminal staining at the most.

Genetics

Data are limited. One case was reported to have a complex translocation including t(7;22),[100] but very recently a similar t(1;3) translocation was reported in two cases, suggesting that this may be a recurrent abnormality characteristic of EHE.[101]

Angiosarcoma

Angiosarcoma is the designation for rare malignant neoplasms with endothelial cell differentiation and showing various degrees of vasoformation. According to our estimate they comprise no more than 1% to 2% of all sarcomas. This group includes several clinical and site-related subsets. The most important are cutaneous angiosarcoma of scalp and face, angiosarcoma arising in lymphedematous extremities, angiosarcoma of the breast, angiosarcoma of deep soft tissue, angiosarcoma of spleen and liver, postradiation angiosarcoma (cutaneous or deep), and angiosarcoma developing around a foreign body. The definition of angiosarcoma is more strict now, and the diagnosis is often based on immunohistochemical identification of endothelial differentiation.

Cutaneous Angiosarcoma of Scalp and Face

This is the most common form of angiosarcoma. It mainly occurs in old patients and forms violaceous nodules or plaques, sometimes with several satellite lesions. Occurrence in the scalp is more common than in the face. The tumor margin is often grossly deceptive, which leads to difficulties in complete surgery and results in recurrence. Distant metastases often develop, and the overall prognosis is poor.[102–105] One study identified tumor size less than 5 cm and lymphoid infiltration as prognostically favorable signs.[105]

Angiosarcoma Following Radiation

Probably the most common form of postirradiation angiosarcoma is now the one occurring in the skin or subcutis of the breast or chest wall following conservative or radical surgery and local radiation for breast carcinoma.[106–109] These tumors vary from well-differentiated and favorable to high-grade malignant ones. External beam radiation for other cancers, most often gynecologic carcinoma, may also be complicated angiosarcoma. Angiosarcomas may also follow radiation for benign conditions, such as hemangiomas. In such circumstances the interval from radiation to tumor formation is longer.

Angiosarcoma Arising in Lymphedematous Extremities

This rare condition, also named Stewart-Treves syndrome according to the authors of the first report, is estimated to develop in less than 1% of women who undergo mastectomy and lymphadenectomy. The incidence is decreasing due to less radical practices in breast cancer surgery. Although these tumors were previously called lymphangiosarcomas, there is no evidence of lymphatic vascular origin. Most commonly, the angiosarcomas arise in the upper arm or chest wall of middle-aged or elderly women with long-standing lymphedema on average 10 years after mastectomy and lymphadenectomy. Radiation has been thought to have a contributory role in many cases, although not all patients received any. Occurrence based on congenital (Milroy disease) or filarial infection-associated lymphedema, has also been reported.[110,111]

The angiosarcomas arising in lymphedematous extremities are highly malignant and, in the absence of radical surgery, tend to spread distally and proximally and to the chest wall. Most patients have died in 2 to 3 years. According to two studies, early amputation improves the chances for long-term survival, which is observed in only 10% to 15% of patients.[110,111]

Grossly, these tumors form multiple purplish cutaneous plaques or nodules. Histologically, they show a spectrum from well-differentiated vasoformative tumors to solid sheets of undifferentiated tumor cells, often in the same patient. The tumors often involve both skin, subcutis, and deep soft tissues. The undifferentiated components have been historically thought to represent recurrent carcinoma, but immunohistochemical studies have verified the endothelial differentiation.

Angiosarcoma of the Breast Parenchyma

These angiosarcomas occur predominantly in young to middle-aged women at the median age of 35 years. They present clinically as breast masses with often purplish discoloration of skin. The mammary angiosarcomas usually require at least subcutaneous mastectomy for complete removal. Despite radical surgery, metastases are common and are most commonly seen in the lungs, liver, bones, and soft tissues, including the contralateral breast.[112–115] Survival has been shown to depend on tumor differentiation. The examples composed entirely or mostly of vascular channels had a 5-year survival of 70% to 76%, whereas the ones composed of solid sarcomatous areas had a 5-year survival rate of only 15%, based on one series.[115]

Grossly, mammary angiosarcomas are typically large, hemorrhagic intraparenchymal masses that may grossly simulate a hematoma. Histologically, the tumors vary from well to poorly differentiated and infiltrate interstitially in the stroma and diffusely in the fat. The well-differentiated components often have a deceptively benign appearance. On the other hand, the occurrence of a wide variety of benign hemangiomas in the breast should be recognized based on well-organized vascular pattern, lobulation, and lack of atypia.[116]

Angiosarcoma of Deep Soft Tissue

This is a heterogeneous group of tumors. According to a recent large series they occur in an extremely wide age range from childhood to old age with the peak incidence in the seventh decade and a moderate (5:3) male predominance.[117] The most common locations are extremities, especially thigh (54%), trunk, especially retroperitoneum (35%), and head and neck (11%).[118] Over half of the patients develop distant metastases and die of tumor. The prognosis is poorer with older patients and intra-abdominal tumors.

Hepatic, Splenic, and Other Internal Angiosarcomas

Hepatic angiosarcomas are remarkable for several known occupational and iatrogenic etiologic connections; many of these tumors also involve spleen and vice versa. Because the circulating carcinogens pass through the liver and may be metabolically activated there, the hepatic sinusoidal endothelia are exposed more to carcinogens than any other endothelia. The carcinogens specifically associated with hepatic angiosarcoma are vinyl chloride (chemical used in rubber manufacturing), thorium oxide (radioactive compound Throrotrast used as a radiologic contrast medium until the 1940s), and arsenic compounds that were used as pesticides.[119–123]

The rare occurrence of hepatic angiosarcomas in children has also been reported. These tumors occurred mostly in small children (mean age, 4 years). They tended to have a spindle cell pattern with eosinophilic globules, and the prognosis was poor.[124]

Splenic angiosarcomas vary from well-differentiated tumors to those anaplastic tumors that may be difficult to recognize as angiosarcomas. They occur in adult patients, sometimes together with hepatic angiosarcoma, and most are highly malignant.[125,126] Angiosarcomas from other locations may also metastasize to the spleen. The splenic hemangiomas and littoral cell angiomas can be distinguished from angiosarcoma based on their organized vascular pattern and lack of endothelial proliferation (piling up) and atypia.

Angiosarcomas have been reported as primary tumors in many other locations including the brain,[127] thyroid,[128] adrenal gland,[129] gastrointestinal tract,[130] and on all serous surfaces; in the latter context angiosarcoma may clinically, grossly, and even histologically simulate a diffuse epithelial mesothelioma.[131,132]

Angiosarcoma Arising in a Malignant Peripheral Nerve Sheath Tumor

This peculiar coincidence has been reported in occasional cases of neurofibromatosis 1-associated tumors.[133]

Angiosarcoma Arising Around a Foreign Body

Angiosarcoma developing around a foreign body, such as a bullet, shrapnel, metallic surgical implant, or accidentally retained surgical sponge has been reported on rare occasions. In some cases, the latency has been over 50 years. Chronic carcinogenic nature of long-standing metal implants has also been suspected. These angiosarcomas are almost invariably high-grade tumors with unfavorable prognosis.[134]

Pathology

Grossly, the cutaneous angiosarcomas, such as postmastectomy angiosarcoma arising in lymphedematous extremity, form multiple purple papules and nodules (Fig. 14–15*A*). The deep angiosarcomas are typically large hemorrhagic masses (Fig. 14–15*B*). Histologically, these tumors commonly have extensive necrosis and fibrin deposition that may lead to erroneous impression of a benign lesion on biopsy.

The histologic spectrum of angiosarcomas includes several overlapping patterns that may occur in the same tumor (Fig. 14–16). A well-differentiated vasoformative pattern that dissects between collagen fibers and fat often occurs in the skin, breast, and soft tissue, including angiosarcomas arising in lymphedema. A solid poorly differentiated pattern that may resemble a carcinoma, melanoma, or lymphoma may be seen in any poorly differentiated angiosarcoma. In many angiosarcomas, there is a mixture of well- and poorly differentiated patterns. Epithelioid cytology with significant atypia and large nucleoli (epithelioid angiosarcoma) is present in approximately 20% to 30% of tumors, especially those in deep soft tissue. A spindle cell pattern somewhat reminiscent of Kaposi sarcoma may occur in any angiosarcoma, but seems to be more common in angiosarcomas of spleen and liver.

A common cytologic pattern for deep angiosarcomas is the epithelioid one. Such tumors differ from epithelioid hemangioendothelioma by the lack of semiorganized corded pattern and the presence of greater nuclear atypia and prominent nucleoli.[118] Thus, the poorly differentiated variants of epithelioid angiosarcoma can be easily confused with carcinoma or melanoma.

Most angiosarcomas are high-grade tumors, and some tumors previously considered low-grade angiosarcomas have been renamed borderline malignant tumors (hemangioendotheliomas).

Differential Diagnosis

Several features allow for the distinction of angiosarcoma from florid benign or reactive vascular proliferations. Angiosarcomas tend to have a randomly oriented (never entirely lobulated) vascular pattern infiltrating between connective or adipose tissue elements. The presence of cytologic atypia in the endothelial cells, tendency to at least focally multilayered growth, and lack of vascular pericytes, recognizable as actin-positive cells, are additional features typical of angiosarcoma. Mitotic activity and atypical mitoses are often present, but regular mitoses may also occur in benign proliferating endothelia. High-grade tumors often have significant hemorrhage and necrosis sometimes obscuring the neoplastic nature.

Clinical context is very helpful in separating Kaposi sarcoma from spindle cell angiosarcoma.

Many other malignant tumors (e.g., renal carcinoma, various undifferentiated carcinomas, epithelioid sarcoma, melanoma) may be highly vascular and hemorrhagic. These tumors should not be mistaken for angiosarcoma, which almost always shows true vasoformation by tumor cells, at least focally; immunohistochemistry for CD31 and S-100 protein is very helpful.

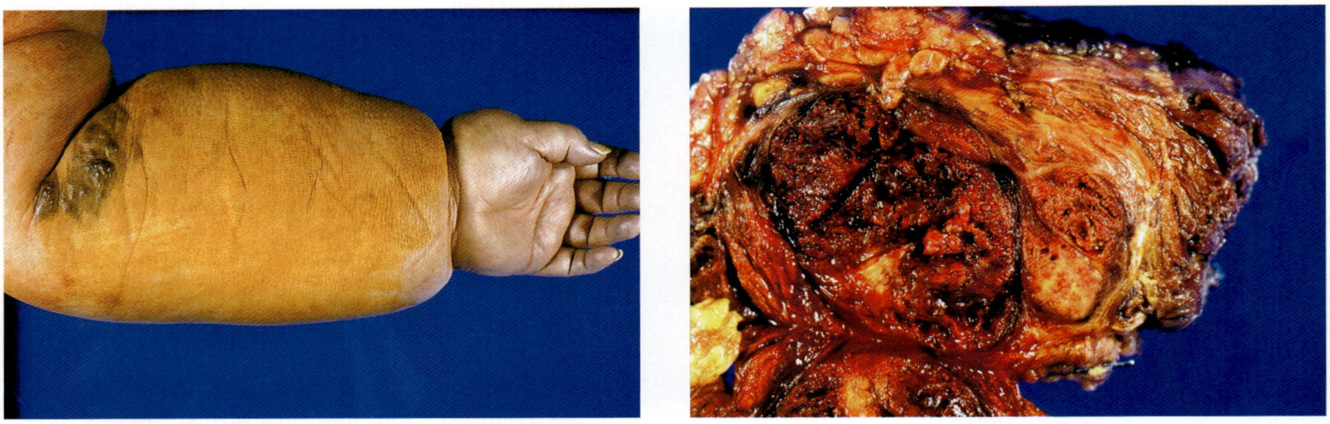

A B

Figure 14–15. *A*, Postmastectomy angiosarcoma arising in a lymphedematous arm shows multiple purple cutaneous nodules. *B*, Angiosarcoma in deep soft tissue presents as a hemorrhagic mass.

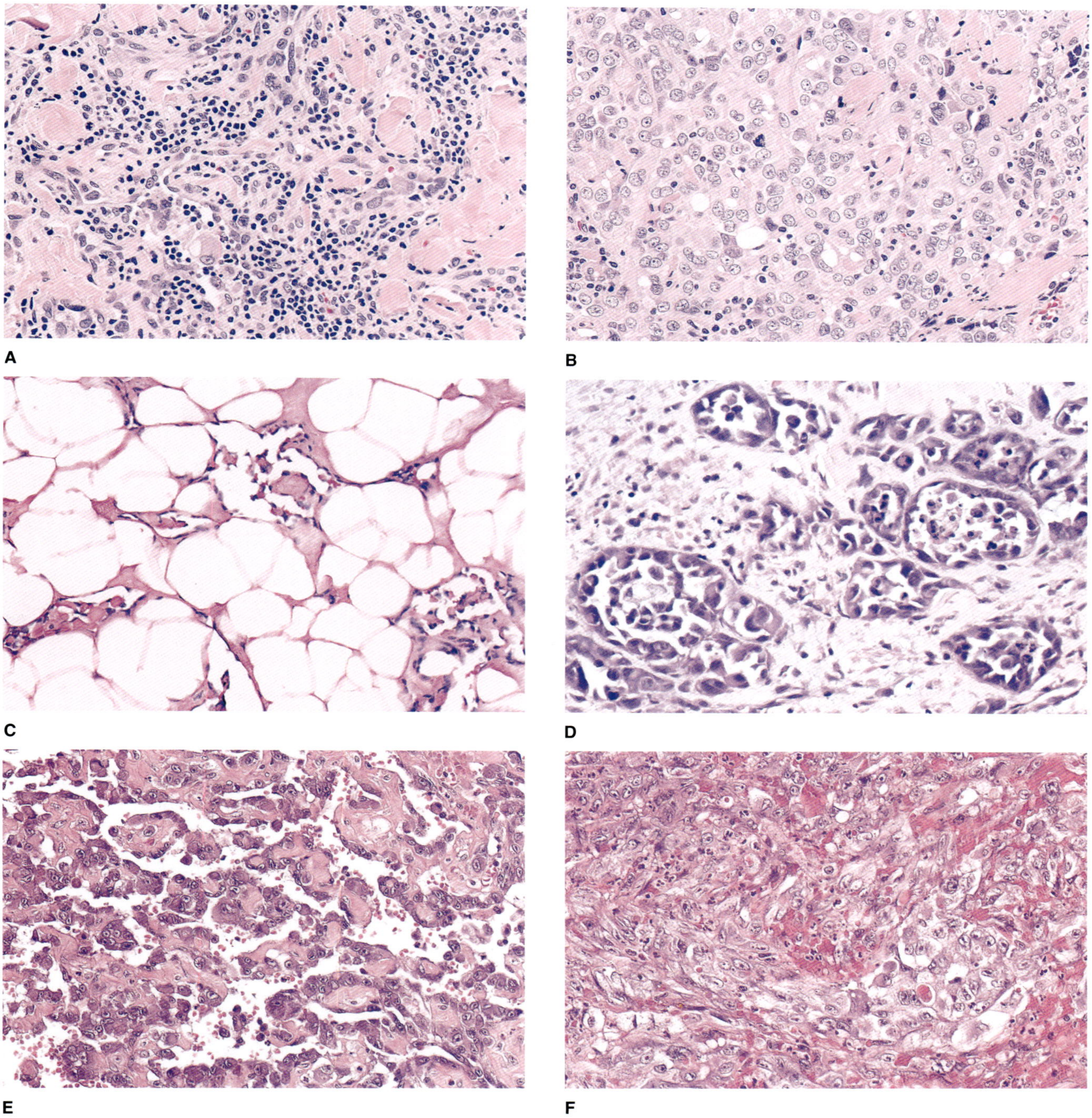

Figure 14–16. Different histologic appearances of angiosarcoma. *A,* Well-differentiated example is composed of narrow vascular slits that dissect through the dermis. Note the endothelial atypia and accompanying lymphoid infiltration. *B,* Poorly differentiated area of the same tumor shows nearly solid sheets of malignant endothelia. *C,* Angiosarcoma of breast demonstrates diffusely dissecting blood vessel formations lined by atypical endothelia. *D,* A peritoneal angiosarcoma in a patient previously radiated for Hodgkin disease shows glandlike vascular formations simulating a peritoneal mesothelioma. *E,* Epithelioid angiosarcoma of the adrenal showing anastomosing channels lined by malignant epithelioid endothelia. *F,* Solid area in the same epithelioid angiosarcoma.

Immunohistochemistry

CD31 is the most reliable marker, seen with a membrane staining pattern in over 90% of angiosarcomas (Fig. 14–17*A*). The positivity of platelets, plasma cells, and histiocytes should not be confused with endothelial reactivity.[135–137]

CD34 is expressed in approximately 50% of angiosarcomas somewhat unpredictably;[136–139] both well and poorly differentiated tumors can be negative.

Von Willebrand factor (factor VIII-related antigen) can be demonstrated in well-differentiated angiosarcomas but only focally if at all in less differentiated tumors, especially the nonepithelioid variants. Positivity typically appears as granular cytoplasmic staining.

Ulex europeaus lectin and BNH9 antibody recognizing similar sugar residues are quite sensitive, but the specificity is low, because these markers also react with many carcinomas, including squamous cell and adenocarcinomas.[139]

Expression of thrombomodulin (CD141) has been suggested useful for angiosarcoma.[140] This marker is shared by endothelia and mesothelia, but according to our experience, expression is variable and inconsistent (only 30% of angiosarcomas positive).

Vascular endothelial growth factor receptor 3 can be demonstrated in approximately 70–80% of angiosarcomas (Fig. 14–17*B*), less commonly so in the epithelioid variants.[141] Another endothelial marker normally expressed in lymphatics, podoplanin, is also present in subsets of angiosarcomas but experience is limited.[142]

Transcriptional regulator gene *Fli-1,* involved in the most common variant of Ewing sarcoma translocation, is constitutionally expressed in endothelial cells and has been suggested as an auxiliary marker for malignant vascular tumors; its expression seems conserved in angiosarcomas.[143]

Keratins, especially K18, and to a lesser degree K7 and K8, are present in 20% to 50% of angiosarcomas, more often in the epithelioid ones. Epithelial membrane antigen can also be present, making it challenging in some cases to differentiate angiosarcoma and carcinoma, and emphasizing interpretation of all clinicopathologic data together. The expression of K7 and K18 in angiosarcoma may reflect the phenotypic features of normal endothelia, which also express these keratins, whereas the presence of K8 more likely reflects neoexpression in transformed endothelia.[144]

Approximately 50% to 60% of angiosarcomas are positive for CD117 (KIT), similar to fetal endothelial cells suggesting oncofetal expression of CD117.[145] This may be significant for the potential of treatment of these tumors with KIT tyrosine kinase inhibitors.

Lack of a well-defined actin-positive pericytic layer may be helpful in differentiating angiosarcoma from benign vascular proliferations, which tend to have preserved pericytes.

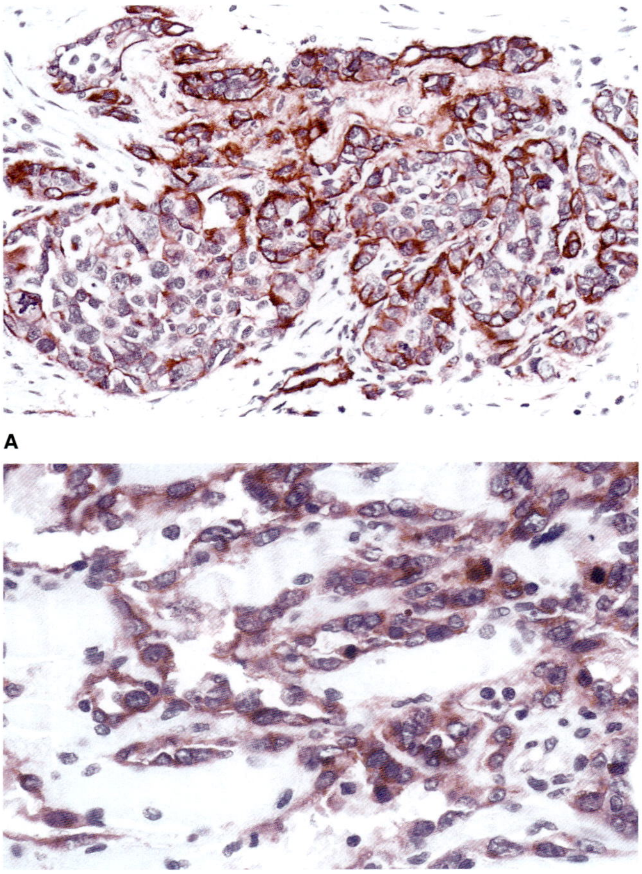

A

B

Figure 14–17. Immunohistochemical documentation of angiosarcoma. *A,* Significant proportion of tumor cells in the peritoneal angiosarcoma are positive for CD31 in a membrane pattern. *B,* Postmastectomy angiosarcoma cells infiltrating skeletal muscle are positive for VEGFR3.

Genetics

All cytogenetic studies on angiosarcomas including cutaneous, postmastectomy, deep soft tissue angiosarcomas, and tumors with epithelioid morphology have shown complex changes. Abnormalities seen more than once include losses of chromosome 22 and 7pter-p15 and gains of 5pter-p11 and 8p12-qter, and 20pter-q12.[146–148]

Kaposi Sarcoma

Kaposi sarcoma (KS) was named after an Austro-Hungarian dermatologist Moritz Kaposi, who reported the first examples of this tumor. KS is a primarily cutaneous malignant vascular tumor, but it can also involve internal organs. It occurs in four clinicopathologically distinctive forms: classic, epidemic form associated with AIDS, endemic in Africa, and iatrogenic, immunosuppression associated.[149,150] The histologic features of the different forms are essentially identical.

Etiology and Pathogenesis

The uniformly strong association with KS and HHV8 (formerly known as Kaposi sarcoma-associated herpesvirus) indicates that this virus is the key etiologic factor for KS; this is perhaps the best demonstrated connection between a virus and human mesenchymal neoplasia. HHV8 is a γ-herpesvirus that can be demonstrated by polymerase chain reaction in all forms of KS. Sexual and parenteral transmission of HHV8 is a likely route of infection, and immunosuppression is a factor promoting its manifestation in AIDS and transplantation patients. HHV8 has also been implicated in certain body cavity-based B-cell lymphomas and multicentric Castleman disease, and it may have a role in multiple myeloma.[151–153]

The mechanism of HHV8 tumorigenesis probably relates to interference of the viral proteins, such as cyclin and bcl-2 analogs, with the host tumor suppressor pathways. Endothelial growth promoting cytokine/growth factor analogs are also produced by the tumor. Viral interferon regulatory factor in turn causes overexpression of the endogenous c-myc (onco)gene.[150]

Clinical Features

Classic (chronic) KS presents in older patients usually over 60 years with a marked (over 10:1) male predominance. The populations most commonly affected as those of Ashkenazi Jewish or Mediterranean origin; the latter also appear to have a higher seroprevalence of HHV8 infection. In the classic form, single or multiple purple to reddish skin lesions develop predominantly in the distal parts of lower extremities, sometimes in the hands and occasionally in other peripheral sites, such as the penile skin. Significant association with other malignancies, especially lymphomas and leukemias, has been demonstrated. The disease is clinically indolent, although the tumors are often multifocal and recur locally. Local excisions and radiation therapy usually give long remissions.[149,150]

Epidemic KS, which is associated with AIDS, is probably the most common form of KS globally. It occurs especially in male homosexual AIDS patients and is rare in those who contracted AIDS by transfusion. Its incidence in AIDS patients is higher in some major urban areas, but appears now to be decreasing. In addition to skin, it involves a wide variety of body sites, especially lymph nodes and oral and gastrointestinal mucosa. In fulminant disease, there may be massive involvement of lungs, liver, peritoneum, and other internal organs. Disseminated KS historically occurred in 10% to 20% of patients with AIDS-KS. The overall survival of AIDS-KS was only 17 months in the early 1990s before the modern treatment. Some evidence indicates that the new antiretroviral treatment also helps against AIDS-KS.

Endemic KS occurs in sub-Saharan equatorial Africa, where it is a common cancer type in many countries. It involves both children and adults and ranges from indolent disease with peripheral skin disease to fulminant multiorgan involvement. The latter typically involves lymph nodes (lymphadenopathic KS). Systemic chemotherapy combined with radiation have been the most important forms of treatment.

Iatrogenic, immunosuppression-associated KS usually occurs in transplant patients, most commonly renal and liver transplant patients, who receive immunosuppressive therapy to counter rejection. In this setting, the KS develops on average 16 months after the transplantation and has less striking male predominance than other forms of KS.[154–156] In transplant patients KS appears to be a reactivation of smoldering HHV8 infection triggered by the immunosuppression. This is supported by a markedly higher incidence of KS in patients from areas or ethnic groups with a higher incidence of KS. The disease usually regresses after cessation of immunosuppression, although often at the cost of a renal transplant. It may involve skin, mucosal surfaces, and internal organs.

Pathology

Grossly, the skin lesions develop through several stages: patch, plaquelike, and nodular. The early lesion is grossly a macular nonpalpable lesion that develops into a palpable plaque and then to a red elevated nodule that may be ulcerated.

Histologically, the earliest patch lesions are often difficult to diagnose because they mainly consist of dilated, irregularly shaped vascular channels, perivascular lymphocytes, and plasma cells. However, there is capillary neovascularization arising from dilated vessels, mainly involving the upper or entire reticular dermis. The presence of small numbers of atypical spindle cells around the neovascularization is diagnostically helpful.[157,158]

A plaquelike lesion contains atypical spindle cells dissecting between the collagen fibers and dispersed throughout the dermis and often extending to the subcutis. Neovascular channels, hemorrhage, hemosiderin, and lymphoplasmacytic infiltration are also present (Fig. 14–18). A peculiar feature often seen in developing KS lesions is the presence of apoptotic endothelial cells.

The nodular lesion typically forms an exophytic growth surrounded by an epithelial collar, similar to that seen in lobular capillary hemangioma. The lesion is composed of sheets of atypical spindle cells in an irregular fascicular, sarcomatous pattern. The background usually contains extravasated erythrocytes. Typical are cytoplasmic pink hyaline globules seen in at least some cells in most lesions, although a small number of globules can also be seen in the earlier stages of the lesion (Fig. 14–18). These globules that can be highlighted with periodic acid-Schiff stain appear to represent partially digested intralysosomal remains of erythrocytes.[159]

A rare form of cutaneous KS lesion, the lymphangiomatous variant, contains permeative infiltration of lymphatic-like vessels and scant if any spindle cell component, inflammation, or hyaline globules making the distinction of this variant from lymphangioma very difficult.

Lymph node involvement may be focal and only seen in the subcapsular area, but when extensive it may cause nodal effacement. Its cellular composition is similar to that of cutaneous KS.

Immunohistochemistry and Cell of Origin

The spindle cells in KS lesions are positive for endothelial cell markers CD31, CD34,[160] whereas they are typically negative for von Willebrand factor, S-100 protein, actins, desmin, keratins, and endothelial membrane antigen. These findings help to separate KS from smooth muscle and myofibroblastic tumors.

The origin of KS has been suggested to be the lymphatic endothelium because of shared enzyme histochemical positivity for 5′-nucleotidase.[161] Shared

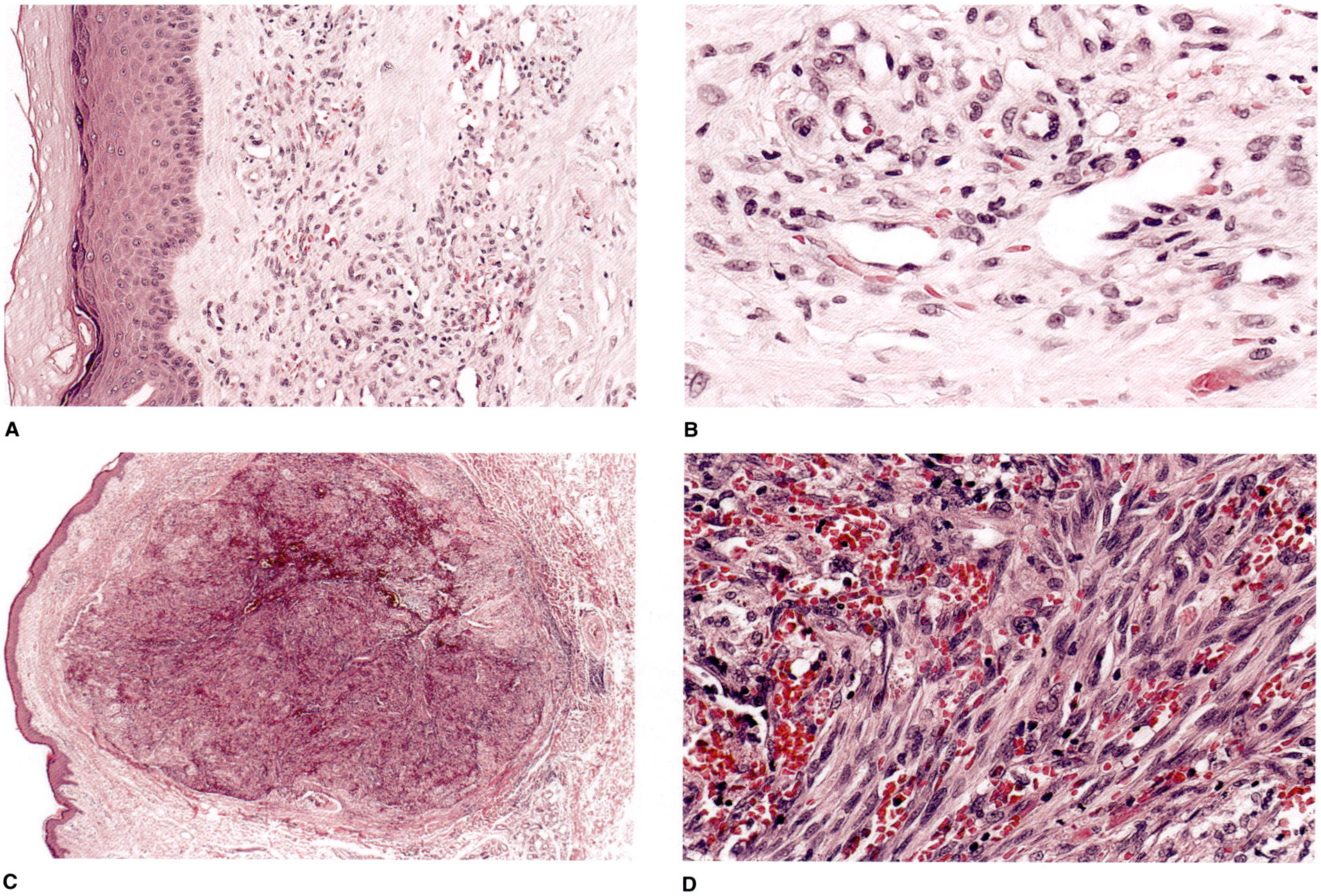

Figure 14–18. Kaposi sarcoma. *A,* An early lesion forms a dermal patch or plaque containing increased number of capillaries surrounded by spindle cells and scattered lymphocytes or plasma cells. *B,* Higher magnification of the early lesion shows atypia spindle cells and a few lymphocytes around the capillaries. *C,* A well-developed lesion forms a circumscribed dermal nodule. *D,* Histologically typical is the hemorrhagic spindle cell proliferation with foci of intracytoplasmic eosinophilic hyaline globules.

expression of VEGFR3 in lymphatic endothelia and KS has also been interpreted to suggest lymphatic origin,[162] although more recently VEGFR3 has been shown in a variety of nonlymphatic endothelia in hemangiomas and neovascular endothelia of tumors.[141]

Differential Diagnosis: KS versus Angiosarcoma

The clinical setting and generally less developed vasoformation separates KS from angiosarcoma, but advanced and systemic lesions may morphologically approach angiosarcoma. Although early reports to the contrary exist,[163] angiosarcomas of liver[164] and soft tissue and skin[165] have been found negative for HHV8 by polymerase chain reaction.

Vascular Tumors of Nonendothelial Origin

Hemangiopericytoma

Despite the name, there is no convincing evidence that hemangiopericytoma is a pericytic tumor. Although original cell culture and ultrastructural observations seemed to support a pericytic derivation, this has not been confirmed by immunohistochemistry (almost always smooth muscle actin negative). Hemangiopericytoma conceptually overlaps with solitary fibrous tumors of soft tissue, and morphologic evidence suggests that these tumors represent a continuum (see Chapter 5). However, a genetic link will be necessary to fully establish or refute their relationship, and this is still missing.

Some sarcomas (especially synovial sarcoma and mesenchymal chondrosarcoma) and certain carcinomas can have a hemangiopericytoma-like pattern.[166,167] Therefore, other specific tumors have to be ruled out before a diagnosis of malignant hemangiopericytoma is made. Most tumors in small children with a hemangiopericytoma-like pattern represent infantile myofibromas (see Chapter 6).

Sinonasal hemangiopericytoma is a peculiar site-specific tumor that differs from ordinary hemangiopericytoma clinically and histologically; it will be discussed separately.

Clinical Features

Hemangiopericytoma usually occurs in adult patients in a wide age range and wide variety of locations. The larger series of peripheral hemangiopericytomas showed a median age of 45 years and no sex predilection. Rare familial occurrence has been reported.[168–171]

The most common locations are the meninges, orbit, lower extremity (thigh), retroperitoneum, pelvis, and other peripheral soft tissues. The location is usually deep, intramuscular, but subcutaneous presentation is also possible. The tumors generally present as space-occupying lesions and in the pelvis and retroperitoneum they often reach a considerable size (>10-15 cm). Hypoglycemia has been documented in some cases, similar to solitary fibrous tumor, further suggesting a conceptual relationship. Surgically, hemangiopericytomas are notable by their tendency to bleed massively. Therefore, preoperative embolization of tumor vessels with particles is often performed to reduce operative bleeding.

Meningeal hemangiopericytomas, previously called angioblastic meningiomas, have been well studied. They are difficult to control surgically and tend to recur repeatedly and some ultimately metastasize, often after long intervals. Metastases develop especially to bones and lungs. Long-term cure is achieved in only 25% of patients.[172–174]

In contrast to their meningeal counterparts, the majority of peripheral hemangiopericytomas have a benign behavior. This is especially true for the tumors that show fewer than 4 mitoses/10 HPF. The largest series documented a 70% 10-year survival.[168] Metastases rarely develop, sometimes long after primary surgery, and sometimes following spindle cell sarcomatous transformation, which may be seen in the primary tumor as well as in the recurrence. The metastases develop in bones and lungs, similar to meningeal hemangiopericytoma.

Pathology

Grossly, hemangiopericytomas are circumscribed oval tumors surrounded by a fibrous pseudocapsule. On sectioning they may have a spongy appearance because of vascular slits and vary from yellowish tan to reddish. Yellowish green zones of necrosis may be present. The tumors in peripheral soft tissues vary from small subcutaneous nodules of 1 to 3 cm to large, deep intramuscular and retroperitoneal masses that are commonly over 10 cm and may reach the size of 20 cm.

Histologically, hemangiopericytomas have a prominent vascular pattern with gaping vessels lined by a single layer of normal-appearing or attenuated endothelia (Fig. 14–19*A* and *B*). Some vessels are surrounded by a zone of perivascular hyalinization. Continuous intercellular network is typically highlighted with a reticulin stain, used in the classical definition of hemangiopericytoma.

Cytologically, the tumor cells are typically uniform, oval to slightly spindled, with round or oval nuclei

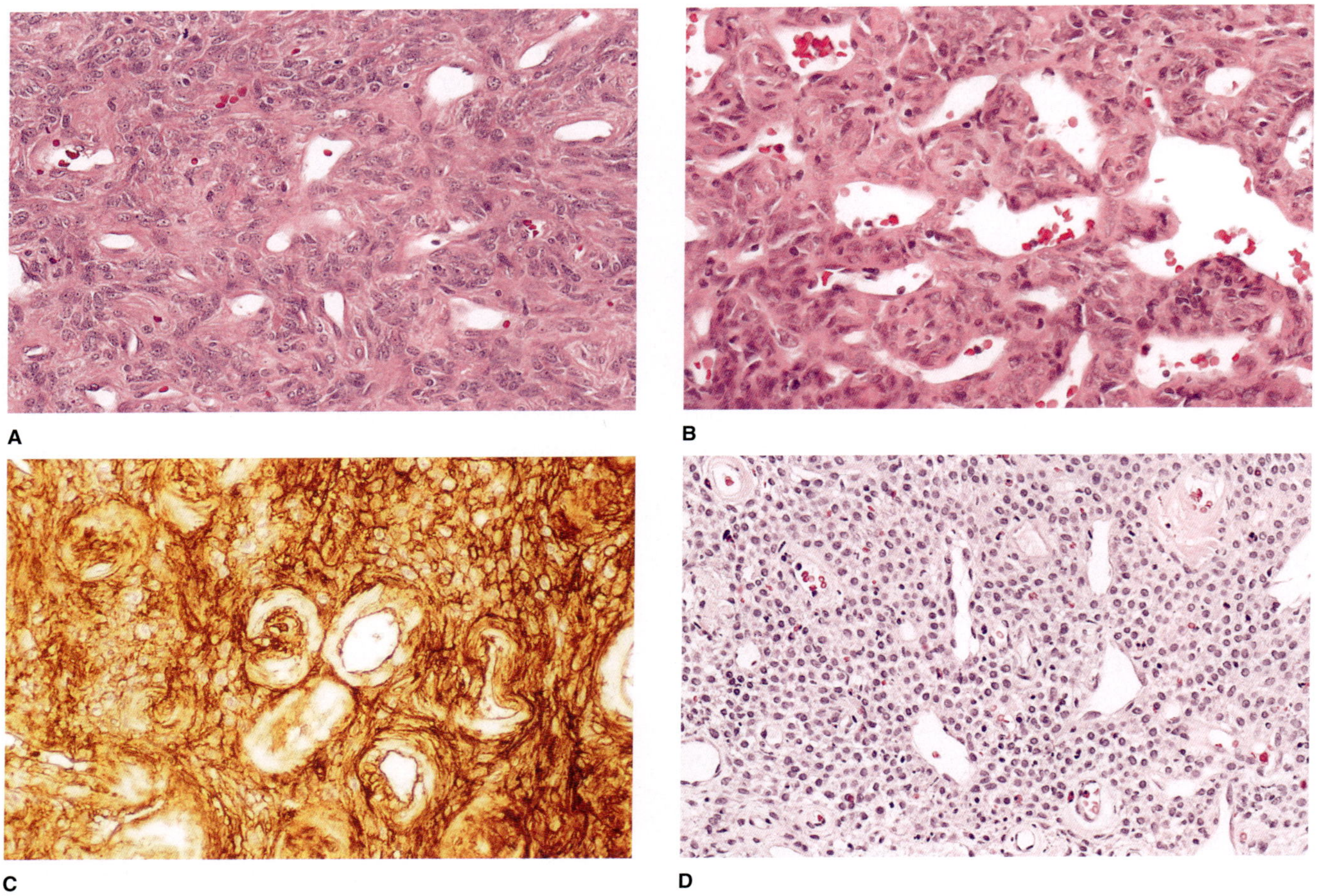

Figure 14–19. Variants of hemangiopericytoma. *A* and *B,* Typical examples with a staghorn-like vascular pattern and proliferation of uniform interstitial cells. *C,* Prominent CD34 positivity in a hemangiopericytoma with perivascular sclerosis. *D,* Sinonasal hemangiopericytoma is a histologically different tumor showing pericellular clearing.

and poorly visible cell borders. Mitotic rate is generally low (up to 3/10 HPF). A mitotic rate of 4 or more per 10 HPF and presence of coagulative necrosis, nuclear pleomorphism, and areas of spindle cell sarcomatous transformation are signs indicating malignancy.

Histologic Variant—Lipomatous Hemangiopericytoma

A peculiar variant with a mature fat component in a histologically typical hemangiopericytoma has been termed lipomatous hemangiopericytoma. Its clinicopathologic features seem to be similar to ordinary hemangiopericytoma,[175,176] but no malignant examples have been documented.

Immunohistochemistry and Ultrastructure

The tumor cells are mesenchymal cells that are typically positive for vimentin and CD34 (Fig. 14–19C) and negative for markers of endothelia (FVIIIRAg, CD31), desmin, and keratins. With rare exceptions, they do not have phenotypic features of mature pericytes and are negative for smooth muscle actin. One study compared meningeal hemangiopericytomas with solitary fibrous tumors of the same location and found the immunophenotypes similar, except that hemangiopericytomas had a less prominent (patchy) CD34 expression.[177] However, others have found widespread CD34 expression.[178]

Ultrastructurally, hemangiopericytoma seems to show evidence of pericyte-like differentiation with the tumor cells showing cytoplasmic processes, basal lamina material, and intimate relationship with complex capillaries. However, phenotypically the tumor cells are not fully comparable with adult pericytes, but rather with immature, developing pericytes.[179]

Differential Diagnosis

Many other tumors can have a hemangiopericytoma-like histologic pattern. Notable sarcomas with such features are monophasic and poorly differentiated synovial sarcoma, mesenchymal chondrosarcoma, and certain liposarcomas. Epithelial tumors that can have a hemangiopericytoma-like pattern include variants of thymomas and poorly differentiated thyroid carcinomas. These diagnoses should be ruled out before a diagnosis of thymic or thyroid hemangiopericytoma is made. The separation from solitary fibrous tumor is based on the prominent vascular pattern and more ovoid versus spindle cell pattern, but in many cases this distinction is arbitrary.

Genetics

Data are scant. A recurrent t(12;19) translocation has been reported in several cases. The occurrence of this translocation in both meningeal and peripheral tumors supports their relationship;[180,181] other translocations such as t(13;22) have also been reported.[182] Meningeal tumors do not have similar *NF2* gene mutations as seen in meningiomas, supporting different pathogenesis and lack of relationship between these tumors.[183]

Sinonasal Hemangiopericytoma

Clinical Features

This hemangiopericytoma subtype, or hemangiopericytoma-like tumor, as it is sometimes called, is a rare tumor that usually occurs in adults in the sixth and seventh decades. The tumor may involve the paranasal sinuses and protrude to the nasal cavity, or primarily involve the latter. Clinically, it can resemble a nasal inflammatory polyp. The tumor is usually relatively small, 2 to 3 cm, but occasionally has been larger than 5 cm.[184,185] It has a high tendency for recurrence (40–50%), often after a long interval, but it is questionable whether bona fide examples ever metastasize. It should be noted that conventional hemangiopericytomas/solitary fibrous tumors may also occur in the sinonasal area.

Pathology

Grossly, the tumor is a polypoid submucosal lesion. Histologically, the tumor is composed of sheets of markedly uniform spindled to oval cells. The tumor is highly vascularized, but the vessels have a less developed gaping profile, as typically observed in ordinary hemangiopericytoma. Retraction of the cytoplasm often gives the tumor a clear cell appearance. Mitotic rate is usually low (Fig. 14–19*D*). Immunohistochemical studies have demonstrated actin expression, but the tumor is negative for keratins, desmin, endothelial cell markers, and CD34; negativity for the latter differs from peripheral hemangiopericytoma.

Glomus Tumor

Glomus tumor is a mesenchymal tumor with cell differentiation similar to the specialized smooth muscle cells of the glomus bodies that regulate peripheral blood flow. The normal glomus bodies can be found in fingers and in the coccygeal region; such structures measuring 1 to 3 mm in diameter can be seen as incidental findings in surgical excisions from those locations and should not be confused with tumors. A great majority of glomus tumors are benign, but atypical and malignant examples exist. The designation "glomus tumor" has historically also been applied to jugulotympanic paragangliomas (glomus jugulare, glomus tympanicum); paraganglioma is the proper designation for these tumors.

Clinical Features

Glomus tumors are more commonly diagnosed in young adults, but they occur in a wide age range. Female predominance has been documented for subungual lesions.[186] Glomus tumors arise in a variety of superficial soft tissue locations, but most distinctive is their occurrence in the nailbed area, consistent with the concept that they are related to the perivascular glomus cells that regulate blood flow in distal extremities. Glomus tumors may also occur in more proximal parts of the extremities and sometimes in the trunk.

The subungual glomus tumors are typically small, only a few millimeters in diameter, and they typically are painful, as are glomus tumors of other soft tissue sites.[186] Benign glomus tumors may recur, and rare malignant variants occur. They most commonly metastasize to the lungs and sometimes to intestines or mesenteries.

The stomach is the origin of nearly all gastrointestinal glomus tumors,[187] where multiple apparently intravascular tumors have also been reported.[188] According to our experience, these tumors occur in adult patients of a wide age range, with a significant female predominance. Nearly all follow a benign clinical course, despite that many have apparent vascular invasion and that many have focal cytologic atypia. However, rare malignant gastric glomus tumors may metastasize to the liver. In our experience, malignant behavior is a rare and unpredictable occurrence in a gastric glomus tumor.[189]

Pathology

Most glomus tumors are circumscribed ovoid or round superficial yellowish to tan-red nodules that measure a few millimeters in diameter. Some reach a larger size, usually less than 2 cm. Most of them are located in the dermis or subcutis, and rare examples are intramuscular. The tumor may be solid or mucoid on sectioning, and some examples are cystic and others surrounded by a fibrous capsule.

Histologically, the peripheral glomus tumors of the skin and soft tissues are composed of uniform, round or slightly polygonal, epithelioid-like cells with sharp cellular borders and eosinophilic cytoplasm. Some tumors have cytoplasmic vacuolization, and others have alternating areas of smaller and larger cells. The cells may be embedded in a myxoid

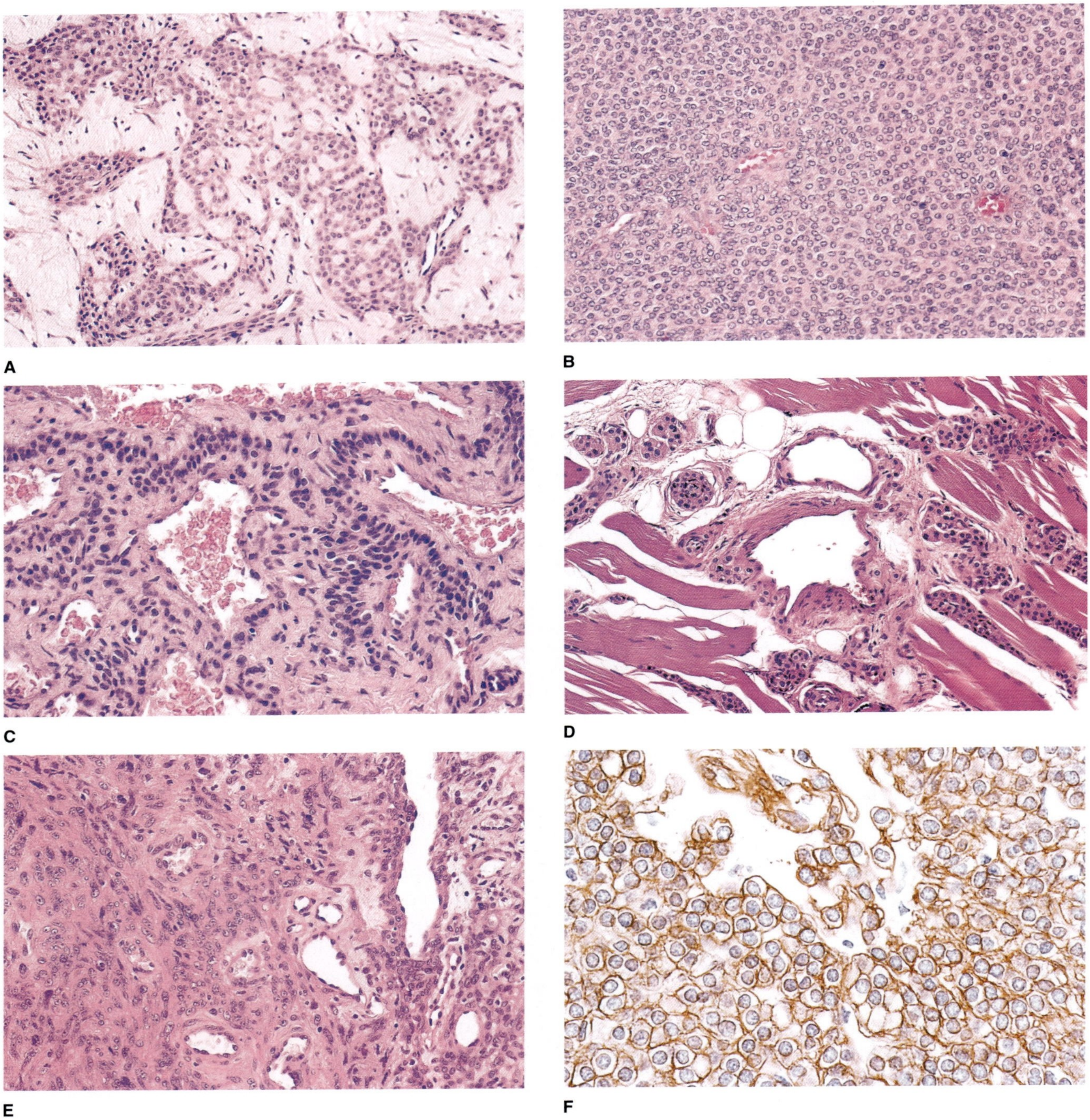

Figure 14-20. Different appearances of a glomus tumor. *A,* Glomus tumor composed of cords of tumor cells in a myxoid stroma. *B,* Glomus tumor with a solid pattern. *C,* Glomangioma with prominent blood vessels. *D,* A rare glomus tumor diffusely involving the skeletal muscle. *E,* Glomangiosarcoma arising in a glomus tumor as an atypical spindle cell proliferation. *F,* Prominent pericellular laminin positivity typically forms a netlike pattern around the glomus cells.

stroma, present as solid sheets (Fig. 14–20) or as a thin layer around cavernously dilated vascular spaces. The latter variant has also been called glomangioma. Some glomus tumors are dispersed as small clusters in fibrous stroma, and many have areas of hemorrhage with focal hemosiderin.

Gastric glomus tumors are usually relatively small (2–4 cm), but they occasionally exceed 5 cm. Histologically, they have a tendency to have significant solid components, often with hemangiopericytoma-like pattern, but are otherwise similar to their peripheral counterparts. Despite the presence of apparent vascular invasion (intravascular growth) in some cases, most tumors behave in a benign manner.[189] It is uncertain at present which criteria may predict malignant behavior of a gastric glomus tumor, but the presence of atypia or increased mitotic rate (>5/50 HPF) have to be viewed as similarly worrisome, similar to the criteria used for the gastrointestinal stromal tumors.

Very rarely glomus tumors occur intramuscularly, and such lesions may be diffuse (glomangiomatosis, Fig. 14–20*D*). Glomangiomatosis thus represents angiomatosis with a glomus cell component; it is clinically benign.

Atypical and Malignant Glomus Tumors

The cytologically atypical, mitotically active, or overtly sarcomatous glomus tumors are rare, probably much less than 5% of all glomus tumors. The recognition of such sarcomatous tumors has to be based on the presence of foci conventional glomus tumor in the periphery. The proposed definitions, based on a recent large series[190] are:

- Glomus tumor with nuclear atypia (symplastic glomus tumor) is a small tumor with marked focal atypia but low mitotic rate. Tumors with these features do not have increased risk for recurrence.
- Glomus tumors with risk for malignant behavior (malignant glomus tumor, glomangiosarcoma) are the ones that are intramuscular and over 2 cm, or the ones with atypical mitoses or marked atypia with regular mitoses (>5/50 HPF); 38% of such tumors were found to metastasize. The malignant glomus tumor may have a round cell (glomus cell) or spindle cell morphology (Fig. 14–20*E*). Vascular invasion may also occur; however, this feature may also be seen in benign glomus tumors.
- Glomus tumors with superficial location but mitotic activity more than 5/50 HPF and all large and deep tumors have to be considered as having an uncertain malignant potential.
- Infiltrative glomus tumors in deep locations often recur locally, but they do not seem to metastasize.[191]

Immunohistochemistry and Ultrastructure

The glomus tumor cells are positive for vimentin and smooth muscle actin, and 20% to 30% are focally or extensively positive for CD34. Laminin and collagen IV-positive basement membranes are surrounding the tumor cells in a netlike pattern (Fig. 14–20*F*). Expression of heavy caldesmon and calponin is variable. Almost all glomus tumors are negative for desmin. They are also negative for keratins and S-100 protein.[192,193]

Electron microscopic studies have documented smooth muscle features in the glomus cells: prominent actin bundles, pinocytic vesicles, and basement membranes.[194] Genetic changes in glomus tumor are unknown.

Differential Diagnosis

Glomus tumors can resemble certain skin adnexal tumors, especially more solid variants of eccrine acrospiroma. Presence of ductular structures, more clear cytoplasm, and keratin expression help to identify the latter. The superficial variants of Ewing family tumors can be distinguished by their much higher cellularity and scant cytoplasm.

Hemangiopericytoma is composed of less differentiated cells with scant cytoplasm. This tumor almost uniformly lacks markers for smooth muscle cells, in contrast to glomus tumor.

REFERENCES

Classification of Vascular Tumors

1. Enzinger FM, Weiss SW: Soft Tissue Tumors, 3rd ed. St. Louis, Mosby, 1995:579–676.
2. Requena L, Sangueza OP: Cutaneous vascular proliferations. Part II. Hyperplasias and benign neoplasms. J Am Acad Dermatol 1997;37:887–919.
3. Kempson RL, Fletcher CDM, Evans HL, Hendrickson MR, Sibley RK: Vascular tumors. In Atlas of Soft Tissue Tumors, Armed Forces Institute of Pathology, Washington, DC, 2001:307–370.

Biology of Endothelia and Angiogenesis

4. Cines DB, Pollak ES, Buck CA, et al: Endothelial cells in physiology and in the pathophysiology of vascular disorders. Blood 1998;91:3527–3561.
5. Cotran RS, Mayadas-Norton T: Endothelial adhesion molecules in health and disease. Pathol Biol (Paris) 1998;46:164–170.
6. Carmeliet P: Mechanisms of angiogenesis and arteriogenesis. Nat Med 2000;6:389–395.
7. Folkman J: Angiogenesis and angiogenesis inhibition: An overview. EXS 1997;79:1–8.

8. Ferrara N, Alitalo K: Clinical applications of angiogenic growth factors and their inhibitors. Nat Med 1999;5:1359–1364.

Bacillary Angiomatosis

9. Stoler MH, Bonfiglio TA, Steigbigel RT, Pereira M: An atypical subcutaneous infection associated with acquired immunodeficiency syndrome. Am J Clin Pathol 1983;80:714–718.
10. LeBoit PE, Berger TG, Egbert BM, Beckstead JH, Yen TS, Stoler MH: Bacillary angiomatosis. The histopathology and differential diagnosis of a pseudoneoplastic infection in patients with human immunodeficiency virus disease. Am J Surg Pathol 1989;13:909–920.
11. Schinella RA, Greco MA: Bacillary angiomatosis presenting as a soft-tissue tumor without skin involvement. Hum Pathol 1990;21:567–569.
12. Cockerell CJ, Tierno PM, Friedman-Kien AE, Kim KS: Clinical, histologic, micro-biologic, and biochemical characterization of the causative agent of bacillary (epithelioid) angiomatosis: A rickettsial illness with features of bartonellosis. J Invest Dermatol 1991;97: 812–817.
13. Tsang WY, Chan JK: Bacillary angiomatosis. A "new" disease with a broadening clinicopathologic spectrum. Histol Histopathol 1992;7:143–152.
14. Koehler JE, Sanchez MA, Garrido CS, et al: Molecular epidemiology of bartonella infections in patients with bacillary angiomatosis-peliosis. N Engl J Med 1997; 337:1876–1883.
15. Reed JA, Brigati DJ, Flynn SD, et al: Immunocytochemical identification of *Rochalimaea henselae* in bacillary (epithelioid) angiomatosis, parenchymal bacillary peliosis, and persistent fever with bacteremia. Am J Surg Pathol 1992;16:650–657.

Verruga Peruana

16. Arias-Stella J, Lieberman PH, Erlandson RA, Arias-Stella J Jr: Histology, immunohistochemistry, and ultrastructure of the verruga in Carrion's disease. Am J Surg Pathol 1986;10:595–610.
17. Arias-Stella J, Lieberman PH, Garcia-Caceres U, Erlandson RA, Kruger H, Arias-Stella J Jr: Verruga peruana mimicking malignant neoplasms. Am J Dermatopathol 1987;9:279–291.
18. Garcia FU, Wojta J, Broadley KN, Davidson JM, Hoover RL: Bartonella bacilliformis stimulates endothelial cells in vitro and is angiogenic in vivo. Am J Pathol 1990; 136:1125–1135.

Syndromes Related to Hemangiomas

19. Fernandes S, Silva A, Coelho A, Campos M, Pontes F: Blue rubber bleb nevus: Case report and literature review. Eur J Gastroenterol Hepatol 1999;11:455–457.
20. Couch V, Lindor NM, Karnes PS, Michels VV: von Hippel-Lindau disease. Mayo Clin Proc 2000;75: 265–272.
21. You CK, Rees J, Gillis DA, Steeves J: Klippel-Trenaunay syndrome: A review. Can J Surg 1983;26:399–403.
22. Paller AS: The Sturge-Weber syndrome. Pediatr Dermatol 1987;4:300–304.
23. El'Dessouky M, Azmy AF, Raine PAM: Kasabach-Meritt syndrome. J Pediatr Surg 1988;23:109–111.
24. Lewis RJ, Ketcham AS: Mafucci's syndrome. Functional and neoplastic significance. J Bone Joint Surg 1973:55A:1465–1479.

Capillary Hemangioma, Including Cellular Type

25. Weiss SW: Vascular tumors: A deductive approach to diagnosis. Surg Pathol 1989;2:185–201.
26. Coffin CM, Dehner LP: Vascular tumors in children and adolescents: A clinicopathologic study of 228 tumors in 222 patients. Pathol Annu 1993;1:97–120.
27. Gonzalez-Crussi F, Reyes-Mugica M: Cellular hemangiomas of infancy ("hemangioendotheliomas"). Light microscopic, immunohistochemical, and ultrastructural observations. Am J Surg Pathol 1991;15:769–778.
28. Enjolras O, Riche MC, Merland JJ, Escande JP: Management of alarming hemangiomas of infancy: A review of 25 cases. Pediatrics 1990;85:491–498.
29. Hunt SJ, Santa Cruz DJ, Barr RJ: Microvenular hemangioma. J Cutan Pathol 1991;18:235–240.
30. Kumakiri M, Muramoto F, Tsukinaga I, Yoshida T, Ohura T, Miura Y: Crystalline lamellae in the endothelial cells of a type of hemangioma characterized by the proliferation of immature endothelial cells and pericytes-angioblastoma. J Am Acad Dermatol 1983; 8:68–75.
31. North PE, Waner M, Mizeracki A, Mihm M Jr: GLUT1: A newly discovered immunohistochemical marker for juvenile hemangiomas. Hum Pathol 2000; 31:11–22.

Pyogenic Granuloma (Lobular Capillary Hemangioma)

32. Patrice SJ, Wiss K, Mulliken JB: Pyogenic granuloma (lobular capillary hemangioma) pathologic study of 178 cases. Pediatr Dermatol 1991;8:267–276.
33. Mills SE, Cooper PH, Fechner RE: Lobular capillary hemangioma: The underlying lesion of pyogenic granuloma. Am J Surg Pathol 1980:4:471–479.
34. Warner J, Wilson-Jones E: Pyogenic granuloma with multiple satellites: A report of 11 cases. Br J Dermatol 1968;80:218–227.
35. Cooper PH, McAllister HA, Helwig EB: Intravenous pyogenic granuloma. A study of 18 cases. Am J Surg Pathol 1979;3:221–228.
36. Ulbright TM, Santa-Cruz DJ: Intravenous pyogenic granuloma. Cancer 1980;45:1646–1652.

Acquired Tufted Angioma (Angioblastoma of Nakagawa)

37. Wilson-Jones E, Orkin M: Tufted angioma (angioblastoma). A benign progressive angioma not to be confused with Kaposi's sarcoma or low-grade angiosarcoma. J Am Acad Dermatol 1989;20:214–225.

38. Alessi E, Bertani E, Sala F: Acquired tufted angioma. Am J Dermatopathol 1986;8:426–429.
39. Padilla RS, Orkin M, Rosai J: Acquired "tufted" angioma (progressive capillary hemangioma). A distinctive clinicopathologic entity related to lobular capillary hemangioma. Am J Dermatopathol 1987; 9:292–300.
40. Cho KH, Kim SH, Park KC, et al: Angio-blastoma (Nakagawa)—Is it the same as tufted angioma? Clin Exp Dermatol 1991;16:110–113.

Targetoid Hemosiderotic Hemangioma and Hobnail Hemangioma

41. Santa-Cruz DJ, Aronberg J: Targetoid hemosiderotic hemangioma. J Am Acad Dermatol 1988;19:550–558.
42. Guillou L, Calonje E, Speight P, Rosai J, Fletcher CD: Hobnail hemangioma: A pseudomalignant vascular lesion with a reappraisal of targetoid hemosiderotic hemangioma. Am J Surg Pathol 1999;23:97–105.
43. Mentzel T, Partanen T, Kutzner H: Hobnail hemangioma ("targetoid hemosiderotic hemangioma"): Clinicopathologic and immunohistochemical analysis of 62 cases. J Cutan Pathol 1999;26:279–286.

Cavernous and Intramuscular Hemangioma and Angiomatosis

44. Calonje E, Fletcher CDM: Sinusoidal hemangioma. A distinctive benign vascular neoplasm within the group of cavernous hemangiomas. Am J Surg Pathol 1991; 14:1130–1135.
45. Allen PW, Enzinger FM: Hemangiomas of skeletal muscle: An analysis of 89 cases. Cancer 1972;29:8–23.
46. Beham A, Fletcher CDM: Intramuscular angioma: A clinicopathological analysis of 74 cases. Histopathology 1991;18:53–59.
47. Howat AJ, Campbell PE: Angiomatosis: A vascular malformation of infancy and childhood. Pathology 1987;19:377–382.
48. Rao VK, Weiss SW: Angiomatosis of soft tissue: An analysis of the histological features and clinical outcome in 51 cases. Am J Surg Pathol 1992;16:764–771.

Littoral Cell Angioma of the Spleen and Other Splenic Angiomas

49. Falk S, Stutte HJ, Frizzera G: Littoral cell angioma. A novel splenic vascular lesion demonstrating histiocytic differentiation. Am J Surg Pathol 1991;15:1023–1033.
50. Bisceglia M, Sickel JZ, Giangaspero F, Gomes V, Amini M, Michal M: Littoral cell angioma of the spleen: An additional report of four cases with emphasis on the association with visceral organ cancers. Tumori 1998; 84:595–599.
51. Arber DA, Stricker JG, Chen YY, Weiss LM: Splenic vascular tumors: A histologic, immunophenotypic, and virologic study. Am J Surg Pathol 1997;21:827–835.
52. Zukerberg LR, Kaynor BL, Silverman ML, Harris NL: Splenic hamartoma and capillary hemangioma are distinct entities: Immunohistochemical analysis of CD68 expression by endothelial cells. Hum Pathol 1991;22: 1258–1261.

Epithelioid Hemangioma and Kimura Disease

53. Kung ITM, Gibson JB, Bannatyne PM: Kimura's disease: A clinicopathologic study of 21 cases and its distinction from angiolymphoid hyperplasia with eosinophilia. Pathology 1984;16:39–44.
54. Urabe A, Tsuneyoshi M, Enjoji M: Epithelioid hemangioma versus Kimura's disease. A comparative clinicopathologic study. Am J Surg Pathol 1987;11: 758–766.
55. Chan JK, Hui PK, Ng CS, Yuen NW, Kung IT, Gwi E: Epithelioid hemangioma (angiolymphoid hyperplasia with eosinophilia) and Kimura's disease in Chinese. Histopathology 1989;15:557–574.
56. Kuo TT, Shih LY, Chan HL: Kimura's disease. Involvement of regional lymph nodes and distinction from angiolymphoid hyperplasia with eosinophilia. Am J Surg Pathol 1988;12:843–854.
57. Motoi M, Wahid S, Horie Y, Akagi T: Kimura's disease: Clinical, histological and immunohistochemical studies. Acta Med Okayama 1992;46:449–455.
58. Li TJ, Chen XM, Wang SZ, Fan MW, Semba I, Kitano M: Kimura's disease: A clinicopathologic study of 54 Chinese patients. Oral Surg Oral Med Oral Pathol Oral Radiol Endod 1996;82:549–555.

Epitheloid Hemangioma

59. Rosai J: Angiolymphoid hyperplasia with eosinophilia of the skin. Its nosological position in the spectrum of histiocytoid hemangioma. Am J Dermatopathol 1982; 4:175–184.
60. Olsen TG, Helwig EB: Angiolymphoid hyperplasia with eosinophilia: A clinicopathologic study of 116 patients. J Am Acad Dermatol 1985;12:781–796.
61. Fetsch JF, Weiss SW: Observations concerning the pathogenesis of epithelioid hemangioma (angiolymphoid hyperplasia). Mod Pathol 1991;4:449–455.
62. Kitamura H, Ito S, Kuwana N, Yutani C: Epithelioid hemangioma of the temporal artery clinically mimicking temporal arteritis. Pathol Int 1999;49:831–835.
63. Banks ER, Mills SE: Histiocytoid (epithelioid) hemangioma of the testis. The so-called vascular variant of "adenomatoid tumor." Am J Surg Pathol 1990;14: 584–589.
64. Luthringer DJ, Virmani R, Weiss SW, Rosai J: A distinctive cardiovascular lesion resembling histiocytoid (epithelioid) hemangioma. Evidence suggesting mesothelial participation. Am J Surg Pathol 1990;14:993–1000.

Glomeruloid Hemangioma

65. Soubrier MJ, Dubost JJ, Sauvezie, BJ: POEMS syndrome: A study of 25 cases and a review of the literature. French study Group on POEMS syndrome. Am J Med 1994;97:543–553.

66. Chan JK, Fletcher CD, Hicklin GA, Rosai J: Glomeruloid hemangioma. A distinctive cutaneous lesion of multicentric Castleman's disease associated with POEMS syndrome. Am J Surg Pathol 1990;14: 1036–1046.
67. Kanitakis J, Roger H, Soubrier M: Cutaneous angiomas in POEMS syndrome. An ultrastructural and immunohistochemical study. Arch Dermatol 1988;124:695–698.
68. Belec L, Mohamed AS, Authier FJ, et al: Human herpesvirus 8 infection in patients with POEMS syndrome-associated multicentric Castleman's disease. Blood 1999;93:3643–3653.

Papillary Endothelial Hyperplasia (Masson Tumor)

69. Kuo TT, Salyers CP, Rosai J: Masson's "vegetant intravascular hemangioendothelioma." A lesion often mistaken for angiosarcoma. A study of seventeen cases located in the skin and soft tissues. Cancer 1976; 38:1227–1236.
70. Clearkin KP, Enzinger FM: Intravascular papillary endothelial hyperplasia. Arch Pathol Lab Med 1976; 100:441–444.
71. Hashimoto H, Daimaru Y, Enjoji M: Intravascular papillary endothelial hyperplasia: A clinicopathologic study of 91 cases. Am J Dermatopathol 1983;5:539–546.
72. Amerigo J, Berry CL: Intravascular papillary endothelial hyperplasia in the skin and subcutaneous tissue. Virchows Arch A Pathol Anat Histopathol 1980;387; 81–90.
73. Weiss SW, Enzinger FM: Spindle cell hemangioendothelioma. A low-grade angiosarcoma resembling a cavernous hemangioma and Kaposi's sarcoma. Am J Surg Pathol 1986;10:521–530.
74. Perkins P, Weiss SW: Spindle cell hemangioendothelioma. An analysis of 78 cases with reassessment of its pathogenesis and biologic behavior. Am J Surg Pathol 1996;20:1196–1204.

Spindle Cell Hemangioma (Hemangioendothelioma)

75. Fanburg JC, Meis-Kindblom JM, Rosenberg AE: Multiple enchondromas associated with spindle cell hemangioendotheliomas. An overlooked variant of Maffucci's syndrome. Am J Surg Pathol 1995;19:1029–1038.
76. Fletcher CD, Beham A, Schmid C: Spindle cell hemangioendothelioma: A clinicopathological and immunohistochemical study indicative of a non-neoplastic lesion. Histopathology 1991;18:291–301.
77. Scott GA, Rosai J: Spindle cell hemangioendothelioma. Report of seven additional cases of a recently described vascular neoplasm. Am J Dermatopathol 1988;10:281288.
78. Ding J, Hashimoto H, Imayama S, Tsuneyoshi M, Enjoji M: Spindle cell haemangioendothelioma: Probably a benign vascular lesion not a low-grade angiosarcoma. A clinicopathological, ultrastructural and immunohistochemical study. Virchows Arch A Pathol Anat Histopathol 1992;420:77–85.
79. Fukunaga M, Ushigome S, Nikaido T, Ishikawa E, Nakamori K: Spindle cell hemangioendothelioma: An immunohistochemical and flow cytometric study of six cases. Pathol Int 1995;45:589–595.

Lymphangioma and Related Tumors

80. Flanagan BP, Helwig EB: Cutaneous lymphangioma. Arch Dermatol 1977;113:24–30.
81. Byrne J, Blanc WA, Warburton D, Wigger J: The significance of cystic hygroma in fetuses. Hum Pathol 1984;15:61–67.
82. Kim KM, Choi KY, Lee A, Kim BK: Lymphangioma of large intestine: Report of ten cases with endoscopic and pathologic correlation. Gastrointest Endosc 2000; 52:255–259.
83. Guillou L, Fletcher CDM: Benign lymphangioendothelioma (acquired progressive lymphangioma): A lesion not to be confused with well-differentiated angiosarcoma and patch stage Kaposi's sarcoma. Am J Surg Pathol 2000;24:1047–1057.

Kaposiform Hemangioendothelioma

84. Niedt GW, Greco MA, Wieczorek R, Blanc WA, Knowles DM: Hemangioma with Kaposi's sarcoma-like features: Report of 2 cases. Pediatr Pathol 1989; 9:567–575.
85. Tsang WYW, Chan JKC: Kaposi-like infantile hemangioendothelioma: A distinctive vascular neoplasm of the retroperitoneum. Am J Surg Pathol 1991;15: 982–989.
86. Zukerberg LR, Nickoloff BJ, Weiss SW: Kaposiform hemangioendothelioma of infancy and childhood. An aggressive neoplasm associated with Kasabach-Merritt syndrome and lymphangiomatosis. Am J Surg Pathol 1993;17:321–328.
87. Sarkar M, Mulliken JB, Kozakewich HP, Robertson RL, Burrows PE: Thrombocytopenic coagulopathy (Kasaback-Merritt phenomenon) is associated with kaposiform hemangioendothelioma and not with common infantile hemangioma. Plastic Reconstr Surg 1997;100:1377–1386.

Dabska Tumor (Papillary Intralymphatic Angioendothelioma) and Retiform Hemangioendothelioma

88. Dabska M: Malignant endovascular papillary angioendothelioma of the skin in childhood. Clinicopathologic study of six cases. Cancer 1969;24:503–510.
89. Fanburg-Smith JC, Michal M, Partanen TA, Alitalo K, Miettinen M: Papillary intralymphatic angioendothelioma (PILA). A report of twelve cases of a distinctive vascular tumor with phenotypic features of lymphatic vessels. Am J Surg Pathol 1999;23:1004–1010.
90. Calonje E, Fletcher CD, Wilson-Jones E, Rosai J: Retiform hemangioendothelioma. A distinctive form of low-grade angiosarcoma delineated in a series of 15 cases. Am J Surg Pathol 1994;18:115–125.
91. Duke D, Dvorak AM, Harris TJ, Cohen LM: Multiple retiform hemangioendotheliomas. A low grade angiosarcoma. Am J Dermatopathol 1996;18:606–610.

Epithelioid Hemangioendothelioma

92. Weiss SW, Enzinger FM: Epithelioid hemangioendothelioma: A vascular tumor often mistaken for a carcinoma. Cancer 1982;50:970–981.
93. Weiss SW, Ishak KG, Dail DH, Sweet DE, Enzinger FM: Epithelioid hemangioendothelioma and related lesions. Semin Diagn Pathol 1986;3:259–287.
94. Mentzel T, Beham A, Calonje E, Katenkamp D, Fletcher CD: Epithelioid hemangioendothelioma of skin and soft tissues: Clinicopathologic and immunohistochemical study of 30 cases. Am J Surg Pathol 1997;21:363–374.
95. Ishak KG, Sesterhenn IA, Goodman ZD, Rabin L, Stromeyer FW: Epithelioid hemangioendothelioma of the liver: A clinicopathologic and follow-up study of 32 cases. Hum Pathol 1984;15:839–852.
96. Kelleher MB, Iwatsuki S, Sheahan DG: Epithelioid hemangioendothelioma of liver. Clinicopathological correlations of 10 cases treated by orthotopic liver transplantation. Am J Surg Pathol 1989;13:999–1008.
97. Makhlouf HR, Ishak KG, Goodman ZD: Epithelioid hemangioendothelioma of the liver. A clinicopathologic study of 137 cases. Cancer 1999;85:562–582.
98. Dail DH, Liebow AA, Gmelich JT: Intravascular bronchioloalveolar tumor of lung: An analysis of twenty cases of a peculiar sclerosing endothelial tumor. Cancer 1983;51:452–464.
99. Verbeken E, Beyls J, Moerman P, Knoackaert D, Goddeeris P, Lauweryns JM: Lung metastasis of malignant epithelioid hemangioendothelioma mimicking a primary intravascular bronchioalveolar tumor. A histologic, ultrastructural, and immunohistochemical study. Cancer 1985;55:1741–1746.
100. Boudousquie AC, Lawce HC, Sherman R, Olson S, Magenis RE, Corless CL: Complex translocation [7;22] identified in an epithelioid hemangioendothelioma. Cancer Genet Cytogenet 1996;92:116–121.
101. Mendlick MR, Nelson M, Pickering D, et al: Translocation t(1;3)(p36.3;q25) is a nonrandom aberration in epithelioid hemangioendothelioma. Am J Surg Pathol 2001;25:684–687.

Cutaneous Angiosarcoma

102. Maddox JC, Evans HL: Angiosarcoma of skin and soft tissue: A study of forty-four cases. Cancer 1981; 51:1907–1921.
103. Cooper PH: Angiosarcomas of the skin. Semin Diag Pathol 1987;4:2–17.
104. Holden CA, Spittle MF, Jones EW: Angiosarcoma of the face and scalp: Prognosis and treatment. Cancer 1987;59:1046–1057.
105. Hodgkinson DJ, Soule EH, Woods JE: Cutaneous angiosarcoma of the head and neck. Cancer 1979;44: 1106–1113.

Postradiation Angiosarcoma, Angiosarcoma in Lymphedematous Extremities

106. Moskaluk CA, Merino MJ, Danforth DN, Medeiros LJ: Low-grade angiosarcoma of the skin of the breast: A complication of lumpectomy and radiation therapy for breast carcinoma. Hum Pathol 1992;23:710–714.
107. Otis CN, Perschel R, Mckhann C, Merino MJ, Duray PH: The rapid onset of cutaneous angiosarcoma after radiotherapy for breast cancer. Cancer 1986;57: 2130–2134.
108. Sessions SC, Smink RD: Cutaneous angiosarcoma of the breast after segmental mastectomy and radiation therapy. Arch Surg 1992;127:1362–1363.
109. Edeiken S, Russo DP, Knecht J, Parry LA, Thompson RM: Angiosarcoma after tylectomy and radiation therapy for carcinoma of the breast. Cancer 1992; 70:644–647.
110. Woodward AH, Ivins JC, Soule EH: Lymphangiosarcoma arising in chronic lymphedematous extremities. Cancer 1972;30:562–572.
111. Sordillo P, Chapman R, Hajdu SI, Magill GB, Golbey RB: Lymphangiosarcoma. Cancer 1981;48:1674–1679.

Angiosarcoma of Breast and Deep Soft Tissues

112. Steingaszner LC, Enzinger FM, Taylor HB: Hemangiosarcoma of the breast. Cancer 1965;18:352–361.
113. Merino MJ, Berman M, Carter D: Angiosarcoma of the breast. Am J Surg Pathol 1983;7:53–60.
114. Chen KT, Kirkegaard DD, Bocian JJ: Angiosarcoma of the breast. Cancer 1980;46:368–371.
115. Rosen PP, Kimmel M, Ernsberger D: Mammary angiosarcoma. The prognostic significance of tumor differentiation. Cancer 1988;62:2145–2151.
116. Jozefczyk MA, Rosen PP: Vascular tumors of the breast. II. Perilobular hemangiomas and hemangiomas. Am J Surg Pathol 1985;9:491–503.
117. Meis-Kindblom JM, Kindblom LG: Angiosarcoma of soft tissue. A study of 80 cases. Am J Surg Pathol 1998;22:683–697.
118. Fletcher CD, Beham A, Bekir S, Clarke AM, Marley NJ: Epithelioid angiosarcoma of deep soft tissue: A distinctive tumor readily mistaken for an epithelial neoplasm. Am J Surg Pathol 1991;15:915–924.

Angiosarcoma in Liver

119. Neshiwat LF, Friedland ML, Suhorr-Lesnick B, Feldman S, Glucksman WJ, Russo RD Jr: Hepatic angiosarcoma. Am J Med 1992;93:219–222.
120. Popper H, Thomas LB, Telles NC: Development of hepatic angiosarcoma in man induced by vinylchloride, thorotrast and arsenic. Am J Pathol 1978;92: 349–376.
121. Alrenga DP: Primary angiosarcoma of the liver. Review article. Int Surg 1975;60:198–203.
122. Kojiro M, Nakashima T, Ito Y: Thorium dioxide-related angiosarcoma of the liver. Pathomorphologic study of 29 autopsy cases. Arch Pathol Lab Med 1985;109:853–857.
123. Lander JJ, Stanley RJ, Sumner HW: Angiosarcoma of the liver associated with Fowler's solution (potassium arsenate). Gastroenterology 1975;68:1582–1586.
124. Selby DM, Stocker JT, Ishak KG: Angiosarcoma of the liver in childhood: A clinicopathologic and follow-up study of 10 cases. Pediatr Pathol 1992;12:485–498.

Angiosarcoma in Spleen and Miscellaneous Sites

125. Falk S, Krishnan J, Meis JM: Primary angiosarcoma of the spleen. A clinicopathologic study of 40 cases. Am J Surg Pathol 1993;17:959–970.
126. Neuhauser T, Derringer G, Thompson LDR, et al: Splenic angiosarcoma. A clinicopathologic and immunohistochemical study of 27 cases. Mod Pathol 2000;13:978–987.
127. Mena H, Ribas JL, Enzinger FM, Parisi JE: Primary angiosarcoma of the central nervous system. Study of eight cases and review of the literature. J Neurosurg 1991;75:73–76.
128. Eusebi V, Carcangiu ML, Dina R, Rosai J: Keratin-positive epithelioid angiosarcoma of thyroid. A report of four cases. Am J Surg Pathol 1990;14:737–747.
129. Wenig BM, Abbondanzo SL, Heffess CS: Epithelioid angiosarcoma of the adrenal glands. A clinicopathologic study of nine cases with a discussion of the implications of finding "epithelial-specific" markers. Am J Surg Pathol 1994;18:62–73.
130. Taxy JB, Battifora H: Angiosarcoma of the gastrointestinal tract. A report of three cases. Cancer 1988;62:210–216.
131. McCaughey WTE, Dardick I, Barr R: Angiosarcoma of serous membranes. Arch Pathol Lab Med 1983;107:304–307.
132. Lin BT, Colby T, Gown AM, Hammar SP, Mertens RB, Churg A, Battifora H: Malignant vascular tumors of the serous membranes mimicking mesothelioma. A report of 14 cases. Am J Surg Pathol 1996;20:1431–1439.
133. Riccardi VM, Wheeler TM, Pickard LR, King B: The pathophysiology of neurofibromatosis: II. Angiosarcoma as a complication. Cancer Genet Cytogenet 1984;12:275–280.
134. Jennings TA, Peterson L, Axiotis CA, Friedlander GE, Cooke RA, Rosai J: Angiosarcoma associated with foreign body material. A report of three cases. Cancer 1988;62:2436–2444.

Angiosarcoma—Immunohistochemistry

135. Kuzu I, Bicknell R, Harris AL, Jones M, Gatter KC, Mason DY: Heterogeneity of vascular endothelial cells with relevance to diagnosis of vascular tumours. J Clin Pathol 1992;45:143–148.
136. Miettinen M, Lindenmayer AE, Chaubal A: Endothelial cell markers CD31, CD34, and BNH9 antibody to H- and Y-antigens: Evaluation of their specificity and sensitivity in the diagnosis of vascular tumors and comparison with von Willebrand's factor. Mod Pathol 1994;7:82–90.
137. deYoung BR, Swanson PE, Angenyi ZB, et al: CD31 immunoreactivity in mesenchymal neoplasms of the skin and subcutis: Report of 145 cases and review of putative immunohistologic markers of endothelial cell differentiation. J Cutan Pathol 1995;22:215–222.
138. Ordonez NG, Batsakis JG: Comparison of *Ulex europaeus* I lectin and factor VIII-related antigen in vascular lesions. Arch Pathol Lab Med 1984;108:129–132.
139. Traweek ST, Kandalaft P, Mehta P, Battifora H: The human progenitor cell antigen (CD34) in vascular neoplasia. Am J Clin Pathol 1991;96:25–31.
140. Appleton MA, Attanoos RL, Jasani B: Thrombomodulin as a marker of vascular and lymphatic tumours. Histopathology 1996;29:153–157.
141. Partanen TA, Alitalo K, Miettinen M: Lack of lymphatic vascular specificity of vascular endothelial growth factor receptor 3 in 185 vascular tumors. Cancer 1999;86:2406–2412.
142. Breiteneder-Geleff S, Soleiman A, Kowalski H, et al: Angiosarcomas express mixed endothelial phenotypes of blood and lymphatic capillaries: Podoplanin as a specific marker for lymphatic endothelium. Am J Pathol 1999;154:385–394.
143. Folpe AL, Chand EM, Goldblum JR, Weiss SW: Expression of Fli-1, a nuclear transcription factor, distinguishes vascular neoplasms from potential mimics. Am J Surg Pathol 2001;25:1061–1066.
144. Miettinen M, Fetsch JF: Distribution of keratins in normal endothelial cells and in a spectrum of vascular tumors: Implications in tumor diagnosis. Hum Pathol 2000;31:1062–1067.
145. Miettinen M, Lasota J: KIT expression in angiosarcomas and in fetal endothelial cells. Lack of c-kit mutations in exons 11 and 17 in angiosarcoma. Mod Pathol 2000;13:536–541.

Angiosarcoma—Genetics

146. Kindblom LG, Stenman G, Angervall L: Morphological and cytogenetic studies on angiosarcoma in Stewart-Treves syndrome. Virchows Arch A Pathol Anat Histopathol 1991;419:439–445.
147. Gill-Benso R, Lopez-Gines C, Soriano P, Almenar S, Vazquez C, Llombart-Bosch A: Cytogenetic study of angiosarcoma of the breast. Genes Chromosom Cancer 1994;10:210–212.
148. Schuborg C, Mertens F, Rydholm A, et al: Cytogenetic analysis of four angiosarcomas from deep and superficial soft tissue. Cancer Genet Cytogenet 1998;100:52–56.

Kaposi Sarcoma

149. Tappero JW, Conant MA, Wolfe SF, Berger TG: Kaposi's sarcoma. Epidemiology, pathogenesis, histology, clinical spectrum, staging criteria and therapy. J Am Acad Dermatol 1993;28:371–395.
150. Antman K, Chang Y: Kaposi's sarcoma. N Engl J Med 2000;342:1027–1038.
151. Chang Y, Cesarman E, Pessin MS, et al: Identification of Herpes virus-like DNA sequences in AIDS-associated Kaposi's sarcoma. Science 1994;266:1865–1869.
152. Moore PJ, Chang Y: Detection of Herpes virus-like DNA sequences in Kaposi's sarcoma patients with and those without HIV-infection. N Engl J Med 1995;332:1181–1185.
153. Ambroziak JA, Blackbourn DJ, Herndier BG, et al: Herpes-like sequences in HIV-infected and uninfected Kaposi's sarcoma patients. Science 1995;268:582–583.
154. Penn I: Kaposi's sarcoma in transplant recipients. Transplantation 1997;64:669–673.

155. Farge D, Lebbe C, Marjanovic Z, et al: Human herpes virus-8 and other risk factors for Kaposi's sarcoma in kidney transplant recipients. Transplantation 1999;67:1236–1242.
156. Fonseca R, Witztig TE, Olson LJ, Edwards BS, Khoor A, Walker RC: Disseminated Kaposi's sarcoma after heart transplantation: Association with Kaposi's sarcoma-associated herpesvirus. J Heart Lung Transplant 1998;17:732–736.
157. Ackerman AB: Subtle clues to diagnosis by conventional microscopy. The patch stage of Kaposi's sarcoma. Am J Dermatopathol 1979;1:165–172.
158. Chor PJ, Santa-Cruz DJ: Kaposi's sarcoma. A clinicopathologic review and differential diagnosis. J Cutan Pathol 1992;19:6–20.
159. Kao G, Johnson FB, Sulica VI: The nature of hyaline (eosinophilic) globules and vascular slits in Kaposi's sarcoma. Am J Dermatopathol 1990;12:256–267.
160. Nickoloff BJ: The human progenitor cell antigen (CD34) is localized on endothelial cells, dermal dendritic cells, and perifollicular cells in formalin-fixed normal skin, and on proliferation endothelial cells and stromal spindle-shaped cells in Kaposi's sarcoma. Arch Dermatol 1991;127:523–529.
161. Beckstead JH, Wood GS, Fletcher V: Evidence for the origin of Kaposi's sarcoma from lymphatic endothelium. Am J Pathol 1985;119;294–300.
162. Jussila L, Valtola R, Partanen TA, et al: Lymphatic endothelium and Kaposi's sarcoma spindle cells detected by antibodies against the vascular endothelial growth factor receptor-3. Cancer Res 1998;58: 1599–1604.
163. McDonagh DP, Liu J, Gaffey MJ, Layfield LJ, Azumi N, Traweek ST: Detection of Kaposi's sarcoma-associated herpesvirus-like DNA sequence in angiosarcoma. Am J Pathol 1996;149:1363–1368.
164. Ishak KG, Bijwaard KE, Makhlouf HR, Taubenberger JK, Lichy JH, Goodman ZD. Absence of human herpesvirus 8 DNA sequences in vascular tumors of the liver. Liver 1998;18:124–127.
165. Lasota J, Miettinen M: Absence of Kaposi's sarcoma-associated virus (human herpesvirus-8 sequences in angiosarocma. Virchows Arch 1999;434:51–56.

Hemangiopericytoma—Clinicopathologic

166. Tsuneyoshi M, Daimaru Y, Enjoji M: Malignant hemangiopericytoma and other sarcomas with hemangiopericytoma-like pattern. Pathol Res Pract 1984; 178:446–453.
167. Nappi O, Ritter JH, Pettinato G, Wick MR: Hemangiopericytoma: Histopathological pattern or clinicopathologic entity? Semin Diagn Pathol 1995;12: 221–232.
168. Enzinger FM, Smith BH: Hemangiopericytoma. An analysis of 106 cases. Hum Pathol 19736;7:61–82.
169. McMaster MJ, Soule EJ, Ivins JC: Hemangiopericytoma: A clinicopathologic study and long-term follow-up of 60 patients. Cancer 1975;36:2232–2244.
170. Spitz FR, Bouvet M, Pisters PW, Pollock RE, Feig BW: Hemangiopericytoma: A 20-year single-institution experience. Ann Surg Oncol 1998;5:350–355.
171. Plukker JT, Koops HS, Molenaar I, Vermey A, Kate LP, Oldhoff J: Malignant hemangiopericytoma in three kindred members of one family. Cancer 1988;61:841–844.
172. Jaaskelainen J, Servo A, Haltia M, Wahlstrom T, Valtonen S: Intracranial hemangiopericytoma: Radiology, surgery, radiotherapy, and outcome in 21 patients. Surg Neurol 1985;23:227–236.
173. Mena H, Ribas JL, Pezeshkpour GH, Cowan DN, Parisi JE: Hemangiopericytoma of the central nervous system: A review of 94 cases. Hum Pathol 1991;22:84–91.
174. Guthrie BL, Ebersold MJ, Scheithauer BW, Shaw EG: Meningeal hemangiopericytoma: Histopathological features, treatment, and long-term follow-up of 44 cases. Neurosurgery 1989;25:514–522.
175. Nielsen GP, Dickersin GR, Provenzal JM, Rosenberg AE: Lipomatous hemangiopericytoma. A histologic, ultrastructural and immunohistochemical study of a unique variant of hemangiopericytoma. Am J Surg Pathol 1995;19:748–756.
176. Folpe AL, Devaney K, Weiss SW: Lipomatous hemangiopericytoma: A rare variant of hemangiopericytoma that may be confused with liposarcoma. Am J Surgical Pathol 1999;23:1201–1207.
177. Perry A, Scheithauer BW, Nascimento AG: The immunophenotypic spectrum of meningeal hemangiopericytoma: A comparison with fibrous meningioma and solitary fibrous tumor of meninges. Am J Surg Pathol 1997;21:1354–1360.
178. Middleton LP, Duray PH, Merino MJ: The histological spectrum of hemangiopericytoma: Application of immunohistochemical analysis including proliferative markers to facilitate diagnosis and predict prognosis. Hum Pathol 1998;29:636–640.
179. Dardick I, Hammar SP, Scheithauer BW: Ultrastructural spectrum of hemangiopericytoma: A comparative study of fetal, adult, and neoplastic pericytes. Ultrastruct Pathol 1989;13:111–154.

Hemangiopericytoma—Genetics

180. Streekantaiah C, Bridge JA, Rao UN, Neff JR, Sandberg AA: Clonal chromosomal abnormalities in hemangiopericytoma. Cancer Genet Cytogenet 1991;54:173–181.
181. Henn W, Wullich B, Thonnes M, Steudel WI, Feiden W, Zang KD: Recurrent t(12;19)(q13;q13.3) in intracranial and extracranial hemangiopericytoma. Cancer Genet Cytogenet 1993;71:151–154.
182. Limon J, Rao U, Dal Cin P, Gibas Z, Sandberg AA. Translocation (13;22) in a hemangiopericytoma. Cancer Genet Cytogenet 1986;21:309–318.
183. Joseph JT, Lisle DK, Jacoby LB, et al: NF2 gene analysis distinguishes hemangiopericytoma from meningioma. Am J Pathol 1995;147:1450–1455.

Sinonasal Hemangipericytoma

184. Compagno J, Hyams VJ: Hemangiopericytoma-like intranasal tumors. A clinicopathologic study of 23 cases. Am J Clin Pathol 1976;66:672–683.
185. Eichhorn JH, Dickersin GR, Bhan AK, Goodman ML: Sinonasal hemangipericytoma. A reassessment with

electron microscopy, immunohistochemistry, and long-term follow-up. Am J Surg Pathol 1990;14:856–866.

Glomus Tumor

186. Tsuneyoshi M, Enjoji M: Glomus tumor. A clinicopathologic and electron microscopic study. Cancer 1982;50:1601–1607.
187. Appelman HD, Helwig EB: Glomus tumor of the stomach. Cancer 1969;23:203–213.
188. Haque S, Modlin IM, West AB. Multiple glomus tumors of the stomach with intravascular spread. Am J Surg Pathol 1992;16:291–299.
189. Miettinen M, Paal E, Lasota J, Sobin LH: Gastrointestinal glomus tumors. A clinicopathologic, immunohistochemical, and molecular genetic study of 32 cases. Am J Surg Pathol 2002;26:301–311.
190. Folpe AL, Fanburg-Smith JC, Miettinen M, Weiss SW: Atypical and malignant glomus tumors: Analysis of 52 cases with a proposal for the reclassification of glomus tumors. Am J Surg Pathol 2001;25:1–12.
191. Gould EW, Manivel JC, Albores-Saavedra J: Locally infiltrative glomus tumors and glomangiosarcomas. A clinical, ultrastructural, and immunohistochemical study. Cancer 1990;65:310–318.
192. Miettinen M, Lehto VP, Virtanen I: Glomus tumor cells: Evaluation of smooth muscle and endothelial cell properties. Virchows Arch B Cell Pathol 1983; 43:139–149.
193. Porter PL, Bigler SA, McNutt M, Gown AM: The immunophenotype of hemangipericytomas and glomus tumors, with special reference to muscle protein expression: An immunohistochemical study and review of the literature. Mod Pathol 1991;4:46–52.
194. Murad TJ, Von Hasam Z, Murthy MSN: The ultrastructure of hemangiopericytoma and glomus tumor. Cancer 1968;22:1239–1249.

Nerve Sheath Tumors

CHAPTER 15

The common benign nerve sheath tumors include neurofibroma, schwannoma, and granular cell tumor and the rare ones are perineurial cell tumors (perineuriomas) and nerve sheath myxoma. Malignant peripheral nerve sheath tumor (MPNST) is the preferred term for malignant tumors arising in nerve sheaths or showing differentiation toward nerve sheath cells. Nerve sheath tumors occur in both peripheral and cranial nerves.[1,2] Their classification applied here is listed in Table 15–1.

Alterations in the neurofibromatosis type 1 (*NF1*) gene are the basis of the neurofibromatosis 1 (NF1) syndrome and associated neurofibromas, and somatic *NF1* gene mutations are probably responsible for sporadic neurofibromas. Neurofibromatosis type 2 (*NF2*) gene is involved in the pathogenesis of the neurofibromatosis 2 (NF2) syndrome with bilateral vestibular schwannomas, meningiomas, and certain gliomas, and this gene is also involved in the pathogenesis of sporadic schwannomas.

True neural tumors, such paraganglioma and related tumors, and neuroectodermal tumors, such as malignant melanoma and clear cell sarcoma, are discussed in Chapter 16. Gastrointestinal autonomic nerve tumor (GANT) is now classified among the gastrointestinal stromal tumors (GISTs) as their ultrastructural variants (see Chapter 11). Although GANTs and GISTs are not nerve sheath tumors, they have a weak association with NF1 syndrome.

Neuroblastoma, a primitive childhood tumor with sympathetic nerve differentiation, peripheral primitive neuroectodermal tumor (PNET) and peripheral neuroepithelioma of the Ewing sarcoma family, will be discussed among small, round cell tumors (Chapter 18).

Cellular Components of Nerve Sheaths and Their Significance for Tumorigenesis

The peripheral nerves contain long axons that originate from the spinal ganglia. The larger nerves form nerve trunks, which are composed of multiple nerve fascicles. Each fascicle is surrounded by perineurium. The fascicles contain numerous axons immediately surrounded by Schwann cells. The nerve fascicles are separated by endoneurium, a fibrous matrix containing fibroblasts. The nerve trunks are surrounded by epineurium. Small nerves seen in skin and peripheral soft tissues represent nearly bare nerve fascicles that are separated from the surrounding tissue by perineurium and an inconspicuous epineurium.

Autonomic nerves of visceral organs originate from the visceral ganglions. In the gastrointestinal (GI) tract, there are two neural plexuses with ganglia: the submucous (Auerbach) and myenteric plexus (Meissner) between the muscle layers. Both of these contain ganglion cells and nerves. In addition, numerous small nerves dispersed between the smooth muscle cells can be highlighted, for example, with S-100 protein immunostaining.

All components of the nerve sheath have been implicated in the pathogenesis of nerve sheath

Table 15–1. Classification of Nerve Sheath Tumors

Nonneoplastic conditions
Neuromuscular hamartoma
Morton neuroma
Traumatic neuroma
Mucosal neuroma
Pacinian neuroma (neurofibroma)
Palisaded encapsulated neuroma
Neurofibroma (NF)
Cutaneous
Cellular
Intraneural including plexiform NF as a variant
Diffuse, including pigmented NF as a variant
Epithelioid
Schwannoma
Conventional
Cellular
Plexiform
Epithelioid
With rosettes
Sarcomatous transformation
Gastrointestinal
Psammomatous melanotic schwannoma
Nerve sheath myxoma
Cellular neurothekeoma
Perineurioma
Intraneural
Sclerosing
Retiform
Granular cell tumor
Malignant granular cell tumor
Malignant peripheral nerve sheath tumor
With heterologous differentiation
Triton tumor
Glandular
Epithelioid

tumors. Schwann cells are spindled cells with elongated, complex, intertwining cell processes and well-developed basement membranes (external laminas). The myelinated Schwann cells provide the myelin for the myelinated nerves, and the nonmyelinated ones surround nonmyelinated nerves. They are immunohistochemically recognized as S-100 protein-positive cells surrounded by laminin and collagen type IV-positive sheaths. They are the principal cells of schwannomas and are an essential cellular component in neurofibromas.

Endoneurium inside the nerve fascicles contains fibroblasts, many of which belong to the specific subset of $CD34^+$ fibroblasts. They participate in the genesis of neurofibromas, together with Schwann cells.

Perineurial cells are usually seen as a multilamellar sheath of spindled, elongated cells around the nerve fascicles. They represent a peripheral continuation of the pia arachnoid membrane of the central nervous system and are identified as slender epithelial membrane antigen (EMA)-positive and S-100 protein-negative cells that are surrounded by basement membranes. Perineuriomas are rare tumors that show perineurial cell differentiation.

Epineurium does not contain cell types specific for nerves. It consists of loose connective tissue containing fibroblasts, mast cells, histiocytes, lymphatics, and blood vessels. These components are the likely origin for nonschwannian, nonperineurial mesenchymal tumors of the peripheral nerves. All these conditions are very rare and include hemangiomas, lipomas, and ganglion cysts of the nerve.

Neuromuscular Hamartoma (Neuromuscular Choristoma)

This very rare lesion contains an intimate admixture of peripheral nerves and skeletal muscle cells. The majority of cases have been reported in children and young adults as a mass that may involve a major nerve or nerve plexus and can cause neurologic signs.[1–4]

Histologically typical is the intermingling of peripheral nerves and clusters of skeletal muscle fibers (Fig. 15–1*A*). Although the components are usually readily apparent in hematoxylin-eosin staining, the neural component can be highlighted as paler staining areas and the muscle as red foci in Masson trichrome staining (Fig. 15–1*B*). The nerves can also be visualized as S-100 protein positive and the skeletal muscle as desmin positive.

Neuromuscular hamartoma is different from "benign Triton tumor," a designation that more appropriately applies to neurofibroma with skeletal muscle differentiation, a very rare event.[5]

Morton Neuroma (Localized Interdigital Neuritis)

This term refers to a peculiar reactive condition involving one of the digital nerves around the distal metatarsal. Similar lesions rarely occur in the hand. The term "localized interdigital neuritis" is used in the Armed Forces Institute of Pathology (AFIP) fascicle of peripheral nerve tumors.[1]

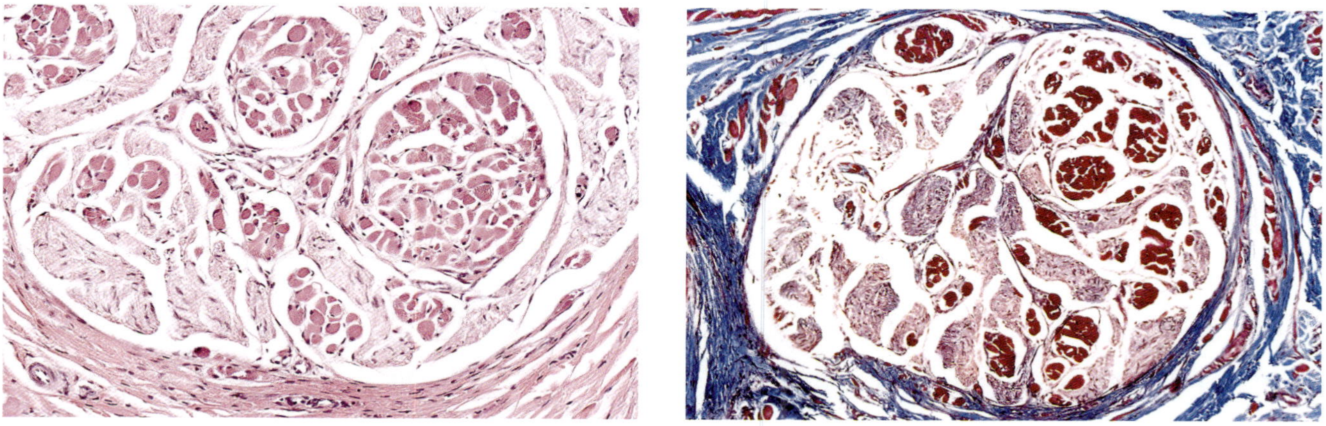

A

B

Figure 15-1. *A*, Neuromuscular hamartoma is composed of a nerve containing clusters of mature skeletal muscle cells. *B*, Trichrome staining highlights the nerve as pale and the muscle as red structures.

The lesion typically presents with a swelling and paroxysmal pain between the second and third or third and fourth metatarsal bones. It is believed to result from minor chronic, repetitive trauma combined with local ischemia, probably related to mechanical factors such as unphysiologically compressing shoes, and most commonly occurs in middle-aged women. Surgical excision of the fibrous nodule may be necessary for pain relief and is curative.[6,7]

Histologically, the nodule consists of fibrofatty tissue with marked epineurial fibrosis (Fig. 15–2*A*). The number of axons and Schwann cells may be reduced reflecting nerve damage. Fibrous thickening of the blood vessel walls is common, and some vessels may have thrombosis.[6–10]

Traumatic Neuroma (Amputation Neuroma)

Traumatic neuroma represents an attempted but insufficient reparative process of a severed nerve that fails to re-establish the axonal connection following the transsection. It may follow an amputation (hence, the old term amputation neuroma), other surgery, or traumatic nerve damage. Clinically, it appears as a small, painful nodule in the amputation stump or site of trauma, most commonly in the extremities. Similar lesions may occur around the cystic duct stump after cholecystectomy and some have been symptomatic.[1,11]

Histologically, the traumatic neuroma consists of tangled, disorganized nerve fascicles containing axons and Schwann cells and surrounded by perineurial cells. Densely collagenous scarring is common between the neural elements. The lesion is often microscopically ill-defined (Fig. 15–2*B*).

Mucosal Neuromas and Ganglioneuromatosis

These lesions usually occur in connection with multiple endocrine neoplasia type 2b (MEN2b), together with medullary thyroid carcinoma and pheochromocytoma in various parts of the GI tract.[12] They are easily visible in the lips and tongue as micronodular elevations, but such lesions are only rarely seen as surgical specimens. In some cases, mucosal biopsies of the GI tract have been helpful in the diagnosis of MEN2b syndrome.

The neuromas of tongue represent histologically numerous hyperplastic nerves that can occur singly or as clusters. The GI lesions may involve diffusely the submucous and myenteric plexuses in a bandlike manner, and typically have both a neural and ganglionic component representing ganglioneuromatosis. Solitary ganglioneuromas may also occur sporadically (see Chapter 16).

Pacinian Neuroma (Pacinian Neurofibroma)

This designation refers to an uncommon hyperplastic process of the pacinian corpuscles, the specialized nerve endings functioning as pressure receptors. The lesion typically occurs in the fingers or hands of middle-aged adults and causes chronic pain. It does not recur following simple excision. There is no association with the neurofibromatoses.

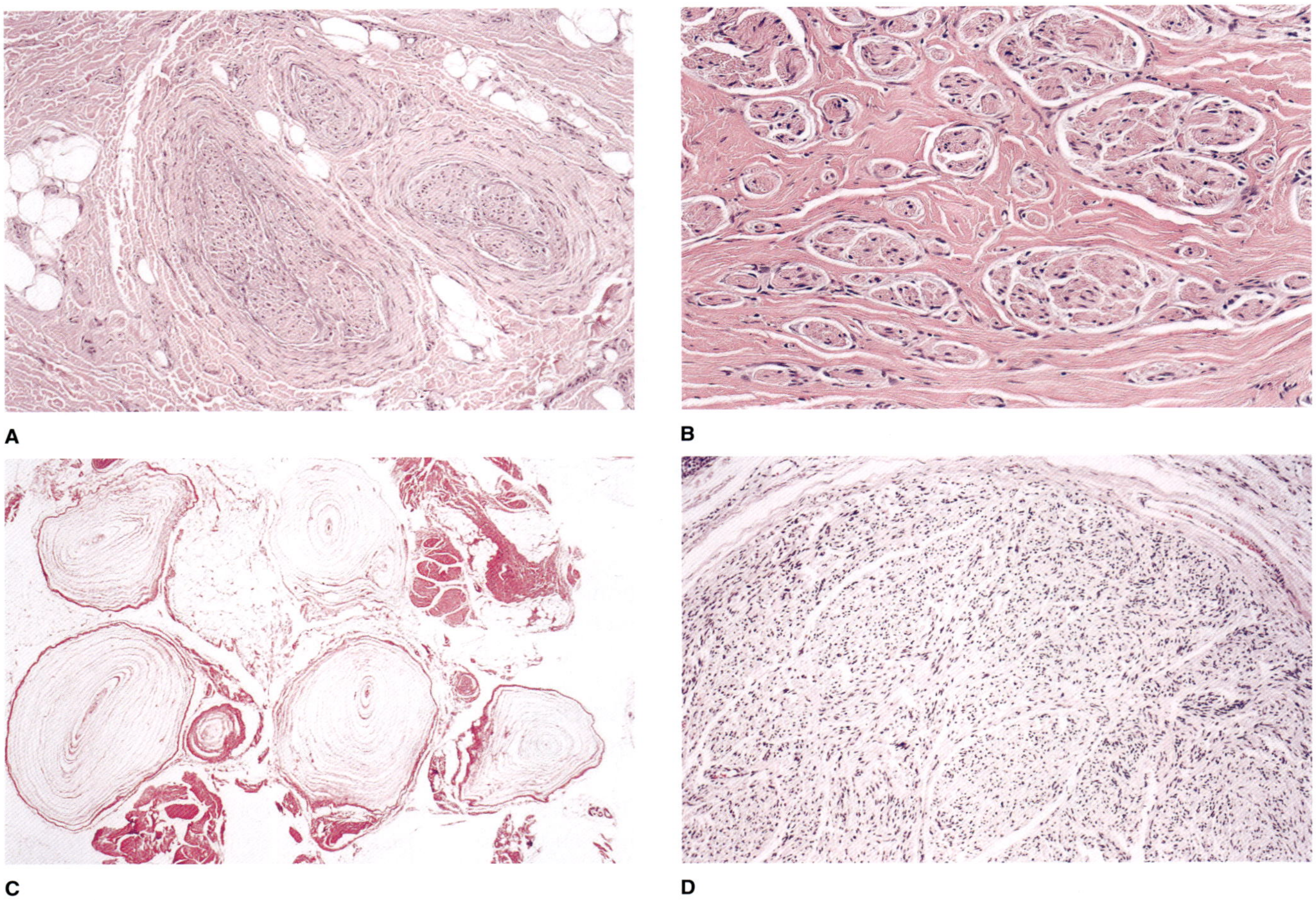

Figure 15–2. Tumors commonly referred to as neuromas. *A,* Morton neuroma shows histologically nerves surrounded by marked perineurial fibrosis. *B,* Traumatic neuroma is composed of bundles of disorganized axons surrounded by scarlike fibrosis. *C,* Pacinian neuroma is composed of a cluster of pacinian corpuscles. *D,* Palisaded encapsulated neuroma forms a round, well-circumscribed, spindle cell lesion that shows bundles of spindled Schwann cells.

Microscopically, pacinian neurofibroma is composed of multiple, clustered pacinian corpuscles (Fig. 15–2C), or occasionally of a single enlarged one. The lamellar units are EMA^+ perineurial cells, and the center contains an S-100 protein-positive schwannian core and a small axon, similar to a normal pacinian corpuscle.[13–15]

Palisaded Encapsulated Neuroma (Solitary Circumscribed Neuroma)

This designation applies to small, circumscribed Schwann cell tumors that are generally considered hyperplastic rather than neoplastic.[16–21] Because palisading and true encapsulation are not consistent features, the name solitary circumscribed neuroma has been suggested as a perhaps more accurate designation.[17]

Clinical Features

This small, benign cutaneous tumor most commonly occurs in middle-aged adults, affecting men and women equally. The vast majority of the lesions occur in the face, most commonly in the nose, cheek, and perioral region. The tumor presents as a small, solitary flesh-colored, dome-shaped papule or nodule. Association with acnelike changes was found in one study,[18] and traumatic origin has been occasionally suspected, based on the presence of numerous axons within the lesion.

The tumor has a benign behavior following simple excision. There is no association with neurofibromatoses or multiple endocrine neoplasia (mucosal neuromas are associated with the latter). Multiple lesions are very uncommon.

Pathology

On sectioning, the tumor is a small whitish nodule usually measuring 5 mm or less. Histologically, it is usually limited to the dermis, but occasionally extends to the subcutis (Fig. 15–2*D*). The lesion consists of one or more spherical to ovoid nodules, and some are composed of multiple nodules and have a plexiform appearance. The nodules contain spindled Schwann cells often arranged in fascicles and sometimes separated by narrow clefts. Focal palisading is often present, whereas typical Verocay bodies are rare. Adjacent peripheral nerve can be identified in many cases.

Immunohistochemically, the lesional cells are positive for S-100 protein and CD57. Large numbers of entrapped axons can be demonstrated by neurofilament immunostaining, and EMA^+ perineurial cells are seen in the perineurium of nerves and also in the periphery of the lesion. The tested examples have been negative for glial fibrillary acidic protein (GFAP).[22,23]

Neurofibroma and Neurofibromatosis Type 1

Neurofibroma is a designation for a group of common, closely related benign nerve sheath tumors that, according to present evidence, have a similar molecular pathogenesis. It seems likely that loss of function-alterations in the *NF1* gene play a role in both *NF1*-associated and sporadic neurofibromas. Neurofibromas are composed of a dual population of Schwann cells and fibroblasts, and entrapped axons are often present in intraneural lesions.

Neurofibromas are most commonly diagnosed in young adults between 20 and 30 years of age, but may occur in adults of all ages. There is a slight male predominance. They may present in superficial or deep soft tissues, and each subtype can present in a wide variety of anatomic locations. The most common form is solitary cutaneous neurofibroma. Other forms discussed here are intraneural neurofibroma, which is called plexiform when forming a complex tortuous mass. Cellular, diffuse, pigmented, and epithelioid are designations given to histologically distinctive less common subtypes of neurofibroma.[1,2]

Plexiform, cutaneous, and diffuse neurofibromas are associated with NF1 and may also occur in children, although they rarely present before the age of 5 years. Commonly associated with the NF1 syndrome are intraneural neurofibromas, which when forming complex masses, are referred to as plexiform neurofibromas. The intraneural neurofibromas may cause neurologic symptoms when involving major nerves. Diffuse neurofibromas, including pigmented variants, may be massive and usually occur in NF1 patients.[24–27]

Cutaneous (and Subcutaneous) Neurofibroma

Cutaneous neurofibroma more commonly forms a small solitary nodule, but in patients with NF1, innumerable lesions may occur. The lesion may present as dome-shaped or polypoid elevation of skin and may grossly resemble a fibroepithelial polyp. It usually measures from a few millimeters to less than 2 cm.

Grossly, neurofibroma is rubbery, gray, and glistening on sectioning. Histologically, cutaneous neurofibroma shows a mixture of elongated spindled Schwann cells and fibroblasts in a background of wavy collagenous fibers. The degree of cellularity may vary (Fig. 15–3*A* and *B*). The Schwann cells have small, oval-to-elongated, irregular nuclei with a dense chromatin. Varying numbers of mast cells are commonly present. There is no association with nerves, unless an intraneural neurofibroma component is present. Entrapped skin adnexal structures occur in some lesions; such epithelial elements were once considered heterologous epithelial differentiation.

A peculiar histologic variant of cutaneous neurofibroma was recently described that contains large ganglion-like cells with dendritic processes (Fig. 15–3*C*), surrounded by ordinary Schwann cells.[28] Both components are positive for S-100 protein (Fig. 15-3*D*). These tumors are usually sporadic and solitary.

Cellular Neurofibroma

This rare variant usually presents in the skin and subcutis, where it forms a solid, rubbery, white 2- to 4-cm nodule. The tumor is more highly cellular than typical neurofibroma and often lacks the typical wavy appearance of collagen. Because of its high cellularity, this neurofibroma can be easily confused with low-grade sarcomas, especially dermatofibrosarcoma protuberans. Focal atypia can also be present, but mitotic activity is very low (Fig. 15–4*A* to *C*). Immunohistochemical demonstration of the S-100 protein and $CD34^+$ schwannian and fibroblastic populations is the key to the diagnosis of cellular neurofibroma (Fig. 15–4*D*).

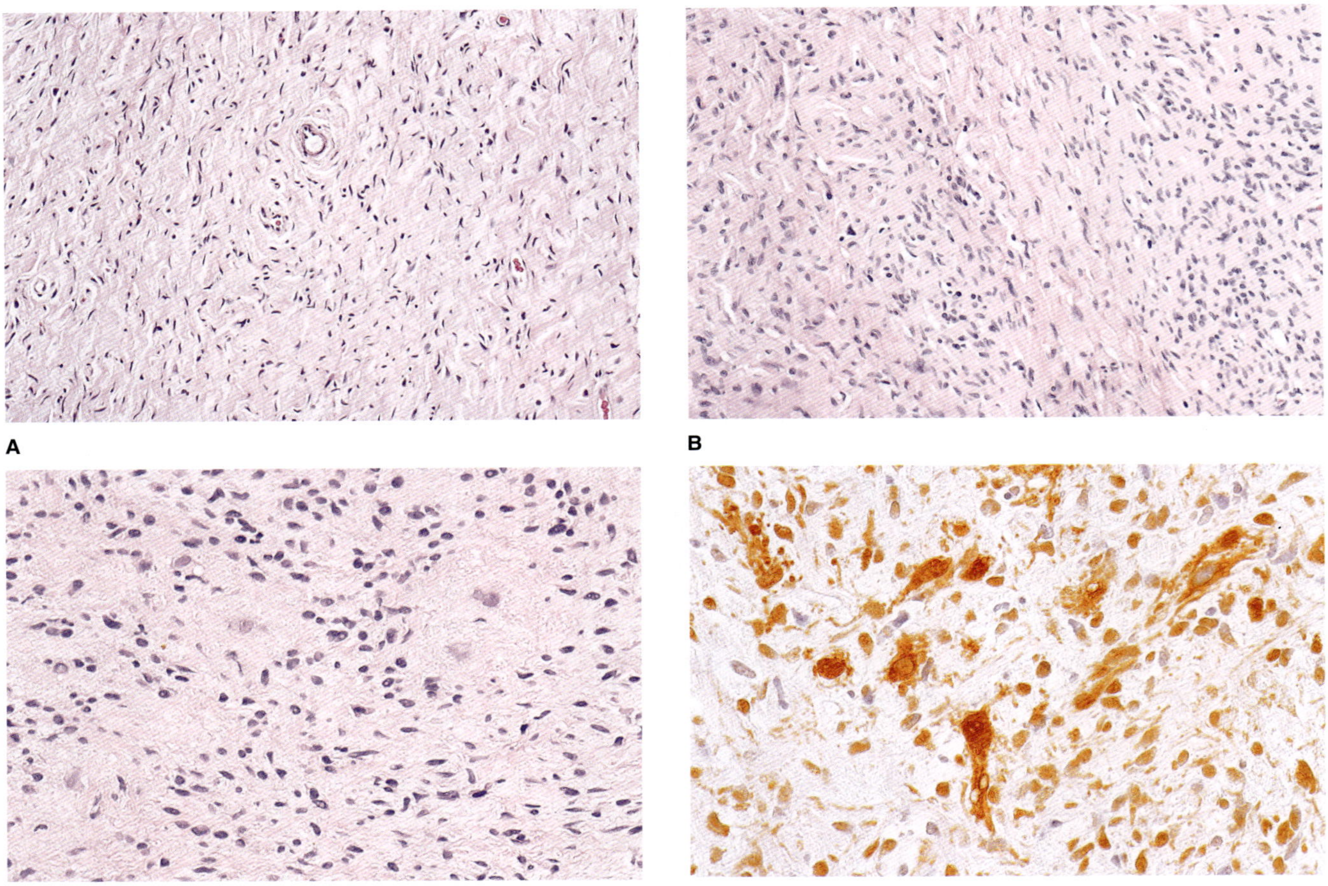

A B C D

Figure 15–3. Variants of superficial neurofibromas. *A* and *B,* Cutaneous neurofibroma is composed of bland Schwann cells and fibroblasts in a collagenous background. *C,* A variant of cutaneous neurofibroma with large dendritic ganglion cell-like Schwann cells. *D,* Significant S-100 protein positivity is not noted in the large dendritic cells and surrounding spindle cells.

Intraneural Neurofibroma

Intraneural neurofibroma is confined to the epineurium and is therefore truly encapsulated. It may involve superficial small nerves, deep somatic and visceral nerves, or major nerve trunks. Grossly, the solitary intraneural neurofibromas are typically fusiform, well-defined lesions that are confined within a nerve, and therefore the lesions involving larger nerves are sharply circumscribed; those involving smaller cutaneous nerves blend with dense dermal collagen. Grossly, the lesions vary from minute nodules to large masses. On sectioning they are gray-white and vary from mucoid to rubbery or gelatinous.

Histologically, intraneural neurofibroma typically has elongated spindle cells diffusely dispersed in a myxoid matrix or around collagen-rich bundles (Fig. 15–5*A* and *B*). The Schwann cells can be spindled or rounded; the latter superficially resemble lymphocytes. Focal atypia in the schwannian elements with enlarged, hyperchromatic nuclei is common and has no specific significance (Fig. 15–5*C*), unless accompanied by marked increase in cellularity and mitotic activity.[29]

As with the cutaneous neurofibromas, there is a mixture of S-100 protein-positive Schwann cells and $CD34^+$ fibroblasts, the latter often seen in a netlike pattern. Residual axons can often be demonstrated with immunostaining for neurofilament proteins in intraneural neurofibromas (Fig. 15–5*D*).

Plexiform Neurofibroma

The clinical significance of this variant lies in its consistent association with NF1 syndrome, and that it has some although low potential for malignant transformation to MPNST. Plexiform neurofibroma is a gross pathologic or low-magnification histologic distinction. It represents a complex aggregate of

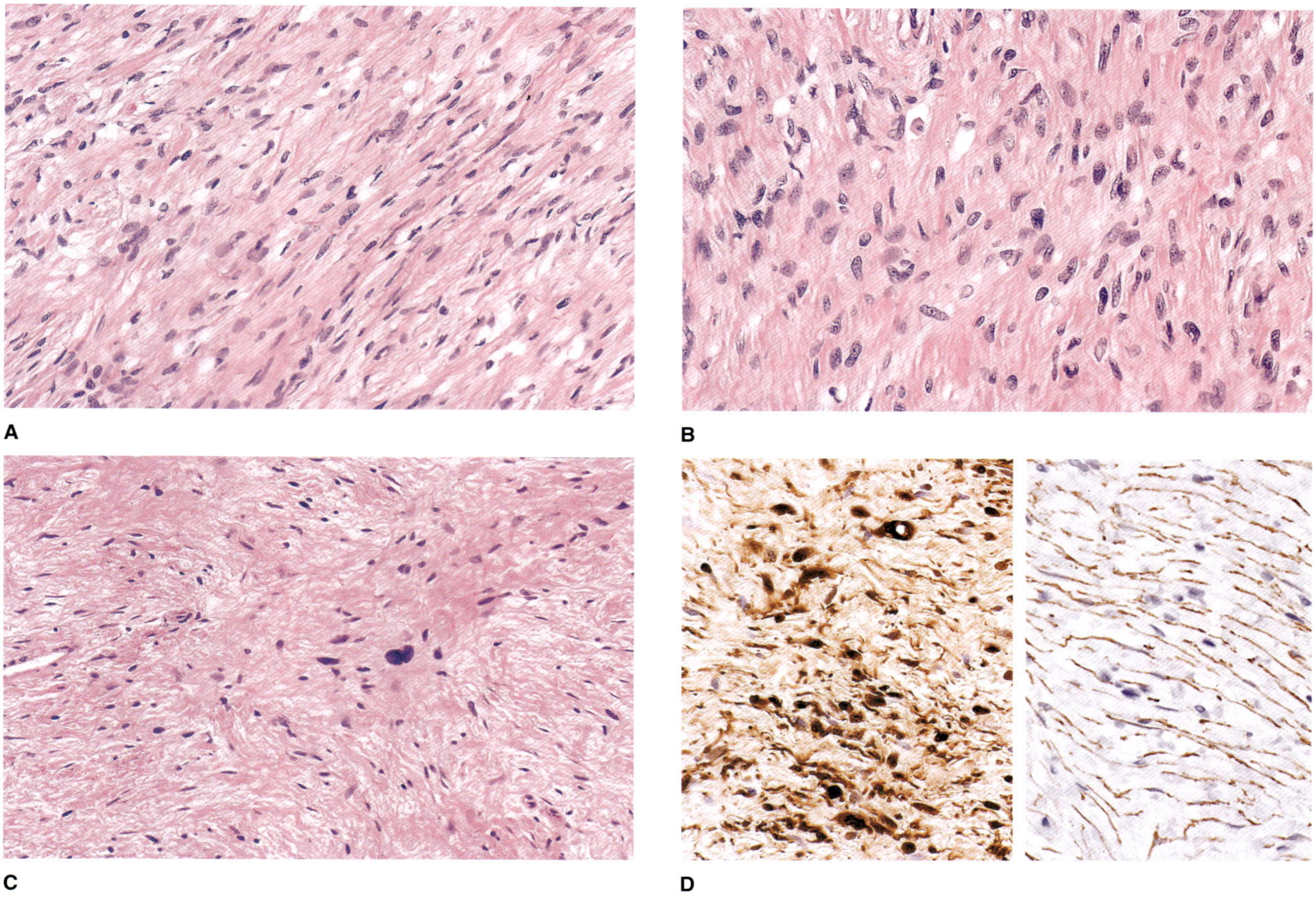

Figure 15–4. Cellular neurofibroma. *A* and *B,* Sheets of spindle cells in a mildly collagenous background is the typical histology. *C,* Focal nuclear atypia is common. *D,* Cellular neurofibroma is positive for S-100 protein (*left*) and also contains large numbers of $CD34^+$ fibroblasts in a netlike pattern (*right*).

intraneural neurofibromas, that is, transformation of multiple adjacent nerves into complex tortuous masses, or a ropelike diffuse thickening of a large nerve trunk, especially when involving the sciatic nerve. Some tumors reach a large size, up to several kilograms. Such lesions may grossly resemble "a bag of worms."

Histologically, plexiform neurofibroma is similar to the usual type of intraneural neurofibroma, except that it is composed of multiple juxtaposed structural units (Fig. 15–6).

Diffuse Neurofibroma

This subtype often occurs in the head and neck area, but may also be seen in trunk and extremity locations. It often occurs in patients with the NF1 syndrome starting from the latter part of the first decade. Malignant transformation of diffuse neurofibroma is very rare.

Grossly, the lesions are plaquelike or form larger contiguous masses, which may reach disfiguring proportions. On sectioning they lack texture and are gray-white and vary from soft, slightly mucoid to firm and rubbery. The excised tumor from locations such as eyelids is often relatively small, but in the trunk and extremity, the lesion often measures 5 cm or more, and may reach massive proportions in NF1 patients. The lesion typically has indistinct borders, and it is primarily subcutaneous.

Histologically, diffuse neurofibroma resembles cutaneous neurofibroma, but it has prominent, diffuse fat infiltration (Fig. 15–7*A*). In some cases, the abundance of fat may mask the neurofibromatous component and simulate a fibrolipoma (Fig. 15–7*B*). A common histologic feature of diffuse neurofibromas is the presence of Wagner-Meissner-like tactile corpuscles[30] (Fig. 15–7*C*). Some lesions are more highly cellular and some may contain elements of intraneural/plexiform neurofibroma. The highly cellular examples can be separated from MPNST based on a very low mitotic activity and limited atypia.

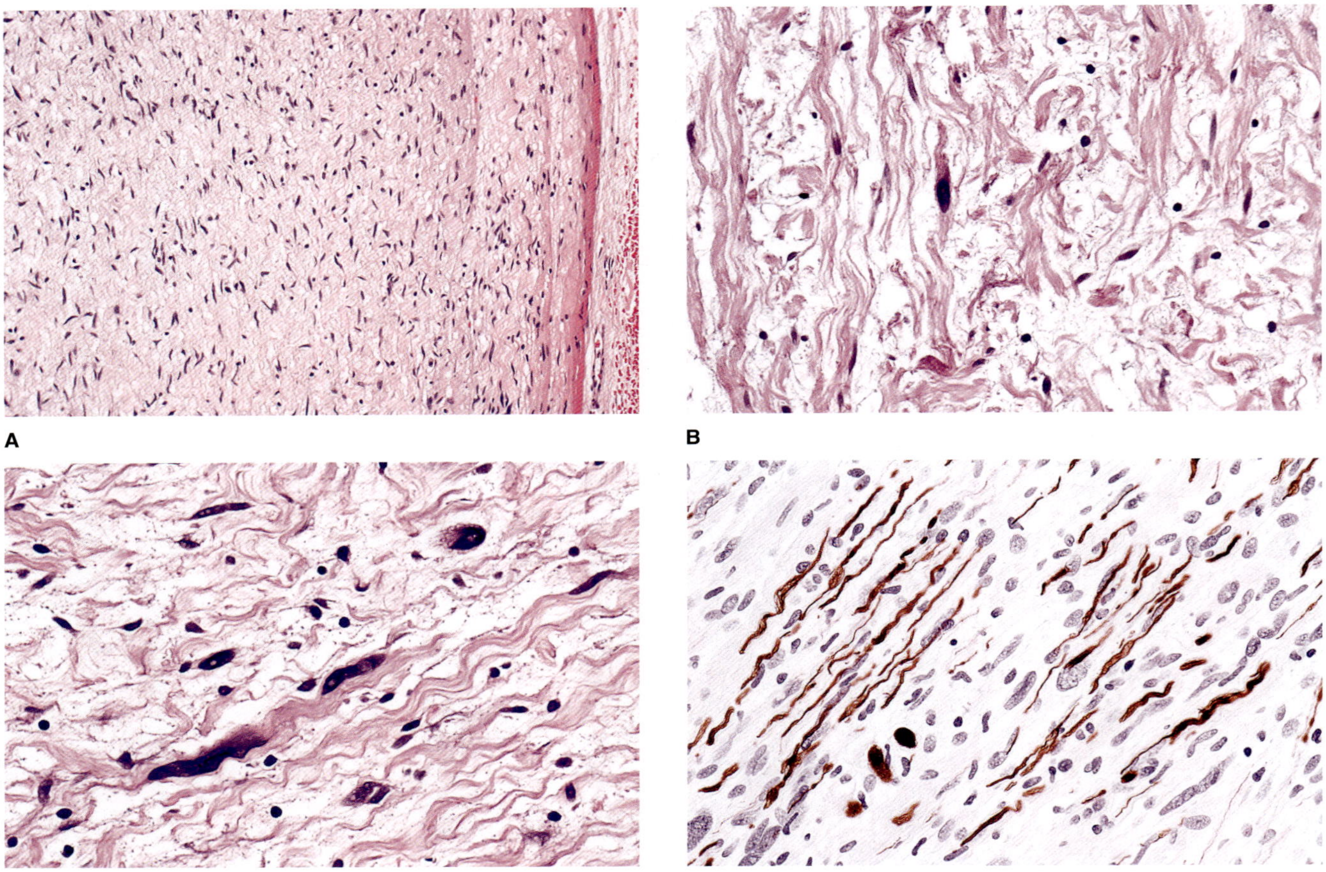

Figure 15–5. *A,* Intraneural neurofibroma is a spindled schwannian proliferation confined in the nerve trunk, and therefore encapsulated. *B,* The spindled Schwann cells, wavy collagen, and myxoid background are typical elements of intraneural neurofibroma. *C,* Focal nuclear atypia is relatively common in intraneural neurofibroma. *D,* Intraneural neurofibromas typically contain numerous neurofilament-positive residual axons.

Pigmented Neurofibroma

Pigmented neurofibroma is a rare variant of diffuse neurofibroma with focal melanocytic differentiation (pigmented or melanocytic neurofibroma). These tumors predominantly occur in blacks in a wide age range. The most common locations are head and neck and buttock or leg. Similar to other diffuse neurofibromas, association of NF1 is common. Behavior is similar to diffuse neurofibroma.[31]

The pigmented neurofibroma most commonly involves subcutis and skin, but occasionally it extends to skeletal muscle. Its features are generally similar to diffuse neurofibroma. In addition, there are scattered or larger clusters of dendritic-shaped pigmented cells (Fig. 15–7*D*). These cells have melanocytic markers HMB45, tyrosinase, and melan A, and like the nonpigmented cells, they are also positive for S-100 protein.[31]

Critical review on historic reports on pigmented neurofibroma reveals that many older cases are more likely pigmented dermatofibrosarcomas (Bednar tumors). Actually Bednar's series on what are now classified as pigmented dermatofibrosarcoma protuberans (DFSPs) were originally published as pigmented neurofibromas.

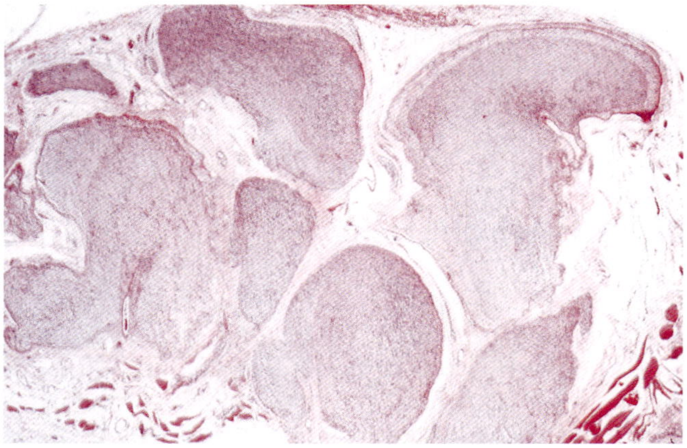

Figure 15–6. Plexiform neurofibroma is an intraneural neurofibroma composed of multiple tortuous nerve profiles.

Epithelioid Neurofibroma

This very rare variant primarily occurs in the dermis. It is typically composed of rounded clusters of epithelioid Schwann cells with abundant cytoplasm (Fig. 15–8). Lesions with small size, limited atypia, and lack of mitotic activity may be diagnosed as epithelioid neurofibroma, especially when combined with spindled more typical areas of neurofibroma. If significant atypia and mitotic activity are present, the diagnoses of malignant epithelioid peripheral nerve sheath tumor is appropriate. Malignant melanoma has to be considered in the differential and should be evaluated with melanoma markers such as HMB45 and tyrosinase.

Immunohistochemistry and Ultrastructure of Neurofibroma

The neurofibromas are typically composed of a dual population of wavy Schwann cells that typically have elongated S-100 protein-positive cytoplasmic processes and nuclei. The Wagner-Meissner-like bodies are typically strongly positive for S-100 protein. There is a variably prominent CD34$^+$ fibroblastic population.[32–34] These cells also have elongated cytoplasmic processes and are typically intermingled with the schwannian component, often in a netlike pattern. CD57 (Leu7) also marks the schwannian component.[35] Neurofilament protein-positive residual axons can be demonstrated especially in intraneural neurofibromas, but axons are not always present and are not required for the diagnosis. EMA$^+$ perineurial cells may be present, usually in the periphery of intraneural neurofibromas. Basement membrane proteins laminin and collagen IV surround the Schwann cells, but positivity in neurofibroma is usually less prominent than that in schwannoma.[36]

It has been suggested that a low Ki-67 analog score and negativity for p53 are features distinguishing neurofibroma from malignant peripheral nerve sheath

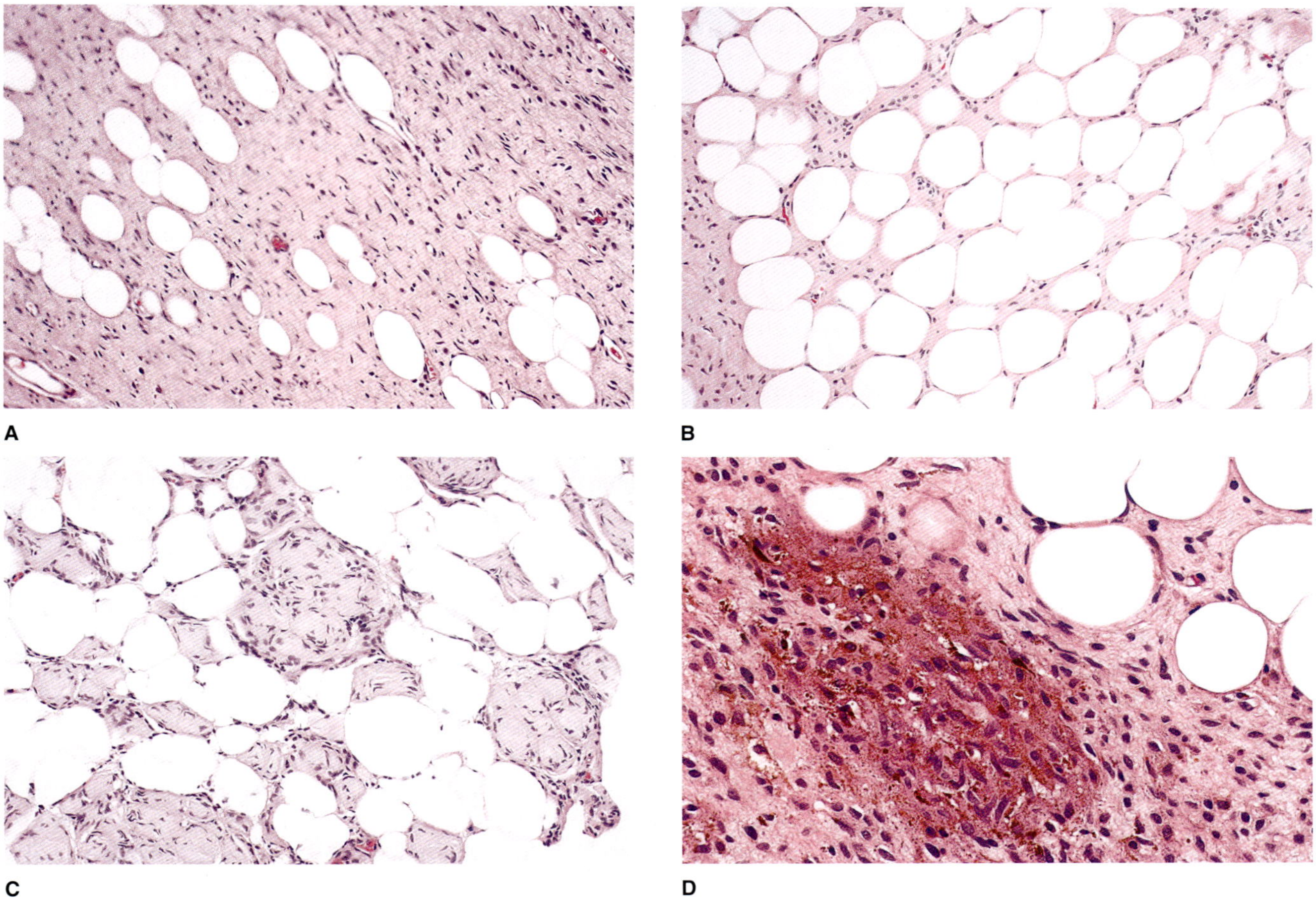

Figure 15–7. *A,* Diffuse neurofibroma typically infiltrates in the subcutaneous fat. *B,* A lesion with a predominant fatty component may appear as fatty tumors at first glance. *C,* Wagner-Meissner-like bodies are commonly seen in diffuse neurofibroma. *D,* Some diffuse neurofibromas have focal areas with melanin pigmentation; these are designated as pigmented neurofibromas.

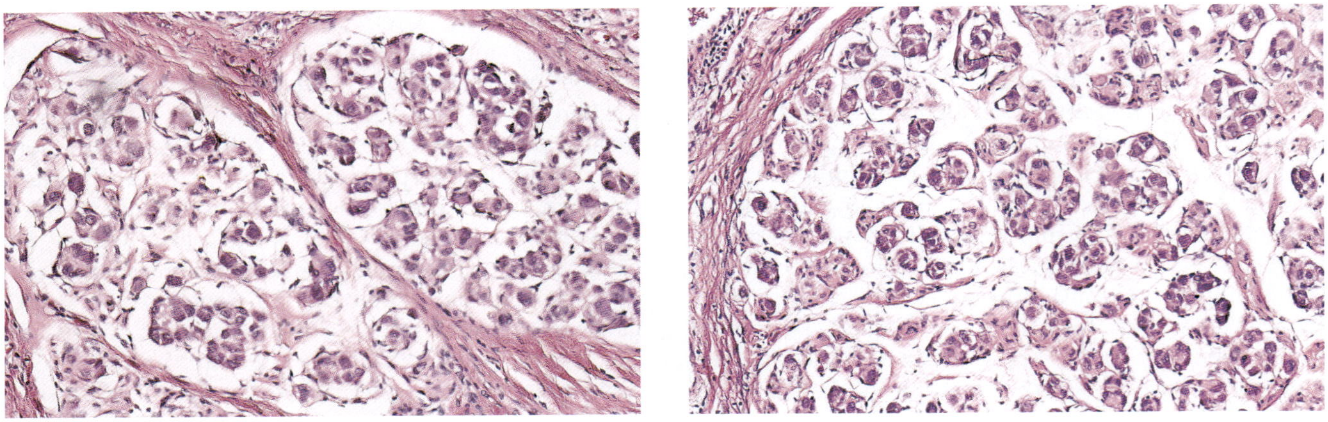

A B

Figure 15–8. *A* and *B,* Epithelioid neurofibroma is composed of lobules of epithelioid Schwann cells with limited atypia and very low mitotic activity.

tumor.[37,38] However, it has not been convincingly demonstrated that these features are useful in borderline tumors, and therefore information from these markers should be evaluated with caution.

Ultrastructural studies have also shown the dual composition of neurofibromas of basement membrane positive Schwann cells and negative fibroblasts.[39]

Transformation and Differential Diagnosis of Neurofibroma

Transformation

The NF1 syndrome carries a risk of malignant transformation of neurofibroma to MPNST, which has been estimated to occur in 2% to 4% of patients.[40] If the development of central nervous system tumor is taken into account, the frequency of development of a malignancy in NF1 patients is around 5%. The risk seems to be greatest for intraneural neurofibromas, especially the plexiform ones.

The transformation of neurofibroma to MPNST is a biologic continuum, and therefore the line between neurofibroma and MPNST is not always clear, and there are no absolute criteria for this distinction. Atypia by itself is not indicative of malignancy, because it is commonly seen in many variants of neurofibromas. Indicative of malignancy are atypia with high cellularity together with significantly elevated mitotic rate (>1–2 mitoses found in a small area). What size of foci with increased mitotic rare indicate malignancy is not clear. In the practical setting, the areas suspicious of malignancy in a neurofibroma should be described. Clinical significance of early malignant transformation of neurofibroma and what constitutes it needs to be addressed in clinicopathologic studies. However, tumors with histologically suspicious features should be excised completely, and preferably widely to prevent local disease progression.

Differential Diagnosis

Differentiation of neurofibroma from schwannoma is sometimes problematic. Most tumors that are difficult in this respect turn out to be neurofibromas. As a general rule, neurofibromas can have schwannoma-like areas, but generally, schwannomas do not have neurofibroma-like areas. Content of residual axons and presence of dual schwannian S-100 protein-positive and fibroblastic CD34^{+} cell populations are features of neurofibroma, often useful in the differential diagnosis.

Whereas the typical cutaneous, intraneural, and plexiform neurofibromas are histologically highly distinctive, the diffuse and cellular types can be easily confused with other tumors.

The pattern of diffuse subcutaneous infiltration of diffuse neurofibroma resembles that of DFSP, but the tumor cells of neurofibroma less commonly have a storiform pattern. In neurofibroma, immunohistochemical studies reveal the dual population of S-100 protein-positive Schwann cells and CD34^{+} fibroblasts (occasionally, the latter is absent). DFSP lesions are typically negative for S-100 protein and positive for CD34. However, some variants (Bednar tumor) may contain isolated S-100 protein-positive tumor cells.

Cellular neurofibroma may be confused with low-grade sarcoma, especially DFSP and low-grade fibromyxoid sarcoma. Immunohistochemical demonstration of a dual population of S-100 protein-positive and CD34^{+} cells is one of the most helpful features to identify these neurofibromas. Myofibroblastic and smooth muscle tumors are usually structurally more homogeneous, and their principal components are myofibroblasts and smooth muscle cells positive for muscle markers.

The specific myxoid neoplasms of the vulvovaginal region (see Chapter 12) have prominent vascular patterns and are generally negative for S-100 protein.

NF1 Tumor Syndrome

Neurofibromatosis type 1 (NF1, von Recklinghausen disease) is caused by loss-of-function mutations and deletions of the *NF1* gene. It is one of the most common autosomal dominant disorders with the birth incidence of 1:3000. Approximately half of the cases of NF1 result from new germline mutations in the *NF1* gene, and the other half are inherited.[41–44] Diagnostic criteria of NF1 based on a National Institutes of Health (NIH)-sponsored consensus conference are the following:[41]

1. Two or more neurofibromas of any type, or one of plexiform type
2. Six or more lightly pigmented macules (cafe au lait spots): more than 5 mm in prepubertal patients, more than 15 mm in postpubertal patients
3. Freckling in axilla or inguinal regions
4. Optic glioma
5. Two or more iris hamartomas (Lisch nodules)
6. Osseous lesions: skeletal dysplasia, cortical thinning of a long bone
7. A first-degree relative with NF1

The presence of two or more of these clinical criteria defines the NF1. Many other tumors occur with increased frequency in NF1 patients. Such tumors especially include GI stromal tumors, duodenal carcinoid with psammoma bodies, and adrenal pheochromocytoma. The severity of NF1 manifestations in different patients vary in a very wide range.

NF1 Gene Alterations

The *NF1* gene is located pericentromerically at chromosome 17q11.2. It encodes for a protein named neurofibromin, which is nearly ubiquitously expressed and is believed to have an inhibitory role in the RAS signal transduction pathway. The *NF1* gene is large, and the distribution and patterns of germline mutations and other changes in the *NF1* gene are yet incompletely characterized.[43,44]

Tumorigenesis in NF1 has been assumed to follow a two-hit hypothesis for recessive tumor suppressor genes. Neurofibroma lesions presumably arise when both alleles are inactivated, by a mutation or an allelic loss.[45,46] In neurofibroma, the Schwann cells, but not the fibroblasts, seem to have the *NF1* gene alterations.[47]

The large size of the *NF1* gene (60 exons spanning 350 kb of genomic DNA) and the existence of homologous pseudogene sequences elsewhere in the genome make the comprehensive analysis of mutations tedious and difficult. Nevertheless, exhaustive analysis of NF1 sequences has allowed a high frequency of mutation detection.[48–50]

Schwannoma (Neurilemoma) and NF2

Schwannoma is a common peripheral nerve sheath tumor that occurs in wide variety of locations. Certain schwannomas, especially the bilateral vestibular ones, are associated with NF2 syndrome and hereditary *NF2* gene mutations. Somatic alterations in this gene seem to be key events for the tumorigenesis of sporadic schwannoma. The rare syndrome with multiple peripheral schwannomas without vestibular tumors is called schwannomatosis.

This text will separately discuss classical schwannoma and variants and review the NF2 syndrome. The GI schwannomas differ from the peripheral ones and will be discussed separately. The rare psammomatous melanotic schwannoma is not associated with NF2.

Conventional Schwannoma

Clinical Features

Schwannomas occur in all ages, although rarely in children. Most commonly they occur in middle-aged individuals without a clear sex predilection. Schwannomas usually present in superficial soft tissues of the extremities and often in the head and neck region, around the spinal column at the spinal nerve roots, mediastinum, and retroperitoneum, where they can reach a large size. Typical schwannoma can also primarily involve visceral sites such as the kidney.[25,51,52]

More commonly peripheral schwannomas present as asymptomatic nodules, but some patients experience nerve-related symptoms such as mild twinge or pain if the tumor is touched. Most schwannomas originate from sensory nerves. Schwannomas of cranial nerves present in the head and neck area and intracranially, especially those of the eighth cranial nerve, where a bilateral one is diagnostic of NF2 tumor syndrome.

Gross Pathology

Schwannomas typically arise in the peripheral aspect of the nerve and are encapsulated by a fibrous band. Although normal nerve can usually be surgically identified in the periphery of the tumor, it is rarely present in the surgical specimen because nerve sacrifice is avoided. On sectioning schwannomas are firm and elastic and may be slightly mucoid. The color varies from gray-tan to yellowish, and many have yellow foci or are homogeneously yellow. Hemorrhagic foci are common, and cystic change may be seen especially in larger tumors (Fig. 15–9). Some schwannomas are extensively cystic, with only a peripheral rim of preserved tumor tissue.

The schwannomas in superficial soft tissue are usually relatively small measuring 1 to 5 cm, whereas the mediastinal and retroperitoneal tumors often reach a large size, the latter often over 10 cm.

Microscopic Pathology

Histologically, schwannomas are spindle cell neoplasms that typically have two components: compact spindle cell Schwann cell components ("Antoni A areas"), and loosely textured histiocyte-rich component ("Antoni B areas"). The schwannian component has a syncytial pattern, and at least focal nuclear palisading with adjacent light microscopically amorphous-appearing pool of cellular processes (Verocay bodies); some tumors show a palisading pattern throughout, and some are essentially composed of cellular palisading areas only (Fig. 15–10*A*), whereas some tumors have focal palisading only (Fig. 15–10*B*). The nuclei vary from oval and blunt ended to elongated, and focal atypia may occur. The tumor cells may have nuclear vacuolization. Tumors with prominent benign atypia have been referred to as "ancient schwannomas."[53] The presence of slight mitotic activity in an otherwise typical, encapsulated schwannoma is acceptable. Necrosis may occur, possibly representing ischemic infarction of an encapsulated tumor under pressure; it is not an alarming feature in a cytologically regular schwannoma.

The histiocyte-rich component contains sheets of xanthoma cells sprinkled with lymphocytes, and these areas may correspond the grossly deeply yellow foci (Fig. 15–10*C*). Many schwannomas have thick-walled vessels with fibrinoid and hyaline changes in the vessel walls (Fig. 15–10*D*).

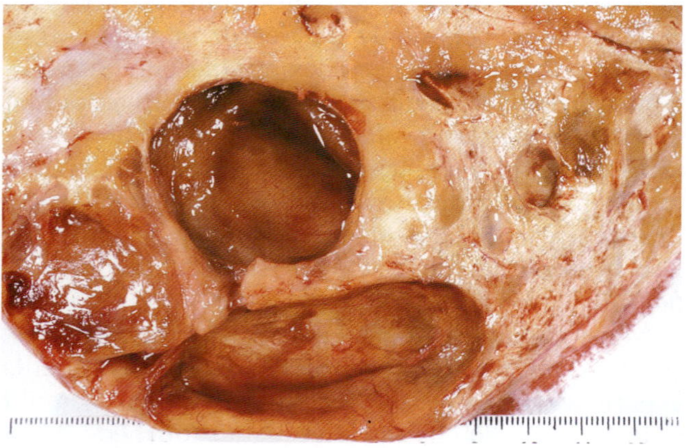

Figure 15–9. A large retroperitoneal schwannoma has a yellowish surface on sectioning and shows multiple cysts.

Immunohistochemistry

Schwannoma cells are strongly and uniformly positive for S-100 protein with both nuclear and cytoplasmic staining (Fig. 15–11*A*). Scattered EMA^+ perineurial cells are often seen in the capsular area, whereas the tumor cells are negative. There are $CD34^+$ fibroblasts especially adjacent to the capsule in the tumor periphery, perivascularly and associated with the degenerative areas, but the cellular areas are $CD34^-$. Schwannomas are consistently positive for vimentin, and about half of them have $GFAP^+$ Schwann cells (Fig. 15–11*B*).[54–56] Keratin positivity (detected for example with AE1 antibody or cocktails) is quite common; its significance is yet to be determined.[56] Schwannoma cells may be positive for CD68 because of their high lysosomal content.[57] The strong immunoreactivity for laminin and collagen type IV reflects the presence of abundant basement membrane material.[58]

Ultrastructure

The cellular areas of schwannoma are composed of Schwann cells with prominent, continuous basal laminas, and the complex cellular processes are also surrounded by them. Many tumors have extracellular foci of banded collagen, the so-called long-spacing collagen.[38,59,60]

Cellular Schwannoma

Highly cellular schwannomas with a solid cellular pattern without typical Verocay bodies have been designated as cellular schwannomas. The greatest significance of this variant is its recognition as a benign nerve sheath tumor and its separation from

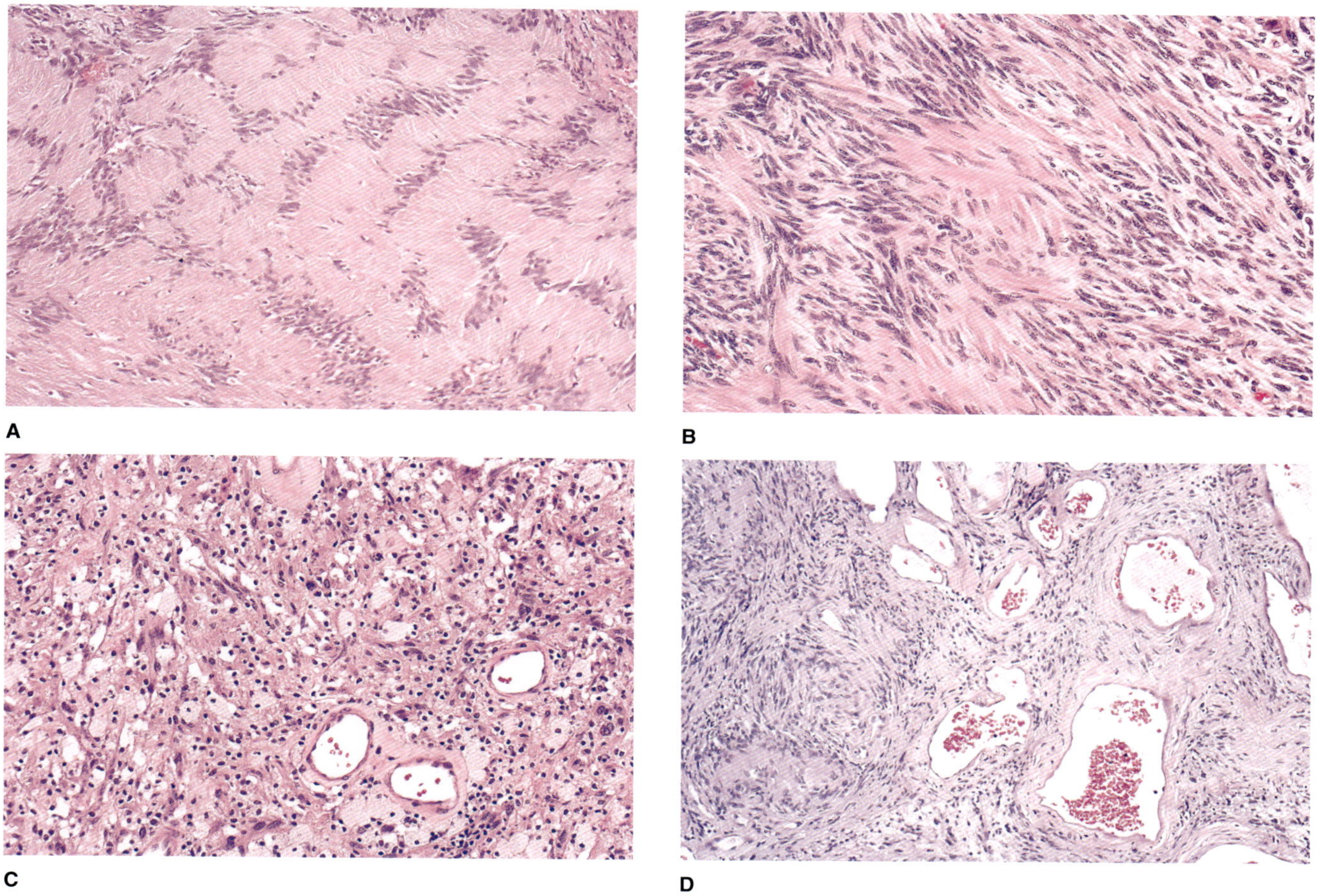

Figure 15-10. Typical appearances of classical schwannoma. *A,* Extensive nuclear palisading. *B,* Focal palisading in a moderately cellular spindle cell tumor. Note the elongated and tapered nuclei. *C,* Schwannoma rich in foamy histiocytes, which impart the yellow gross appearance. *D,* Dilated vessels with hyalinized walls are common in schwannoma.

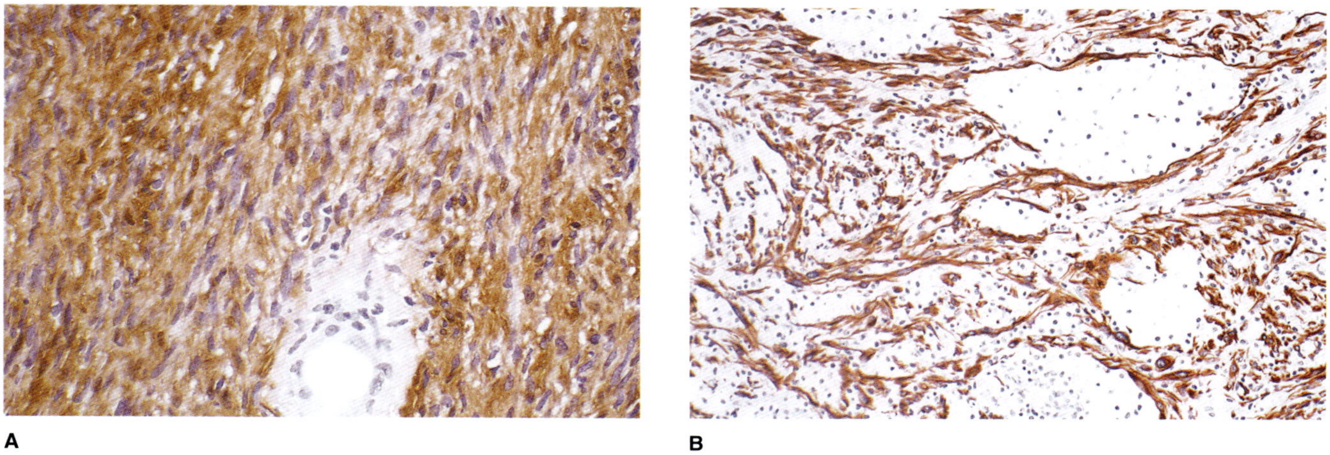

Figure 15-11. *A,* Schwannoma shows global, strong S-100 protein positivity. *B,* A subset of tumor cells is positive for GFAP.

malignant peripheral nerve sheath tumors; apparently many of these tumors have been earlier diagnosed as malignant schwannomas.

Clinical Features

According to three largest clinicopathologic series,[61–64] cellular schwannomas occur in a wide age range with a predominance in young and middle-aged adults, with the peak incidence in the fourth decade and median and mean ages between 40 and 54 years. The two largest series report a significant (63–72%) female predominance.[62,63] A majority of cellular schwannomas occur in the retroperitoneum and posterior mediastinum, whereas few are seen in the head and neck and the extremities. Tumors adjacent to spine or ribs may cause bone erosion. Although the behavior is benign, local recurrence rate of 23% was reported in one series.[64]

Pathology

Grossly, cellular schwannomas are well-demarcated and usually encapsulated spherical or ovoid masses, similar to conventional schwannomas. They tend to be grayish white on sectioning and more homogeneous than ordinary schwannomas, but yellow histiocytic foci may be present. The tumor size varies in a wide range (1–20 cm), with the median size 6 cm in the largest series.

Histologically, the tumors are composed of sheets and fascicles of spindle cells that are more slender than smooth muscle cells and sometimes form perivascular whorls (Fig. 15–12). A majority of tumors have foci of loose texture with xanthomatous histiocytes. Lymphoid clusters may be seen in the capsular region. Mitotic activity is present but is usually limited to 4/10 high-power fields (HPF); however foci of higher mitotic activity may be present. Necrosis occurs rarely, and when present is limited to small foci. Pleomorphism is not a feature of cellular schwannoma.

Immunohistochemically, cellular schwannomas are similar to the ordinary ones with strong S-100 protein positivity. This is one distinguishing feature from MPNST, which are usually much less positive for S-100 protein than are cellular schwannomas.

Differential Diagnosis

Lack of atypia and significant necrosis and the presence of elements seen in the context of ordinary schwannoma (vascular changes, xanthoma cells) support the diagnosis of cellular schwannoma over MPNST. Proliferation marker studies showed that the Ki67 index was 6% to 8% in both nonrecurrent and recurrent tumors, and this parameter was not helpful to predict recurrence. Focal p53 positivity was also common, despite benign nature.[64]

Other tumors with variable nuclear palisading pattern include GI stromal tumors, which are KIT$^+$ (see Chapter 11), and monophasic synovial sarcomas (see Chapter 19). None of these is an encapsulated tumor.

Plexiform Schwannoma

Clinical Features

This designation refers to a rare, multinodular schwannoma that usually presents as a small solitary cutaneous or subcutaneous nodule, most commonly in the extremities. Some examples occur in other peripheral locations and isolated cases have been reported in the GI tract, where the tumor may reach a larger size. There is a predilection to young adults.[65–69]

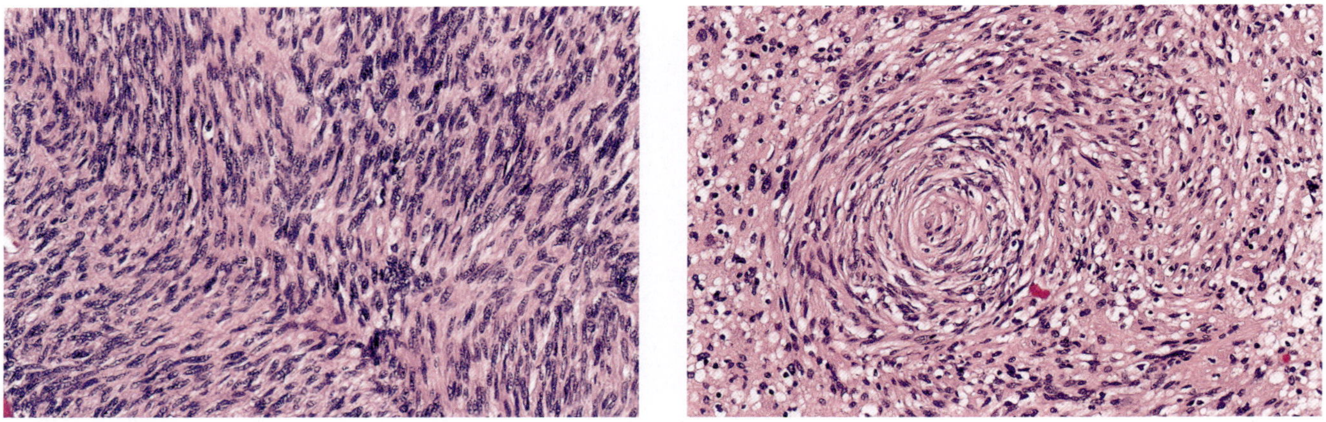

A B

Figure 15–12. *A*, Cellular schwannoma is composed of solid sheets of spindle cells, with occasional palisading. *B*, Perivascular whorling in a cellular schwannoma.

Some association with NF2 syndrome has been reported.[70] Local recurrences have occurred in some cases, but otherwise the behavior is benign.

Pathology

Grossly, the lesion is multinodular, gray or yellowish gray. Histologically, it consists of multiple round-to-oval nodules composed of spindled Schwann cells. Nuclear palisading and Verocay bodies are usually present, but xanthoma cells and lymphocytic infiltration are uncommon (Fig. 15–13*A*). Diagnosis is supported by identification of a purely S-100 protein-positive Schwann cell population. Some plexiform neurofibromas may have areas resembling schwannoma, but these tumors can be diagnosed as neurofibroma by the typical areas elsewhere in the tumor and by the presence of prominent $CD34^+$ cellular component.

Epithelioid Schwannoma

This rare variant of schwannoma with epithelioid cellular morphology has been reported in peripheral soft tissues and the neck of urinary bladder in adult patients; we have seen similar tumors in the peripheral soft tissues and in the submucosa of colon (Fig. 15–13*B* and *C*). These tumors are typically small (<1–2 cm) and have a benign course.[71]

Immunohistochemical identification of S-100 protein-positive pure Schwannian element is a key feature, and lack of atypia and significant mitotic activity help to distinguish this tumor from malignant epithelioid MPNST and melanoma; the latter can be identified based on expression of melanoma-specific markers. When intestinal, lack of neuroendocrine markers and keratins help to separate it from carcinoid.

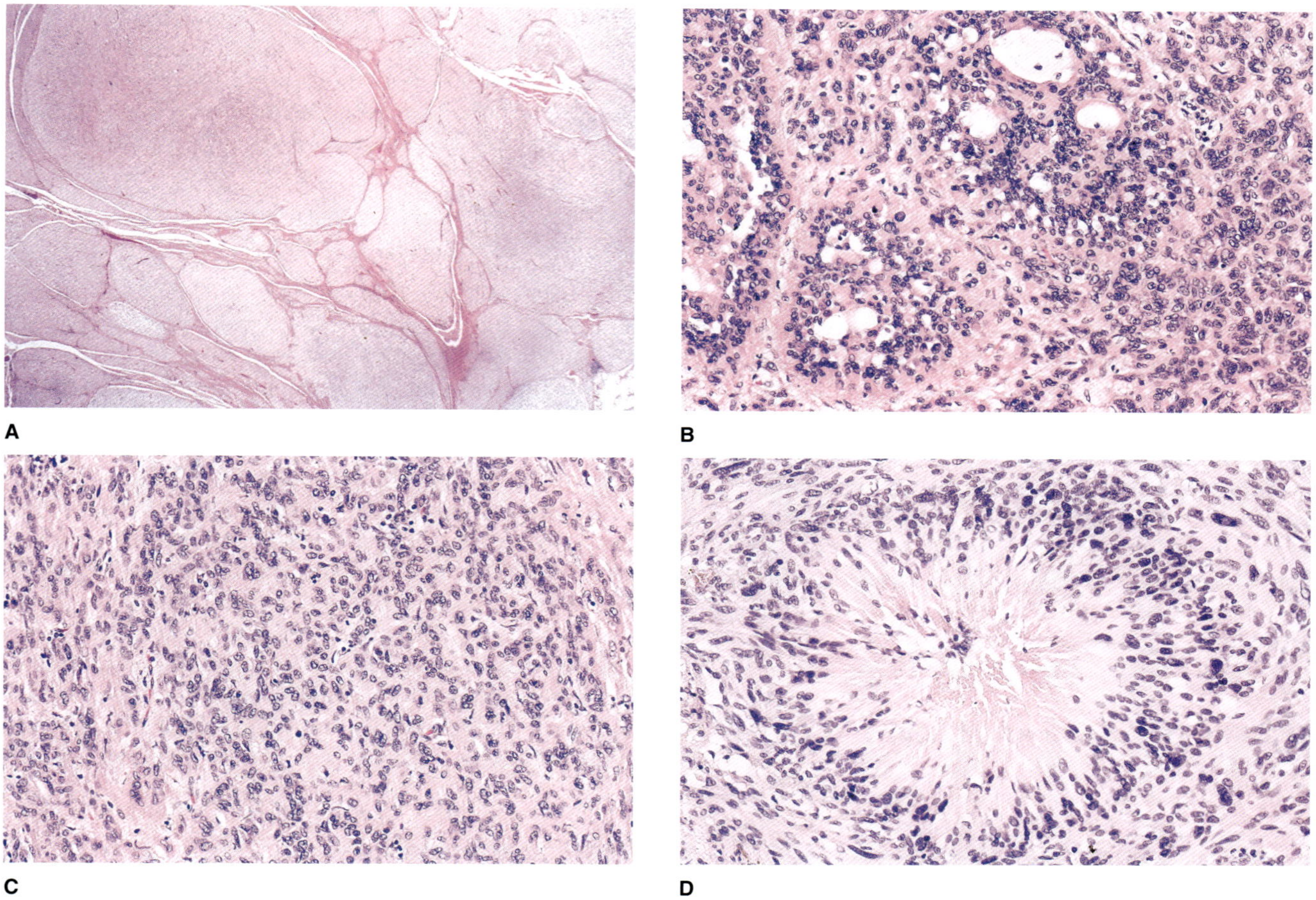

Figure. 15–13. Unusual variant of schwannomas. *A*, A plexiform schwannoma is composed of multiple units of schwannian proliferation separated by delicate septa. This tumor was gastric. *B* and *C*, Epithelioid schwannoma is composed of polygonal cells, which may form pseudoglandular spaces. *D*, A giant rosette in a schwannoma with rounded cells.

Schwannoma with Rosettes and Neuroblastoma-like Features

Schwannomas composed of densely packed oval cells with rosette-like structures have been called neuroblastoma-like schwannomas.[72] The reported three tumors occurred in young or middle-aged adults. Such tumors show high cellularity, areas of tumor cells with oval-to-round cell morphology, and peculiar rosettes surrounding amorphous material, somewhat resembling Homer-Wright rosettes of neuroblastoma (Fig. 15–13*D*). However, immunophenotypic features are those of schwannoma with uniform and strong S-100 protein positivity and negativity for the true neural markers. The tumor appears benign, although follow-up of the reported cases has been short.

Sarcoma Arising in Schwannoma

Malignant transformation of an ordinary schwannoma is an extremely rare event, but isolated cases and small series have been reported. As defined by Woodruff et al.,[73] such a diagnosis requires documented origin of the malignant component from a pre-existing schwannoma, proof of malignant behavior of the transformed component, and exclusion of the possibility that the malignant component is metastasis from another source.

According to review of well-documented cases, schwannomas with malignant transformation occur in middle-aged patients and have a high tumor-related mortality, commonly with liver and lung metastases. Histologically, they are high-grade tumors, usually with epithelioid morphology. Keratin positivity is common, and S-100 protein positivity is patchy rather than diffuse.[73]

Angiosarcoma may arise in schwannoma. The reported tumors have often occurred in the neck region in older men, and many of them originated from the vagus nerve, and some clinically simulated a carotid body tumor. Most were histologically epithelioid angiosarcomas.[74–76]

NF2 and NF2 Gene Alterations

Neurofibromatosis type 2 is an autosomal dominant disorder caused by a germline mutation in the *NF2* gene, located in the pericentromeric region chromosome arm 22q11.2.[77,78] NF2 syndrome is much less common than NF1, with the birth incidence of 1:40,000. Like with NF1, half the NF2 cases result from new mutations.[79,80] NF2 predominantly involves the central nervous system, and bilateral vestibular schwannomas are typical and diagnostic; NF2 have been synonymously called central neurofibromatosis or bilateral vestibular neurofibromatosis. Multiple meningiomas and gliomas, especially spinal ones, and meningoangiomatosis, are also manifestations of NF2 syndrome.

Diagnosis of NF2 Syndrome

Bilateral vestibular schwannomas are diagnostic of NF2. According to the NIH consensus conference,[81] additional diagnostic criteria of the NF2 are the following:

1. Family history of NF2 and unilateral vestibular schwannoma below the age of 30
2. Family history of NF2 and two of the following in any combinations: glioma, meningioma, schwannoma, juvenile cortical cataract (posterior eye lens opacities)

Probable diagnosis (requiring further evaluations) is based on both of the preceding findings without family history of NF2. Also multiple meningiomas either with unilateral vestibular schwannoma below the age of 30 or any of the sign of point 2 is suspicious of NF2 and requires further evaluation. Demonstration of a germline mutation in *NF2* gene from peripheral blood can confirm the diagnosis.

Pathogenesis in NF2 Syndrome and NF2-Associated Tumors

The key event in pathogenesis of both NF2-associated and sporadic schwannomas (and many types of meningiomas) seems to be loss of function of the NF2 encoded protein merlin (schwannomin), following a two-hit mechanism. This occurs by a combination of inactivating *NF2* mutations and allelic losses, analogous to the changes in *NF1* gene in NF1 syndrome.[82] Experimental expression of the mutant NF2 protein causes Schwann cell hyperplasia and tumors supporting the direct role of abrogation of this protein.[83] There seems to be a molecular correlation with severity of disease. Truncation of *NF2* (premature stop codons) results in a more severe phenotype than missense mutations.[84,85] In addition to mutation, calcium-activated proteolytic degradation of NF2 protein may be an alternative disease mechanism in some cases.[86]

Schwannomatosis

Schwannomatosis is the designation for a very rare and so far incompletely characterized condition that manifests as multiple peripheral schwannomas. These tumors have been reported in superficial soft tissues and in the spinal region. The patients do not have bilateral vestibular tumors and lack the other criteria for NF2.[87–89] However, overlap with NF2 syndrome in some cases has been suggested.[90]

The syndrome only rarely has a hereditary basis, and no germline mutations in the *NF2* gene have been identified.[91,92] However, propensity to somatic mutations in the *NF2* gene may be a key to the pathogenesis because the multiple schwannomas carry truncating somatic *NF2* mutations, similar to those seen in peripheral sporadic schwannomas.[91]

GI Schwannoma

This rare tumor differs sufficiently from conventional schwannoma to be placed in a separate clinicopathologic category, and its pathogenesis may also be different from that of schwannoma.

Clinical Features

Schwannomas in the GI tract most commonly occur in the stomach (60–70%). The next most common site is the colon, whereas only isolated cases have been reported in the esophagus and small intestine.[93–95] GI schwannomas are much rarer than GISTs, occurring in a ratio of approximately 1 schwannoma to 50 GISTs in our estimate.

The GI schwannomas occur in a wide age range most commonly in older adults, similar to GISTs. There is no clear sex predilection. Many patients present with GI bleeding, but some tumors are incidental findings during endoscopy or imaging studies for cancer surveillance. Follow-up studies indicate a uniformly benign clinical course. There is no association with NF1 or NF2.

Pathology

Grossly, the GI schwannomas are typically ovoid, yellowish nodules that appear sharply demarcated, although unencapsulated. The tumor usually measures 2 to 4 cm, and usually less than 5 cm. In the stomach, schwannomas usually present as circumscribed submucosal tumors, whereas many colonic ones appear as polypoid intraluminal masses, although with transmural involvement.

Histologically, the most common variant of GI schwannoma is a spindle cell tumor at least focally surrounded by a lymphoid cuff, often with germinal centers that may extend in the peripheral portion of the tumor (Fig. 15–14*A*). The tumor cells are often arranged in fascicles in a microtrabecular pattern between thick vascular septa, and focal nuclear atypia and mild lymphoplasmacytic infiltration is common throughout the tumor and the vascular septa. Focal nuclear atypia is a regular feature, but mitotic activity almost never exceeds 5/50 HPF. Vascular hyaline changes, nuclear palisading, and xanthoma cells are not prominent features, in contrast to peripheral schwannomas (Fig. 15–14*B* and *C*).

Plexiform and epithelioid schwannomas, similar to those seen in peripheral soft tissues, may also occur

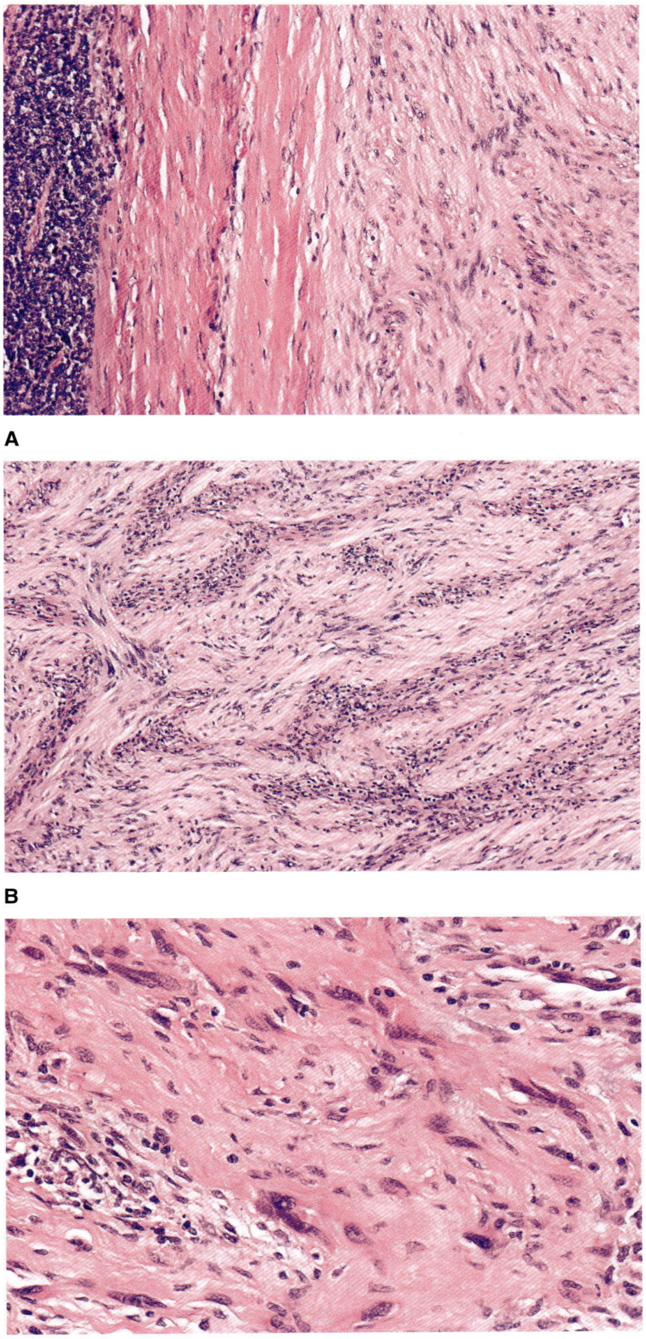

Figure 15–14. *A,* Gastrointestinal schwannomas typically have a peripheral lymphoid cuff, often with a zone of dense fibrosis. *B,* A trabecular microscopic pattern is typical. *C,* Focal nuclear atypia is common in GI schwannomas.

in the GI tract. The former present as multinodular masses and may reach a considerable size. The latter may form small intraluminal polyps, especially in the colon.[95]

Immunohistochemically, the tumor cells are typically strongly positive for S-100 protein and usually for GFAP and nerve growth factor receptor (NGFR)/p75. Most tumors are negative for CD34, and these tumors are uniformly negative for KIT (CD117).

Genetically, GI schwannomas differ from the peripheral ones by the lack of *NF2* gene alterations. Instead, many of these tumors show allelic losses in *NF1*, indicating that the GI schwannomas may be genetically more related to neurofibromas than schwannomas.[96]

Differential Diagnosis

The GISTs are KIT$^+$ GI mesenchymal tumors, and a minority of them (10–15%) are also S-100 protein positive. Many GISTs show prominent nuclear palisading, which should not lead to confusion with schwannoma. True neurofibromas occur in the GI tract in two different clinical contexts: plexiform and diffuse neurofibromas in young patients with NF1 and sporadic small polypoid mucosal neurofibromas in adults. Most if not all highly malignant, strongly S-100 protein-positive spindle cell and epithelioid tumors of the intestines are metastatic melanomas; some of them are polypoid. The diagnosis is aided by the use of melanoma-specific markers and clinical history.

Psammomatous Melanotic Schwannoma

This rare Schwann cell tumor combines the features of schwannoma (schwannian differentiation) and melanoma (presence of melanosomes and melanin pigmentation). Common association with the Carney complex is notable.

Clinical Features

In half the cases, this tumor occurs as a part of a heritable syndrome, named the Carney complex based on its first description by Carney in 1985. The other manifestations of Carney complex include spotty cutaneous hyperpigmentation, cutaneous myxoma (superficial angiomyxoma), cardiac myxoma, and endocrine overactivity (Cushing syndrome, acromegaly, calcifying Sertoli cell tumor). According to Carney, 14% of patients with Carney complex have a psammomatous melanotic schwannoma. There is no association with neurofibromatoses.[97]

This tumor usually presents at a relatively young age, between 20 and 40 years. The patients with Carney complex are almost 10 years younger (average 23 years) than those without it (average 33 years). The lesions often occur near midline in the skin,[98] subcutis, or deep soft tissues or viscera. The three most common locations are spinal nerve roots (back) and the soft tissues of the trunk and extremities. Destructive bone involvement is also possible, and isolated tumors have occurred in the heart, liver, and bronchus. Some patients have multiple tumors, a feature potentially difficult to distinguish from metastatic disease. Primary bone tumors of this type have been reported.[99]

A majority of pigmented melanotic schwannomas are benign. Complete excision with tumor-free margins is believed to be the optimal treatment. Recurrence may occur after incomplete excision, but truly malignant behavior is rare. In Carney's series, 3 of 31 patients died of metastatic disease between 2 and 7 years. Metastases developed in lungs, pleura, liver, and spleen.

Pathology

Melanotic schwannoma ranges from a small nodule less than 1 cm to a bulky tumor over 20 cm; most examples are larger than 5 cm. Grossly, melanotic schwannomas are less often encapsulated than the typical ones, but some are surrounded by a thick capsule. Like conventional schwannomas, the tumors are often fusiform, sausage, or dumbbell shaped. On sectioning, they typically have a gray to black surface with paler foci due to variable melanin pigmentation. Larger tumors may have cysts.

Histologically, the tumor may have a solid, fascicular, or whorled pattern. It is composed of spindled to variably epithelioid cells with moderate to abundant cytoplasm, and spindled cells with dendritic processes also occur. Schwannoma-like nuclear palisading is not prominent but may be present. The occurrence of spherical, periodic acid-Schiff (PAS)-positive multilaminated psammomatous calcifications in variable numbers is unique to this tumor (Fig. 15–15). Pigmentation varies from zones of dark melanin-laden histiocytes to fine, cytoplasmic punctate melanin. Over half the tumors have mature adipose tissue component, and multivacuolated lipoblasts may be present.

Cytologically, most tumor cells have limited atypia with mildly atypical nuclei having a small nucleolus. The spindle cells may have a dendritic morphology. Nuclear pseudoinclusions, similar to those seen in other schwannian tumors, may be present. Some tumors cells have large, sometimes multiple nuclei with prominent nucleoli. Increased nuclear atypia with prominent nucleoli and tumor necrosis are features seen in malignant variants. However, DNA aneuploidy does not appear to be predictive.

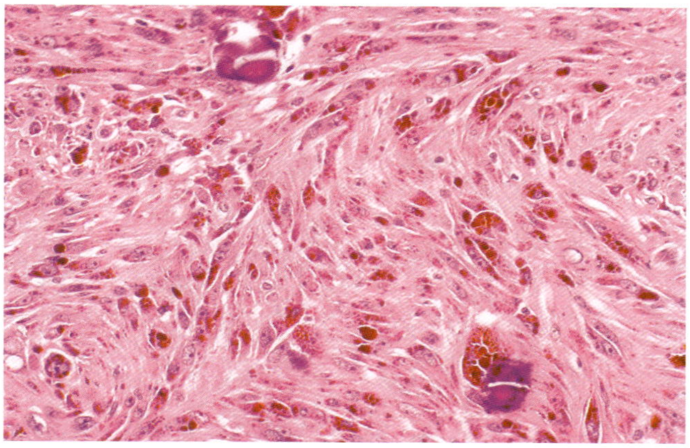

Figure 15–15. Pigmented melanocytic schwannoma is highly cellular and contains abundant melanin pigment and scattered psammoma bodies.

Ultrastructurally, the tumors combine schwannian features, such as complex cell processes and well-developed basement membranes, with the presence of melanosomes.

Specific genetic information is not available for this tumor.

Immunohistochemistry

The pigmented melanotic schwannomas are typically positive for both S-100 protein and HMB45. Like ordinary schwannomas, the melanotic ones are positive for basement membrane components laminin and collagen type IV. According to our experience, they may be positive for GFAP, similar to many conventional schwannomas.

Differential Diagnosis

Tumors that may resemble psammomatous melanotic schwannoma include metastatic melanoma, clear cell sarcoma, and pigmented neurofibroma. The presence of dendritic, bipolar cytologic features are more typical of melanotic pigmented schwannoma than melanoma. Both psammoma bodies and fatty component are specific of melanocytic schwannoma and do not occur in other melanocytic tumors. Clear cell sarcoma typically shows a compartmental pattern, and pigmented neurofibroma shows areas typical of neurofibroma elsewhere in the tumor.

Some cellular schwannomas may have focal melanin pigmentation. These melanotic schwannomas do not have psammoma bodies are not related to psammomatous melanotic schwannoma. Such tumors have been mainly reported from the paraspinal region.[100] There is no association with Carney complex.

Nerve Sheath Myxoma (Myxoid Neurothekeoma)

The tumors originally described as neurothekeomas[101] can be now be divided into two histogenetically unrelated categories: the true nerve sheath myxomas that are schwannian tumors and cellular neurothekeomas, which do not have schwannian features and are rather of fibroblastic or myofibroblastic derivation. These tumors have some clinicopathologic differences and can be separated immunohistochemically, and in most cases, also by morphology.

Clinical Features

Nerve sheath myxoma occurs in peripheral superficial soft tissues in a wide age range but has a predilection to young adults equally in men and women. The tumor occurs in a wide variety of locations, most commonly in the extremities, with a predilection to distal parts. The tumor has a uniformly benign behavior, and local excision is sufficient.[102–105]

Pathology

This dermal or subcutaneous tumor typically appears as a multinodular mucoid mass that usually measures 0.5 to 2 cm. Histologically, the tumor is typically composed of multiple myxoid nodules separated by dense collagenous septa (Fig. 15–16*A*). The nodules are hypocellular, and are composed of loosely arranged cords or bundles of spindle cells surrounded by myxoid material. Some tumor cells have large, hyperchromatic nuclei or are multinucleated. Some lesions have more compact areas that can have spindle cells forming Verocay bodies (Fig. 15–16*B*). Mitotic activity is inconspicuous.

Immunohistochemically, the tumor cells are positive for S-100 protein, GFAP, and NGFR (p75). A $CD34^+$ fibroblastic component is present, similar to neurofibromas (Fig. 15–16C).

Cellular Neurothekeoma

Clinical Features

This rare tumor usually occurs in the head and neck region in children and young adults with a female predominance. It usually forms a relatively small subcutaneous nodule but may also occur in the buccal soft tissues.[105–108]

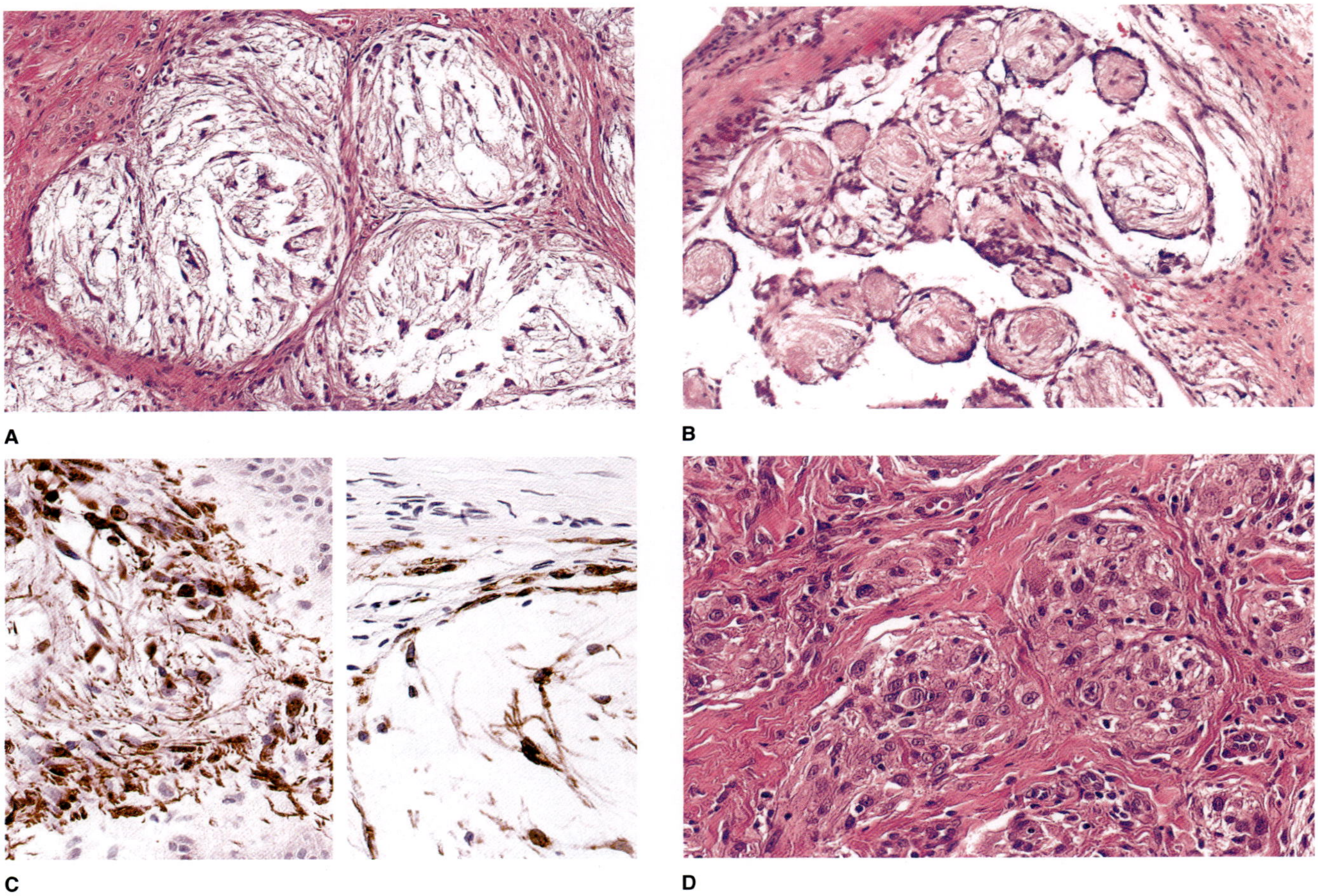

Figure 15–16. *A,* Nerve sheath myxoma is composed of multiple myxoid lobules composed of narrow bundles of elongated cells, some of which show mild nuclear atypia. *B,* Schwannoma-like features in a nerve sheath myxoma. *C,* Nerve sheath myxoma cells are positive for S-100 protein (*left*), and some cells are positive for GFAP (*right*). *D,* In comparison, cellular neurothekeoma also has a nodular compartmental pattern, but there is no myxoid stroma and the cytology is epithelioid.

Pathology

Grossly, cellular neurothekeoma presents as a small 1- to 2-cm oval nodule, which may be rubbery or hard. Microscopically, the lesion is composed of multiple, often ill-defined or partly coalescent, highly cellular nodules partly separated by narrow collagenous bands. In contrast to nerve sheath myxoma, the nodules are highly cellular and have no or only a minimal amount of myxoid background. The tumor cells have an epithelioid morphology with well-defined cell borders. The atypia is usually minimal and mitotic activity is rare (Fig. 15–16*D*).

Immunohistochemically, the cells are negative for S-100 protein, GFAP, NGFR (p75), and CD34, but they are positive for smooth muscle actin and calponin, probably indicating myofibroblastic differentiation. Positivity for CD63/NK1/C3, an antigen also expressed in melanoma, has been reported as a typical feature.[109] Based on the antigenic profile, cellular neurothekeoma appears unrelated to true nerve sheath myxoma, and it is not a true nerve sheath tumor, but is rather related to fibrohistiocytic tumors.

Differential Diagnosis

The multinodularity and the cytologic features resemble those of plexiform fibrohistiocytic tumor, although giant cells are not present. The cytologic resemblance to epithelioid variant of fibrous histiocytoma has led to the suggestion that these tumors are related.[110] A relationship with epithelioid variant of pilar leiomyoma has also been considered, but this is not supported by only weak actin positivity and negativity for desmin.[109]

Perineurioma—Tumor of Perineurial Cells

Perineurial cells form the outer cellular lining around the peripheral nerve fascicles and small nerves. These cells represent the peripheral continuation of the meningeal cells in the pia-arachnoid membranes. The normal perineurial cells are typically elongated mesenchymal cells that are often stacked in a lamellar fashion. Their typical ultrastructural features include elongated cell processes, basement membranes, and pinocytic vesicles. Immunohistochemically, the perineurial cells are positive for vimentin and EMA and negative for S-100 protein.[111-113]

Perineuriomas (perineurial cell tumors) are very rare nerve sheath tumors that display pure perineurial cell differentiation without Schwann cell components. The group is clinically and histologically heterogeneous and contains two main types: intraneural and soft tissue perineurioma. Although many of these tumors are histologically very distinctive, the diagnosis of soft tissue perineuriomas is usually based on immunohistochemical demonstration of EMA positivity, ultrastructural analysis, or both. Because immunohistochemical positivity for EMA is not specific for perineurial cells, any tumors not conforming with the known variants of perineurioma should not be diagnosed solely based on EMA positivity; the identification of unusual variants of soft tissue perineurioma also requires ultrastructural documentation.

Electron microscopically perineurial cells and perineuriomas show elongated cells with partial basal lamina and prominent pinocytic vesicles. Rough endoplasmic reticulum is less prominent than in fibroblasts.[114,115]

Intraneural Perineurioma

This very rare tumor was previously variably referred to as localized hypertrophic neuropathy, hypertrophic mononeuropathy,[116] localized hypertrophic neurofibrosis, hypertrophic interstitial neuritis, and intraneural neurofibroma. The tumor occurs in children and young adults and causes motor or sometimes sensory neurologic deficits. Because the condition is benign, conservation of the involved nerve is generally advocated and treatment should be limited to biopsy only. Excision of the lesion should be reserved to nonfunctional nerves.[117]

Intraneural perineurioma forms a fusiform, symmetric expansion of the involved nerve that usually measures 2 to 10 cm. Histologically, it consists of innumerable expanded nerve fascicles surrounded by concentric, onion bulblike spindled perineurial cell proliferation. A central degenerating axon and small amounts of Schwann cells remain in the core of each concentric unit (Fig. 15–17*A*).

Immunohistochemically, the tumor cells are positive for EMA and negative for S-100 protein. Small numbers of residual Schwann cells are S-100 protein positive and neurofilament-positive central axon can usually be demonstrated.

The presence of clonal chromosomal changes, namely the loss of chromosome 22,[117] supports neoplastic nature of this lesion, which earlier was uniformly considered a hyperplastic process.

Sclerosing Perineurioma

This is a characteristic, probably the most common clinicopathologic variant of soft tissue perineurioma.[118] Based on the series of 19 cases from the AFIP, this tumor typically occurs as a circumscribed, small (usually <2 cm), painless nodule in the fingers and hands. The tumor has a strong predilection to young adults in the third and fourth decades with a 2:1 male predominance. Single cases have been seen in children and in older adults. There is often a long history of a tumor that remains stationary or slowly growing over the observation period of up to 40 years. The tumor is benign and does not have a significant tendency to recur.

Grossly, the tumor forms a well-circumscribed nodule. On sectioning it is off-white with a rubbery, occasionally cartilage-like consistency. The lesion usually measures less than 1 cm to over 3 cm (median, 1.5 cm). Histologically, sclerosing perineurioma is a densely collagenous mass. It contains clusters, cords, or concentric arrangements of small, cuboidal, epithelioid-appearing tumor cells in a densely collagenous background (Fig. 15–17*B* and *C*), sometimes around small nerves.

Immunohistochemically, the tumor cells are strongly positive for EMA (Fig. 15–17*D*) and basement membrane proteins laminin and collagen IV. They are negative for S-100 protein, and CD34, and only occasionally positive for keratins. Muscle actin expression has been noted in nearly half of the cases.

A cryptic *NF2* gene deletion has recently been described in one case of sclerosing perineurioma.[119] Missense *NF2* mutations and allelic losses of *NF2* gene have been found in sclerosing perineuriomas, suggesting two-hit involvement of *NF2* gene in a manner similar to meningiomas and schwannomas.[120]

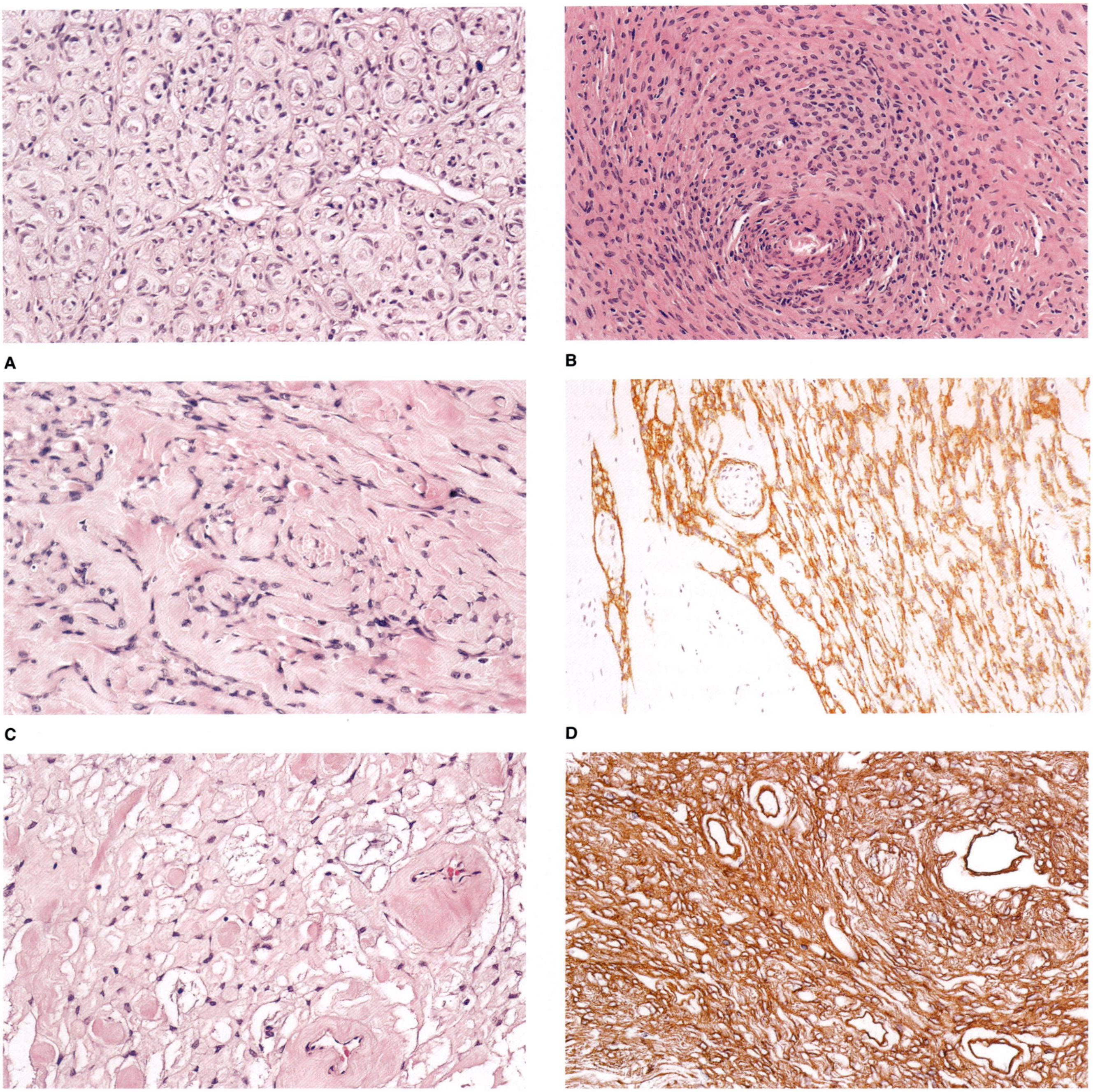

A B C D E F

Figure 15–17. Variants of perineuriomas. *A,* Intraneural perineurioma features innumerable nerve fascicles surrounded by proliferating, multilamellar perineurial cells. *B* and *C,* Sclerosing perineurioma contains streaks and arcades of epithelioid tumor cells in a dense collagenous stroma. *D,* The tumor cells of sclerosing perineurioma are EMA^+. *E,* Retiform perineurioma is composed of spindled cells that form a netlike pattern in loose stroma. *F,* Strong laminin positivity is typical of all perineuriomas, as seen in this cellular retiform variant.

Differential Diagnosis

Sclerosing glomus tumor and mixed tumor of the skin may resemble sclerosing perineurioma by histologic pattern. However, the former is a smooth muscle tumor strongly positive for SMA and with vascular association, and the latter usually shows evidence of epithelial differentiation and is keratin positive.

Other Soft Tissue Perineuriomas

This is a somewhat heterogeneous group of tumors with pure perineurial cell differentiation. The first soft tissue perineurioma was described by Lazarus and Trombetta in 1978[114] based on ultrastructural features of perineurial cells in a deep soft tissue tumor.

Soft tissue perineuriomas present in a wide variety of body sites in adult patients. Histologically, these tumors typically have a spindle cell pattern, often with a storiform, meningioma-like architecture. They have been generally identified as hypocellular spindle cell tumors of the skin or subcutis based on their concentric lamellar pattern, EMA positivity, meningioma-like architecture, and ultrastructural features.[121-123]

A histologically distinctive retiform variant was recently described. The reported four tumors measured 1.5 to 2 cm and occurred in the upper extremity of young women. Similar tumors have been reported in other soft tissue locations.[124,125] The tumor cells form a netlike pattern and are separated by alternating myxoid matrix and dense collagen (Fig. 15–17*E*). The tumor cells are positive for EMA and basement membrane proteins, collagen IV, and laminin (Fig. 15–17*F*). At least some soft tissue perineuriomas have losses in chromosome 22,[126] but *NF2* gene mutations have not been found as a universal feature.[120]

Malignant Perineurioma

Although perineuriomas are generally benign tumors, occasional malignant examples have been described. The seven cases reported by Hirose et al[127] occurred in a wide range of ages and locations and varied from a small nodule to a 30-cm tumor. Histologically, they showed whorling light microscopic pattern, concentric lamellar pattern by electron microscopy, and EMA positivity and S-100 protein negativity by immunohistochemistry. Although most tumors were high grade histologically, they had a better prognosis than MPNSTs. Rare similar tumors have been reported by others.[128]

Differential Diagnosis

The identification of malignant perineurioma is based on compatible morphology and EMA positivity, ideally supported by electron microscopy. Many unrelated malignant spindle cell tumors can be focally EMA$^+$, and they should not be confused with perineurioma. Some dedifferentiated liposarcomas have meningothelial-like whorls; these tumors can be properly identified by their atypical lipomatous component and common bony metaplasia, which are not features of perineurioma.

Granular Cell Tumor

Granular cell tumor (GCT), historically called "granular cell myoblastoma" is a S-100 protein-positive Schwann cell-related neoplasm usually presenting in superficial soft tissues and less commonly in the respiratory and GI tracts; rare malignant variants occur. Gingival granular cell tumor in infants ("congenital epulis") is a separate entity clinically and histogenetically unrelated to ordinary GCT.

Clinical Features

According to the AFIP data on over 1800 GCTs of all sites, these tumors occur in all age groups, although they are very rare in children under the age of 5 years and are uncommonly removed after the eighth decade. Otherwise the age distribution roughly parallels that of the general population. There is a mild female predominance (5:4) and relative predilection to blacks.

The GCTs occur in a wide variety of sites, of which tongue and superficial soft tissues are the most common. The soft tissues sites especially include hands, forearm, chest wall, back, thigh, and anogenital area. GCTs of the breast may clinically and radiologically simulate breast carcinoma. In peripheral soft tissues, the tumor is rarely intramuscular. Internal organ sites include esophagus, external hepatobiliary tract, larynx, and bronchi and neurohypophysis. Multiple lesions may occur in peripheral soft tissues and internal sites and are not to be taken as a sign of malignancy.[129-135] In one patient, 52 separate GCTs were reported in a colectomy specimen.[135]

Pathology

The majority of GCTs are 1 to 2 cm in diameter, and occasional ones reach the size of 5 cm or more. Grossly, the tumor typically forms an oval nodule that varies from sharply circumscribed to an ill-defined mass, typically with a yellow surface on sectioning.

Microscopically, GCTs are composed of polygonal or slightly elongated cells with well-defined cell borders. The cytoplasm is abundant and granular and the nuclei are usually small with a dense chromatin. Focal atypia may occur, but mitoses are rare. In some cases, the tumor cells form solid compact sheets (Fig. 15–18*A*). In others, clusters of granular cells are diffusely dispersed between collagen fibers (Fig. 15–18*B*). In the tongue, the tumor cells may form a checkerboard pattern with the entrapped skeletal muscle cells. The granular cytoplasm is variably positive on PAS staining. In some cases, the granular cells are surrounding small nerves, in accordance with their relationship with peripheral nerve tumors. Proximity of granular cell tumor of an epithelial surface, especially in the tongue and perineum, may induce pseudoepitheliomatous hyperplasia, which should not be confused with squamous cell carcinoma.

Immunohistochemistry and Ultrastructure

Immunohistochemically, GCTs are consistently positive for S-100 protein and neuron-specific enolase (NSE) and negative for muscle cell and epithelial markers. Due to the high lysosomal content, the tumor cells are also positive for CD68.[136–138] The intermediate filaments are composed of vimentin only, and basement membrane proteins can typically be demonstrated around cell clusters.[139] Recently, granular cell tumors of the hepatobiliary areas were shown to be inhibin positive.[140] According to our experience, this also applies to peripheral granular cell tumors but not to neurofibromas and schwannomas, setting GCTs apart from other peripheral nerve tumors (Fig. 15–18C).

Ultrastructurally, the granular cytoplasm contains numerous phagolysosomes (autophagic vacuoles), and some cells also contain large boat-shaped cytoplasmic crystals referred to as angulated bodies.[141]

Differential Diagnosis

The true GCTs are believed to be Schwann cell related and consistently S-100 protein positive, which separates them from most other granular cell lesions including those of histiocytic, fibroblastic, or smooth muscle derivation. Some smooth muscle tumors have a granular cell appearance; their diagnosis is based on other features of smooth muscle tumors and immunohistochemical demonstration of actins, desmin, or both.[142]

Granular cell histiocytic reaction usually contains more conventional histiocytes and multinucleated ones. Epithelial tumors, such as jaw ameloblastomas and carcinomas with granular cell features, should not be confused with true GCTs.

Malignant GCT

Malignant behavior of GCT is rare (<1%), and it may be impossible to predict histologically. Compared with their benign counterparts, these tumors tend to be larger and occur in slightly older patients.[143] Malignant GCTs may recur locally with multiple skin satellite nodules and some metastasize, especially to liver and lungs, and may be fatal.

According to the largest published series, the following features are associated with an increased metastatic risk: mitotic rate 2 or more per 10 HPF, increased nuclear atypia, high nucleocytoplasmic ratio, prominent nucleoli, cell spindling, and tumor necrosis (Fig. 15–18*D*). It was found that tumors with three or more of these features had a high frequency of malignant behavior, with half of the patients developing distant metastases.[143]

Gingival GCT

The gingival GCT is not a nerve sheath tumor, but has fibroblastic or pericytic origin. It is a clinicopathologically distinctive tumor of infants.

Clinical Features

This rare tumor has also been referred to as "gingival epulis of newborn." It predominantly (90%) occurs in female infants and typically presents as a polypoid pale to pinkish mass bulging from the anterior alveolar ridge, more commonly in the maxilla than mandible. It may reach a considerable size and interfere with feeding. The average size is 2.0 to 2.5 cm, and the largest examples have been over 5 cm. Multiple tumors occur in 10% of cases, and there is no racial predilection. Conservative excision sparing the unerupted teeth is sufficient because incompletely removed tumors do not have tendency to recur, and the tumor may involute with time.[144]

Disseminated congenital GCT has been reported. In addition to gingiva, it involved most major internal organs, pituitary, and leptomeninges of a stillborn fetus, and similar to the gingival tumors, it was negative for S-100 protein.[145]

Pathology

Histologically, the gingival GCT is composed of sheets of ovoid or rounded granular cells surrounding a prominent network of branching capillaries (Fig. 15–19). The cells typically have well-defined cell borders. The nuclei are small and centrally located, and mitotic activity and atypia are absent.

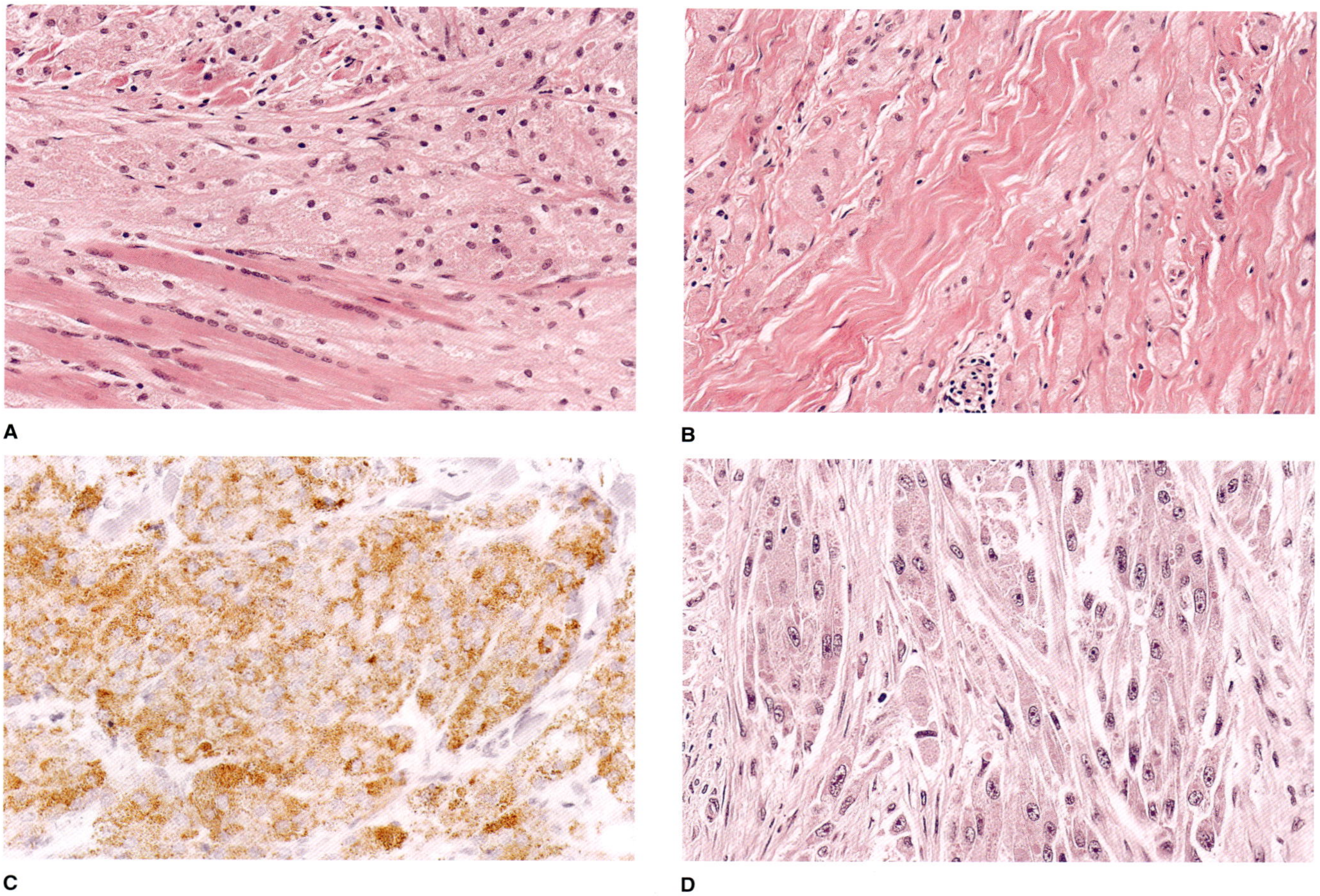

Figure 15-18. Different appearances of granular cell tumor. *A,* A variant with a solid pattern. *B,* A variant with scattered tumor cells in a fibrous stroma. *C,* Granular cell tumors are inhibin positive. *D,* Granular cell tumor that metastasized to the lungs shows spindling, atypia, and mitotic activity.

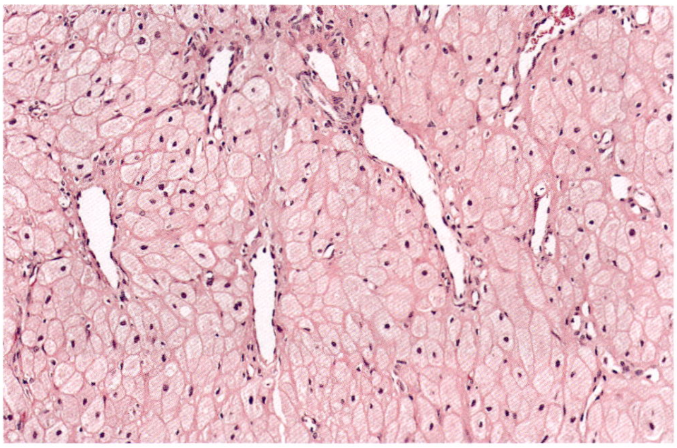

Figure 15-19. A gingival granular cell tumor is a non-Schwann cell-related lesion with a prominent capillary pattern.

In contrast to the GCTs of soft tissues, the gingival ones are negative for S-100 protein. They are of fibroblastic, pericytic, or primitive mesenchymal cell origin, based on ultrastructural and immunohistochemical features.[145-149] Smooth muscle differentiation has been suggested in some cases based on actin positivity.[150]

MPNST

The designation, malignant peripheral nerve sheath tumor, has replaced the old terms of neurofibrosarcoma and malignant schwannoma. When applied strictly, the diagnosis should be used only for malignant tumors that originate from a neurofibroma, nerve, or in connection with NF1. Some tumors can be identified as probable examples by their histologic similarity with tumors belonging to the preceding groups. This especially includes epithelioid MPNST, a histologic subgroup, which is discussed separately. Excluded from the definition are sarcomas arising from benign schwannoma and other types of sarcomas in NF1 patients; both are rare. So far, no genetic markers have been defined specific for MPNST.

Clinical Features

This tumor occurs in all ages from early childhood but it is most common in early middle age, with the median ages in the largest series varying between 35 and 45 years. Most series show a mild female predominance. This is especially true for the patients with NF1, who also have a younger age at presentation.[151–161] A small percentage of MPNSTs arise on the site of previous irradiation (postirradiation sarcoma), and radiation may accelerate the development of MPNST in patients with NF1.[162,163]

The tumor most commonly presents as a mass, often with pain, and a minority of patients have focal neurologic deficits or tingling. The most common sites are the proximal parts of lower and upper extremities, paraspinal region of the trunk, and the head and neck region. Five-year survival varies from 15% to 40%, and patients with NF1 have a poorer prognosis. Other adverse factors are tumor size over 5 cm, mitotic rate over 20/10 HPF, central location, and incomplete resection. The local recurrence rate is high, and metastases develop in over half the patients. Most commonly they occur in the lungs, bones, pleura, and liver; spread by the meningeal route is also possible.

Pathology

Grossly, the tumor typically forms an oval or fusiform mass arising from a nerve, often involved by intraneural, often plexiform neurofibroma (Fig. 15–20*A*). The tumor often measures over 10 cm, sometimes over 25 cm. It typically shows a variegated surface on sectioning with areas of hemorrhage and necrosis. Elements of the pre-existing neurofibroma may be visible as focal rubbery or fibromyxoid areas either in the periphery of the tumor or in the ends of a fusiform tumor (Fig. 15–20*B*).

Identification of elements of pre-existing neurofibroma helps the identification of those MPNSTs that are not arising from a major nerve; such elements and the MPNST often show a sharp demarcation.

Histologically, most MPNSTs are high-grade tumors with high mitotic rate and commonly necrosis. The tumor cells may be seen as rounded perivascular collars surrounded by extensive necrosis (Fig. 15–21*A*). The most common histologic patterns include a high-grade fibrosarcomatous one composed of densely packed sheets of plump but relatively uniform spindle or oval cells (Fig. 15–21*B*), and a herringbone pattern may also be present. Many tumors have geographic necrosis and vascular proliferation resembling those commonly seen in glioblastoma multiform (Fig. 15–21*C*), and some have plump, slightly epithelioid spindle cells (Fig. 15–21*D*). Pleomorphic malignant fibrous histiocytoma-like pattern is seen in some cases, and there may be a prominent vascular pattern slightly reminiscent of hemangiopericytoma. Myxoid matrix may be seen. The tumor cells have often spindled, bent nuclei with diffuse hyperchromasia. The pathology epithelioid MPNST will be discussed separately later.

Plexiform MPNST is the designation given for a subset of childhood MPNSTs. The reported tumors mainly occurred in peripheral soft tissues and measured 1.5 to 8 cm. Histologically, they were composed

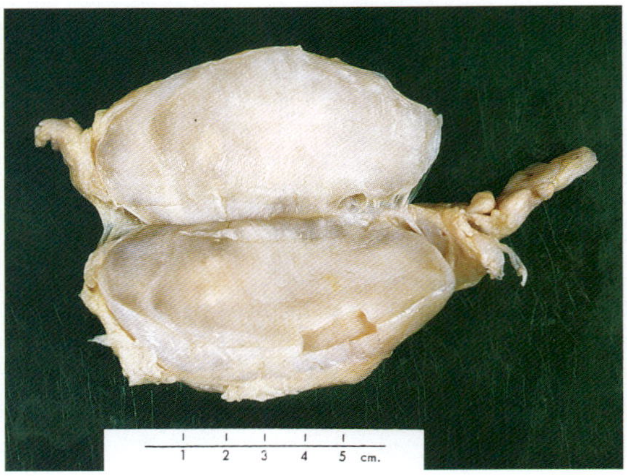

A

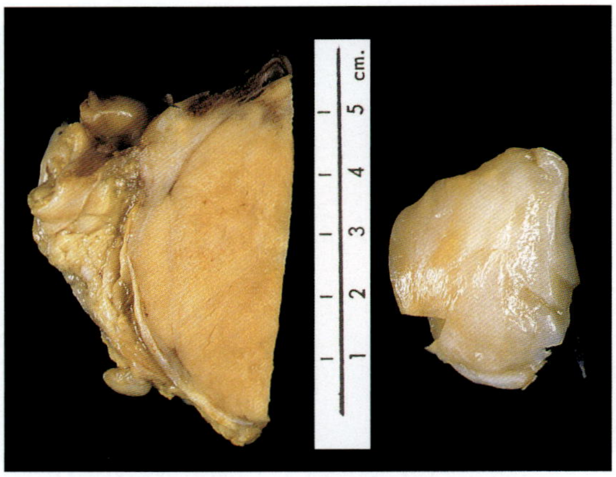

B

Figure 15–20. *A*, Malignant peripheral nerve sheath tumor arising in an intraneural neurofibroma is a fusiform enlargement of a nerve trunk. *B*, Areas of pre-existing neurofibroma are grossly mucoid, gray, and glistening (*right*), whereas the MPNST is yellowish and has a firm texture (*left*).

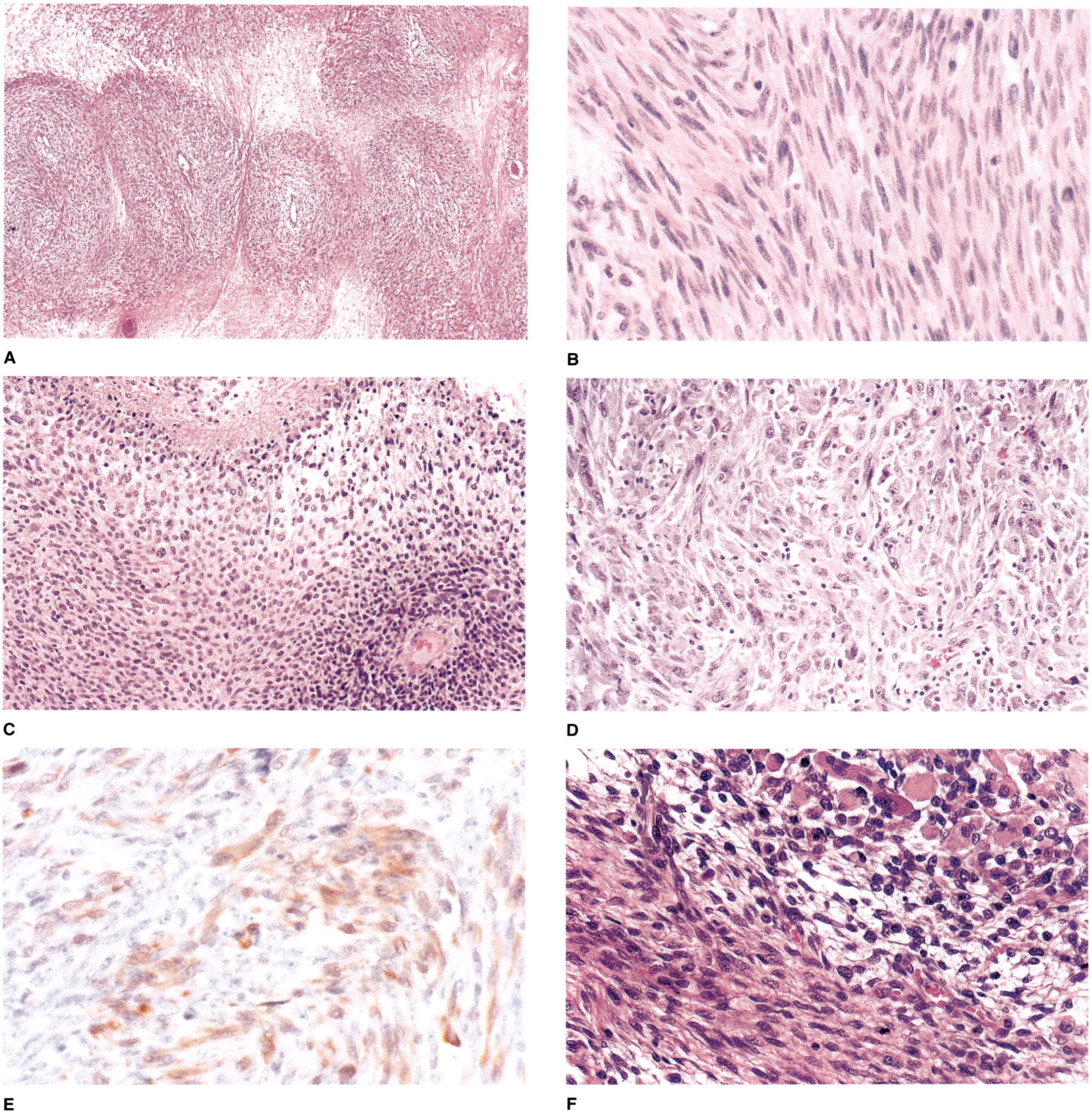

Figure 15-21. Histologic spectrum of MPNST. *A,* Tumor with a perivascular collar-like pattern surrounded by extensive necrosis. *B,* A high-grade fibrosarcoma-like appearance. *C,* Geographic necrosis is common. *D,* A slightly more epithelioid appearance in an MPNST arising in neurofibroma. *E,* Significant S-100 protein positivity is seen in less than half of the MPNSTs. *F,* Triton tumor combines the features of spindled MPNST and focal rhabdomyoblastic differentiation.

of bundles of spindle cells giving the tumor a microscopically plexiform architecture. The cellularity was high and mitotic rate varied from 1 to 18/10 HPF; however, only one tumor was fatal.[164] Because of the generally good prognosis and plexiform histology, these tumors have been reinterpreted as cellular plexiform schwannomas by others.[165]

Immunohistochemistry

The MPNSTs often show nonspecific or less commonly schwannian immunohistochemical features. Only a minority of them are extensively S-100 protein positive, whereas many are focally positive (Fig. 15-21*E*); in some cases the latter reflects intermingled remnants of residual nerve or neurofibroma.[166,167] In contrast to neurofibroma, CD34 expression is uncommon. In our experience, focal keratin (K) K8 and K18 positivity is quite common, but K7 and K19 are absent. Presence of desmin and actins usually reflects the presence of a heterologous rhabdomyoblastic component (Triton tumor, see following). Considering that synovial sarcoma can also be S-100 protein positive, immunohistochemical results have to be interpreted with caution.

Ultrastructure

Some MPNSTs show schwannian differentiation, such as complex cell processes and variably developed basal laminas. However, many of these tumors have no specific ultrastructural features.[168] The role of electron microscopy in defining a poorly differentiated sarcoma as MPNST is dubious.

Differential Diagnosis

Synovial sarcoma that arises close to nerves, contains benign neural proliferation, or has nuclear palisading should not be confused with MPNST. These tumors, when of monophasic spindle cell type, can often be identified by scattered EMA^+ and keratin-positive cells. In problematic cases, demonstration of the SYT-SSX fusion transcript is helpful. Such synovial sarcomas may account for some tumors reported as $SYT\text{-}SSX^+$ MPNSTs. Histologic distinction between MPNST and fibrosarcoma is more difficult, and the identification of MPNST in this context usually requires the proper context (NF1, nerve, or neurofibroma origin).

Cellular schwannoma should be seriously considered in well-differentiated tumors with sparse mitotic activity and extensive S-100 protein positivity. These tumors are encapsulated and often contain xanthoma cells.

Metastatic (or primary large) malignant melanoma should be ruled out in the case of strongly S-100 protein-positive spindled or epithelioid malignant tumor, especially when seen in a lymph node. Additional melanoma markers and clinical correlation (information on previous melanoma) are helpful.

In the GI tract, a large majority of sarcomas are GISTs, even when associated with NF1; our review has not identified any bona fide GI MPNSTs in the AFIP files.

Genetics

Cytogenetic studies have shown complex clonal abnormalities in most cases.[169–171] Rare cases have had single abnormalities, such as +7 and −22, neither of which is diagnostically specific.[171] Homozygous deletion of the *INK4A/CDKN2A* gene at 9p, encoding for cyclin-dependent kinase inhibitor-cell cycle regulators such as p16 and p19, has been shown typical of MPNST, but not of neurofibromas. Mutations or methylation of this gene were not observed in two studies.[172,173]

MPNST with Divergent Differentiation

The most common divergent differentiation (heterologous elements) of MPNST is rhabdomyosarcomatous differentiation (malignant Triton tumor). Malignant glandular MPNST with epithelial elements is very rare. Additional heterologous elements include cartilaginous and osteosarcomatous ones, which may occur together with the other heterologous components. Heterologous elements more commonly occur in tumors of NF1 patients and may be associated with more malignant tumor behavior.

Origin of angiosarcoma in the MPNST has been reported on occasion.[1,2] This event may represent an extreme level of tumor angiogenesis with malignant transformation.

Malignant Triton Tumor

Triton tumor is the designation for MPNST with rhabdomyosarcomatous differentiation. The name is derived from Triton salamander, in which development of both myoid and neural elements from transplanted sciatic nerve were experimentally demonstrated.[174]

Clinical Features

Triton tumors are clinically similar to other MPNSTs, except that they are more often associated with NF1 (60–70%). They also occur at a younger age (mean, 33 years) when associated with NF1, whereas the patients without NF1 have been slightly older (mean, 42 years). The tumors present in a wide variety of locations, with the head and neck and trunk being among the most common. The clinicopathologic series show a highly malignant behavior, with the 5-year survival being 10% to 20%.[174–177]

Pathology

Characteristic of this tumor is focal rhabdomyosarcomatous differentiation occurring in the background of a high-grade spindle cell or pleomorphic MPNST (Fig. 15–21*F*). Well-differentiated rhabdomyoblastic components are scattered between the spindle cells or seen in clusters. They are positive for desmin, myoglobin, and MyoD1. S-100 protein positivity is variable, and remnants of neurofibroma can often be demonstrated. Electron microscopy is also useful in verifying the skeletal muscle differentiation.

Malignant Glandular MPNST

This variant of MPNST with heterologous epithelial differentiation is extremely rare. Many of the reported cases have been associated with NF1 syndrome. The tumors have occurred in children or young adults in a wide variety of locations, and most have shown a malignant behavior.[178,179]

Histologically remarkable is the occurrence of glandular elements in the background of MPNST, generally with a spindle cell sarcomatous pattern. The glandular elements have often been mucin-producing and contained goblet cells, and squamous differentiation is also possible. Other heterologous elements, such as cartilage, may also occur in glandular MPNST.

Differential Diagnosis

Glandular differentiation of MPNST has to be separated from entrapped sweat glands in nerve sheath tumors; some earlier reports on "glandular schwannoma" might have included such tumors.

Pseudoglandular spaces may occur in MPNST, but they are not lined by true epithelial cells. Also, those biphasic synovial sarcomas that are S-100 protein positive should not be confused with malignant glandular MPNST. In synovial sarcoma, the epithelial elements are prominently K7 positive, whereas those in glandular MPNST tend to be negative. K20 can be present in both.

Epithelioid MPNST

This histologically distinctive, rare variant of MPNST often arises in a nerve and has a predilection to young adults; in contrast to the other types of MPNST, association with the NF1 syndrome is weak.

Clinical Features

Based on data presented in three clinicopathologic series, epithelioid MPNST occurs from childhood to old age, but has a predilection to young adults, with the median ages in the three series between 29 and 39 years. The combined data do not suggest any sex predilection.[180–182]

Sixty percent of reported cases have occurred in a nerve, including small superficial nerves, sciatic nerve, and brachial plexus as the most common locations. The most common involved sites are thigh and the upper extremity, with most tumors being proximally located and only a few in the hands and feet. Despite frequent nerve involvement, neurologic symptoms are rare. Only occasional cases have been associated with neurofibromatosis type I.

The tumors have a significant risk for metastasis to lungs, pleura, and liver, but superficial tumors may have a better prognosis. However, long-term follow-up data is relatively limited.[182]

Pathology

Grossly, the tumor forms a white nodule or mass that usually varies from 1 to 15 cm (median, 4–5 cm); the superficial tumors are smaller than the deep ones (Fig. 15–22*A*). Histologically, the tumor is typically composed of multiple nodules of polygonal epithelioid cells separated by fibrovascular septa. In some cases, the tumor cells spread in the enlarged nerve fascicles. The tumor cells often form trabeculae or cords separated by variably myxoid stroma (Fig. 15–22*B* and *C*), but they may also form solid areas. Cytologically, the tumor cells have large nuclei with prominent nucleoli and a moderate amount of eosinophilic or amphophilic cytoplasm. Focal fatlike vacuolization and rhabdoid tumor-like cytoplasmic eosinophilic inclusions may be present.

Immunohistochemically, the tumors are usually strongly positive for S-100 protein (Fig. 15–22*D*) and NSE, but negative for HMB45 and tyrosinase; the latter findings are useful in distinguishing these tumors from metastatic melanoma. The tumors have been reported as negative for keratins.

MPNSTs Arising from Ganglioneuroma and Pheochromocytoma

A small number of MPNSTs have been reported to have arisen from a ganglioneuroma, ganglioneuroblastoma, or pheochromocytoma, mostly in the adrenal glands.[183–187]

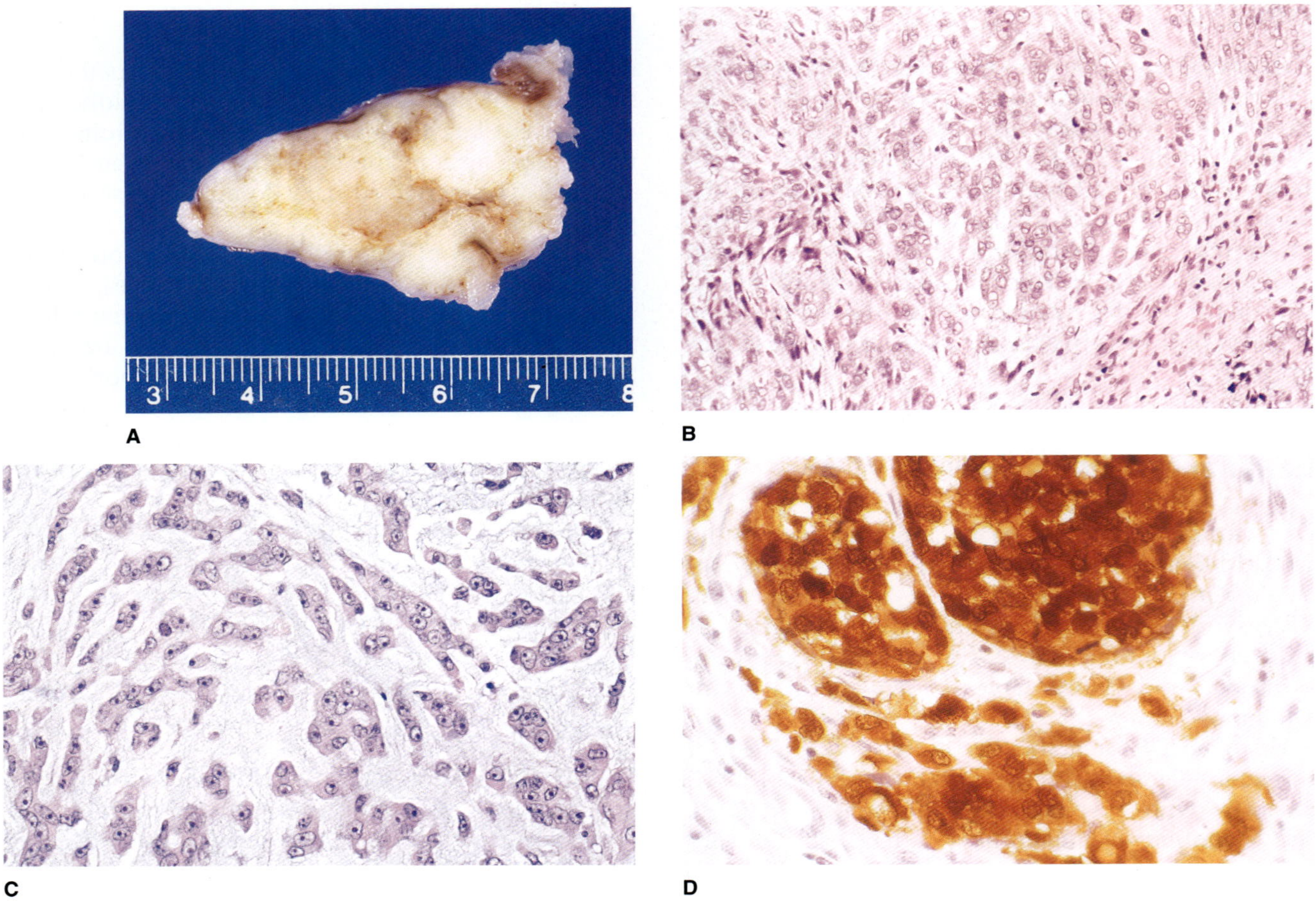

Figure 15–22. Epithelioid MPNST. *A,* Grossly, the tumor is a white, multinodular homogeneous mass. *B,* This epithelioid MPNST has a nearly solid histologic pattern. *C,* This tumor has a trabecular architecture with myxoid background. *D,* The tumor cells are strongly and uniformly S-100 protein positive.

These tumors have mostly been large, occurred in young adults, and had an unfavorable course. Histologically, they have been high-grade spindle cell sarcomas, and the specific diagnosis has been based on the immunohistochemical demonstration of S-100 protein.

REFERENCES

General

1. Scheithauer BW, Woodruff JM, Erlandson RA: Tumors of the Peripheral Nervous System. Washington, DC, Armed Forces Institute of Pathology, 1999.
2. Weiss SW, Goldblum JR (eds): Nerve sheath tumors. In Soft Tissue Tumors, 4th ed. Mosby, St. Louis, 2001.

Neuromuscular Hamartoma

3. Louhimo I, Rapola J: Intraneural muscular hamartoma: A report of two cases in small children. J Pediatr Surg 1972;7:696–699.
4. Markel SF, Enzinger FM: Neuromuscular hamartoma—A benign "Triton" tumor composed of mature neural and striated muscle elements. Cancer 1982;49: 140–144.
5. Azzopardi JG, Eusebi V, Tison V, Betts BM: Neurofibroma with rhabdomyomatous differentiation: Benign "Triton" tumor of the vagina. Histopathology 1983;7: 561–572.

Morton Neuroma

6. Wu KK: Morton neuroma and metatarsalgia. Curr Opin Rheumatol 2000;12:131–142.
7. Bennett GL, Graham CE, Mauldin DM: Morton's interdigital neuroma: A comprehensive treatment protocol. Foot Ankle Int 1995;16:760–763.
8. Reed RJ, Bliss BO: Morton's neuroma. Regressive and productive intermetatarsal elastofibrositis. Arch Pathol 1973;95:123–129.
9. Lassmann G, Lassmann H, Stockinger L: Morton's metatarsalgia. Light and electron microscopic observations and their relation to entrapment neuropathies. Virchows Arch Pathol Anat Histopathol 1976;370: 307–321.

10. Bourke G, Owen J, Machet D: Histological comparison of the third interdigital nerve in patients with Morton's metatarsalgia and control patients. Aust NZ J Surg 1994;64:421–424.

Traumatic Neuroma

11. Larson DM, Storsteen KA: Traumatic neuroma of the bile ducts with intrahepatic extension causing obstructive jaundice. Hum Pathol 1984;15:287–289.

Mucosal Neuroma and Ganglioneuroma(tosis)

12. Carney JA, Sizemore GW, Hayles AB: Multiple endocrine neoplasia type 2b. Pathobiol Annu 1978;8: 105–153.

Pacinian Neurofibroma

13. MacDonald DM, Wilson-Jones E: Pacinian neurofibroma. Histopathology 1977;1:247–255.
14. Fletcher CD, Theaker JM: Digital pacinian neuroma: A distinctive hyperplastic lesion. Histopathology 1989; 15:249–256.
15. Reznik M, Thiry A, Fridman V: Painful hyperplasia and hypertrophy of pacinian corpuscles in the hand: Report of two cases with immunohistochemical and ultrastructural studies, and a review of the literature. Am J Dermatopathol 1998;20:203–207.

Palisaded Encapsulated Neuroma

16. Reed RJ, Fine RM, Meltzer HD: Palisaded encapsulated neuromas of the skin. Arch Dermatol 1972;1-6: 865–870.
17. Fletcher CD: Solitary circumscribed neuroma (so-called palisaded encapsulated neuroma). A clinicopathologic and immunohistochemical study. Am Surg Pathol 1989;13:574–580.
18. Dover JS, From L, Lewis A: Palisaded encapsulated neuromas. A clinicopathologic study. Arch Dermatol 1989;125:386–389.
19. Dakin MC, Leppard B, Theaker JM: The palisaded encapsulated neuroma (solitary circumscribed neuroma). Histopathology 1992;20:405–410.
20. Chauvin PJ, Wysocki GP, Daley T, Pringle GA: Palisaded encapsulated neuroma of oral mucosa. Oral Surg Oral Med Oral Pathol 1992;73:71–74.
21. Argenyi ZB, Cooper PH, Santa Cruz D: Plexiform and other unusual variants of palisaded encapsulated neuroma. J Cutan Pathol 1993;20:34–39.
22. Albrecht S, Kahn HJ, From L: Palisaded encapsulated neuroma: An immunohistochemical study. Mod Pathol 1989;2:403–406.
23. Argenyi ZB: Immunohistochemical characterization of palisaded, encapsulated neuroma. J Cutan Pathol 1990; 17:329–335.

Neurofibroma—Clinicopathologic and Histopathologic Studies

24. Reed ML, Jacoby RA: Cutaneous neuroanatomy and neuropathology. Am J Dermatopathol 1983;5:335–362.
25. Fletcher CD: Peripheral nerve sheath tumors. A clinicopathologic update. Pathol Annu 1990;25 Part 1: 53–74.
26. Megahed M: Histopathological variants of neurofibroma. A study of 114 lesions. Am J Dermatopathol 1994;16:486–495.
27. Requena L, Sangueza OP: Benign neoplasms with neural differentiation. A review. Am J Dermatopathol 1995;17:75–96.
28. Michal M, Fanburg-Smith JC, Mentzel T, et al: Dendritic cell neurofibroma with pseudorosettes. A report of 18 cases of a distinct and hitherto unrecognized neurofibroma variant. Am J Surg Pathol 2001;25: 587–594.
29. Lin BT, Weiss LM, Medeiros LJ: Neurofibroma and cellular neurofibroma with atypia: A report of 14 tumors. Am J Surg Pathol 1997;21:1443–1449.
30. Kaiserling E, Geerts ML: Tumour of Wagner-Meissner touch corpuscles. A Wagner-Meissner neurilemmoma. Virchows Arch Pathol Anat Histopathol 1986;409: 241–250.
31. Fetsch JF, Michal M, Miettinen M: Pigmented (melanotic) neurofibroma: A clinicopathologic and immunohistochemical analysis of 19 lesions from 17 patients. Am J Surg Pathol 2000;24:331–343.

Neurofibroma—Immunohistochemistry and Ultrastructure

32. Weiss SW, Langloss JM, Enzinger FM: Value of S100-protein in the diagnosis of soft tissue tumors with particular reference to benign and malignant Schwann cell tumors. Lab Invest 1983;49:299–308.
33. Weiss SW, Nickoloff BJ: CD34 is expressed by a distinctive cell population in peripheral nerve, nerve sheath tumors and related lesions. Am J Surg Pathol 1993;17:1039–1045.
34. Chaubal A, Paetau A, Zoltick P, Miettinen M: CD34 immunoreactivity in nervous system tumors. Acta Neuropathol 1994;88:454–458.
35. Perentes E, Rubinstein LJ: Immunohistochemical recognition of human nerve sheath tumors by anti-Leu 7 antibodies (HNK-1) monoclonal antibody. Acta Neuropathol 1986;69:227–233.
36. Chanoki M, Ishii M, Fukai K, et al: Immunohistochemical localization of type I, III, IV, V and VI collagens and laminin in neurofibroma and neurofibrosarcoma. Am J Dermatopathol 1991;13:365–373.
37. Kindblom LG, Ahlden M, Meis-Kindblom JM, Stenman G: Immunohistochemical and molecular analysis of p53, MDM2, proliferating cell nuclear antigen and Ki-67 in benign and malignant nerve sheath tumors. Virchows Arch 1995;427:19–26.
38. Halling KC, Scheithauer BW, Halling AC, et al: p53 expression in neurofibroma and malignant peripheral nerve sheath tumor. An immunohistochemical study of sporadic and NF1-associated tumors. Am J Clin Pathol 1996;106:282–288.
39. Erlandson RA, Woodruff JM: Peripheral nerve sheath tumors: An electron microscopic study of 43 cases. Cancer 1982;49:273–287.

Genetics of Neurofibroma and NF1

40. Sorensen SA, Mulvihill JJ, Nielsen A: Long-term follow-up of von Recklinghausen neurofibromatosis. Survival and malignant neoplasms. N Engl J Med 1986;314:1010–1015.
41. Mulvihill JJ, Parry DM, Sherman JL, Pikus A, Kaiser-Kupfer MI, Eldridge R: NIH conference. Neurofibromatosis 1 (Recklinghausen disease) and neurofibromatosis 2 (bilateral acoustic neurofibromatosis). An update. Ann Intern Med 1990;113:39–52.
42. Gutmann DH, Aylsworth A, Carey JC, et al: The diagnostic evaluation and multidisciplinary management of neurofibromatosis 1 and neurofibromatosis 2. JAMA 1997;278:51–57.
43. Shen MH, Harper PS, Upadhyay M: Molecular genetics of neurofibromatosis type 1 (NF1). J Med Genet 1996;22:2–17.
44. Rasmussen SA, Friedman JM: NF1 gene and neurofibromatosis 1. Am J Epidemiol 2000;151:33–40.
45. Serra E, Puig S, Otero D, et al: Confirmation of a double-hit model for the NF1 gene in benign neurofibromas. J Med Genet 1997;61:512–519.
46. Sawada S, Florell S, Purandare SM, Ota M, Stephens K, Viskochil D: Identification of NF1 mutations in both alleles of a dermal neurofibroma. Nat Genet 1996;14:110–112.
47. Kluwe L, Friedrich R, Mautner VF: Loss of NF1 allele in Schwann cells but not in fibroblasts derived from an NF1-associated neurofibroma. Genes Chromosomes Cancer 1999;24:283–285.
48. Eisenbarth I, Beyer K, Krone W, Assum G: Toward a survey of somatic mutation of the NF1 gene in benign neurofibromas of patients with neurofibromatosis type 1. Am J Hum Genet 2000;66:393–401.
49. John AM, Ruggieri M, Ferner R, Upadhyaya M: A search for evidence of somatic mutations in the NF1 gene. J Med Genet 2000;37:44–49.
50. Messiaen LM, Callens T, Mortier G, et al: Exhaustive mutation analysis of the NF1 gene allows identification of 95% of mutations and reveals a high frequency of unusual splicing defects. Hum Mutat 2000; 15:541–555.

Classical Schwannoma (Neurilemoma)—Clinicopathologic Studies and Immunohistochemistry

51. Das Gupta TK, Brasfield RD, Strong EW, Hajdu SI: Benign solitary schwannomas (neurilemomas). Cancer 1969;24:255–366.
52. Alvarado-Cabrero I, Folpe AL, Srigley JR, et al: Intrarenal schwannoma: A report of four cases including three cellular variants. Mod Pathol 2000;13: 851–856.
53. Dahl I: Ancient neurilemmoma (schwannoma). Acta Pathol Microbiol Scand A 1977;85:812–818.
54. Gould VE, Moll R, Moll I, Lee I, Schwechheimer K: The intermediate filament complement of the spectrum of nerve sheath neoplasms. Lab Invest 1986; 55:463–474.
55. Kawahara E, Oda Y, Ooi A, Katsuda S, Nakanishi I, Umeda S: Expression of glial fibrillary acidic protein (GFAP) in peripheral nerve sheath tumors. A comparative study of immunoreactivity of GFAP, vimentin, S100-protein and neurofilament in 38 schwannomas and 18 neurofibromas. Am J Surg Pathol 1988;12: 115–120.
56. Kaiserling E, Xiao JC, Ruck P, Horny HP: Aberrant expression of macrophage-associated antigens (CD68 and Ki-M1P) by Schwann cells in reactive and neoplastic neural tissue. Mod Pathol 1994;6:463–468.
57. Gray MH, Rosenberg AE, Dickersin GR, Bhan AK: Glial fibrillary acidic protein and keratin expression by benign and malignant nerve sheath tumors. Hum Pathol 1989;20:1089–1096.
58. Oda Y, Kawahara E, Minamoto T, Tsuenyoshi M: Immunohistochemical studies on the tissue localization of collagen types I, III, IV, V and VI in schwannomas. Virchows Arch Pathol Anat Histol 1988;56: 153–163.
59. Waggener JD: Ultrastructure of benign peripheral nerve sheath tumors. Cancer 1966;19:699–709.
60. Dickersin GR: The electron microscopic spectrum of nerve sheath neoplasms. Ultrastruct Pathol 1987;11: 103–146.

Variants of Schwannoma and Malignant Transformation

61. Woodruff JM, Godwin TA, Erlandson RA, Susin M, Martini N: Cellular schwannoma: A variety of schwannoma sometimes mistaken for a malignant tumor. Am J Surg Pathol 1981;5:733–744
62. Lodding P, Kindblom LG, Angervall L, Stenman G: Cellular schwannoma. A clinicopathologic study of 29 cases. Virchows Arch [A] 1990;416:237–244.
63. White W, Shiu MH, Rosenblum MK, Erlandson RA, Woodruff JM: Cellular schwannoma. A clinicopathologic study of 57 patients and 58 tumors. Cancer 1990;66:1266–1275.
64. Casadei GR, Scheihauer BW, Hirose T, Manfrini M, Van Houton C, Wood MB: Cellular schwannoma. A clinicopathologic, DNA flow-cytometric and proliferation marker study of 71 cases. Cancer 1995;75: 1109–1119.
65. Woodruff JM, Marshall ML, Goodwin TA, Funkhouser JW, Thompson NJ, Erlandson RA: Plexiform (multinodular) schwannoma: A tumor simulating plexiform neurofibroma. Am J Surg Pathol 1983;7:691–697.
66. Fletcher CDM, Davies SE: Benign plexiform (multinodular) schwannoma: A rare tumor unassociated with neurofibromatosis. Histopathology 1986;10:971–980.
67. Iwashita T, Enjoji M: Plexiform neurilemoma: A clinicopathological and immunohistochemical analysis of 23 tumors from 20 patients. Virchows Arch 1987;411: 305–309.
68. Kao GR, Laskin WB, Olsen TG: Solitary cutaneous plexiform neurilemmoma (schwannoma): A clinicopathologic, immunohistochemical, and ultrastructural study of 11 cases. Mod Pathol 1989;2:20–26.
69. Hirose T, Scheithauer BW, Sano T: Giant plexiform schwannoma. A report of two cases with soft tissue

and visceral involvement. Mod Pathol 1997;10: 1075–1081.
70. Ishida T, Kuroda M, Motoi T, Oka T, Imamura T, Machinami R: Phenotypic diversity of neurofibromatosis 2: Association with plexiform schwannoma. Histopathology 1998;32:264–270.
71. Kindblom LG, Meis-Kindblom JM, Havel G, Busch C: Benign epithelioid schwannoma. Am J Surg Pathol 1998;22:762–770.
72. Goldblum JR, Beals TF, Weiss SW: Neuroblastoma-like neurilemoma. Am J Surg Pathol 1994;18:266–273.
73. Woodruff JM, Selig AM, Crowley K, Allen RW: Schwannoma (neurilemmoma) with malignant transformation. A rare, distinctive peripheral nerve tumor. Am J Surg Pathol 1994;18:882–895.
74. Mentzel T, Katenkamp D: Intraneural angiosarcoma and angiosarcoma arising in benign and malignant peripheral nerve sheath tumours: Clinicopathological and immunohistochemical analysis of four cases. Histopathology 1999;35:114–120.
75. Ruckert RI, Fleige B, Rogalla P, Woodruff JM: Schwannoma with angiosarcoma. Report of a case and comparison with other types of nerve sheath tumors with angiosarcoma. Cancer 2000;89: 1577–1585.
76. McMenamin ME, Fletcher CD: Expanding the spectrum of malignant change in schwannomas: Epithelioid malignant change, epithelioid malignant peripheral nerve sheath tumor, and epithelioid angiosarcoma: A study of 17 cases. Am J Surg Pathol 2001;25:13–25.

NF2 and Genetics of Schwannoma

77. Rouleau GA, Merel P, Lutchman M, et al: Alteration in a new gene encoding a putative membrane-organizing protein causes neurofibromatosis type 2. Nature 1993; 363:515–521.
78. Trofatter JA, MacCollin MM, Rutter JL, et al: A novel moesin-, ezrin-, radixin-like gene is a candidate for the neurofibromatosis 2 tumor suppressor. Cell 1993; 72:791–800.
79. Louis DN, Ramesh V, Gusella JF: Neuropathology and molecular genetics of neurofibromatosis 2 and related tumors. Brain Pathol 1995;5:163–172.
80. Evans DG, Sainio M, Baser ME: Neurofibromatosis type 2. J Med Genet 2000;37:897–904.
81. Giovannini M, Robanus-Maandag E, Niwa-Kawakita M, et al: Schwann cell hyperplasia and tumors in transgenic mice expressing a naturally occurring mutant NF2 protein. Genes Dev 1999;15: 978–986.
82. Ruttledge MH, Andermann AA, Phelan CM, et al: Type of mutation in the neurofibromatosis 2 gene frequently determines severity of disease. Am J Hum Genet 1996;59:331–342.
83. Parry DM, McCollin MM, Kaiser-Kupfer MI, et al: Germ-line mutations in the neurofibromatosis 2 gene: Correlations with disease severity and retinal abnormalities. Am J Human Genet 1996;59:529–539.
84. Kimura Y, Saya H, Nakao M: Calpain-dependent proteolysis of NF2 protein: Involvement in schwannomas and meningiomas. Neuropathology 2000;20: 153–160.
85. Gutmann DH, Aylsworth A, Carey JC, et al: The diagnostic evaluation and multidisciplinary management of neurofibromatosis 1 and neurofibromatosis 2. JAMA 1997;278:51–57.
86. De Vitis LR, Tedde A, Vitelli F, et al: Analysis of the neurofibromatosis type 2 gene in different human tumor of neuroectodermal origin. Hum Genet 1996; 97:638–641.

Schwannomatosis

87. Purcell SM, Dixon SL: Schwannomatosis. An unusual variant of neurofibromatosis or a distinct clinical entity. Arch Dermatol 1989;125:390–393.
88. MacCollin M, Woodfin W, Kronn D, Short MP: Schwannomatosis: A clinical and pathologic study. Neurology 1996;46:1072–1079.
89. Wolkenstein P, Benchikhi H, Zeller J, Wechsler J, Revuz J: Schwannomatosis: A clinical entity distinct from neurofibromatosis type 2. Dermatology 1997;195:228–231.
90. Evans DG, Mason S, Huson SM, Ponder M, Harding AE, Starchan T: Spinal and cutaneous schwannomatosis is a variant form of type 2 neurofibromatosis: A clinical and molecular study. J Neurol Neurosurg Psychiatr 1997;62:361–366.
91. Jacoby LB, Jones D, Davis K, et al: Molecular analysis of NF2 tumor-suppressor gene in schwannomatosis. Am J Hum Genet 1997;61:1293–1302.
92. Seppälä MT, Sainio MA, Haltia MJ, Kinnunen JJ, Setälä KH, Jääskeläinen JE: Multiple schwannomas: Schwannomatosis or neurofibromatosis type 2? J Neurosurg 1998;89:36–41.

GI Schwannoma

93. Daimaru Y, Kido H, Hashimoto H, Enjoji M: Benign schwannoma of the gastrointestinal tract: A clinicopathologic and immunohistochemical study. Hum Pathol 1988;19:257–264.
94. Prevot S, Bienvenu L, Vaillant JC, de Saint-Maur PP: Benign schwannoma of the digestive tract. A clinicopathologic and immunohistochemical study of five cases, including a case of esophageal tumor. Am J Surg Pathol 1999;23:431–436.
95. Miettinen M, Shekitka KM, Sobin LH: Schwannomas in the colon and rectum. Clinicopathologic and immunohistochemical study of 20 cases. Am J Surg Pathol 2001;25:846–855.
96. Lasota J, Wasag B, Miettinen M: Lack of NF2 gene alterations and LOH of NF1 in gastrointestinal schwannomas [abstract]. Mod Pathol 2002;15:134A.

Psammomatous Melanotic Schwannoma

97. Carney JA: Psammomatous melanotic schwannoma. A distinctive, heritable tumor with special associations, including cardiac myxoma and the Cushing syndrome. Am J Surg Pathol 1990;14:206–222.

98. Thornton CM, Handley J, Bingham EA, Toner PG, Walsh MY: Psammomatous melanotic schwannoma arising in the dermis in a patient with Carney's complex. Histopathology 1992;20:71–73.
99. Myers JL, Bernreuter W, Dunham W: Melanotic schwannoma of bone. Clinicopathologic, immunohistochemical and ultrastructural features of a rare primary bone tumor. Am J Clin Pathol 1990;93:424–429.
100. Lowman RM, Livolsi VA: Pigmented (melanotic) schwannomas of the spinal canal. Cancer 1980;46: 391–397.

Nerve Sheath Myxoma and Cellular Neurothekeoma

101. Gallager RL, Helwig EB: Neurothekeoma—A benign cutaneous tumor of neural origin. Am J Clin Pathol 1980;74:759–764.
102. Holden CA, Wilson-Jones E, MacDonald DM: Cutaneous lobular neuromyxoma. Br J Dermatol 1982;106: 211–215.
103. Angervall L, Kindblom LG, Haglid K: Dermal nerve sheath myxoma. A light and electron microscopic, histochemical and immunohistochemical study. Cancer 1984;53:1752–1759.
104. Pulitzer DR, Reed RJ: Nerve sheath myxoma (perineurial myxoma). Am J Dermatopathol 1985;7: 409–421.
105. Argenyi ZB, LeBoit PE, Santa Cruz D, Swanson PE, Kutzner H: Nerve sheath myxoma (neurothekeoma) of the skin: Light microscopic and immunohistochemical reappraisal of the cellular variant. J Cutan Pathol 1993;20:294–303.
106. Laskin WB, Fetsch JF, Miettinen M: The "neurothekeoma." Immunohistochemical analysis distinguishes the true nerve sheath myxoma from its mimics. Hum Pathol 2000;31:1230–1241.
107. Rosati LA, Fratamico CM, Eusebi V: Cellular neurothekeoma. Appl Pathol 1986;4:186–191.
108. Barnhill RL, Dickersin GR, Nickeleit V, et al: Studies on the cellular origin of neurothekeoma: Clinical, light microscopic, immunohisto-chemical, and ultrastructural observations. J Am Acad Dermatol 1991;25:80–88.
109. Calonje E, Wilson-Jones E, Smith NP, Fletcher CDM: Cellular "neurothekeoma": An epithelioid variant of pilar leiomyoma? Morphological and immunohistochemical analysis of a series. Histopathology 1992;20: 397–404.
110. Zelger BG, Steiner H, Kutzner H, Maier H, Zelger B: Cellular "neurothekeoma": An epithelioid variant of dermatofibroma? Histopathology 1998;32:414–422.

Perineurioma

111. Perentes E, Nakagawa Y, Ross GW, Stanton C, Rubinstein LJ: Expression of epithelial membrane antigen in perineurial cells and their derivatives: An immunohistochemical study with multiple markers. Acta Neuropathol 1987;75:160–165.
112. Ariza A, Bilbao JM, Rosai J: Immunohistochemical detection of epithelial membrane antigen in normal perineurial cells and perineurioma. Am J Surg Pathol 1988;12:678–683.
113. Theaker JM, Fletcher CD: Epithelial membrane antigen expression by the perineurial cell: Further studies of peripheral nerve lesions. Histopathology 1989;14: 581–591.
114. Lazarus SS, Trombetta LD: Ultrastructural identification of a benign perineurial cell tumor. Cancer 1978; 41:1823–1829.
115. Erlandson RA: The enigmatic perineurial cell and its participation in tumors and tumorlike entities. Ultrastruct Pathol 1991;15:335–351.
116. Bilbao JM, Khoury NJS, Hudson AR, Briggs SJ: Perineurioma (localized hypertrophic neuropathy). Arch Pathol Lab Med 1984;108:557–560.
117. Emory TS, Scheithauer BW, Hirose T, Wood M, Onofrio BM, Jenkins RB: Intraneural perineurioma: A clonal neoplasm associated with abnormalities of chromosome 22. Am J Clin Pathol 1995:103:696–704.
118. Fetsch JF, Miettinen M: Sclerosing perineurioma. A clinicopathologic study of 19 cases of a distinctive soft tissue lesion with a predilection for the fingers and palms of young adults. Am J Surg Pathol 1997;21: 1433–1442.
119. Sciot R, Dal Cin P: Cutaneous sclerosing perineurioma with cryptic NF2 gene deletion. Am J Surg Pathol 1999;23:849–853.
120. Lasota J, Fetsch JF, Wozniak A, Wasag B, Sciot R, Miettinen M: The neurofibromatosis type 2 gene is mutated in perineurial cell tumors: A molecular genetic study of eight cases. Am J Pathol 2001;158: 1223–1229.
121. Ushigome S, Takakuwa T, Hyuga M, Tadokoro M, Shinagawa T: Perineurial cell tumor and the significance of the perineurial cells in neurofibroma. Acta Pathol Jpn 1986;36:973–987.
122. Tsang WY, Chan JKC, Chow LTC, Tse CCH: Perineurioma: An uncommon soft tissue neoplasm distinct from localized hypertrophic neuropathy and neurofibroma. Am J Surg Pathol 1992;16:756–763.
123. Mentzel T, dei Tos AP, Fletcher CDM: Perineurioma (storiform perineurial fibroma): Clinicopathological analysis of four cases. Histopathology 1994;25: 261–267.
124. Michal M: Extraneural retiform perineuriomas. A report of four cases. Path Res Pract 1999;195:759–763.
125. Graadt van Roggen JF, McMenamin ME, Belchis DA, Nielsen GP, Rosenberg AE, Fletcher CD: Reticular perineurioma: A distinctive variant of soft tissue perineurioma. Am J Surg Pathol 2001;25:485–493.
126. Giannini C, Scheithauer BW, Jenkins RB, et al: Soft tissue perineurioma. Evidence for an abnormality of chromosome 22, criteria for diagnosis, and review of the literature. Am J Surg Pathol 1997;21:164–173.
127. Hirose T, Scheithauer BW, Sano T: Perineurial malignant peripheral nerve sheath tumor (MPNST). A clinicopathologic, immunohistochemical, and ultrastructural study of seven cases. Am J Surg Pathol 1998;22:1368–1378.
128. Zamecnik M, Michal M: Malignant peripheral nerve sheath tumor with perineurial cell differentiation (malignant perineurioma). Pathol Int 1999;49:69–73.

Granular Cell Tumor of Soft Tissues

129. Lack EE, Worsham GF, Callihan MD, et al: Granular cell tumor: A clinicopathologic study of 110 patients. J Surg Oncol 1980;13:301–316.
130. Compagno J, Hyams VJ, Sainte-Marie P: Benign granular cell tumors of the larynx: A review of 36 cases with clinicopathologic data. Ann Otol Rhinol Laryngol 1975;84:308–314.
131. Chaudhry AP, Jacobs MS, Sunder Raj M, Yamane GM, Jain R, Scharlock SE: A clinico-pathologic study of 50 adult oral granular cell tumors. J Oral Med 1984;39: 97–103.
132. Johnston J, Helwig EB: Granular cell tumors of the gastrointestinal tract and perianal region: A study of 74 cases. Dig Dis Sci 1981;26:807–816.
133. Damiani S, Koerner FC, Dickersin GR, Cook MG, Eusebi V: Granular cell tumour of the breast. Virchows Arch A Pathol Anat Histol 1992;420:219–226.
134. Ordonez NG: Granular cell tumor: A review and update. Adv Anat Pathol 1999;6:186–203.
135. Melo CR, Melo IS, Schmitt FC, Fagundes R, Amendola D: Multicentric granular cell tumor of the colon: Report of a patient with 52 tumors. Am J Gastroenterol 1993;88:1785–1787.
136. Nakazato Y, Ishizeki J, Takahashi K, Yamaguchi H: Immunohistochemical localization of S100-protein in granular cell myoblastoma. Cancer 1982;49:1624–1628.
137. Mazur MT, Schultz JJ, Myers JL: Granular cell tumor. Immunohistochemical analysis of 21 benign tumors and one malignant tumor. Arch Pathol Lab Med 1990;114:692–696.
138. Filie AC, Lage JM, Azumi N: Immunoreactivity of S100-protein, alpha-1-antitrypsin, and CD68 in adult and congenital granular cell tumors. Mod Pathol 1996;9:888–892.
139. Miettinen M, Lehtonen E, Lehtola H, Ekblom P, Lehto VP, Virtanen I: Histogenesis of granular cell tumour—An immunohistochemical and ultrastructural study. J Pathol 1984;142:221–229.
140. Murakata LA, Ishak KG: Expression of inhibin-alpha by granular cell tumors of the gallbladder and extrahepatic bile ducts. Am J Surg Pathol 2001;25:1200–1203.
141. Carstens PH, Yacoub O: Importance of the angulate bodies in the diagnosis of granular cell tumors (schwannomas). Ultrastruct Pathol 1993;17:271–278.
142. Mentzel T, Wadden C, Fletcher CD: Granular cell change in smooth muscle tumours of skin and soft tissue. Histopathology 1994;24:223–231.
143. Fanburg-Smith JC, Meis-Kindblom JM, Fante R, Kindblom LG: Malignant granular cell tumor of soft tissue: Diagnostic criteria and clinicopathologic correlation. Am J Surg Pathol 1998;22:779–794.

Gingival Granular Cell Tumor

144. Lack EE, Worsham GF, Callihan MD, Crawford BE, Vawter GF: Gingival granular cell tumors of the newborn (congenital "epulis"). A clinical and pathologic study of 21 patients. Am J Surg Pathol 1981;5:37–46.
145. Park SH, Kim TJ, Chi JG: Congenital granular cell tumor with systemic involvement. Immunohistochemical and ultrastructural study. Arch Pathol Lab Med 1991;115:934–938.
146. Lack EE, Perez-Atayde AR, McGill TJ, Vawter GF: Gingival granular cell tumors of the newborn (congenital "epulis"): Ultrastructural observations relating to histogenesis. Hum Pathol 1982;13:686–689.
147. Rohrer MD, Young SK: Congenital epulis (gingival granular cell tumor): Ultrastructural evidence of origin from pericytes. Oral Surg Oral Med Oral Pathol 1982;53:56–63.
148. Zarbo RJ, Lloyd RV, Beals TF, McClatchey KD: Congenital gingival granular cell tumor with smooth muscle cytodifferentiation. Oral Surg Oral Med Oral Pathol 1983;56:512–520.
149. Takahashi H, Fujita S, Satoh H, Okade H: Immunohistochemical study of congenital gingival granular cell tumor (congenital epulis). J Oral Pathol Med 1990;19:492–496.
150. Tucker MC, Rusnock EJ, Azumi N, Hoy GR, Lack EE: Gingival granular cell tumors of the newborn. An ultrastructural and immunohistochemical study. Arch Pathol Lab Med 1990;114:895–898.

Malignant Peripheral Nerve Sheath Tumor

151. Ghosh BC, Ghosh L, Huvos AG, Fortner JG: Malignant schwannoma. A clinicopathologic study. Cancer 1973;31:184–190.
152. Guccion JG, Enzinger FM: Malignant schwannoma associated with von Recklinghausen's neurofibromatosis. Virchows Arch Pathol Anat Histol [A] 1979; 383:43–57.
153. Tsuneyoshi M, Enjoji M: Primary malignant peripheral nerve tumors (malignant schwannomas). A clinicopathologic and electron microscopic study. Acta Pathol Jpn 1979;29:363–375.
154. Matsunou H, Shimoda T, Kakimoto S, Yamashita H, Ishikawa E, Mukai M: Histopathologic and immunohistochemical study of malignant tumors of peripheral nerve sheaths (malignant schwannoma). Cancer 1985;56:2269–2279.
155. Ducatman BS, Scheithauer BW, Piepgras DW, Reiman HM, Ilstrup DM: Malignant peripheral nerve sheath tumors: A clinicopathologic study of 120 cases. Cancer 1986;57:2006–2021.
156. Vauthey JN, Woodruff JM, Brennan MF: Extremity malignant peripheral nerve sheath tumors (neurogenic sarcomas): A 10-year experience. Ann Surg Oncol 1995;2:126–131.
157. Hruban RH, Shiu MH, Senie RT, Woodruff JM: Malignant peripheral nerve sheath tumors of the buttock and lower extremity. A study of 43 cases. Cancer 1990;66:1253–1265.
158. Ducatman BS, Scheithauer BW, Piepgras DG, Reiman HM: Malignant peripheral nerve sheath tumors in childhood. J Neurooncol 1984;2:241–248.
159. Meis JM, Enzinger FM, Martz KL, Neal JA: Malignant peripheral nerve sheath tumors (Malignant schwannomas) in children. Am J Surg Pathol 1992;16:694–707.

160. Ramanathan RC, Thomas JM: Malignant peripheral nerve sheath tumors associated with von Recklinghausen's neurofibromatosis. Eur J Surg Oncol 1999;25: 190–193.
161. Kourea HP, Bilsky MH, Leung DHY, Lewis JJ, Woodruff JM: Subdiaphragmatic and intrathoracic paraspinal malignant peripheral nerve sheath tumors. A clinicopathologic study of 25 patients and 26 tumors. Cancer 1998;82:2191–2203.
162. Foley KM, Woodruff JM, Ellis FT, Posner JB: Radiation-induced malignant and atypical peripheral nerve sheath tumors. Ann Neurol 1980;7:311–318.
163. Ducatman BS, Scheithauer BW: Postirradiation neurofibrosarcoma. Cancer 1983;51:1028–1033.
164. Meis-Kindblom JM, Enzinger FM: Plexiform malignant peripheral nerve sheath tumor of infancy and childhood. Am J Surg Pathol 1994;18:479–485.
165. Woodruff JM, Erlandson RA, Scheithauer BW: Nerve sheath tumors [letter to the editor]. Am J Surg Pathol 1995;19:608–609.
166. Daimaru Y, Hashimoto H, Enjoji M: Malignant peripheral nerve sheath tumors (malignant schwannomas): An immunohistochemical study of 29 cases. Am J Surg Pathol 1985;9:434–444.
167. Wick MR, Swanson PE, Scheithauer BW, Manivel JC: Malignant peripheral nerve sheath tumors: An immunohistochemical study of 62 cases. Am J Clin Pathol 1987:87:425–433.
168. Herrera GA, de Moraes PH: Neurogenic sarcoma in patients with neurofibromatosis (von Recklinghausen's disease). Light, electron microscopy and immunohistochemistry study. Virchows Arch A Pathol Anat Histol 1984;403:361–376.

MPNST—Genetics

169. Jhanwar SC, Chen Q, Li FP, Brennan MF, Woodruff JM: Cytogenetic analysis of soft tissue sarcomas. Recurrent chromosome abnormalities in malignant peripheral nerve sheath tumors (MPNST). Cancer Genet Cytogenet 1994;78:138–144.
170. Plaat BEC, Molenaar WM, Mastik MF, Hoekstra HJ, Te Meerman GJ, Van den Berg E: Computer-assisted cytogenetic analysis of 51 malignant peripheral-nerve-sheath tumors: Sporadic vs. neurofibromatosis-type-1 associated malignant schwannomas. Int J Cancer 1999;83:171–178.
171. Mertens F, Dal Cin P, de Wever I, et al: Cytogenetic characterization of peripheral nerve sheath tumours: A report of the CHAMP study group. J Pathol 2000; 190:31–38.
172. Kourea HP, Orlow I, Scheithauer BW, Cordon-Cardo C, Woodruff JM: Deletions of the INK4A gene occur in malignant peripheral nerve sheath tumors but not in neurofibromas. Am J Pathol 1999;155:1855–1860.
173. Nielsen GP, Stemmer-Rachamimov AO, Ino Y, Moller MB, Rosenberg AE, Louis DN: Malignant transformation of neurofibromas in neurofibromatosis 1 is associated with CDKN2A/p16 inactivation. Am J Pathol 1999;155:1879–1884.

MPNSTs with Divergent Differentiation

174. Brooks JSJ, Freeman M, Enterline HT: Malignant "Triton" tumors. Natural history and immunohistochemistry of nine new cases with literature review. Cancer 1985;55:2543–2549.
175. Woodruff JM, Chernik NL, Smith MC, Millett WB, Foote FW: Peripheral nerve tumors with rhabdomyosarcomatous differentiation (malignant "Triton" tumors). Cancer 1973;32:426–439.
176. Daimaru Y, Hashimoto H, Enjoji M: Malignant "Triton" tumors: A clinicopathologic and immunohistochemical study of nine cases. Hum Pathol 1984;15: 768–778.
177. Ducatman BS, Scheithauer BW: Malignant peripheral nerve sheath tumors with divergent differentiation. Cancer 1984;54:1049–1057.
178. Woodruff JM: Peripheral nerve sheath tumors showing glandular differentiation (glandular schwannomas). Cancer 1976;37:2399–2413.
179. Christensen WN, Strong EW, Bains MS, Woodruff JM: Neuroendocrine differentiation in glandular peripheral nerve sheath tumor. Pathologic distinction from the biphasic synovial sarcoma with glands. Am J Surg Pathol 1988;12:417–426.

Epithelioid MPNSTs

180. Lodding P, Kindblom LG, Angervall L: Epithelioid malignant schwannoma. A study of 14 cases. Virchows Arch A Pathol Anat Histopathol 1986;409:433–451.
181. DiCarlo EF, Woodruff JM, Bansal M, Erlandson RA: The purely epithelioid malignant peripheral nerve sheath tumor. Am J Surg Pathol 1986;10:478–490.
182. Laskin WB, Weiss SW, Bratthauer GL: Epithelioid variant of malignant peripheral nerve sheath tumor (malignant epithelioid schwannoma). Am J Surg Pathol 1991;15:1136–1145.

MPNSTs Arising from Ganglioneuroma and Pheochromocytoma

183. Ricci A, Parham DM, Woodruff JM, Callihan T, Green A, Erlandson RA: Malignant peripheral nerve sheath tumors arising from ganglioneuromas. Am J Surg Pathol 1984;8:19–29.
184. Fletcher CD, Fernando IN, Braimbridge MV, McKee PH, Lyall JR: Malignant nerve sheath tumor arising in a ganglioneuroma. Histopathology 1988;12:445–448.
185. Damiani S, Manetto V, Carrillo G, DiBlasi A, Nappi O, Eusebi V: Malignant peripheral nerve sheath tumor arising in a de novo ganglioneuroma. Tumori 1991;77: 90–93.
186. Min KW, Clemens A, Bell J, Dick H: Malignant peripheral nerve sheath tumor and pheochromocytoma. A composite tumor of the adrenal. Arch Pathol Lab Med 1988;112:266–270.
187. Miettinen M, Saari A: Pheochromocytoma combined with malignant schwannoma: Unusual neoplasm of the adrenal medulla. Ultrastruct Pathol 1988;12:513–527.

Neuroectodermal and Neural Tumors

CHAPTER 16

The neuroectodermal tumors discussed here include metastatic melanoma, desmoplastic melanoma, and clear cell sarcoma of tendons and aponeuroses. For discussions of cutaneous nevi and ordinary cutaneous melanoma, the reader is referred to dermatopathology texts. Pigmented neuroectodermal tumor of infancy is an uncommon tumor of the facial skeleton. Melanocytes are generally regarded as cells of neural crest origin. Glial tumors and meningiomas that rarely present in soft tissues will also be discussed.

The true neural tumors included here are paragangliomas, including pheochromocytoma and related tumors showing autonomic neural differentiation. Gastrointestinal autonomic nerve tumors (GANTs) are now classified among the gastrointestinal stromal tumors (GISTs, see Chapter 11). Neuroblastoma, a primitive childhood tumor with sympathetic nerve differentiation, and peripheral primitive neuroectodermal tumor (PNET) of the Ewing sarcoma family, will be discussed among small, round cell tumors (see Chapter 18).

Metastatic Melanoma

Metastatic malignant melanoma is a common problem in soft tissue pathology. Melanoma metastases can present at almost any surgical site, often a long time (10–20 years or more) after the primary diagnosis. This often makes it difficult to connect the metastasis with the primary tumor. The wide variety of morphologic appearances contributes to the problem.[1] Metastatic melanoma always has to be considered in the differential diagnosis of problematic poorly differentiated tumors.

Clinical Features

Melanoma metastases occur equally in men and women of all ages; they are uncommon in children and rare in persons with dark skin color. They are common in the lymph nodes, skin, and subcutis at almost any site. Axillary and inguinal lymph node metastasis may develop into massive tumor conglomerates with combined nodal and extranodal involvement. Cerebral, gastrointestinal (GI), hepatic, ovarian, osseous, and pulmonary metastases are relatively common, whereas other parenchymal metastases are rarely encountered as surgical specimens. Some metastatic melanomas have no apparent primary tumor. Explanations offered for this include regression of the cutaneous primary tumor and hypothetical origin from melanocytic rests of nodal capsules.

Paradoxically, large primary cutaneous melanomas may be difficult to identify as such, and they can be confused with soft tissue sarcomas whenever junctional involvement is not detected.

Pathology

Grossly, melanoma metastases form fleshy nodules and masses that vary from pigmented to nonpigmented. In some cases, the entire lesion may be pigmented, whereas in others, small pigmented areas are present. When nonpigmented, the lesions are commonly brownish tan, but they may also be bright white.

The histologic variation in metastatic melanoma is extensive (Fig. 16–1). Architecturally, a trabecular compartmental pattern is common, especially seen in metastases with epithelioid cytology. Diffuse sheets may also be seen. The cellular cohesion varies from good to poor, from carcinoma-like to formation of alveolar spaces. Eosinophilic coagulation necrosis is common and may be extensive, only leaving preserved tumor cells as narrow perivascular collars. Glomeruloid vascular proliferation similar to that often seen in malignant peripheral nerve sheath tumors (MPNSTs), glioblastoma, and neuroendocrine tumors may occur.[2] The pigmentation seen in tumor cells or streaks of melanophages is helpful if present.

The several cytologic patterns encountered in metastatic melanoma include epithelioid (carcinoma-like), spindle cell (spindle cell sarcoma-like), pleomorphic (malignant fibrous histiocytoma-like), and round cell (lymphoma-like) and combinations thereof. By these patterns melanomas can simulate almost any other poorly differentiated tumor. A combination of the epithelioid and spindle cell patterns is perhaps the most common. The spindle cell metastases may have solid sheets of tumor cells resembling a spindle cell sarcoma, especially an MPNST.[3,4] Rhabdoid cytologic features with inclusion-like cytoplasm may be encountered. Signet ring carcinoma-like, adenoid pseudopapillary, hemangiopericytoma-like, and myxoid patterns have also been reported.[1]

Cytologically, metastatic melanoma cells often have well-defined borders. The cytoplasm varies from pale, variably basophilic to deeply eosinophilic. The nuclei typically have complex outlines with grooves and cleavages sometimes resulting in nuclear pseudoinclusions (cytoplasmic invaginations), similar to those seen in Schwann cell tumors. Multinucleated forms may occur. The nucleoli may be prominent.

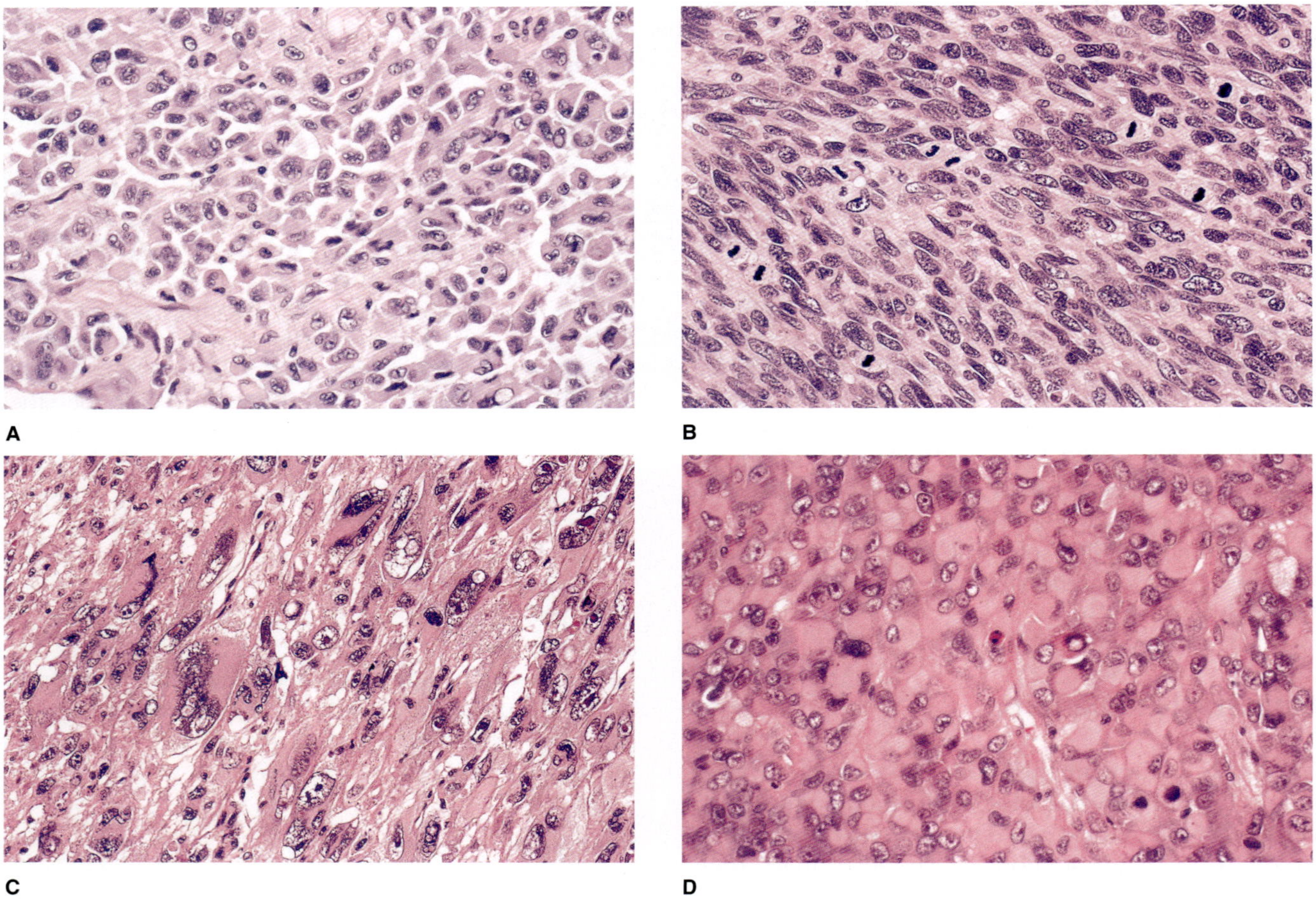

Figure 16–1. Histologic spectrum of metastatic melanoma. *A*, Epithelioid pattern. *B*, Spindle cell pattern resembling MPNST. *C*, Pleomorphic malignant fibrous histiocytoma-like pattern. *D*, Rhabdoid cytologic pattern.

Immunohistochemistry

When evaluating a strongly S-100 protein-positive malignant soft tissue tumor, malignant melanoma has to be considered. Nearly all metastatic melanomas are strongly and globally S-100 protein positive, but a small portion of them show reduced or no S-100 protein expression. HMB45$^+$ cells are present in 60% to 70% of cases, but often only focally. Tyrosinase is probably the best marker in terms of sensitivity and specificity, because it is rarely present in other tumors (except the related clear cell sarcoma).[5,6] Melan A is somewhat less sensitive (75%). Microphthalmia transcription factor is present in most metastatic melanomas, although is typically absent in desmoplastic melanomas (similar to HMB45, melan A, and tyrosinase).[6]

In some metastases, S-100 protein may be the only positive marker, and in some cases foci of more differentiated tyrosinase-positive components are present (Fig. 16–2).

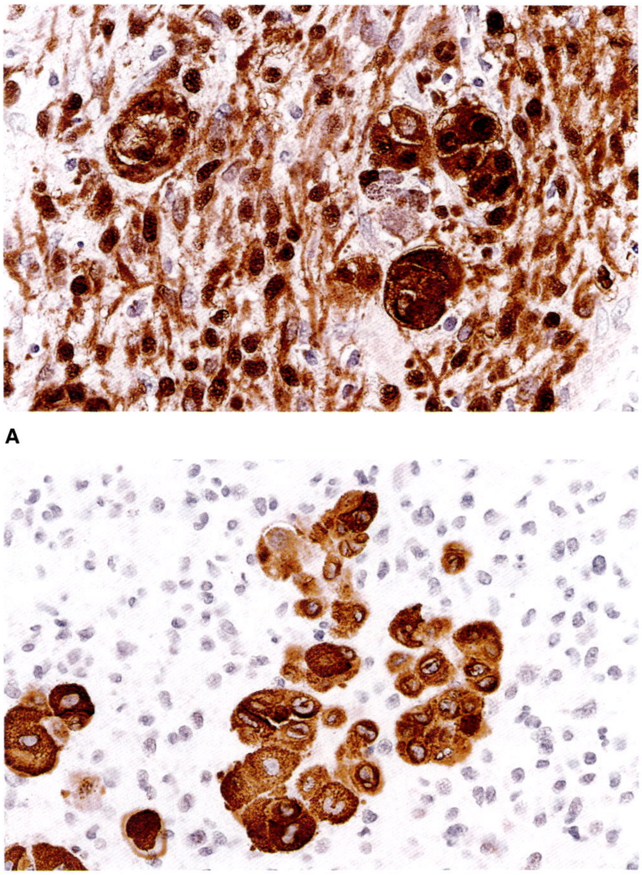

A

B

Figure 16–2. Immunohistochemical features of metastatic melanoma. *A,* All tumors cells are S-100 protein positive in this melanoma combining spindle cell and epithelioid components. *B,* Only the epithelioid clusters are positive for tyrosinase.

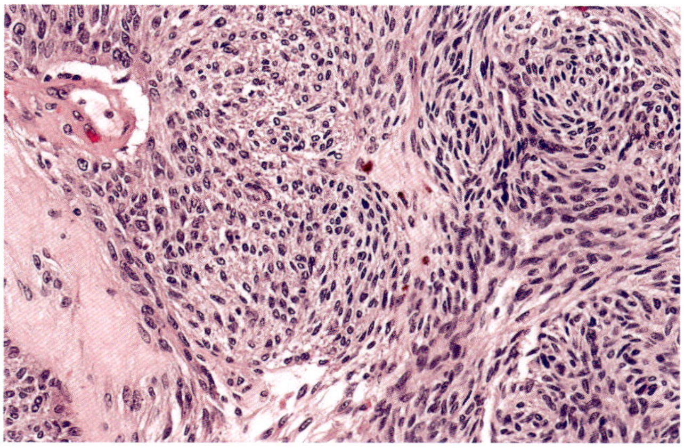

Figure 16–3. Cellular blue nevus shows a microlobulated pattern. Note pigmented melanophages and limited atypia in tumor cells.

Keratin positivity, especially keratin 18, is seen in 20% of metastatic melanomas, but there is no keratin 19, which may be helpful in the differential diagnosis between melanoma and metastatic carcinoma. The presence of keratins 8 and 18 in metastatic melanoma has also been confirmed by Western blotting.[7] Similar to many carcinomas, the melanoma metastases are often positive for E-cadherin.

The common expression of histiocytic markers in melanomas, such as α_1-antitrypsin and CD68, should not lead to confusion with histiocytic tumors. Microphthalmia transcription factor also can be expressed in mononuclear histiocytes, although it is more commonly expressed in osteoclast-like histiocytes.

Differential Diagnosis

Cellular blue nevus is a benign cutaneous or subcutaneous tumor that often occurs in the buttocks and back of young adults.[8,9] It is a circumscribed lesion composed of tapered spindle cells, often arranged in vague compartments and foci of pigmented melanophages. It lacks the atypia typically seen in melanoma metastases (Fig. 16–3). Extremely rare malignant transformation has been reported.

Metastatic melanoma has to be ruled out before a superficial epithelioid MPNST is diagnosed.

Clear cell sarcoma is a clinically and histologically distinctive related tumor, which typically has an organoid pattern divided by fibrous septa.

Psammomatous melanotic schwannoma and certain variants of MPNSTs may phenotypically closely simulate melanoma by their S-100 protein positivity. However, the latter do not express HMB45. Clinical context of the lesion may be decisive in some cases.

Epithelioid sarcoma has typically large cells with abundant, eosinophilic cytoplasm. In contrast to melanoma, S-100 protein positivity is rare, and keratin positivity is nearly uniform.

Genetics

Malignant melanomas typically show complex cytogenetic changes, and no specific diagnostic features have emerged. They do not have the t(12;22) translocation seen in clear cell sarcoma.

Desmoplastic Melanoma

Desmoplastic melanoma is a rare melanoma subtype, which typically occurs in the dermis and subcutis and contains dense fibrous stroma. Its variant neurotropic melanoma has a propensity to infiltrate along small nerves. Approximately one third of desmoplastic melanomas do not contain an atypical junctional component, and they appear as primary soft tissue tumors. A great majority of desmoplastic melanomas are amelanotic.

Clinical Features

Desmoplastic melanoma generally occurs at an older age than conventional melanoma. The patient median ages in the largest series have been around 60 years. Occasional cases have been reported in children. The largest series show a to 2:1 male predominance. The tumor has a predilection to head and neck region (50–80%) in different series.[10–19] The most common sites are cheek and neck. Thirty to 50% of tumors have occurred in the trunk and extremities, more commonly in the upper than lower ones. Presentation in mucosal sites, oral in particular, has been reported rarely.[20]

Clinically, the lesion often develops from a superficial lentigo maligna type melanoma, which may precede the desmoplastic melanoma for 10 to 20 years. However, in one third of cases, no preceding or simultaneous melanocytic lesion is present, and the desmoplastic melanoma is considered arising de novo. The lesion typically forms a shallow elevation and induration below an intact skin.

Earlier reports showed recurrence rate over 50%, which is down to 10% to 15% with wide excision. Lymph node metastasis is less common than in conventional melanoma.[18] Distant metastasis to lungs, liver, and central nervous system may develop. Although the original series showed a grim prognosis, probably because many tumors were diagnosed at an advanced stage, the latest series show a 5-year survival rates as high as 70% to 75%, and demonstrate better survival than for conventional melanoma of similar thickness. Female patients may have better survival.[17,18]

Pathology

On sectioning, the lesion appears as a dense, plaque-like dermal-subcutaneous expansion that is usually classified having Clark level IV to V. The reported tumors have usually been 2 to 10 mm thick, and laterally measured 1 to 3 cm, but early lesions are being recognized. Despite their small overall dimensions (5 mm maximum diameter), microscopic deep extension around adnexa and nerves is common.[21]

Histologically, desmoplastic melanoma typically forms a dermal thickening extending to subcutis as fibrous streaks. The lesion is often deceptively bland, and it can resemble a scar or an inflammatory process with the tumor cells dispersed in a fibrous desmoplastic stroma (Fig. 16–4). The tumor cells often form curved, narrow fascicles or a sheetlike pattern similar to that of conventional spindle cell melanoma. In some cases, the stromal collagen has a keloid-like appearance. Lymphoplasmacytic infiltration is typical and may mask the neoplastic population.

Cytologically at least the tumor cells show mild to moderate atypia, but many lesions show at least some markedly atypical cells with hyperchromatic irregularly shaped nuclei. The mitotic rate varies widely, and atypical mitoses may be seen.

Unfavorable histologic features are increasing tumor thickness and presence of stromal mucin, which has been thought to promote tumor invasion.[17]

Immunohistochemistry

The tumor cells of desmoplastic melanoma are almost always strongly positive for S-100 protein and vimentin (Fig. 16–4*D*). Most series have found these tumors uniformly negative for HMB45,[6,22] whereas others have found a minority of cases to be positive.[16,23] Tyrosinase and melan A are typically absent, but the results on microphthalmia transcription factor expression vary from 5% to 50% in two series[6,24] seen in the epithelioid components when present.[6] The tumor cells are also more consistently positive for the low-affinity nerve growth factor receptor p75 than conventional melanoma.[25] Keratin positivity is less common than in conventional melanoma. The significant smooth muscle actin-positive spindle cell component has been demonstrated to represent an

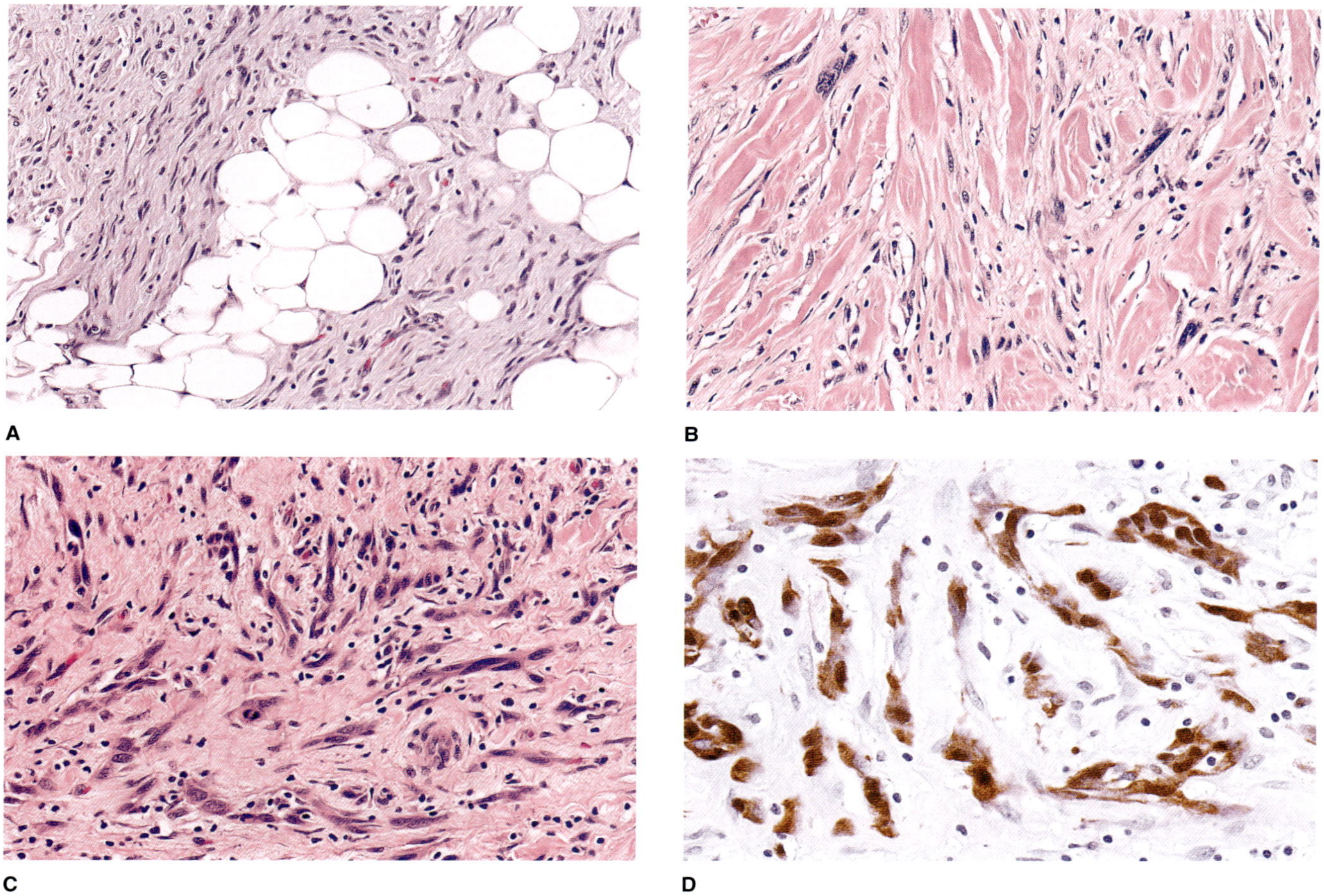

Figure 16–4. Histologic spectrum of desmoplastic melanoma. *A,* Tumor involves dermis and infiltrates as broad streaks into the subcutaneous fat. *B,* This example shows scattered atypical nuclei in a sclerosing spindle cell infiltrate. *C,* Typical bundles of tumor cells. *D,* Immunostaining for S-100 protein highlights the bundles of tumor cells.

S-100 protein-negative reactive myofibroblastic population on double staining.[22]

Differential Diagnosis

A high index of suspicion should be maintained, and plaquelike scarring dermal lesions with any atypia should be tested for S-100 protein to rule out desmoplastic melanoma. Benign nerve sheath tumors are typically more organized and cytologically bland. It may be difficult to distinguish desmoplastic melanoma from a superficial malignant nerve sheath tumor; actually most tumors with this differential diagnostic dilemma are desmoplastic melanomas.

Genetics

Allelic losses of the neurofibromatosis 1 (*NF1*) gene have been reported to be common in desmoplastic melanoma.[26]

Clear Cell Sarcoma

This histologically distinctive rare tumor typically presents in the distal lower extremity of young adults. It comprises approximately 1% of all sarcomas. Although clear cell sarcoma has many histologic similarities with melanoma, this tumor is genetically different from melanoma by its unique t(12;22) translocation. Therefore the term clear cell sarcoma is preferable to "malignant melanoma of soft parts." The so-called clear cell sarcoma of the kidney refers to an unrelated childhood tumor, which may show primitive epithelial differentiation.

Clinical Features

Clear cell sarcoma occurs predominantly in young adults aged 20 to 35 years, and there is a 3:2 female predominance in the largest series. Nearly half of the tumors occur in the foot and ankle. Less common sites include leg and proximal lower extremity, hand, forearm, and shoulder region, whereas presentation in the head and neck area is less common.[27–33] Well-documented cases positive for the clear cell sarcoma translocation or fusion transcript have been reported in small intestine in the ileum,[34] colon,[35] and kidney.[36]

The tumor shows highly malignant behavior, and recurrences are common. Metastases develop to lymph nodes, liver, bones, and lungs, and the two largest series both report a 5-year survival of approximately 54%.[32,33]

Pathology

The tumor typically occurs as a small elevated and palpable nodule around the tendons of foot and ankle usually measuring 1 to 3 cm. The proximally located tumors tend to be larger and commonly measure 5 to 10 cm. Grossly, the mass is ill-defined and may merge with tendons. On sectioning, the tumor varies from white to gray. Larger tumors may contain necrosis.

Histologically typical is division into compartments separated by dense collagenous septa (Fig. 16–5). Oval cellular compartments, fascicles of tumor cells, or and alveolar pattern may be seen, although some tumors, especially recurrent and metastatic ones, may show a lesser degree of organization. The tumor cells are spindled or polygonal, and have a moderate amount of cytoplasm that varies from slightly clear to mildly or moderately eosinophilic. The nuclei are round and uniform and often have large nucleoli that vary from amphophilic to deeply eosinophilic. Some tumor cells are multinucleated with a Touton-like or wreathlike nuclear arrangement (Fig. 16–5C). Nuclear pseudoinclusions, similar to those seen in melanoma, may be present. The clarity of the cytoplasm results from the prominent glycogen content (periodic acid-Schiff positive, diastase sensitive). The mitotic rate is usually low

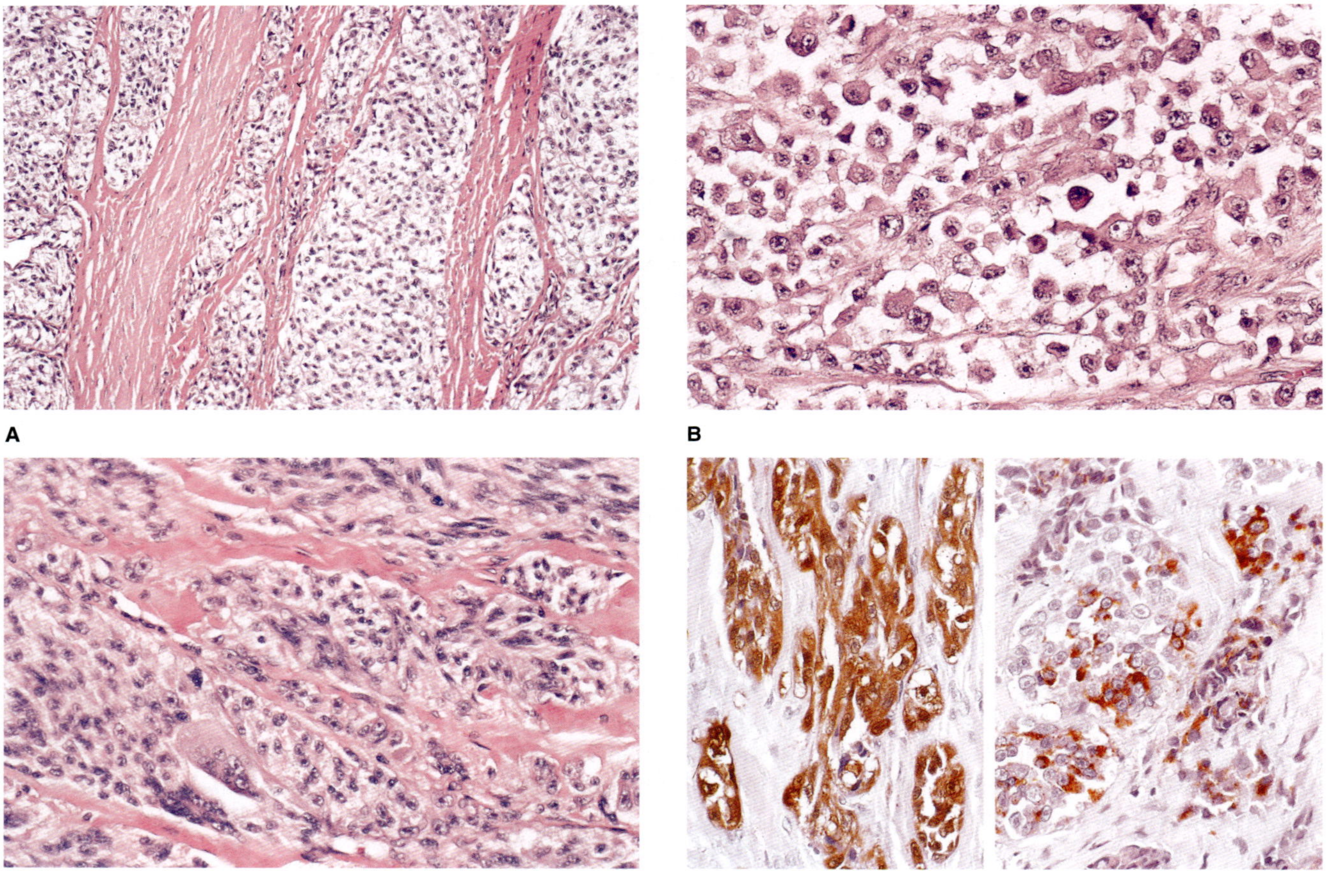

A B C D

Figure 16–5. Histologic spectrum of clear cell sarcoma. *A,* Trabeculae and clusters of tumors cells are surrounded by fibrous septa. *B,* Some cases have a loose, alveolar pattern. Note prominent nucleoli. *C,* Multinucleated tumor giant cells are often present. *D,* The tumor cells are strongly positive for S-100 protein (*left*) and moderately positive for HMB45 (*right*).

(<5/10 high-power field). However, recurrent and metastatic tumors may show greater atypia and less specific histologic features. Melanin pigmentation occurs in some cases, and melanosomes have been demonstrated by electron microscopy.

Adverse histologic prognostic factors are tumor size over 5 cm, presence of tumor necrosis, and high proliferation index.[30–32]

Immunohistochemistry

Immunohistochemically, clear cell sarcoma is similar to and virtually indistinguishable from malignant melanoma (Fig. 16–5*D*). The tumor cells are positive for S-100 protein, HMB-45, neuron-specific enolase (NSE), CD57, and vimentin[37] and in our experience often (but variably) for tyrosinase, microphthalmia transcription factor, and CD117 (KIT). The level of positivity for S-100 and HMB45 varies from case to case. The tumor cells are negative for keratins, epithelial membrane antigen (EMA), muscle actins, and desmin, although occasional keratin positivity has been reported.[38]

Differential Diagnosis

Primary or metastatic malignant melanoma should be ruled out. Typical tumor location, architectural and histologic features with compartmentalization and fibrous septa, lack of cutaneous involvement, and history of melanoma are helpful.

Cellular blue nevus usually presents as a well-circumscribed cutaneous or subcutaneous nodule. It is almost always at least focally pigmented with melanophages, and there are more spindled cellular components, typically with smaller nuclei and less prominent nucleoli.

Skin adnexal and metastatic clear cell tumors may simulate clear cell sarcoma, but they show histologic signs or markers for epithelial differentiation, and usually have a more prominent clear cell pattern than seen in an average clear cell sarcoma.

Cytogenetic or molecular genetic verification is highly desirable, especially in tumors that present at unusual sites.

Recently, Folpe and colleagues reported a series of myomelanocytic tumors in the hepatic falciform ligament in children and young adults. These tumors showed similar compartmentalization to clear cell sarcoma, but were S-100 protein negative and had dual expression of HMB45 and muscle cell markers, similar to the tumors of the angiomyolipoma family. Although most tumors were benign, one metastasized.[39]

Genetics

The typical diagnostic genetic change is t(12;22)(q13;q12) translocation that was demonstrated by several investigators in the early 1990s.[40–43] The involved regions were cloned and found to lead to fusion of genes *ATF1* (activating transcription factor 1) in 12q13 and *EWS* (Ewing sarcoma) in the 22q12.[44] The fusion transcript can be demonstrated by reverse transcription-polymerase chain reaction.[44–46] The fusion protein leads to constitutive activation of *ATF1* and has been shown important for tumor cell viability.[47] Limited number of cytogenetic changes, diploid pattern on flow cytometry, lack of microsatellite instability, and paucity of loss of heterozygosity (LOH) suggest lack of complex genetic changes in most cases of clear cell sarcoma.[48] The clear cell sarcoma translocation has not been found in malignant melanomas.[49]

Pigmented Neuroectodermal Tumor of Infancy (Melanotic Progonoma, Retinal Anlage Tumor)

Clinical Features

This rare pediatric tumor usually occurs in infants during the first 6 months of life and rarely in children over the age of 1 year; all series show male predominance. The tumor presents as a rapidly growing mass in the maxilla or less commonly in the mandible, where it commonly measures 1 to 2 cm in diameter.[50–53] Rare examples have occurred intracranially in the dura or brain[54,55] and in the epididymis of male infants where the tumor has reached a size of 2 to 3 cm and typically resulted in orchiectomy.[56–58] One bone tumor was reported in femur;[51] some reports in peripheral soft tissues have been disputed.

In some cases, serum metanephrine levels have been elevated. Despite its histologically immature appearance, this tumor is usually benign. However, local recurrences, lymph node metastases, and even distant metastasis with fatal outcome have been reported. Based on review of literature, the rate of malignancy has been estimated as 3% to 4%.[50]

Pathology

Histologically, the tumor is composed of cellular nests spaced by fibrous septa with prominent, thick-walled capillaries. The cellular nests contain small, undifferentiated round cells in the center, and larger, somewhat epithelioid, finely pigmented cells in the

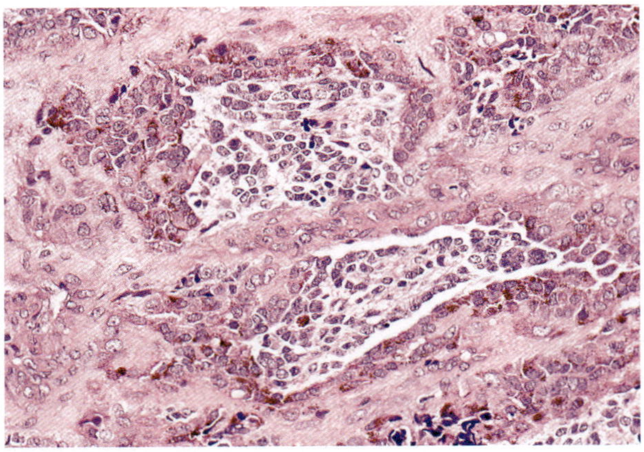

Figure 16–6. Pigmented melanotic neuroectodermal tumor of infancy is composed of clusters with a central small round cell component surrounded by larger epithelioid cells with melanin pigmentation.

periphery. These components are sometimes separated by clefts, and the proportions of components may vary (Fig. 16–6). Foci of eosinophilic rhabdomyoblasts may also be present. No clear criteria exist for prediction of malignancy.

This tumor has to be differentiated from malignant teratomas with pigmented neuroectodermal components and from pigmented melanotic schwannoma.

Immunohistochemically, the small cells are positive for neuroendocrine and neural markers such as NSE, synaptophysin, microtubule-associated protein 2, and occasionally for chromogranin, and variably for neurofilaments. The large epithelioid cells are variably positive for neuroendocrine markers, but are consistently positive for keratins and HMB45, similar to retinal pigment epithelium, which these tumor cells appear to simulate. The large cells may also be focally positive for glial fibrillary acidic protein (GFAP). In contrast to melanoma and related tumors, the tumor cells are negative for S-100 protein. Desmin is present in the rhabdomyoblastic components.[53,59]

Histogenesis

Similarities with fetal pineal gland have been noted and interpreted to suggest pineal-like differentiation in this tumor[60] that ultrastructurally combines neuroblastic and melanocytic differentiation.[61]

Molecular Genetics

Studies on three typical maxillary tumors revealed lack of MYCN amplification and no losses in chromosome 1p. The lack of these alterations commonly seen in neuroblastoma suggests no relationship between these tumors. Lack of t(11;12) translocations similar to those in Ewing sarcoma and small round cell desmoplastic tumor was also noted.[62]

Ectopic Meningiomas and Related Lesions

Clinical Features

Meningioma-like nodules and tumors can present outside the central nervous system at least in three different locations: skin of scalp (meningothelial hamartoma, ectopic meningioma), paranasal sinuses (ectopic meningioma), and in the lung and pleura (meningothelial nodules). Common to all of them is phenotypic similarity to meningiomas of the central nervous system, including histologic appearance and positivity for EMA. By definition, extension from an intracranial meningioma has to be ruled out.[63–70] Although most of these tumors are benign, some can cause potentially fatal local complications, similar to intracranial meningiomas.[70]

Primary cutaneous meningiomas (cutaneous heterotopic meningeal nodules) occur in the scalp or back of children, and some lesions are congenital. Connection with defects of spinal closure suggest that some of these tumors may be comparable to rudimentary meningocele.

Minute pulmonary meningothelial nodules are small 1 to 3 mm tan to yellow nodules in the visceral pleura or lung parenchyme that may not be grossly appreciated. In one study, most cases were incidental autopsy findings. Microscopically, these nodules are composed of meningothelial whorls, and immunohistochemically they are positive for EMA and vimentin, similar to meningiomas. These lesions, previously called minute pulmonary chemodectomas, clearly differ from paraganglioma (chemodectoma).[69]

Pathology

Histologically, ectopic meningiomas resemble their intracranial counterparts, and typically contain whorls of syncytially arranged meningothelial cells and often have psammoma bodies. A large series of sinonasal meningiomas documented meningothelial histology in the majority of cases, and also metaplastic variants with lipomatous components. Immunohistochemically ectopic meningiomas are usually at least focally positive for EMA (Fig. 16–7).

Hamartoma of the scalp with ectopic meningothelial nodules is the designation given by Suster and Rosai[68] to small solitary subcutaneous nodules of the scalp. The lesions occur in children or young adults. Histologically typical is infiltration of clustered epi-

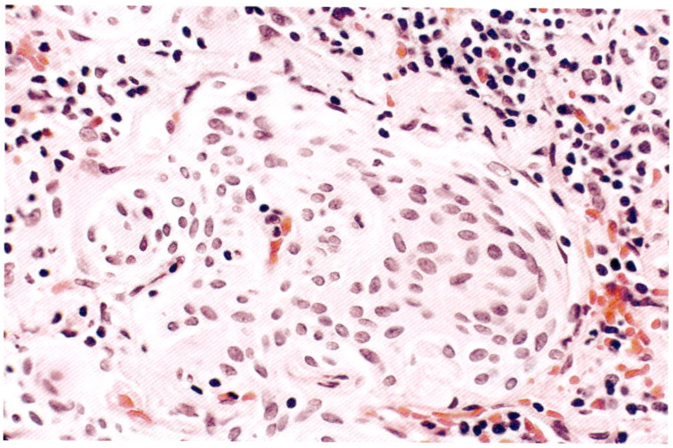

A

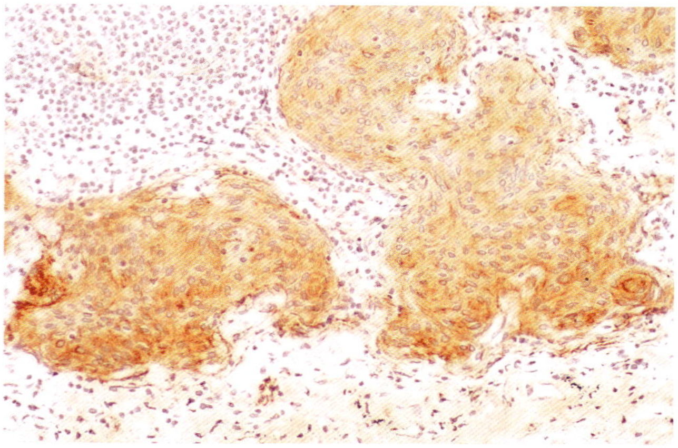

B

Figure 16–7. *A,* Minute pulmonary meningothelial nodule from the visceral pleura. This was an incidental finding in a wedge resection specimen containing a low-grade mucosa-associated lymphoid tissue lymphoma. *B,* The meningothelial nodules are strongly positive for EMA.

thelioid meningothelial cells between collagen fibers; such a lesion may histologically mimic angiosarcoma or an epithelioid vascular tumor of other type. The meningothelial cells in this hamartoma are positive for vimentin and EMA and show desmosomes, similar to the features of true meningioma.

Tumors that should not be confused with ectopic meningiomas include dedifferentiated liposarcomas with meningothelial whorls (see liposarcoma) and dendritic reticulum cell sarcomas. Both of these tumors especially occur intra-abdominally.

Ectopic Glial Tissue—Nasal Glioma and Soft Tissue Gliomatosis

Ectopic glial tissue most commonly occurs in the nasal region ("glioma nasi") in small children. The lesion may be located inside the nose or in the nasal skin or subcutis, and it probably always is congenital. Nasal glioma has been viewed as a disconnected (sequestered) encephalocele, a congenital malformation. True encephaloceles, lesions connected with brain, may also occur. The possible communication with the liquor space must be considered in the surgical treatment.[71–73]

Rare examples of cutaneous and subcutaneous glial lesions, termed soft tissue gliomatosis, have been reported in nonnasal sites. Most reported cases have occurred as solitary masses in the chest wall of infants and children younger than 2 years.[74,75]

Occasional examples in scalp have been considered sequestered encephaloceles, and occurrence in the sacrococcygeal region has been explained as a manifestation of sacrococcygeal teratoma with glial elements. Peritoneal gliomatosis represent multifocal peritoneal growth of ruptured ovarian teratoma with glial elements. All reported cases of peripheral soft tissue gliomatosis have been clinically benign.

Histologically, the ectopic glial elements are seen as pale staining, small, irregularly shaped nests surrounded by fibrous tissue (Fig. 16–8). There is no atypia or mitotic activity. The glial elements are positive for GFAP and S-100 protein.

Myxopapillary Ependymoma

Clinical Features

More commonly known as a central nervous system tumor virtually specific to the terminal part of the spinal cord, the filum terminale and cauda equina, this form of ependymoma rarely occurs as a primary soft tissue tumor in the subcutis of lower back. These tumors are not connected with the

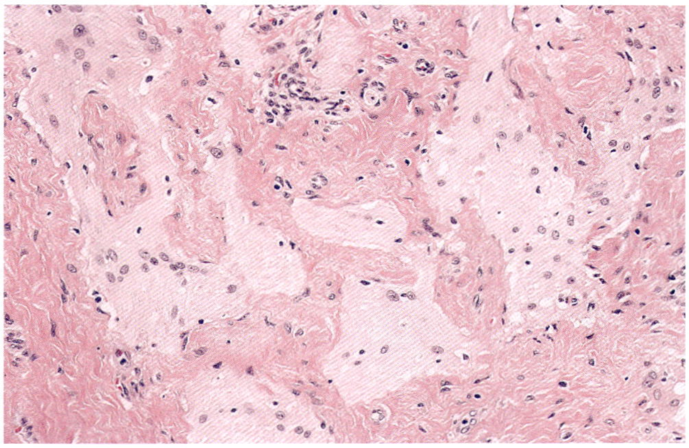

Figure 16–8. Soft tissue gliomatosis is composed of streaks of glial cells in fibrous background.

spinal cord. The myxopapillary ependymomas of soft tissues have to be considered at least potentially malignant, because 15% of them eventually develop distant metastases, most commonly to the lungs. In some cases the metastasis has occurred 20 years after the primary tumor.[76–79]

Pathology

Grossly, myxopapillary ependymomas form sharply circumscribed masses. They appear friable and gelatinous on sectioning. Histologically, myxopapillary ependymoma is composed of cuboidal epithelioid tumor cells lining papillary projections with a central vascular core (Fig. 16–9*A*). The papillary units are dispersed in a myxoid matrix. The tumor cells are strongly positive for GFAP (Fig. 16–9*B*).

Minute ependymal rests may also occur in the same locations; these lesions that may be microscopic incidental findings, measure only a few millimeters; they are benign and may represent precursors of myxopapillary ependymoma.[80]

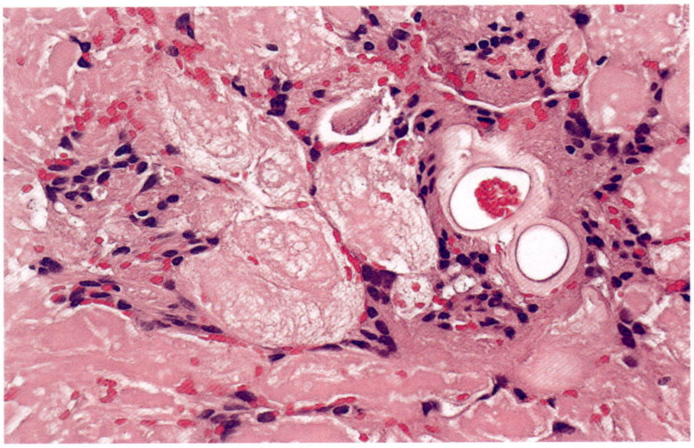

A

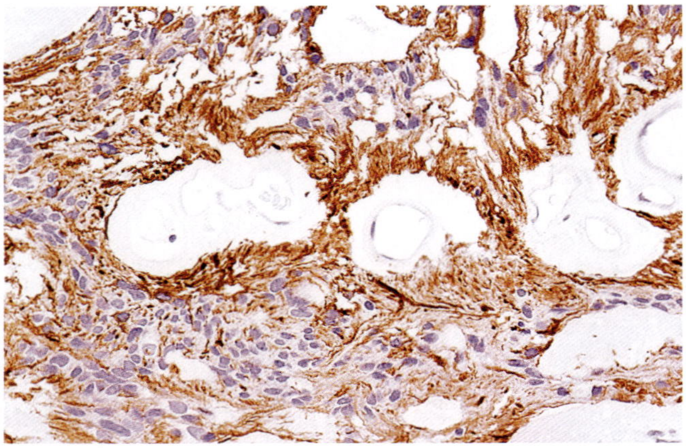

B

Figure 16–9. *A,* Myxopapillary ependymoma shows tumor cells as perivascular pseudorosettes in a myxoid stroma. *B,* The tumor cells are uniformly GFAP^{+}.

Genetics

Clonal chromosomal changes identified in these tumors include telomeric fusions and chromosome instability.[81]

Paraganglioma

Overview on Paraganglia

Paraganglia represent collections of specialized neural cells, which serve neurosecretory and neuroreceptive functions at various sites. Paraganglioma is the designation for closely related neural tumors that originate in paraganglia and occur in several clinical settings.[82]

Normal paraganglia are composed of neural cells, the chief cells that are typically clustered as spherical collections "Zellballen." They are surrounded by Schwann cell-like elongated cells, the so-called sustentacular cells. The chief cells are positive for neural markers including NSE, chromogranin, and synaptophysin and neurofilament protein, whereas the spindled Schwann cell-like sustentacular cells are positive for S-100 protein and sometimes for GFAP.

Overview on Paragangliomas

The most common are adrenal medullary paragangliomas (pheochromocytomas), which are usually hormonally active with catecholamine production. Extra-adrenal retroperitoneal paragangliomas, those arising in the posterior mediastinum adjacent to the sympathetic chain (aortosympatethic paragangliomas) and urinary bladder paragangliomas are closely related to the adrenal ones.

Another group is formed by the head and neck paragangliomas (those of carotid body, glomus jugulare, and vagal body). These tumors are usually hormonally inactive. Duodenal gangliocytic paraganglioma is a unique tumor that combines elements of paraganglioma with epithelial, ganglionic, and schwannian components; paraganglioma of cauda equina is related to this type.

Most paragangliomas are well-differentiated tumors that show a close homology to the corresponding normal structures, the adrenal medulla, extra-adrenal paraganglia, and paraganglia of the head and neck. A majority are clinically benign, but prediction of behavior is notoriously difficult in this group of tumors.

Pheochromocytoma (Paraganglioma) of the Adrenals

Paragangliomas of adrenal medullary origin are called pheochromocytomas. The adrenal pheochromocytomas are catecholamine-secreting tumors, and they outnumber the closely related extra-adrenal retroperitoneal counterparts by a margin of 9:1.

Clinical Features

A majority of pheochromocytomas occur sporadically, and the population incidence based on studies from several countries varies between 2 and 8 per million. The tumor is most common in middle age, but occurs from childhood to old age without a clear sex predilection. A minority of pheochromocytomas occur on a hereditary basis in patients with multiple endocrine neoplasia (MEN) 2A or MEN2B, von Hippel Lindau disease, NF1, or familially on a yet unknown genetic basis.[82,83]

The sporadic tumors are often discovered based on hormonal symptoms such as sustained or paroxysmal hypertension or paroxysms of sweating, headaches, or attacks of anxiety. Some are incidentally discovered in asymptomatic patients. In clinically suspected cases, the diagnosis is aided by measurement of urine metanephrines, the most relevant catecholamine metabolites in this context. Computed tomography and scintigraphy with radioiodine-labeled metaiodobenzyl-guanidine, a catecholamine analogue taken up by the tumors, are used to localize the suspected tumors in patients with elevated catecholamine secretion.

The hereditary tumors in patients with MEN2A/MEN2B syndromes are more often asymptomatic and are often found in imaging studies of patients under tumor surveillance. The tumors that occur in the syndromes tend to be smaller and bilateral and they are often diagnosed in younger patients.

Before modern detection and treatment, many patients died of stroke or hypertensive crisis attributed to catecholamine release from the tumor.[84]

Malignancy is rare (2–5%) in the adrenal pheochromocytoma, but it is difficult to predict histologically. Metastases develop in the liver, lungs, bones, or sometimes in lymph nodes. Some patients with metastatic disease have had a long survival with the disease.

Pathology

Grossly, pheochromocytomas are usually circumscribed, nodular tumors that expand the adrenal medulla. They vary from small 1- to 2-cm nodules to bulky masses that can exceed 20 cm in diameter and 2 kg in weight. Residual normal adrenal cortex is usually found in careful search as a yellow rim around the tumor. On sectioning, the tumors are soft and often hemorrhagic. The color is usually homogeneously brown to dark brown, but is occasionally pale with brown foci. After being a few days in formalin, the fixative typically turns brown, a feature quite unique to pheochromocytoma.

Histologically, pheochromocytomas vary (Fig. 16–10). They typically have an "organoid" structure being composed of cells arranged in compartments separated by thin vascular septa. Some of the compartments are round (referred to as Zellballen), and others are irregularly shaped, trabecular, or poorly developed with the tumor showing a more solid pattern. The cell size varies from small to large, and shapes vary from round to epithelioid and are occasionally spindled. The cytoplasm varies from eosinophilic to basophilic; the latter variants often have a granular cytoplasm. Nuclear pleomorphism is not uncommon, and some tumors have nuclear pseudoinclusions (cytoplasmic invaginations). Eosinophilic cytoplasmic globules occur in some cases, and a minority have lipofuscin (neuromelanin) pigmentation. Extensive hemorrhage or stromal fibrosis may be present.

Pheochromocytoma-ganglioneuroma composite tumors are rare, and there are isolated reports of spindle cell sarcomas, usually MPNSTs, arising in pheochromocytoma.[82,85]

Prediction of Malignancy

Histologic assessment of malignancy is notoriously difficult in these tumors. In one study, tumors that were malignant were larger and had coarse nodularity, but vascular invasion and increased mitotic activity were not reliable indicators.[86] In another study, presence of more than one of the following features was predictive of malignancy: coarse nodularity, tumor necrosis, and absence of hyaline globules.[85]

Immunohistochemistry

Immunohistochemically, the chief cells of pheochromocytoma are consistently positive for panneuroendocrine markers NSE, chromogranin, and synaptophysin. Neurofilaments of 68 kd can be typically demonstrated in frozen sections, but only inconsistently in paraffin-embedded tissue. All components are almost invariably negative for keratins.

The neuropeptides leu-encephalin and metencephalin, somatostatin, and pancreatic polypeptide have been found in the majority of tumors, and other neuropeptides (adrenocorticotropic hormone, calcitonin, bombesin) in a minority of tumors.[87–89]

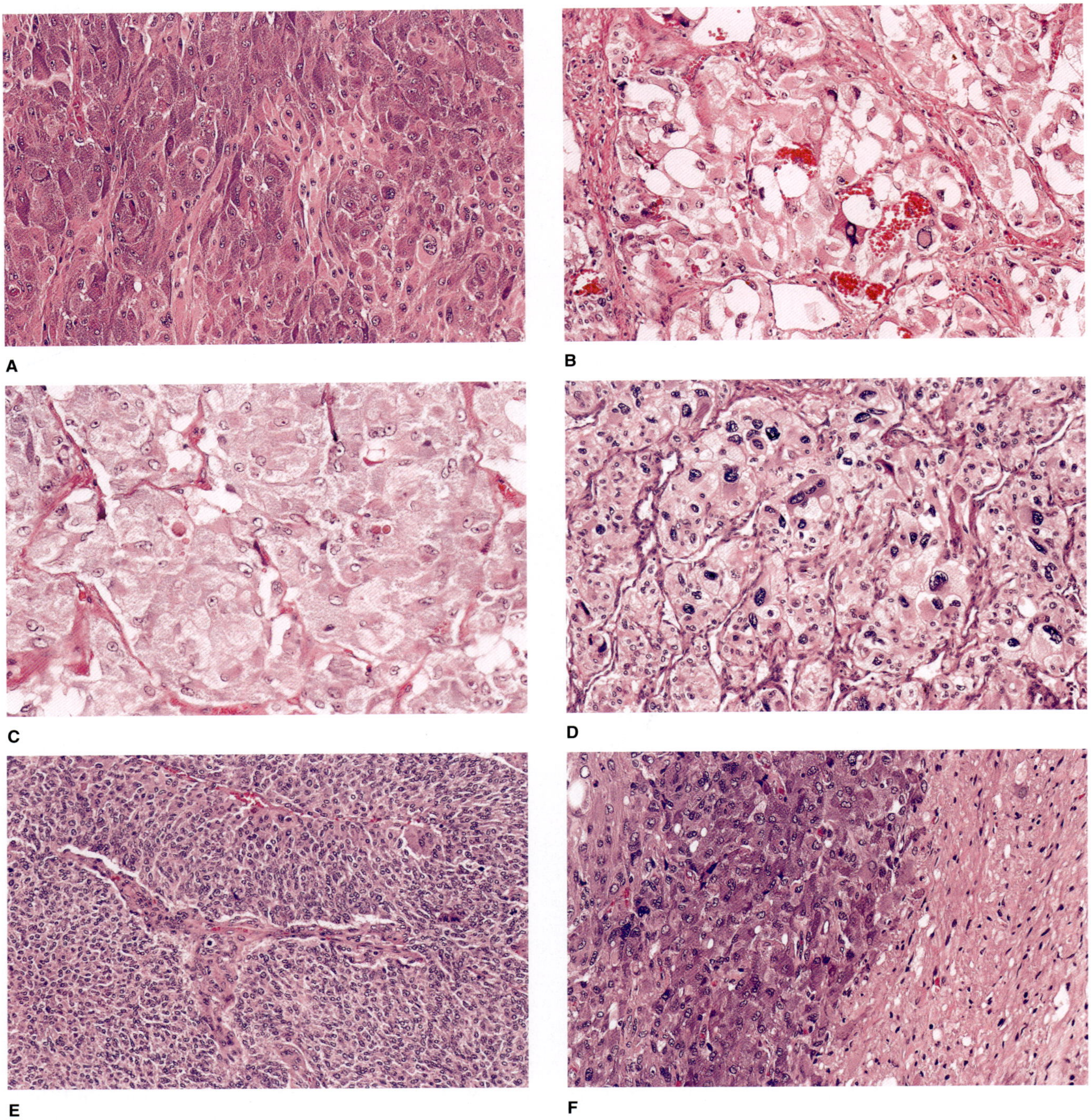

Figure 16–10. Histologic spectrum of adrenal and extra-adrenal paraganglioma. *A,* Tumor composed of solid sheets of polygonal cells with granular basophilic cytoplasm. *B,* Nuclear pseudoinclusions and organoid pattern. *C,* Cytoplasmic hyaline globules. *D,* Nuclear pleomorphism. *E,* Spindled variant. *F,* Paraortic paraganglioma with ganglioneuroma.

Reduced expression of neuropeptides has been observed in malignant variants.[89]

A Schwann cell-like S-100 protein-positive spindled sustentacular cell component is variably present around the chief cell compartments.[90] This cell population is often less prominent in pheochromocytoma than carotid body paraganglioma. In contrast to head and neck paragangliomas, the adrenal ones do not have GFAP$^+$ sustentacular cells.[91] The sustentacular cell component appears to be reduced or absent in malignant tumors. Pheochromocytomas in patients with MEN have been reported to have a greater number of S-100 protein-positive sustentacular cells than those associated with NF1 syndrome.[90]

A proliferative index greater than 2%[89] or 2.5% by MIB-1-immunostaining has been suggested to be indicative of malignancy.[92,93] Because the differences are small between benign and malignant tumors, such results may not reproducible and practically useful.

Ultrastructure

Pheochromocytoma cells are rich in dense core granules of 150 to 250 nm. Among them there are granules filled with electron dense substance and those with an empty halo-like space. The morphologic correlation with secretion type seems to be incomplete.[86]

Genetics

Mutations leading in the ligand-independent activation of RET tyrosine kinase seem to be a central mechanism in MEN syndrome-associated pheochromocytoma. Germline mutations occur in patients with MEN2A and MEN2B syndromes,[94,95] and somatic mutations have been found in some sporadic pheochromocytomas, but not in sporadic extra-adrenal paragangliomas, according to one study.[96] Patients with von Hippel-Lindau syndrome have germline mutations in the *VHL* gene, but such mutations have not been found in sporadic tumors.[97,98] *SDHD* gene mutations, similar to carotid body paragangliomas, have been recently described. Some these were germline mutations, and these patients had the occult hereditary paraganglioma syndrome, but some were somatic.[99]

Losses in chromosomes 1p and 3q have been detected by comparative genomic hybridization in the majority of pheochromocytomas in two independent studies.[100,101] Similar changes have been documented in extra-adrenal paragangliomas.[100]

Extra-Adrenal Retroperitoneal Paragangliomas

Pheochromocytoma-like paragangliomas may occur paraortally in the retroperitoneum and mediastinum, but they are much rarer than in the adrenals.[102,103] In the retroperitoneum some arise from the aortic paraganglia (organ of Zuckerkandl).

The retroperitoneal paragangliomas typically occur in young adults with a female predominance. A higher percentage of these tumors are malignant than of the adrenal paragangliomas; in nonselected series the percentage of malignancy is approximately 10%, much higher than that of adrenal pheochromocytoma.[102] Histologic predictive features are the same as found for adrenal paragangliomas: confluent tumor necrosis, extensive soft tissue of vascular invasion, and lack of hyaline globules. Malignant variants may have low mitotic activity, and the architectural patterns have no discriminatory value.[85]

The gross, histologic, and immunohistochemical features are generally similar to those of adrenal tumors (Fig. 16–10). Pronounced fibrosis occurs more often in the retroperitoneal tumors. Pigmented variants have been described. They contain melanin-like pigment but are negative for HMB45.[104] Similar to adrenal tumors, some have combined features of pheochromocytoma and ganglioneuroma.[82,85]

Paraganglioma (Pheochromocytoma of the Urinary Bladder)

Normal paraganglia were demonstrated in over half of the bladders examined in one autopsy study.[105] Paragangliomas of the urinary bladder are rare and fewer than 100 cases have been reported. These tumors occur in a wide age range with a 3:1 female predominance based on the largest series.[106] Some tumors manifest by hematuria and others are diagnosed based on hormonal symptoms caused by paroxysmal catecholamine secretion on micturition. Most tumors can be treated by transurethral resection. The frequency of malignancy is approximately 10% to 15%. Late recurrences and metastases may occur indicating the necessity of long-term follow-up.[106,107]

Histologically and immunohistochemically paragangliomas of the bladder resemble their adrenal counterparts. Tumor aneuploidy appears to have no prognostic significance and is also found in the benign tumors.[107] The same difficulties in predicting tumor behavior histologically apply, as for other paragangliomas.

Paragangliomas of the Head and Neck

Clinical Features

The most common are paragangliomas of the carotid body, followed by jugulotympanic and vagal tumors. Occasional cases have been reported in the laryngeal paraganglia and elsewhere. Head and neck paragangliomas generally occur in middle-aged patients, and many reports show 2:1 female predominance. These tumors are usually hormonally silent and become symptomatic by their space-occupying nature. However, catecholamine-secreting examples have been reported.[82,108]

A minority of head and neck paragangliomas occur on a hereditary basis, and such patients may have multiple paragangliomas in different locations.

Carotid Body Paraganglioma (Carotid Body Tumor, Chemodectoma)

The carotid body paraganglia are located in the carotid bifurcation and act as chemoreceptors for oxygen tension. Chronic hypoxia, such as living at high altitudes or from chronic obstructive pulmonary disease, cause hyperplasia of the chief cells, and living at a high altitude may also predispose to a carotid body tumor. In Peru, the incidence of carotid body tumors has been estimated as 10 times higher in the high altitudes than at sea level.[109–111]

Most tumors measure between 2 and 6 cm. They are usually benign, but metastases develop in 5% to 10% of cases, most commonly in bones, lung, and liver.[112–115] Prediction of metastasis is difficult.

Jugulotympanic Paragangliomas

Jugulotympanic paragangliomas have been often referred to as "glomus tumors" or "glomus jugulare tumors" in the earlier literature. They typically occur in middle-aged to older patients with a female predominance and cause hearing loss or tinnitus.[116]

Most of these tumors are small middle ear nodules less than 1 cm, attached to the tympanic membrane, and they are easily excised. Larger masses invading the petrous bone are difficult to manage, and complications of the tumor excision have to be weighed against risks of a conservative approach or radiation.[117]

Vagal Body Paragangliomas

Vagal body paragangliomas occur in the lower neck arising from the vagal body paraganglia, most commonly in middle-aged patients with a 2:1 female predominance. They are usually benign, but can reach a size of 5 cm or more. Tumors extending to the skull basis are difficult to manage and may cause lethal complications.[118] Occasional metastasizing examples have been reported.[119]

Pathology

Grossly, the carotid body and vagal body paragangliomas are typically fleshy, red to brownish homogenous oval or dumbbell-shaped pseudoencapsulated masses (Fig. 16–11). In carotid body tumors, the organoid clustering with compartments (Zellballen) is typically well-developed, but the compartment sizes vary greatly. The tumors are highly vascular and may have foci of hemosiderin and fibrosis and sometimes have a hemangioma or hemangiopericytoma-like overall pattern (Fig. 16–12). Some tumors have wide fibrous septa. Jugulotympanic paragangliomas often have a more diffuse histologic appearance.

Cytologically, the tumor cells have variably clear to basophilic to eosinophilic cytoplasm. The nuclei have usually finely distributed chromatin, but atypical, hyperchromatic, bizarre nuclei may occur and do not indicate malignancy (Fig. 16–12*D*). Nuclear pseudoinclusions similar to those seen in adrenal tumors, may occur. Mitotic activity is usually inconspicuous.

It is difficult to predict tumor behavior histologically, but vascular invasion and tumor necrosis have been suggested as features correlating with malignant behavior.[112–115]

Immunohistochemistry

All head and neck paragangliomas, similar to the adrenal tumors, are positive for neuroendocrine markers NSE, chromogranin, and synaptophysin, and negative for keratins. PGP9.5 has also been consistently shown in all paragangliomas.[120,121] S-100 protein- and GFAP-positive sustentacular cells can be identified at least in the carotid body and

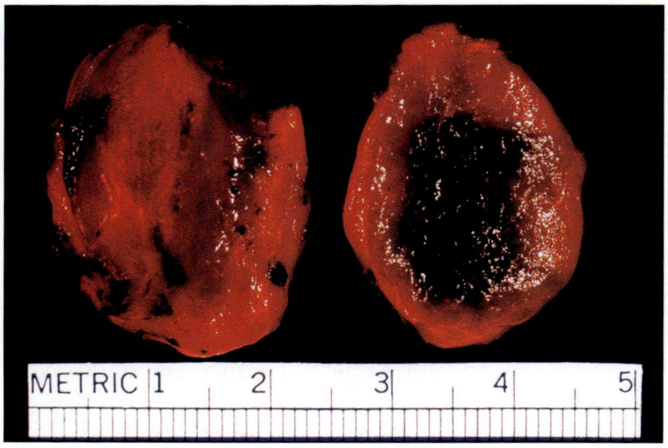

Figure 16–11. Grossly, carotid body paraganglioma is a sharply circumscribed nodule with a brownish cut surface.

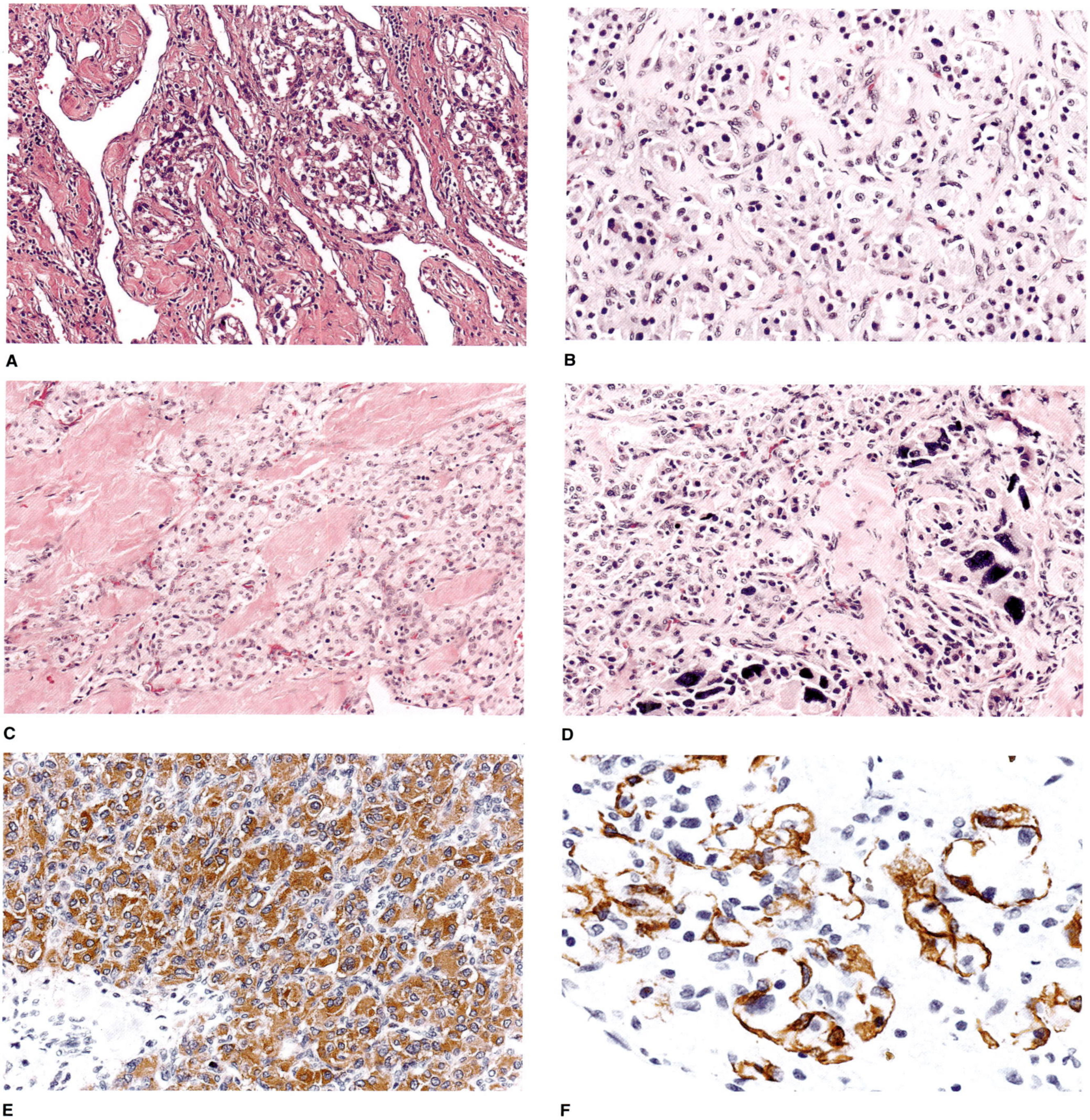

Figure 16–12. Histologic spectrum of carotid body paraganglioma. *A,* This tumor is highly vascular and contains organoid clusters of neuroendocrine cells. *B,* A well-developed organoid Zellballen pattern. *C,* Tumor with thick fibrous septa. *D,* Marked nuclear pleomorphism is not uncommon. *E,* The chief cells are strongly positive for synaptophysin. *F,* The sustentacular cells demonstrate GFAP immunoreactivity.

jugulotympanic tumors. This component may be less prevalent in the malignant tumors.[122]

Differential Diagnosis

The differential diagnosis is site dependent. Neuroendocrine carcinomas with an organoid appearance are composed of epithelial neuroendocrine cells that are positive for keratins and synaptophysin. Meningioma and epithelioid smooth muscle tumors may have an organoid appearance not to be confused with that of paraganglioma.

Alveolar soft part sarcoma, originally believed to be a paraganglioma variant, may structurally simulate the organoid or solid variants of paraganglioma. In this tumor, the cells are larger with ample, eosinophilic cytoplasm, and neuroendocrine markers are absent.

The most common middle ear tumor is middle ear adenoma, carcinoid tumor primary in this location. In contrast to paraganglioma, this tumor is composed of ribbons of cells that are epithelial neuroendocrine cells positive for keratins.

Genetics

Three genetic loci relevant to hereditary paragangliomas have been identified at 11q23 and named as PGL1, PGL2, and PGL3 (paraganglioma loci 1–3). Imprinting has been noted in the *PGL* genes, and disease occurs when the paternal allele is inherited, with autosomal dominant pattern with an incomplete penetrance.[123–125] Gene *SDHD* encoding a subunit of cytochrome B of the mitochondrial electron transport system has been identified in the PGL1 locus. This gene shows germline mutations in patients with hereditary paranganglioma, and allelic losses have been seen in the tumors, in line with a recessive tumor suppressor gene model. Both missense and nonsense mutations have been identified in the involved families. The *SDHD* gene mutations are believed to cause permanent hypoxic signal, which leads to hyperplasia and neoplasia via an unknown mechanism, possibly similar to high altitude hypoxia.[126]

Gangliocytic Paraganglioma of the Duodenum

The gangliocytic paraganglioma is a rare neuroendocrine tumor almost specific to the duodenum, originally described as duodenal ganglioneuroma.[127–131] Similar histologic features may occur in paragangliomas of the cauda equina. The presence of pancreatic-like ducts and expression of pancreatic polypeptide has led to the suggestion that this tumor is histogenetically related to ectopic pancreatic tissue.[129]

Clinical Features

Gangliocytic paraganglioma occurs in adults in a wide age range with a median age around 50 to 55 years and a male predominance. Association with NF1 is rare. The vast majority of the tumors occur in the second part of the duodenum, and a small number of cases have been reported in the third, first, and fourth parts of the duodenum and the pylorus. Some patients present with GI bleeding, few with biliary obstruction, and some tumors are incidental findings during surgery or autopsy. The behavior is almost invariably benign, but local recurrences and lymph node metastases have been reported on rare occasions.[131–133] Complete conservative excision and follow-up are felt to be adequate.

Pathology

Grossly, the tumor forms a relatively small 1- to 3-cm intraluminal pedunculated or sessile polyp, which may be ulcerated; bigger examples up to 10 cm are on record. The tumor involves submucosa and often infiltrates in muscularis propria. Histologically, it often shows an organoid Zellballen or trabecular pattern. The tumor is composed of three components that are present in various proportions: epithelial cells often with spindled morphology, spindled Schwann-like cells resembling those seen in ganglioneuroma, and polygonal ganglion cell components. Some tumors contain psammoma bodies more commonly seen in duodenal carcinoids. The epithelial component is often prevalent, and forms solid sheets or ribbons (Fig. 16–13). Mitotic activity is low.

The epithelial elements are positive for keratins, which are rarely seen in other paragangliomas. The spindle cell component with a Schwann cell-like appearance is S-100 protein positive; S-100 protein-positive sustentacular cells may also be seen around the epithelial elements.[129–131,134] The ganglion cells are scattered in and adjacent to the epithelial and schwannian elements, and they are positive for neural markers (NSE, synaptophysin, neurofilament proteins). Synaptophysin and chromogranin can also be demonstrated in the epithelial component. Like pancreatic neuroendocrine tumors, the epithelial component in gangliocytic paraganglioma can be positive for neurofilament NF68.[133] The neuropeptides and neurotransmitters often detected include pancreatic

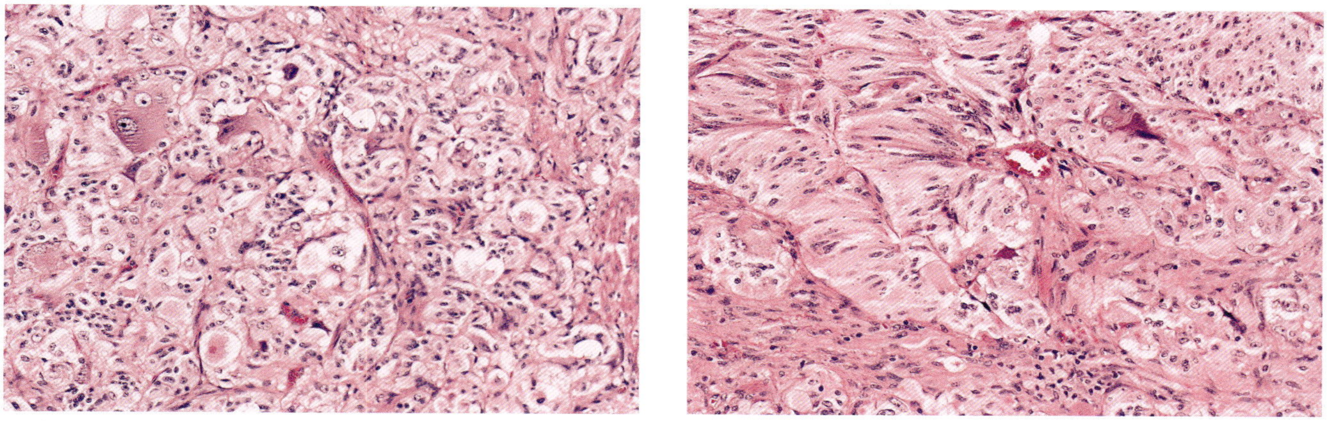

A B

Figure 16–13. Different areas of duodenal gangliocytic paraganglioma. *A,* Organoid clusters with ganglion cells. *B,* Spindled neuroendocrine cells and Schwann cell-like elements.

polypeptide, somatostatin, and serotonin; others have been found sporadically.

Paraganglioma of the Cauda Equina

Clinical Features

This rare paraganglioma occurs in adult patients and usually causes sciatica symptoms and sometimes paraplegia (cauda equina syndrome). The largest series reported an 18:13 male predominance. The tumor is usually well-circumscribed and limited to filum terminale. It is almost always benign, but local complications including paraplegia are possible.[82,135]

Pathology

Grossly, the tumor is typically an encapsulated intradural, extraspinal mass and measures 1.5 to 4 cm in maximum diameter. The histologic appearance may resemble that of a carotid body tumor. Nearly half of the cases have ganglion cell differentiation, and some cases bear a striking resemblance to gangliocytic paraganglioma of the duodenum.

Immunohistochemically, the tumor cells are positive for neuroendocrine markers. The largest series found consistent positivity for NSE in the chief cells and S-100 protein in the sustentacular cells, which were variably positive for GFAP in half of the cases. Neurotransmitters and neuropeptides 5-hydroxytryptamine (serotonin) and somatostatin were present in most cases.[135] In our experience, chromogranin and synaptophysin also can be demonstrated, similar to other paragangliomas. The tumor is often keratin positive, similar to duodenal gangliocytic paraganglioma and different from most other paragangliomas.

Differential Diagnosis

The paraganglioma of cauda equina has to be separated from ependymoma, which in this location is usually of myxopapillary, less commonly of solid type. Ependymomas lack the organoid structure, are globally positive for GFAP; they do not show biphasic structure with chief cell and sustentacular cell components, and ganglion cells are not present.

Ganglioneuroma

Ganglioneuroma is a benign sympathetic nervous system tumor, and it can be considered a fully mature counterpart of neuroblastoma. Solitary ganglioneuromas occur in soft tissues in the body cavities, and ganglioneuromatous polyps and ganglioneuromatosis occur almost exclusively in the lower GI tract.

Clinical Features

Solitary ganglioneuromas occur in children and young adults with a female predominance, and half of them are diagnosed in the first decade. The most common locations are retroperitoneum, pelvis, posterior mediastinum, and the adrenals. Some cases occur in patients with NF1. The tumor is benign and treated by simple excision.[136,137] A rare variant with Leydig cells has been described; this produces testosterone and may cause virilization.[82,138]

Gastrointestinal ganglioneuromas can be divided into three clinicopathologic groups.[139–141] Polypoid ganglioneuroma occurs sporadically in adults of all ages, usually in the colon and rectum without syndrome association. It is usually an incidental finding at

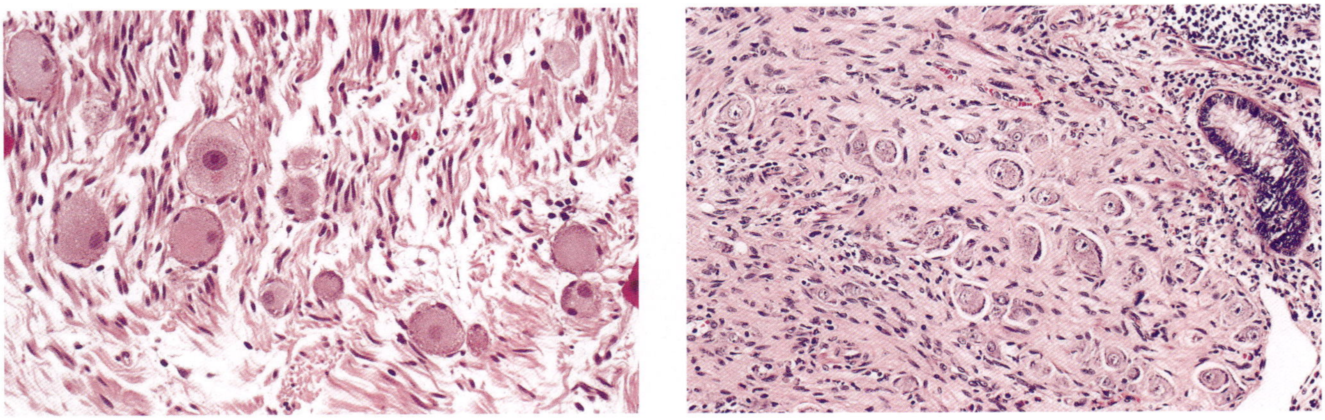

A B

Figure 16–14. *A,* Solitary ganglioneuroma is composed of a predominant neurofibroma-like fibrous component and scattered ganglion cells. *B,* Mucosal ganglioneuroma forms a focus of ganglion and a neurofibroma-like spindle cell component.

endoscopy or surgery. Multiple ganglioneuromatous polyps and diffuse ganglioneuromatosis mainly occur in the colon and rectum of young and middle-aged adults with MEN2B syndrome or NF1; the diffuse form may also involve the appendix, ileum, and stomach. The lesions may cause lower GI bleeding. The diffuse ganglioneuromatosis may cause megacolon.

Pathology

Grossly, solitary ganglioneuroma of soft tissues is an encapsulated tumor usually measuring 3 to 10 cm. It is white to yellowish on sectioning, and some tumors have a lipoma-like slightly mucoid gross appearance. Histologically, it is composed of tightly bundled fascicles of neurofibroma-like fibrous component, which contains nerves and scattered ganglion cells, often seen in small clusters (Fig. 16–14*A*). The fibrous component is highly collagenous and may have a myxoid component. The ganglion cells tend to be large and they may be multinucleated. They may or may not have surrounding satellite cells.

The GI polypoid ganglioneuroma may resemble a juvenile polyp with multiple epithelial cysts and is usually smaller than 2 cm. The ganglioneuromatosis polyposis may form small filiform lesions and multiple polyps similar to polypoid ganglioneuroma. The diffuse ganglioneuromatosis may involve extensively the entire intestinal wall forming large stricture-like lesions that can measure over 15 cm. Histologically, mucosal ganglioneuromas show patchy involvement with mucosal and submucosal ganglion cells and schwannian spindle cell elements (Fig. 16–14*B*). The diffuse variants infiltrate muscularis propria and contain neurofibromatous components with scattered ganglion cells and typically include neural proliferation.

Malignant peripheral nerve sheath tumors developing in a ganglioneuroma have been occasionally reported; some of these were documented as S-100 protein positive.[142] All tumors occurred in children or young adults, and in some cases, there was a previous history of neuroblastoma. Radiation could have contributed to the genesis of sarcoma in one case, which was diagnosed 17 years after the history of radiated neuroblastoma.[143]

Differential Diagnosis

The solitary ganglioneuromas in children have to be sampled thoroughly, in order not to miss less differentiated foci of neuroblastoma or ganglioneuroblastoma. The immature components may be grossly recognizable or reddish or hemorrhagic foci; if present, the tumor has to be diagnosed as ganglioneuroblastoma. Neurofibromas involving sympathetic ganglia have to separated from ganglioneuromas. In such instances, the ganglion cells are consistently surrounded by normal satellite cells, whereas such cells are variably present in ganglioneuromas. Ganglion cells in ganglioneuroma may appear immature, but neuropil should not be present; this is a sign of ganglioneuroblastoma.

REFERENCES

Metastatic Melanoma and Its Differential Diagnosis

1. Nakhleh RE, Wick MR, Rocamora A, Swanson PE, Dehner LP: Morphologic diversity in malignant melanomas. Am J Clin Pathol 1990;93:731–740.
2. Gaudin P, Rosai J: Florid vascular proliferation associated with neural and neuroendocrine neoplasms. A

diagnostic clue and potential pitfall. Am J Surg Pathol 1995;19:642–652.

3. Lodding P, Kindblom LG, Angervall L: Metastases of malignant melanoma simulating soft tissue sarcoma. A clinicopathological, light and electron microscopic and immunohistochemical study of 21 cases. Virchows Arch Pathol Anat Histopathol [A] 1990;417:377–388.
4. King R, Busam K, Rosai J: Metastatic malignant melanoma resembling malignant peripheral nerve sheath tumor: Report of 16 cases. Am J Surg Pathol 1999;23:1499–1505.
5. Kaufmann O, Koch S, Burghardt J, Audring H, Dietel M: Tyrosinase, melan-A, KBA62 as markers for the immunohistochemical identification of metastatic amelanotic melanomas on paraffin sections. Mod Pathol 1998;11:740–746.
6. Miettinen M, Fernandez M, Franssila KO, Gataliza Z, Lasota J, Sarlomo-Rikala M: Microphthalmia transcription factor in the immunohistochemical diagnosis of metastatic melanoma: Comparison with four other melanoma markers. Am J Surg Pathol 2001;25:205–211.
7. Zarbo RJ, Gown AM, Nagle RB, Visscher DW, Crissman JD: Anomalous cytokeratin expression in malignant melanoma: One- and two-dimensional Western blot analysis and immunohistochemical survey of 100 melanomas. Mod Pathol 1990;3:494–501.
8. Rodriguez H, Ackerman LV: Cellular blue nevus. Cancer 1968;21:393–405.
9. Temple-Camp CR, Saxe N, King H: Benign and malignant cellular blue nevus. A clinicopathologic study of 30 cases. Am J Dermatopathol 1988;10:289–296.

Desmoplastic Melanoma

10. Conley J, Lattes R, Orr W: Desmoplastic malignant melanoma (a rare variant of spindle cell melanoma). Cancer 1971;28:914–936.
11. Reed RJ, Leonard DD: Neurotropic melanoma. A variant of desmoplastic melanoma. Am J Surg Pathol 1979;3:301–311.
12. Reiman HM, Goellner JR, Woods JE, Mixter RC: Desmoplastic melanoma of the head and neck. Cancer 1987;60:2269–2274.
13. Egbert B, Kempson R, Sagebiel R: Desmoplastic malignant melanoma. A clinicohistopathologic study of 25 cases. Cancer 1988;62:2033–2041.
14. Jain S, Allen PW: Desmoplastic malignant melanoma and its variants. A study of 45 cases. Am J Surg Pathol 1989;13:358–373.
15. Smithers BM, McLeod GR, Little JH: Desmoplastic, neural transforming and neurotropic melanoma: A review of 45 cases. Aust N Z J Surg 1990;60:967–972.
16. Carlson JA, Dickersin GR, Sober AJ, Barnhill RL: Desmoplastic neurotropic melanoma. A clinicopathologic analysis of 28 cases. Cancer 1995;75:478–494.
17. Skelton HG, Smith KJ, Laskin WB, et al: Desmoplastic malignant melanoma. J Am Acad Dermatol 1995;32:717–725.
18. Tsao H, Sober AJ, Barnhill RL: Desmoplastic neurotropic melanoma. Semin Cutan Med Surg 1997;16:131–136.
19. Quinn MJ, Crotty KA, Thompson JF, Coates AS, O'Brien CJ, McCarthy WH: Desmoplastic and desmoplastic neurotropic melanoma: Experience with 280 patients. Cancer 1998;83:1128–1135.
20. Kilpatrick SE, White WL, Browne JD: Desmoplastic malignant melanoma of the oral mucosa. An underrecognized diagnostic pitfall. Cancer 1996;78:383–389.
21. Wharton JM, Carlson JA, Mihm MC: Desmoplastic malignant melanoma: Diagnosis of early clinical lesions. Hum Pathol 1999;30:537–542.
22. Longacre TA, Egbert BM, Rouse RV: Desmoplastic and spindle-cell malignant melanoma. An immunohistochemical study. Am J Surg Pathol 1996;20:1489–1500.
23. Antey A, Cerio R, Ramnarain N, Orchard G, Smith N, Wilson-Jones E: Desmoplastic malignant melanoma. An immunocytochemical study of 25 cases. Am J Dermatopathol 1994;16:14–22.
24. Koch MB, Shih IM, Weiss SW, Folpe AL: Microphthalmia transcription factor and melanoma cell adhesion molecule expression distinguish desmoplastic/spindle cell melanoma from morphologic mimics. Am J Surg Pathol 2001;25:58–64.
25. Kanik AB, Yaar M, Bhawan J: p75 nerve growth factor receptor staining helps identify desmoplastic and neurotropic melanoma. J Cutan Pathol 1996;23:205–210.
26. Gutzmer R, Herbst RA, Mommert S, et al: Allelic loss at the neurofibromatosis type 1 (NF1) gene locus is frequent in desmoplastic neurotropic melanoma. Hum Genet 2000;107:357–361.

Clear Cell Sarcoma—Clinicopathologic Studies and Differential Diagnosis

27. Enzinger FM: Clear cell sarcoma of tendons and aponeuroses: An analysis of 21 cases. Cancer 1965;18:1163–1174.
28. Chung EM, Enzinger FM: Malignant melanoma of soft parts: Reassessment of clear cell sarcoma. Am J Surg Pathol 1983;7:405–413.
29. Kindblom LG, Lodding P, Angervall L: Clear cell sarcoma of tendons and aponeuroses. An immunohistochemical and electron microscopic analysis indicating neural crest origin. Virchows Arch A Pathol Anat Histopathol 1983;401:109128.
30. Sara AS, Evans HL, Benjamin RS: Malignant melanoma of soft parts (clear cell sarcoma): A study of 17 cases, with emphasis on prognostic factors. Cancer 1990;65:367–374.
31. Lucas DR, Nascimento AG, Sim FH: Clear cell sarcoma of soft tissues. Mayo Clinic experience with 35 cases. Am J Surg Pathol 1992;16:1197–1204.
32. Montgomery EA, Meis JM, Ramos AG, Martz KL: Clear cell sarcoma of tendons and aponeuroses. A clinicopathologic study of 58 cases with analysis of prognostic factors. Int J Surg Pathol 1993;1:89–100.
33. Deenik W, Mooi WJ, Rutgers EJ, Peterse JL, Hart AA, Kroon BB: Clear cell sarcoma (malignant melanoma)

of soft parts. A clinicopathologic study of 30 cases. Cancer 1999;86:969–975.
34. Donner LR, Trompler RA, Dubin S: Clear cell sarcoma of the ileum: The crucial role of cytogenetics for the diagnosis. Am J Surg Pathol 1998;22:121–124.
35. Fukuda T, Kakihara T, Baba K, Yamaki T, Yamaguchi T, Suzuki T: Clear cell sarcoma arising in the transverse colon. Pathol Int 2000;50:412–416.
36. Rubin BP, Fletcher JA, Renshaw AA: Clear cell sarcoma of soft parts: Report of a case primary in the kidney with cytogenetic confirmation. Am J Surg Pathol 1999;23:589–594.
37. Swanson PE, Wick MR: Clear cell sarcoma: An immunohistochemical analysis of six cases and comparison with other epithelioid neoplasms of soft tissue. Arch Pathol Lab Med 1989;113:55–60.
38. Graadt van Roggen JF, Mooi WJ, Hogendoorn PC: Clear cell sarcoma of tendons and aponeuroses (malignant melanoma of soft parts) and cutaneous melanoma: Exploring the histogenetic relationship between these two clinicopathological entities. J Pathol 1998;186:3–7.
39. Folpe AL, Goodman ZD, Ishak KG, et al: Clear cell myomelanocytic tumor of the falciform ligament/ligamentum teres: A novel member of the perivascular epithelioid cell clear cell family of tumors with a predilection for children and young adults. Am J Surg Pathol 2000;24:1239–1246.

Clear Cell Sarcoma—Genetics

40. Peulve P, Michot C, Vannier JP, Tron P, Hemet J: Clear cell sarcoma with t(12;22)(q13-14;q12). Genes Chromosomes Cancer 1991;3:400–402.
41. Stenman G, Kindblom LG, Angervall L: Reciprocal translocation t(12;22)(q13;q13) in clear cell sarcoma of tendons and aponeuroses. Genes Chromosomes Cancer 1992;4:122–127.
42. Reeves BR, Fletcher CD, Gusterson BA: Translocation t(12;22)(q13;q13) is a nonrandom rearrangement in clear cell sarcoma. Cancer Genet Cytogenet 1992;64:101–103.
43. Mrozek K, Karakousis CP, Perez-Mesa C, Bloomfield CD: Translocation t(12;22)(q13;q12.2-12.3) in a clear cell sarcoma of tendons and aponeuroses. Genes Chromosomes Cancer 1993;6:249–252.
44. Fujimura Y, Ohno T, Siddique H, Lee L, Rao VN, Reddy ES: The EWS-ATF-1 gene involved in malignant melanoma of soft parts with t(12;22) chromosome translocation encodes a constitutive transcriptional activator. Oncogene 1996;4:159–167.
45. Pellin A, Monteagudo C, Lopez-Gines C, Carda C, Boix J, Llombart-Bosch A: New type of chimeric fusion product between the EWS and ATFI genes in clear cell sarcoma (malignant melanoma of soft parts). Genes Chromosomes Cancer 1998;23:358–360.
46. Sonobe H, Taguchi T, Shimizu K, Iwata J, Furihata M, Ohtsuki Y: Further characterization of the human clear cell sarcoma cell line HS-MM demonstrating a specific t(12;22)(q13;q12) translocation and hybrid EWS/ATF-1 transcript. J Pathol 1999;187:594–597.
47. Bosilevac JM, Olsen RJ, Bridge JA, Hinrichs SH: Tumor cell viability in clear cell sarcoma requires DNA binding activity of the EWS/ATF1 fusion protein. J Biol Chem 1999;274:34811–34818.
48. Aue G, Hedges LK, Schwartz HS, Bridge JA, Neff JR, Butler MG: Clear cell sarcoma or malignant melanoma of soft parts: Molecular analysis of microsatellite instability with clinical correlation. Cancer Genet Cytogenet 1998;105:24–28.
49. Langezaal SM, Graadt van Roggen JF, Cleton-Jansen AM, Baelde JJ, Hogendoorn PC: Malignant melanoma is genetically distinct from clear cell sarcoma of tendons and aponeuroses (malignant melanoma of soft parts). Br J Cancer 2001;84:535–538.

Pigmented Neuroectodermal Tumor of Infancy

50. Cutler LS, Chaudry AP, Topazian R: Melanotic neuroectodermal tumor of infancy: An ultrastructural; study, literature review, and re-evaluation. Cancer 1981;48:257–270.
51. Johnson RE, Scheithauer BW, Dahlin DC: Melanotic neuroectodermal tumor of infancy. A review of seven cases. Cancer 1983;52:661–666.
52. Pettinato G, Manivel JC, d'Amore ES, Jaszcz W, Gorlin RL: Melanotic neuroectodermal tumor of infancy. A re-examination of a histogenetic problem based on immunohistochemical, flow cytometric, and ultrastructural study of 10 cases. Am J Surg Pathol 1991; 15:233–245.
53. Kapadia SB, Frisman DM, Hitchcock CL, Ellis GL, Popek EJ: Melanotic neuroectodermal tumor of infancy. Clinicopathological, immunohistochemical, and flow cytometric study. Am J Surg Pathol 1993;17:566–573.
54. Pierre-Kahn A, Cinalli G, Lellouch-Tubiana A, et al: Melanotic neuroectodermal tumor of the skull and meninges in infancy. Pediatr Neurosurg 1992;18:6–15.
55. Yu JS, Moore MR, Kupsky WJ, Scott RM: Intracranial melanotic neuroectodermal tumor of infancy: Two case reports. Surg Neurol 1992;37:123–129.
56. Ricketts RR, Majmuddar B: Epididymal melanotic neuroectodermal tumor of infancy. Hum Pathol 1985; 16:416–420.
57. Calabrese F, Danieli D, Valente M: Melanotic neuroectodermal tumor of the epididymis in infancy: Case report and review of the literature. Urology 1995;46:415–418.
58. Kobayashi T, Kunimi K, Imao T, et al: Melanotic neuroectodermal tumor of infancy in the epididymis. Case report and literature review. Urol Int 1996;57:262–265.
59. Raju U, Zarbo RJ, Regezi JA, Krutchkoff D, Perrin E: Melanotic neuroectodermal tumor of infancy: Intermediate filaments, neuroendocrine and melanoma-associated antigen profiles. Appl Immunohistochem 1993;1:69–76.
60. Dooling EC, Chi JG, Gilles FH: Melanotic neuroectodermal tumor of infancy: Its histological similarities to fetal pineal gland. Cancer 1977;39:1535–1541.
61. Navas-Palacios JJ: Malignant melanotic neuroectodermal tumor: Light and electron microscopic study. Cancer 1980;46:529–536.

62. Khoddami M, Squire J, Zielenska M, Thorner P: Melanotic neuroectodermal tumor of infancy: A molecular genetic study. Pediatr Dev Pathol 1998;1:295–299.

Ectopic Meningioma

63. Lopez DA, Silvers DN, Helwig EB: Cutaneous meningiomas: A clinicopathologic study. Cancer 1974;34: 728–744.
64. Hirakawa E, Kobayashi S, Terasaka K, Ogino T, Terai Y, Ohmori M: Meningeal hamartoma of the scalp. A variant of primary cutaneous meningioma. Acta Pathol Jpn 1992;42:353–357.
65. Miyamoto T, Mihara M, Hagari Y, Shimao S: Primary cutaneous meningioma on the scalp: Report of two siblings. J Dermatol 1995;22:611–619.
66. Argenyi ZB, Thieberg MD, Hayes CM, Whitaker DC: Primary cutaneous meningioma associated with von Recklinghausen's disease. J Cutan Pathol 1994;21: 549–556.
67. Theaker JM, Fletcher CD, Tudway AJ: Cutaneous heterotopic meningeal nodules. Histopathology 1990;16: 475–479.
68. Suster S, Rosai J: Hamartoma of the scalp with meningothelial elements. A distinctive benign soft tissue lesion that may simulate angiosarcoma. Am J Surg Pathol 1990;14:1–11.
69. Gaffey MJ, Mills SE, Askin FB: Minute pulmonary meningothelial-like nodules. A clinicopathologic study of the so-called minute pulmonary chemodectoma. Am J Surg Pathol 1988;12:167–175.
70. Thompson LD, Guyre K: Extracranial sinonasal tract meningiomas: A clinicopathologic study of 30 cases with a review of the literature. Am J Surg Pathol 2000;24:640–650.

Nasal Glioma and Soft Tissue Gliomatosis

71. Hirsh LF, Stool SE, Langfitt RF, Schut L: Nasal glioma. J Neurosurg 1977;46:85–91.
72. Azumi N, Matsuno T, Tateyama M, Inoue K: So-called nasal glioma. Acta Pathol Jpn 1984;34:215–220.
73. Fletcher CD, Carpenter G, McKee PH: Nasal glioma. A rarity. Am J Dermatopathol 1986;8:341–346.
74. Shepherd NA, Coates PJ, Brown AA: Soft tissue gliomatosis—Heterotopic glial tissue in the subcutis: A case report. Histopathology 1987;11:655–660.
75. McDermott MB, Glasner SD, Nielsen PL, Dehner LP: Soft tissue gliomatosis. Morphologic unity and histogenetic diversity. Am J Surg Pathol 1996;20:148–155.

Subcutaneous Sacrococcygeal Ependymoma

76. Wolff M, Santiago H, Duby MM: Delayed distant metastasis from a subcutaneous sacrococcygeal myxopapillary ependymoma. Case report, with tissue culture, ultrastructural observations, and review of the literature. Cancer 1972;30:1046–1067.
77. Helwig EB, Stern JB: Subcutaneous sacrococcygeal myxopapillary ependymoma. A clinicopathologic study of 32 cases. Am J Clin Pathol 1984;81:156–161.
78. Kindblom LG, Lodding P, Hagmar B, Stenman G: Metastasizing myxopapillary ependymoma of the sacrococcygeal region. A clinicopathologic, light- and electron microscopic, immunohistochemical, tissue culture, and cytogenetic analysis of a case. Virchows Arch Pathol Anat Histol 1986;94:79–90.
79. Sonneland PR, Scheithauer BW, Onofrio BM: Myxopapillary ependymoma. A clinicopathologic and immunocytochemical study of 77 cases. Cancer 1985;56:883–893.
80. Pulitzer DR, Martin PC, Collins PC, Ralph DR: Subcutaneous sacrococcygeal ("myxopapillary") ependymal rests. Am J Surg Pathol 1988;12:672–677.
81. Sawyer JR, Miller JP, Ellison DA: Clonal telomeric fusions and chromosome instability in a subcutaneous sacrococcygeal myxopapillary ependymoma. Cancer Genet Cytogenet 1998;100:169–175.

Pheochromocytoma—Adrenal and Extra-Adrenal

82. Lack EE: Tumors of the adrenal gland and extra-adrenal paraganglia. Armed Forces Institute of Pathology, Third series, Fascicle 19. Washington, DC, 1997.
83. Pacak K, Lineham WM, Eisenhofer G, McClellan W, Goldstein DS: Recent advances in genetics, diagnosis, localization, and treatment of pheochromocytoma. Ann Int Med 2001;134:315–329.
84. Melicow MM: One hundred cases of pheochromocytoma (107 tumors) at the Columbia-Presbyterian Medical Center, 1926–1976. Cancer 1977;40:1987–2004.
85. Linnoila RI, Keiser HR, Steinberg SM, Lack EE: Histopathology of benign versus malignant sympathoadrenal paragangliomas: Clinicopathologic study of 120 cases including unusual histologic features. Hum Pathol 1990;21:1168–1180.
86. Medeiros LJ, Wolf BC, Balogh K, Federman M: Adrenal pheochromocytoma. A clinicopathologic review of 60 cases. Hum Pathol 1985;16:580–589.
87. Hassoun J, Monges G, Giraud B, Henry JF, Charpin C, Payan H, Toga M: Immunohistochemical study of pheochromocytomas: An investigation of methinonine-enkephalin, vasoactive intestinal polypeptide, somatostatin, corticotropin, β-endorphin, and calcitonin in 16 tumors. Am J Pathol 1984;114:56–63.
88. Hacker GW, Bishop AE, Terenghi G, et al: Multiple peptide production and presence of general neuroendocrine markers detected in 12 cases of human phaechromocytoma and in mammalian adrenal glands. Virchows Arch A Pathol Anat Histopathol 1988;412: 399–411.
89. Linnoila RI, Lack EE, Steinberg SM, Keiser HR: Decreased expression of neuropeptides in malignant paragangliomas: An immunohistochemical study. Hum Pathol 1988;19:41–50.
90. Lloyd RV, Blaivas M, Wilson BS: Distribution of chromogranin and S100 protein in normal and abnormal adrenal medullary tissues. Arch Pathol Lab Med 1985;109:633–635.
91. Achilles E, Padberg BC, Holl K, Klöppel G, Schröder S: Immunocytochemistry of paragangliomas—Value of staining for S-100 protein and glial fibrillary acid pro-

tein in diagnosis and prognosis. Histopathology 1991; 18:453–458.

92. Nagura S, Katoh R, Kawaoi A, Kobayashi M, Obara T, Omata K: Immunohistochemical estimations of growth activity to predict biological behavior of pheochromocytomas. Mod Pathol 1999;12:1107–1111.
93. van der Harst E, Bruining HA, Jaap Bonjer H, et al: Proliferative index in pheochromocytomas: Does it predict the occurrence of metastases? J Pathol 2000; 191:175–180.

Pheochromocytoma—Genetics

94. Eng C: RET proto-oncogene in the development of human cancer. J Clin Oncol 1999;17:380–393.
95. Komminoth P, Kunz E, Hiort O, et al: Detection of RET proto-oncogene point mutations in paraffin-embedded pheochromocytoma specimens in non-radioactive single-strand conformational polymorphism and direct sequencing. Am J Pathol 1994;145:922–929.
96. Krijger RR, Harst EV, Muletta-Feurer S, et al: RET is expressed but not mutated in extra-adrenal paragangliomas. J Pathol 2000;191:264–268.
97. Bar M, Friedman E, Jakobovitz O, et al: Sporadic pheochromocytomas are rarely associated with germline mutations in the von Hippel-Lindau and RET genes. Clin Endocrinol 1997;47:707–712.
98. Hes F, Zewald R, Peeters T, et al: Genotype-phenotype correlations in families with deletions in the von Hippel-Lindau (VHL) gene. Hum Genet 2000;106:425–431.
99. Gimm O, Armanios M, Dziema H, Neumann HP, Eng C: Somatic and occult germ-line mutations in SDHD, a mitochondrial complex II gene, in nonfamilial pheochromocytomas. Cancer Res 2000;60:6822–6825.
100. Edstrom E, Mahlamaki E, Nord B, et al: Comparative genomic hybridization reveals frequent losses of chromosomes 1p and 3q in pheochromocytomas and abdominal paragangliomas, suggesting a common genetic etiology. Am J Pathol 2000;156:651–659.
101. Danenberg H, Speel EJ, Zhao J, et al: Losses of chromosomes 1p and 3q are early genetic events in the development of sporadic pheochromocytomas. Am J Pathol 2000;157:353–359.

Extra-Adrenal Pheochromocytoma (Retroperitoneal, Mediastinal of Urinary Bladder)

102. Lack EE, Cubilla AL, Woodruff JM, Lieberman PH: Extra-adrenal paragangliomas of the retroperitoneum: A clinicopathologic study of 12 tumors. Am J Surg Pathol 1980;4:109–120.
103. Moran CA, Suster S, Fishback N, Koss MN: Mediastinal paragangliomas. A clinicopathological and immunohistochemical study of 16 cases. Cancer 1993;72: 2358–2364.
104. Moran CA, Albores-Saavedra J, Wenig BM, Mena H: Pigmented extraadrenal paragangliomas. A clinicopathologic and immunohistochemical study of five cases. Cancer 1997;79:398–402.
105. Honma K: Paraganglia of the urinary bladder. An autopsy study. Zentralbl Pathol 1994;139:465–469.
106. Grignon DJ, Ro JY, Mackay B, et al: Paraganglioma of the urinary bladder: Immunohistochemical, ultrastructural, and DNA flow cytometric studies. Hum Pathol 1991;22:1162–1169.
107. Cheng L, Leibovich BC, Cheville JC, et al: Paraganglioma of the urinary bladder: Can biologic potential be predicted? Cancer 2000;88:844–852.

Paragangliomas of the Head and Neck—Clinicopathologic Studies

108. Tannir NM, Cortas N, Allam C: A functioning catecholamine secreting vagal body tumor. A case report and review of literature. Cancer 1983;52:932–935.
109. Saldana MJ, Salem LE, Travezan R: High altitude hypoxia and chemodectomas. Hum Pathol 1973;4: 251–263.
110. Arias-Stella J, Valcarcel J: Chief cell hyperplasia in the human carotid body at high altitudes. Physiologic and pathologic significance. Hum Pathol 1976;7:361–373.
111. Rodriguez-Cuevas S, Lopez-Garza J, Labastida-Almendaro S: Carotid body tumors in inhabitants of altitudes higher than 2000 meters above sea level. Head Neck 1998;20:374–378.
112. Shamblin WR, ReMine WH, Sheps SG, Harrison EG: Carotid body tumor (chemodectoma): Clinicopathologic analysis of 90 cases. Am J Surg 1971;122: 732–739.
113. Lack EE, Cubilla AL, Woodruff JM: Paragangliomas of the head and neck region. A pathologic study of tumors from 71 patients. Hum Pathol 1979;10:191–218.
114. Hodge KM, Byers RM, Peters LJ: Paragangliomas of the head and neck. Arch Otolaryngol Head Neck Surg 1988;114:872–877.
115. Nora JD, Hallett JW Jr, O'Brien PC, Naessens JM, Cherry KJ Jr, Pairolero PC: Surgical resection of carotid body tumors. Long-term survival, recurrence and metastasis. Mayo Clin Proc 1988;63:348–352.
116. Brown JS: Glomus jugulare tumors revisited: A ten year statistical follow-up of 231 cases. Laryngoscope 1985;95:284–288.
117. van der Mey AG, Frijns JH, Cornelisse CJ, et al: Does intervention improve the natural course of glomus tumors? A series of 108 patients seen in a 32-year period. Ann Otol Rhinol Laryngol 1992;101:635–642.
118. Netterville JL, Jackson CG, Miller FR, Wanamaker JR, Glasscock ME: Vagal paraganglioma: A review of 46 patients treated during a 20-year period. Arch Otolaryngol Head Neck Surg 1998;124:1133–1140.
119. Heinrich MC, Harris AE, Bell WR: Metastatic intravagal paraganglioma. Case report and review of the literature. Am J Med 1985;78:1017–1024.
120. Warren WH, Lee I, Gould VE, Memoli VA, Jao W: Paragangliomas of the head and neck. Ultrastructural and immunohistochemical analysis. Ultrastruct Pathol 1985;8:333–343.
121. Hamid Q, Varndell IM, Ibrahim NB, Mingazzini P, Polak JM: Extraadrenal paragangliomas. An immunocytochemical and ultrastructural report. Cancer 1987; 60:1776–1781.

122. Kliewer KE, Wen DR, Cancilla PA, Cochran AJ: Paragangliomas. Assessment of prognosis by histologic, immunohistochemical, and ultrastructural techniques. Hum Pathol 1989;20:29–39.

Head and Neck Paraganglioma—Genetics

123. Heutink P, van der Mey AG, Sandkuijl LA et al: A gene subject to genomic imprinting and responsible for hereditary paragangliomas maps to chromosome 11q23-qter. Hum Mol Genet 1992;1:7–10.
124. Hegarty JL, Lalwani AK: Paragangliomas of the head and neck: Implications of molecular genetics in clinical medicine. Curr Opin Otolaryngol Head Neck Surg 2000;8:384–390.
125. Bikhazi PH, Messina L, Mhatre AN, Goldstein J, Lalwani AK: Molecular pathogenesis in sporadic head and neck paraganglioma. Laryngoscope 2000;110: 1346–1348.
126. Baysal BE, Ferrell RE, Willet-Brozick JE, et al: Mutations in SDHD, a mitochondrial complex II gene, in hereditary paraganglioma. Science 2000;287:848–851.

Gangliocytic Paraganglioma

127. Kepes JJ, Zacharias DL: Gangliocytic paraganglioma of the duodenum: A report of two cases with light and electron microscopic examination. Cancer 1971; 27:61–70.
128. Reed RJ, Daroca PJ Jr, Harkin JC: Gangliocytic paraganglioma. Am J Surg Pathol 1977;1:207–216.
129. Perrone T, Sibley RK, Rosai J: Duodenal gangliocytic paraganglioma. An immunohistochemical and ultrastructural study and hypothesis concerning its origin. Am J Surg Pathol 1985;7:31–41.
130. Scheithauer BW, Nora FE, Lechago J, et al: Duodenal gangliocytic paraganglioma. Clinicopathologic and immunohistochemical study of 11 cases. Am J Clin Pathol 1986;86:559–565.
131. Burke AP, Helwig EB: Gangliocytic paraganglioma. Am J Clin Pathol 1989;92:1–9.
132. Inai K, Kobuke T, Yonehara S, Tokuoka S: Duodenal gangliocytic paraganglioma with lymph node metastasis in a 17-year-old boy. Cancer 1989;63:2540–2545.
133. Dookhan DB, Miettinen M, Finkel G, Gibas Z: Recurrent duodenal gangliocytic paraganglioma with lymph node metastases. Histopathology 1993;22:399–401.
134. Hamid QA, Bishop AE, Rode J, et al: Duodenal gangliocytic paragangliomas: A study of 10 cases with immunocytochemical neuroendocrine markers. Hum Pathol 1986;17:1151–1157.

Other Paragangliomas

135. Sonneland PRL, Scheithauer BW, Lechago J, Crawford BG, Onofrio BM: Paraganglioma of the cauda equina region. Clinicopathologic study of 31 cases with special reference to immunocytology and ultrastructure. Cancer 1986;58:1720–1735.

Ganglioneuroma

136. Carpenter WB, Kernohan JW: Retroperitoneal ganglioneuromas and neurofibromas. A clinicopathological study. Cancer 1963;16:788–797.
137. Abell MR, Hart WR, Olson JR: Tumors of the peripheral nervous system. Hum Pathol 1970;1:503–551.
138. Aquirre P, Scully RE: Testosterone-secreting adrenal ganglioneuromas containing Leydig cells. Am J Surg Pathol 1983;7:699–705.
139. d'Amore ESG, Manivel JC, Pettinato G, Niehans GA, Snover DC: Intestinal ganglioneuromatosis: Mucosal and transmural types. A clinicopathologic and immunohistochemical study of six cases. Hum Pathol 1991;22:276–286.
140. Shekitka KM, Sobin LH: Ganglioneuromas of the gastrointestinal tract. Relation to von Recklinghausen's disease and other multiple tumor syndromes. Am J Surg Pathol 1994;18:250–257.
141. Weidner N, Flanders DJ, Mitros FA: Mucosal ganglioneuromatosis associated with multiple colonic polyps. Am J Surg Pathol 1984;8:779–786.
142. Ricci A Jr, Callihan T, Parham DM, Green A, Woodruff JM: Malignant peripheral nerve sheath tumors arising from ganglioneuromas. Am J Surg Pathol 1984;8:19–29.
143. Fletcher CD, Fernando IN, Braimbridge MV, McKee PH, Lyall JR. Malignant nerve sheath tumors arising in a ganglioneuroma. Histopathology 1988;12: 445–448.

Julie C. Fanburg-Smith

Cartilage- and Bone-Forming Tumors and Tumor-like Lesions

CHAPTER 17

Introduction

This chapter discusses a heterogeneous group of cartilage- and bone-forming lesions in soft tissue, including the bone-forming tumor ossifying fibromyxoid tumor. Many of these lesions have an intraosseous counterpart that is often more common in bone than in soft tissue. However, clinicopathologic features and genetic changes may vary between the intraosseous and counterpart extraskeletal lesions.

From an historical viewpoint, most of these lesions have been well defined since at least the last one to five decades. Lichtenstein[1] was the first author to describe *chondroma of soft parts* in the hands and feet in 1964; this tumor had been previously described by Jaffe[2] in 1958 in para-articular and intracapsular locations. *Synovial chondromatosis* was first described in 1558 by Abroise Pare in Monsters and Prodigies; in 1900, it was identified in the German literature by Reichel.[3] Although Stout and Verner[4] described extraskeletal chondrosarcomas in 1953, the most common variant, *extraskeletal myxoid chondrosarcoma,* was defined by Enzinger and Shiraki in 1972.[5] *Mesenchymal chondrosarcoma* was first identified by Lichtenshein and Berstein in 1959.[6] *Parachordoma,* originally thought to be the soft tissue counterpart to chordoma, that is, called "chordoma perphericum"[7] in 1951, was given the name "parachordoma" by Dabska in 1977.[8] Although *tumoral calcinosis* has been recognized since 1899 by Duret, it was first described as "tumoral calcinosis" in 1943 by Inclan.[9] Although calcium pyrophosphate dihydrate (CPPD) deposition disease was originally recognized in 1958,[10] McCarty linked pseudogout due to crystals of calcium pyrophosphate deposition in 1962.[11] Furthermore, the term *tophaceous pseudogout* was first seen in the literature in 1982.[12] The development of a mass after trauma has been known since the 18th century and clinical descriptions were found as early as 1692; however, *myositis ossificans* was first described as a clinicopathologic entity by Ackerman in 1958.[13] The first known description of *fibrodysplasia ossificans progressiva* was in 1962, by a French physician Guy-Patin in a letter to a colleague.[14] One of the earliest reports of *extraskeletal osteosarcoma* was that of Fine and Stout in 1956.[15] Finally, *ossifying fibromyxoid tumor,* the most recent addition to the spectrum of cartilage- and bone-forming tumors, was first defined by Enzinger and coworkers in 1989.[16]

Chondroma of Soft Parts (Extraskeletal Chondroma and Soft Part Chondroma)

Clinical Features

Soft tissue chondromas usually occur in adults between the ages of 30 and 60, with a male predominance.[17–21] They typically present as a small painless mass of the hands (especially the fingers) or sometimes feet (especially the toes). Intraosseous, periosteal, or juxtacortical chondromas are more common than their soft tissue counterparts. Chondromas also occur in para-articular or intracapsular[21] locations of large joints, usually the knee. The pulmonary chondromas are usually asymptomatic chest x-ray findings. The intracapsular or para-articular lesions are associated with pain and decreased motion.[22]

No clinical syndromes are known to be associated with soft tissue chondromas, whereas bone enchondromas may be associated with Ollier disease or Maffucci syndrome. However, pulmonary chondroma may be associated with the Carney triad: pulmonary chondroma, gastrointestinal stromal tumor, and functioning extra-adrenal paraganglioma.[23–25] This rare syndrome, with at least two of the three components of the triad, occurs predominantly in young women[24] and the chondromas may be multiple.

Extraskeletal chondroma may locally recur (10–30%)[17,18] but it is benign; there have been no reports of chondrosarcomatous transformation, which may occur in intraosseous tumors. Complete local excision is the treatment of choice for all variants.

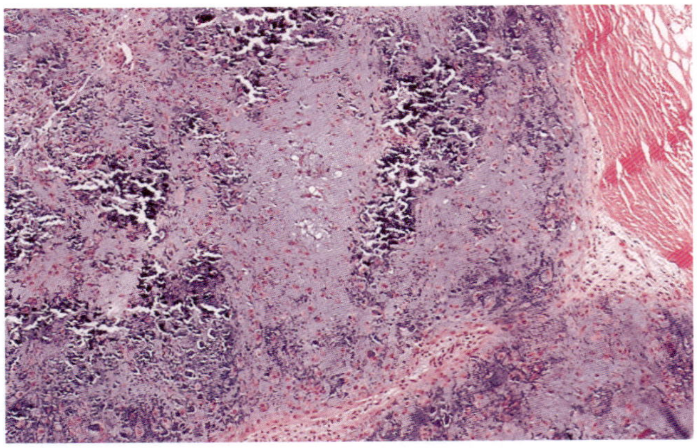

Figure 17–2. Typical chondroma composed of lobules of hyaline cartilage with variable amounts of calcification, fibrous tissue, and myxoid change.

Pathology

Grossly, soft tissue chondromas are well circumscribed and small, usually less than 3 cm, and may be lobulated. They are associated with the tendon, tendon sheath, or joint capsule of the hands or feet. The intracapsular or para-articular variant averages 5 cm and is usually in an infrapatellar location. Both the soft tissue and the pulmonary variants may have extensive peripheral calcification, which can be identified radiographically. On sectioning, they may be firm and glistening or gelatinous or myxoid (Fig. 17–1).

Histologically, soft tissue chondromas are composed of lobules of hyaline cartilage with variable amounts of ossification (Fig. 17–2), fibrosis, and myxoid change (Fig. 17–3). Occasionally residual fat is seen at the periphery of the lesion. One theory for development of these lesions is that fat undergoes myxoid change, then chondromyxoid change, and finally chondroid changes, with different stages of cartilage development. Variants of extraskeletal chondroma include those with granuloma-like areas with epithelioid chondrocytes and multinucleated giant cells, comprising approximately 10% of cases (Figs. 17–4 and 17–5), and those with immature chondroblasts and prominent myxoid change (Fig. 17–6). Increased cellularity, slight pleomorphism, and binucleation are acceptable as part of the cytologic spectrum and do not indicate malignancy. These changes are particularly common in the myxoid subtype of chondroma.

Immunohistochemically, extraskeletal chondromas are positive for S-100 protein and vimentin. Nonspecific markers neuron-specific enolase (NSE) and CD57 may also be present in cartilaginous tumors.

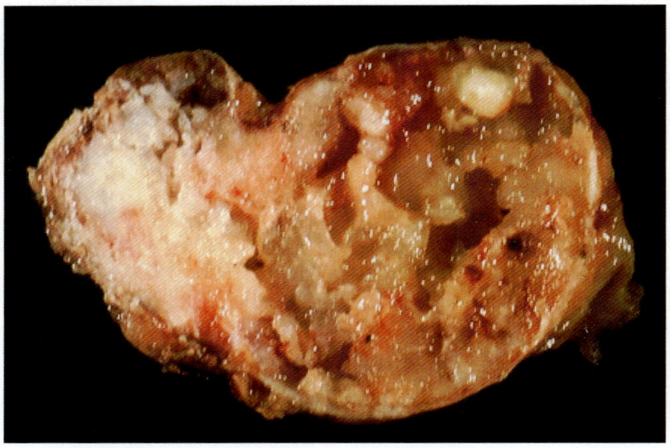

Figure 17–1. Grossly, chondroma of soft parts is sharply circumscribed and shows chondroid and myxoid elements.

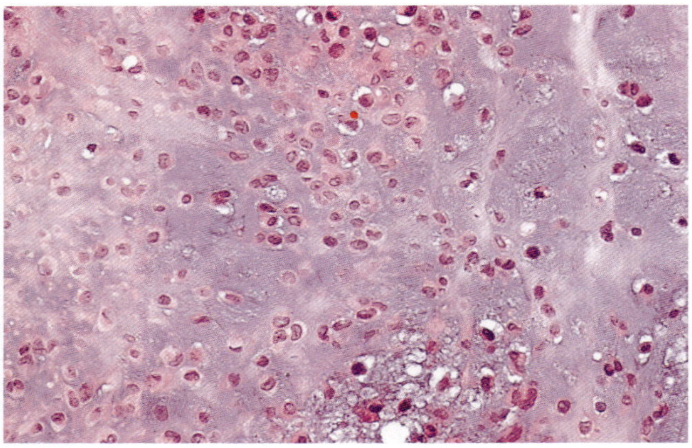

Figure 17–3. Ten percent of extraskeletal chondromas are "granulomatous" or osteoblastoma-like with epithelioid features of the chondrocytes.

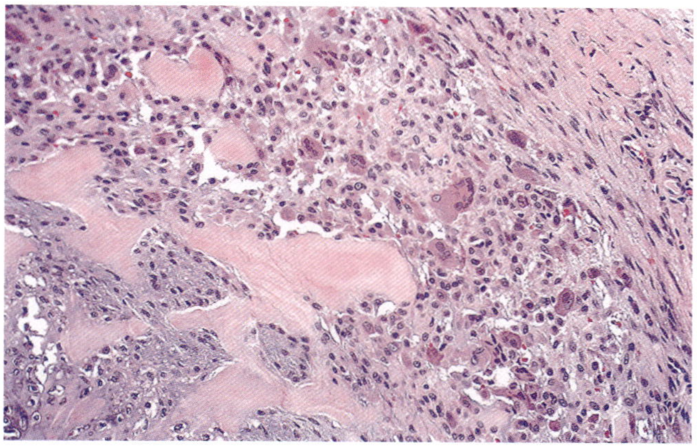

Figure 17-4. This granulomatous subtype of chondroma contains osteoclast-like multinucleated giant cells. Variable amounts of fibrosis are seen in all chondromas.

Differential Diagnosis

The differential diagnosis for chondroma most importantly includes chondrosarcoma. However, extraskeletal hyaline cartilage chondrosarcomas are exceedingly rare to nonexistent; most extraskeletal chondrosarcomas are the myxoid type. Extraskeletal myxoid chondrosarcomas can be distinguished from myxoid chondromas by their cellularity and linear arrangement, proximal or axial locations, and lack of hyaline cartilage. Synovial chondromatosis typically occurs in large joints and is surrounded by a synovial lining. Myxomas are much less cellular than myxoid chondromas and lack hyaline cartilage. The peripheral location of giant cells and presence of hyaline cartilage separates the granuloma-like soft tissue chondroma from tenosynovial giant cell tumors.

Genetics

Monosomy of chromosomes 6 and rearrangement of chromosome 11q13 have been reported for chondroma. Changes reported in a periosteal chondroma included a nonrandom occurrence of the 12q13-q15 involvement.[26,27] Pulmonary chondromas have cytogenetic changes that include a 6p rearrangement involving the *HMGI(Y)* gene that encodes for a transcriptional regulator.[28,29]

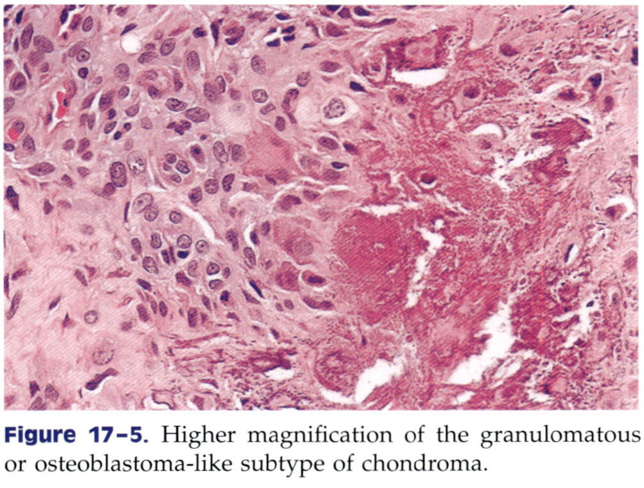

Figure 17-5. Higher magnification of the granulomatous or osteoblastoma-like subtype of chondroma.

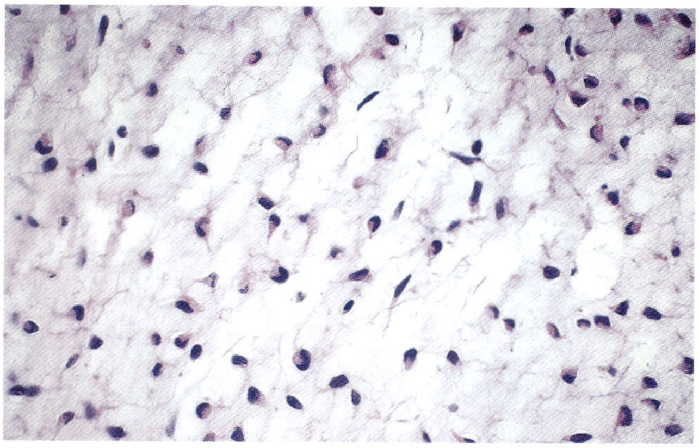

Figure 17-6. Another subtype of chondroma is the myxoid type, seen here. Hyaline cartilage was observed in other parts of the tumor. Note the mild pleomorphism and myxoid change, yet the cellularity and atypia are not as striking as seen in EMCHSA.

Synovial Chrondromatosis

Various synonyms for this condition are synovial osteochondromatosis, synovial chondrometaplasia, synovial osteochondrosis, Reichel disease, and Henderson-Jones disease.

Clinical Features

Synovial chondromatosis typically occurs in the third to fifth decade with a mean age of about 40 years.[30–33] It is twice as common in men as women. Two thirds involve the knee, followed by the hip, the elbow, and other synovial joints. Presenting symptoms include pain, swelling, palpable loose bodies, joint clicking and locking, and loss of joint movement. Osteoarthritis is a frequent complication.[34]

Synovial chondromatosis is a benign condition, although recurrence is possible in approximately 17% of cases. There is an estimated 6% potential for malignant transformation to chondrosarcoma,[35] typically after multiple recurrences. However, true malignancy is rare, because there is usually only bone invasion, and metastases do not develop.[31] Treatment includes removal of the loose bodies with a synovectomy, to decrease the potential for local recurrence.

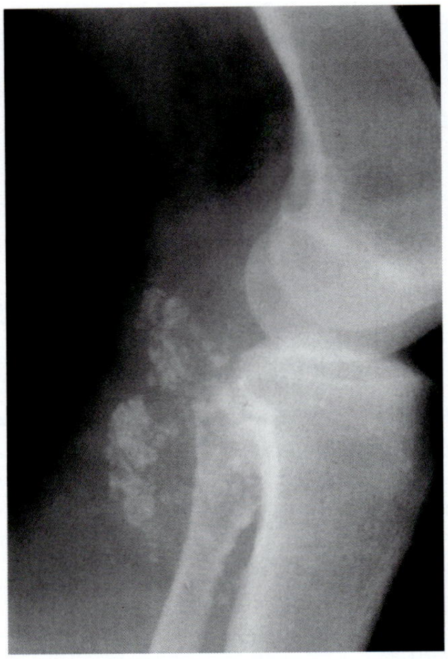

Figure 17–7. Radiographic features of synovial chondromatosis with popcorn-like or stippled calcification.

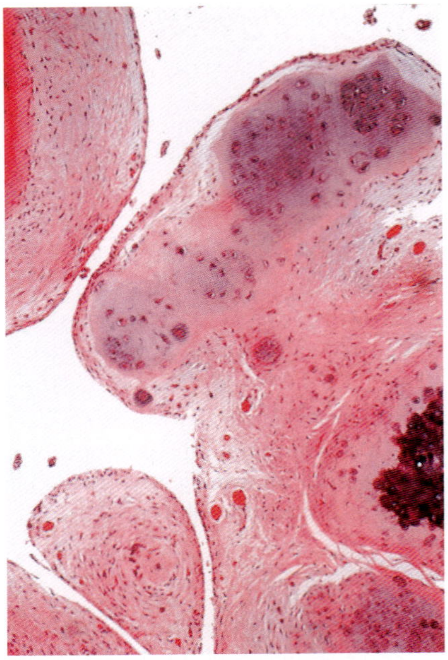

Figure 17–9. Synovial chondromatosis with microscopic islands of hyaline cartilage surrounded by a synovial lining.

Pathology

Grossly, multiple white-gray cartilaginous nodules are seen in synovial-lined locations, both within the joint and extra-articularly (Fig. 17–7).[32] Large calcified lesions (up to >20 cm), formed by fusion of multiple synovial chondromatoses, are termed "giant" or "massive" synovial osteochondromatosis. Synovial chondromatosis may invade bone (Fig. 17–8).

Histologically, synovial chondromatosis is composed of lobules of hyaline cartilage surrounded by a synovial lining (Fig. 17–9), within the joint, bursae, or tendon sheath. Cellularity and pleomorphism (Fig. 17–10) in synovial chondromatosis may be striking, with double and multiple nuclei within individual chondrocytes, but mitotic activity is rare. Calcification and disorganized ossification may be present, but usually represents less than 10% of the lesion. Sheets of atypical chondrocytes, marked myxoid stromal change, necrosis, mitotic figures, and

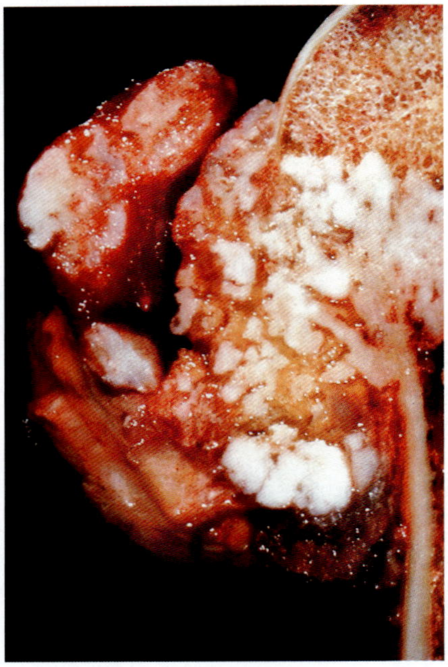

Figure 17–8. The gross appearance of a synovial chondromatosis adjacent to the humerus with multiple cartilaginous nodules in synovial lined tissue and bony invasion.

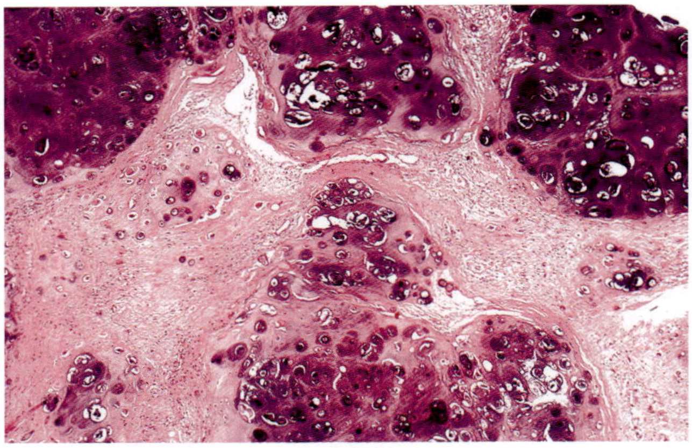

Figure 17–10. Higher magnification of synovial chondromatosis; the nuclear pleomorphism and cellularity is acceptable in this benign lesion.

crowding and spindling of the nuclei at the periphery of the lobules have been suggested to indicate malignancy. However, even the malignant-appearing lesions are only locally aggressive with potential for bone invasion and no metastases.[21,35,36]

Immunohistochemically, synovial chondromatosis is S-100 and vimentin positive.[37] The differential diagnosis would include soft part chondroma, as discussed previously.

Genetics

Clonal chromosomal changes suggest that synovial chondromatosis is a true neoplastic lesion.[38,39] These include complex changes with multiple translocations and loss of chromosome copies. Common findings are the loss of band 10q26 and rearrangements of 1p13 and 12q13. Among them the 12q13-15 segment is recurrently rearranged in a variety of chondromatous tumors, such as pulmonary chondromas and other benign tumors.[40]

Extraskeletal Myxoid Chondrosarcoma

Extraskeletal myxoid chondrosarcoma (EMCHSA) was previously referred to as chordoid sarcoma.[41,42]

Clinical Features

Most patients with extraskeletal myxoid chondrosarcomas[5] are middle-aged adults, with a median age in the fifth decade and a slight male predominance. This tumor can also occur in children.[43] The most common location is the deep thigh. Other sites include the hand, retroperitoneum, and head and neck. Most EMCHSAs present as a painful mass.

Prognosis for EMCHSA was originally thought to be favorable. However, there is a late onset of metastases in patients with long-term follow-up.[44] High-grade variants[45] and high-grade transformation[46] of a low-grade tumor may occur. In some series the metastatic potential for high-grade tumors is as high as 82%.[47] Metastases are generally to the lung, lymph nodes, or soft tissue. The estimated 5-, 10-, and 15-year survival rates are 90%, 70%, and 60%, respectively. High cellularity, pleomorphism, high mitotic activity, older patient age, larger tumor size, metastases, and proximal location have been cited as adverse prognostic factors.[48] Wide local excision, with consideration to adjuvant therapy in dedifferentiated high-grade tumors, is the treatment of choice.

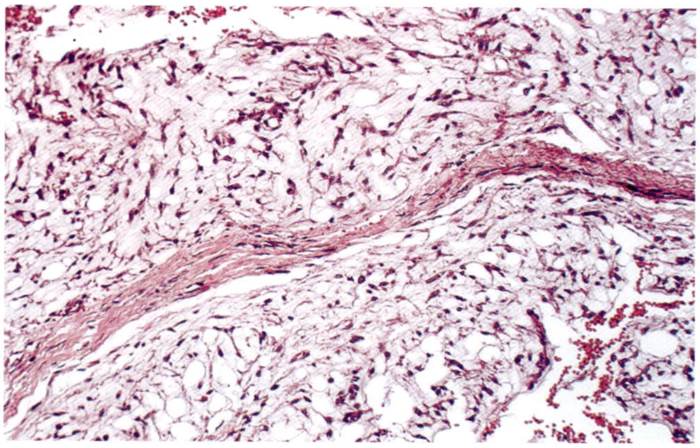

Figure 17–11. EMCHSA with a lobular growth pattern, separated by fibrous septa, and a fishnet stocking-like corded arrangement of tumor cells.

Pathology

Most EMCHSAs are intramuscular, but 25% are located in the subcutis.[5] The median tumor size is approximately 11 cm (range, 5–15 cm). Grossly, the tumors are gelatinous and often hemorrhagic; they may simulate hematomas.[5]

Histologically, the tumors are typically composed of multiple lobules, separated by fibrous septa (Fig. 17–11). The tumor cells are arranged in cords or strands in a netlike or linear pattern, from the periphery into the center of the lobules (Fig. 17–12), with central 4- to 10-cell clustered nests (Fig. 17–13), embedded in a myxoid background. The cells are round to stellate with hyperchromatic round nuclei and scant to moderately abundant eosinophilic cytoplasm. Mitotic activity is generally low, and the usual type is a low-grade tumor. However, highly cellular, less myxoid areas may occur in higher

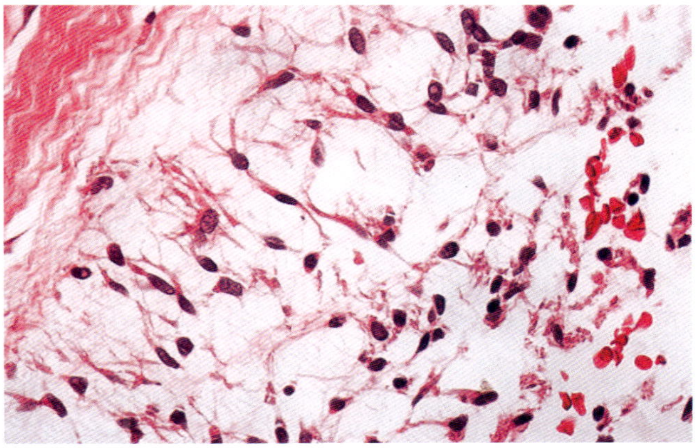

Figure 17–12. The periphery of the lobules of EMCHSA shows the malignant chondrocytes arranged in a "string of pearls"-like manner.

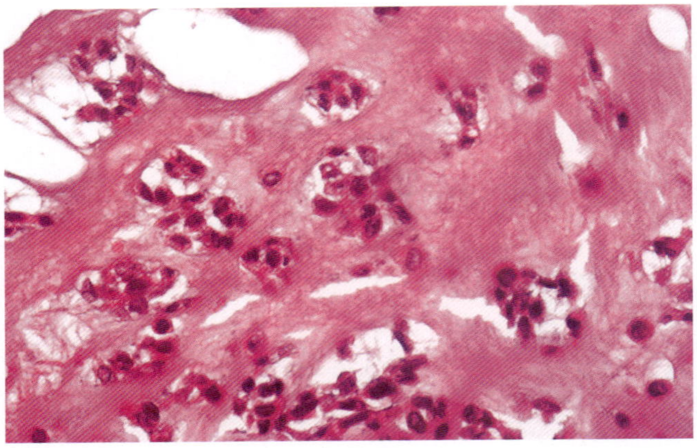

Figure 17–13. In the center of the lobules, the clusters of 4 to 10 tumor cells are pathoneumonic for EMCHSA and separate it from intraosseous myxoid chondrosarcoma.

grade tumors, with epithelioid or malignant fibrous histiocytoma-like areas.

Immunohistochemically, EMCHSA has variable positivity for S-100 protein[48–50] and vimentin.[49] These tumors may be positive for Leu7 and epithelial membrane antigen (EMA),[51] but are generally negative for cytokeratin,[51] with exceedingly rare exceptions with Cam5.2,[52,53] and glial fibrillary acidic protein (GFAP).

Differential Diagnosis

The differential diagnosis includes soft part chondroma, parosteal chondrosarcoma, metastatic chordoma, parachordoma, mixed tumors of the salivary or sweat glands, myxoma, myxoid liposarcoma, myxoid malignant fibrous histiocytoma, myxoid malignant peripheral nerve sheath tumors, and myxopapillary ependymomas. Site and the presence of hyaline cartilage can easily separate the first two lesions. Chordomas and mixed tumors are generally positive for cytokeratin, Cam5.2, and EMA.[52,53] Chordomas and parachordomas have larger cells with more abundant cytoplasm that wrap around each other rather than form a "string of pearls" of netlike pattern, as in extraskeletal myxoid chondrosarcoma. Myxoma lacks the cellularity of EMCHSA, and GFAP positivity and site would separate myxopapillary ependymoma from EMCHSA.

Genetics

Extraskeletal myxoid chondrosarcoma is marked by a nonrandom reciprocal translocation: t (9;22) (q22;q12) generating an *EWS/TEC* gene fusion,[54–59] in at least 75% of cases.[47] Although most osseous myxoid chondrosarcomas are pathologically and genetically different and do not have this translocation, there are rare bone tumors similar to EMCHSA with this translocation.[60] A variant t (9;17) translocation with a novel fusion product TAF2N (an *EWS*-related gene)-TEC[61] and additional novel variants (see Chapter 4) for EMSCHSA have also been recently identified.

Mesenchymal Chondrosarcoma

Clinical Features

This tumor usually occurs in young adults (ages 15–35 years), with a female predilection, in the head and neck (brain, orbit, meninges) or lower extremities, especially the thigh.[62–64] This tumor occurs three to four times more frequently in bone than in soft tissue.[65] Mesenchymal chondrosarcoma is a high-grade tumor with a poor survival (10-year survival rate is 25%).[66] Metastases are generally to the lungs. Treatment of choice includes surgery and adjuvant therapy.

Pathology

The size may range from 2.5 to over 30 cm. Grossly, the tumors are circumscribed and fleshy, sometimes with visible chondroid foci (Fig. 17–14).

Histologically, mesenchymal chondrosarcoma is characterized by primitive small round or slightly spindled cells, often with a hemangiopericytic growth pattern (Fig. 17–15), with usually an abrupt transition to single or coalescing lobules of well-differentiated hyaline cartilage (Fig. 17–16).

Immunohistochemically, the intracartilaginous chondrocytes and some immediately adjacent round cells are positive for S-100 protein;[67–69] however,

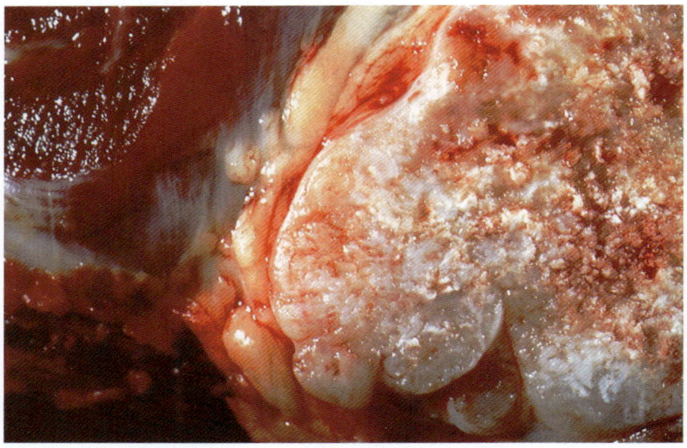

Figure 17–14. Extraskeletal mesenchymal chondrosarcoma shows fleshy soft gray-white tissue and foci of cartilage and even bone.

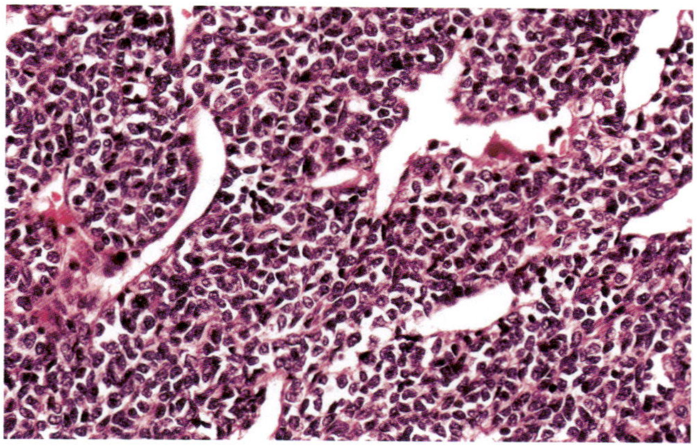

Figure 17–15. The primitive round cells in mesenchymal chondrosarcoma are typically arranged in a hemangiopericytoma-like growth pattern.

most of the small round cells are negative for S-100 protein. CD99 positivity has been rarely reported in the small cell component of mesenchymal chondrosarcoma.[67] All components of the tumor (small cells, lacunar chondroblasts, and chondroid matrix) stain for Leu7. NSE is identified in some small and some lacunar cells. None of the tumor cells are immunoreactive with desmin, actin, cytokeratin, EMA, or synaptophysin. The immunophenotype of mesenchymal chondrosarcoma resembles that of embryonic cartilage, consistent with the premise that mesenchymal chondrosarcoma may be the neoplastic counterpart of fetal-like chondroid tissues.

Differential Diagnosis

The differential diagnosis includes small round cell tumors such as Ewing/primitive neuroectodermal tumor (PNET), small cell osteosarcoma, and rhabdomyosarcoma, poorly differentiated synovial sarcoma, and hemangiopericytoma. The cytokeratins and EMA in synovial sarcoma are unlikely to be found in mesenchymal chondrosarcoma. Ewing sarcoma and hemangiopericytoma lack metaplastic hyaline cartilage. Small cell osteosarcoma would, by definition, have neoplastic bone. Desmin positivity in rhabdomyosarcoma would distinguish it from mesenchymal chondrosarcoma.

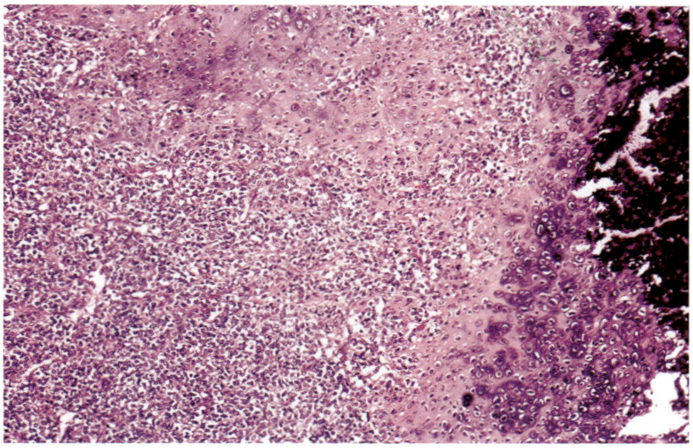

Figure 17–16. The fairly abrupt transition of the primitive cells to hyaline cartilage is typical of mesenchymal chondrosarcoma.

Genetics

Cytogenetic analysis of extraskeletal mesenchymal chondrosarcoma has shown complex karyotypes with numerous translocations and other chromosomal rearrangements. Reciprocal translocation (11;22)(q24;q12) was reported in one case.[70–73]

Parachordoma

Parachordoma is a controversial lesion, believed by many pathologists to represent a variant of a (malignant) mixed tumor or myoepithelioma of soft tissue.[74,75] However, it differs from cartilage tumors, chordoma, and EMCHSA.

Clinical Features

Parachordomas are asymptomatic deep extremity lesions in adults. They are classified as low-grade malignant, although metastasis is exceptional.[76]

Pathology

Grossly, the lesions are circumscribed, but unencapsulated, lobular masses.

Histologically, these tumors are composed of variable epithelioid to spindled cells with glomoid round cells and a myxoid to hyaline, not chondroid, background.[51,77]

Immunohistochemically, these lesions are positive for CK8/18 (Cam 5.2), EMA, S-100 protein, and vimentin.

Differential Diagnosis

The differential diagnosis would include EMCHSA, which lacks the spindled and glomoid cell population of parachordoma, shows a chondroid matrix, and is only rarely positive for Cam 5.2. Chordoma, a tumor arising from notochordal elements in an axial location (clivus and sacrum are the most common locations) metastasizes in 20% to 40% of cases. Chordoma may metastasize to soft tissue and therefore be in the differential diagnosis for parachordoma.

However, chordoma can be distinguished from parachordoma by its lack of a glomoid cell population, its presence of chondroid matrix, and its positivity for high-molecular-weight cytokeratins and 19.[51] Ossifying fibromyxoid tumor (see later) may be in the differential diagnosis for parachordoma, but it can be distinguished by its peripheral rim of bone, its morphologic lack of large cells, its high vascularity, and its immunohistochemical lack of keratins. Parachordoma may indeed represent a variant of mixed tumor or myoepithelioma, because parachordoma may express calponin[51] and the actins and GFAP are not present in all mixed tumors/myoepitheliomas. However, additional comparisons must be made.

Genetics

Cytogenetic analysis of parachordoma has not yet yielded recurrent change.[76,78]

Tumoral Calcinosis

Other names for this condition include tumoral calcinosis-like, calcifying collagenolysis, calcifying bursitis, tumoral lipocalcinosis, pseudotumoral calcinosis, and hip stone disease.

Clinical Features

This is the designation for an extraskeletal soft tissue hydroxyapatite calcification with a granulomatous response that develops in patients with secondary hyperparathyroidism or hypercalcemia, usually due to end-stage kidney disease. It is less commonly idiopathic. Clinical classification of these lesions into three types has been proposed: solitary lesion without hyperphosphatemia, multiple lesions with hyperphosphatemia but not hypercalcemia as a familial disease, and lesions associated with hypercalcemia secondary to renal disease.[79,80]

In the first group, the solitary lesions occur in patients without hyperphosphatemia, generally from tropical or subtropical areas, and are suspected to be parasite-related granulomas.[80]

In the second group, the familial multiple lesions usually occur in black adolescents with hyperphosphatemia and elevated serum 1,25-dihydroxyvitamin D levels. It is inherited as an autosomal recessive or dominant pattern.[81,82]

The third group, tumoral calcinosis-like, is most common. In this group, the lesions occur with secondary hypercalcemia or hyperphosphatemia, often linked to end-stage chronic renal disease. These patients are older, do not have familial disease, and may have visceral involvement. Less commonly, it is associated with a hypercalcemia state with massive bone destruction by metastases, hypervitaminosis D, or other causes.

Tumoral calcinosis, in general, is thought to arise from an error in phosphorus metabolism that leads to extracellular deposition of calcium hydroxyapatite crystals.[83] This is thought to be due to a defect in the regulation of 25-hydroxy-1-α-hydrolase in the kidney, an enzyme participating in vitamin D metabolism. These patients will also have dental abnormalities, transient periosteal thickenings, and eye lesions.[84]

Tumoral calcinosis typically involves the periarticular areas of shoulder, scapulae, hips, buttocks, and elbows, but it is not intra-articular. Symptoms include a firm nontender mass, often with signs of inflammation. Sinus tracts with excretion of white creamy material may occur.[84] The natural history for tumoral calcinosis is one of progressive slow growth and disfigurement, with limitation of joint function.[85] Treatment is difficult because local excision of a large mass is often impossible and results in rapid recurrence. The first group may be treated with surgical treatment alone.[86] There has been some success with surgical treatment in the second group as well.[86] Treatment of the third group is mainly medical aimed at correction of the metabolic error by dietary restriction of phosphorus, use of phosphate binders to lower the serum phosphorus levels, a low-calcium dialysate for dialysis, renal transplantation, and parathyroidectomy.[79,87–90] Administration of sodium thiosulfate and vinpocentine has also reduced the mass size.[91–93]

Pathology

The lesions vary, but may reach as large as 30 cm in diameter. Grossly, the lesion is a single, firm, multiloculated, cystic mass with a rubbery texture that contains milky white to gritty yellow fluid. Cutaneous ulceration may develop over subcutaneous deposits. The radiographic picture, with fluid–fluid levels, is classic (Fig. 17–17).

Histologically, both tumoral calcinosis and tumoral calcinosis-like lesions have the same findings (i.e., all three groups).[94,95] Central calcification with calcosperites, surrounding mononuclear and multinucleated (foreign body and Langerhans type) histiocytes, and multiloculation with surrounding granulation tissue or fibrosis (Fig. 17–18). The cyst walls are composed of dense hyalinized fibrous tissue with plasma cells and lymphocytes, as well as histiocytes. Minimal cytologic atypia is observed. Slavin and coworkers divide the microscopic findings into three stages:

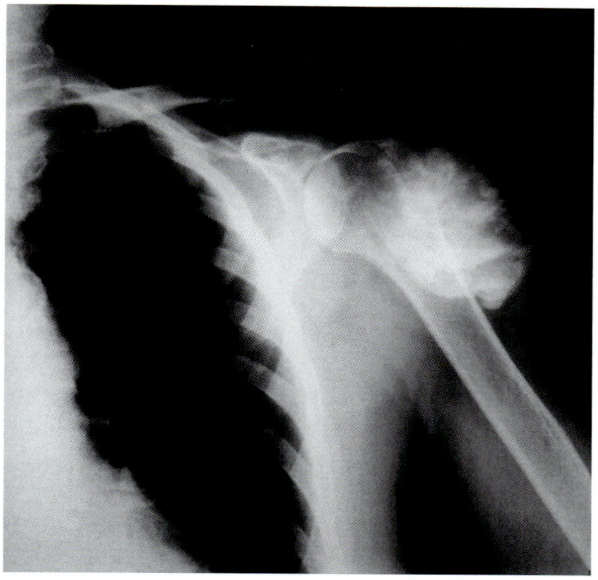

Figure 17–17. Characteristic radiographic fluid–fluid levels in a tumoral calcinosis-like lesion around proximal humerus.

(1) cellular acalcific lesions with nodular and linear aggregates of foamy histiocytes dissecting between collagen bundles with foci of acute hemorrhage, (2) cellular cystic calcific lesions with a cavity composed of multinucleated osteoclast type (with cytoplasmic vacuoles containing minute calcifications) and mononuclear histiocytes with central fibrin, histiocytes, and calcified spherules, and (3) inactive calcifying lesions with calcification and osseous metaplasia surrounded by hyalinized fibrous tissue.[82]

Immunohistochemically, the histiocytes stain with CD68 and MAC 387; an antibody to parathyroid hormone may be positive in the intralocular debris in patients with end-stage renal disease.[79] α-1-Antichymotrypsin and α-1-antitrypsin have also been found within the cytoplasmic vacuoles of the multinucleated osteoclast-type histiocytes.[82]

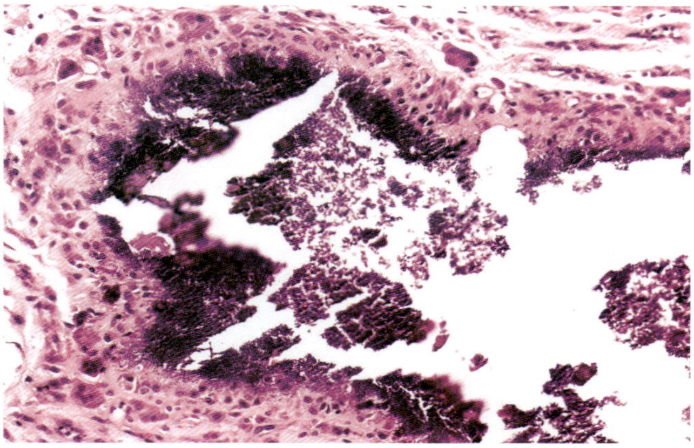

Figure 17–18. Microscopic central hydroxyapatite crystalline material surrounded by a granulomatous (histiocytoid) response, with multinucleated giant cells.

The differential diagnosis may include the formation of soft tissue calcium deposits due to milk alkali syndrome, collagen vascular diseases, and other causes.[95] Occasionally, tumoral calcinosis may be confused with a calcified soft tissue chondroma with granuloma-like features; the presence of hyaline cartilage (in chondroma) and clinical history (of renal disease for tumoral calcinosis) will separate the two lesions.

Genetics

No genetic abnormalities have been identified for tumoral calcinosis, even for the hereditary type.[96]

Tophaceous Pseudogout (Focal Tumoral CPPD Deposition or Crystal Deposition Disease)

Clinical Features

This rare condition forms a solitary, large mass with abundant calcium pyrophosphate crystals. It is distinctive from polyarticular chondrocalcinosis and calcium pyrophosphate deposition disease. It typically occurs in middle-aged and older adults with a female predominance. Locations include the temporomandibular, metcarpophalangeal, first metatarsophalangeal joints, and large joints, in descending order of frequency.[97] Presenting symptoms include swelling, pain, or neurovascular compromise. The clinical, radiographic, and pathologic features may resemble chondrosarcoma.[97,98] Although some authors believe that the calcium phosphate deposition is secondary to breakdown of fibrocartilage,[98] the etiology of the formation of a mass of calcium pyrophosphate with a cartilaginous response is unknown. This benign process may be destructive of bone.[97,99] Local recurrence may occur after complete or incomplete surgical excision,[97,98] but generally local excision is curative.

Pathology

Grossly, tophaceous pseudogout is a whitish gray mass with a chalky appearance. Involvement of the adjacent bone, due to pressure erosion, is common.[97] The radiographic (Fig. 17–19), gross, and microscopic features may mimic a benign or malignant chondroid neoplasm.

Histologically, the crystals of tophaceous pseudogout are rhomboid (Fig. 17–20) and weakly positively birefringent by polarization; they may be detected by

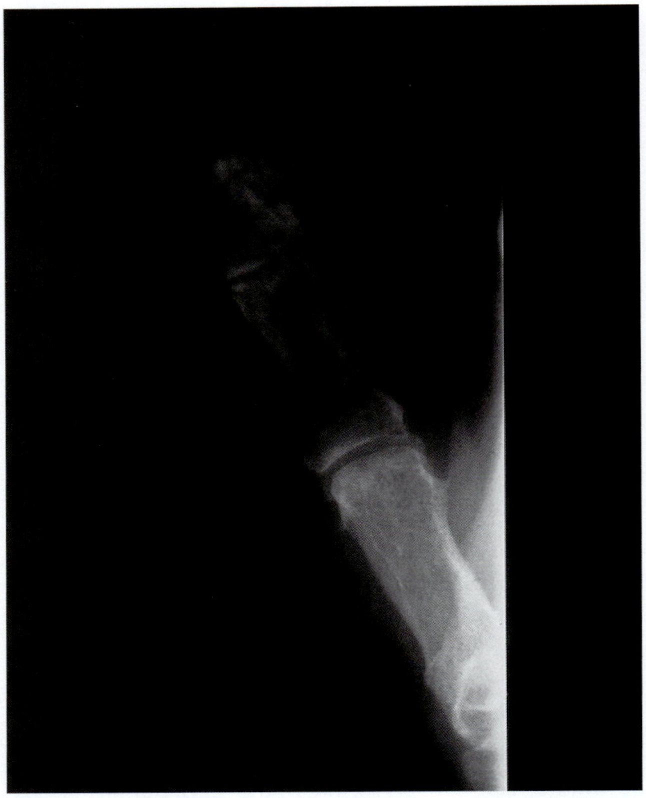

Figure 17–19. Radiograph of tophaceous pseudogout adjacent to the finger. Note the cartilage popcorn-like or stippled features of the lesion.

alizarin red stain. A foreign body granulomatous response is often observed. Hyaline and fibrocartilage surround the crystals and may often exhibit cellular atypia, mimicking benign and malignant chondroid neoplasms (Figs. 17–21 through 17–23).

The differential diagnosis includes benign and malignant chondroid neoplasms. The chalky gross

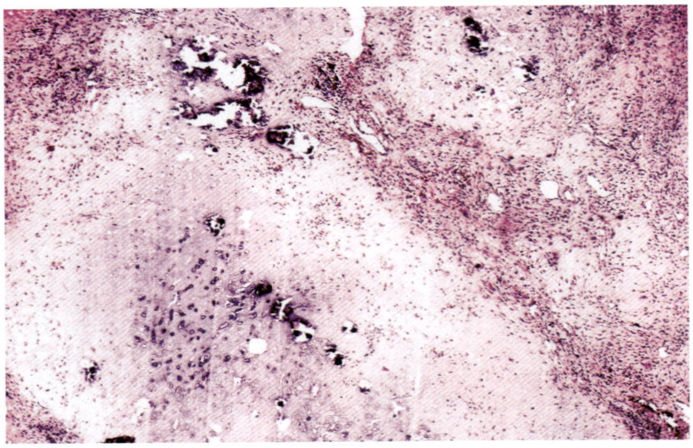

Figure 17–21. The low-power appearance of tophaceous pseudogout, with a large cartilaginous response; this mimics chondroid neoplasms.

appearance and presence of a granulomatous response and the crystals (or their spaces after being lost in decalcification processes) separate this lesion from true chondrosarcoma. Similarly, the crystals separate this from chondroma of soft parts, although a case has been reported of soft tissue chondroma with calcium pyrophosphate.[100] Tumoral calcinosis is composed of hydroxyapatite crystals, rather than calcium pyrophosphate, and has a different clinical history. Synovial chondromatosis also lacks the rhomboid crystals of tophaceous pseudogout.

Myositis Ossificans

Myositis ossificans has also been known as myositis ossificans circumscripta, pseudomalignant heterotopic ossification, pseudomalignant osseous tumor of soft tissue, and heterotopic ossification.

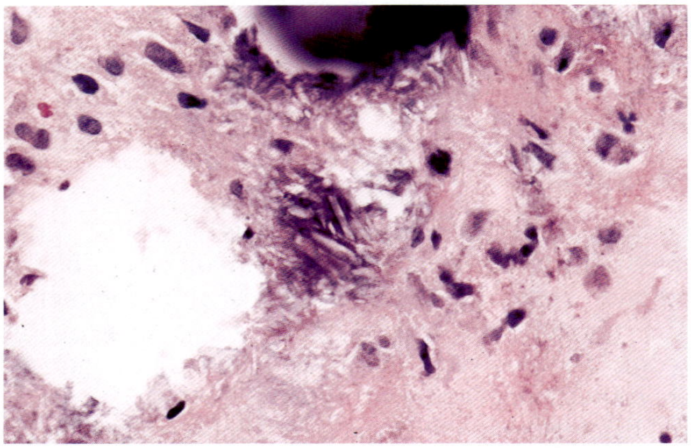

Figure 17–20. Microscopically, tophaceous pseudogout is composed of rhomboid crystals of calcium pyrophosphate.

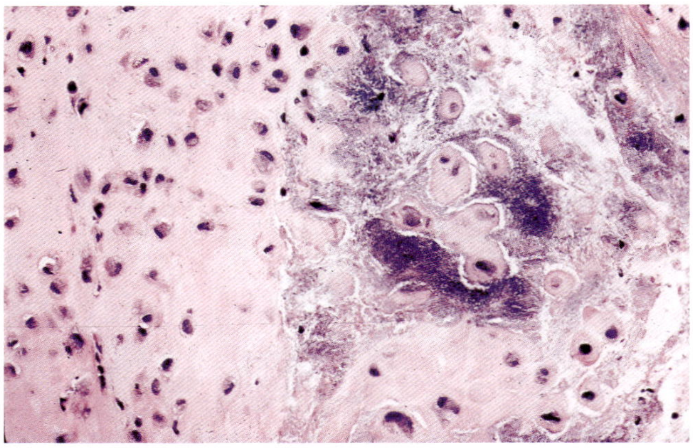

Figure 17–22. The chondrocytes in tophaceous pseudogout look like epithelioid histiocytes in some areas.

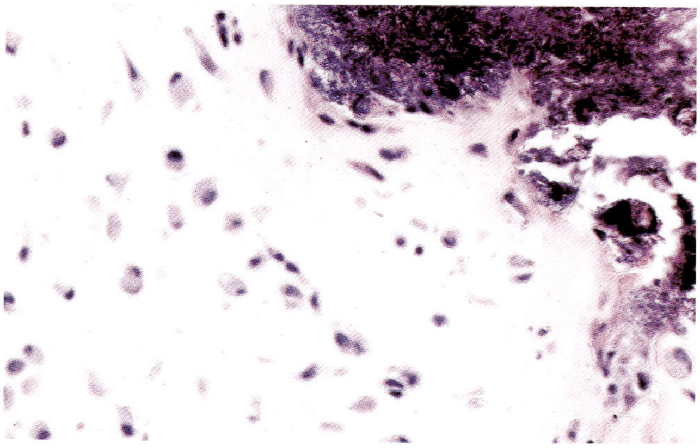

Figure 17–23. Mildly hypercellular cartilage and dense deposition of calcium pyrophosphate in tophaceous pseudogout. The cartilaginous response makes this difficult to distinguish from chondroid neoplasms.

Clinical Features and Related Lesions

Myositis ossificans is a solitary pseudomalignant heterotopic ossification with a zone configuration from central cellular areas with random, less mature bone to peripheral more mature and organized bone. This lesion typically occurs in children[101] and young adults, in the second and third decades of life. Most studies show an equal sex distribution. The most common locations are the anterior muscles of the thigh or the buttocks.

Panniculis ossificans (Fig. 17–24) is located in the upper extremity subcutis of mainly females and demonstrates a less prominent zoning phenomenon than myositis ossificans.[102] Fascial lesions are termed *fasciitis ossificans. Small reactive heterotopic ossifications* (considered by some to be "osteomas"[21,102]), other than myositis ossificans, may be seen in sites of trauma (e.g., tendon avulsion) as a posttraumatic ossifying lesion. These heterotopic calcifications are intramembranous and endochondral. They are metaplastic bone that lack the zone and clinicopathologic features of myositis ossificans, composed primarily of mature lamellar bone with a well-defined haversian system with bone marrow and myxoid, vascular, and fibrous connective tissue between bony trabuculae. Sites include the posterior tongue and the thigh.[103]

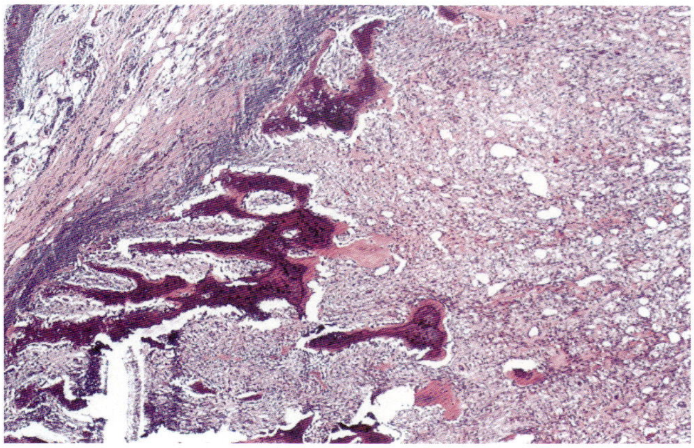

Figure 17–24. Panniculitis ossificans, a less organized form of myositis ossificans, involving the panniculitic fat.

Myositis ossificans is associated with trauma in 75% cases. It is a rapidly growing painful mass that expands for 6 to 8 weeks, often with prodromal viral-like symptoms. After active growth, the pain ceases and the lesion matures during several months. It may shrink and sometimes regress in 35% of cases.[104,105]

Surgical excision may be necessary if the lesions are unusually large, painful, or restrictive of motion, or if the diagnosis is uncertain.[106] The occurrence of malignant transformation is questionable, and many pathologists view such cases as well-differentiated extraskeletal osteosarcoma from the inception.

Pathology

The radiographic image is very helpful regarding the gross pathology (Fig. 17–25).[107] If the lesion is well-developed, 3 to 6 weeks after trauma, then it will have a mature rim of bone at the periphery (eggshell-like), both radiographically and grossly, which can separate this lesion from an osteosarcoma. Unlike myositis ossificans, osteosarcoma has central bone formation and infiltration into soft tissue. Also myositis ossificans is usually seen over the shaft of

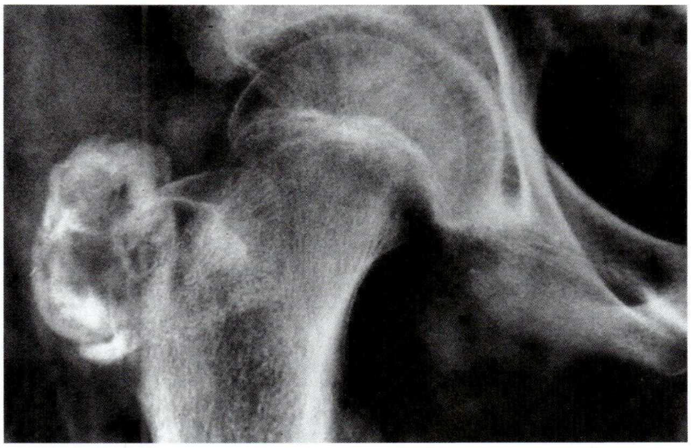

Figure 17–25. Typical radiographic features of myositis ossificans with a peripheral eggshell-like mature calcification distinguishes this lesion from osteosarcoma, which has central mature ossification and invasion of immature areas into soft tissue.

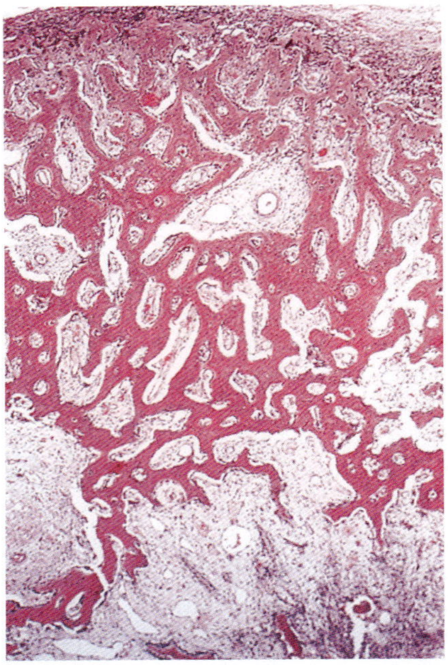

Figure 17–26. Microscopically, myositis ossificans has a zone phenomenon, with mature bone at the periphery to less mature areas in the center. Figures 17–26 to 17–28 are sequential from periphery to center, respectively. This picture depicts the mature outer bone at the periphery.

the bone, not at the metaphyseal junction, as with osteosarcoma.[106] Grossly, the lesion is white and glistening or gritty cut surface, rarely larger than 6 cm. Spicules of trabeculae radiate inward toward a less mature zone.

Histologically, zonal maturing of the bone from the center to the periphery is the pathognomonic feature (Figs. 17–26 through 17–28). The center often has a cellular fibroblastic proliferation with abundant mitoses and osteoclast type giant cells and there may be osteoid bone that has not yet undergone maturation to woven bone (Fig. 17–28). The center may initially be worrisome for osteosarcoma; waiting several weeks to rebiopsy would lead to the correct diagnosis. Cartilage may also be present as part of the endochondral ossification.

Differential Diagnosis

The differential diagnosis may include fibrodysplasia ossificans progressive (FOP), an autosomal dominant disease and osteosarcoma. FOP may be separated by its multifocality and specific hypoplasia of the first metacarpal and metatarsal bones. Osteosarcoma may be distinguished by its "backward" zone phenomenon, most mature bone in the center with woven bone at the periphery, produced by malignant osteoblasts.

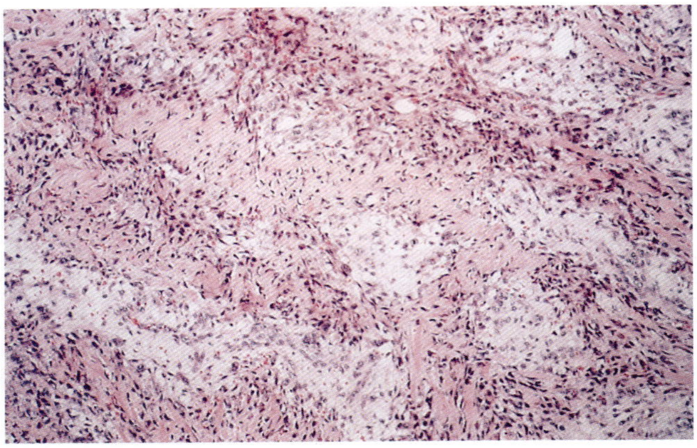

Figure 17–27. This less mature area is adjacent to the center of myositis ossificans.

Genetics

By molecular methods, myositis ossificans traumatica expresses bone morphogenetic proteins 1,4,6, and c-fos mRNAs, but not c-jun mRNA.[108] However, no specific genetic abnormalities have been identified.

Fibrodysplasia Ossificans Progressiva

This condition was previously referred to as myositis ossificans progressiva; it is called Munchmeyer disease in the French literature.

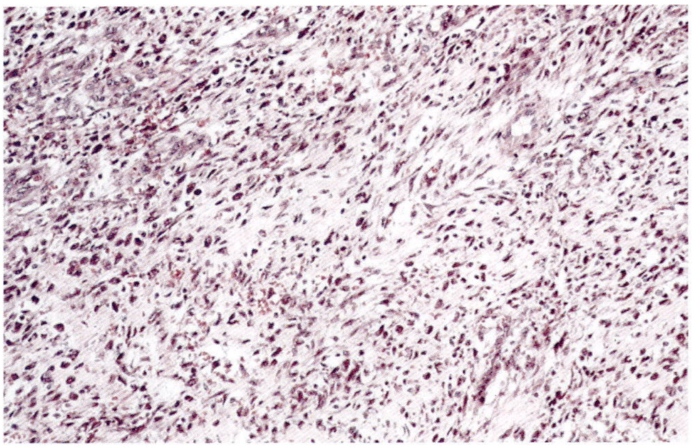

Figure 17–28. This central area of myositis ossificans has the most immature bone and cellular fibroblastic stroma; this may be confused with osteosarcoma; waiting a few weeks to rebiopsy this lesion would show that it becomes more mature with time and makes the diagnosis of myositis ossificans easier.

Clinical Features

This is a very rare disease of children with progressive ectopic endochondral ossification of the soft tissue that ultimately leads to immobilization of the entire body. Much of the new information of this disease is derived from the studies by the International Center for FOP located at the Department of Orthopedic Surgery of the University of Pennsylvania, Philadelphia (Director Dr. Fred Kaplan, MD, website: www.med.upenn.edu/ortho/fop).

Fibrodysplasia ossificans progressiva has been estimated to affect approximately 1/2,000,000 people.[109] The disease is now mainly sporadic because affected patients are often not able to reproduce,[110] but 5% of patients have autosomal dominant transmission.

The signs of disease usually appear by 5 years of age, but may be present at birth.[109] Half the patients have some evidence for the disease by age 2 years. Early lesions may be associated with classic signs of inflammation and systemic symptoms such as low-grade fever and elevated erythrocyte sedimentation rate.[111] The patients typically have skeletal malformations including short, deviated, and monophalangic big toes, broad femoral necks, fusion of the cervical vertebrae, hypoplasia of the vertebral bodies, and short first metacarpal bones (short thumbs).[112] The ectopic endochondral ossification has a predilection for the paraspinal and scalp muscles, the jaw muscles, and the extremity musculature in a proximal-to-distal gradient. The patient with this entity can develop endochondral ossification of ligaments, tendons, or muscles that have undergone the slightest injury, resulting in fusion of the spine, limbs, rib cage, and jawbones and complete immobilization.

The lesions many grow rapidly and may be mistaken for soft tissue lesions and biopsied. However, surgical treatment is contraindicated, because it exacerbates the ectopic bone formation. The patient usually develops severe scoliosis and ankylosis of all major joints of the axial and appendicular skeleton by early adulthood, and is usually confined to a wheelchair by age 20 years. Starvation may occur secondary to ankylosis of the jaw, and pneumonia may develop secondary to fixation of the chest wall. Although there are no current effective means for prevention or treatment, steroids have been used during the early myositis phase, as well as analgesics, until the acute phase subsides. Other trial medical therapies have been largely unsuccessful.[109,113–115]

The pathogenesis of FOP has been suggested to involve overexpression of bone morphogenetic protein 4 (BMP-4), a growth factor (cytokine) of the transforming growth factor-β superfamily that promotes chondro-osteogenesis in mesenchymal cells. The *BMP-4* gene mRNA, indicating activity, was present in the lymphocytes of 26 of 32 FOP patients, compared to 1 of 12 normal controls.[116] BMP-4 has also been found in fibroblast-like cells of the preosseous lesions of patients with FOP.[116,117]

Pathology

Histologically, the earliest changes include lymphocyte infiltration and muscle degeneration,[118] followed by a granulation-like tissue and endochondral ossification with woven bone that remodels into mature lamellar bone with marrow elements.[110] The bone formation is central.

Immunohistochemically, the early spindled cells are fibroblastic and stain with vimentin and BMP-2/BMP-4;[118,119] the cartilage of the endochondral ossification stains with S-100 protein.

Differential Diagnosis

The differential diagnosis includes nodular or cranial fasciitis and aggressive juvenile fibromatosis. Nodular fasciitis may be in the differential diagnosis of extremity or trunk lesions and cranial fasciitis may be in the differential of a skull lesion, particularly in a young child. The presence of toe abnormalities, multiple lesions, and BMP-2/BMP-4 in the lesions would easily distinguish FOP from nodular or cranial fasciitis. Similarly, early FOP lesions may mimic aggressive juvenile fibromatosis; however, the elongate vessels of fibromatosis and the toe abnormalities and BMP-2/BMP-4 in FOP will distinguish the two entities. Unlike cranial fasciitis and fibromatosis, FOP lesions will undergo endochondral ossification. Other causes for ectopic ossification, such as an entity called progressive osseous heteroplasia, or focal cutaneous ossification secondary to acne, burns, hemorrhage, infection, and connective tissue diseases must also be clinically distinguished from FOP. The specific toe anomalies of FOP are absent in these other clinical entities. The lesions of progressive osseous heteroplasia are random and not predictably symmetrical as in FOP. Albright hereditary osteodystrophy can also be distinguished on clinical grounds; the ossification involves the skin only and not the deeper tissues as in FOP.[120]

Genetics

Although BMP-4 has been mapped to chromosome 14q22-23,[121,122] only heterologous molecular findings in these patients have been identified.[123] It is difficult to study the genetics of this disease, due to lack of tissue available, because it is best not to biopsy these lesions, and the paucity of families with this entity because the patients rarely are physically able to procreate.

Fibro-osseous Pseudotumor of the Digits

Fibro-osseous pseudotumor of the digits (FOPD) is also known as florid reactive periostitis of the tubular bones of hands and feet[124,125] and parosteal nodular fasciitis.[126]

Clinical Features

This is a heterotopic ossification of the subcutis of the digits, closely related to myositis ossificans, but not as organized; some consider this a form of myositis ossificans.

Fibro-osseous pseudotumor of the digits is a painful or nonpainful swelling of the proximal phalangeal area of the fingers (usually the middle or index finger), less frequently of the toes, in young adults (median age, 33 years), with a female predominance.[102,127–130] A history of trauma can be elicited in approximately 40% of patients.[125,131] One study proposed an infectious etiology because elevated white blood cell counts and increased streptolysin O titers were found in some patients. Symptoms include a firm mass that does not impair function. Complete local excision is curative.

Pathology

Radiography will show an ill-defined soft tissue mass overlying the proximal or middle phalanges with evidence of calcification, well separated from the adjacent bone, without a periosteal reaction.

Histologically, FOPD is composed of irregular nodules of fibroblasts, sometimes atypical appearing, and benign bone, within a fibrous to myxoid matrix (Fig. 17–29). There is often intramembranous ossification, with both woven and lamellar bone. Bony trabeculae show osteoid seams and are rimmed by the osteoblasts (Fig. 17–30). Osteoclasts are infrequent and no bone marrow elements are apparent.

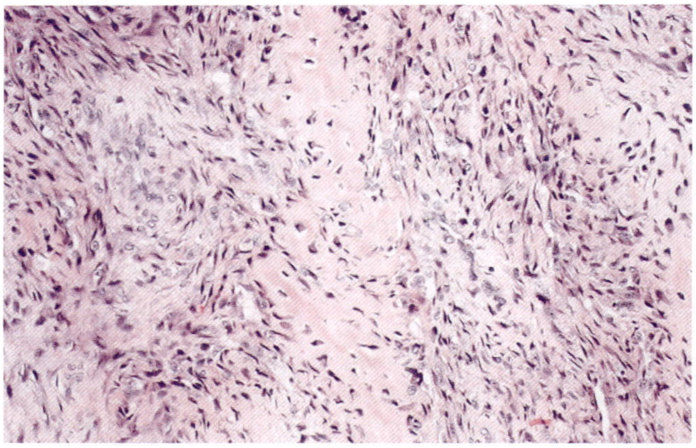

Figure 17–29. FOPD is histologically similar to myositis ossificans, but is less organized. Either the bone or fibroblastic spindled components may predominate.

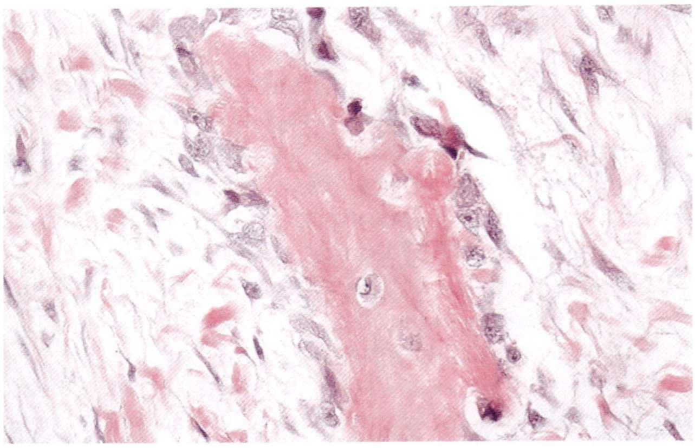

Figure 17–30. The bone in FOPD is rimmed by osteoblasts, a benign sign.

Differential Diagnosis

The differential diagnosis primarily includes osteosarcoma; however, osteoblastic rimming of bony trabeculae (a benign sign) and absence of atypical mitoses in fibroosseous pseudotumor of the digits help to distinguish this lesion from osteosarcoma.

Metaplastic Bone

Metaplastic bone may be present in a variety of unrelated soft tissue tumors, including ossifying fibromyxoid tumor (OFT), calcifying aponeurotic fibroma, calcifying fibrous pseudotumor, lipoma, liposarcoma, synovial sarcoma, malignant fibrous histiocytoma (MFH; in this tumor, it must be distinguished from osteoid), and malignant peripheral nerve sheath tumor.

Calciphylaxis (Systemic Calcinosis or Metastatic Calcification)

Clinical Features

Calciphylaxis refers to metastatic calcification associated with a hypersensitivity reaction to hypercalcemia, usually in end-stage renal disease or other causes of hyperparathyroidism.

The patients typically present with symmetrical superficial skin necrosis of the extremities after painful, pruritic violaceous skin discolorations in a livedo reticularis pattern.[132] Visceral organs may be involved, and there is a high mortality rate, 60% to 80%,[132,133] usually from sepsis. Treatment is largely supportive with removal of the potential sensitizer or challenger. Parathyroidectomy has been beneficial in some cases.[133-135]

Pathology

Grossly, this condition involves soft tissue, especially diffuse calcification of the medial layer of small to medium-sized vessels. The calcifications may be picked up radiographically as "pipe stem" calcifications of large vessels and metastatic calcifications.

Histologically, the vessels show medial calcification and endovascular fibrosis.

Extraskeletal Osteosarcoma (Extraskeletal Osteogenic Sarcoma, Extraosseous Osteosarcoma)

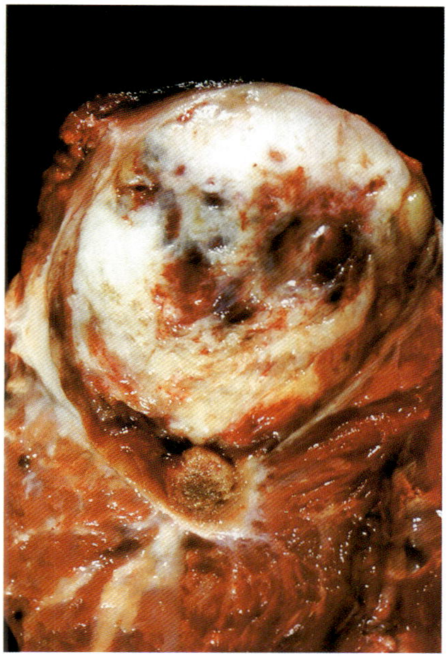

Figure 17-31. Extraskeletal osteosarcoma may have grossly evident bony matrix.

Clinical Features

Extraskeletal osteosarcomas comprise 1% to 2% of all soft tissue sarcomas; they represent approximately 4% to 5% of all osteosarcomas.[15,136-138] Mechanical injury, such as injection site or fracture, radiation therapy, and heterotopic ossification or stromal metaplasia have been proposed as etiologies. Patients are generally older than 40 years, with a male predominance in most series; the most common locations include the thigh and retroperitoneum. Extraskeletal osteosarcoma can occur in other sites, such as the breast.[139,140]

Prognosis and therapy depend on tumor grade and size.[141] Most extraskeletal osteosarcomas are high grade; therefore adjuvant therapy, following surgery, is usually clinically indicated. Metastases are generally to the lung, lymph nodes, bone, and soft tissue. Mortality rates are approximately 80%.[141-144]

Pathology

Tumor sizes are generally greater than 5 cm, but range from a few to several centimeters. The musculature, subcutis, or dermis may be involved. The lesions are generally well defined. Ossification may be evident radiographically or grossly (Fig. 17-31).

Histologically, by definition an extraskeletal osteosarcoma is composed of malignant cells of osteoblastic phenotype that produce malignant bone (osteoid; Figs. 17-32 and 17-33). Diagnosis also depends on identification of extraskeletal location. Extraskeletal osteosarcoma is subclassified similar to intraosseous osteosarcoma.[145,146] The most common subtype is osteoblastic osteosarcoma, which is high grade with marked atypia and mitotic activity. On the other side of the spectrum is the rare well-differentiated, parosteal-like osteosarcoma, characterized by parallel spicules of more mature bone with abundant, relatively bland stroma. High-grade fibroblastic osteosarcoma has lesser amounts of bone and more spindled stroma. MFH-like type is designated for a tumors that resemble MFH, with a storiform, spindle cell pattern and pleomorphism, yet has any amount of osteoid. The giant cell-rich type has scattered benign-appearing osteoclasts in addition to malignant osteoblasts and malignant bone. Small cell osteosarcoma (Fig. 17-34) is characterized by small round blue cells

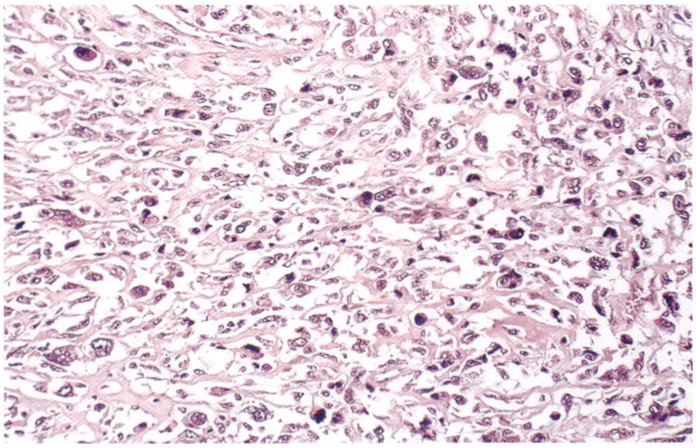

Figure 17-32. The bone in extraskeletal osteosarcoma may be lacelike, delicate, and spiculated, as seen here. Note the marked cytologic atypia.

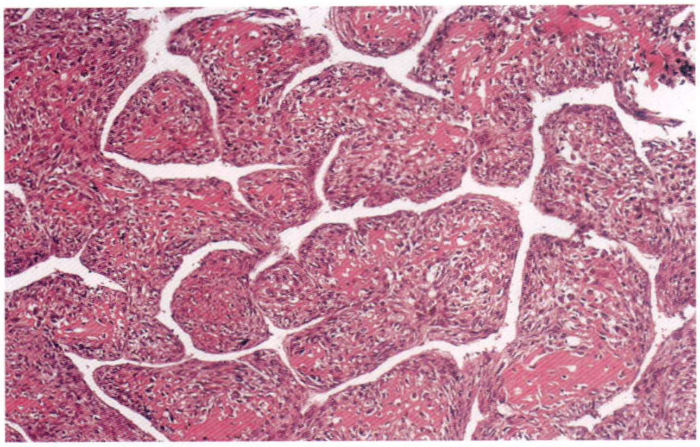

Figure 17-33. Highly vascular pattern of an extraskeletal osteosarcoma with cytologic atypia and bone production by the tumor.

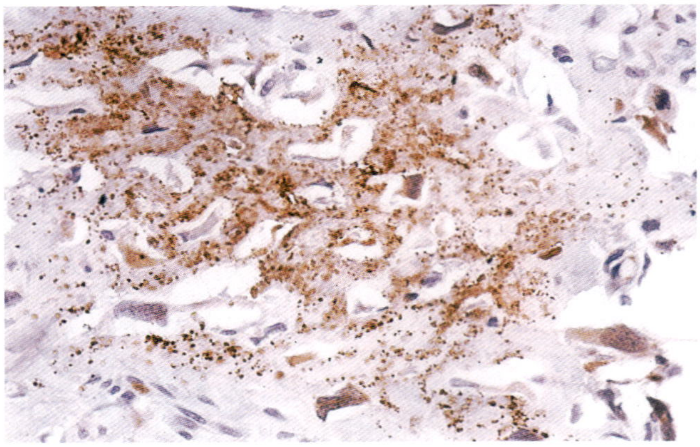

Figure 17-35. Osteocalcin immunoreactivity in an extraskeletal osteosarcoma is present in the cells and matrix, specifically identifying osteoblastic phenotype and noncollagen or noncartilage matrix, respectively.

with osteoid production, and telangiectatic osteosarcoma has abundant ectatic spaces lined by giant cell rich osteoblasts with osteoid formation.

Immunohistochemically, osteocalcin is an abundant human bone protein that can be used as a marker for osteoblastic phenotype (Fig. 17–35).[147,148] Although osteonectin, another abundant bone protein, is not specific for cells of osteoblastic phenotype, both antiosteocalcin and antiosteonectin can mark bone (i.e., neoplastic bone/osteoid) and distinguish it from dense collagen and cartilage matrix.[147,148]

Differential Diagnosis

The differential diagnosis depends on the subtype of osteosarcoma, but includes malignant melanoma, carcinoma, lymphoma, other sarcomas, and benign bone-forming tumors. The absence of malignant bone and specific immunostains help separate these entities from osteosarcoma. *Malignant mesenchymoma,* a term rarely now used, was a concept introduced by Stout to refer to soft tissue tumors with two different sarcoma types, in addition to a nonspecific fibrosarcoma. An example would be a case with osteosarcoma, chondrosarcoma, rhabdomyosarcoma, and fibrosarcoma. This occurs because of divergent differentiation of pluripotential primitive mesenchymal cells.

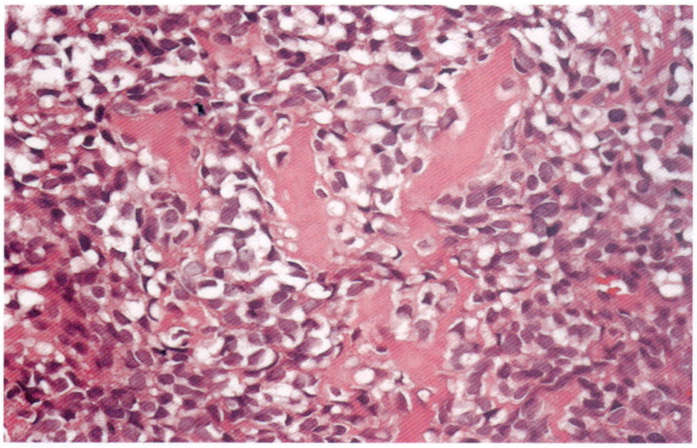

Figure 17-34. Small cell osteosarcoma has a differential diagnosis of other small round cell tumors; small cell osteosarcoma seems to be immunophenotypically different from the other osteosarcoma subtypes.[147,148]

Genetics

Intraosseous osteosarcomas are known to have multiple complex chromosomal abnormalities, but there is little information on specific features of extraskeletal osteosarcoma.

Ossifying Fibromyxoid Tumor

Clinical Features

Ossifying fibromyxoid tumor (OFT) of soft parts, first described by Enzinger et al[15] is typically a well-circumscribed lobulated mass of the extremities, upper trunk, or head and neck region of adults.[16,149,150]

The tumor behavior is generally benign, but local recurrence may occur in up to one third of patients. Malignant cases with metastases seem to only occur in those patients with multiple recurrences or increased cellularity, increased mitotic activity, or presence of central osteoid.[151,152] The latter feature, however, conceptually overlaps with osteosarcoma. Complete excision with careful long-term patient follow-up appears to be the treatment of choice; the malignant cases may require more aggressive treatment.

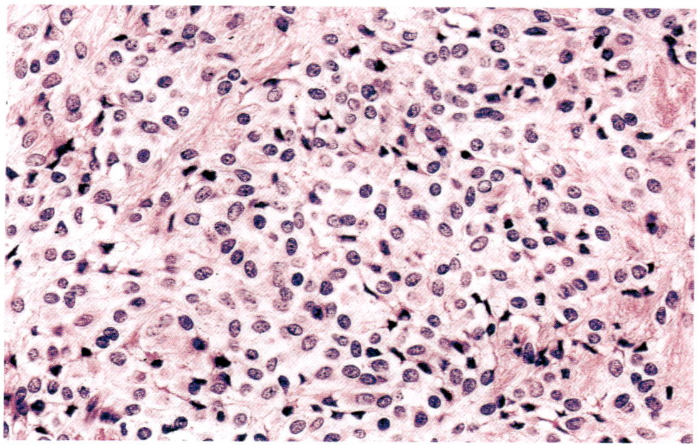

Figure 17–36. The indistinct cytoplasmic borders of the vesicular cells of this OFT are offset by their peripheral cytoplasmic clearing.

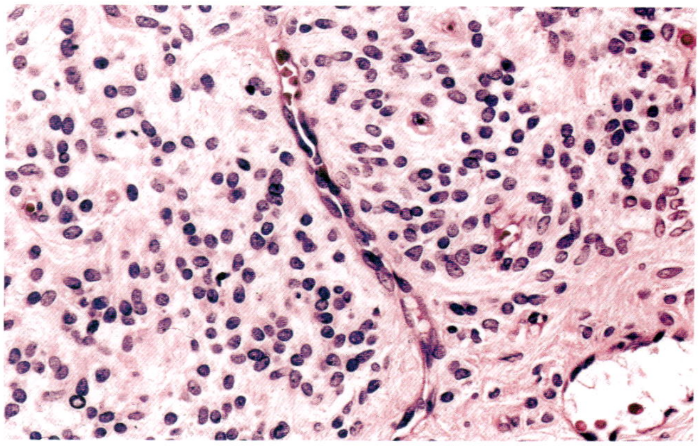

Figure 17–38. Higher magnification of the characteristic prominent vascularity.

Pathology

Grossly, these are small, superficial, well-defined, lobulated lesions, with an incomplete peripheral rim of bone in 80% of cases.[153]

Histologically, the lesion is composed of uniform polygonal to round cells with indistinct cytoplasmic borders, frequent peripheral clearing (Fig. 17–36), and vesicular nuclei, arranged in cords, trabeculae, and nests within a richly vascularized (Figs. 17–37 and 17–38), variable hyalinized, fibrous to myxoid stroma. The incomplete rim of bone is present in most cases (Fig. 17–39); it may show central marrow. Highly cellular, cytologically atypical, and mitotically active variants have been observed (Figs. 17–40), and warrant consideration as potentially malignant.

Immunohistochemically, this tumor demonstrates both cartilaginous and neural phenotypes, due to the positivity of these lesions for S-100 protein, and occasional positivity for Leu7 and GFAP. Ultrastructural features, such as presence of cell processes and basement membranes, are interpreted as reminiscent of Schwann cell origin.[154] Desmin and smooth muscle actin positivity in these lesions has also been reported.[149]

Differential Diagnosis

The differential diagnosis includes nerve sheath myxoma, epithelioid nerve sheath tumors, and EMCHSA. Lack of involvement of nerves, related neurofibromatosis, or presence of collagen type II rules out these diagnoses. Furthermore the abundant vessels of OFT are absent in EMCHSA. OFT is negative for cytokeratins and HMB-45, separating it from cutaneous mixed tumor and clear cell sarcoma, respectively.

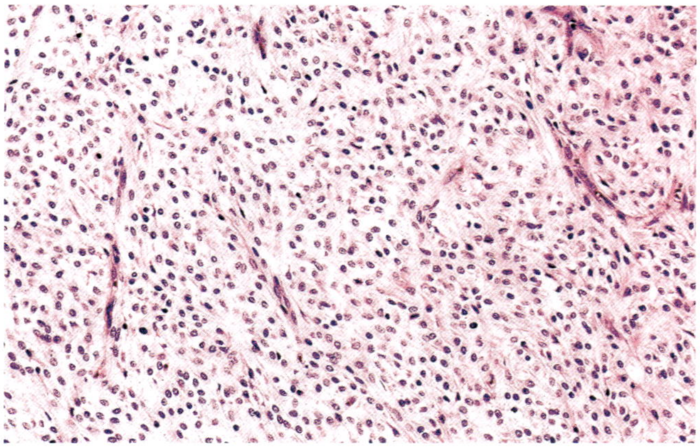

Figure 17–37. Low magnification showing the high vascularity of OFT, a feature that distinguishes it from EMCHSA.

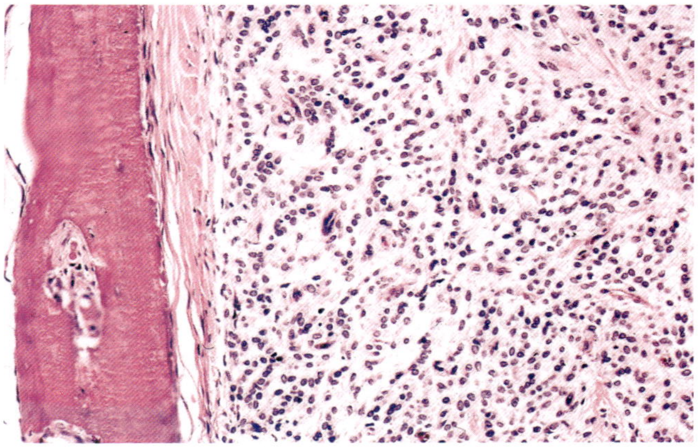

Figure 17–39. Approximately 80% of OFTs have an incomplete peripheral rim of bone. The corded or trabecular pattern of the cells of OFT is distinctive.

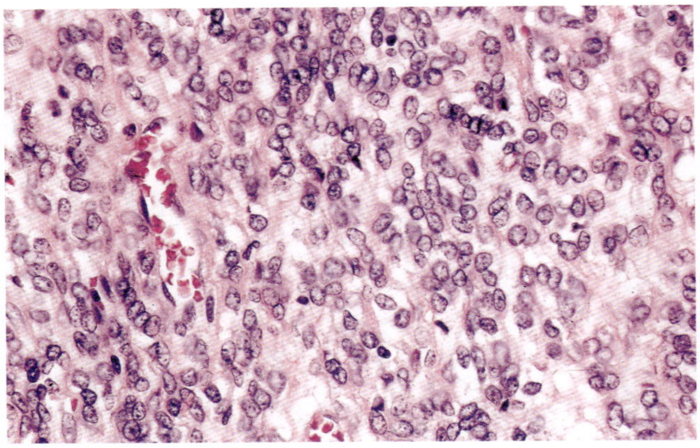

A

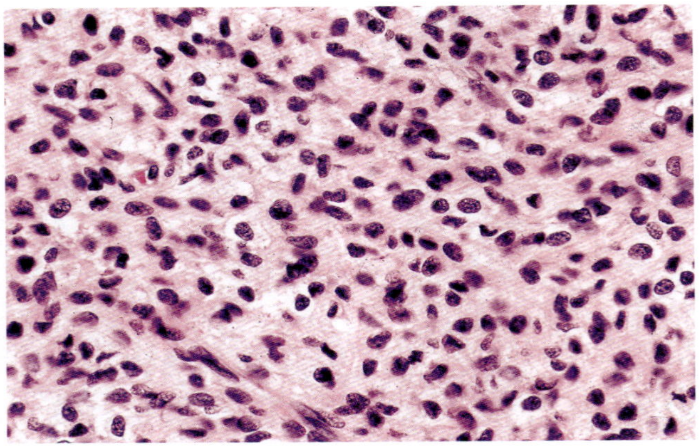

B

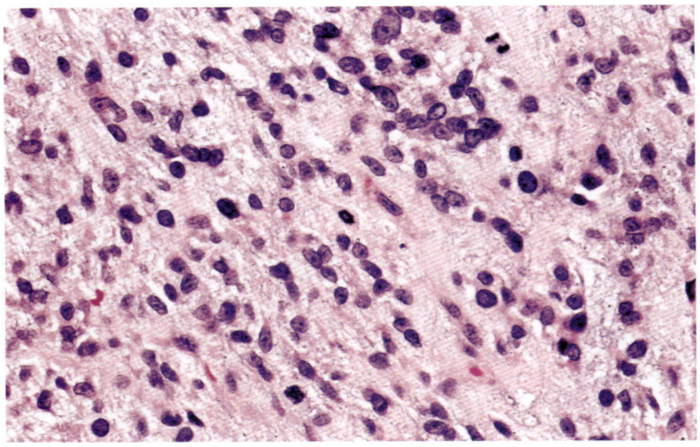

C

Figure 17-40. The combination of increased cellularity (*A*), cytologic atypia (*B*), and increased mitotic activity (*C*) are worrisome for recurrence and malignancy.

Genetics

No specific chromosomal abnormalities are known for OFT to date.

REFERENCES

General History

1. Lichtenstein L, Goldman RL: Cartilage tumors in soft tissues, particularly in the hand and foot. Cancer 1964;17:1203–1208.
2. Jaffe HL: Synovial chondromatosis and other benign articular tumors. In Tumor and Tumorous Conditions of the Bone and Joints. Philadelphia: Lea & Febiger 1958:558–566.
3. Reichel PF: Chrondmatose der Kniegelenkkapsel. Arch Klin Chir 1900;61:717–724.
4. Stout AP, Verner EW: Chondrosarcoma of the extraskeletal soft tissues. Cancer 1953;6:581–590.
5. Enzinger FM, Shiraki M: Extraskeletal myxoid chondrosarcoma: An analysis of 34 cases. Hum Pathol 1972; 3:421–435.
6. Lichtenstein L, Berstein D: Unusual benign and malignant chondroid tumors of bone; survey of some mesenchymal cartilage tumors and malignant chondroblastic tumors including few multicentric ones as well as many atypical benign chondroblastomas and chondromyxoid fibromas. Cancer 1959;12: 1142–1157.
7. Laskowski J: Zarys onkologii. In Kolodziejska H, ed.: Pathology of Tumors. Warsaw, PZWL, 1955:91–99.
8. Dabska M. Parachordoma. A new clinical entity. Cancer 1977;40:1586–1592.
9. Inclan A: Tumoral calcinosis. JAMA 1943;121:490.
10. Zitnan D, Sitaj S: Multiple familial calcification of articular cartilages. Bratisl Lek Listy 1958;38: 217–228.
11. McCarty D, Kohn N, Faires J: The significance of calcium phosphate crystals in the synovial fluid of arthritic patients: The "pseudogout syndrome." II. Identification of crystals. Ann Intern Med 1962;56: 738–745.
12. Ling D, Murphy WA, Kyriakos M: Tophaceous pseudogout. AJR Am J Roentgenol 1982;138:162–165.
13. Ackerman LV: Extraosseous localized non-neoplastic bone and cartilage formation (so-called myositis ossificans). J Bone Joint Surg 1958;40A:279–298.
14. Shore EM, Gannon FH, Kaplan FS: Fibrodysplasia ossificans progressiva: Why do some people have two skeletons? Expansion Scientifique Publications 1999: 192S-97S.

15. Fine G, Stout AP: Osteogenic sarcoma of the extraskeletal soft tissues. Cancer 1956;9:1027–1043.
16. Enzinger FM, Weiss SW, Liang CY: Ossifying fibromyxoid tumor of soft parts. A clinicopathologic analysis of 59 cases. Am J Surg Pathol 1989;13:817–827.

Extraskeletal (Soft Tissue) Chondroma

17. Dahlin DC, Salvador AH: Cartilaginous tumors of the soft tissues of the hands and feet. Mayo Clin Proc 1974;49:721–726.
18. Chung EB, Enzinger FM: Chondroma of soft parts. Cancer 1978;41:1414–1424.
19. Zlatkin MB, Lander PH, Begin LR, Hadjipavlou A: Soft-tissue chondroma. AJR Am J Roentgenol 1985; 144:1263–1267.
20. Humphreys H, Pambakian PH, Fletcher CDM: Soft tissue chondroma—A study of 15 tumors. Histopathology 1986;10:147–159.
21. Reiman HM, Dahlin DC: Cartilage- and bone-forming tumors of the soft tissues. Semin Diagn Pathol 1986;3:288–305.
22. Steiner GC, Meushar N, Norman A, Present D: Intracapsular and paraarticular chondromas. Clin Orthop 1994;303:231–236.
23. Mendes W, Ayoub A, Chapchap P, Antoneli CBG, Sredni ST, de Camargo B. Association of gastrointestinal stromal tumor (leiomyosarcoma), pulmonary chondroma, and non-functional retroperitoneal paraganglioma. Med Pediatr Oncol 1998;31:537–540.
24. Carney JA. Gastric stromal sarcoma, pulmonary chondroma, and extra-adrenal paraganglioma (Carney's triad): Natural history, adrenocortical component and possible familial occurrence. Mayo Clin Proc 1999; 74:543–552.
25. Carney JA, Sheps SG, Go VL, Gordon H: The triad of gastric leiomyosarcoma, functioning extra-adrenal paraganglioma and pulmonary chondroma. N Engl J Med 1977;296:1517–1518.
26. Dal Cin P, Qi H, Sciot R, Van den Berghe H: Involvement of chromosomes 6 and 11 in a soft tissue chondroma. Cancer Genet Cytogenet 1997;93:177–178.
27. Mandahl N, Willen H, Rydholm A, Heim S, Mitelman F: Rearrangement of band q13 on both chromosomes 12 in a periosteal chondroma. Genes Chromosomes Cancer 1993;6:121–123.
28. Fletcher JA, Pinkus GS, Donovan K, et al: Clonal rearrangement of chromosome band 6p21 in the mesenchymal component of pulmonary chondroid hamartoma. Cancer Res 1992;52:6224–6228.
29. Xiao S, Lux ML, Reeves R, Hudson TJ, Fletcher JA: HMGI(Y) activation by chromosome 6p21 rearrangements in multilineage mesenchymal cells from pulmonary hamartoma. Am J Pathol 1997;150:911–918.

Synovial Chondromatosis

30. Crotty JM, Monu JUV, Pope TL Jr: Synovial osteochondromatosis. Radiol Clin North Am 1996;34:327–342.
31. Milgram JW, Addison RG: Synovial osteochondromatosis of the knee. Chondromatous recurrence with possible chondrosarcomatous degeneration. J Bone Joint Surg [Am] 1976;58;264–266.
32. Sim FH, Dahlin DC, Ivins JC: Extra-articular synovial chondromatosis. J Bone Joint Surg Am 1977;59A: 492–495.
33. Sviland L, Malcolm AJ: Synovial chondromatosis presenting as painless soft tissue mass. A report of 19 cases. Histopathology 1995;27:275–279.
34. Lagier R: Primary synovial osteochondromatosis of the knee with extensive bone formation observed over a period of 13 years. Skeletal Radiol 1987;16:660–665.
35. Hermann G, Klein M, Abdelwahab IF, Kenan S: Synovial chondrosarcoma arising in synovial chondromatosis of the right hip. Skeletal Radiol 1997;26: 366–369.
36. Davies RI, Hamilton A, Biggart JD: Primary synovial chondromatosis: A clinicopathologic review and assessment of malignant potential. Human Pathol 1998;29:683–688.
37. Saotome K, Tamai K, Koguchi Y, Sakai H, Yamaguchi T: Growth potential of loose bodies: An immunohistochemical examination of primary and secondary synovial osteochondromatosis. J Orthopaed Res 1999;17: 73–79.
38. Sciot R, Dal Cin P, Bellemans J, Samson I, Van den Berghe H, Van Damme B: Synovial chondromatosis clonal chromosome changes provide further evidence for a neoplastic disorder. Virchows Arch 1998;433: 189–191.
39. Mertens F, Jonsson K, Willen H, et al: Chromosome rearrangements in synovial chondromatous lesions. Br J Cancer 1996;74:251–254.
40. Mitelman F. Chromosomes, genes, and cancer [editorial]. Cancer J Clin 1994;4:133–135.

Extraskeletal Myxoid Chondrosarcoma

41. Weiss SW: Ultrastructure of the so-called "chordoid sarcoma." Evidence supporting cartilagenous differentiation. Cancer 1978;41:2250–2266.
42. Wick MR, Burgess JH, Manivel JC: A reassessment of chordoid sarcoma: Ultrastructural and immunohistochemical comparison with chordoma and skeletal myxoid chondrosarcoma. Modern Pathol 1988;1:433–443.
43. Hachitanda Y, Tsuneyoshi M, Daimaru Y, et al: Extraskeletal myxoid chondrosarcoma in young children. Cancer 1988;61:2521–2526.
44. Saleh G, Evans HL, Ro JY, Ayala AG: Extraskeletal myxoid chondrosarcoma. A clinicopathologic study of ten patients with long-term follow-up. Cancer 1992;70: 2827–2830.
45. Lucas DR, Fletcher CD, Adsay NV, Zalupski MM: High-grade extraskeletal myxoid chondrosarcoma: A high-grade epithelioid malignancy. Histopathology 1999;35:201–208.
46. Ramesh K, Gahukamble L, Sarma NH, Al Fituri OM: Extraskeletal myxoid chondrosarcoma with dedifferentiation. Histopathology 1995;27:381–382.
47. Rubin BP, Fletcher JA: Skeletal and extraskeletal myxoid chondrosarcoma: Related or distinct tumors? Adv Anat Pathol 1999;6:204–212.

48. Meis-Kindblom JM, Bergh P, Gunterberg B, Kindblom L-G: Extraskeletal myxoid chondrosarcoma. A reappraisal of its morphologic spectrum and prognostic factors based on 117 cases. Am J Surg Pathol 1999;23:636–650.
49. Fletcher CDM, Powell G, McKee PH: Extraskeletal myxoid chondrosarcoma: A histochemical and immunohistochemical study. Histopathology 1986;10:489–499.
50. Dei Tos AP, Wadden C, Fletcher CDM: Extraskeletal myxoid chondrosarcoma: An immunohistochemical reappraisal of 39 cases. Appl Immunohistochem 1997;5:73–77.
51. Folpe AL, Agoff SN, Willis J, Weiss SW: Parachordoma is immunohistochemically and cytogenetically distinct from axial chordoma and extraskeletal myxoid chondrosarcoma. Am J Surg Pathol 1999;23:1059–1067.
52. Antonescu CR, Argani P, Erlandson RA, Healey JH, Ladanyi M, Huvos AG: Skeletal and extraskeletal myxoid chondrosarcoma. A comparative clinicopathologic, ultrastructural, and molecular study. Cancer 1998;83:1504–1521.
53. O'Hara B, Paetau A, Miettinen M: Keratin subsets and monoclonal antibody HBME-1 in chordoma: Immunohistochemical differential diagnosis between tumors simulating chordoma. Hum Pathol 1998;29:119–126.
54. Brody RI, Ueda T, Hamelin A, et al: Molecular analysis of the fusion of EWS to an orphan nuclear receptor gene in extraskeletal myxoid chondrosarcoma. Am J Pathol 1997;150:1049–1058.
55. Labelle Y, Bussieres J, Courjal F, Goldring MB: The EWS/TEC fusion protein encoded by the t(9;22) chromosomal translocation in human chondrosarcomas is a highly potent transcriptional activator. Oncogene 1999;18:3303–3308.
56. Hibshoosh H, Lattes R: Immunohistochemical and molecular genetic approaches of soft tissue tumor diagnosis: A primer. Semin Oncol 1997;24:515–525.
57. Stenman G, Andersson H, Mandahl N, Meis-Kindblom JM, Kindblom LG: Translocation t(9;22)(q22;q12) is a primary cytogenetic abnormality in extraskeletal myxoid chondrosarcoma. Int J Cancer 1995;62:398–402.
58. Hirabayashi Y, Ishida T, Yoshida MA, Kohima T, Eihara Y, Machinami R, Ikeuchi T: Translocation (9;22)(q22;q12). A recurrent chromosome abnormality in extraskeletal myxoid chondrosarcoma. Cancer Genet Cytogenet 1995;81:33–37.
59. Sciot R, Dal Cin P, Fletcher C, et al: t(9;22)(q22-31;q11-12) is a consistent marker of extraskeletal myxoid chondrosarcoma: Evaluation of three cases. Mod Pathol 1995;8:765–768.
60. Kilpatrick SE, Inwards CY, Fletcher CD, Smith MA, Gitelis S: Myxoid chondrosarcoma (chordoid sarcoma) of bone: A report of two cases and review of the literature. Cancer 1997;79:1903–1910.
61. Sjogren H, Meis-Kindblom J, Kindblom L-G, Aman P, Stenman G: Fusion of the EWS-related gene TAF2N to TEC in extraskeletal myxoid chondrosarcoma. Cancer Res 1999;59:5064–5067.

Extraskeletal Mesenchymal Chondrosarcoma

62. Guccion JG, Font RL, Enzinger FM, Zimmerman LE: Extraskeletal mesenchymal chondrosarcoma. Arch Pathol 1973;95:336–340.
63. Nakashima Y, Unni KK, Shives TC, Swee RG, Dahlin DC: Mesenchymal chondrosarcoma of bone and soft tissue. A study of 111 cases. Cancer 1986;57:2444–2453.
64. Salvador AH, Beabout JW, Dahlin DC: Mesenchymal chondrosarcoma—observations on 30 new cases. Cancer 1971;28:605–615.
65. Bertoni F, Picci P, Bacchini P, et al: Mesenchymal chondrosarcoma of bone and soft tissues. Cancer 1983;2:533–541.
66. Shapeero LG, Vanel D, Couanet D, Contesso G, Ackerman LV: Extraskeletal mesenchymal chondrosarcoma. Radiology 1993;186:819–826.
67. Aramburu-Gonzalez J-A, Rodriquez-Justo M, Jimenez-Reyes J, Santonja C: A case of soft tissue mesenchymal chondrosarcoma metastatic to skin, clinically mimicking keratoacanthoma. Am J Surg Dermatopathol 1999;21:392–294.
68. Swanson PE, Lillemoe TJ, Manivel JC, Wick MR: Mesenchymal chondrosarcoma. An immunohistochemical study. Arch Pathol Lab Med 1990;114:943–948.
69. Rushing EJ, Armonda RA, Ansari Q, Mena H: Mesenchymal chondrosarcoma: A clinicopathologic and flow cytometric study of 13 cases presenting in the central nervous system. Cancer 1996;77:1884–1891.
70. Szymanska J, Taarkkanen M, Wiklund T, et al: Cytogenetic study of extraskeletal mesenchymal chondrosarcoma. A case report. Cancer Genet Cytogenet 1996;86:170–173.
71. Sainati L, Scapinello A, Montaldi A, et al: A mesenchymal chondrosarcoma of a child with the reciprocal translocation (11;22)(q24;q12). Cancer Genet Cytogenet 1993;71:144–147.
72. Stenger AM, Garre ML, Andreussi L, et al: Expression of histone H3 cell cycle-related gene, vimentin and MYC genes in pediatric brain tumors. A preliminary analysis showing the different malignant cell growth potential. Brain Res Mol Brain Res 1992;13:273–275.
73. Castresana JS, Barrios C, Gomez L, Kreicbergs A: Amplification of the c-myc proto-oncogene in human chondrosarcoma. Diagn Mol Pathol 1992;1:235–238.

Parachordoma

74. Michal M, Miettinen M: Myoepitheliomas of the skin and soft tissues. Report of 12 cases. Virchows Arch 1999;434:393–400.
75. Kilpatrick SE, Hitchcock MG, Kraus MD, Calonje E, Fletcher CDM: Mixed tumors and myoepitheliomas of soft tissue. A clinicopathologic study of 19 cases with a unifying concept. Am J Surg Pathol 1997; 21:13–22.
76. Limon J, Babinska M, Denis, A, Rys J, Niezabitowski A: Parachordoma: A rare sarcoma with clonalchromosomal changes. Cancer Genet Cytogenet 1998;102:78–80.
77. Fisher C, Miettinen M: Parachordoma: A clinicopathologic and immunohistochemical study of four cases of an unusual soft tissue neoplasm. Ann Diagnostic Pathol 1997;1:3–10.

78. Tihy F, Scott P, Russo P, Champagne M, Tabet J-C, Lemieux N: Cytogenetic analysis of a parachordoma. Cancer Genet Cytogenet 1998;105:14–19.

Tumoral Calcinosis

79. McGregor D, Burn J, Lynn K, Robson R: Rapid resolution of tumoral calcinosis after renal transplantation. Clinical Nephrology 1999;51:54–58.
80. Smack D, Norton SA, Fitzpatrick JE: Proposal for a pathogenesis-based classification of tumoral calcinosis. Int J Dermatol 1996;35:265–271.
81. Narchi H: Hyperostosis with hyperphosphatemia: Evidence of familial occurrence and association with tumoral calcinosis. Pediatrics 1997;99:745–748.
82. Slavin RE, Wen J, Kumar D, Evans EB: Familial tumoral calcinosis. A clinical, histopathologic and ultrastructural study with an analysis of its calcifying process and pathogenesis. Am J Surg Pathol 1993;17:788–802.
83. Chew FS, Crenshaw WB: Idiopathic tumoral calcinosis. AJR Am J Roentgenol 1992;158:330.
84. Albraham Z, Rozner I, Rozenbaum M: Tumoral calcinosis: Report of a case and brief review of the literature. J Dermatopathol 1996;23:545–550.
85. Vogt BA, Myers MT: Clinical quiz. Pediatr Nephrol 1999;13:362–364.
86. Noyez JF, Murphree SM, Chen K: Tumoral calcinosis, a clinical report of eleven cases. Acta Orthopaed Belg 1993;59:249–254.
87. Tezelman S, Siperstein AE, Duh Q-Y, Clark OH: Tumoral calcinosis. Controversies in the etiology and alternatives in the treatment. Arch Surg 1993;128: 737–743.
88. Thakur A, Hines OJ, Thakur V, Gordon HE: Tumoral calcinosis regression after subtotal parathyroidectomy: A case presentation and review of the literature. Surgery 1999;126:95–98.
89. Kuriyama S: Successful treatment of tumoral calcinosis using CAPD combined with hemodialysis with low-calcium dialysate. Blood Purif 1998;16:43–48.
90. Fernandez E, Montoliu J: Successful treatment of massive uraemic tumoral calcinosis with daily haemodialysis and very low calcium dialysate. Nephrol Dial Transplant 1994;9:1207–1209.
91. Kyriakopoulos G, Kontogianni K: Sodium thiosulfate treatment of tumoral calcinosis in patient with end-stage renal disease. Ren Fail 1990;12:213–219.
92. Papadakis JT, Patrikarea A, Digenis GE, et al: Sodium thiosulfate in the treatment of tumoral calcifications in a hemodialysis patient without hyperparathyroidism. Nephron 1996;72:308–312.
93. Ueyoshi A, Ota K: Clinical appraisal of vinpocentine for the removal of intractable tumoral calcinosis in haemodialysis patients with renal failure. J Int Med Res 1992;20:435–443.
94. Pakasa NM, Kalengyai RM: Tumoral calcinosis. A clinicopathological study of 111 cases with emphasis on the earliest changes. Histopathology 1997;31:18–24.
95. McKee PH, Liomba NG, Hutt MSR: Tumoral calcinosis: A pathological study of fifty-six cases. Br J Dermatol 1982;107:669–674.
96. Todesco S, Venturi Pasini C, Glorioso S, Fagiolo U: Family occurrence and HLA system in tumoral calcinosis. Int Surg 1983;68:89–90.

Tophaceous Pseudogout

97. Ishida T, Dorfman HD, Bullough PG: Tophaceous pseudogout (tumoral calcium pyrophosphate dihydrate crystal deposition disease. Hum Pathol 1995; 26:587–593.
98. Shun-Iu Y, Rui-zong L, Zhao-han B: Tumoral calcium pyrophosphate dihydrate deposition disease. Chin Med J 1992;105:780–784.
99. Grant GA, Wener MH, Yaziji H, et al: Destructive tophaceous calcium hydroxyapatite tumor of the infratemporal fossa. Case report and review of the literature. J Neurosurg 1999;90:148–152.
100. Athanasou NA, Caughey M, Burge P, Eta L: Deposition of calcium pyrophosphate dihydrate crystals in a soft tissue chondroma. Ann Rheum Dis 1991;50:950–952.

Myositis Ossificans

101. Akgun I, Erdogan F, Aydingoz O, Kesmezacar H: Myositis ossificans in early childhood. J Arthroscopic Rel Surg 1998;15:522–526.
102. Kransdorf MJ, Meis JM: From the archives of the AFIP. Extraskeletal osseous and cartilaginous tumors of the extremities. Radiographics 1993;13:853–884.
103. Schweitzer ME, Greenway G, Resmick D, Haghighi P, Snoots WE: Osteoma of soft parts. Skeletal Radiol 1992;21:177–180.
104. Goldman AB: Myositis ossificans circumscripta: A benign lesion with a malignant differential diagnosis. Am J Roentgenol 1976;126:32–40.
105. Kaplan FS, Gannon FH, Hahn GV, Wollner N, Rauner R: Pseudomalignant heterotopic ossification. Differential diagnosis and report of two cases. Clin Orthop 1998;346:134–140.
106. Luc-Jouve J, Cottalorda J, Bollini G, Scheiner C, Daoud A: Myositis ossificans: Report of seven cases in children. J Pediatr Orthop (Part B) 1997;6:33–41.
107. Hanquinet S, Ngo L, Anooshiravani M, Garcia J, Bugman P: Magnetic resonance imaging helps in the early diagnosis of myositis ossificans in children. Pediatr Surg Int 1999;15:287–289.
108. Shafritz AB, Kaplan FS: Differential expression of bone and cartilage related genes in fibrodysplasia ossificans progressiva, myositis ossificans traumatica, and osteogenic sarcoma. Clin Orthop 1998;346:46–52.

Fibrodysplasia Ossificans Progressiva

109. Smith R, Athanasou NA, Vipond SE: Fibrodysplasia (myositis) ossificans progressiva: Clinicopathological features and natural history. Q Med J 1996;89: 445–456.
110. Kaplan FS, Taas JA, Gannon FH, Finkel G, Hahn GV, Zasloff MA: The histopathology of fibrodysplasia ossificans progressiva. J Bone Joint Surg Am 1993;75: 220–230.

111. Cohen RB, Hahn GV, Tabas JA, et al: The natural history of heterotopic ossification in patients who have fibrodysplasia ossificans progressiva. A study of forty-four patients. J Bone Joint Surg Am 1993;75(2):215–219.
112. Connor JM, Evans DA: Fibrodysplasia ossificans progressiva: The clinical features and natural history of 34 patients. J Bone J Surg Br 1982;64:76–83.
113. Zasloff MA, Rocke DM, Crofford LJ, Hahn GV, Kaplan FS: Treatment of patients who have fibrodysplasia ossificans progressiva with isoretinoin. Clin Orthop 1998;346:121–129.
114. Brantus JF, Meunier PJ: Effects of intravenous etidronate and oral corticosteroids in fibrodysplasia ossificans progressiva. Clin Orthop 1998;346:117–120.
115. Palhares DB: Myositis ossificans progressive. Calcif Tissue Int 1997;60:394.
116. Shafritz AB, Kaplan FS: Differential expression of bone and cartilage related genes in fibrodysplasia ossificans progressiva, myositis ossificans traumatic, and osteogenic sarcoma. Clin Orthop 1998;346:46–52.
117. Olmsted EA, Gannon FH, Wang Z-Q, et al: Embryonic overexpression of the c-Fos protooncogene. A murine stem cell chimera applicable to the study of fibrodysplasia ossificans progressiva in humans. Clinical Orthop 1988;346:81–94.
118. Gannon FH, Valentine BA, Shore EM, Zasloff MA, Kaplan FS: Acute lymphocytic infiltration in an extremely early lesion of fibrodysplasia ossificans progressiva. Clin Orthop 1998;346:19–25.
119. Gannon FH, Kaplan FS, Olmsted E, Finkel GC, Zasloff MA, Shore E: Bone morphogenetic protein 2/4 in early fibromatous lesions of fibrodysplasia ossificans progressiva. Hum Pathol 1997;28:339–343.
120. Kaplan FS, Craver R, MacEwen GD, et al: Progressive osseous heteroplasia: A distinct developmental disorder of heterotopic ossification. Two new case reports and follow-up of three previously reported cases. J Bone Joint Surg Am 1994;76:425–436.
121. Van den Wijngaard A, Wedhuis DO, Boersma CJC, van Zoelen EJJ, van Kesssel AG, Olijve W: Fine mapping of the human bone morphogenetic protein 4 gene (BMP4) to chromosome 14q22-q23 by in situ hybridization. Genomics 1995;27:559–560.
122. Van den Wijngaard A, van Kraay M, van Zoelen EJJ, Olijve W, Boersma CJC: Genomic organization of the human bone morphogenetic protein 4 gene: Molecular basis for multiple transcripts. Biochem Biophys Res Commun 1996;219:789–794.
123. Virdi AS, Shore EM, Oreffo ROC, et al: Phenotypic and molecular heterogeneity in fibrodysplasia ossificans progressiva. Calcif Tissue Int 1999;65:250–255.

Fibro-osseous Pseudotumor

124. Spjut HJ, Dorfman HD: Florid reactive periostitis of the tubular bones of the hands and feet: A benign lesion which may simulate osteosarcoma. Am J Surg Pathol 1981;5:423–433.
125. Kovach JC, Truong L, Kearns RJ, et al: Florid reactive periostitis. J Hand Surg 1986;11:902–905.
126. McCarthy EF, Ireland DCR, Sprague BL, Bonfiglio M: Periosteal (nodular) fasciitis of the hand. J Bone Joint Surg 1976;58A:714–716.
127. Angervall L, Stener B, Stener I, et al: Pseudomalignant osseous tumor of soft tissue. J Bone Joint Surg 1969;51B:654–663.
128. Carpenter EB, Lublin B: An unusual osteogenic lesion of a finger. J Bone Joint Surg 1967;49A:527–531.
129. Tang J-B, Gu YQ, Xia RG: Fibro-osseous pseudotumor that may be mistaken for a malignant tumor in the hand: A case report and review of the literature. J Hand Surg 1996;21A:714–716.
130. Sleater J, Mullins D, Chun K, Hendricks J: Fibro-osseous pseudotumor of the digit: A comparison to myositis ossificans by light microscopy and immunohistochemical methods. J Cutan Pathol 1995;23: 373–377.
131. Dupree WB, Enzinger FM: Fibro-osseous pseudotumor of the digits. Cancer 1986;58:2103–2109.

Calciphylaxis

132. Fischer AH, Morris DJ: Pathogenesis of calciphylaxis: Study of three cases with literature review. Hum Pathol 1995;26:1055–1064.
133. Oh DH, Eulau D, Tokugawa DA, McGuire JS, Kohler S: Five cases of calciphylaxis and a review of the literature. J Am Acad Dermatol 1999;40:979–987.
134. Hafner J, Keusch G, Wahl C, et al: Uremic small-artery disease with medial calcification and intimal hyperplasia (so-called calciphylaxis): A complication of chronic renal failure and benefit from parathyroidectomy. J Am Acad Dermatol 1995;33:954–962.
135. Khafif RA, DeLima C, Silverberg A, Frankel R: Calciphylaxis and systemic calcinosis. Arch Intern Med 1990;150:956–959.

Extraskeletal Osteosarcoma

136. Huvos AG: Osetogenic sarcoma of bones and soft tissue in older persons. A clinicopathologic analysis of 117 patients older than 60 years. Cancer 1986;57: 1442–1449.
137. Rao U, Cheng A, Didolkar MS: Extraosseous osteogenic sarcoma: Clinicopathological study of eight cases and review of the literature. Cancer 1978;41: 1488–1496.
138. Jensen ML, Schumacher B, Jensen OM, Nielsen OS, Keller J: Extraskeletal osteosarcomas. A clinicopathologic study of 25 cases. Am J Surg Pathol 1998;22: 588–594.
139. Silver SA, Tavassoli FA: Primary osteogenic sarcoma of the breast. A clinicopathologic analysis of 50 cases. Am J Surg Pathol 1998;22:925–933.
140. Cook PA, Murphy MS, Innis PC, Yu JS: Extraskeletal osteosarcoma of the hand. J Bone Joint Surg 1998; 80A:725–729.
141. Bane BL, Evans HL, Ro JY, et al: Extraskeletal osteosarcoma. A clinicopathologic review of 26 cases. Cancer 1990;66:2762–2770.

142. Chung EB, Enzinger FM: Extraskeletal osteosarcoma. Cancer 1987;60:11132–1142.
143. Allen CJ, Soule EH: Osteogenic sarcoma of the somatic soft tissues: Clinicopathologic study of 26 cases and review of the literature. Cancer 1971;27: 1121–1133.
144. Sordillo PP, Hajdu SI, Magill GB, Golbey RB: Extraosseous osteogenic sarcoma: A review of 48 patients. Cancer 1983;51:727–734.
145. Lee, JSY, Fetsch JF, Wasdhal DA, Lee BP, Pritchard DJ, Nascimento AG: A review of 32 patients with extraskeletal osteosarcoma. Cancer 1995;76:2253–2259.
146. Yi ES, Shmookler BM, Malawer MM, Sweet DE: Well-differentiated extraskeletal osteosarcoma. A soft-tissue homologue of parosteal osteosarcoma. Arch Pathol Lab Med 1991;115:906–909.
147. Fanburg JC, Rosenberg AE, Weaver DL, et al: Osteocalcin and osteonectin immunoreactivity in the diagnosis of osteosarcoma. J Clin Pathol 1997;108: 464–473.
148. Fanburg-Smith JC, Bratthauer GL, Miettinen M: Osteocalcin and osteonectin immunoreactivity in extraskeletal osteosarcoma. A study of 28 cases. Human Pathol 1999;30:32–38.

Ossifying Fibromyxoid Tumor

149. Schofield JB, Krausz T, Stamp GW, Fletcher CD, Fisher C, Azzopardi JG: Ossifying fibromyxoid tumour of soft parts: Immunohistochemical and ultrastructural analysis. Histopathology 1993;22(2):101–112.
150. Miettinen M: Ossifying fibromyxoid tumor of soft parts. Additional observations of a distinctive soft tissue tumor. Am J Clin Pathol 1991;95:142–149.
151. Kilpatrick SE, Ward WG, Mozes M, Miettinen M, Fukunaga M, Fletcher CDM: Atypical and malignant variants of ossifying fibromyxoid tumor. Clinicopathologic analysis of six cases. Am J Surg Pathol 1995;19:1039–1046.
152. Zamecnik M, Michal M, Simpson RH, et al: Ossifying fibromyxoid tumor of soft parts: A report of 17 cases with emphasis on unusual histologic features. Ann Diagn Pathol 1997;1:73–81.
153. Thompson J, Castillo M, Reddick RL, Smith K, Shockley W: Nasopharyngeal nonossifying variant of ossifying fibromyxoid tumor: CT and MR findings. Am J Neuroradiol 1995;16:1132–1134.
154. Donner LR: Ossifying fibromyxoid tumor of soft parts: Evidence supporting Schwann cell origin. Human Pathol 1992;23:200–202.

David M. Parham

Small Round Cell Tumors

CHAPTER 18

"Small round blue cell tumor" is the name given to a group of highly malignant neoplasms that largely occur in the pediatric age group. Although this term could also apply to some adult neoplasms, notably small cell carcinoma of the lung, the term has become widely associated with childhood cancer.[1] The name derives from the primitive, highly cellular nature of these lesions, which typically present a vast sea of dark blue nuclei on hematoxylin-based stains. Cytoplasmic abundance roughly correlates with cellular differentiation, which is often modest. Although cytoplasmic landmarks allow for cell type identification in some cases, ancillary techniques, such as immunohistochemistry, electron microscopy, and genetics, have become important in the diagnosis of these tumors.

Although childhood cancer comprises a relatively small proportion of all malignancies, it causes a large proportion of pediatric mortality, being second only to accidents as a cause of death in industrialized nations.[2] It also differs from adult cancer in the great percentage of cases treated on multi-institutional protocols.[3] Despite success in treatment,[2] more than 100,000 person are lost each year to this group of cancers.[3]

Types of Round Cell Tumors and Their Differential Diagnosis

Leukemias and brain tumors comprise the majority of childhood cancers. Although leukemias can present as solid masses, these lesions do not typically enter into the differential diagnosis of small round cell tumors. Table 18–1 lists the most common lesions in this tumor group. Of these tumors, neuroblastoma, rhabdomyosarcoma, lymphoma, and Wilms tumor are most common. This chapter will discuss neuroblastoma, Ewing sarcoma/peripheral primitive neuroectodermal tumor (PNET), desmoplastic small cell tumor (DSCT), and extrarenal rhabdoid tumor. Rhabdomyosarcoma and lymphoma will be discussed elsewhere.

The majority of small round blue cell tumors, such as neuroblastoma and Wilms tumor are "organ-specific blastomas." These embryonal tumors recapitulate the embryogenesis of their organs of origin. Another portion of them, rhabdomyosarcomas and Ewing sarcomas, are primarily soft tissue and bone lesions, the former representing a neoplastic attempt at embryonic muscle development. Often, however, the embryonic tissue differentiation of small round blue cell tumors is undetectable at light microscopic level, necessitating ancillary techniques for diagnosis. These techniques historically included histochemical stains and electron microscopy, and now usually comprise immunohistochemistry and cytogenetics, and more recently molecular genetic techniques, especially reverse transcription-polymerase chain reaction (RT-PCR) and fluorescence in situ hybridization (FISH).

Genetic Factors

Epidemiologic studies of Wilms tumors found no maternal factors of note. Some paternal occupations

Table 18–1. Pediatric Small Round Blue Cell Tumors

Neuroblastoma
Rhabdomyosarcoma
Lymphoma
Ewing sarcoma/primitive neuroectodermal tumor (PNET)
Desmoplastic small cell tumor (DSCT)
Melanotic neuroectodermal tumor
Mesenchymal chondrosarcoma
Rhabdoid tumor
Germ cell tumors
Organ-specific blastomas
Wilms tumor (nephroblastoma)
Hepatoblastoma
Sialoblastoma
Pancreatoblastoma
Pleuropulmonary blastoma

appeared to place offspring at risk,[4] raising speculation on the relationship of this association with the well-described phenomenon of genetic imprinting in Wilms tumor genes.[5] There is no doubt that certain inherited conditions, such as Beckwith-Wiedemann syndrome,[6] Li-Fraumeni syndrome, and neurofibromatosis 1[7] place one at increased risk for small cell tumors such as rhabdomyosarcoma.

The discovery of genetic and oncoviral factors in small round cell tumorigenesis has implicated a number of acquired gene rearrangements and epigenetic lesions in the causation of these diseases. Foremost are translocations, in which gene fusion products alter transcription control leading to unrestrained cellular proliferation. Perhaps the best known is the t(11;22)(q24;q12), which fuses the *FLI1* proto-oncogene with the *EWS* gene and creates a chimeric protein that exhibits abnormal binding to DNA and leads to tumor induction.[8] Indeed, it was the discovery of this cytogenetic aberration that led to subsequent discoveries proving two morphologically disparate lesions, Ewing sarcoma and PNETs, to be biologically and clinical identical neoplasms.[9] These translocations are not only a basis for a disease mechanism, but they also serve as diagnostic markers.

Gene deletions that predispose to embryonal cancers include those of the *APC* gene, which is associated with hepatoblastoma,[10] the *patched* gene, which is associated with medulloblastoma,[11] and the *TP53* gene, which is associated with rhabdomyosarcoma.[12] These all may represent acquired mutations in the Knudson-Strong "two-hit" hypothesis,[13] or they may occur as a constitutional lesion, as with polyposis coli, basal cell-nevus syndrome, or Li-Fraumeni syndrome, respectively.[14]

Our persistent failure to isolate a single embryonal rhabdomyosarcoma-associated locus, as well as a single locus responsible for Beckwith-Wiedemann syndrome,[15] leads one to suspect that epigenetic mechanisms may be responsible for some of these tumors. Epigenetic mechanisms produce alterations of the DNA sequence without mutation, and they are responsible for diverse biologic phenomena such as imprinting, X-inactivation, and aging.[16,17] Recent reports of methylation alterations in rhabdomyosarcoma genes[18] furnish evidence that epigenetic aberrations are associated with these tumors.

Ewing Sarcoma Family of Tumors

History

Skeletal tumors of adolescents and young adults, now known as Ewing sarcoma, were initially named by James Ewing as endothelioma of bone. Arthur Purdy Stout reported a sarcoma of the ulnar nerve, which he termed a peripheral neuroepithelioma. Although a similar age group was affected, these tumors differed in their histologic appearance and site of origin; Ewing's endothelioma was an undifferentiated small cell tumor of bones whose histogenesis was obscure, and Stout's peripheral neuroepithelioma was a soft tissue lesion that displayed definite neural characteristics similar to those of neuroblastomas as described James Homer Wright. Bone pathologists agreed that the Ewing sarcoma existed, but there was debate as to whether it was truly a primary lesion or a metastasis from an undiscovered adrenal neuroblastoma. A key observation came from Stout, who noted that Ewing sarcomas at times appeared to have vague neural features, such as he had described for the peripheral neuroepithelioma (for reviews, see Dehner[19] and Yunis[20]).

By the 1960s, the question of whether Ewing sarcoma was a primary or metastatic lesion was resolved, but the histogenesis of the lesion remained obscure. Besides Stout's suggestion that these were neural lesions, previous and subsequent authors hypothesized that these were of hematopoietic, mesenchymal, and other origins.[20] Proof of any of these hypotheses was lacking. Then, in the 1970s, several key reports appeared of a soft tissue lesion having morphologic features similar to Ewing sarcoma.[21,22] These tumors also appeared in young adults and were composed of sheets of primitive small cells. By the 1970s, ultrastructural studies showed that both the skeletal[23] and extraskeletal[24] forms of Ewing sarcoma sometimes contained neural organelles.

Reports of soft tissue lesions resembling Stout's peripheral neuroepithelioma, known as PNETs,[25] included the study by Askin and colleagues of a series of tumors that arose in the chest wall of adolescents and young adults.[26] In the early 1980s, Jaffe and others reported PNETs of bone and demonstrated neural proteins by immunohistochemistry.[27] At this juncture, there appeared to be two separate entities, PNET and Ewing sarcoma, that could arise within either bone or soft tissue, although the former appeared more common in soft tissue and the latter in bone.

Cytogenetic studies showed that Ewing sarcoma, Askin tumor, and PNET contained a common karyotypic change: a translocation between the long arms of chromosomes 11 and 22, known as the t(11;22)(q24;q12).[28,29] Other methods later confirmed that the majority of these neoplasms had the same chromosomal abnormality showing genetic identity of these morphologically dissimilar lesions.[30,31]

Cavazzana and coworkers[32] then demonstrated that neural differentiation could be induced in vitro in Ewing sarcoma cells, which began sprouting neurites similar to those described by Murray and Stout in peripheral neuroepithelioma cultures.[33] Cavazzana and colleagues demonstrated expression of neural proteins indicative of neural differentiation, a finding subsequently verified by others. These experiments showed that Ewing sarcoma and PNET were closely related, if not the same entity, now known as the Ewing sarcoma family of tumors.[34]

Clinical Features

The Ewing sarcoma family of tumors primarily arises in adolescents and young adults, and occasionally occurs in young children and in older adults. There is a striking ethnic predilection, because the disease is distinctly uncommon in blacks.[35] Like rhabdomyosarcomas, Ewing sarcomas have a slight predilection for males.[36]

Ewing sarcoma family tumors most commonly present as bone lesions and can affect any bone in the skeleton. On the other hand, there has been increased recognition of the soft tissue lesions as a result of standardized reviews,[37] better techniques of diagnosis, and greater awareness of these tumors. Currently, Ewing sarcoma family of tumors is the second most common soft tissue malignancy in children and adolescents, following rhabdomyosarcoma. For example, in the Kiel Pediatric Tumor Series, comprised of 1687 childhood sarcomas, 45% of cases were rhabdomyosarcomas and 23% were PNETs or extraosseous Ewing sarcomas.[38]

Geographic predilection for Ewing sarcoma family tumors, independent of racial proclivity, has not been described. However, cluster outbreaks have occurred,[39] raising the question of an infectious etiology. Familial clusters have also been reported.[40] Cases have also been described in individuals with acquired immunodeficiency syndrome,[41] again raising the possibility of infection as an initiating event. However, no infectious agent has been proven from Ewing family tumors in humans. Nevertheless, human adenovirus may induce embryonic neuroepithelial tumors resembling PNET in rodents.[42] Some investigators claim that adenovirus genes can induce the Ewing translocation,[42A] but others refute this data.[42B]

Patients affected with Ewing sarcoma family tumors may have symptoms of inflammation of the affected extremity. As a result, it is not uncommon for delay of diagnosis to occur, as physicians attempt to treat a presumably infected joint, bone, or soft tissue mass with a long course of immobilization and antibiotics. Therefore, it is important for radiologists to be able to recognize the signs of these tumors, particularly when they occur in bones. Otherwise, the symptoms are primarily those of a mass, sometimes with pathologic fracture.

A variety of anatomic locations have been described as the sites of origin for these tumors. Both axial and extremity bones can be affected, but diaphyseal tumors predominate.[43] The most common soft tissue locations are the paravertebral region, retroperitoneum, and chest wall, followed by extremities (Fig. 18–1).[44,45] Of note is the increasing number of reports of these tumors occurring as renal neoplasms,[46] and also skin tumors are being described.[47,48] Another unusual but possible location is the epidural space of both the cranium and the spine.[49] In these regions and other soft tissue sites, origin from peripheral nerves or nerve roots may occur, as with Stout's original description. This

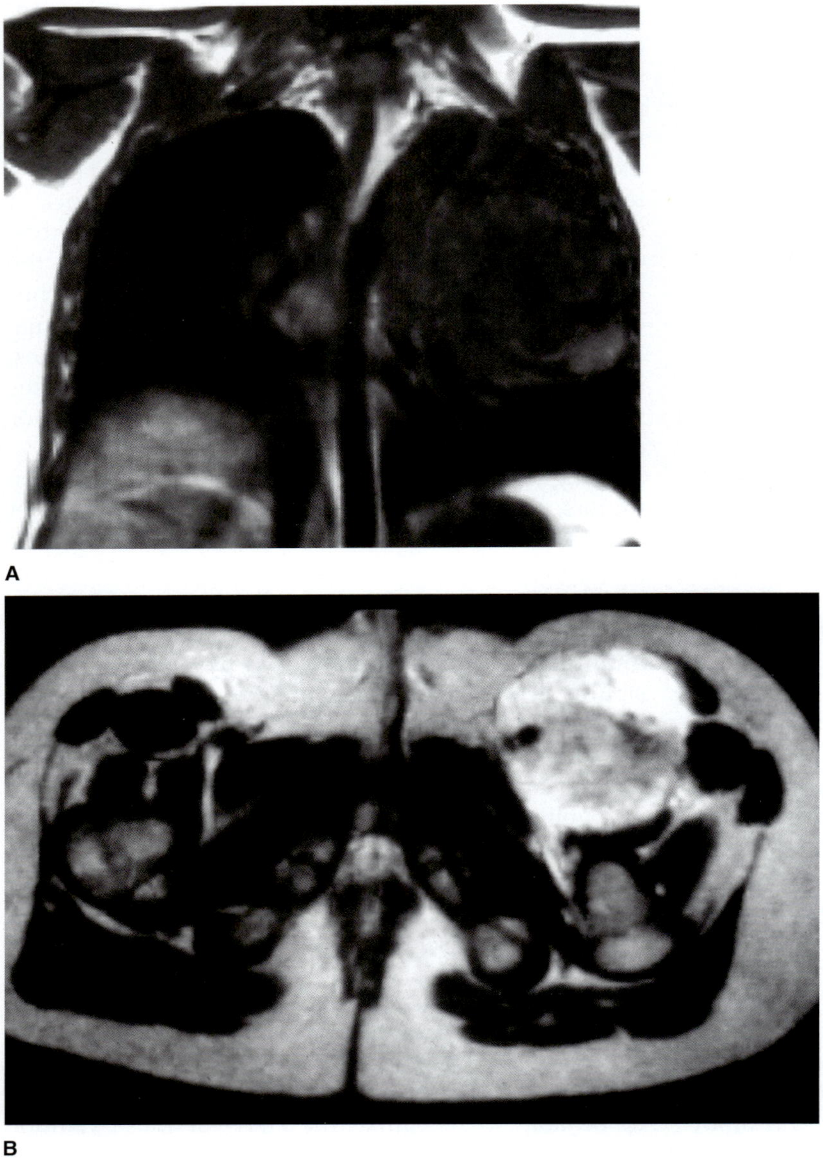

Figure 18–1. Nuclear magnetic images of Ewing sarcoma family tumors. *A,* A large chest wall mass protrudes into the left hemithorax, causing a marked mediastinal shift. *B,* An ovoid soft tissue mass arises from the muscles of the inguinal region. (Courtesy of Dr. Sue Kaste, St. Jude Children's Research Hospital, Memphis, TN.)

phenomenon creates diagnostic and biologic confusion with malignant peripheral nerve sheath tumors, as the latter may contain PNET-like foci.[50]

Radiologic studies can help to determine whether a Ewing family tumor arises in the bone or the soft tissue. Bony lesions are typically permeative, destructive lesions that may greatly resemble osteomyelitis. There is often a large, associated soft tissue mass that overshadows the bony component. Lesions arising in the kidney are usually large, invasive masses that have no radiographic distinction from other related neoplasms. Paraspinal tumors may present dumbbell-shaped masses with intraspinal invasion, reminiscent of neuroblastoma. Radiographs were used to separate the soft tissue lesions of the chest wall described by Askin[26] from bony Ewing sarcomas arising in the ribs, but this has no practical diagnostic utility today.

Gross Pathology

Ewing sarcoma family tumors are usually large, fleshy masses that may contain extensive necrosis. Bone tumors are typically permeative and destructive. They commonly show periosteal breakthrough and elevation, often with multilamination that creates an onion skin appearance on plain radiographs. Soft tissue lesions may be pseudoencapsulated. The viable portions of the soft tissue masses have a yellow-tan, fleshy appearance. The adjacent muscle may be massively edematous, creating an erroneous impression on magnetic resonance images of tissue

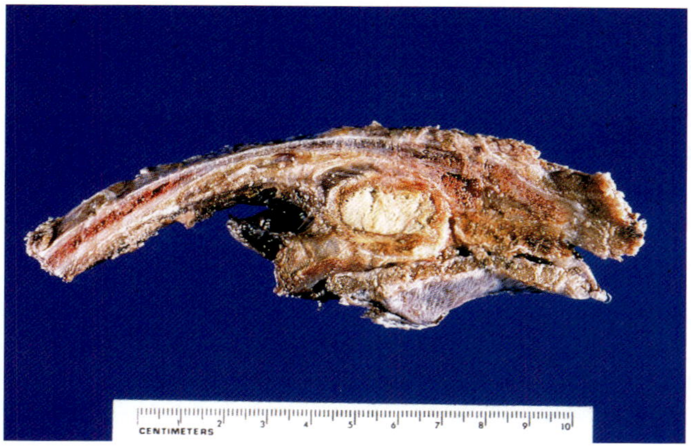

A

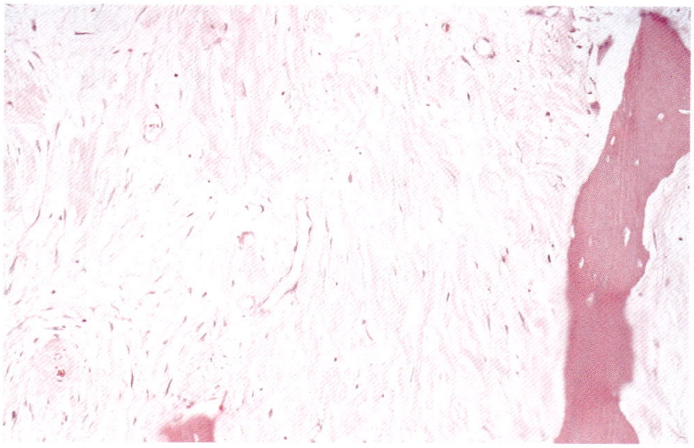

B

Figure 18–2. Ewing sarcoma posttreatment. *A,* Gross photograph of lesion involving rib and thoracic soft tissues, with marked necrosis in soft tissue lesion. *B,* Photomicrograph of bony component, illustrating loose fibrosis and absence of tumor (hematoxylin and eosin, ×25).

extension.[51] After a course of multiagent chemotherapy, there is usually dense fibrosis, hemorrhage, and necrosis, often without macroscopic evidence of tumor (Fig. 18–2). Adjacent bone marrow often loses its fatty quality and becomes more serous creating abnormal radiographic images.[52]

Microscopic Pathology

The majority of Ewing sarcoma family tumors present a relatively monotonous pattern of sheets of small blue cells with round to oval, hyperchromatic nuclei, modest amounts of cytoplasm, and inconspicuous cellular boundaries (Fig. 18–3). A number of subtle cytologic and histologic features have been used to separate these tumors into three major histologic categories: (1) typical Ewing sarcoma, (2) atypical Ewing sarcoma, and (3) peripheral PNET.[53] This distinction has been cited in a number of studies as having prognostic value, but the majority of more recent studies have failed to confirm this observation, as will be discussed later. However, familiarity with the histologic varieties of Ewing sarcoma family tumors aids in their proper diagnosis and distinction from other similar round cell neoplasms.

Typical Ewing Sarcoma

This constitutes the most common category of Ewing sarcoma family tumor. There are usually two cell types present: those with round nuclear contours, smooth, even chromatin, and clear to vacuolated cytoplasm, and those with more angulated nuclear contours, hyperchromatic chromatin, and lightly eosinophilic cytoplasm. These have been respectively termed "light" cells and "dark" cells (Fig. 18–4). The light and dark cells are often intermingled, with no

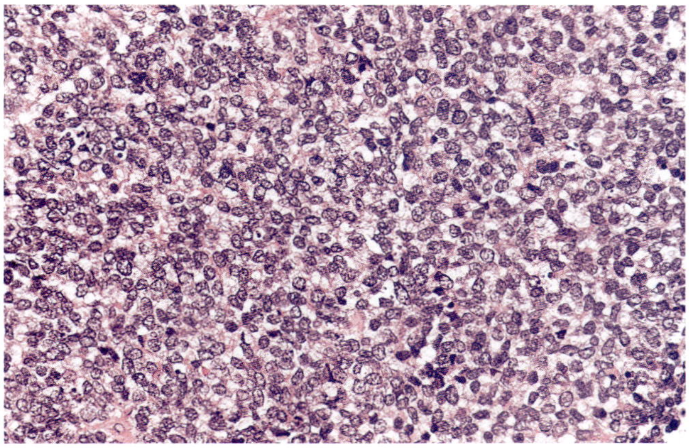

Figure 18–3. Photomicrograph of Ewing sarcoma, comprising a highly cellular sheet of relatively featureless small cells, with round, dark nuclei and inconspicuous cytoplasm (hematoxylin and eosin, ×50).

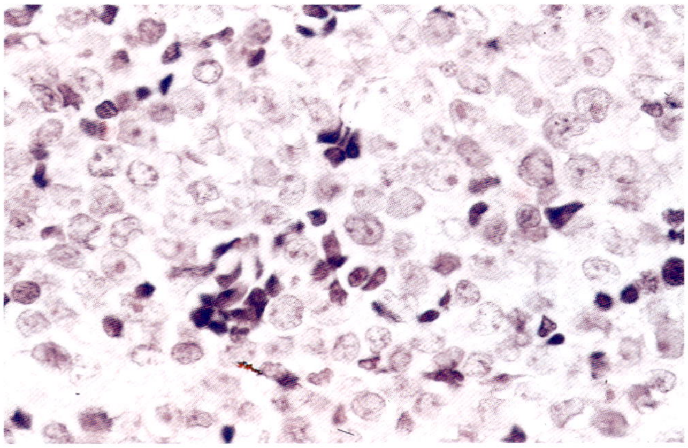

Figure 18–4. High power photomicrograph of Ewing sarcoma, illustrating mixture of cells with smooth, lightly staining nuclear chromatin ("light" cells) and darkly staining nuclear chromatin ("dark" cells) (hematoxylin and eosin, ×100).

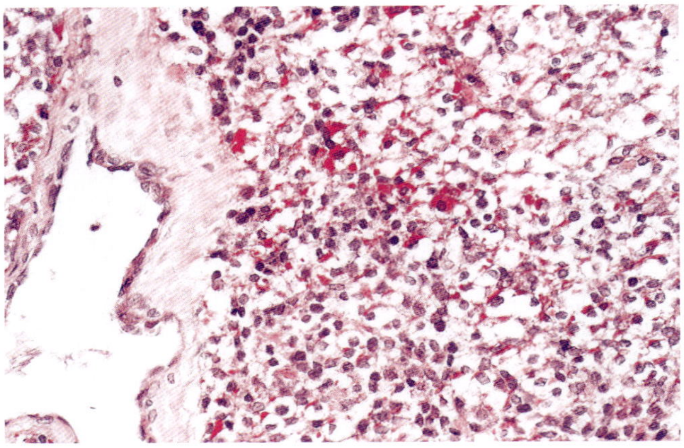

Figure 18–5. Periodic acid-Schiff stain of Ewing sarcoma, illustrating cytoplasmic positivity indicative of glycogen (PAS/hematoxylin, ×50).

discernible pattern, or the dark cells may present a streaming pattern among the lighter elements.

Neither light nor dark cells contain conspicuous nucleoli, a property that aids in the distinction of typical Ewing sarcoma from the atypical variant. A somewhat ironic feature of the typical lesions, in view of their rapid, destructive growth, is their paucity of mitotic figures, usually less than one per high-power field. The clear, vacuolated cytoplasm reflects a high content of glycogen demonstrable by periodic acid-Schiff (PAS) stain (Fig. 18–5). Although PAS staining is usually strongly positive, glycogen dissolves in water-based fixatives, such as formalin, so that only focal staining or negative results may occur. Other round cell tumors, such as rhabdomyosarcoma, germinoma, and lymphoblastic lymphoma, may also contain glycogen. Another oft-cited feature in the older literature is the paucity of fibers in reticulin stains. This feature aided the previous generation of pathologists in distinction of Ewing sarcoma from large cell lymphoma (also called reticulum cell sarcoma in the older literature). The tendency of some B-cell lymphomas to produce fibrosis is well described,[54] but this is not a uniform feature of all lymphomas, particularly the lymphoblastic ones that are easily confused with Ewing tumors.[55]

Atypical Ewing Sarcomas

These tumors have several features that distinguish them from typical tumors, as recounted in Table 18–2. Foremost among these is their pleomorphism, exhibited by irregular nuclear contours and prominent nucleoli (Fig. 18–6). These characteristics and larger cell size make large cell lymphoma a diagnostic consideration. Some cases display a nodular pattern on low-power examination, reminiscent of alveolar rhabdomyosarcoma or neuroendocrine tumors (Fig. 18–7). Despite their worrisome features, atypical Ewing sarcomas are similar to typical lesions in clinical behavior.[56] However, they tend to exhibit nascent neural differentiation, as shown by neuron-specific enolase (NSE) positivity and ultrastructural characteristics.[53] For this reason, they may be considered the "missing link" between Ewing sarcoma and PNET. In Intergroup Rhabdomyosarcoma Study publications, typical and atypical forms of Ewing sarcoma were termed type 1 and type 2 extraosseous Ewing sarcomas, respectively.[37]

Peripheral PNETs

These tumors are the differentiated form of Ewing sarcoma family tumors, and Homer Wright rosettes comprise the major light microscopic criterion for their recognition (see Table 18–2). Homer Wright

Table 18–2. Distinguishing Features of Ewing Sarcoma Family Tumors

Feature	Typical	Atypical	PNET
Nuclear size	Small (roughly the size of histiocytes)	Large (larger than histiocytes)	Small or large
Mitotic index	Low (<1/400×field)	High (>1/400×field)	Generally high
Nuclear contours	Regular	Irregular	Variable
Rosettes	No	No	Yes
Nucleoli	Inconspicuous	Prominent	Prominent
NSE positivity	Negative	Positive	Positive, along with at least one other neural marker
Electron microscopic features	No differentiation; pools of glycogen; scattered free ribosomes; few other organelles	Blunt processes, increased numbers of organelles, e.g., mitochondria	Well-defined dendritic processes, microtubules, neurosecretory granules

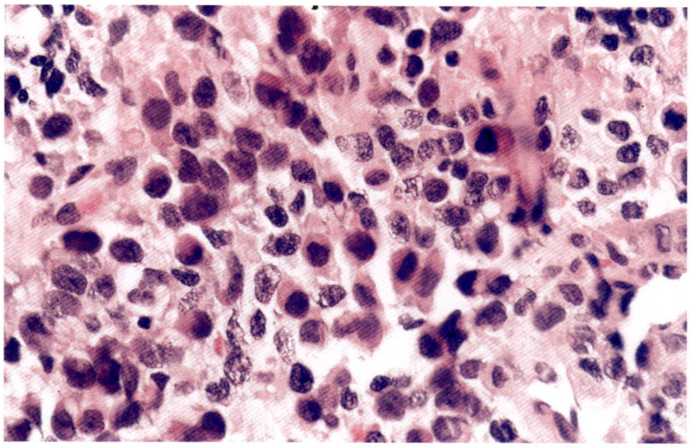

Figure 18–6. Atypical Ewing sarcoma. The tumor cells display larger size, greater nuclear variability, and occasionally prominent nucleoli (hematoxylin and eosin, ×100).

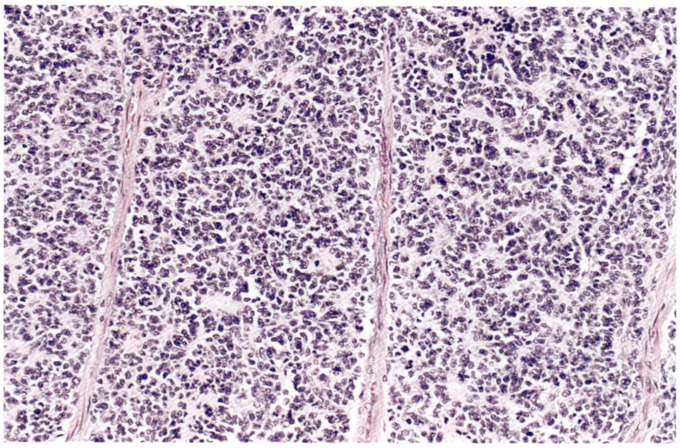

Figure 18–8. PNET, containing numerous, conspicuous Homer Wright rosettes (hematoxylin and eosin, ×50).

rosettes should be easily recognizable, with a lightly eosinophilic, fibrillary core surrounded by a circular wreath of round to oval nuclei (Fig. 18–8). Other features that may be apparent include a "lobular" pattern reminiscent of alveolar rhabdomyosarcoma (see Fig. 18–7),[36] a pericytomatous pattern resembling neuroectodermal or pericytic tumors, and a spindle cell pattern recapitulating nerve sheath lesions (Fig. 18–9).[57] In rare tumors, ganglionic differentiation may be seen and can be strikingly similar to ganglioneuroma (Fig. 18–9).[58] In fact, the range of potential differentiation shown by PNETs parallels that of neural crest cells, and in the case of ectomesenchymoma it even includes mesenchymal derivatives. Ectomesenchymoma most typically comprises PNET and rhabdomyosarcoma-like elements, replete with rhabdomyoblasts and rosettes.[59–60] Thus, the phenotypic range of PNET is surprisingly broad.[61]

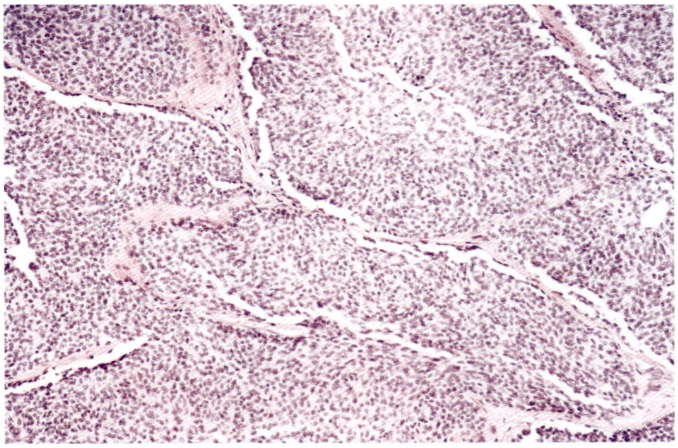

Figure 18–7. Atypical Ewing sarcoma. On low-power examination, this lesion contains lobules of tumor cells invested by a fine fibrovascular stroma, creating a nodular pattern (hematoxylin and eosin, ×25).

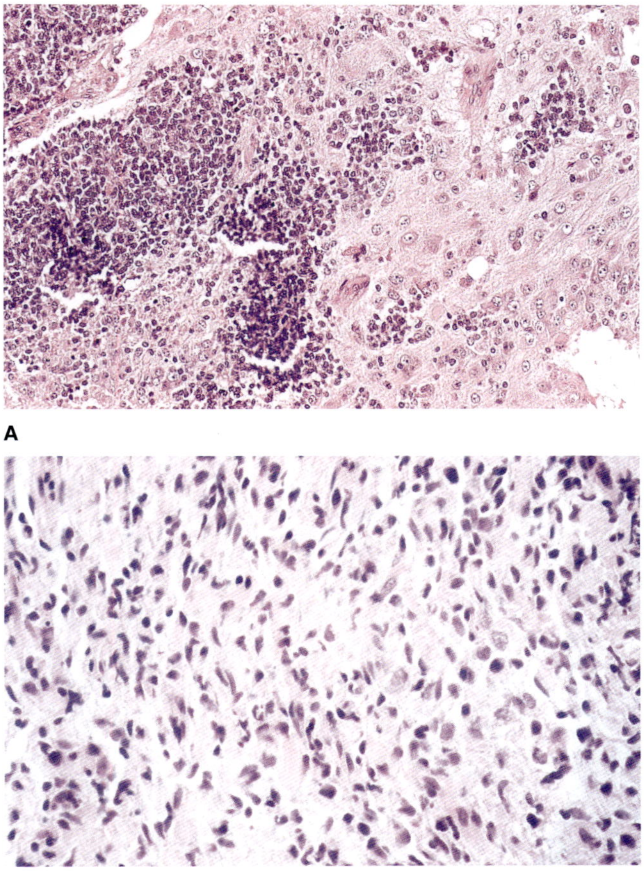

A

B

Figure 18–9. Unusual patterns in peripheral PNET. *A,* An anterior chest wall lesion contains an admixture of primitive cells and differentiated ganglionic cells (hematoxylin and eosin, ×50). *B,* A *FLI1;EWS*–positive tumor composed of spindle cells is reminiscent of malignant peripheral nerve sheath tumor (hematoxylin and eosin, ×50).

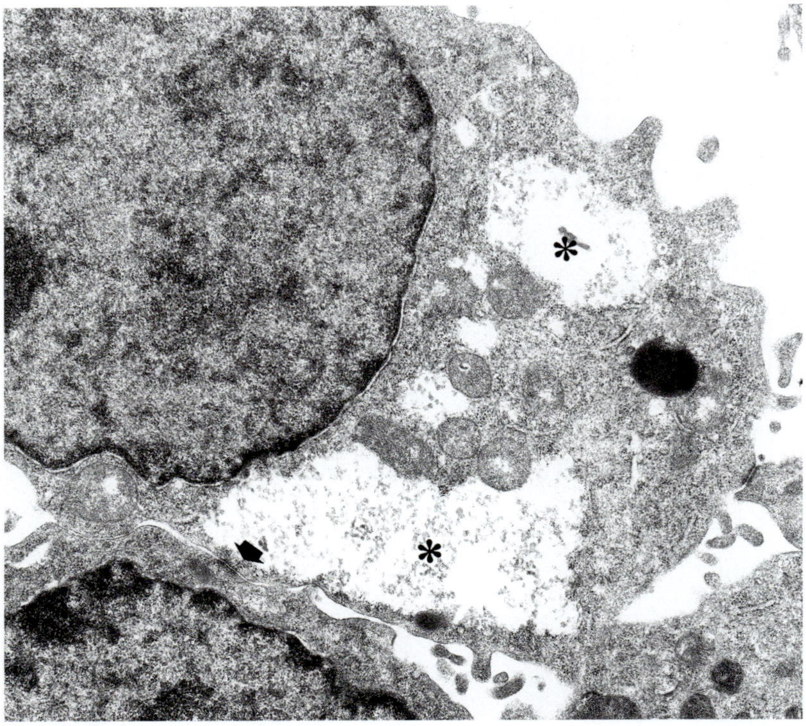

Figure 18–10. Electron micrograph of Ewing sarcoma cell. There is a dearth of cytoplasmic organelles, but pools of cytoplasmic glycogen *(asterisks)* are prominent. Note the simple intercellular junction *(arrow)* ×13,000.

Electron Microscopy

Typical Ewing sarcoma ultrastructurally displays a dearth of cytoplasmic organelles, principally free ribosomes, occasional mitochondria, and short profiles of endoplasmic reticulum. The presence of primitive intercellular junctions of the zonula occludens type helps to differentiate this tumor from lymphoma.[62] The most striking feature is the prominence of cytoplasmic pools of β-glycogen, which may be recognizable only as irregular electron-lucent zones in poorly preserved cells (Fig. 18–10). However, other primitive tumors, such as rhabdomyosarcoma, lymphoblastic lymphoma, and neuroblastoma may also be glycogen-rich.[63]

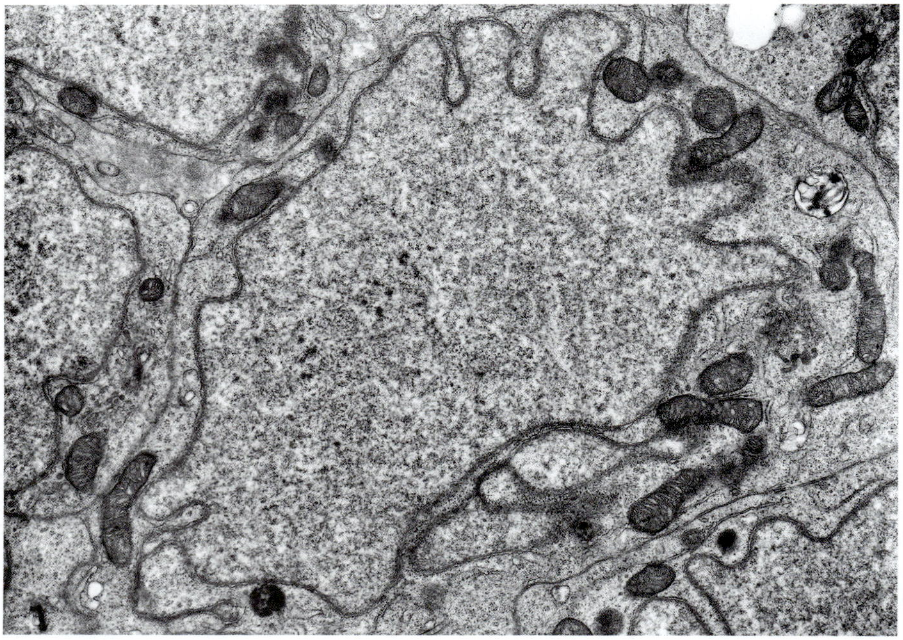

Figure 18–11. Electron micrograph of atypical Ewing sarcoma. Irregularities of the nuclear and cytoplasmic membranes are prominent, with formation of blunt processes, and there are increased numbers of organelles (see Fig. 18–10) (×7000). (Courtesy of Ms. Cindy Hastings and Dr. Francine Tryka, University of Arkansas for Medical Sciences, Little Rock, AR.)

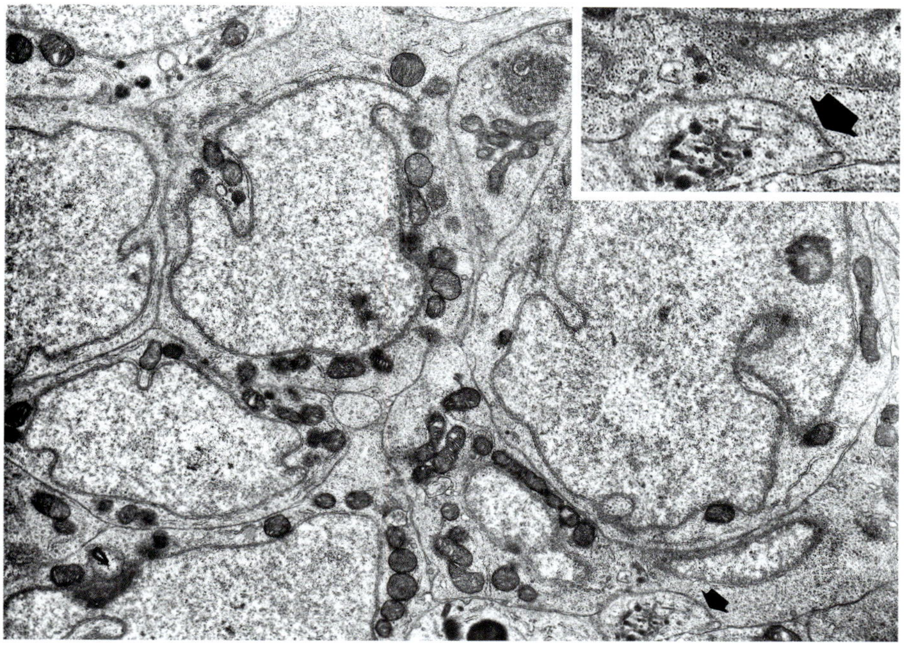

Figure 18–12. Electron micrograph of PNET. Besides the features noted in Figure 18–11, a cytoplasmic process *(arrow, inset)* contains somewhat pleomorphic neurosecretory granules (×4400). (Courtesy of Ms. Cindy Hastings and Dr. Francine Tryka, University of Arkansas for Medical Sciences, Little Rock, AR.)

Atypical Ewing sarcoma shows greater cytoplasmic diversity. There may be clusters of mitochondria and globoid concentrations of intermediate filaments akin to those in rhabdoid tumor.[53,62] Blunted elongations of the cellular periphery exemplifies the submicroscopic boundary between atypical Ewing sarcoma and PNET (Fig. 18–11).[53]

The ultrastructural diagnosis of PNET requires intertwining bundles of dendritic processes with discrete neurosecretory granules (Fig. 18–12). These granules should contain a central dense core surrounded by an electron-lucent halo wrapped in a trilaminar membrane. They are most commonly found in the cell processes comprising the central portions of Homer Wright rosettes. Primary lysosomes may be mistaken for neurosecretory granules, but they more typically lie within the perikaryon, often near Golgi apparatus, and intermingle with phagolysosomes. The neurosecretory granules of PNETs may be pleomorphic and dumbbell-shaped (Fig. 18–12), creating the possibility of confusion.[53] Ultrastructural histochemical identification of neurosecretory granules by the uranaffin reaction may help in the distinction.[64]

Immunohistochemistry

Immunohistochemical features of the Ewing sarcoma family are listed on Table 18–3. For a long time, the only positive marker of note was vimentin, which is common not only in mesenchymal tumors but also in epithelial lesions.[65] Concomitantly, PNET was recognized as exhibiting an

Table 18–3. Immunohistochemical Markers of Ewing Family Tumors

Marker	Comment
β_2-microglobulin	Seen in PNET; not seen in neuroblastoma
CD57 (Leu7)	Seen in PNET and some atypical Ewing sarcomas
CD99	Characteristic of all Ewing sarcoma family tumors, but may be negative in unusual examples
Chromogranin	Uncommon in PNET; more typical of neuroblastoma
Cytokeratin	Low molecular weight keratins (e.g., as stained with CAM5.2) often seen with Ewing sarcoma; occasional strong positivity in PNET
Desmin	Rare but occasionally seen in PNET, more typical of ectomesenchymoma
FLI1	Characteristic of all Ewing sarcoma family tumors
NSE	More frequent in atypical Ewing sarcoma; usual in PNET
Synaptophysin	More frequent in PNET; occasional in atypical Ewing sarcoma
Vimentin	Characteristic of typical Ewing sarcoma

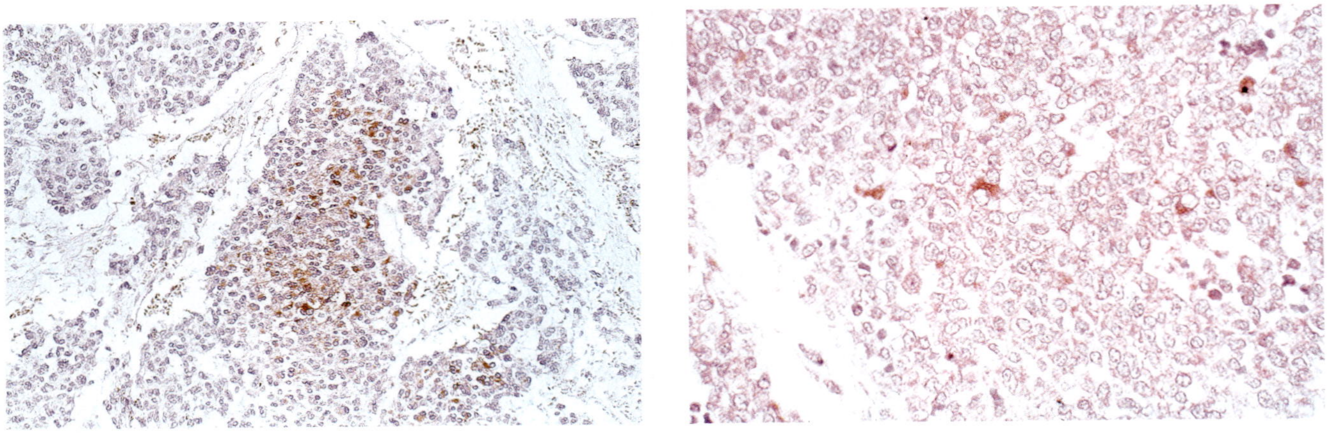

A B

Figure 18–13. Immunohistochemical evidence of neural differentiation in Ewing sarcoma, with cytoplasmic staining for NSE *(A)* and synaptophysin *(B)*. (Avidin-biotin-complex method with hematoxylin counterstain; *A*, anti-NSE, ×50; *B*, antisynaptophysin, ×50).

immunostaining profile that largely paralleled that of other neural tumors, such as neuroblastoma.[66] With the description of PNETs of bone,[27] more studies of the neural phenotypic profile of Ewing sarcomas were undertaken, culminating in the observation that NSE and even CD57 (Leu7) staining of these tumors was not uncommon in the entire group (Fig. 18–13).[67] Stains of low-molecular-weight keratins and desmosomal proteins were positive in a surprising number of cases,[68,69] paralleling the primitive junctions and rare tonofilaments seen with electron microscopy (Fig. 18–14). The epithelial nature of some Ewing sarcoma family tumors has been underscored by description of cases that strongly resemble adamantinoma.[70]

The greatest advance to date in the immunohistochemical characterization of Ewing sarcoma family tumors has been their reactivity for CD99 (or MIC2) antigen (Fig. 18–15).[71] CD99 is the protein product of a pseudoautosomal gene present on both the X and Y chromosomes. It decreases proliferation of both Ewing sarcoma cells and thymocytes by a negative action on insulin-like growth factor-I.[72] As recognized by monoclonal antibody clones O13, HBA71, and 12E7, CD99 was originally discovered in immunologic studies of T-cell leukemia,[73] and it was subsequently found to mark the great majority of both typical Ewing sarcomas and PNETs.[74,75] It is a sensitive marker positive in over 95% of these tumors. However, CD99 is not specific, as it has been

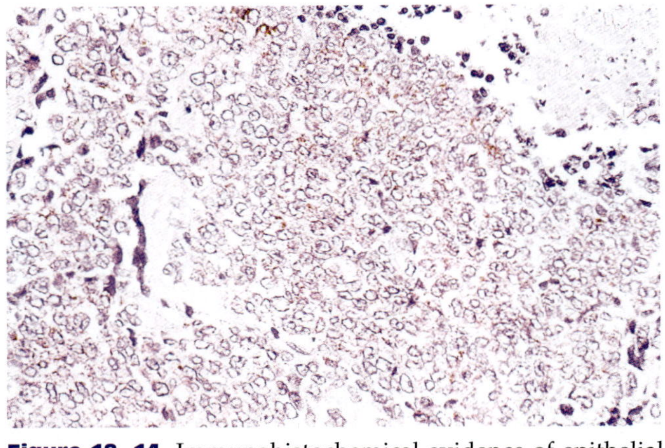

Figure 18–14. Immunohistochemical evidence of epithelial differentiation in Ewing sarcoma, with weak, patchy cytokeratin positivity (avidin-biotin-complex method with hematoxylin counterstain, anticytokeratin clone CAM5.2, ×50).

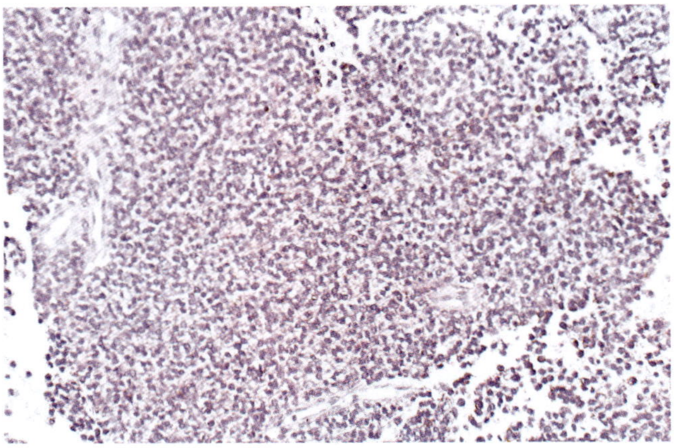

Figure 18–15. Ewing sarcoma with immunostain positivity for CD99. There is weak but diffuse membranous staining (Avidin-biotin-complex method with hematoxylin counterstain, anti-CD99 clone HBA71, ×25).

reported in rhabdomyosarcoma, synovial sarcoma, small cell carcinoma, sex cord tumors, and a variety of other cancers.[74] It is also positive in lymphoblastic lymphoma. Lymphoblastic lymphomas, which can arise in bone, may show little or no reactivity to CD45 (leukocyte common antigen) and strong staining with CD99, creating a diagnostic dilemma.[76,77] It is thus prudent to use CD99 with a panel of lymphoid markers, such as CD3, terminal deoxynucleotidyl transferase (TdT), or CD43. On the other hand, CD99 has not been reported to date in neuroblastomas, so that it remains a useful marker in their distinction from PNETs.[74,78] Conversely, the neural cell adhesion molecule (NCAM) is usually negative in Ewing sarcomas and positive in neuroblastoma.[79–81]

Rare desmin positivity of PNETs creates potential confusion with rhabdomyosarcoma.[82] Some PNET-like tumors, however, do contain myogenous elements and are termed ectomesenchymomas, as mentioned previously (Fig. 18–16). Ectomesenchymomas contain a myogenic component recognizable by light microscopy or electron microscopy, in addition to the neural component.[59–60] Their histogenesis is currently speculative, but the myogenic potential of the neural crest has been documented.[83] Abnormal transcriptional signals resulting from helix-loop-helix protein heterodimers[84] might also be responsible. Ectomesenchymomas are currently treated as rhabdomyosarcomas by the Intergroup Rhabdomyosarcoma Study Group, and their clinical behavior seems to be related to the histologic variety of rhabdomyosarcoma that comprises the myogenic component.[59A] Genetic studies (see following section) have offered us a new immunostain marker for the Ewing sarcoma family. FLI1, which forms part of the usual gene fusion, is expressed by all members of this group. Like CD99, some lymphomas are also positive for FLI1 and it also stains normal endothelium.[85]

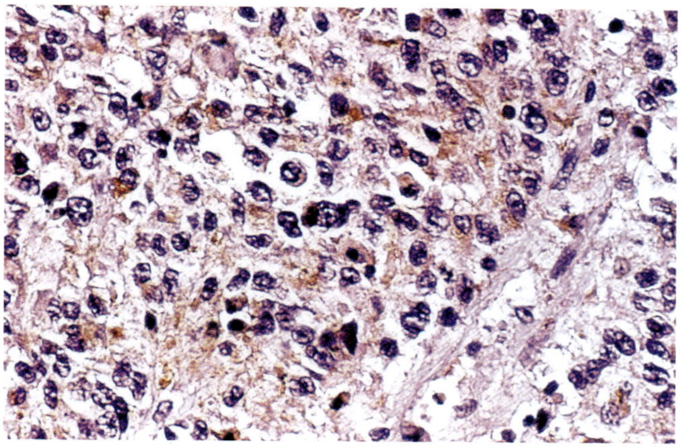

A

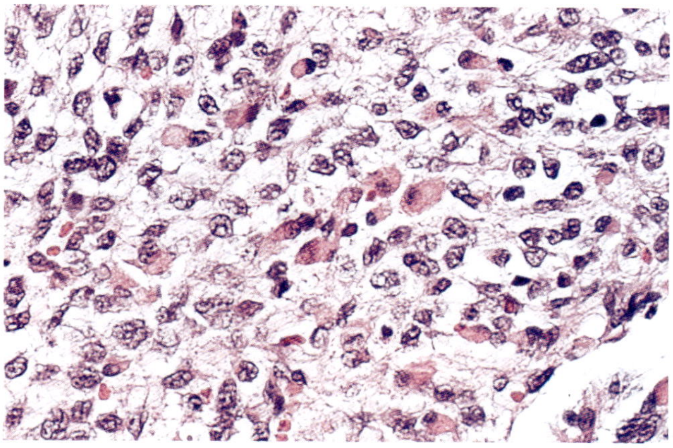

B

Figure 18–16. Ectomesenchymoma. There is a mixture of neural elements, as evidenced by synaptophysin-positive fibrillary stroma *(A)*, and myogenous elements, evidenced by scattered rhabdomyoblasts *(B)* (*A*, avidin-biotin-complex method with hematoxylin counterstain, ×100; *B*, hematoxylin and eosin, ×100).

Genetics

Cytogenetic studies typically reveal a reciprocal translocation between chromosomes 11 and 22, the t(11;22)(q24;q12) (Fig. 18–17). This karyotypic aberration has been found in the entire morphologic spectrum of typical Ewing sarcomas, atypical Ewing sarcomas, Askin tumors, and PNETs,[9] forming a theoretic basis for relatedness of these lesions.[34,86] Subsequent analyses have revealed additional cytogenetic abnormalities, such as the der(16)t(1;16)(q21;q13)[87] and trisomy 8 and 12 (Fig. 18–17),[88,89] in both Ewing sarcomas and PNETs, but these are not a consistent feature and appear to represent secondary events.[90,91] Frequency of their detection ranges from around 40% by karyotyping and FISH[88] to around 75% by comparative genomic hybridization.[91]

The t(11;22)(q24;q12) in Ewing sarcoma represents a fusion between the *FLI1* gene, located on chromosome 11q, and the *EWS* gene on chromosome 22q12 (Fig. 18–18).[92] The *FLI1* gene is the human homologue of a proto-oncogene whose murine counterpart produces erythroleukemia, and the *EWS* (from *EW*ing *S*arcoma) gene is a newly discovered locus. *FLI1* contains sequences identifying it as an ETS family gene, distinguished by production of a highly conserved DNA-binding region known as the Ets domain. On the EWS protein is an RNA-binding region that is replaced by the FLI1 DNA-binding region resulting in abnormal transcription control.[93] The chimeric transcript can produce tumors in mice and transform cultured cells. Because its antisense RNA represses this tumorigenicity,[94] the abnormal

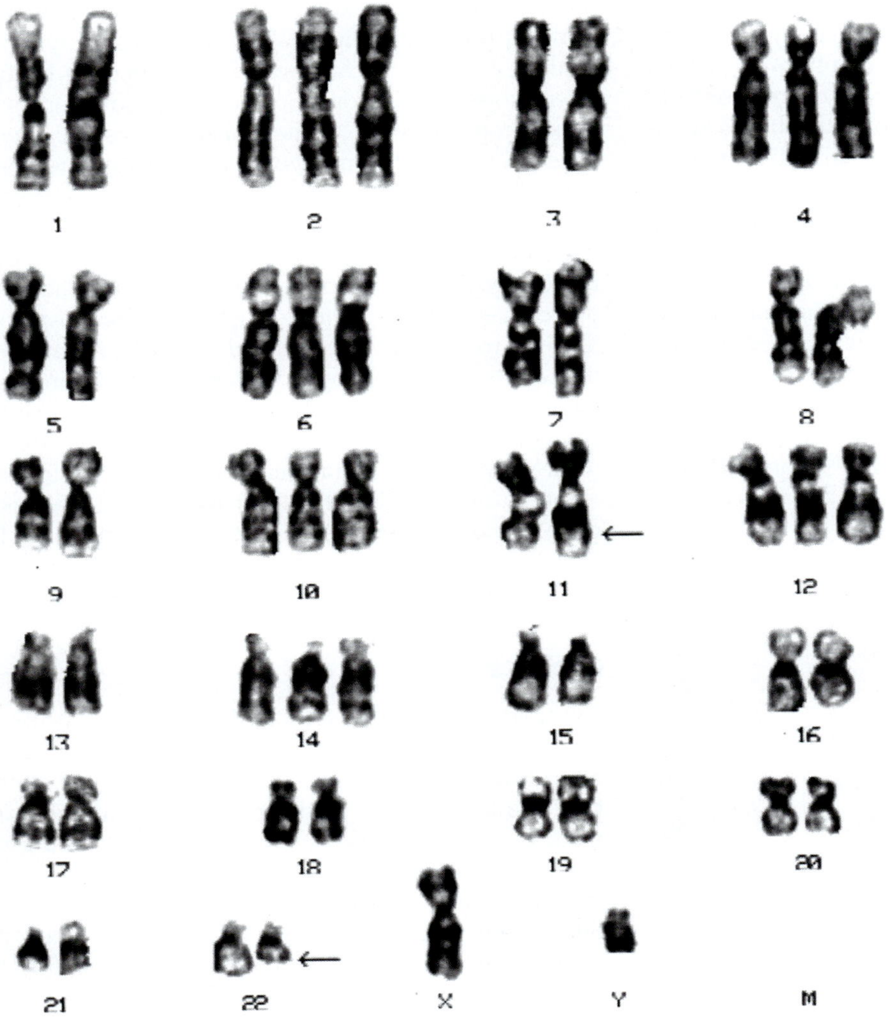

Figure 18–17. Karyotype of Ewing sarcoma. There is a reciprocal translocation involving the long arms of chromosomes 11 and 22 *(arrow)*. Note also the multiple trisomies, including trisomy 12, a common secondary change. (Courtesy of Mr. Charles Swanson and Dr. Jeff Sawyer, Arkansas Children's Hospital, Little Rock, AR.)

transcript appears to be the key biologic event in the tumorigenesis of Ewing sarcoma.

Other ETS family genes may produce morphologically identical lesions. The first "alternate partner" discovered for the *EWS* was the *ERG* gene on chromosome 21, with an *ERG/EWS* fusion resulting from a t(21;22)(q22;q12) (Fig. 18–19).[95] About 10% of Ewing sarcoma family tumors contain this alternate translocation.[35] Like FLI1, the ERG product has an ETS motif with a similar DNA transcription region. This translocation produces a fusion product resembling the one in the FLI1/EWS fusion protein and possessing

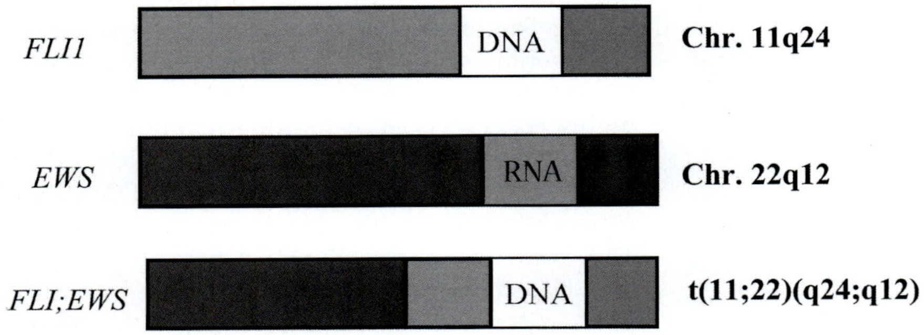

Figure 18–18. Drawing of *FLI1;EWS* genetic fusion resulting from translocation of portions of chromosome (chr) 11 and 22. Note that in the fusion gene *(lowest panel)*, a sequence on *EWS* that transcribes an RNA-binding region is replaced by one on *FLI1* that transcribes a DNA-binding region.

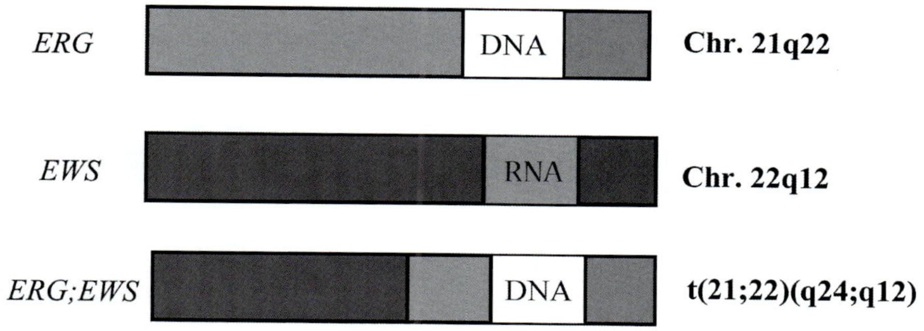

Figure 18–19. Drawing of *ERG; EWS* genetic fusion resulting from translocation of portions of chromosome (chr) 21 and 22. Like the *FLI;EWS* fusion, the *ERG;EWS* fusion *(lowest panel)* replaces a sequence transcribing an RNA-binding region on EWS with one transcribing a DNA-binding region.

matching tumorigenic properties. More recently, additional alternate translocations have been described for Ewing sarcoma family tumors, including a t(7;22) that fuses *EWS* with *ETV1*,[96] a t(2;22) that fuses *EWS* with *FEV*,[97] and a t(17;22) that fuses *EWS* with *E1AF*.[98]

Molecular genetic methods for demonstrating fusion transcripts have been developed.[99,100] Although these tests are most reliable with snap-frozen tissue, formalin-fixed material may be used with mixed results.[101] The FLI1/EWS molecule exhibits a number of different fusion points, because of so-called "combinatorial fusion."[102] Because of this variability, a relatively long sequence of complementary DNA (cDNA) is required for the PCR process to span the various breakpoints. Thus, successful RT-PCR may be problematic if only short strands of RNA are available in paraffin-embedded tissues, and the sensitivity of the assay varies according to the procedure used.[103] The extreme sensitivity of this test in fresh tissue, however, allows for detection of circulating tumor cells in peripheral blood.[104]

The variability of the *FLI1;EWS* breakpoint results in two major types of fusion proteins, termed type 1 and 2. The type of fusion protein possessed by a given Ewing tumor is related to its clinical behavior, with type 1 lesions having a better prognosis.[105] There appears to be no clinical significance to date for the alternate fusions.

Other genetic features of Ewing family sarcomas include losses of p16[106] and amplification of *MDM2* and *CDK4* genes in 12q.[107] One interesting observation, considering the neuroectodermal connection of these tumors, is gastrin-releasing peptide expression, also noted in neuroendocrine carcinomas.[108]

Prognosis and Outcome

Although initial studies showed poorer prognosis for PNETs as compared to typical Ewing sarcoma,[109] current studies based on prospective trials have failed to confirm this,[110] so that PNET is no longer considered inherently more aggressive than Ewing sarcoma. A new biologic marker suggested for aggressiveness is the presence of type 2 fusions of FLI1/EWS.[105] Another feature of aggressiveness, confirmed in several centers, is lack of responsiveness to preoperative chemotherapy, as histologically measured in resection specimens.[111,112] Secondary cytogenetic changes, such as deletions of chromosome 1p, also signify adverse tumor behavior.[90]

A variety of clinical parameters correlate with aggressive behavior. Foremost among these is the presence of metastatic disease at diagnosis.[113,114] Current trials using agents such as ifosfamide show improved survival with localized tumors but not with metastatic lesions.[114] Another prognostic parameter is tumor size, with lesions greater than 100 ml in volume having 3-year disease-free survivals of 32%, compared to that of 80% for smaller tumors.[115] Pelvic tumors show more aggressive behavior than nonpelvic lesions, perhaps because they also are often larger at diagnosis and nonresectable.[115] Other related factors are completeness of surgical excision and local tumor control.[116,117]

Differential Diagnosis

Entities that enter in the differential diagnosis of Ewing sarcoma depend on patient age, because tumors in older patients may be confused with small cell carcinoma, and lesions in younger patients may be mistaken for rhabdomyosarcoma, neuroblastoma, and Wilms tumor. Distinction of PNET from Ewing sarcoma is less of an issue than in previous years, but the presence of rosettes by light microscopy, neurosecretory granules by electron microscopy, and multiple neural proteins by immunohistochemistry defines the former.

Ancillary studies are often necessary to confirm the diagnosis of Ewing sarcoma family tumors. The most important marker from a surgical pathology standpoint is CD99, because this it is almost universally present in Ewing tumors but is negative in neuroblastomas.[78] Molecular genetic methods such as FISH or RT-PCR offer turnaround times and specificity comparable to immunohistochemistry, with occasional exceptions.[118]

Neuroblastoma

Clinical Features

Neuroblastoma and Ewing sarcoma family of tumors share a number of pathologic features, such as rosettes and primitive histology, and are sometimes lumped together as part of the PNET family.[119] One of the most distinctive differences between them is the age of presentation, which is generally below the age of 5 years in neuroblastoma, compared to the young adult and adolescent predilection of Ewing family sarcomas. In fact, neuroblastoma is the most common solid tumor of children under 1 year of age.[120] It typically presents as an abdominal mass (Fig. 18–20), although it may also arise from sympathetic ganglia of the neck, thorax, and pelvis. The adrenal gland is the most common site of origin, and neuroblastoma may rightly be considered a tumor of the sympathetic nervous system, with production of catecholamines, their precursors, their byproducts, and the enzymes responsible for their production.

Catecholamine secretion is a key diagnostic feature for neuroblastoma. Twenty-four-hour urine specimens should be tested for homovanillic acid (HVA) and vanillylmandelic acid (VMA) before or soon after excision of these tumors, because serum levels drop quickly. The ratio of the precursor molecule, HVA, to its product, VMA, correlates with the degree of tumor differentiation and survival.[121] Other hormonal substances produced by neuroblastoma, such as vasoactive intestinal polypeptide, may cause a paraneoplastic syndrome such as watery diarrhea and hypokalemia.[122]

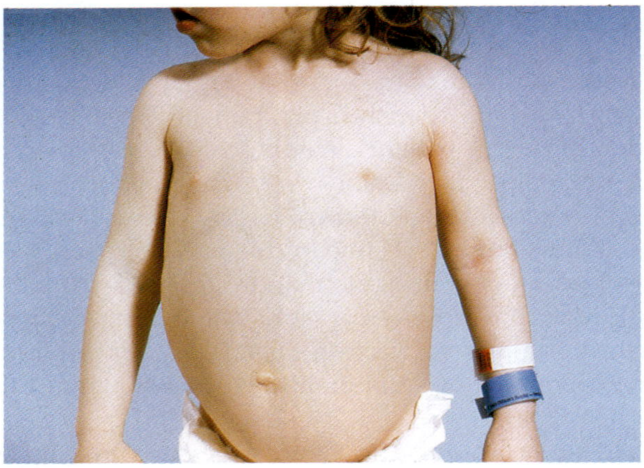

Figure 18–20. Young child with abdominal mass, later proven to be neuroblastoma.

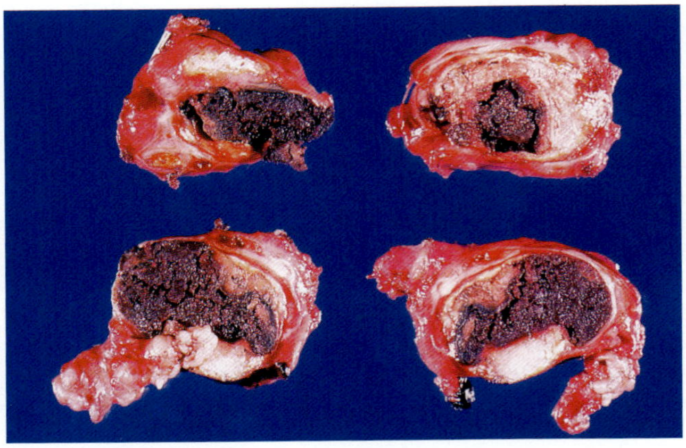

Figure 18–21. Adrenal neuroblastoma, transversely sectioned to reveal masses of bright yellow calcification and dark gray-brown hemorrhagic necrosis. This lesion was resected following combination chemotherapy.

Other paraneoplastic syndromes can result from immune phenomena. In the myoclonus-opistonus syndrome, antibodies produced against the tumor cause cerebellar ataxia and rapid eye movements. Horner syndrome, Ondine curse, and a host of other unusual clinical symptoms may also occur.[122] Maternal antibodies in pregnancy serum are capable of tumor cytolysis and possibly cause tumor regression.[123] The histologic presence of lymphocytes in excised, pretreated tumors is another manifestation of the immunogenicity of these tumors.

The clinical behavior of aggressive neuroblastoma differs distinctly from that of PNET. Neuroblastoma only rarely metastasizes to the lung, and those lesions that do have unusual features.[124] Conversely, aggressive PNETs typically exhibit pulmonary metastases. Both tumors may show bone marrow metastases, but this phenomenon is more typical of neuroblastoma. Neuroblastoma also commonly spreads to regional and even distant lymph nodes, an unusual metastatic site in Ewing family sarcomas except in widespread disease.[125]

Another key characteristic of neuroblastoma is its stippled calcification (Fig. 18–21), easily visible on abdominal radiographs. This feature may be recognizable on prenatal ultrasonography and lead to diagnosis of congenital tumors. In some countries, predominately Japan, widespread population screening using this technology has led to the diagnosis of early tumors. However, because many congenital tumors mature spontaneously, the effect this procedure has had on reducing mortality has been debatable.

The presence of metastatic disease in the bone marrow, a calcified suprarenal mass, or catecholamine secretion are assuring signs for neuroblastoma in cytologic specimens, and may obviate the need for open biopsy.[126]

Pathology—Gross and Microscopic Features

Grossly, neuroblastomas typically display a lobulated, encapsulated, ovoid surface that on sectioning is often grossly hemorrhagic and punctuated by flecks of calcification (Fig. 18–22). Geographic necrosis may obscure these features and render the diagnosis difficult on small biopsies. Paravertebral neuroblastomas may invade the intervertebral foramina and encroach on the spinal epidural space in a dumbbell fashion. In adrenal lesions, a small yellow focus of intact glandular tissue may be flattened against the fibrous capsule. After combination chemotherapy, there is often extensive posttreatment effect, with fibrosis, calcification, and necrosis (see Fig. 18–21) creating an appearance dissimilar to untreated lesions.

Microscopically, the diagnostic requirement is the presence of primitive neural cells that are identical to the migratory neural crest elements that normally invade the fetal adrenal gland. In fact, adrenal neuroblastic foci may be numerous and large at birth and may be termed "congenital neuroblastomas," but they usually involute as the glands mature.[127] Neuroblastic elements in true neuroblastomas commonly appear to float within a sea of hemorrhagic detritus and aggregate into fibrillary balls known as Homer Wright rosettes (Fig. 18–23). Homer Wright rosettes are composed of lightly eosinophilic, neurofibrillary cores surrounded by wreaths of round, hyperchromatic nuclei with coarsely granular chromatin and inconspicuous nucleoli. Neurofibrillary material may be focally abundant and form a scaffolding within which the oval nuclei are suspended. One characteristic feature is the tendency of neuroblasts to undergo varying degrees of cell maturation, characterized by the acquisition of increased cytoplasm with Nissl substance and the vacuolation of nuclei with increased prominence of nucleoli. Tumors with this feature are known as "differentiating neuroblastomas." This process continues to the point of creation of fully mature ganglion cells, indistinguishable from nonneoplastic neurons, at which point the combination of neuroblasts and mature ganglion cells is termed a *ganglioneuroblastoma* (Fig. 18–24).

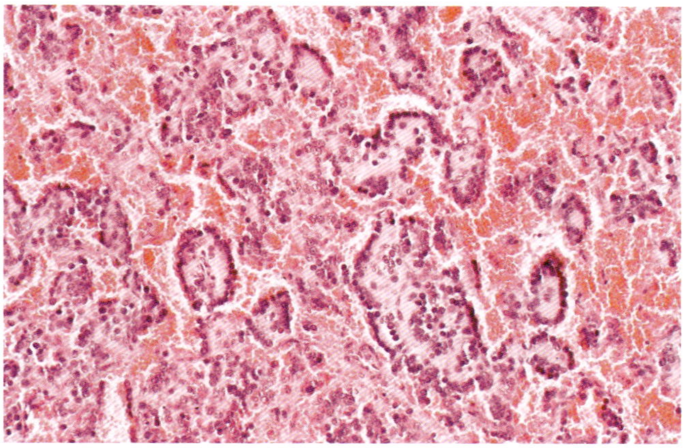

Figure 18–23. Neuroblastoma, comprising well-formed Homer Wright rosettes with fibrillary cores, floating in a sea of hemorrhage (hematoxylin and eosin, ×50).

At the fully differentiated end of the histologic spectrum lies the *ganglioneuroma,* a benign tumor comprised of mature, neoplastic ganglion cells enmeshed in a prominent spindle cell stroma derived from

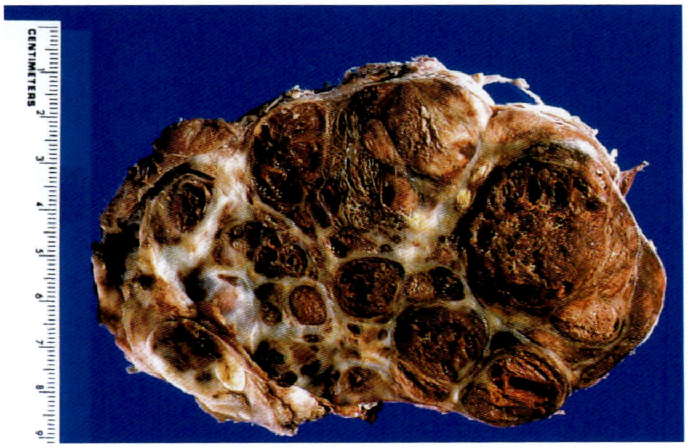

Figure 18–22. Mediastinal neuroblastoma, before treatment, composed of lobules of fleshy, hemorrhagic tissue circumscribed by a fibrous stroma.

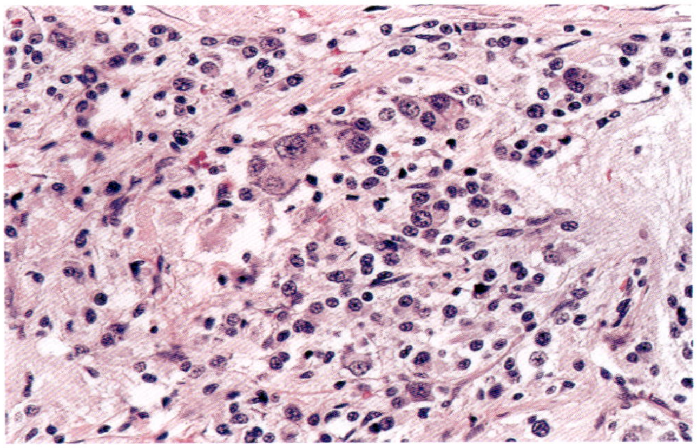

Figure 18–24. Ganglioneuroblastoma, containing mature ganglion cells in addition to immature neuroblastic elements (hematoxylin and eosin, ×50).

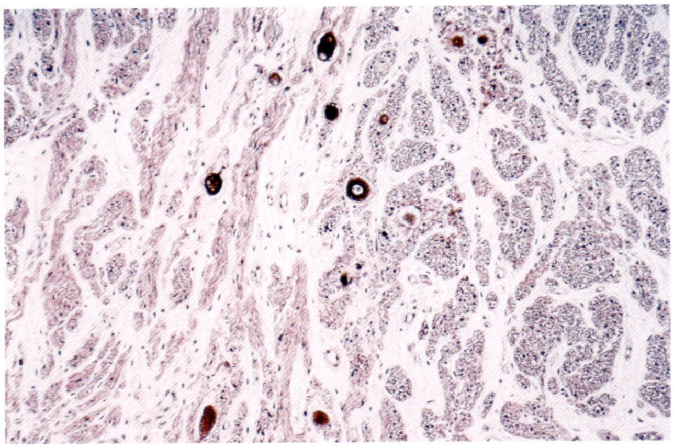

Figure 18–25. Ganglioneuroma, composed entirely of mature neural elements, including bundles of Schwann cells and strongly neurofilament-positive ganglion cells (avidin-biotin-complex method with hematoxylin counterstain and monoclonal antineurofilament protein, ×25)

Schwann cell elements (Fig. 18–25). These lesions have a whorled, fibrous cut surface rather than a hemorrhagic one (Fig. 18–26). Ganglioneuromas often arise in the posterior mediastinum rather than the abdomen. They may represent evidence of spontaneous maturation of previous neuroblastomas, a process occasionally noted in exceptionally fortunate patients, or alternatively, they may occur as metastatic, matured lesions in previously treated children.

Possible ganglioneuromas should grossly be carefully examined for hemorrhagic nodules, which denote nodular foci of residual neuroblastoma. These mixed tumors are referred to as "nodular neuroblastomas" or "composite ganglioneuroblastomas," and they are malignant lesions capable of metastatic behavior. Ganglioneuromas should also be liberally sectioned and microscopically examined for neuroblastic foci. Lesions containing a few immature cells have been termed "borderline ganglioneuroblastomas" by Joshi and coworkers,[128] but are now considered "maturing ganglioneuromas."[129]

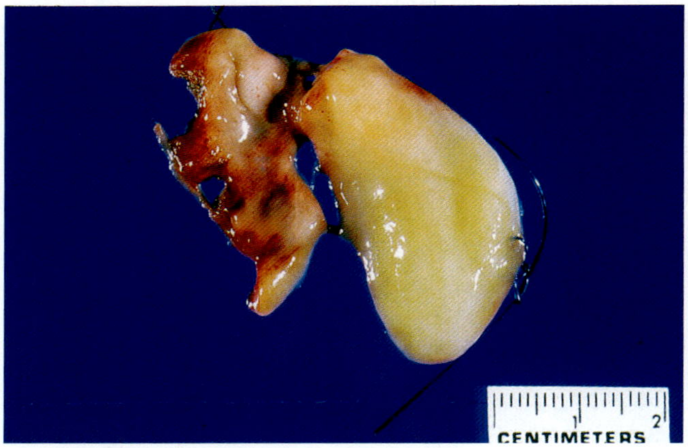

Figure 18–26. Ganglioneuroma. On cut surface, the mass has a homogeneous, pale yellow, fibrous appearance.

Shimada and colleagues have created a grading scheme for neuroblastomas known as the Shimada classification.[130] This classification is independently predictive of clinical behavior and is now used as an internationally accepted standard.[131] It is outlined in Table 18–4. Several terms used in this schema require explanation. First, the term "stroma" refers to Schwann cell elements and not neurofibrillary material, so that "stroma-rich" tumors are actually "intermixed ganglioneuroblastomas," as per the classification created by Joshi and coworkers.[128] Secondly, the mitosis/karyorrhexis index (MKI) is a numerical, semiquantitative value derived from counting the number of mitotic figures and fragmented, karyorrhectic nuclei among 5000 cells. This onerous chore can be greatly simplified by estimating the total number of cells in a ×40 objective, high-power field. Used in this manner, the Shimada classification is a reproducible and easily learned technique that is clinically useful and prognostically accurate.

Unusual histologic variants of neuroblastic tumors include "anaplastic neuroblastomas" having prominent large neoplastic cells with bizarre, hyperchromatic nuclei.[132] This finding appears to have no

Table 18–4. The International Neuroblastoma Pathology Classification (Shimada System)

Good Prognosis

Ganglioneuroblastoma, intermixed (stroma-rich) type, any age

Differentiating neuroblastomas with low MKI,* age 1.5–5 y

Undifferentiated/poorly differentiated neuroblastomas with low or intermediate MKI,* age <1.5 y

Ganglioneuroma, any age

Poor Prognosis

Ganglioneuroblastomas, nodular type, any age

Neuroblastomas with high MKI,* any age

Undifferentiated/poorly differentiated neuroblastomas, age 1.5–5 y

Neuroblastomas with intermediate MKI,* age 1.5–5 y

Neuroblastoma, any type, age >5 y

*MKI, mitosis/karyorrhexis index: low, <100/5000 cells; intermediate, 100–200/5000 cells; high, >200/5000 cells.

(From Shimada H, Ambros IM, Dehner LP, et al: The International Neuroblastoma Pathology Classification (the Shimada system). Cancer 1999;86:364.)

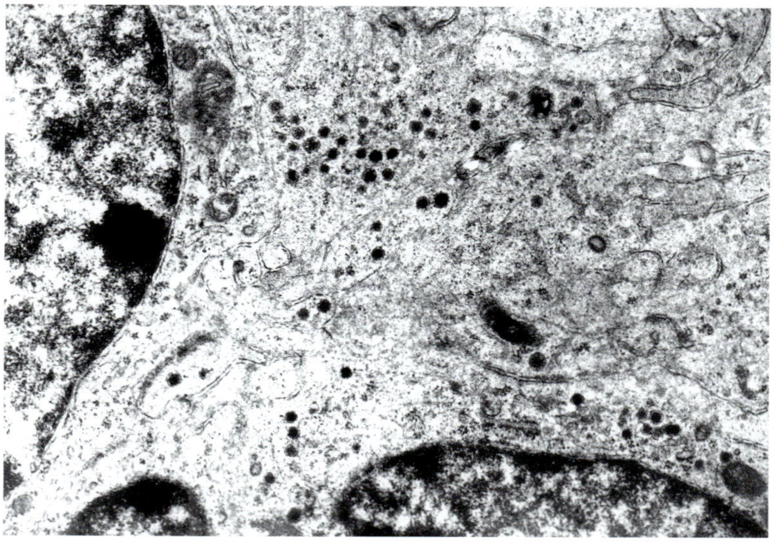

Figure 18-27. Electron micrograph of neuroblastoma containing prominent clusters of 80- to 100-nm neurosecretory granules (×25,000).

clinical significance.[128] Rhabdoid cells with abundant eosinophilic cytoplasm and hyaline inclusions may also be seen.[128] Other neural crest differentiation, particularly melanocytic[133,134] or paragangliomatous[135] may also occur. Tumors with the latter features are more accurately classified as pheochromocytomas with a prominent ganglioneuromatous component.

Ancillary Diagnostic Techniques

Neuroblastomas usually present less of a diagnostic challenge than the Ewing sarcoma family of tumors, because they tend to be more differentiated and to have a better defined clinical picture. However, undifferentiated forms may occur, older patients may be affected,[136] and paravertebral, nonadrenal primaries can broaden the differential diagnosis. In addition, extremely rare examples of PNETs contain differentiated areas similar to ganglioneuroblastoma (see preceding discussion). In nonadrenal locations and older patients, it is important to rule out PNET, using ancillary techniques, because neuroblastomas are treated differently and display a vastly dissimilar clinical behavior.

Ultrastructurally, the neural features of neuroblastomas are prominent and comprise clusters of dense core granules (Fig. 18–27), elongated, intertwining dendritic processes, neurosecretory vesicles, and parallel arrays of microtubules (Fig. 18–28). The neurofibrillary material that constitutes the cores of

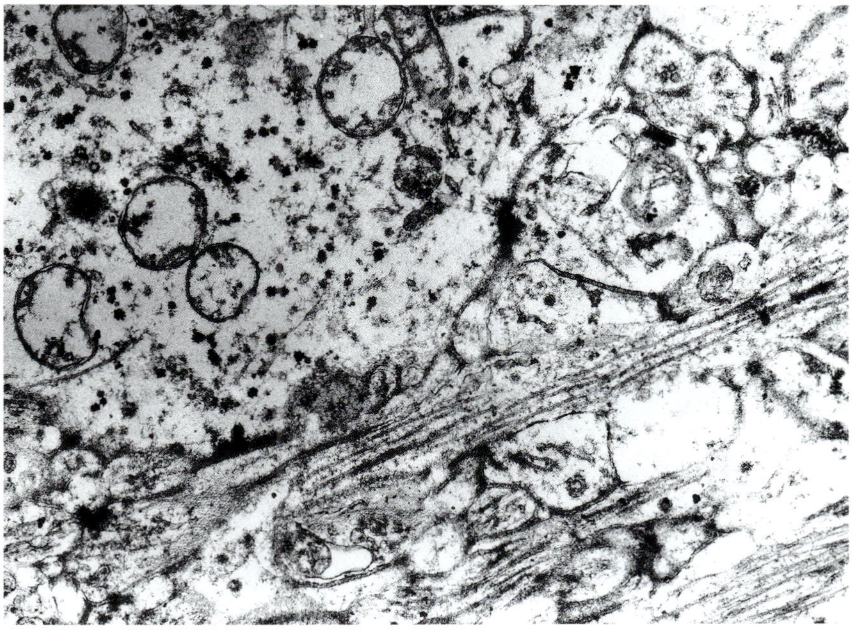

Figure 18-28. Electron micrograph of neuroblastoma containing intricate interweaving of neuritic processes and parallel arrays of microtubules (×34,000).

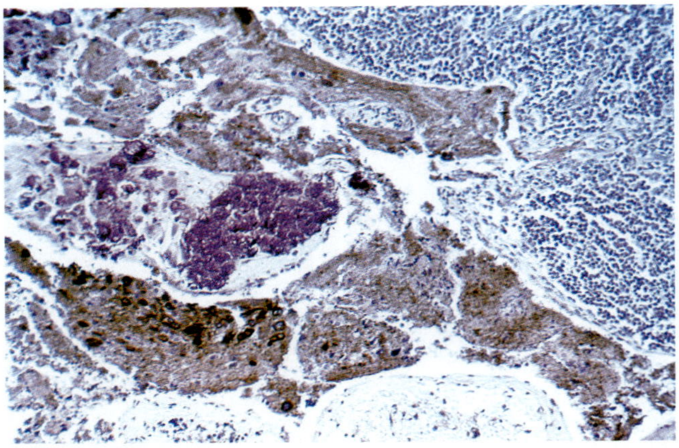

Figure 18–29. Strongly NSE-positive metastatic neuroblastoma distends the sinuses of an involved lymph node. Note the central microcalcification (avidin-biotin-complex method with hematoxylin counterstain, polyclonal anti-NSE, ×25).

rosettes is composed of intricately entwined neuritic processes (Fig. 18–28). Although PNETS also contain these structures, experienced electron microscopists note a distinction in their prominence in neuroblastomas that assists in diagnosis (see Fig. 18–12).[137]

Another key diagnostic feature separating neuroblastoma from other neural neoplasms is the presence of catecholamine secretion, as measured in pre-excisional urine specimens. A biochemical distinction is *MYCN* (or N-*myc*) expression and amplification (discussed following), typical of neuroblastoma, whereas PNETs overexpress *c-myc*.[138] However, the occasional *MYCN* amplification seen in alveolar rhabdomyosarcoma[139,140] excludes use of this phenomenon to differentiate rhabdomyoblastic tumors from neuroblastic ones.

Immunohistochemistry is often of great assistance in the diagnosis of primitive neuroblastic tumors. These lesions are typically positive for neural proteins, such as NSE (Fig. 18–29), synaptophysin, neurofilaments (see Fig. 18–25), and chromogranin, usually separating them from nonneural embryonal lesions. Unlike PNETs, they are CD99$^-$ and β_2-microglobulin negative, so that these latter stains can be extremely useful (see preceding discussion). An important observation is that although it is a sensitive marker, NSE is relatively nonspecific.[141] Other markers are also available.[141A]

Genetics

Neuroblastomas are typified by three cytogenetic abnormalities: deletions of chromosome 1, double minute (dm) chromosomes, and homogeneous staining regions (hsrs). The former alterations reflect the loss of an as yet undefined tumor suppressor gene, and the latter ones reflect amplification of the *N-myc* gene (also known as the *MYCN* gene).

Alterations of chromosome 1 in neuroblastoma (Fig. 18–30) represent the single most common cytogenetic event[142] and usually result in loss of a large segment of the short arm (1p). The addition of an

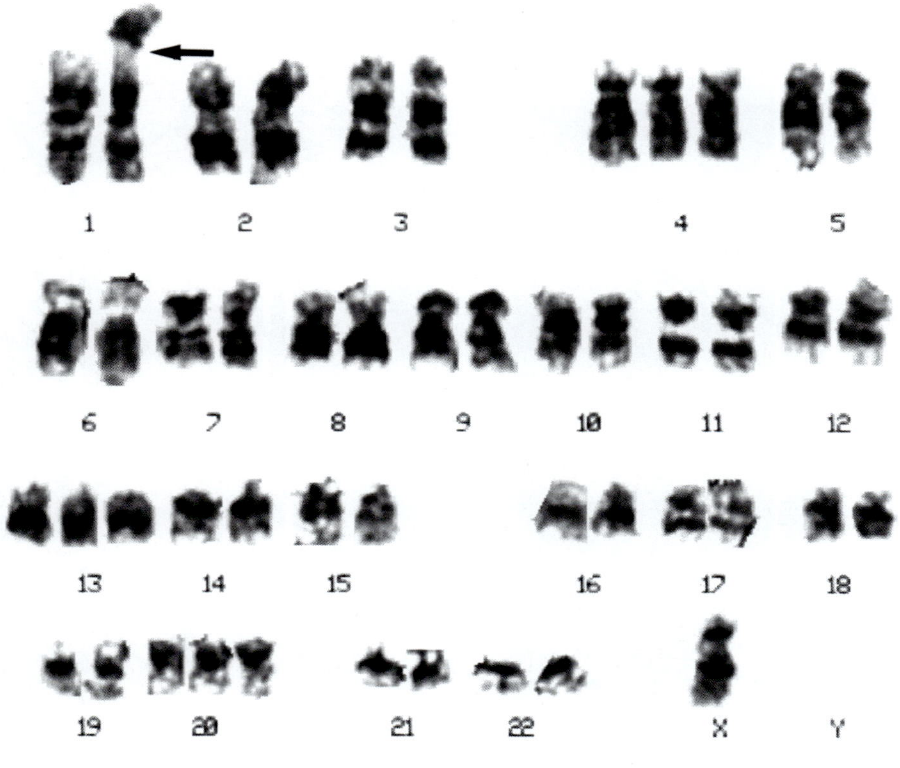

Figure 18–30. Karyotype of neuroblastoma with an unbalanced translocation affecting the distal short arm of chromosome 1 *(arrow).* Near-diploidy is also present. (Courtesy of Mr. Charles Swanson and Dr. Jeffrey Sawyer, Arkansas Children's Hospital, Little Rock, AR.)

intact chromosome 1 suppresses the tumorigenicity of neuroblastomas, indicating the tumor suppressor function of this region. A common locus affected in all tumors is a distal region of 1p including 1p36.2 and 1p36.3.[143] The exact gene responsible for the tumor suppressor function of this region remains unproven, but candidates include a p53 homologue, a CDK2 homologue, transcription factors, a transcription elongation factor, and members of the tumor necrosis family.[143] Although a strong correlation exists between the presence of losses in 1p and high-risk clinical features such as older age and N-myc amplification, it is debatable whether 1p deletions have an independent effect on outcome.[143]

The dm chromosomes are short, bipartite chromosome fragments that are separate from the major chromosomes and are usually multiple. The hsrs are uniformly staining elongations of the genome that are inserted into major chromosomes in a spanner fashion (Fig. 18–31). Both of these phenomena were noted on cytogenetic studies of neuroblastoma explants that were readily immortalized into cell lines. It became apparent that those tumors that could easily be transferred to an in vitro existence were associated with poor clinical outcome in vivo, and cytogenetic studies of these cells were noteworthy for both dms and hsrs. Cloning experiments of these regions revealed that they were composed of amplified segments of *MYCN*, a gene located on chromosome 2p24 and having homology to the c-myc proto-oncogene.[143] Thus, the ready immortalization of cells in vitro and the aggressive clinical behavior in vivo result from multiplied segments of a tumor-causing gene, with high levels of production of the resultant protein. Amplification of *MYCN* typically ranges from 50 to 400 copies of this usually single segment.

MYCN is normally expressed in the developing nervous system. The gene product is a DNA-binding protein. It contains a helix-loop-helix/leucine zipper motif that mediates its interactions with DNA and related proteins like Max and Mad. Amplification of *MYCN* causes an imbalance between its product and the proteins and DNA sequences with which it interacts, resulting in unrestrained cell proliferation. Forced overexpression of *MYCN* in transgenic mice causes neuroblastic tumors, further indicating the relationship of this gene and the tumorigenesis of neuroblastomas.[143]

Detection of *MYCN* amplification has a marked relationship to clinical outcome and is therefore used to stratify patients for treatment purposes. Testing generally requires fresh tissue, so that portions should be frozen in all suspected neuroblastomas, before their submersion in fixatives. Initially, Southern blots were used to detect this phenomenon, but interphase FISH is generally used today.[144] By FISH

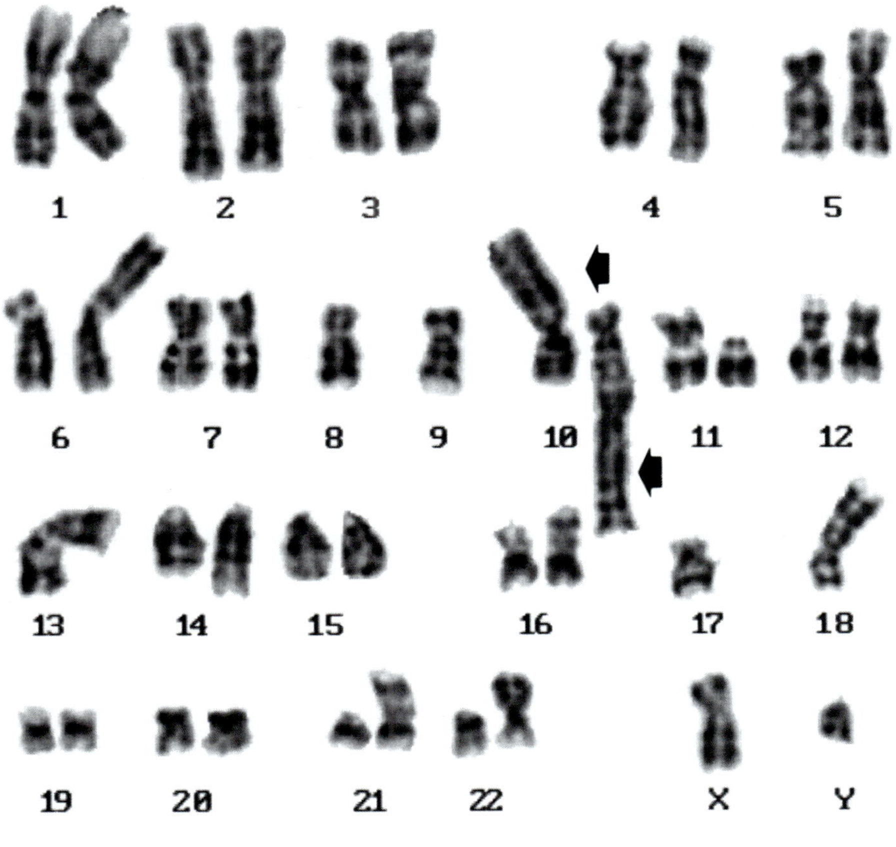

Figure 18–31. Karyotype of neuroblastoma with homogeneous staining regions found in the short and long arms of chromosomes 10 *(arrows)*. These markedly elongated genetic segments represent amplification of the *MYCN* gene and are a marker of a poor prognosis. (Courtesy of Mr. Charles Swanson and Dr. Jeffrey Sawyer, Arkansas Children's Hospital, Little Rock, AR.)

analysis, *MYCN* amplification is apparent in cells with dms as multiple, randomly distributed sites of fluorescence, whereas hsrs are indicated by the presence of long, contiguous strands of fluorescence.

Another cytogenetic feature that is related to clinical outcome of neuroblastomas is aneuploidy.[145,146] Paradoxically, hyperdiploidy is usually indicative of poor outcome in adult tumors, but in neuroblastoma it is a favorable finding. The presence of aneuploidy in these tumors denotes a genomic instability that renders them more susceptible to cancer chemotherapy and usually separates them from the poor-prognosis, *MYCN*-amplified group.

Newer genetic features of neuroblastoma to consider include *TRK* and telomerase expression. The trk family is a group of receptor proteins that are critical in the transfer of extracellular signals from nerve growth and differentiation factors, or neurotrophins, into the intracellular milieu of neural cells. Three relevant neurotrophin receptors, or trk proteins, are identified, trkA, trkB, and trkC. TrkA and trkC are differentiation-inducing proteins whose expression is inversely related to neuroblastoma stage and *N-myc* amplification.[147] TrkB, on the other hand, is overexpressed in advanced tumors.[143] Telomerase is an enzyme that has been associated with cell immortalization. Increased telomerase expression is related to greater neuroblastoma aggressiveness.[148]

Table 18–5. International Neuroblastoma Staging System

Stage	Definition
1	Localized tumor, complete gross excision, lymph nodes negative*
2A	Localized tumor, incomplete gross excision, lymph nodes negative*
2B	Localized tumor, with or without complete gross excision, ipsilateral lymph nodes positive*
3	Unresectable tumor with midline extension,† either by primary tumor or lymph node metastasis
4	Metastatic lesions involving distant lymph nodes, bone, bone marrow, liver, skin, or other (except as defined for stage 4S)
4S	Localized, stage 1, 2A, or 2B tumors with dissemination limited to skin, liver, and/or bone marrow, and in patients <1 y old

*Lymph nodes attached to and removed with the tumor specimen may be positive in lower stages. To upstage the patient, the lymph node must be separately sampled.
†Defined by the vertebral column.
(From Brodeur GM, Pritchard J, Berthold F, et al: Revisions of the international criteria for neuroblastoma: Diagnosis, staging, and response to treatment. J Clin Oncol 1993;11:1466.)

Prognosis and Clinical Outcome

Prognosis of neuroblastoma is a rather complicated affair related to its clinical, histologic, and genetic features. Three distinct genetic subgroups, a low-risk group, an intermediate-risk group, and a high-risk group, have been identified by Brodeur and colleagues.[149] The low-risk group comprises hyperdiploid tumors with few rearrangements, generally occurring in infants with localized tumors. The intermediate-risk group comprises near-diploid tumors with no consistent abnormality; these usually are seen in older patients with more advanced disease. The high-risk group comprises lesions with a near-diploid or tetraploid karyotype, with deletions or loss of heterozygosity (LOH) for 1p36, amplification of *MYCN*, or both, and occurs in older patients with rapidly progressive lesions.

Staging is important to management, although low-stage tumors that show high-risk biologic factors must be aggressively treated. Staging is based on the adequacy of excision, extension of disease across the midline, and presence of metastatic tumor, as indicated in Table 18–5.[126] One paradoxical group is stage IVS, typically comprised of infants with apparent metastatic disease but relatively good outcome. Of note is the lesser frequency of *MYCN* amplification in these tumors as compared to stage IV tumors.[150]

Differential Diagnosis

Diagnosis of neuroblastoma generally presents less of a problem than that of its less differentiated Ewing sarcoma family cousins. In the presence of a calcified adrenal mass and catecholamine secretion, identification of clusters of primitive cells in fine needle aspirates or bone marrow is sufficient (Fig. 18–32).[126] In patients with primitive, nonadrenal tumors, particularly older children and adolescents, PNET should be strongly considered, requiring the ancillary techniques discussed previously. One particularly important caveat is not to overinterpret *MYCN* amplification as definitive evidence of neuroblastoma in these cases, because this phenomenon also occurs in alveolar rhabdomyosarcoma. Positivity for MyoD or myogenin and the presence of the PAX/FRKHR fusion are sufficient to make the latter diagnosis. Another abdominal tumor that should be considered in the differential diagnosis is the desmoplastic small

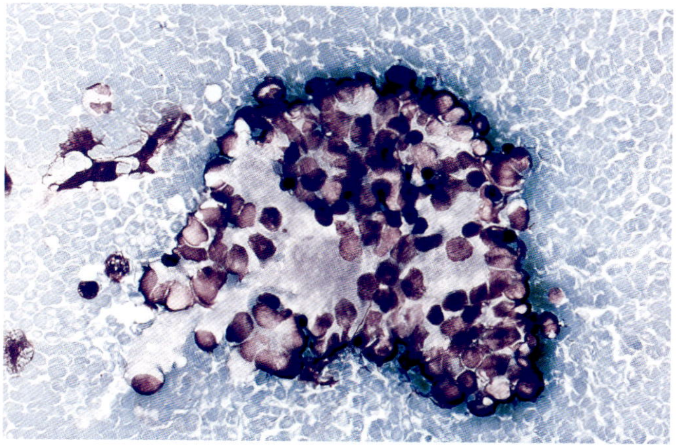

Figure 18–32. Fine needle aspirate sample of neuroblastoma, containing clusters of small round tumor cells with a wispy neurofibrillary "stroma" (Wright-Giemsa, ×100).

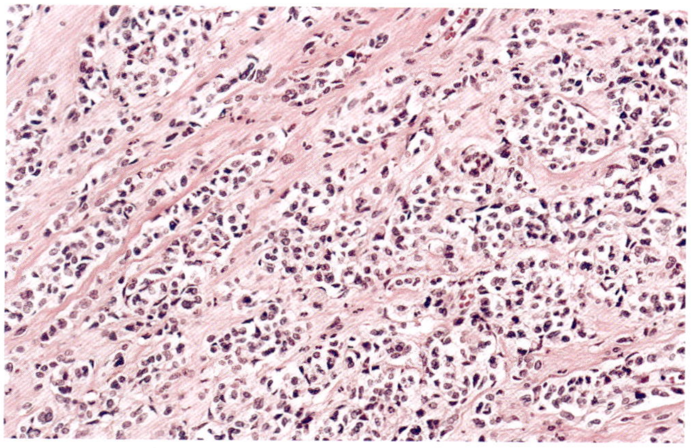

Figure 18–33. Desmoplastic small cell tumor. A fibrous stroma encloses nests and cords of tumor cells with no discernible differentiation (hematoxylin and eosin, ×50).

cell tumor. This lesion may involve the retroperitoneum and could potentially lead to confusion in large tumors that involve the adrenals, as rosettes have been described in them.[149]

Small Cell Desmoplastic Tumor

Clinical Features

Small cell desmoplastic tumor (SCDT) is predominately an intra-abdominal lesion that usually occurs in male adolescents, as reflected by its original name, "intra-abdominal desmoplastic small round cell tumor."[151] It typically occurs as an intraperitoneal, retroperitoneal, or pelvic mass that may arise in different parts of the abdominal cavity. Because of the continuity of the peritoneum and the scrotal sac via the processus vaginalis, SCDTs may also arise as intrascrotal lesions.[152,153] The site diversity of SCDTs has been broadened in recent years by discovery of these neoplasms in sites such as the pleura, cranium, and hand.[154-156] Clinically, these tumors are usually discovered as nonsymptomatic abdominal masses, similar to ovarian tumors, although complications from intestinal or biliary tract obstruction may signal some lesions. Unfortunately, a relatively large percentage exhibit peritoneal spread coincident or soon after the time of their clinical detection.[157]

Pathology—Gross and Microscopic Features

Small cell desmoplastic tumors are gritty, yellow-gray lesions that have a firm fibrous cut surface. They are usually not encapsulated and invade adjacent organs, such as the pancreas. Evidence of peritoneal studding should be carefully investigated at the time of surgery.

Histologically, the fibroplasia of SCDTs is a key diagnostic feature. Nests of small primitive cells punctuate this framework of dense collagen, scattered fibroblasts, and small blood vessels (Fig. 18–33). In some areas the small round cells may fuse into larger aggregates and form ribbons or trabeculae. The small round cell component of these tumors is comprised of primitive, cohesive cells with hyperchromatic, round-to-oval nuclei and minimal cytoplasm. Scattered tumor cells may have an epithelioid appearance, as exemplified by modest amounts of lightly eosinophilic cytoplasm and increased cohesiveness. Other foci may have a vague neural appearance, forming ill-defined rosettes.[150] Some tumors have focal pleomorphism, and others contain rhabdoid cells with large amounts of eosinophilic cytoplasm, intracytoplasmic hyaline inclusions, and eccentric nuclei with prominent nucleoli. Because of this latter feature, SCDTs must be included among the differential diagnosis, "pseudorhabdoid tumors."

Immunohistochemistry and Electron Microscopy

A defining feature of SCDTs, which aids in their distinction from rhabdomyosarcomas, is their polyphenotypia. They usually display positivity for keratins, vimentin, desmin, epithelial membrane antigen, NSE, and, often, CD57 (Fig. 18–34). WT1 is often expressed as strong nuclear positivity.[158] CD99 may be positive in some cases, but MyoD and myogenin stains are nonreactive. One should avoid overinterpretation of cytoplasmic MyoD staining as evidence for rhabdomyosarcoma; this pattern is nonspecific. This is important because SCDT may resemble alveolar rhabdomyosarcoma and usually shows desmin positivity. A list of immunohistochemical findings in

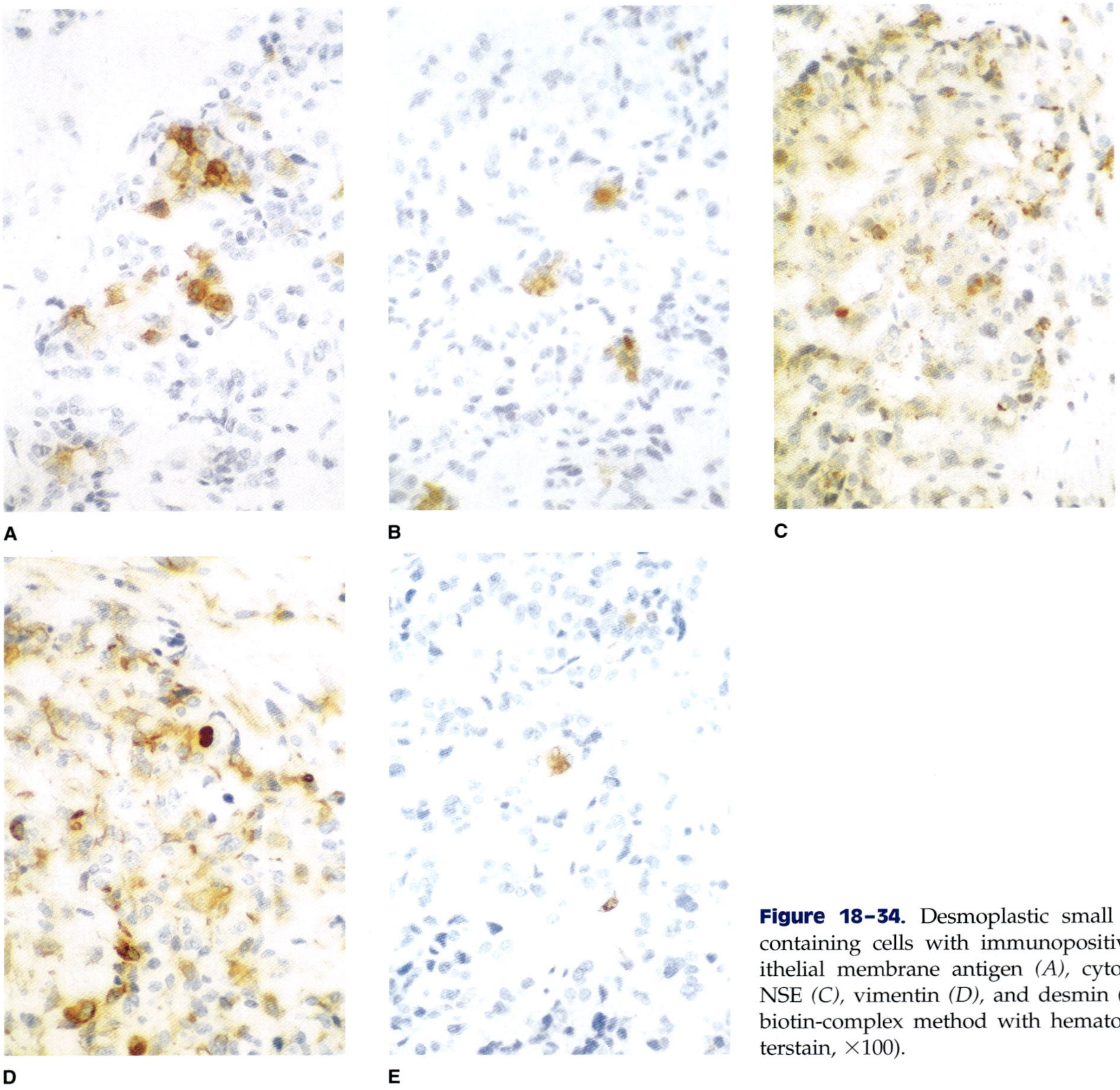

Figure 18–34. Desmoplastic small cell tumor, containing cells with immunopositivity for epithelial membrane antigen *(A)*, cytokeratin *(B)*, NSE *(C)*, vimentin *(D)*, and desmin *(E)*, (avidin-biotin-complex method with hematoxylin counterstain, ×100).

SCDT is given in Table 18–6. Another caveat is that occasional cases may be keratin negative.[159]

Ultrastructural features of SCDTs include intercellular junctions and tonofilaments, representing the epithelial component. Microtubules and neurosecretory granules are compatible with a neural phenotype, and correlate with staining for markers such as synaptophysin.[150] Myogenous organelles such as thick and thin filaments or Z-bands are absent.

Cytogenetics and Molecular Biology

Like Ewing sarcoma and alveolar rhabdomyosarcoma, SCDT is cytogenetically defined by a reciprocal translocation: the t(11;22)(p13;q12).[160] This translocation creates a fusion gene that transcribes a chimeric protein containing portions of the WT1 protein and the EWS protein (Fig. 18–35).[161] In this fashion, a gene whose deletion is associated with Wilms tumor development *(WT1)* is combined with the gene whose fusion with an alternate partner, *FLI1*, is causative of Ewing sarcoma. This anomaly may explain some phenotypic features of this neoplasm, because the propensity for it to occur in the peritoneal cavity may be related to the strong expression of *WT1* by developing mesothelium.[162,163] It also may be responsible for the WT1 immunostaining of these tumors.[158] In like manner, some lesions previously diagnosed as "extrarenal Wilms tumor"[164] may represent examples of SCDT. The epithelial and mesenchymal polyphenotypia of the latter tumor is reminiscent of Wilms tumor, and the neural phenotype is similar to that of Ewing sarcoma family tumors. The fusion protein produced by the *WT1/ EWS* gene is capable of inducing the expression

Table 18-6. Immunohistochemical Markers Reported to Be Positive in Desmoplastic Small Cell Tumor

Mesenchymal
Vimentin
Desmin
Smooth muscle actin
Muscle-specific actin
Epithelial
Keratins
Epithelial membrane antigen
Neural
NSE
CD57 (Leu7)
Synaptophysin
Chromogranin
NB84
Miscellaneous
CD15
WT1
CD99
CA125
BerEP4

(From Ordonez NG: Desmoplastic small round cell tumor. II: An ultrastructural and immunohistochemical study with emphasis on new immunohistochemical markers. Am J Surg Pathol 1998;2:1314.)

of endogenous platelet-derived growth factor A, which is a powerful mitogen and chemoattractant whose DNA contains WT1-binding sites in its promoter region.[165] Thus, by fusion with *EWS, WT1* is converted from a tumor suppressor gene into an oncogene.

Besides its provocative associations with Ewing sarcoma and Wilms tumor, the *WT1/EWS* fusion offers a means of ancillary diagnosis. This may be accomplished by either RT-PCR or FISH,[159,166,167] and it can be used for confirmation of diagnosis in limited samples such as obtained via fine-needle aspiration biopsy.[155] One caveat should be noted: occasional cases that clinically and phenotypically appear to be SCDTs may show the Ewing sarcoma genotype, FLI1/EWS, by these ancillary studies.[168] The effectiveness of chemotherapeutic agents active against Ewing sarcoma would dictate that lesions that genetically represent Ewing sarcoma presently be treated as such.

Prognosis and Clinical Outcome

The SCDTs are aggressive neoplasms with a penchant for intra- and extraperitoneal dissemination. As with ovarian neoplasms, the peritoneal metastases are associated with complications such as ascites, serosal adhesions, and intestinal and ureteral obstructions. Modern combination chemotherapy may induce temporary remissions, but the ultimate outcome remains dismal with these aggressive neoplasms.[152,169]

Diagnostic Summary and Differential Diagnosis

The diagnosis of SCDT should be considered in all intra-abdominal and intrascrotal small cell neoplasms, particularly those with a prominent fibrous stroma. However, the latter feature does not exclude other small neoplasms, such as alveolar rhabdomyosarcoma, PNET, and extrarenal Wilms tumor. Demonstration of polyphenotypia by expression of epithelial, neural, and mesenchymal markers is key to the diagnosis. If well-formed tubules or glomeruli are present, a diagnosis of extrarenal Wilms tumor should be rendered.[164,170] In limited biopsies, demonstration of the *WT1/EWS* or the t(11;22)(p13;q12) is particularly helpful. In all such cases, it is important to save frozen material for the optimal demonstration of the fusion gene.[167] WTI immunostains also offer good discrimination between SCDT and Ewing sarcoma.[170A]

Extrarenal Rhabdoid Tumor

History and Controversies

Although the eosinophilic rhabdoid cells, filled with whorled eosinophilic filaments, are morphologically highly distinctive, rhabdoid tumor is a problematic entity, because many other tumor types can have cells with rhabdoid cytoplasm.[171,172] Recent biologic

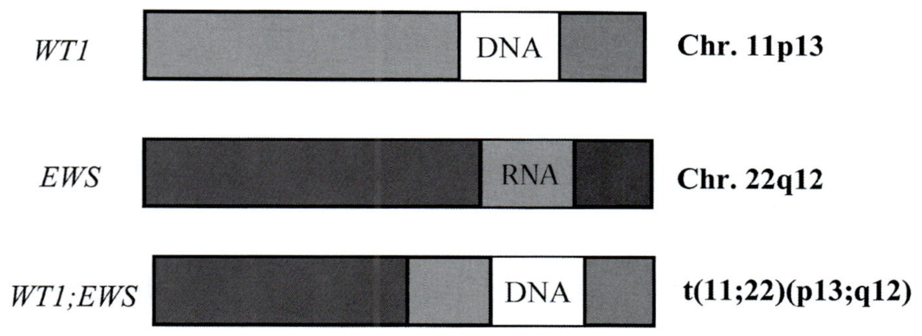

Figure 18-35. Illustration of the *WT1;EWS* gene fusion. Note that like Ewing translocations, the sequence transcribing a putative RNA-binding region of the *EWS* gene is replaced by one encoding a DNA-binding region *(lowest panel).*

observations indicate that some of these tumors do indeed share genetic alterations that would define a specific disease entity.[173,174]

The rhabdoid tumor was introduced in 1978 by Beckwith and Palmer, who described new categories of aggressive pediatric renal neoplasms based on a cohort entered on the first National Wilms Tumor Study.[175] These tumors included anaplastic Wilms tumors and the clear cell, hyalinizing, and rhabdomyosarcomatoid variants of Wilms tumor; the latter subsequently were labeled as distinct entities known as rhabdoid tumors and clear cell sarcomas of the kidney.

Subsequent to Beckwith and Palmer's discovery of malignant rhabdoid tumors of the kidney, others described rhabdoid tumors of the soft tissues, liver, brain, genitourinary tract, and skin.[176-178] In retrospect, lesions such as "malignant histiocytoma"[179,180] and "rhabdomyoblastoma,"[181] described prior to Beckwith and Palmer's report, also had rhabdoid features. However, reports from Japan and the Intergroup Rhabdomyosarcoma Study found that although some soft lesions could be characterized as discrete entities,[178,182] others were actually different tumors that contained a rhabdoid component.[171,183,184] Also, remarkable polyphenotypia was noted,[171,185] similar to that seen in "teratoid-rhabdoid tumors" of brain.[186]

Clinical Features

One prominent feature of rhabdoid tumors of all sites is their predilection to occur in infants and very young children. Rhabdoid tumors comprise a large percentage of infantile renal tumors,[187] and most of the extrarenal tumors without other apparent histologies also arise in the very young.[171] Thus, origin of an "extrarenal rhabdoid tumor" from an older child or adult should raise suspicion that another tumor diagnosis may be in order.

Extrarenal rhabdoid tumors have been reported in a variety of sites, but variable documentation makes the data difficult to interpret. Nevertheless, hepatic and soft tissue lesions are well reported. Among favored sites are axial and paravertebral lesions,[171] as well as extremity lesions.[180,188] Superficial lesions may arise in the dermis and subcutis,[177] but appropriate imaging studies are essential to rule out a renal primary.[189] Some cutaneous rhabdoid tumors are associated with hamartomas, such as sebaceous nevi.[171,190]

Hypercalcemia has been reported as a paraneoplastic phenomenon with rhabdoid tumors of the kidney.[191,192] This has been associated with secretion of parathormone and parathormone-like substances.[193] Another clinical feature described in both renal and extrarenal rhabdoid tumors is the coexistence of PNETs of the central nervous system.[194,195] Although these brain tumors may mistakenly be considered to be metastases by radiologic reports, they actually represent PNETs like medulloblastoma or ependymoma.

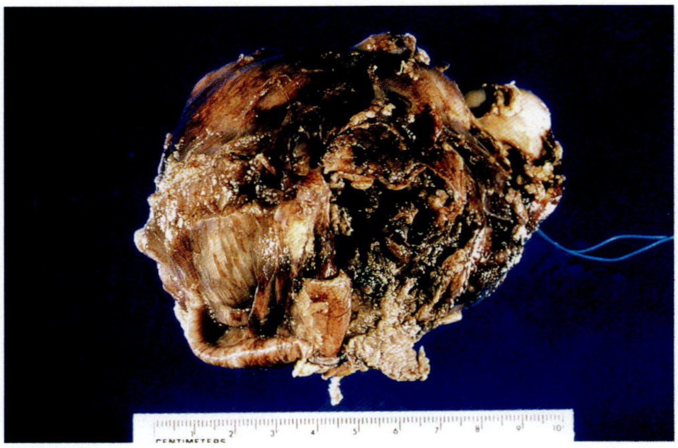

Figure 18–36. Rhabdoid tumor of kidney, with friable, necrotic, hemorrhagic material exuding from a surgical rupture.

Pathology—Gross and Microscopic Features

Grossly, the typical invasive, nonencapsulated appearance of rhabdoid tumors, accented by a soft, fleshy, focally necrotic cut surface, underscores their malignant nature at any site (Fig. 18–36). Because of their invasiveness, rhabdoid tumors are often incompletely excised. Documentation of the surgical margins can be an arduous task, due to the soupy consistency of the tumors.

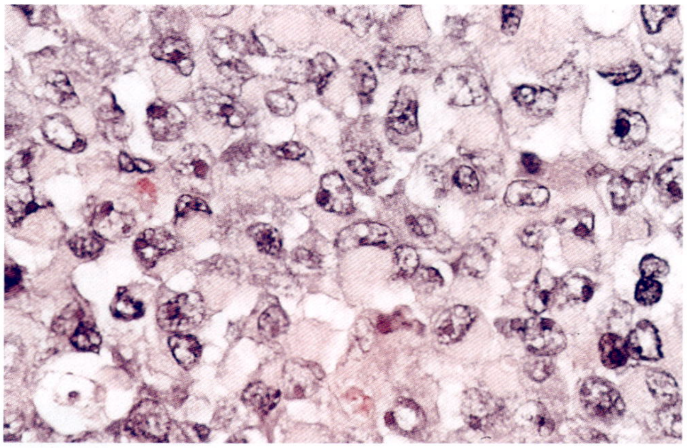

Figure 18–37. Rhabdoid tumor, composed of poorly cohesive cells with large, "owl's eye" nuclei, eosinophilic cytoplasm, and hyaline intracytoplasmic inclusions (hematoxylin and eosin, ×100).

Microscopically, the rhabdoid cells have eccentric nuclei with prominent nucleoli and abundant cytoplasm with round, hyaline inclusions (Fig. 18–37). Some lesions have less abundant cytoplasm potentially simulating a hematopoietic neoplasm.[196] Weeks and coworkers described hemangiopericytomatous, spindle cell, and carcinoid-like morphologies in renal rhabdoid tumors,[196] which may also be seen in extrarenal examples. The occurrence of paraganglioma-like patterns raises the question of neuroectodermal differentiation, and gene expression profiles seem to support this.[197]

Electron Microscopy

The key ultrastuctural feature in rhabdoid tumors is the presence of the paranuclear, spherical intermediate filament aggregates, that correspond to the hyaline inclusions seen by light microscopy (Fig. 18–38). These inclusions are not specific, and other features

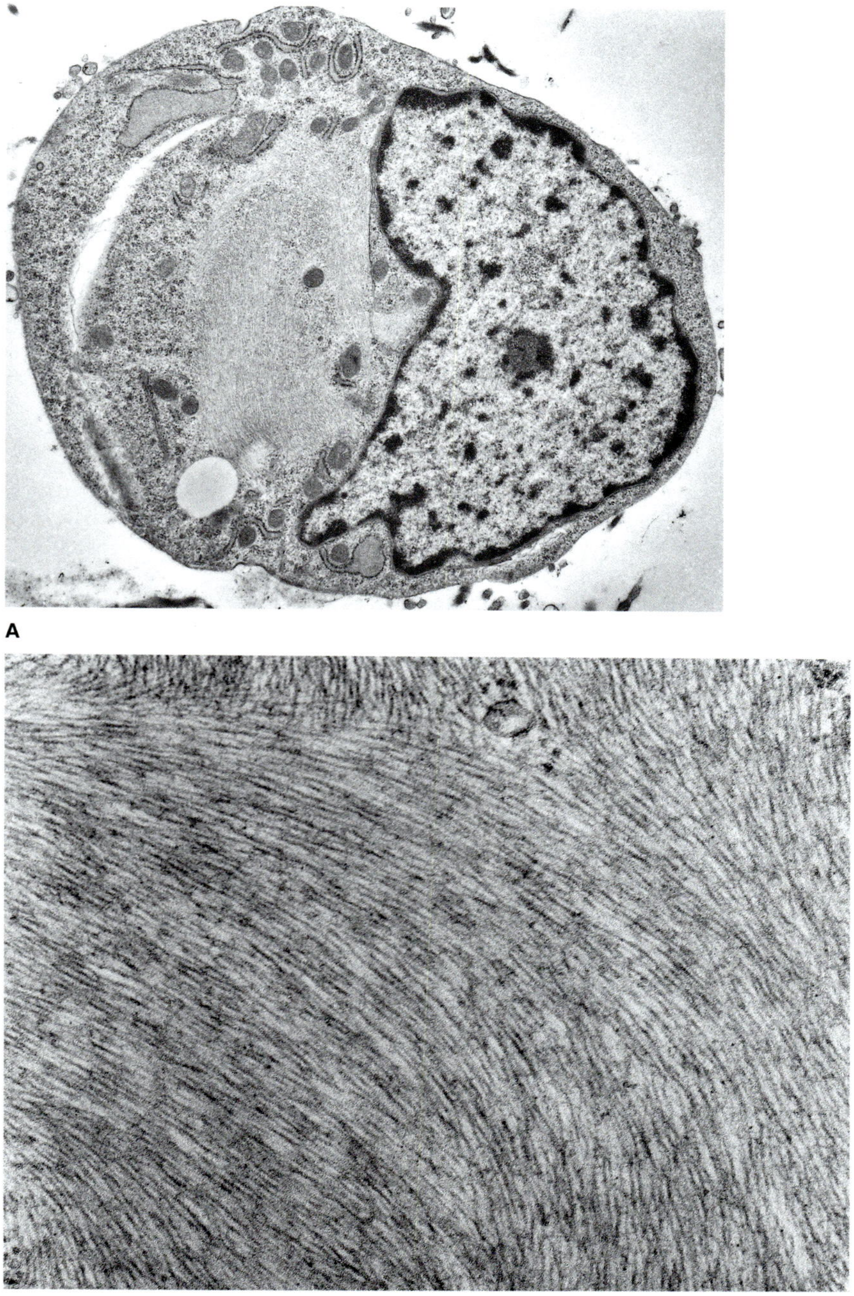

A

B

Figure 18–38. *A,* Electron micrograph of rhabdoid cell with eccentric nucleus and paranuclear inclusion (×7000). *B,* Higher magnification of cytoplasmic inclusion, composed of intermingled mass of filaments measuring 10 nm in diameter (×30,000).

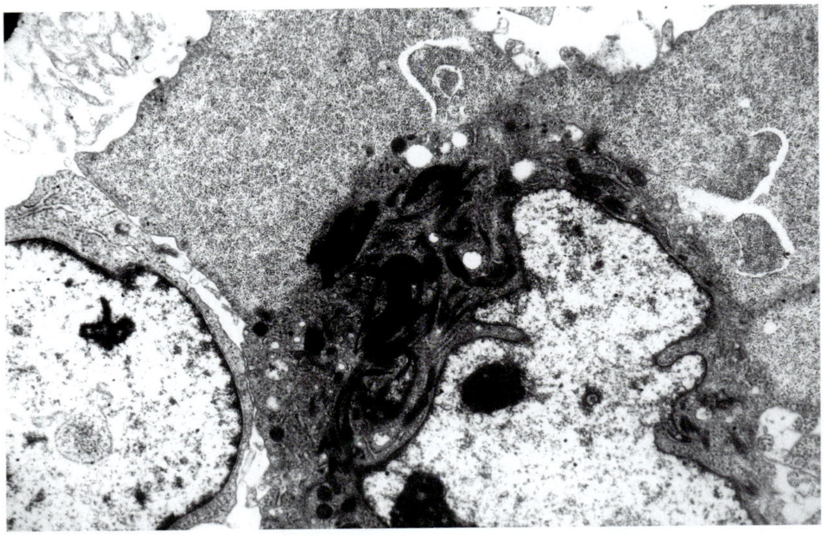

Figure 18–39. Electron micrograph of putative rhabdoid tumor explant. A tumor cell contains prominent cytoplasmic bundles of tonofilaments, suggestive of a diagnosis of epithelioid sarcoma (×7000).

may lead to another diagnosis. Tonofilaments indicate epithelioid sarcoma (Fig. 18–39), thick and thin filaments rhabdomyosarcoma, and neurosecretory granules and processes PNET or neuroendocrine carcinoma (Fig. 18–40).[171]

Immunohistochemistry

The intermediate filaments in rhabdoid tumors consist of keratins and vimentin (Fig. 18–41). The keratin types vary, and immunoreactivity may depend on antibody. Rhabdoid tumors are also positive for epithelial membrane antigen (Fig. 18–42). A variety of other markers may be positive, including myogenous and neural markers, and the seeming nonspecificity of these stains has led some to postulate that the staining might be artefactual.[196] Nevertheless, this phenomenon correlates with the diverse organelles that may be observed by careful electron microscopy.[171]

Cytogenetics

Early studies of the cytogenetics of rhabdoid tumors were disappointing because of their lack of any apparent karyotypic abnormality.[198] However, it was noted that atypical teratoid-rhabdoid tumors of the brain consistently exhibited a monosomy 22.[199,200]

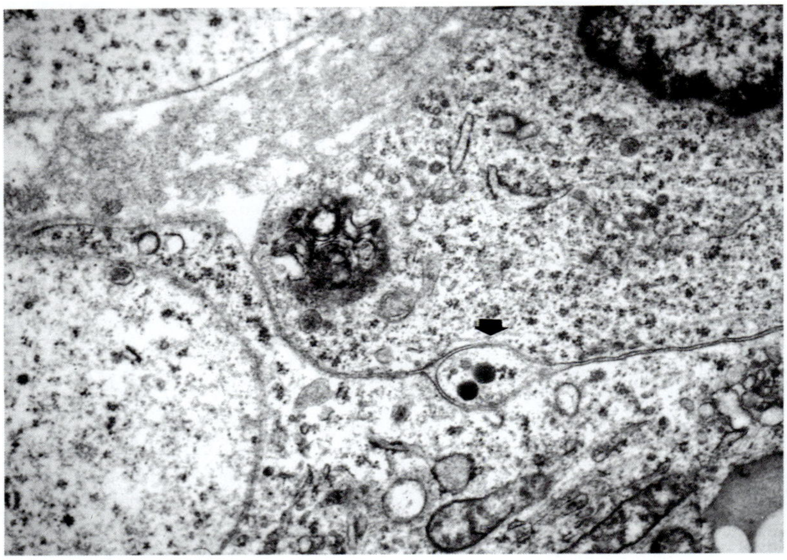

Figure 18–40. Electron micrograph of putative rhabdoid tumor. A small, discrete cytoplasmic process contains dense core granules *(arrow)*, suggestive of a diagnosis of PNET (×25,000).

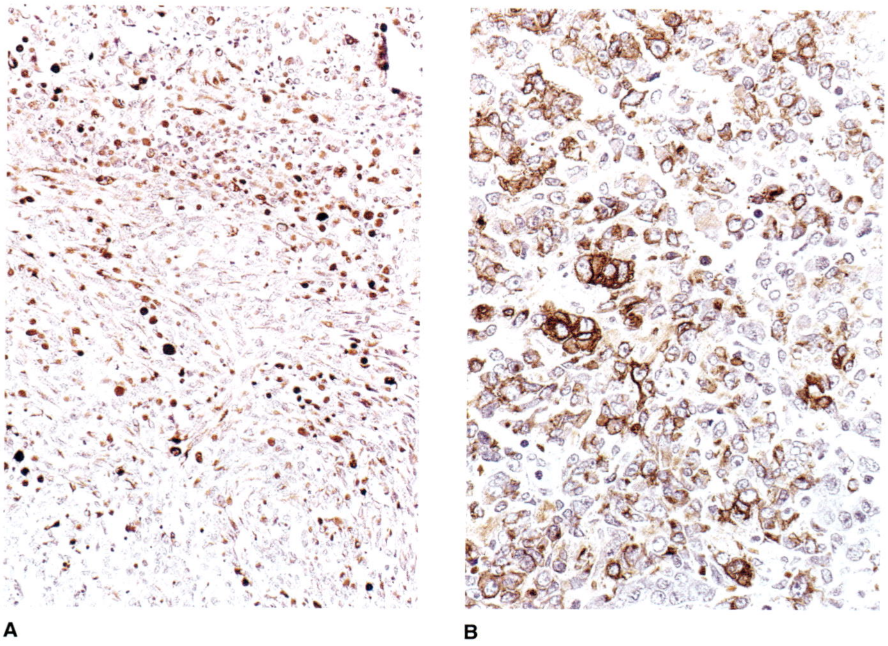

Figure 18-41. Rhabdoid tumor with immunohistochemical evidence of vimentin *(A)* and cytokeratin *(B)* coexpression. Note the globular vimentin staining, corresponding to cytoplasmic intermediate filament inclusions (see Fig. 18–38) (avidin-biotin-complex method with hematoxylin counterstain; *A,* ×25; *B,* ×50).

Subsequent studies of rhabdoid tumors have focused on chromosome 22, with resultant discovery of a region of common deletion at 22q11 in both renal and extrarenal cases (Fig. 18–43).[201] This region does not involve the *EWS* or *NF2* loci but appears to overlap with the *BCR* gene, which is involved in chronic myelogenous leukemia and some cases of acute lymphoblastic leukemia.[202] The most recent studies have delimited a putative tumor suppressor gene locus, termed the *hSNF5/INI1* gene.[203] Genetic studies of chromosome 22 have recently been used as a means of ancillary diagnosis of extrarenal rhabdoid tumor.[173,174]

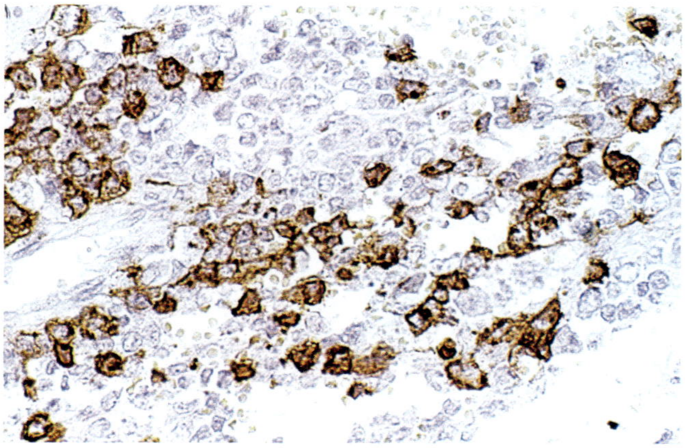

Figure 18-42. The epithelial nature of rhabdoid tumor is confirmed by its epithelial membrane positivity, seen here in a typical membranous pattern (avidin-biotin-complex method with hematoxylin counterstain, ×50).

Another phenomenon of note in rhabdoid tumor cytogenetics is their association with alterations of the short arm with chromosome 11. The mistaken identity of a rhabdoid cell line as Wilms tumor led to its use in biologic studies of the latter lesion, demonstrating that tumorigenesis could be reversed by implantation of a normal chromosome 11.[204] Genetic alterations are also described in this region that suggest a molecular kinship between rhabdoid tumor and rhabdomyosarcoma.[205,206]

Mutation analysis of rhabdoid tumors has revealed alteration of the cytokeratin (CK8) gene in areas that relate to protofilament interactions. This observation might explain the intermediate filament abnormality typical of these tumors.[207]

Differential Diagnosis

Rhabdoid tumor is a diagnosis by exclusion, and other neoplasms with rhabdoid cytoplasm must be ruled out (Table 18–7 and Fig. 18–44). This is especially true for extrarenal lesions in adults. Some tumors, such as epithelioid sarcoma,[207] show more aggressive behavior if rhabdoid cells are prominent. MyoD or myogenin expression defines a rhabdomyosarcoma.[208] Genetic testing for 22q deletions holds promise as a diagnostic aid,[173,174] but the specificity of this finding awaits confirmation.

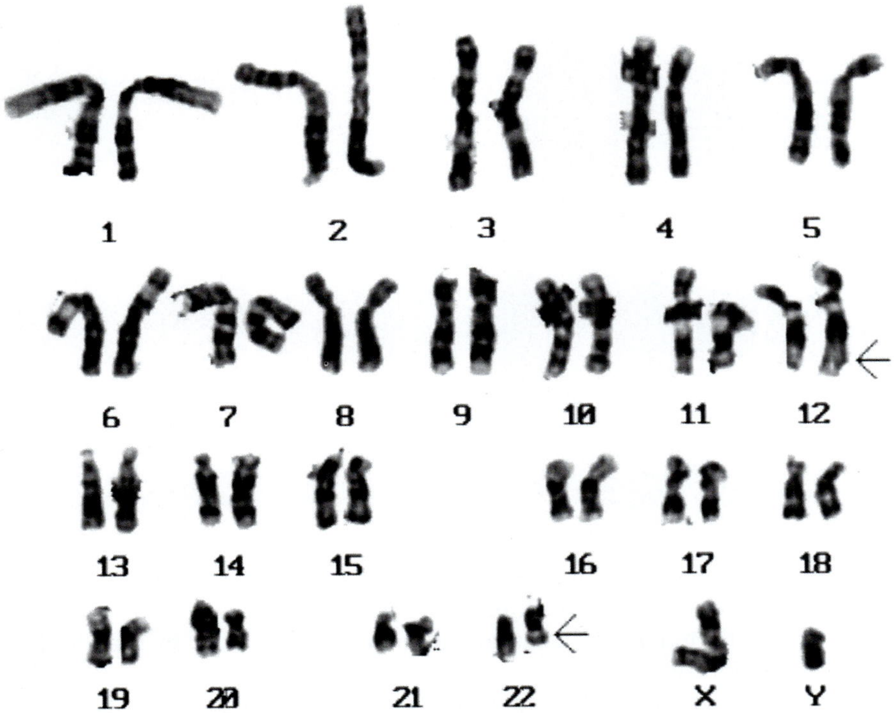

Figure 18–43. Karyotype of rhabdoid tumor, with translocation involving chromosomes 12q and 22q *(arrows)*. Although this appears to be a balanced translocation, portions of a tumor suppressor gene 22q11 might be missing at a molecular level. (Courtesy of Mr. Charles Swanson and Dr. Jeffrey Sawyer, Arkansas Children's Hospital, Little Rock, AR.)

Table 18–7. Tumors Reported to Contain Rhabdoid Cells

Rhabdomyosarcoma	Salivary gland tumors
Synovial sarcoma	Adenocarcinoma
Paraganglioma	PNET
Neuroendocrine carcinoma	Myofibrosarcoma
Melanoma	Myoepithelioma
Transitional cell carcinoma	Merkel cell carcinoma
Epithelioid sarcoma	Leiomyosarcoma
Desmoplastic small cell tumor	Lung carcinoma
Neuroblastoma	Thyroid carcinoma
Glioma	Meningioma

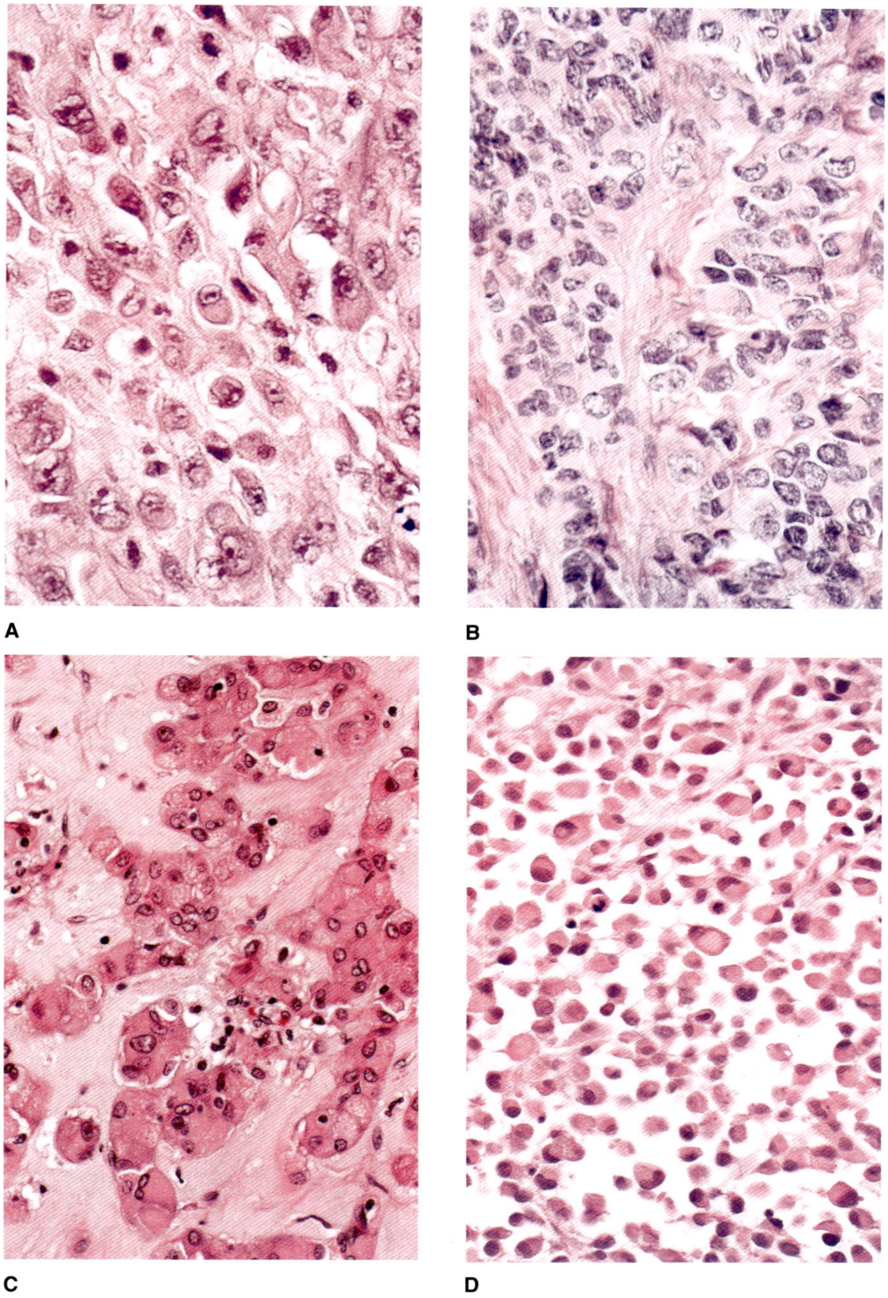

Figure 18–44. "Pseudorhabdoid" tumors, including epithelioid sarcoma *(A)*, rhabdomyosarcoma *(B)*, neuroendocrine carcinoma *(C)*, and myofibrosarcoma *(D)*, may contain rhabdoid cells with cytoplasmic inclusions (hematoxylin and eosin; *A*, *B*, and *C*, ×100; *D*, ×50).

REFERENCES

General

1. Triche TJ, Askin FB: Neuroblastoma and the differential diagnosis of small-, round-, blue-cell tumors. Hum Pathol 1983;14:569.
2. Donaldson SS: Lessons from our children. Int J Radiat Oncol Biol Phys 1993;26:739.
3. Ross JA, Severson RK, Pollock BH, et al: Childhood cancer in the United States: A geographical analysis of cases from the Pediatric Cooperative Clinical Trials Groups. Cancer 1996;77:201.
4. Olshan AF, Breslow NE, Daling JR, et al: Wilms' tumor and paternal occupation. Cancer Res 1990;50:3212.
5. Grundy P, Wilson B, Telzerow P, et al: Uniparental disomy occurs infrequently in Wilms tumor patients. Am J Hum Genet 1994;54:282.
6. Koufos A, Hansen MF, Copeland NG, et al: Loss of heterozygosity in three embryonal tumours suggests a common pathogenetic mechanism. Nature 1985; 316:330.

7. Heyn R, Haeberlen V, Newton WA, et al: Second malignant neoplasms in children treated for rhabdomyosarcoma. J Clin Oncol 1993;11:262.
8. May WA, Lessnick SL, Braun BS, et al: The Ewing's sarcoma *EWS/FLI-1* fusion gene encodes a more potent transcriptional activator and is a more powerful transforming gene than *FLI-1*. Mol Cell Biol 1993;13:7393.
9. Whang-Peng J, Triche TJ, Knutsen T, et al: Cytogenetic characterization of selected small round cell tumors of childhood. Cancer Genet Cytogenet 1986;21:185.
10. Oda H, Imai Y, Nakatsuru Y, et al: Somatic mutations of the *APC* gene in sporadic hepatoblastomas. Cancer Res 1996;56:3320.
11. Raffel C, Jenkins RB, Frederick L, et al: Sporadic medulloblastomas contain PTCH mutations. Cancer Res 1997;57:842.
12. Felix CA, Chavez Kappel C, Mitsudomi T, et al: Frequency and diversity of p53 mutations in childhood rhabdomyosarcoma. Cancer Res 1992;52:2243.
13. Knudsen AG, Strong LC: Mutation and cancer. A model for Wilms' tumor of the kidney. J Natl Cancer Inst 1972;48:313.
14. Knudson AG: Antioncogenes and human cancer. Proc Natl Acad Sci USA 1993;90:10914.
15. Hoovers JM, Kalikin LM, Johnson LA, et al: Multiple genetic loci within 11p15 defined by Beckwith-Wiedemann syndrome rearrangement breakpoints and subchromosomal transferable fragments. Proc Natl Acad Sci USA 1995;92:12456.
16. Jones PA, Laird PW: Cancer epigenetics comes of age. Nat Genet 1999;21:163.
17. Baylin SB: Tying it all together: Epigenetics, genetics, cell cycle, and cancer. Science 1997;277:1948.
18. Chen B, Dias P, Jenkins JJ, et al: Methylation alterations of the MyoD1 upstream region are predictive of subclassification of human rhabdomyosarcomas. Am J Pathol 1998;152:1071.

Ewing Family of Tumors

19. Dehner LP: Primitive neuroectodermal tumor and Ewing's sarcoma. Am J Surg Pathol 1993;17:1.
20. Yunis EJ: Ewing's sarcoma and related small round cell neoplasms in children. Am J Surg Pathol 1986; 10(suppl 1):54.
21. Angervall L, Enzinger FM: Extraskeletal neoplasm resembling Ewing's sarcoma. Cancer 1975;36:240.
22. Tefft M, Vawter GF, Mitus A: Paravertebral "round cell" tumors in children. Radiology 1969;92:1501.
23. Schmidt D, Mackay B, Ayala AG: Ewing's sarcoma with neuroblastoma-like features. Ultrastruct Pathol 1982;3:143.
24. Mierau GW: Extraskeletal Ewing's sarcoma (peripheral neuroepithelioma). Ultrastruct Pathol 1985;9:91.
25. Seemayer TA, Thelmo WL, Bolande RP, et al: Peripheral neuroectodermal tumors. Perspect Pediatr Pathol 1975;2:151.
26. Askin FB, Rosai J, Sibley RK, et al: Malignant small cell tumor of the thoracopulmonary region in childhood: A distinctive clinicopathologic entity of uncertain histogenesis. Cancer 1979;43:2438.
27. Jaffe R, Santamaria M, Yunis EJ, et al: The neuroectodermal tumor of bone. Am J Surg Pathol 1984; 8:885.
28. Turc-Carel C, Philip I, Berger MP, et al: Chromosome study of Ewing's sarcoma (ES) cell lines. Consistency of a reciprocal translocation t(11;22)(q24;q12). Cancer Genet Cytogenet 1984;12:1.
29. Whang-Peng J, Triche TJ, Knutsen T, et al: Chromosome translocation in peripheral neuroepithelioma. N Engl J Med 1984;311:584.
30. Ladanyi M, Lewis R, Garin-Chesa P, et al: EWS rearrangement in Ewing's sarcoma and peripheral neuroectodermal tumor. Molecular detection and correlation with cytogenetic analysis and MIC2 expression. Diagn Mol Pathol 1993;2:141.
31. Pellin A, Boix J, Blesa JR, et al: EWS/FLI-1 rearrangement in small round cell sarcomas of bone and soft tissue detected by reverse transcriptase polymerase chain reaction amplification. Eur J Cancer [A] 1994; 30A:827.
32. Cavazzana AO, Miser JS, Jefferson J, et al: Experimental evidence for a neural origin of Ewing's sarcoma of bone. Am J Pathol 1987;127:507.
33. Stout AP, Murray MR: Neuroepithelioma of radial nerve with study of its behavior in vitro. Rev Can Biol 1942;1:651.
34. Delattre O, Zucman J, Melot T, et al: The Ewing family of tumors—A subgroup of small-round-cell tumors defined by specific chimeric transcripts. N Engl J Med 1994;331:294.
35. Grier HE: The Ewing family of tumors. Ewing's sarcoma and primitive neuroectodermal tumors. Pediatr Clin North Am 1997;44:991.
36. Kissane JM, Askin FB, Foulkes M, et al: Ewing's sarcoma of bone: Clinicopathologic aspects of 303 cases from the Intergroup Ewing's Sarcoma Study. Hum Pathol 1983;14:773.
37. Soule EH, Newton W Jr, Moon TE, et al: Extraskeletal Ewing's sarcoma: A preliminary review of 26 cases encountered in the Intergroup Rhabdomyosarcoma Study. Cancer 1978;42:259.
38. Harms D: Soft tissue sarcomas in the Kiel Pediatric Tumor Registry. Curr Top Pathol 1995;89:31.
39. Holman CDJ, Reynolds PM, Byrne MJJ, et al: Possible infectious etiology of six cases of Ewing's sarcoma in Western Australia. Cancer 1983;52:1974.
40. Hutter RVP, Francis KD, Foote FW: Ewing's sarcoma in siblings: Report of the second known occurrence. Am J Surg 1964;4:598.
41. Gariepy G, Drouin R, Lemieux N, et al: Ultrastructural, immunohistochemical, and cytogenetic study of a malignant peripheral neuroectodermal tumor in a patient seropositive for human immunodeficiency virus. Am J Clin Pathol 1990;93:818.
42. Ogawa K: Embryonal neuroepithelial tumors induced by human adenovirus type 12 in rodents. 1. Tumor induction in the peripheral nervous system. Acta Neuropathol (Berl) 1989;77:244.

42A. Sanchez-Prieto R, de Alava E, Palomino T, et al: An association between viral genes and human oncogenic alterations: The adenovirus EIA induces the Ewing tumor fusion transcript EWS-FL11. Nat Med 1999;5:1076.
42B. Kovar H, Fallaux FJ, Pribill I, et al: Adenovirus EIA does not induce the Ewing tumor-associated gene fusion EWS-FL11. Cancer Res 2000;6:1557.
43. Mirra JM: Bone Tumors: Clinical, Radiologic, and Pathologic Correlations. Philadelphia, Lea & Febiger, 1989.
44. Marina NM, Etcubanas E, Parham DM, et al: Peripheral primitive neuroectodermal tumor (peripheral neuroepithelioma) in children: A review of the St. Jude experience and controversies in diagnosis and management. Cancer 1989;64:1952.
45. Shimada H, Newton WA Jr, Soule EH, et al: Pathologic features of extraosseous Ewing's sarcoma: A report from the Intergroup Rhabdomyosarcoma Study. Hum Pathol 1988;19:442.
46. Parham DM, Roloson GJ, Feely M, et al: Primary malignant neuroepithelial tumors of the kidney: A clinicopathologic analysis of 146 adult and pediatric cases from the National Wilms' Tumor Study Group Pathology Center. Am J Surg Pathol 2001;25:133.
47. Sexton CW, White WL: Primary cutaneous Ewing's family sarcoma. Report of a case with immunostaining for glycoprotein p30/32 mic2. Am J Dermatopathol 1996;18:601.
48. Smith LM, Adams RH, Brothman AR, et al: Peripheral primitive neuroectodermal tumor presenting with diffuse cutaneous involvement and 7;22 translocation. Med Pediatr Oncol 1998;30:357.
49. Kaspers G-JJL, Kamphorst W, Van de Graaff M, et al: Primary spinal epidural extraosseous Ewing's sarcoma. Cancer 1991;68:648.
50. Meis JM, Enzinger FM, Martz KL, et al: Malignant peripheral nerve sheath tumors (malignant schwannomas) in children. Am J Surg Pathol 1992;16:694.
51. Hanna SL, Fletcher BD, Kaste SC, et al: Increased confidence of diagnosis of Ewing sarcoma using T2-weighted MR images. Magn Reson Imaging 1994; 12:559.
52. Lemmi MA, Fletcher BD, Marina NM, et al: Use of MR imaging to assess results of chemotherapy for Ewing sarcoma. AJR Am J Roentgenol 1990; 155:343.
53. Tsokos M: Peripheral primitive neuroectodermal tumors. Diagnosis, classification, and prognosis. Perspect Pediatr Pathol 1992;16:27.
54. Carr TF, Lockwood L, Stevens RF, et al: Childhood B cell lymphomas arising in the mediastinum. J Clin Pathol 1993;46:513.
55. Riopel M, Dickman PS, Link MP, et al: MIC2 analysis in pediatric lymphomas and leukemias. Hum Pathol 1994;25:396.
56. Nascimento AG, Unni KK, Pritchard DJ, et al: A clinicopathologic study of 20 cases of large-cell (atypical) Ewing's sarcoma of bone. Am J Surg Pathol 1980;4:29.
57. Cavazzana AO, Ninfo V, Roberts J, et al: Peripheral neuroepithelioma: A light microscopic, immunocytochemistry, and ultrastructural study. Mod Pathol 1992;5:71.
58. Williams S, Parham DM, Jenkins JJ: Peripheral neuroepithelioma with ganglion cells: Report of two cases and review of the literature. Pediatr Dev Pathol 1999;2:42.
59. Kawamoto EH, Weidner N, Agostini RM, et al: Malignant ectomesenchymoma of soft tissue: Report of two cases and review of the literature. Cancer 1987;59:1791.
59A. Boué DR, Parham DM, Webber B, Crist WM, Qualman SJ: Clinicopathologic study of ectomesenchymomas from Intergroup Rhabdomysarcoma Study Groups III and IV. Pediatr Devel Pathol 2000;3:290.
60. Tan SY, Burchill S, Brownhill SC: Small round cell tumor with biphenotypic differentiation and variant of t(21;22)(q32;q12). Pediatr Devel Pathol 2001;4:391.
61. Dehner LP: Whence the primitive neuroectodermal tumor. Arch Pathol Lab Med 1990;114:16.
62. Llombart-Bosch A, Peydro-Olaya A: Scanning and transmission electron microscopy of Ewing's sarcoma of bone (typical and atypical variants). Virchows Arch [A] 1983;398:329.
63. Triche TJ, Ross WE: Glycogen-containing neuroblastoma with clinical and histopathologic features of Ewing's sarcoma. Cancer 1978;41:1425.
64. Damjanov I, Tuma B, Dominis M: Electron microscopy of large cell undifferentiated and giant cell tumors. Pathol Res Pract 1989;184:137.
65. Miettinen M, Lehto VP, Virtanen I: Histogenesis of Ewing's sarcoma. An evaluation of intermediate filaments and endothelial cell markers. Virchows Arch [B] 1982;1:277.
66. Llombart-Bosch A, Lacombe MJ, Peydro-Olaya A, et al: Malignant peripheral neuroectodermal tumours of bone other than Askin's neoplasm: Characterization of 14 new cases with immunohistochemistry and electron microscopy. Virchows Arch [A] 1988;412:421.
67. Pinto A, Grant LH, Hayes FA, et al: Immunohistochemical expression of neuron-specific enolase and Leu 7 in Ewing's sarcoma of bone. Cancer 1989;64: 1266.
68. Greco MA, Steiner GC, Fazzini E: Ewing's sarcoma with epithelial differentiation: Fine structural and immunocytochemical study. Ultrastruct Pathol 1988; 12:317.
69. Moll R, Lee I, Gould VE, et al: Immunocytochemical analysis of Ewing's tumors: Patterns of expression of intermediate filaments and desmosomal proteins indicate cell type heterogeneity and pluripotential differentiation. Am J Pathol 1987;127:288.
70. Bridge JA, Fidler ME, Neff JR, et al: Adamantinoma-like Ewing's sarcoma: Genomic confirmation, phenotypic drift. Am J Surg Pathol 1999;23:159.
71. Ambros IM, Ambros PF, Strehl S, et al: MIC2 is a specific marker for Ewing's sarcoma and peripheral primitive neuroectodermal tumors: Evidence for a common histogenesis of Ewing's sarcoma and peripheral primitive neuroectodermal tumors from MIC2 expression and specific chromosome aberration. Cancer 1991;67:1886.

72. Hamilton G, Mallinger R, Hofbauer S, et al: The monoclonal HBA-71 antibody modulates proliferation of thymocytes and Ewing's sarcoma cells by interfering with the action of insulin-like growth factor I. Thymus 1991;18:33.
73. Ramani P, Rampling D, Link M: Immunocytochemical study of 12E7 in small round-cell tumours of childhood: An assessment of its sensitivity and specificity. Histopathology 1993;23:557.
74. Stevenson AJ, Chatten J, Bertoni F, et al: CD99 (p30/32^{MIC2}) neuroectodermal/Ewing's sarcoma antigen as an immunohistochemical marker: Review of more than 600 tumors and the literature experience. Appl Immunohistochem 1994;2:231.
75. Fellinger EJ, Garin-Chesa P, Glasser DB, et al: Comparison of cell surface antigen HBA71 (p30/32^{MIC2}), neuron-specific enolase, and vimentin in the immunohistochemical analysis of Ewing's sarcoma of bone. Am J Surg Pathol 1992;16:746.
76. Weiss LM, Arber DA, Chang KL: CD45: A review. App Immunohistochem 1993;1:166.
77. Ozdemirli M, Fanburg-Smith JC, Hartmann DP, et al: Precursor B-Lymphoblastic lymphoma presenting as a solitary bone tumor and mimicking Ewing's sarcoma: A report of four cases and review of the literature. Am J Surg Pathol 1998;22:795.
78. Pappo AS, Douglass EC, Meyer WH, et al: Use of HBA71 and anti-b2-microglobulin to distinguish peripheral neuroepithelioma from neuroblastoma. Hum Pathol 1993;24:880.
79. Molenaar WM, Muntinghe FL: Expression of neural cell adhesion molecules and neurofilament protein isoforms in skeletal muscle tumors. Hum Pathol 1998;29:1290.
80. Strother DR, Parham DM, Houghton PJ: Expression of the 5.1 H11 antigen, a fetal muscle surface antigen, in normal and neoplastic tissue. Arch Pathol Lab Med 1990;114:593.
81. Garin-Chesa P, Fellinger EJ, Huvos AG, et al: Immunohistochemical analysis of neural cell adhesion molecules: Differential expression in small round cell tumors of childhood and adolescence. Am J Pathol 1991;139:275.
82. Parham DM, Dias P, Kelly DR, et al: Desmin positivity in primitive neuroectodermal tumors of childhood. Am J Surg Pathol 1992;16:483.
83. Le Douarin NM, Ziller C: Plasticity in neural crest cell differentiation. Curr Opin Cell Biol 1993;5:1036.
84. Murre C, McCaw PS, Vaessin H, et al: Interactions between heterologous helix-loop-helix proteins generate complexes that bind specifically to a common DNA sequence. Cell 1989;58:537.
85. Llombart-Bosch A, Navarro S: Immunohistochemical detection of EWS and FLI-1 proteins in Ewing sarcoma and primitive neuroectodermal tumors: Comparative analysis with CD99 (MIC-2) expressions. App Immunohistochem Mol Morphol 2001; 9:255.
86. Navarro S, Cavazzana AO, Llombart-Bosch A, et al: Comparison of Ewing's sarcoma of bone and peripheral neuroepithelioma: An immunocytochemical and ultrastructural analysis of two primitive neuroectodermal neoplasms. Arch Pathol Lab Med 1994; 118:608.
87. Douglass EC, Rowe ST, Valentine M, et al: A second nonrandom translocation, der(16)t(1;16)(q21;q13), in Ewing sarcoma and peripheral neuroectodermal tumor. Cytogenet Cell Genet 1990;53:87.
88. Maurici D, Perez-Atayde A, Grier HE, et al: Frequency and implications of chromosome 8 and 12 gains in Ewing sarcoma. Cancer Genet Cytogenet 1998;100:106.
89. Mugneret F, Lizard S, Aurias A, et al: Chromosomes in Ewing's sarcoma. II. Nonrandom additional changes, trisomy 8 and der(16)t(1;16). Cancer Genet Cytogenet 1988;32:239.
90. Hattinger CM, Rumpler S, Strehl S, et al: Prognostic impact of deletions at 1p36 and numerical aberrations in Ewing tumors. Genes Chromosomes Cancer 1999; 24:243.
91. Armengol G, Tarkkanen M, Virolainen M, et al: Recurrent gains of 1q, 8 and 12 in the Ewing family of tumours by comparative genomic hybridization. Br J Cancer 1997;75:1403.
92. Delattre O, Zucman J, Plougastel B, et al: Gene fusion with an ETS DNA-binding domain caused by chromosome translocation in human tumours. Nature 1992;359:162.
93. Ladanyi M: The emerging molecular genetics of sarcoma translocations. Diagn Mol Pathol 1995;4:162.
94. Ouchida M, Ohno T, Fujimura Y, et al: Loss of tumorigenicity of Ewing's sarcoma cells expressing antisense RNA to EWS-fusion transcripts. Oncogene 1995;11:1049.
95. Ida K, Kobayashi S, Taki T, et al: *EWS-FLI-1* and *EWS-ERG* chimeric mRNAs in Ewing's sarcoma and primitive neuroectodermal tumor. Int J Cancer 1995;63:500.
96. Jeon IS, Davis JN, Braun BS, et al: A variant Ewing's sarcoma translocation (7;22) fuses the EWS gene to the ETS gene ETV1. Oncogene 1995;10:1229.
97. Peter M, Couturier J, Pacquement H, et al: A new member of the ETS family fused to EWS in Ewing tumors. Oncogene 1997;14:1159.
98. Ishida S, Yoshida K, Kaneko Y, et al: The genomic breakpoint and chimeric transcripts in the EWSR1-ETV4/E1AF gene fusion in Ewing sarcoma. Cytogenet Cell Genet 1998;82:278.
99. Downing JR, Head DR, Parham DM, et al: Detection of the t(11;22)(q24;q12) translocation of Ewing's sarcoma and peripheral neuroectodermal tumor by reverse transcription polymerase chain reaction. Am J Pathol 1993;143:1294.
100. Desmaze C, Zucman J, Delattre O, et al: Interphase molecular cytogenetics of Ewing's sarcoma and peripheral neuroepithelioma t(11;22) with flanking and overlapping cosmid probes. Cancer Genet Cytogenet 1994;74:13.
101. Kumar S, Pack S, Kumar D, et al: Detection of EWS-FLI-1 fusion in Ewing's sarcoma/peripheral primitive neuroectodermal tumor by fluorescence in situ

hybridization using formalin-fixed paraffin-embedded tissue. Hum Pathol 1999;30:324.
102. Zucman J, Melot T, Desmaze C, et al: Combinatorial generation of variable fusion proteins in the Ewing family of tumours. EMBO J 1993;12:4481.
103. Meier VS, Kuhne T, Jundt G, et al: Molecular diagnosis of Ewing tumors: Improved detection of EWS-FLI-1 and EWS-ERG chimeric transcripts and rapid determination of exon combinations. Diagn Mol Pathol 1998;7:29.
104. West DC, Grier HE, Swallow MM, et al: Detection of circulating tumor cells in patients with Ewing's sarcoma and peripheral primitive neuroectodermal tumor. J Clin Oncol 1997;15:583.
105. de Alava E, Kawai A, Healey JH, et al: EWS-FLI1 fusion transcript structure is an independent determinant of prognosis in Ewing's sarcoma. J Clin Oncol 1998;16:1248.
106. Kovar H, Jug G, Aryee DN, et al: Among genes involved in the RB dependent cell cycle regulatory cascade, the p16 tumor suppressor gene is frequently lost in the Ewing family of tumors. Oncogene 1997; 15:2225.
107. Ladanyi M, Lewis R, Jhanwar SC, et al: MDM2 and CDK4 gene amplification in Ewing's sarcoma. J Pathol 1995;175:211.
108. Lawlor ER, Lim JF, Tao W, et al: The Ewing tumor family of peripheral primitive neuroectodermal tumors expresses human gastrin-releasing peptide. Cancer Res 1998;58:2469.
109. Schmidt D, Herrmann C, Jurgens H, et al: Malignant peripheral neuroectodermal tumor and its necessary distinction from Ewing's sarcoma. A report from the Kiel Pediatric Tumor Registry. Cancer 1991;68:2251.
110. Parham DM, Hijazi Y, Steinberg SM, et al: Neuroectodermal differentiation in Ewing's sarcoma family of tumors does not predict tumor behavior. Hum Pathol 1999;30:911.
111. Oberlin O, Patte C, Demeocq R, et al: The response to initial chemotherapy as a prognostic factor in localized Ewing's sarcoma. Eur J Cancer Clin Oncol 1985; 21:463.
112. Picci P, Bohling T, Bacci G, et al: Chemotherapy-induced tumor necrosis as a prognostic factor in localized Ewing's sarcoma of the extremities. J Clin Oncol 1997;15:1553.
113. Aparicio J, Munarriz B, Pastor M, et al: Long-term follow-up and prognostic factors in Ewing's sarcoma. A multivariate analysis of 116 patients from a single institution. Oncology 1998;55:20.
114. Wexler LH, Delaney TF, Tsokos M, et al: Ifosfamide and etoposide plus vincristine, doxorubicin, and cyclophosphamide for newly diagnosed Ewing's sarcoma family of tumors. Cancer 1996;78:901.
115. Jürgens H, Exner U, Gadner H, et al: Multidisciplinary treatment of primary Ewing's sarcoma of bone: A 6-year experience of a European cooperative trial. Cancer 1988;61:23.
116. Ozaki T, Hillmann A, Hoffmann C, et al: Significance of surgical margin on the prognosis of patients with Ewing's sarcoma—A report from the cooperative Ewing's sarcoma study. Cancer 1996;78:892.
117. Evans RG: The four S's of Ewing's sarcoma. Int J Radiat Oncol Biol Phys 1991;21:1671.
118. Thorner P, Squire J, Chilton-MacNeill S, et al: Is the *EWS/FLI-1* fusion transcript specific for Ewing sarcoma and peripheral primitive neuroectodermal tumor? A report of four cases showing this transcript in a wider range of tumor types. Am J Pathol 1996;148:1125.

Neuroblastoma

119. Dehner LP: Peripheral and central primitive neuroectodermal tumors. A nosologic concept seeking a consensus. Arch Pathol Lab Med 1986;110:997.
120. Matthay KK: Neuroblastoma: A clinical challenge and biologic puzzle. CA Cancer J Clin 1995;45:179.
121. Evans AE, D'Angio GJ, Propert K, et al: Prognostic factors in neuroblastoma. Cancer 1987;59:1853.
122. Kelly DR, Joshi VV: Neuroblastoma and related tumors. In Parham DM (ed): Pediatric Neoplasia: Morphology and Biology. Philadelphia, Lippincott-Raven, 1996:105.
123. Bolande RP: A natural immune system in pregnancy serum lethal to human neuroblastoma cells: A possible mechanism of spontaneous regression. Perspect Pediatr Pathol 1992;16:120.
124. Graeve JLA, De Alarcon PA, Sato Y, et al: Miliary pulmonary neuroblastoma: A risk of autologous bone marrow transplantation. Cancer 1988;62:2125.
125. Telles NC, Rabson AS, Pomeroy TC: Ewing's sarcoma: An autopsy study. Cancer 1978;41:2321.
126. Brodeur GM, Pritchard J, Berthold F, et al: Revisions of the international criteria for neuroblastoma diagnosis, staging, and response to treatment. J Clin Oncol 1993;11:1466.
127. Acharya S, Jayabose S, Kogan SJ, et al: Prenatally diagnosed neuroblastoma. Cancer 1997;80:304.
128. Joshi VV, Silverman JF, Altshuler G, et al: Systematization of primary histopathologic and fine-needle aspiration cytologic features and description of unusual histopathologic features of neuroblastic tumors: A report from the Pediatric Oncology Group. Hum Pathol 1993;24:493.
129. Shimada H, Ambros IM, Dehner LP, et al: Terminology and morphologic criteria of neuroblastic tumors: Recommendations by the International Neuroblastoma Pathology Committee. Cancer 1999;86:349.
130. Shimada H, Chatten J, Newton WA Jr, et al: Histopathologic prognostic factors in neuroblastic tumors: Definition of subtypes of ganglioneuroblastoma and an age-linked classification of neuroblastomas. J Natl Cancer Inst 1984;73:405.
131. Shimada H, Ambros IM, Dehner LP, et al: The International Neuroblastoma Pathology Classification (the Shimada system). Cancer 1999;86:364.
132. Cozzutto C, Carbone A: Pleomorphic (anaplastic) neuroblastoma. Arch Pathol 1988;112:621.

133. Gonzalez-Crussi F, Hsueh W: Bilateral adrenal ganglioneuroblastoma with neuromelanin. Clinical and pathologic observations. Cancer 1988;61:1159.
134. Tsokos M, Scarpa S, Ross RA, et al: Differentiation of human neuroblastoma recapitulates neural crest development. Study of morphology, neurotransmitter enzymes, and extracellular matrix proteins. Am J Pathol 1987;128:484.
135. Balázs M: Mixed pheochromocytoma and ganglioneuroma of the adrenal medulla: A case report with electron microscopic examination. Hum Pathol 1988;19:1352.
136. Blatt J, Gula MJ, Orlando SJ, et al: Indolent course of advanced neuroblastoma in children older than 6 years at diagnosis. Cancer 1995;76:890.
137. Mierau GW, Berry PJ, Malott RL, et al: Appraisal of the comparative utility of immunohistochemistry and electron microscopy in the diagnosis of childhood round cell tumors. Ultrastruct Pathol 1996;20:507.
138. Thiele CJ: Pediatric peripheral neuroectodermal tumors, oncogenes, and differentiation. Cancer Invest 1990;8:629.
139. Dias P, Kumar P, Marsden HB, et al.: N-myc gene is amplified in alveolar rhabdomyosarcomas (RMS) but not in embryonal RMS. Int J Cancer 1990;45:593.
140. Driman D, Thorner PS, Greenberg ML, et al: *MYCN* gene amplification in rhabdomyosarcoma. Cancer 1994;73:2231.
141. Leader M, Collins M, Patel J, et al: Antineuron specific enolase staining reactions in sarcomas and carcinomas: Its lack of neuroendocrine specificity. J Clin Pathol 1986;39:1186.
141A. Wick MR: Immunohistology of neuroendocrine and neuroectodermal tumors. Semin Diagn Pathol 2000; 17:194.
142. Brodeur GM, Green AA, Hayes FA, et al: Cytogenetic features of human neuroblastomas and cell lines. Cancer Res 1981;41:4678.
143. Maris JM, Matthay KK: Molecular biology of neuroblastoma. J Clin Oncol 1999;17:2264.
144. Shapiro DN, Valentine MB, Rowe ST, et al: Detection of *N-myc* gene amplification by fluorescence in situ hybridization. Diagnostic utility for neuroblastoma. Am J Pathol 1993;142:1339.
145. Look AT, Hayes FA, Nitschke R, et al: Cellular DNA content as a predictor of response to chemotherapy in infants with unresectable neuroblastoma. N Engl J Med 1984;311:231.
146. Look AT, Hayes FA, Shuster JJ, et al: Clinical relevance of tumor cell ploidy and N-*myc* gene amplification in childhood neuroblastoma: A Pediatric Oncology Group study. J Clin Oncol 1991;9:581.
147. Tanaka T, Sugimoto T, Sawada T: Prognostic discrimination among neuroblastomas according to Ha-ras/ trk A gene expression: A comparison of the profiles of neuroblastomas detected clinically and those detected through mass screening. Cancer 1998;83:1626.
148. Maitra A, Yashima K, Rathi A, et al: The RNA component of telomerase as a marker of biologic potential and clinical outcome in childhood neuroblastic tumors. Cancer 1999;85:741.
149. Brodeur GM, Azar C, Brother M, et al.: Neuroblastoma: Effect of genetic factors on prognosis and treatment. Cancer 1992;70(suppl):1685.

Small Cell Desmoplastic Tumor

150. Ordonez NG: Desmoplastic small round cell tumor: I: A histopathologic study of 39 cases with emphasis on unusual histological patterns. Am J Surg Pathol 1998;22:1303.
151. Gerald WL, Miller HK, Battifora H, et al: Intraabdominal desmoplastic small round-cell tumor: Report of 19 cases of a distinctive type of high-grade polyphenotypic malignancy affecting young individuals. Am J Surg Pathol 1991;15:499.
152. Kretschmar CS, Colbach C, Bhan I, et al: Desmoplastic small cell tumor: A report of three cases and a review of the literature. J Pediatr Hematol Oncol 1996;18:293.
153. Ordonez NG, El-Naggar AK, Ro JY, et al: Intraabdominal desmoplastic small cell tumor: A light microscopic, immunocytochemical, ultrastructural, and flow cytometric study. Hum Pathol 1993;24:850.
154. Adsay V, Cheng J, Athanasian E, et al: Primary desmoplastic small cell tumor of soft tissues and bone of the hand. Am J Surg Pathol 1999;23:1408.
155. Bian Y, Jordan AG, Rupp M, et al: Effusion cytology of desmoplastic small round cell tumor of the pleura: A case report. Acta Cytol 1993;37:77.
156. Tison V, Cerasoli S, Morigi F, et al: Intracranial desmoplastic small-cell tumor—Report of a case. Am J Surg Pathol 1996;20:112.
157. Schmidt D, Koster E, Harms D: Intraabdominal desmoplastic small-cell tumor with divergent differentiation: clinicopathological findings and DNA ploidy. Med Pediatr Oncol 1994;22:97.
158. Ordonez NG: Desmoplastic small round cell tumor: II: An ultrastructural and immunohistochemical study with emphasis on new immunohistochemical markers. Am J Surg Pathol 1998;22:1314.
159. Trupiano JK, Machen SK, Barr FG, et al: Cytokeratin-negative desmoplastic small round cell tumor: A report of two cases emphasizing the utility of reverse transcriptase-polymerase chain reaction. Mod Pathol 1999;12:849.
160. Sawyer JR, Tryka AF, Lewis JM: A novel reciprocal chromosome translocation t(11;22)(p13;q12) in an intraabdominal desmoplastic small round-cell tumor. Am J Surg Pathol 1992;16:411.
161. Ladanyi M, Gerald W: Fusion of the EWS and WT1 genes in the desmoplastic small round cell tumor. Cancer Res 1994;54:2837.
162. Park S, Schalling M, Bernard A, et al: The Wilms tumour gene *WT1* is expressed in murine mesoderm-derived tissues and mutated in a human mesothelioma. Nat Genet 1993;4:415.
163. Walker C, Rutten F, Yuan X, et al: Wilms' tumor suppressor gene expression in rat and human mesothelioma. Cancer Res 1994;54:3101.

164. Roberts DJ, Haber D, Sklar J, et al: Extrarenal Wilms' tumors. A study of their relationship with classical renal Wilms' tumor using expression of WT1 as a molecular marker. Lab Invest 1993;68:528.
165. Lee SB, Kolquist KA, Nichols K, et al: The EWS-WT1 translocation product induces PDGFA in desmoplastic small round-cell tumour. Nat Genet 1997;17:309.
166. De Alava E, Ladanyi M, Rosai J, et al: Detection of chimeric transcripts in desmoplasmic small round cell tumor and related developmental tumors by reverse transcriptase polymerase chain reaction—A specific diagnostic assay. Am J Pathol 1995;147:1584.
167. Argatoff LH, O'Connell JX, Mathers JA, et al: Detection of the *EWS/WT1* gene fusion by reverse transcriptase-polymerase chain reaction in the diagnosis of intra-abdominal desmoplastic small round cell tumor. Am J Surg Pathol 1996;20:406.
168. Katz RL, Quezado M, Senderowicz AM, et al: An intra-abdominal small round cell neoplasm with features of primitive neuroectodermal and desmoplastic round cell tumor and a EWS/FLI-1 fusion transcript. Hum Pathol 1997;28:502.
169. Amato RJ, Ellerhorst JA, Ayala AG: Intraabdominal desmoplastic small cell tumor. Report and discussion of five cases. Cancer 1996;78:845.
170. Coppes MJ, Wilson PCG, Weitzman S: Extrarenal Wilms' tumor: Staging, treatment, and prognosis. J Clin Oncol 1991;9:167.
170A. Hill DA, Pfeifer JD, Marley EF, et al: WTI staining reliably differentiates desmoplastic small cell tumor from Ewing sarcoma/primitive neuroectodermal tumor. An immunohistochemical and molecular diagnostic study. Am Clin Pathol 2000;114:345.

Extrarenal Rhabdoid Tumor

171. Parham DM, Weeks DA, Beckwith JB: The clinicopathologic spectrum of putative extrarenal rhabdoid tumors: An analysis of 42 cases studies with immunohistochemistry and/or electron microscopy. Am J Surg Pathol 1994;18:1010.
172. Leong FJ, Leong AS: Malignant rhabdoid tumor in adults—Heterogenous tumors with a unique morphological phenotype. Pathol Res Pract 1996;192:796.
173. White FV, Dehner LP, Belchis DA, et al: Congenital disseminated malignant rhabdoid tumor: Distinct clicopathologic entity demonstrating abnormalities of chromosome 22q11. Am J Surg Pathol 1999;23: 249.
174. Simons J, Teshima I, Zielenska M, et al: Analysis of chromosome 22q as an aid to the diagnosis of rhabdoid tumor: A case report. Am J Surg Pathol 1999;23:982.
175. Beckwith JB, Palmer NF: Histopathology and prognosis of Wilms tumors: Results from the First National Wilms' Tumor Study. Cancer 1978;41:1937.
176. Balaton AJ, Vaury P, Videgrain M: Paravertebral malignant rhabdoid tumor in an adult. A case report with immunocytochemical study. Pathol Res Pract 1987;182:713.
177. Dabbs DJ, Park HK: Malignant rhabdoid skin tumor: An uncommon primary skin neoplasm. Ultrastructural and immunohistochemical analysis. J Cutan Pathol 1988;15:109.
178. Tsuneyoshi M, Daimaru Y, Hashimoto H, et al: Malignant soft tissue neoplasms with the histologic features of renal rhabdoid tumors: An ultrastructural and immunohistochemical study. Hum Pathol 1985; 16:1235.
179. Gonzalez-Crussi F, Goldschmidt RA, Hsueh W, et al: Infantile sarcoma with intracytoplasmic filamentous inclusions: Distinctive tumor of possible histiocytic origin. Cancer 1982;49:2365.
180. Lemos LB, Hamoudi AB: Malignant thymic tumor in an infant (malignant histiocytoma). Arch Pathol Lab Med 1978;102:84.
181. Hajdu SI: Pathology of Soft Tissue Tumors. Philadelphia, Lea & Febiger, 1979.
182. Kodet R, Newton WA Jr, Sachs N, et al: Rhabdoid tumors of soft tissues: A clinicopathologic study of 26 cases enrolled on the Intergroup Rhabdomyosarcoma Study. Hum Pathol 1991;22:674.
183. Tsuneyoshi M, Daimaru Y, Hashimoto H, et al: The existence of rhabdoid cells in specified soft tissue sarcomas: Histopathological, ultrastructural and immunohistochemical evidence. Virchows Arch [A] 1987;411:509.
184. Kodet R, Newton WA, Jr., Hamoudi AB, et al: Rhabdomyosarcomas with intermediate-filament inclusions and features of rhabdoid tumors: Light microscopic and immunohistochemical study. Am J Surg Pathol 1991;15:257.
185. Tsokos M, Kouraklis G, Chandra RS, et al: Malignant rhabdoid tumor of the kidney and soft tissues: Evidence for a diverse morphological and immunocytochemical phenotype. Arch Pathol Lab Med 1989; 113:115.
186. Rorke LB, Packer RJ, Biegel JA: Central nervous system atypical teratoid/rhabdoid tumors of infancy and childhood: Definition of an entity. J Neurosurg 1996;85:56.
187. Chung CJ, Cammoun D, Munden M: Rhabdoid tumor of the kidney presenting as an abdominal mass in a newborn. Pediatr Radiol 1990;20:562.
188. Kent AL, Mahoney DH, Gresik MV, et al: Malignant rhabdoid tumor of the extremity. Cancer 1987; 60:1056.
189. Dominey A, Paller AS, Gonzalez-Crussi F: Congenital rhabdoid sarcoma with cutaneous metastases. J Am Acad Dermatol 1990;22:969.
190. Perez-Atayde AR, Newbury R, Fletcher JA, et al: Congenital "neurovascular hamartoma" of the skin. A possible marker of malignant rhabdoid tumor. Am J Surg Pathol 1994;18:1030.
191. Jayabose S, Iqbal K, Newman L, et al: Hypercalcemia in childhood renal tumors. Cancer 1988;61:788.
192. Mayes LC, Kasselberg AG, Roloff JS, et al: Hypercalcemia associated with immunoreactive parathyroid hormone in a malignant rhabdoid tumor of the kidney (rhabdoid Wilms' tumor). Cancer 1984;54:882.

193. Rousseau-Merck MF, Nogues C, Roth A, et al: Hypercalcemic infantile renal tumors: Morphological, clinical, and biological heterogeneity. Pediatr Pathol 1985;3:155.
194. Bonnin JM, Rubinstein LJ, Palmer NF, et al: The association of embryonal tumours originating in the kidney and in the brain. Cancer 1984;54:2137.
195. Chang CH, Ramirez N, Sakr WA: Primitive neuroectodermal tumor of the brain associated with malignant rhabdoid tumor of the liver: Histologic, immunohistochemical, and electron microscopic study. Pediatr Pathol 1989;9:307.
196. Weeks DA, Beckwith JB, Mierau GW, et al: Rhabdoid tumor of kidney: A report of 111 cases from the National Wilms' Tumor Study Pathology Center. Am J Surg Pathol 1989;13:439.
197. Suzuki A, Ohta S, Shimada M: Gene expression of malignant rhabdoid tumor cell lines by reverse transcriptase-polymerase chain reaction. Diagn Mol Pathol 1997;6:326.
198. Douglass EC, Valentine M, Rowe ST, et al: Malignant rhabdoid tumor: A highly malignant childhood tumor with minimal karyotypic changes. Genes Chromosomes Cancer 1990;2:210.
199. Biegel JA, Rorke LB, Emanuel BS: Monosomy 22 in rhabdoid or atypical teratoid tumors of the brain. N Engl J Med 1989;321:906.
200. Bhattacharjee MB, Armstrong DD, Vogel H, et al: Cytogenetic analysis of 120 primary pediatric brain tumors and literature review. Cancer Genet Cytogenet 1997;97:39.
201. Schofield DE, Beckwith JB, Sklar J: Loss of heterozygosity at chromosome regions 22q11-12 and 11p15.5 in renal rhabdoid tumors. Genes Chromosomes Cancer 1996;15:10.
202. Biegel JA, Allen CS, Kawasaki K, et al: Narrowing the critical region for a rhabdoid tumor locus in 22q11. Genes Chromosomes Cancer 1996;16:94.
203. Versteege I, Sevenet N, Lange J, et al: Truncating mutations of hSNF5/INI1 in aggressive paediatric cancer. Nature 1998;394:203.
204. Garvin AJ, Re GG, Tarnowski BI, et al: The G401 cell line, utilized for studies of chromosomal changes in Wilms' tumor, is derived from a rhabdoid tumor of the kidney. Am J Pathol 1993;142:375.
205. Reid LH, Davies C, Cooper PR, et al: A 1-Mb physical map and PAC contig of the imprinted domain in 11p15.5 that contains TAPA1 and the BWSCR1/WT2 region. Genomics 1997;43:366.
206. Sabbioni S, Barbanti-Brodano G, Croce CM, et al: GOK: A gene at 11p15 involved in rhabdomyosarcoma and rhabdoid tumor development. Cancer Res 1997;57:4493.
207. Shiratsuchi H, Saito T, Sakamoto A, et al: Mutation analysis of himan cytokeratin 8 gene in malignant rhabdoid tumor: A possible association with intracytoplasmic inclusion body formation. Mod Pathol 2002;15:146.
208. Guillou L, Wadden C, Coindre JM, et al: "Proximal-type" epithelioid sarcoma, a distinctive aggressive neoplasm showing rhabdoid features. Clinicopathologic, immunohistochemical, and ultrastructural study of a series. Am J Surg Pathol 1997;21:130.

Soft Tissue Tumors with Epithelial Differentiation

CHAPTER 19

Epithelial tumors presenting in soft tissue form a heterogeneous group of unrelated tumors, common to which is evidence for epithelial differentiation. Such a differentiation is often easily detected histologically, but it is more easily highlighted with immunohistochemical markers for epithelial differentiation (keratins, epithelial membrane antigen [EMA], others). Therefore, unrelated tumors of this group enter in the differential diagnosis of soft tissue tumors that are positive for epithelial markers.

It should be recognized that some other nonepithelial cells and tumors also can express keratins. Examples of these include normal and neoplastic smooth muscle cells, melanomas, and some sarcomas, including epithelioid vascular tumors. These are discussed in the appropriate chapters.

The tumors discussed in this chapter are synovial sarcoma, epithelioid sarcoma, mixed tumor of soft tissues, multicystic peritoneal mesothelioma, malignant mesothelioma, and ectopic hamartomatous thymoma, a rare specific, epithelial soft tissue tumor of the neck. Merkel cell carcinoma and metastatic carcinomas are also discussed.

Synovial Sarcoma

Synovial sarcoma is a specific soft tissue sarcoma demonstrating dual epithelial and mesenchymal differentiation. The tumor is not related to synovial lining cells, and it is only rarely associated with synovial tissue. The name is based on historical reasons only because the epithelial components of the biphasic tumors were once thought to simulate the synovial slits. The typical t(X;18) translocation with *SYT-SSX* gene fusion is diagnostically important, and probably also is a key pathogenetic event.

Clinical Features at Typical Sites

Synovial sarcoma is a relatively common soft tissue sarcoma comprising 7% to 10% of all soft tissue sarcomas. It typically presents in the extremities of young adults with a median age in various series between 30 and 35 years. It may occur in children from first decade on, and it may be seen in older adults in the seventh and eighth decades. Many series show a slight male predominance (55:45). The tumor primarily occurs in deep, intramuscular soft tissue, and has a strong predilection to the extremities (70–80%). The most common sites are the thigh, knee region, ankle and feet, hands, and the other parts of the upper extremity; location in the proximal parts of extremities is slightly more common than distal. Direct synovial involvement is exceptional, but a periarticular tumor may bulge into synovial space from outside.

Small tumors of the hand and wrist often clinically simulate a ganglion cyst or another benign process. Many synovial sarcomas are painful, but otherwise they are not clinically distinctive from other soft tissue tumors.

Local recurrence is rare after adequate wide excision, but occurs in 30% to 50% if the tumor is simply shelled out. Lymph node metastases, rare in other sarcomas, may occur, sometimes long after primary surgery. Distant metastases develop in 40% to 50% of the patients. The most common metastatic site is lung, and massive pleuropulmonary metastasis is the leading cause of death. Liver and brain metastases may also occur. The 5-year survival rate for patients with tumors other than poorly differentiated ones is 60% to 70%, whereas those with the poorly differentiated tumors have a markedly worse 5-year survival, only 20% to 30%. Notably, children and young adults below age 20 years have a better prognosis.[1–10]

Clinical Features at Rare Sites

Less common, nonextremity sites include scalp, neck,[11] orofacial region,[12] upper aerodigestive tract (oropharynx-parapharynx-esophagus), chest wall, mediastinum,[13] pleura and lungs,[14–16] prostate,[17,18] retroperitoneum,[19] and abdominal wall.[20] Intravascular presentation in the femoral vein[21,22] and atrium of heart[23] has also been reported on a few occasions. Recently, tumors originally classified as embryonal sarcomas of the kidney were reclassified as primary renal synovial sarcomas.[24] The tumors at the uncommon sites also tend to occur in young adults. However, the possibility of metastasis from an extremity tumor has to be considered before diagnosing a primary organ-based synovial sarcoma. Many recent reports on organ-based synovial sarcoma are well-documented showing the synovial sarcoma specific t(X;18) translocation.

Pathology

Grossly, synovial sarcoma is rarely diagnostic. Tumor size varies in a broad range. Peripheral tumors may be 1 cm or smaller, whereas these tumors more commonly reach the size of at least 3 to 10 cm in more proximal locations and 10 to 20 cm in the deep thigh. On sectioning the tumor is soft, gray-white,

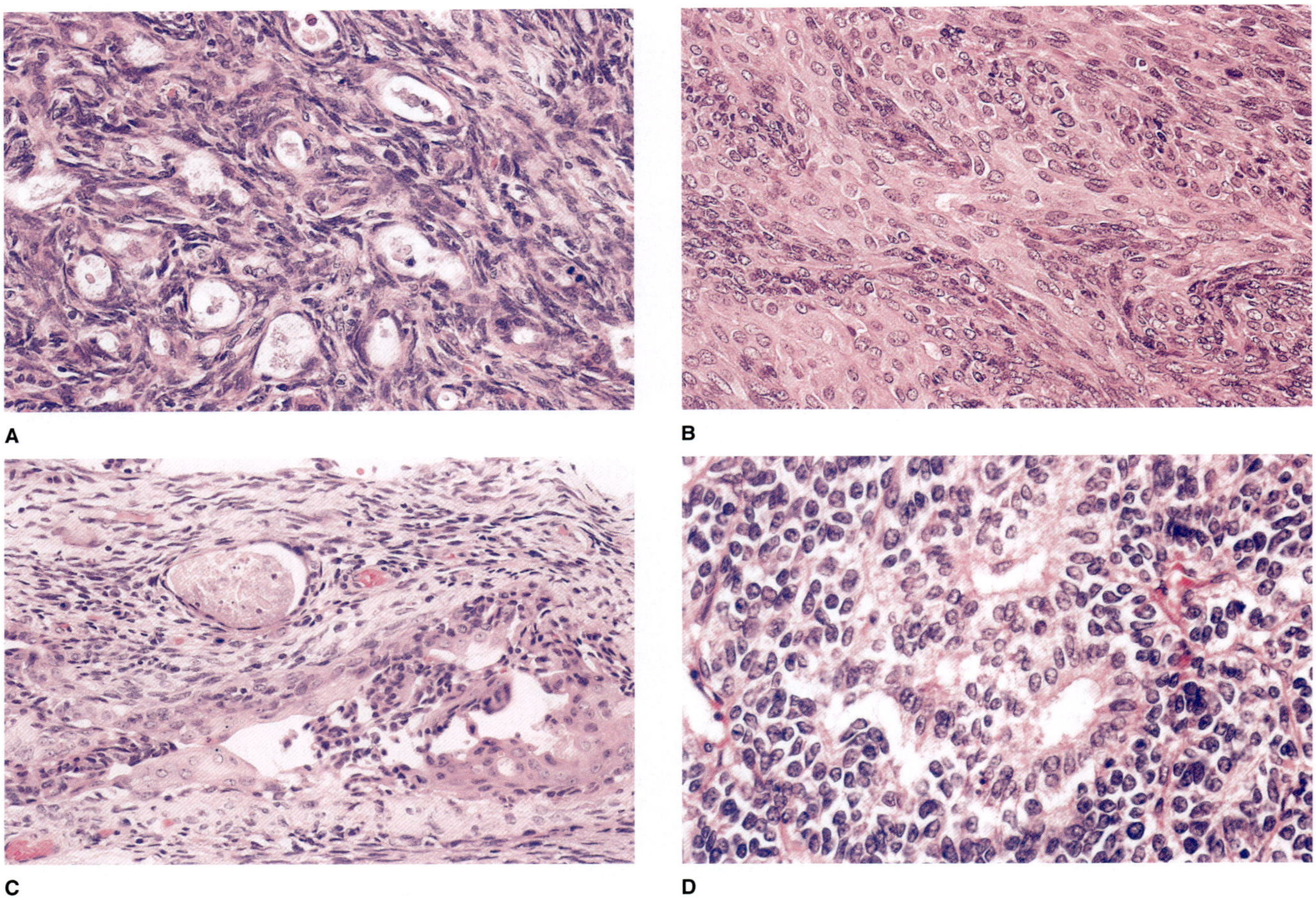

Figure 19–1. Histologic spectrum of biphasic synovial sarcoma. Note different histologic patterns of epithelial differentiation including glandular epithelia with luminal secretion *(A)*, pale staining glandular epithelia with poor lumen formation *(B)*, well-differentiated glands with stratified epithelia *(C)*, and poorly differentiated cells forming primitive glands *(D)*.

and like fish flesh. Some tumors are extensively cystic lined by a narrow rim of tumor tissue. In the past, such tumors have been considered to originate from the bursa, but more likely the cystic nature is unrelated to pre-existing anatomic structures. Gross calcification and ossification may occur.

Synovial sarcoma has a wide histologic spectrum that includes three variants that sometimes coexist in one tumor. Monophasic spindle cell pattern is the most common followed by biphasic synovial sarcoma and poorly differentiated synovial sarcoma.

Pathology of Biphasic Type

Biphasic synovial sarcoma (20–30%) is the most distinctive although not the most common variant. It contains a combination of epithelial and spindle cell elements. The former represent well-formed glandular epithelial structures or solid epithelial sheets surrounded by a basement membrane. The lumen may contain periodic acid-Schiff (PAS)-positive secretion (Fig. 19–1). The appearance of the glandular epithelium varies from cuboidal to tall columnar, and occasionally has squamous features with keratinization.[25] The spindle cell component is similar to that in the monophasic tumors. Some biphasic tumors contain sheets of epithelial cells with poorly differentiated glandular structures. The proportion of the epithelial component varies in a wide range. Some tumors are almost entirely monophasic spindle cell lesions that contain only a few glands, whereas rare cases are composed almost entirely of the epithelial component. In some cases, diagnosis of biphasic histology is very focal requiring extensive sampling.

Pathology of Monophasic Spindle Cell Type

Many spindle cell sarcomas earlier classified as fibrosarcomas are actually monophasic synovial sarcomas, as defined around the early 1980s.[26–28] The monophasic spindle cell variant (50–60%) is composed of relatively uniform spindle cells that may be densely packed or arranged in a matrix that varies from myxoid to densely collagenous, sometimes in an alternating pattern in one tumor (Fig. 19–2). Some tumors have nuclear palisading resembling

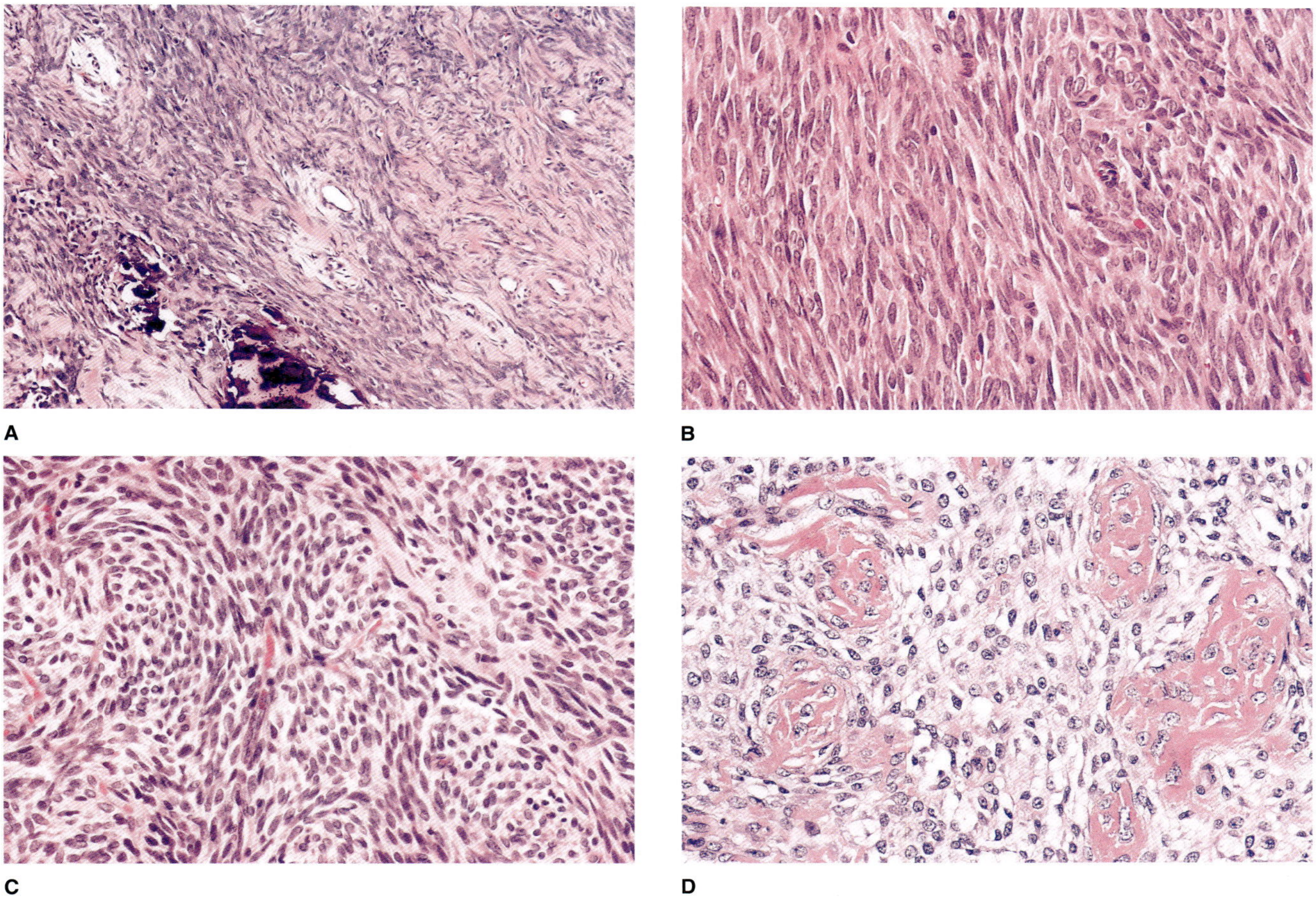

Figure 19–2. Histologic spectrum of monophasic synovial sarcoma. *A,* Moderately cellular spindle cell tumor with focal calcification. *B,* Highly cellular variant with focal whorl formation. *C,* Prominent whorl formation. *D,* A variant with myxoid stroma.

that of schwannoma. Focal calcifications are common in the fibrous matrix and extensive calcification[29] and ossification[30] may also occur. Vague epithelioid differentiation is sometimes seen among spindle cells. Mast cell infiltration is typical. Hemangiopericytoma-like pattern may also occur. Cytologically, the nuclei are elongated with pointed ends and lack of nuclear pleomorphism is most typical of this tumor. The cytoplasm is basophilic and cell borders are inconspicuous.

Pathology of Poorly Differentiated Synovial Sarcoma

Poorly differentiated synovial sarcoma (15–25%) has different histologic patterns. Common to all of them is high-grade sarcomatous appearance with a high mitotic rate (over 15 mitoses/10 high-power fields [HPF]). The tumors may show a hemangiopericytoma-like vascular pattern with sheets of oval tumor cells between the vessels (Fig. 19–3). A high-grade fibrosarcoma-like pattern with fascicular appearance occurs, and some poorly differentiated synovial sarcomas show a small, round cell pattern simulating small round cell tumors such as extraskeletal Ewing sarcoma or peripheral neuroepithelioma. Some cases contain rhabdoid cells with perinuclear cytoplasmic inclusions of intermediate filaments. Recognition of these tumors as synovial sarcomas often requires special studies, unless differentiated components are present in other areas. Extensive sampling is recommended, because it may reveal the diagnosis more easily than any special studies, especially if glands are present.[31]

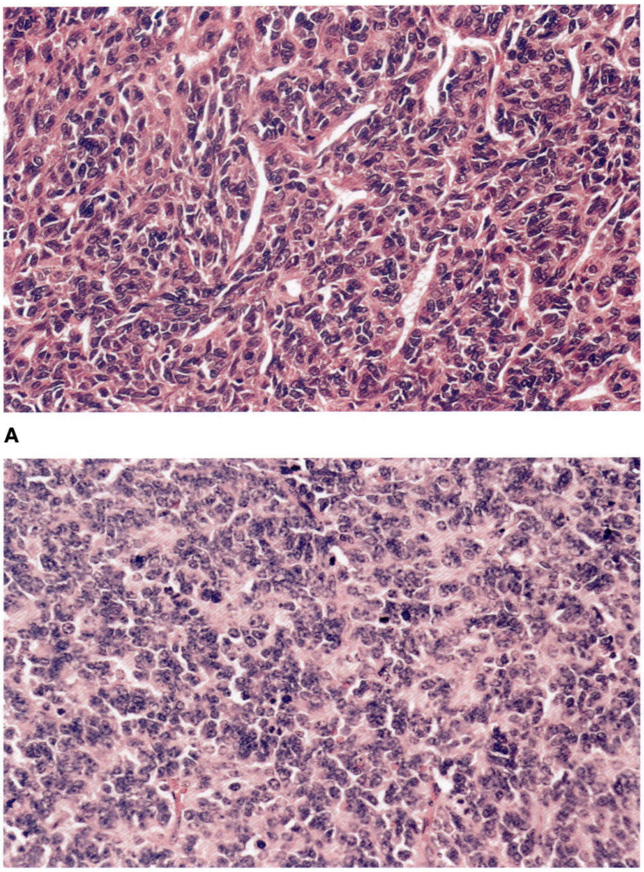

A

B

Figure 19–3. Variants of poorly differentiated synovial sarcoma. *A,* Hemangiopericytoma-like pattern. *B,* Ewing-primitive neuroectodermal tumor-like round cell pattern with pseudorosettes.

Prognostic Factors

Favorable prognostic factors are tumor size less than 5 cm, peripheral location, young age (<20 years), high mast cell content (>20/10 HPF), and extensive calcifications. Unfavorable are mitotic rate more than 15/10 HPF, the presence of a rhabdoid component, tumor necrosis, poorly differentiated histology, high stage, and incomplete primary excision.[3–9]

The prognostic significance of monophasic versus biphasic type is still controversial. Recently, SSX2-type gene fusion of the synovial sarcoma translocation has been found prognostically favorable,[32] with one of the studies showing 89% of metastasis-free survival with this genotype.[33]

Immunohistochemistry

Immunohistochemical analysis is often essential for the diagnosis of monophasic variants, where the demonstration of keratins and EMA is essential.[34–38]

The epithelial cells in the biphasic tumors and scattered cells or nests and small clusters of spindle cells are positive for keratins and EMA, E-cadherin, and BerEp4. The epithelial cells in biphasic synovial sarcomas contain simple epithelial keratins K7, K8, K18, and K19 and additionally high-molecular-weight keratins of complex epithelia K14 and K17, and sporadically K13, K16, and K20 (Fig. 19–4). Examples with squamous differentiation may show K10 in the keratinizing epithelia.[38]

The monophasic tumors contain scattered cells positive for keratins K7, K8, K18, and K19, whereas other keratins are rare in the monophasic tumors. EMA reactivity is seen in patches, and the number of positive cells may be greater than that for keratins (Fig. 19–4). E-Cadherin and N-cadherin are variably expressed, especially in the epithelial component;[39] according to our experience, the former is usually more prevalent.

Some markers often used in the positive identification of mesothelioma ("mesothelial markers") are expressed in synovial sarcoma. In the biphasic tumors, the glandular epithelial cells are HBME1$^+$, whereas

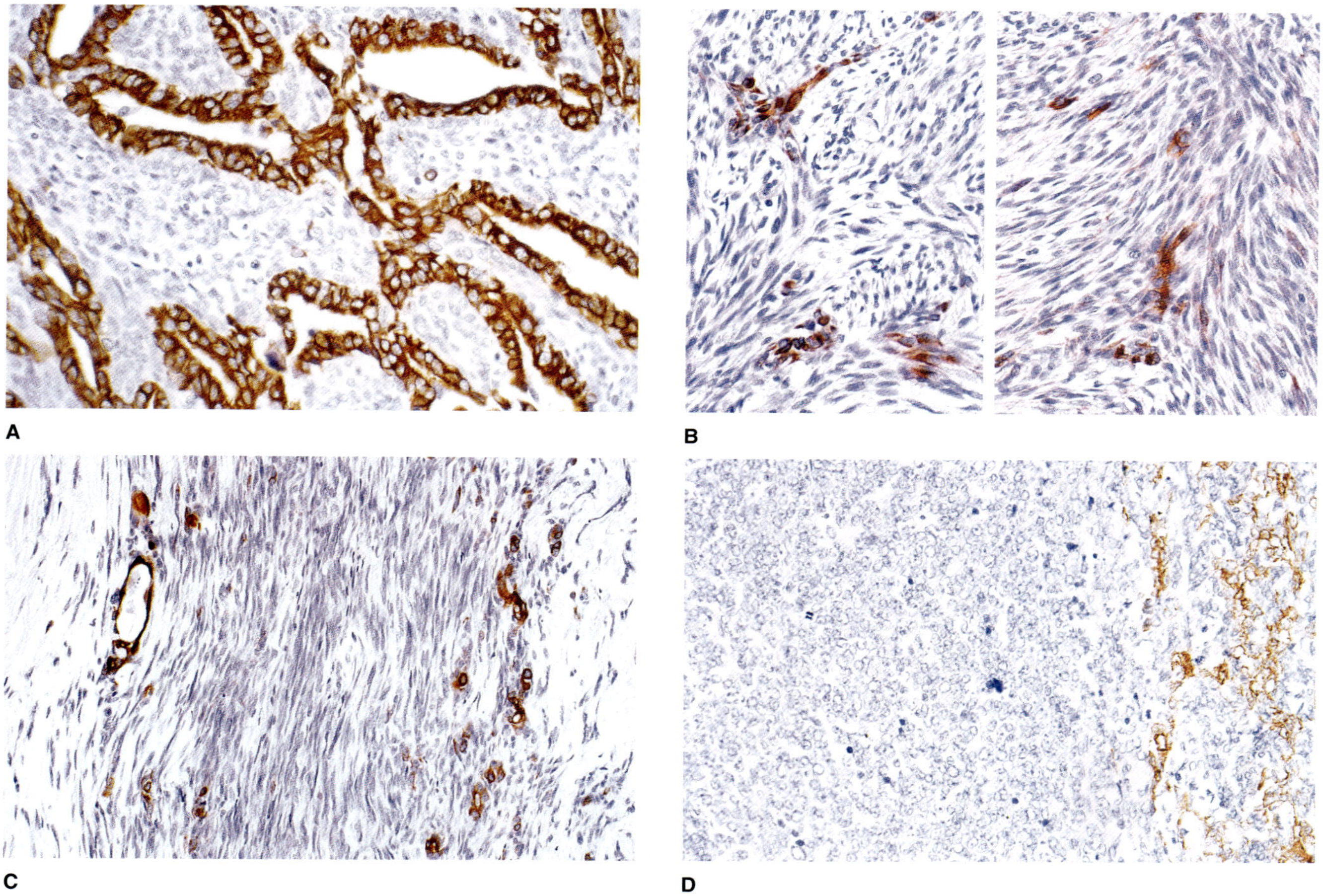

Figure 19–4. Immunohistochemical documentation of synovial sarcoma. *A,* Biphasic tumor with prominent positivity for K14. *B,* Monophasic tumor with focal K19 *(left)* and patchy EMA positivity *(right). C,* Monophasic tumor with streaks of K7 positivity and one positive glandlike structure. *D,* Poorly differentiated area of synovial sarcoma is negative for keratin cocktail AE1/AE3, but an adjacent better-differentiated area shows focal positivity.

the monophasic and poorly differentiated tumors are typically negative. The epithelial cells may also be positive for calretinin, which is more commonly expressed in the spindle cell component, monophasic tumors, and poorly differentiated components; approximately 70% of synovial sarcomas have calretinin-positive cells; this should not lead into confusion with mesothelioma. Of the other mesothelioma markers, CD141 (thrombomodulin) is rarely expressed in synovial sarcoma, whereas these tumors seem to be negative for Wilms tumor 1 protein (WT1).[40]

Positivity for S-100 protein is seen in 30% of synovial sarcomas, sometimes as extensive reactivity in the majority of tumor cells. Positivity may occur in all types of synovial sarcoma, although it is more common in biphasic than monophasic tumors. In addition, small hyperplastic nerve twigs are highlighted, especially in small synovial sarcomas.[41]

Rarely, biphasic tumors have a focally $CD34^+$ spindle cell component, which is practically uniformly negative for smooth muscle actin and desmin.

Vimentin is expressed in both spindle cell and epithelial components, the latter often showing a basal cytoplasmic pattern. Many cases react with CD99; this has to be considered in the differential diagnosis of Ewing sarcoma and related tumors.[42] The spindle cells of synovial sarcoma are typically positive for bcl2, whereas the epithelial component is usually negative.[43]

Poorly differentiated synovial sarcomas may show limited if any keratin and EMA positivity, and immunohistochemistry may be inconclusive. Recognition of the poorly differentiated variant requires cytogenetic or molecular diagnosis, unless better differentiated areas or typical patterns of keratin or EMA expression are present.

Differential Diagnosis

Monophasic synovial sarcoma often resembles fibrosarcoma, and actually a majority of deep fibrosarcoma-like tumors are synovial sarcomas. The tumors with palisades with S-100 positivity may resemble cellular schwannoma. However, monophasic synovial sarcoma is more highly cellular and more homogenous in composition than schwannoma.

Small synovial sarcomas in the peripheral extremities often elicit a significant neural proliferation inside the tumor and should not be misinterpreted as malignant peripheral nerve sheath tumors. The cellular components between the neuroma-like elements are similar to monophasic (or rarely biphasic) synovial sarcoma.

The biphasic tumors can resemble teratomas or mixed tumors. The former do not generally occur in soft tissue locations, and the latter do not have similar biphasic pattern as seen in synovial sarcoma.

The poorly differentiated tumors may simulate Ewing family tumors both histologically and immunohistochemically (CD99$^+$). If no differentiated components are present, the patterns of keratins and EMA may be helpful—synovial sarcoma being more often K7$^+$, K19$^+$, and EMA$^+$. In the cases negative for keratins, molecular diagnosis of specific translocations is often necessary for the definitive diagnosis.

Genetics

Synovial sarcoma typically shows a t(X;18)(p11.2; q11.2) translocation that creates a large derivative X where a major portion of the long arm of chromosome 18 is translocated to the short arm of X chromosome.[44,45] This distinctive chromosomal change appears specific for synovial sarcoma and has not been documented in other sarcomas.

The genes involved in the synovial sarcoma translocation are *SYT* in chromosome 18 and one of the *SSX* genes in X chromosome: *SSX1*, *SSX2*,[46–50] or very rarely, *SSX4*.[51]

The synovial sarcoma translocation creates a gene fusion with a resulting fusion transcript (chimeric transcript) and fusion protein. Both *SYT* and *SSX* gene products are expressed in the nuclei. *SYT* gene apparently is a transcriptional activator and SSX genes are transcriptional repressors. The altered regulatory function of these genes may be the key event in the pathogenesis of synovial sarcoma.[50] The *SSX* genes are normally expressed in testis, and also have been detected in many cancers, representing the so-called testis-cancer antigens.[52]

The translocation can be diagnosed, in addition to the classic cytogenetics, by fluorescence in situ hybridization (FISH)[53–59] or by reverse transcription-polymerase chain reaction (RT-PCR).[32,60–64] FISH studies have expectedly shown that both the epithelial and spindle cells in biphasic tumors carry the translocation.[58] Whether or not *SSX1* or *SSX2* is involved can also be determined by FISH using appropriate probes.[59]

Several series have shown the feasibility of RT-PCR test in both fresh and paraffin-embedded tissue.[32,60–64] It has been shown that a great majority of biphasic tumors have *SSX1* gene involvement, whereas the monophasic ones have either *SSX1* or *SSX2* with an equal frequency.[32,50] Tumors with the *SYT-SSX2* fusion have a longer metastasis-free survival than the ones with *SYT-SSX1* fusion; in one study there was 89% metastasis-free survival in tumors with *SSX2* fusion.[33] The tumors with SSX1 fusion have been shown to have a higher proliferative activity.[64]

Moderately large numbers of other sarcomas have been evaluated for the SYT-SSX fusions, and all have been found negative.[65] Opposite results have been presented, including the apparently common presence of the *SYT-SSX* fusions in neurofibroma and malignant peripheral nerve sheath tumor.[66] However, these results have been viewed with great skepticism because of the uniform lack of t(X;18) translocation in the cytogenetic studies of large numbers of peripheral nerve sheath tumors.[67] Potential reasons for the differences include different diagnostic criteria for tumors, and false-positive results in the translocation assay. Further studies are necessary to clarify this issue.

Additional, secondary genetic changes often produce complex karyotypes, and they probably represent genetic disease progression, as such changes are more common in recurrent tumors.[68] Comparative genomic hybridization has shown no DNA copy number changes in 50% of the cases, apparently representing the cases with balanced translocation only. In the remaining 50% of the cases, the most common additional copy DNA number changes have been gains of 8q and 12q and losses of 13q21-31 and 3p.[69]

Epithelioid Sarcoma

Epithelioid sarcoma, first described by Enzinger in 1970, is a histologically distinctive rare soft tissue tumor predominantly occurring in the distal extremities of young adults; the tumor may histologically simulate a necrotizing granuloma or carcinoma. The normal cell counterpart of epithelioid sarcoma is unknown.[70]

Clinical Features

Most epithelioid sarcomas present in the second to fourth decades, and the tumor has a male predominance. The tumor occasionally occurs in children in the first decade and may occur in old individuals. The most common locations are the fingers, hands, forearm, and foot. Epithelioid sarcoma may also occur in the trunk, especially in the vulva, perineum, and inguinal region. The lesions often involve the tendons and, on occasion, may ulcerate the surface. Especially recurrent tumors infiltrate along tendons and tendon sheath and often extend longitudinally along them beyond the dominant mass. The tumor almost inevitably recurs unless completely excised, and more extensive disease in the hand often necessitates a ray amputation or amputation of a hand. Regional lymph node metastases occur regularly, and distant metastases develop in 20% to 30% of the patients. Typical metastatic sites include the soft tissue of scalp and lungs. Although the 5-year survival rate is 75%, the 10-year survival rate drops to 50% as distant metastases continue to develop.[71–77]

Pathology

Grossly, epithelioid sarcoma may form a sharply circumscribed nodule, usually 2 to 5 cm, or it may be difficult to identify in the resected soft tissues containing tendons and fibrofatty tissue. The nodules typically reveal a gray-white surface on sectioning, and necrosis may be identifiable.

Histologically, the lesions are composed of nodules and clusters of deeply eosinophilic epithelioid or spindled cells. The cellular areas may form central geographic necrosis "garland pattern" or invade as narrow streaks in a dense, fibrous stroma. The tumor cells have complex nuclear outlines and delicate nucleoli with little pleomorphism. The epithelioid sarcoma cells typically have an abundant, strongly eosinophilic cytoplasm (Fig. 19–5).

Large cell variants occur, often in atypical locations, such as the inguinal area and trunk and especially in these cases, the tumor cells may contain "rhabdoid" cytoplasmic inclusions ultrastructurally composed of whorls of intermediate filaments. This has been named "proximal variant" and seems to have a worse prognosis than the typical epithelioid sarcoma.[75]

The angiomatoid variant represents an epithelioid sarcoma with hemorrhagic cysts lined by epithelioid

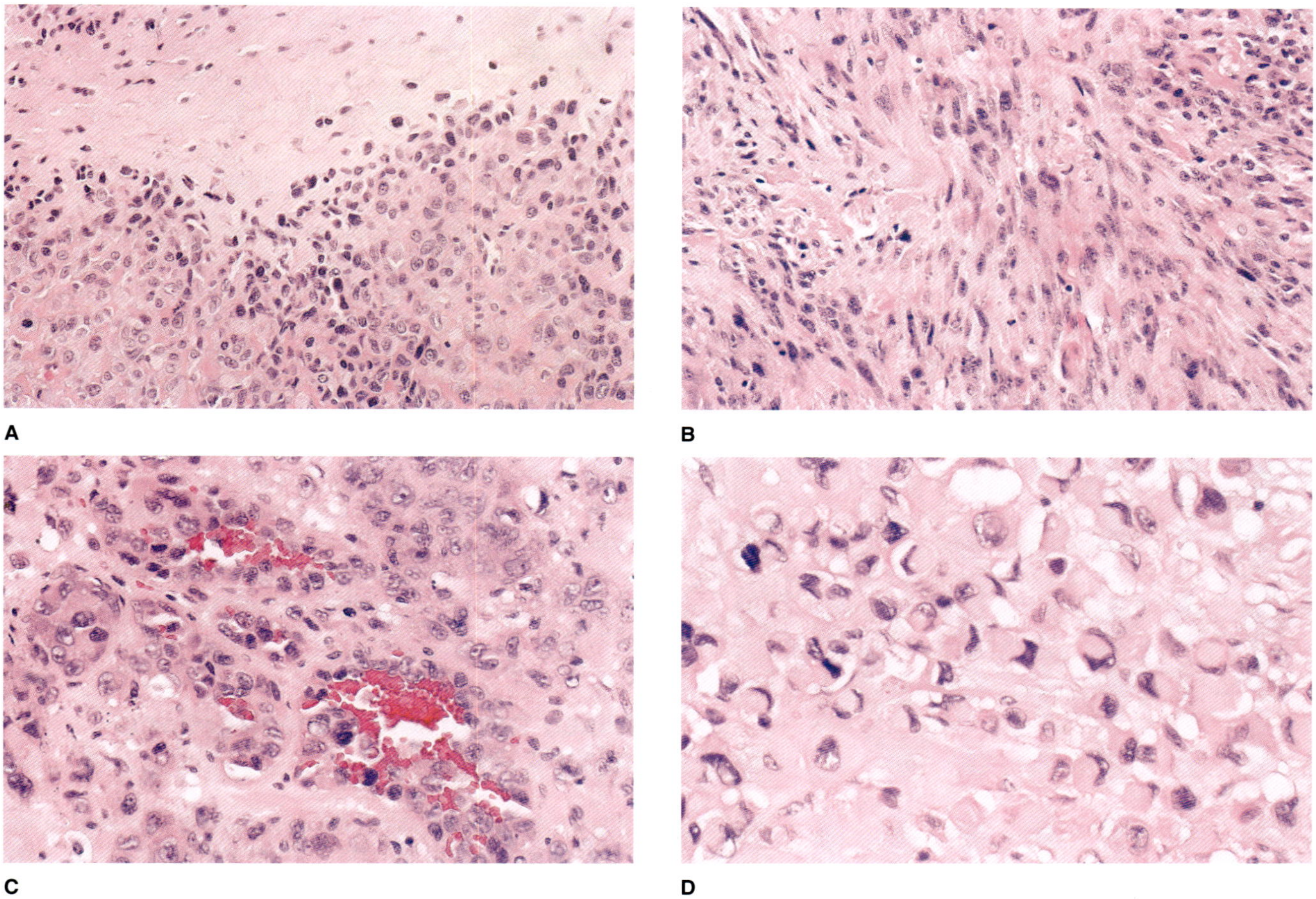

Figure 19–5. Histologic spectrum of epithelioid sarcoma. *A,* Typical variant with clusters of tumor cells bordering fibrous septa *B,* Fibrous histiocytoma-like appearance. *C,* Angiomatoid pattern. *D,* Large cell rhabdoid morphology in a vulvar epithelioid sarcoma.

sarcoma cells; these tumors have to be separated from true vascular tumors such as angiosarcoma.[76]

A fibrohistiocytic variant shows a prominent spindle cell component simulating fibrous histiocytoma, but there is infiltration by the epithelioid tumor cells among the major spindle cell component.[77]

Immunohistochemistry

Epithelioid sarcoma cells are consistently positive for vimentin, and they are nearly always strongly positive for keratins and EMA.[78–84] Among the keratin polypeptides present are K8, K18, and usually K19, typically with the majority of tumor cells strongly positive.[84] According to our experience, K7 is focally present in 20% of cases, K14 often focally, K17 very rarely, and K20 never (Fig. 19–6). Multidirectional differentiation, including expression of neurofilament proteins, has been reported.[85,86] Half the cases are positive for CD34 with a membrane staining pattern,[83,84,87] and approximately one third react with muscle actins (HHF-35). Immunoreactivity for S-100 protein and desmin is very rare. In contrast with many other epithelial tumors, epithelial sarcomas have been reported negative for E-cadherin but positive for V-cadherin (vascular cadherin).[88]

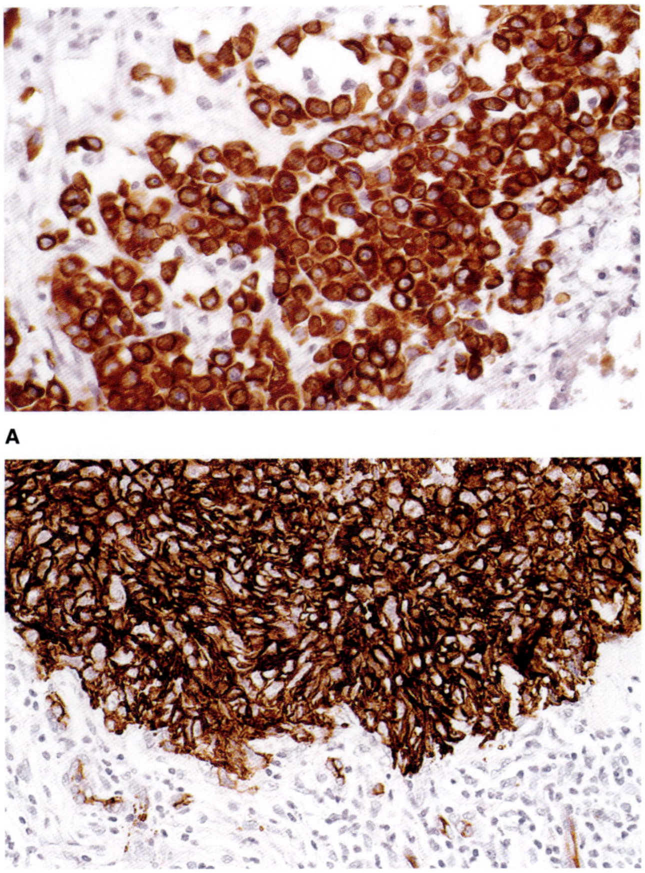

A

B

Figure 19–6. Immunohistochemical documentation of epithelioid sarcoma. Tumor cells are positive for K19 *(A)* and for CD34 *(B)*.

Differential Diagnosis

The rarity of epithelioid sarcoma and its variable histologic patterns can make this diagnosis very difficult and may result in delayed tumor diagnosis. The presence of osteoid spicules should not lead into confusion with panniculitis or myositis ossificans. The distinctive modular pattern, profile of keratin expression (negative for K7) and the CD34 expression, together with the histologic pattern, aid in the distinction from metastatic or skin adnexal carcinoma. The carcinomas that may simulate epithelioid sarcoma include metastatic carcinomas from different sites, especially from lung and kidney. Melanoma cells may have prominently eosinophilic cytoplasm, but this tumor is easily separated by immunohistochemical positivity for melanoma markers. Epithelioid sarcoma has to be a consideration in rhabdoid soft tissue tumors of adults. Furthermore, immunohistochemical expression of epithelial markers distinguish epithelioid sarcoma from necrobiotic granuloma.[89]

Genetics

Cytogenetic studies report heterogeneous changes, and no consistent alterations have been observed in the different studies. Reports of single cases have shown terminal deletion in 1p,[90] translocation t(8;22) (q22;q11) suggesting possible involvement of the Ewing sarcoma gene,[91] translocation t(18;22) (q11;p11.2) together with several numerical aberrations,[92] and complex changes including involvement of 18p in a proximal/large cell rhabdoid variant.[93] Allelic losses in chromosome 22 have been reported with small numbers of markers in a small number of cases.[94] Comparative genomic hybridization has shown gains in 11q13 as the most common recurrent changes, possible including amplification of the cyclin D1 gene.[95]

Mixed Tumor and Myoepithelioma of Soft Tissues

Mixed tumors of skin and soft tissues are analogous to corresponding tumors commonly seen in salivary glands. They may belong to a common spectrum with chondroid syringomas, a name given to mixed tumors of skin usually limited to the dermis. The tumors typically have epithelial and metaplastic cartilage-like components. In the skin mixed tumors most likely originate from the sweat glands or ducts. It is not clear how the occurrence of similar tumors in deep soft tissue can be explained. The available data are essentially based on two published series.[96,97]

Clinical Features

The tumors reported in soft tissue have occurred in a wide age range from 2 to 93 years with the median ages in two series 30 and 59 years and apparent male predominance. Occurrence in children was reported in one of the series.[96] The tumors occur in a wide range of locations, including distal and proximal extremities, trunk, and head and neck. Most tumors involved subcutis, and some also the dermis; four extended to or were located in the skeletal muscle. Both series reported local recurrence with a frequency of approximately 20%, and distant metastases with fatal outcome were reported in one series.[96] The behavior of this tumor may be difficult to predict histologically, and the tumor should be completely excised.

Pathology

Grossly, they form circumscribed, often lobulated masses, which may be mucoid or firm. The reported tumors have measured 1 to 17 cm, but most have been less than 3 cm.

Microscopically, the tumors can be recognized by their similarity to the analogous tumors of the salivary glands and skin. The composition varies from case to case, but most examples show epithelioid tumor cells forming cords, nests, and occasional tubular epithelial structures in a loose myxoid or dense hyaline matrix (Fig. 19–7). Some variants are composed of solid sheets of epithelial cells. The cytoplasm is usually eosinophilic, but some tumors have

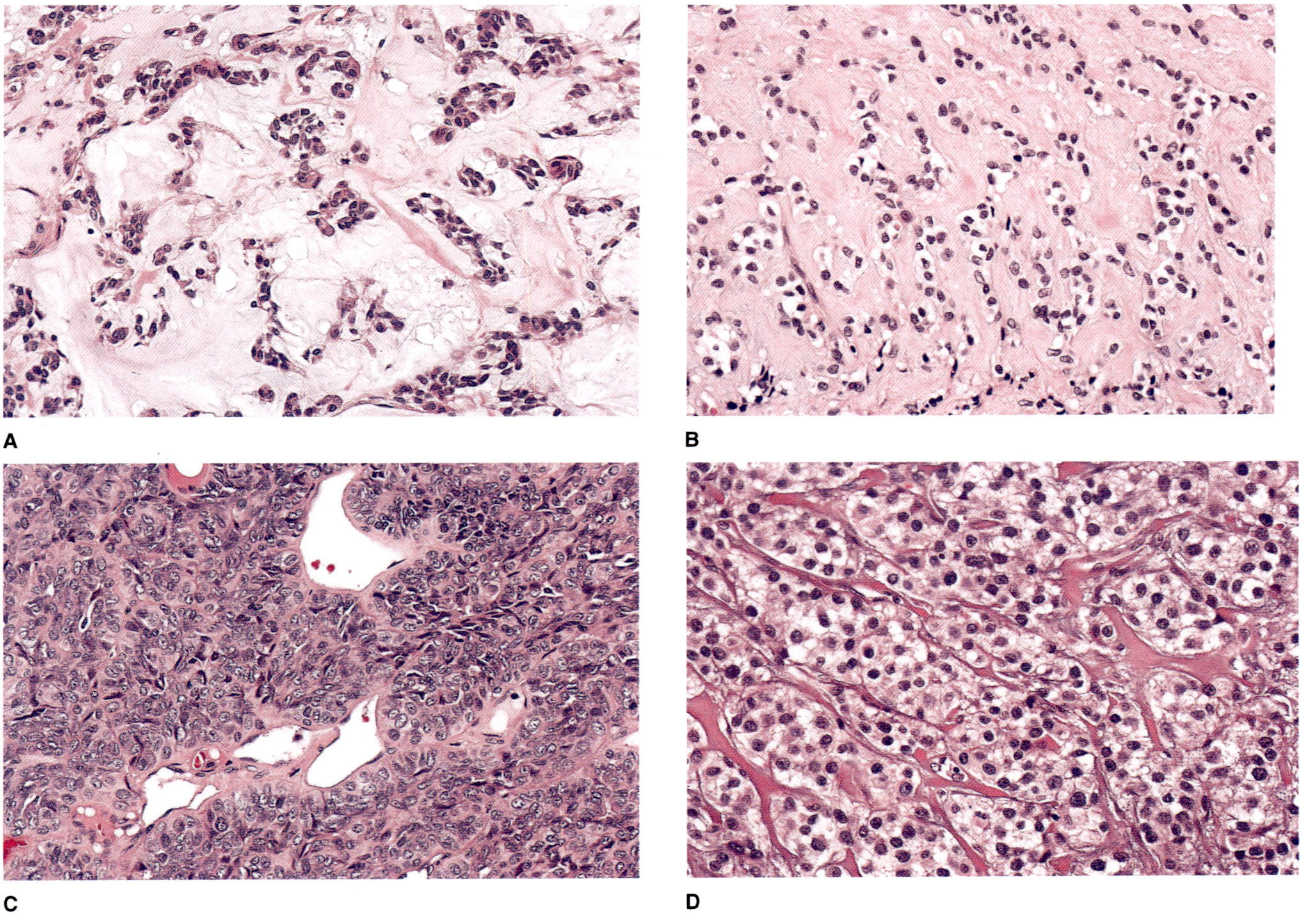

Figure 19–7. Histologic spectrum of mixed tumor of soft tissue. *A*, Myxoid-trabecular pattern. *B*, Trabecular-hyalinizing pattern. *C*, Solid hemangiopericytoma-like pattern. *D*, Clear cell pattern, which can be confused with clear cell sarcoma.

clear cell features. Mitotic activity is typically low, and nuclear atypia is limited.

Immunohistochemistry

Myoepitheliomas are typically positive for keratins, and the great majority of tumors also show significant positivity for S-100 protein. Expression of EMA, glial fibrillary acidic protein, and smooth muscle actin, other determinants seen in myoepithelial cells, has been more variable.

Differential Diagnosis

Although some histologic features may resemble extraskeletal myxoid chondrosarcoma, the latter lacks epithelial differentiation and almost uniformly epithelial markers. Parachordoma may be a related tumor, but is discussed here separately. It tends to show less complex epithelial differentiation with lack of K19, but complete comparison of these tumor types is not available. The diagnoses of metastatic carcinoma and synovial sarcoma have also to be considered in the case of deep soft tissue tumors with epithelial differentiation.

Parachrodoma

Originally named by Dabska,[98] parachordoma is a rare soft tissue tumor and very few series have been published. Histogenesis of this tumor is unresolved, but there are similarities with deep mixed tumors of soft tissues.

Clinical Features

The tumor occurs in all ages, being reported between 4 and 62 years with predilection to young adults; the collective median age of the three largest series was 30 years.[98–100] There is no sex predilection. The tumor typically presents in deep soft tissue of the extremities. Clinical course seems favorable, although data on long-term follow-up is scant.

Pathology

Grossly, parachordoma forms a 1- to 3-cm circumscribed whitish nodule in the subcutis or deep tissue. Histologically, the tumor is typically multinodular. The nodules are composed of cords of epithelioid cells separated from a myxoid stroma (Fig. 19–8). By these features, parachordoma resembles chordoma. Immunohistochemically, the tumor cells are positive for keratins and S-100 protein.

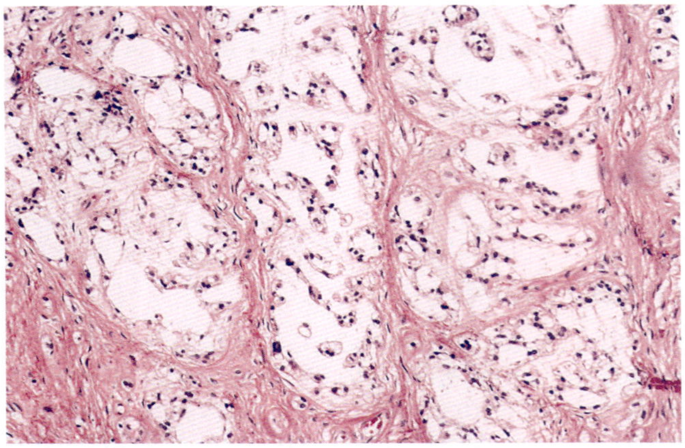

Figure 19–8. Parachordoma is composed of multiple lobules of tumor cells arranged in trabeculae separated by myxoid stroma.

Differential Diagnosis

It is quite apparent that parachordoma differs from chordoma, based on less complex keratin pattern (no K19). It also differs from extraskeletal myxoid chondrosarcoma, which is typically negative for epithelial markers. However, there are many similarities with mixed tumors or myoepitheliomas of soft tissue, and the possible relationship between these tumors cannot be dismissed.

Chordoma

Chordoma is primarily a bone tumor with epithelial differentiation, almost exclusively occurring in spine and skull base, most commonly in the sacrococcygeal region. However, this tumor may metastasize to skin and peripheral soft tissues and cause differential diagnostic difficulties.[101,102] It may also bulge into body cavities (mediastinum, retroperitoneum) and to the skin and subcutis from the primary bone tumor.[103]

Clinical Features

Chordoma occurs predominantly in older adults but is occasionally seen in children. The sacral tumors frequently bulge outward forming a subcutaneous mass. Chordoma may metastasize to the skin and deeper soft tissues.

Pathology

Grossly, chordoma typically forms a pale multinodular mass that often has a mucoid appearance on sectioning. Histologically distinctive is a multinodular pattern of growth, similar to cartilaginous tumors. The tumor cells may form cords in a myxoid matrix or sometimes

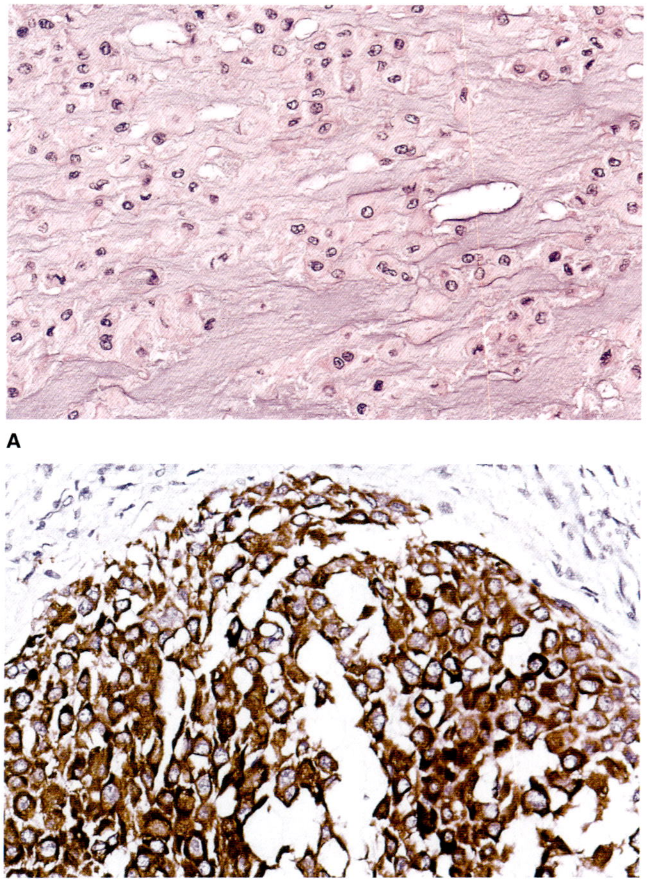

A

B

Figure 19–9. *A,* Chordoma is composed of trabeculae of tumor cells in myxoid background. *B,* The cells are strongly positive for keratins.

as solid sheets of epithelioid cells (Fig. 19–9*A*). The nuclei are usually small, but some chordomas have focal nuclear pleomorphism. Fibrosarcoma-like or malignant fibrous histiocytoma-like transformation may occur.

Immunohistochemically, chordoma cells are typically positive for simple epithelial keratins K8, K18, and K19 (Fig. 19–9*B*), whereas they are usually negative for K7 (focal positivity is possible). Most cases are also positive for EMA. Vimentin positivity is consistent, whereas the chordoma cells are only variably positive for S-100 protein.[104]

Differential Diagnosis

Architectural differences—especially trabecular epithelioid pattern and the presence of epithelial markers, keratins, and EMA—separate chordoma from conventional and extraskeletal myxoid chondrosarcoma. Chordoma metastasis can be separated from mixed tumors of the skin and soft tissues by the structural heterogeneity and the presence of tubular epithelial structures and cartilage-like differentiation in the latter.

Ectopic Hamartomatous Thymoma

This peculiar epithelial and spindle cell tumor is both clinically and pathologically distinctive, although earlier it was variably diagnosed as a variant of mixed tumor or squamous cell carcinoma.

Clinical Features

The tumor occurs specifically in the lower end of the sternocleidomastoid muscle, just above the clavicle. It usually presents as a small 1- to 3-cm painless subcutaneous mass. According to available follow-up information, the tumor is benign.[105–108]

Pathology

Grossly, the tumor is well circumscribed but unencapsulated. The tissue is white to yellow-white on sectioning, and fluid-containing cysts may be recognized by the naked eye.

Histologically, the lesion contains cleftlike and slitlike epithelial structures lined variably by glandular or squamous epithelia. The epithelial structures are surrounded by a spindle cell component, which usually dominates. Foci of adipose tissue may be present (Fig. 19–10).

Both the squamous epithelial and spindle cell components are positive for keratins, and contain both low-molecular-weight, simple epithelial keratins (K8, K18, K19) and higher-molecular-weight keratins, such as K13 and K14.

Multicystic Peritoneal Mesothelioma

This clinicopathologically distinctive, rare, benign mesothelial proliferation may represent a reactive process. Its separation from true mesothelioma is prognostically important.

Clinical Features

Multicystic peritoneal mesothelioma typically occurs in young women in the pelvic peritoneum adjacent to the uterus and other pelvic organs. Less than 20% of the cases have occurred in men. The median age for the largest series was 38 years for women and 47 years for men. Approximately 10% of these tumors occurred in children.[109] Occurrence together with endometriosis has been reported in some cases.

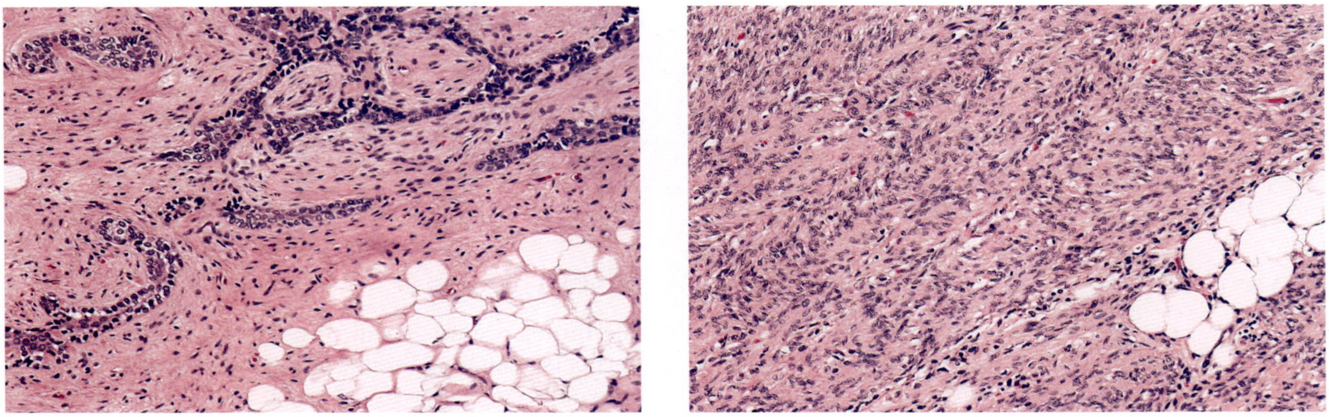

A B

Figure 19–10. Ectopic hamartomatous thymoma. *A,* The tumor shows glandular epithelial elements in a fibrous-like stroma. *B,* This tumor is dominated by spindle cell component and has a focal fatty component.

Lower abdominal pain is the most common presenting symptom. The prognosis has been generally excellent, especially in the cases in which complete excision of the tumor has been performed. However, local recurrences may develop. The two fatalities reported in the largest series were one infant whose tumor also contained areas of typical epithelial mesothelioma and a man who declined treatment.[109]

Pathology

Grossly, the lesions form either multiple, confluent cysts or less commonly as a solitary mass. The lesions contain cysts filled with clear or blood-tinged fluid. The cysts vary from a few millimeters in diameter to several centimeters (Fig. 19–11*A*).

Histologically, the lesions contain multiple mesothelial-lined cysts and intervening stroma with reactive myofibroblasts and, commonly, acute and chronic inflammatory infiltration. The mesothelial cyst lining varies from flattened to cuboidal (Fig. 19–11*B*), and in some cases, may contain proliferative mesothelium with slight papillary change or show adenomatoid tumor-like features (Fig. 19–11*C*). The cyst-lining epithelial components are positive for keratins and calretinin.

Differential Diagnosis

Lymphangioma has similar multicystic quality, but the lining cells are attenuated and express endothelial and not mesothelial markers, although K7 and K18 may be present. Endometriosis lesions rarely have a distinctive multicystic appearance and are often more heterogeneous with hemorrhage, hemosiderin deposition, and fibrosis.

Well-Differentiated Papillary Mesothelioma of Peritoneum

Two series have reported these tumors, one as "benign papillary mesothelioma,"[110] and the other as "well-differentiated papillary mesothelioma."[111] According to the latter series, these tumors occur predominantly in young and middle-aged women as multiple peritoneal nodules, and no relationship with asbestosis could be established. Most lesions are small (0. 5–2 cm) and incidentally found during surgery for other conditions, but some patients have ascites. The possibility cannot be ruled out that there is a continuum between this tumor and well-differentiated, low-grade malignant mesothelioma. In some reported cases, death from tumor could not be ruled out. The largest series concluded that adjuvant treatment is not indicated unless the tumor is clinically progressive.[111]

Histologically, a typical case shows well-differentiated papillary structures lined by a single layer of mesothelial cells with limited atypia (Fig. 19–11*D*). More solid patterns have occurred in some cases with cordlike or glandular features. Any greater atypia in papillary mesothelial proliferation should generally lead to the diagnosis of malignant mesothelioma.

Malignant Mesothelioma and Its Variants

Malignant mesothelioma is an epithelial neoplasm of mesothelial origin. It will be only briefly discussed here for differential diagnostic purposes. It most commonly occurs as a primary pleural neoplasm, but can involve any other serous surfaces, such as

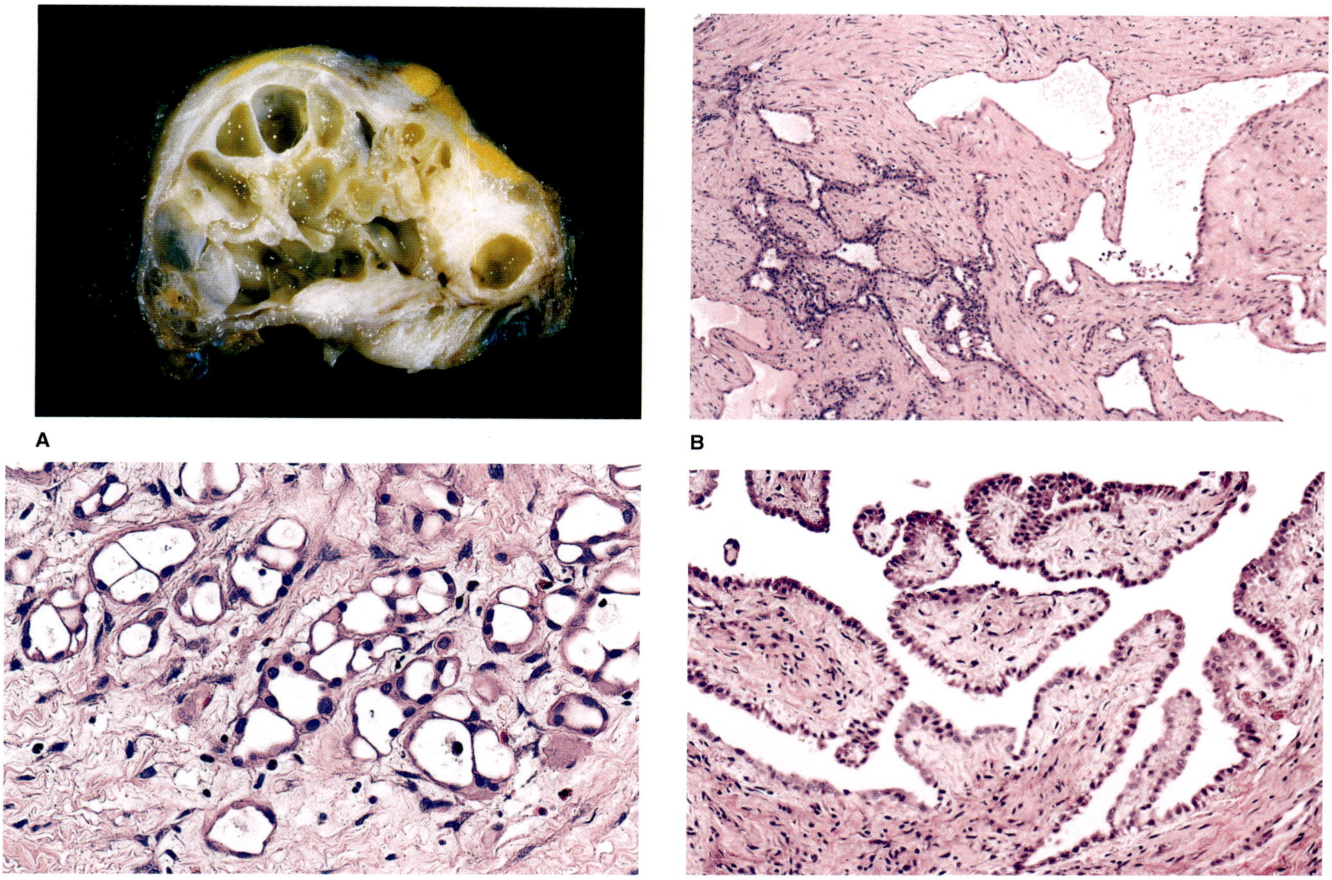

A B C D

Figure 19–11. *A,* Grossly, multicystic peritoneal mesothelioma forms sharply demarcated lesion composed of multiple cysts several millimeters in diameter. *B,* Histologically, the tumor is composed of multiple cystic spaces lined by a thin layer of mesothelial cells with foci of smaller glands with more prominent epithelia. *C,* Adenomatoid tumor-like pattern is focally present. *D,* Well-differentiated papillary mesothelioma is composed of papillae with fibrous cores lined by a monolayer of mesothelial cells with very limited atypia.

pericardium, peritoneal surfaces and the scrotal invaginations of the peritoneum, the tunica vaginalis testis. Mesotheliomas usually occur in middle and older age, and they are three times more common in men than women. Asbestosis exposure is believed to be responsible for the development of mesothelioma in the majority of cases (70%), but is an unlikely cause for the rare mesotheliomas in children and young adults. Asbestosis fibers of the smallest caliber are the most carcinogenic ones. The latency of asbestosis-related carcinogenesis is long (20–40 years, or more). Hemorrhagic pleural effusion is a typical sign of mesothelioma and may precede the diagnosis of tumor by several years. Prognosis is generally poor.[112–115]

Mesothelioma metastases may occur, sometimes as the first presentation, in regional lymph nodes.[116] They can present in superficial and deep soft tissues, especially in the chest wall where pleural mesothelioma may grow as a direct continuation. The histologic problems related to mesothelioma most importantly include differential diagnosis from benign mesothelial proliferations and carcinomas, recognition of unusual variants, such as the deciduoid, desmoplastic, and sarcomatous variants; the latter should be distinguished from sarcomas.

Tumors formerly named benign and malignant fibrous mesotheliomas have been reclassified as benign and malignant solitary fibrous tumors, which are fibroblastic neoplasms (see Chapter 5).

Pathology—Gross Features

Malignant mesothelioma typically starts as multifocal serosal nodules, and later forms a diffuse covering onto pleural and peritoneal surfaces often encasing entire organs. Rare instances have been reported with malignant mesothelioma forming a localized mass, up to 10 cm in diameter.[117] These tumors may have a better prognosis than the diffuse malignant mesotheliomas.

Histopathology

Histologically, mesotheliomas can be classified into epithelial ones with epithelioid morphology. The variants of epithelial mesothelioma include tubulopapillary and deciduoid mesothelioma. The sarcomatoid mesotheliomas have spindle cell (or pleomorphic) patterns and include desmoplastic mesothelioma as a variant. Mixed pattern ("biphasic mesothelioma") refers to a combination of epithelioid and sarcomatoid morphology.

Tubulopapillary Malignant Mesothelioma

Tubular and papillary patterns are common variants of epithelial mesothelioma. The malignant papillary tumors are microscopically invasive and have greater cytologic atypia than the well-differentiated papillary mesotheliomas (Fig. 19–12*A*). A glycogen-rich clear cell pattern is also possible (Fig. 19–12*B*).

Deciduoid Mesothelioma

Deciduoid mesothelioma is a designation for a rare solid variant of epithelial mesothelioma with large, decidua-like epithelial cells. This variant was originally reported in the peritoneum of young women without asbestosis history, but similar tumors have been subsequently reported in the pleura in male patients with history of asbestosis.[118–120]

Histologically, the deciduoid mesothelioma is composed of diffuse sheets of large epithelioid cells with pale staining abundant cytoplasm imparting a decidual cell-like appearance (Fig. 19–12*C*).

Solid variants of epithelial mesothelioma with a less copious cytoplasm are more common than the true deciduoid mesothelioma and represent a structurally poorly differentiated variant of epithelial mesothelioma (Fig. 12*D*).

Desmoplastic Mesothelioma

This variant of sarcomatoid mesothelioma is characterized by atypical spindled cells in a densely collagenous, desmoplastic stroma, often arranged in a slightly storiform pattern (Fig. 19–12*E*). The diagnosis requires demonstration of stromal invasion, overt sarcomatous, atypical component or demonstration of clinically invasive or metastatic behavior. The presence of tumor cell necrosis is supportive of malignancy although is not specific.[121–123]

Sarcomatoid mesotheliomas may be very pleomorphic simulating soft tissue sarcomas such as malignant fibrous histiocytoma. Demonstration of strong keratin

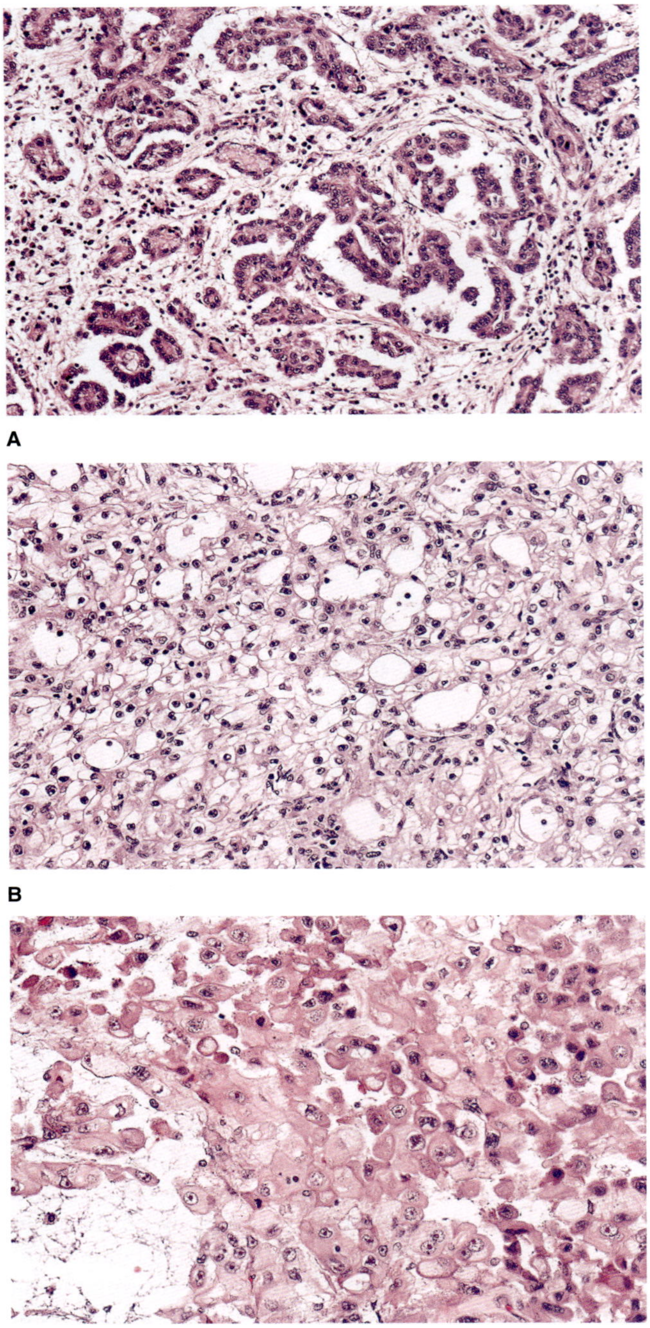

A

B

C

Figure 19–12. Different histologic patterns of epithelial malignant mesothelioma. *A*, Tubulopapillary pattern. *B*, Clear cell pattern in epithelial mesothelioma. *C*, Deciduoid mesothelioma with cells with abundant pale cytoplasm.

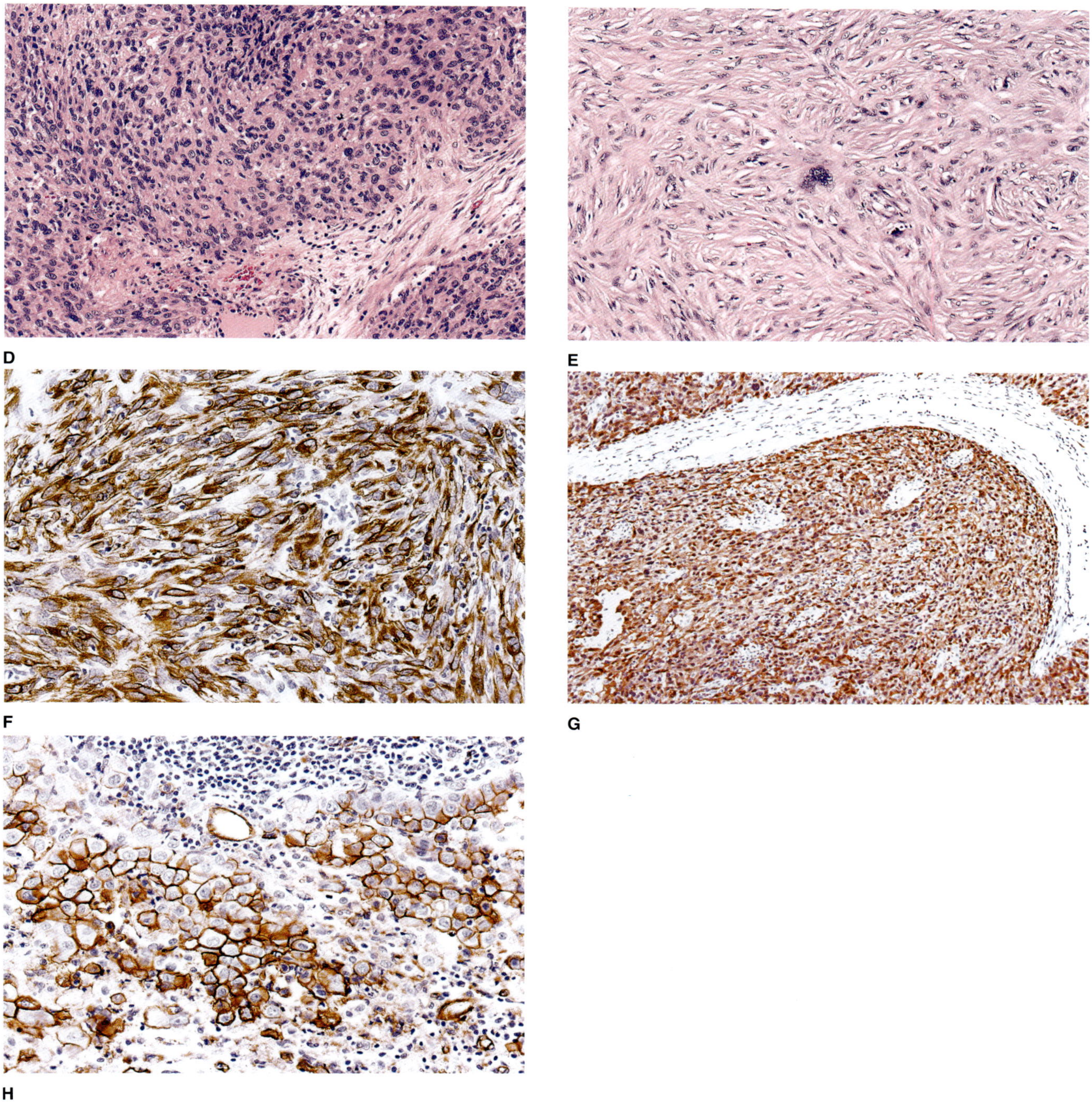

Figure 19–12. *Continued D,* A solid poorly differentiated epithelial mesothelioma. *E,* Desmoplastic mesothelioma with a storiform pattern and one markedly atypical tumor cell. *F,* All tumor cells in desmoplastic mesothelioma are positive for K7. *G,* Strong calretinin positivity in a diffuse, poorly differentiated epithelial mesothelioma. *H,* Membrane staining for thrombomodulin in an epithelial mesothelioma.

expression is diagnostically helpful (Fig. 19–12*F*), whereas many markers typical of mesotheliomas are inconsistently expressed in these tumors.

Immunohistochemistry and Differential Diagnosis of Malignant Mesothelioma

A large number of immunohistochemical markers have been suggested for diagnostic aids, and the general consensus is that none of the markers alone are diagnostic, but they become very useful when used as a panel, including both antigens typically expressed in mesothelioma and those that are more often present in carcinomas.[123A–134]

The markers that are useful in the positive identification of mesothelioma and less commonly expressed in adenocarcinoma, are calretinin, keratins 5/6, thrombomodulin, and the WT1 (Table 19–1). There are specific exceptions. One of these is the common expression of HBME1 and WT1 in serous carcinomas of ovarian and primary peritoneal origin.

Markers typically expressed in adenocarcinoma and not mesothelioma are glycoproteins CEA, CD15, BerEp4, MOC31, and B72.3 (see Chapter 3).

Keratins

All mesotheliomas are epithelial tumors and as such are positive for keratins. This is also true for the sarcomatoid mesotheliomas. Simple epithelial keratins K7, K8, K18, and K19 are expressed in mesothelioma[132] and adenocarcinoma similarly, except that some adenocarcinomas (e.g., intestinal and prostatic ones) are negative for K7. However, K5 (often detected with an antibody also recognizing K6) is more commonly reactive in mesothelioma than adenocarcinoma, and this keratin has been viewed as one of the most useful single markers in the differential diagnosis between mesothelioma and adenocarcinoma.[133,134] However, carcinomas with squamous differentiation are expected to be also positive.

The submesothelial cells and the spindle cells in pleural plaque are also positive for keratins; this should be noted in the differential diagnosis of mesothelioma and reactive conditions. Therefore, demonstration of keratin-positive cells per se has no value in the diagnosis of mesothelioma.[135,136]

Calretinin

This S-100 protein-related marker is expressed in the cytoplasm and nuclei of mesothelial cells and most mesotheliomas (Fig. 19–12*G*). Less than 10% of pulmonary and ovarian adenocarcinomas are positive. Colon carcinomas, especially the poorly differentiated ones, may be positive.[127]

Thrombomodulin (CD141)

Membrane staining for this marker is typically seen in endothelial and mesothelial cells and in mesothe-

Table 19–1. Immunohistochemical Markers in the Differential Diagnosis of Mesothelioma and Adenocarcinoma

Typically Positive in Adenocarcinoma and Negative in Mesothelioma	Typically Positive in Mesothelioma and Negative in Adenocarcinoma
CEA (monoclonal)*	Calretinin†
CD15 (LeuM1)*	Keratins 5/6‡
BerEp4*	Thrombomodulin§
MOC 31	HBME-1 ‖ #
B72.3	WT1 ‖

Note that each marker can be occasionally positive in either tumor. Also expressed in ovarian serous carcinomas and related tumors.
Exceptions to the common staining patterns:
*A small minority of mesotheliomas are focally positive.
†Mesotheliomas typically show strong cytoplasmic and nuclear positivity. A small minority of adenocarcinomas, such as those of breast, lung, and colorectal origin, may be positive, usually focally. Synovial sarcomas often have significant positivity.
‡Some carcinomas, especially adenosquamous ones and squamous carcinomas, are variably positive.
§Some adenocarcinomas are focally positive. Endothelial cells and a minority of malignant vascular tumors are also positive.
‖Serous carcinomas of ovarian of primary peritoneal origin are typically positive for WT1 and HBME-1.
#The carcinomas that are positive for HBME-1 often show more limited membrane positivity than mesotheliomas.

liomas (Fig. 19–12*H*). A minority of adenocarcinomas are focally positive.[128–131]

HBME-1

This monoclonal antibody by Battifora typically shows strong, circumferential, membrane staining in mesothelia and mesotheliomas. Some carcinomas, such as ovarian and peritoneal serous ones, are also consistently positive. Other adenocarcinomas are often focally positive, but rarely show extensive membrane staining, as seen in mesotheliomas.[128,129]

WT1

This transcriptional regulator protein is localized in the nuclei. It is present in mesothelia and well-differentiated mesotheliomas, but is often absent in the sarcomatoid tumors.[126] However, WT1 is also expressed in serous and some other müllerian system carcinomas. [137,138]

Ultrastructure of Mesothelioma

Typical of mesothelioma are tall and thin microvilli on the cell surface. It has been suggested that only microvilli whose length exceeds the width by a margin of 15:1 are diagnostic of mesothelioma.[139] Because the microvilli are often poorly developed in sarcomatoid mesotheliomas, electron microscopy is generally not useful in their diagnosis.

Mesothelioma versus Vascular Tumors

The rare epithelioid vascular tumors of the serous surfaces may histologically simulate mesothelioma. Their diagnosis is significantly based on immunohistochemical demonstration of endothelial markers and strong positivity for vimentin and limited/variable positivity for keratins.[140,141] Vimentin expression does not reliably discriminate between mesothelioma and carcinoma, although the former is more commonly positive.[129,130]

Merkel Cell Carcinoma

Both primary and metastatic carcinomas can involve soft tissues at almost any surgical site. Among the former, Merkel cell carcinoma is the most important, whereas the latter is a heterogeneous and a diagnostically difficult group often calling for a clinical correlation for ultimate diagnosis. In some cases, characteristic histologic features and application of tissue-specific immunohistochemical markers help to determine the primary site.

Merkel cell carcinoma is a distinctive primary cutaneous or subcutaneous high-grade neuroendocrine carcinoma, originally reported as trabecular carcinoma of the skin.[142] It resembles the cutaneous neuroendocrine cells, the Merkel cells, which are scattered basally in the epidermis and hair shafts, by expression of K20, but differs from them in its neurofilament positivity.[143–147]

Clinical Features

Merkel cell carcinoma typically occurs in adults in the seventh and eight decade with no sex predilection, but occurrence in younger adults is also possible.[146] Over half the tumors occur in the head and neck region, and the rest in the extremities and trunk. Immunosuppressed, especially posttransplantation patients, have an increased risk and lower age of presentation for this tumor, and many patients have other skin carcinomas.[148] The tumor may involve both dermis and subcutis, or only either one. Few cases have been reported in inguinal and axillary lymph nodes without primary tumor elsewhere, and were believed to be nodal primary tumors.[149] Metastases may develop to regional lymph nodes and sometimes systemically, sometimes long after the primary tumor. It has been estimated that 30% of the patients die of the tumor. Distally located and small tumors less than 2 cm have a better prognosis.[147]

Pathology

Grossly, Merkel cell carcinomas are typically white and soft masses of 1 to 5 cm in diameter. On sectioning they are soft and white, and often grossly resemble a lymphoma. Histologically, the tumor is composed of sheets of closely packed or trabecularly arranged strikingly uniform medium-sized cells, which often infiltrate diffuse in the dermis and subcutaneous fat. The tumor cells often have precisely round, uniform nuclei with a hypochromatic, stippled chromatin and scant cytoplasm. Mitotic activity is typically high (Fig. 19–13*A* and *B*). A minority of Merkel cell carcinomas exhibit a trabecular pattern (Fig. 19–13*C*).

Some tumors involve epidermis in a pagetoid manner, and some tumors coexist with cutaneous squamous cell carcinoma, or have a focal squamous cell component. Heterologous skeletal muscle differentiation has also been reported.[150]

Ultrastructurally typical is the presence of perinuclear intermediate filament whorls and scattered dense core neuroendocrine granules.

Immunohistochemistry

Immunohistochemically characteristic is positivity for K8 and K18 detected with antibodies to keratin cocktails, and nearly consistent positivity for K20 (Fig. 19–13*D*). Many cases show punctate, perinuclear

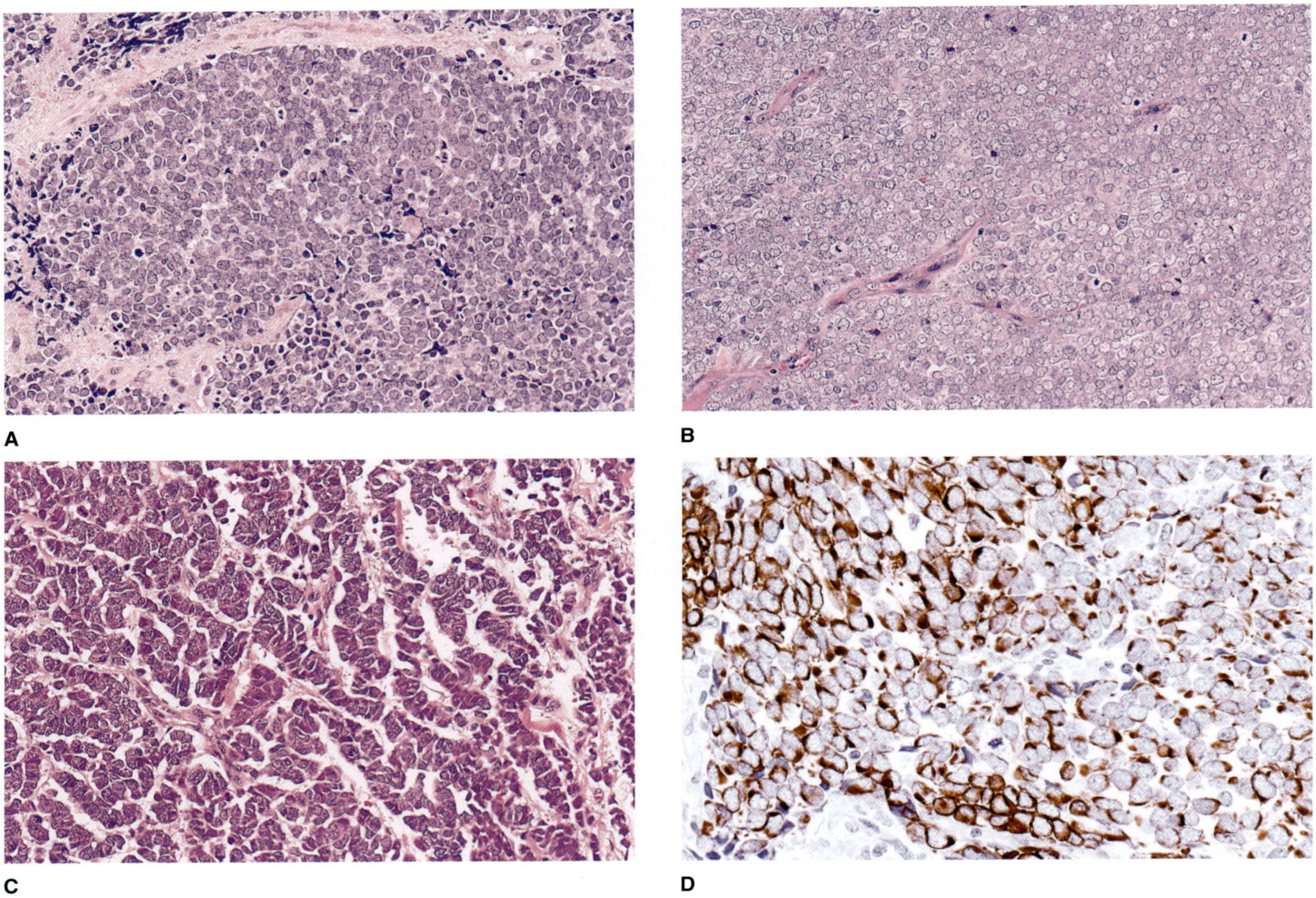

Figure 19-13. Merkel cell carcinoma. *A,* A typical diffuse pattern. *B,* The tumor cells are uniform with round, vesicular nuclei. *C,* A trabecular pattern. *D,* The tumor cells are positive for K20 with a dotlike perinuclear pattern.

positivity, whereas in some cases, the immunoreactivity is seen in the entire cytoplasm. Positivity for neurofilaments (especially NF68) is seen in a similar pattern in most cases. Most tumors are positive for synaptophysin and neuron-specific enolase and variably for chromogranin. Negativity for thyroid transcription factor 1 (TTF-1) helps to distinguish this tumor from metastatic pulmonary small cell carcinoma (SCC).[151-153]

Differential Diagnosis

Pulmonary SCC tends to have a more prominent vascular pattern and often has more spindled and hyperchromatic nuclei. The common presence of TTF-1 and absence of K20 are distinguishing features from Merkel cell carcinoma. Immunohistochemical evaluation for leukocyte markers CD20, CD30, and CD45 are helpful in separating Merkel cell carcinoma from cutaneous lymphomas.

Genetics

Changes in chromosome 1p region also involved in neuroblastoma were initially believed to suggest neural crest origin.[154] Involvement of 1p36 has been confirmed, but specifically involved genes have not been identified.[155]

Metastatic Pulmonary SCC

This high-grade neuroendocrine carcinoma may be seen as metastasis in the skin and subcutis of any location, and in such circumstances, the differential diagnosis from Merkel cell carcinoma may be problematic.

Histologically, the pulmonary SCC usually shows more oval or spindled cell morphology, as opposed to the uniformly round nuclei typically seen in Merkel cell carcinoma.

Immunohistochemical features that strongly favor the pulmonary origin of SCC are positivity for TTF-1

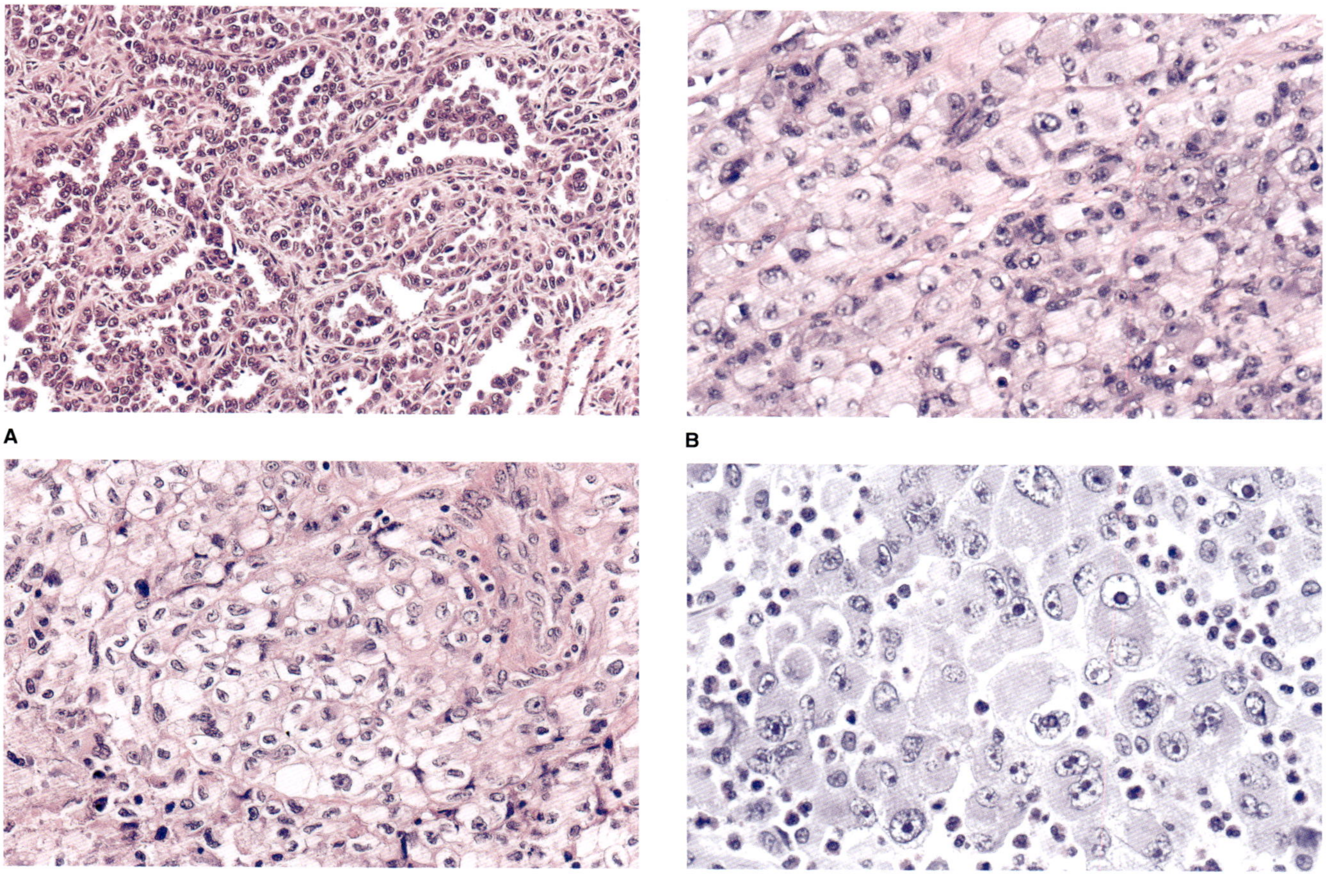

A B C D

Figure 19–14. Metastatic carcinomas in soft tissue simulating a soft tissue sarcoma. *A,* Metastatic pulmonary adenocarcinoma showing an alveolar pattern resembling that of alveolar rhabdomyosarcoma. *B,* A solid epithelioid pattern of metastatic pulmonary adenocarcinoma. *C,* A tumor with a partial clear cell pattern is a metastatic renal cell carcinoma. *D,* This large cell tumor is metastatic hepatocellular carcinoma. Note prominent eosinophil infiltration.

and K7 (the latter is only rarely positive in Merkel cell carcinoma). The pulmonary SCCs are negative for K20, in contrast to Merkel cell carcinoma. They are usually positive for neuron-specific enolase and synaptophysin and are variably positive for chromogranin.

The expression of TTF-1 has been reported in some nonpulmonary SCCs, but not in Merkel cell carcinoma.

Metastatic Pulmonary Non-SCC

Metastatic pulmonary carcinomas (adeno, squamous) commonly involve the subcutis, and sometimes present in deep soft tissues (Fig. 19–14*A* and *B*). Some of these histologic patterns can closely simulate sarcomas. Immunohistochemical findings that are typically positive in these tumors include K7 (nearly all cases) and TTF-1, which can be demonstrated in 60% to 70% of adenocarcinomas.

Metastatic Renal Cell Carcinoma

Renal cell carcinomas (clear cell and other variants) commonly metastasize in peripheral soft tissues in a wide variety of locations, and detection of metastasis before primary tumor is not rare. The sites that are more commonly involved are lower genital tract of women, scalp, and occasionally deep soft tissues. Bones are commonly involved. Because of their high vascularity, renal carcinoma metastases may bleed heavily during surgery.

When the tumor has histologically clear cell features and a high vascularity, renal origin has to be seriously considered (Fig. 19–14*C*). Metastases with sarcomatoid features may be very difficult to link with the renal primary and are more likely confused

Table 19–2. Immunohistochemical Markers Helpful in Determining the Origin for Metastatic Carcinoma

Primary Site	Markers
Breast, endometrium	Estrogen and progesterone receptors (also positive in müllerian stromal tumors)
Lung (adenocarcinoma, small cell carcinoma) Differentiated thyroid carcinomas	Thyroid transcription factor
Thyroid medullary carcinoma	Calcitonin, CEA
Liver	HepPar I
Ovary, serous carcinoma	WT1
Prostate	PSA, PSAP
Lower GI tract Urothelial, transitional cell Merkel cell	K20

CEA, carcinoembryonic antigen; GI, gastrointestinal; PSA, prostate-specific antigen; PSAP, prostate acid phosphatase.

with sarcomas. It may be prudent to clinically rule out the possibility of occult sarcomatoid renal carcinoma before diagnosing a keratin-positive soft tissue or osseous malignant fibrous histiocytoma.

Metastatic Prostatic Carcinoma

When extending to pelvic soft tissues or presenting as cervical lymph node metastasis, metastatic prostatic carcinoma may be difficult to recognize. Many of such metastases are high-grade tumors. They are typically composed of large cells with prominent nucleoli. The tumor cells may be arranged in "neuroendocrine-like" rosette-forming patterns. Immunoreactivity for prostate-specific antigen and prostate acid phosphatase is very helpful for diagnosis.

Carcinomas from Other Specific Sites

A wide variety of other carcinomas may manifest as soft tissue metastases. The identification of the primary source usually requires a clinical correlation. For example, hepatocellular carcinoma in a soft tissue location may be difficult to identify because this is an unexpected occurrence (Fig. 19–14*D*). A summary for immunohistochemical markers to pinpoint the primary site of metastatic carcinoma is shown in Table 19–2.

REFERENCES

Synovial Sarcoma—General Reviews and Clinicopathologic Series

1. Fisher C: Synovial sarcoma. Ann Diagn Pathol 1998;2:401–421.
2. Schmidt D, Thum P, Harms D, Treuner J: Synovial sarcoma in children and adolescents. A report from the Kiel Pediatric Tumor Registry. Cancer 1991;67:1667–1672.
3. Oda Y, Hashimoto H, Tsuneyoshi M, Takeshita S: Survival in synovial sarcoma. A multivariate study of prognostic factors with special emphasis on the comparison between early death and long term survival. Am J Surg Pathol 1993;17:35–44.
4. Pappo AS, Fontanesi J, Luo X, et al: Synovial sarcoma in children and adolescents: The St. Jude Children's Research Hospital experience. J Clin Oncol 1994;12:2360–2366.
5. Singer S, Baldini EH, Demetri GC, Fletcher JA, Corson JM: Synovial sarcoma: Prognostic significance of tumor size, margin of resection, and mitotic activity for survival. J Clin Oncol 1996;14:1201–1208.
6. Bergh P, Meis-Kindblom JM, Gherlinzoni F, et al: Synovial sarcoma: Identification of low and high risk groups. Cancer 1999;85:2596–2607.
7. Machen SK, Fisher C, Gautam RS, Tubbs RR, Goldblum JR: Synovial sarcoma of the extremities: A clinicopathologic study of 34 cases, including semi-quantitative analysis of spindled, epithelial, and poorly differentiated areas. Am J Surg Pathol 1999;23:268–275.
8. Lewis JJ, Antonescu CR, Leung DH, et al: Synovial sarcoma: A multivariate analysis of prognostic factors in 112 patients with primary localized tumors of the extremity. J Clin Oncol 2000;18:2087–2094.
9. Spillane AJ, A'Hern R, Judson IR, Fisher C, Thomas JM: Synovial sarcoma: A clinicopathologic, staging, and prognostic assessment. J Clin Oncol 2000;18:3794–3800.
10. Trassard M, LeDoussal V, Hacene K, et al: Prognostic factors in localized primary synovial sarcoma: A multicenter study of 128 adult patients. J Clin Oncol 2001;19:525–534.

Synovial Sarcoma at Unusual Sites

11. Roth JA, Enzinger FM, Tannenbaum M: Synovial sarcoma of the neck: A follow-up study of 24 cases. Cancer 1975;35:1243–1253.
12. Shmookler BM, Enzinger FM, Brannon RB: Orofacial synovial sarcoma. A clinicopathologic study of 11 new cases and review of the literature. Cancer 1982;50:269–276.

13. Witkin G, Miettinen M, Rosai J: A biphasic tumor of the mediastinum with features of synovial sarcoma. A report of four cases. Am J Surg Pathol 1989;13:490–499.
14. Zeren H, Moran CA, Suster S, Fishback NF, Koss MN: Primary pulmonary sarcomas with features of monophasic synovial sarcoma: A clinicopathological, immunohistochemical and ultrastructural study of 25 cases. Hum Pathol 1995;26:474–480.
15. Kaplan MA, Goodman MD, Satish J, Bhagavan BS, Travis WD: Primary pulmonary sarcoma with morphologic features of monophasic synovial sarcoma and chromosome translocation t(X;18). Am J Clin Pathol 1996;105:195–199.
16. Hisaoka M, Hashimoto H, Iwamasa T, Ishikawa K, Aoki T: Primary synovial sarcoma of the lung: Report of two cases confirmed by molecular detection of SYT-SSX fusion gene transcript. Histopathology 1999; 34:205–210.
17. Iwasaki H, Ishiguro M, Ohjimi Y, et al: Synovial sarcoma of the prostate with t(X;18)(p11.2;q11.2). Am J Surg Pathol 1999;23:220–226.
18. Fritsch M, Epstein JI, Perlman EJ, Watts JC, Argani P: Molecularly confirmed primary prostatic synovial sarcoma. Hum Pathol 2000;31:246–250.
19. Shmookler BM: Retroperitoneal synovial sarcoma. A report of four cases. Am J Clin Pathol 1982;77:686–691.
20. Fetsch JF, Meis JM: Synovial sarcoma of the abdominal wall. Cancer 1993;72:469–477.
21. Miettinen M, Santavirta S, Slatis P: Intravascular synovial sarcoma. Hum Pathol 1987;18:1075–1077.
22. Robertson NJ, Halawa MH, Smith ME: Intravascular synovial sarcoma. J Clin Pathol 1998;51:172–173.
23. Karn CM, Socinski MA, Fletcher JA, Corson JM, Craighead JE: Cardiac synovial sarcoma with translocation (X;18) associated with asbestosis exposure. Cancer 1994;73:74–78.
24. Argani P, Faria PA, Epstein JI, et al: Primary renal synovial sarcoma: Molecular and morphologic delineation of an entity previously included among embryonal sarcomas of the kidney. Am J Surg Pathol 2000;24:1087–1096.

Synovial Sarcoma—Histologic Variants and Prognostic Factors

25. Mirra JM, Wang S, Bhuta S: Synovial sarcoma with squamous differentiation of its mesenchymal glandular elements. A case report with light-microscopic, ultramicroscopic, and immunologic correlation. Am J Surg Pathol 1984;8:791–796.
26. Mckenzie DH: Monophasic synovial sarcoma—A histologic entity? Histopathology 1977;1:151–157.
27. Evans HL: Synovial sarcoma: A study of 23 biphasic and 17 probable monophasic examples. Pathol Annu 1980;15:309–313.
28. Krall RA, Kostianovsky M, Patchefsky AS: Synovial sarcoma: A clinical, pathological and ultrastructural study of 26 cases supporting the recognition of a monophasic variant. Am J Surg Pathol 1981;5:137–151.
29. Varela-Duran J, Enzinger FM: Calcifying synovial sarcoma. Cancer 1982;50:345–352.
30. Milchgrub S, Ghandur-Mnaymneh L, Dorfman HD, Albores-Saavedra J: Synovial sarcoma with extensive osteoid and bone formation. Am J Surg Pathol 1993;17:357–363.
31. van de Rijn M, Barr FG, Xiong QB, Hedges M, Shipley J, Fisher C: Poorly differentiated synovial sarcoma: An analysis of clinical, pathologic, and molecular genetic features. Am J Surg Pathol 1999;23:106–112.
32. Kawai A, Woodruff J, Healey JH, Brennan MF, Antonescu CR, Ladanyi M: SYT-SSX gene fusion as a determinant of morphology and prognosis in synovial sarcoma. N Engl J Med 1998;338:153–160.
33. Skytting B: Synovial sarcoma. A Scandinavian Sarcoma Group project. Acta Orthoped Scand Suppl 2000;291:1–28.

Synovial Sarcoma—Immunohistochemistry

34. Ordonez NG, Mahfouz SM, Mackay B: Synovial sarcoma: An immunohistochemical and ultrastructural study. Hum Pathol 1990;21:733–749.
35. Miettinen M: Keratin subsets in spindle cell sarcomas. Keratins are widespread but synovial sarcoma contains a distinctive keratin polypeptide pattern and desmoplakins. Am J Pathol 1991;138:505–513.
36. Lopes JM, Bjerkehagen B, Holm R, Bruland O, Sobrinho-Simoes M, Nesland JM: Immunohistochemical profile of synovial sarcoma with emphasis on the epithelial-type differentiation. A study of 49 primary tumors, recurrences and metastases. Pathol Res Pract 1994;190:168–177.
37. Folpe AL, Gown AM: Poorly differentiated synovial sarcoma: Immunohistochemical distinction from primitive neuroectodermal tumors and high grade malignant peripheral nerve sheath tumors. Am J Surg Pathol 1998;22:673–682.
38. Miettinen M, Limon J, Niezabitowski A, Lasota J: Patterns in keratin polypeptides in 110 biphasic, monophasic and poorly differentiated synovial sarcomas. Virchows Arch 2000;438:275–283.
39. Sato H, Hasegawa T, Abe Y, Sakai H, Hirohashi S: Expression of E-cadherin in bone and soft tissue sarcomas: A possible role in epithelial differentiation. Hum Pathol 1999;30:1344–1349.
40. Miettinen M, Limon J, Niezabitowski A, Lasota J: Calretinin expression in synovial sarcoma. Analysis of similarities and differences from malignant mesothelioma. Am J Surg Pathol 2001;25:610–617.
41. Guillou L, Wadden C, Kraus MD, Dei Tos AP, Fletcher CDM: S-100 protein reactivity in synovial sarcomas. A potentially frequent diagnostic pitfall. Immunohistochemical analysis of 100 cases. Appl Immunohistochem 1996;4:167–175.
42. Stevenson AJ, Chatten J, Bertoni F, Miettinen M: CD99 (p30/32 -MIC2) neuroectodermal/Ewing sarcoma antigen as an immunohistochemical marker.

Review of more than 600 tumors and the literature experience. Appl Immunohistochem 1994;2:231–240.
43. Suster S, Fisher C, Moran CA: Expression of bcl2 oncoprotein in benign and malignant spindle cell tumors of soft tissue, skin, serosal surfaces, and gastrointestinal tract. Am J Surg Pathol 1998;22:863–872.

Synovial Sarcoma—Genetics

44. Limon J, Mrozek K, Mandahl N, et al: Cytogenetics of synovial sarcoma: Presentation of ten new cases and review of the literature. Genes Chromosomes Cancer 1991;3:338–345.
45. Dal Cin P, Rao U, Jani-Sait S, Karakousis C, Sandberg AA: Chromosome in the diagnosis of soft tissue tumors. I. Synovial sarcoma. Mod Pathol 1992;5:57–62.
46. Clark J, Rocques PJ, Crew AJ, Gill S, et al: Identification of novel genes, SYT and SSX, involved in the t(X;18)(p11.2;q11.2) translocation found in human synovial sarcoma. Nat Genet 1994;7:502–508.
47. de Leeuw B, Balemans M, Olde Weghuis D, Geurts van Kessel A: Identification of two alternative fusion genes, SYT-SSX1 and SYT-SSX2, in t(X;18)(p11.2;q11.2)-positive synovial sarcomas. Hum Mol Genet 1995;4: 1097–1099.
48. Crew J, Clark J, Fisher C, et al: Fusion of SYT to two genes, SSX1 and SSX2, encoding proteins with homology to the Kruppel-associated box in human synovial sarcoma. EMBO J 1995;14:2333–2340.
49. Renwick PJ, Reeves BR, Dal Cin P, et al: Two categories of synovial sarcoma defined by divergent chromosome translocation breakpoints in Xp11.2, with implications for the histologic sub-classification of synovial sarcoma. Cytogenet Cell Genet 1995;70:58–63.
50. dos Santos NR, de Bruijn DRH, van Kessel AG: Molecular mechanisms underlying human synovial sarcoma development. Genes Chromosomes Cancer 2001;30: 1–14.
51. Skytting B, Nilsson G, Brodin B, Xie Y, Lundeberg J, Uhlen M: A novel fusion gene, SYT-SSX4, in synovial sarcoma. J Natl Cancer Inst 1999;91:974–975.
52. Gure AO, Türeci Ö, Sahin U, et al: SSX: A multigene family with several members transcribed in normal testis and human cancer. Int J Cancer 1997;72: 965–971.
53. de Leeuw B, Suijkerbujik, RF, Olde Weghuis D, et al: Distinct Xp11.2 breakpoint regions in synovial sarcoma revealed by metaphase and interphase FISH: relationship to histologic subtypes. Cancer Genet Cytogenet 1994;73:89–94.
54. Poteat HT, Corson JM, Fletcher JA: Detection of chromosome 18 rearrangement in synovial sarcoma by fluorescence in situ hybridization. Cancer Genet Cytogenet 1995;84:76–81.
55. Nagao K, Ito H, Yoshida H: Chromosomal translocation t(X;18) in human synovial sarcomas analyzed by fluorescence in situ hybridization using paraffin-embedded tissue. Am J Pathol 1996;148:601–609.
56. Shipley J, Crew J, Birdsall S, et al: Interphase fluorescence in situ hybridization and reverse transcription polymerase chain reaction as a diagnostic aid for synovial sarcoma. Am J Pathol 1996;148:559–567.
57. Zilmer M, Use of nonbreakpoint DNA probes to detect the t(X;18) in interphase cells from synovial sarcoma: Implications for detection of diagnostic tumor translocations. Am J Pathol 1998;152:1171–1177.
58. Birdsall S, Osin P, Ly YJ, Fisher C, Shipley J: Synovial sarcoma specific translocation associated with both epithelial and spindle cell components. Int J Cancer 1999;82:605–608.
59. Lu YJ, Birdsall S, Summersgill B, et al: Dual colour fluorescence in situ hybridization to paraffin-embedded samples to deduce the presence of the der(x)t (x;18)(p11.2;q11.2) and involvement of either the SSX1 or SSX2 gene: A diagnostic and prognostic aid for synovial sarcoma. J Pathol 1999;187:490–496.
60. Fligman I, Leonardo F, Jhanwar SC, Gerald WL, Woodruff J, Ladanyi M: Molecular diagnosis of synovial sarcoma and characterization of a variant SYT-SSX2 fusion transcript. Am J Pathol 1995;147: 1592–1599.
61. Argani P, Zakowski MF, Klimstra DS, Rosai J, Ladanyi M: Detection of the SYT-SSX chimeric RNA of synovial sarcoma in paraffin-embedded tissue and its application in problematic cases. Mod Pathol 1997;11:65–71.
62. Lasota J, Jasinski M, Debiec-Rychter M, Limon J, Miettinen M: Detection of the SYT-SSX fusion transcripts in formaldehyde-fixed, paraffin embedded tissue: A reverse transcription polymerase chain reaction amplification assay useful in the diagnosis of synovial sarcoma. Mod Pathol 1998;11:626–633.
63. Tsuji S, Hashimoto H: Detection of SYT-SSX fusion transcripts in synovial sarcoma by reverse transcription-polymerase chain reaction using archival paraffin-embedded tissues. Am J Pathol 1998;153:1807–1812.
64. Nilsson G, Skytting B, Xie Y, et al: The SYT-SSX1 variant of synovial sarcoma is associated with a high rate of tumor cell proliferation and poor clinical outcome. Cancer Res 1999;59:3180–3184.
65. van de Rijn M, Barr FG, Collins MH, Xiong QB, Fisher C: Absence of SYT-SSX fusion products in soft tissue tumors other than synovial sarcoma. Am J Clin Pathol 1999;112:43–49.
66. O'Sullivan MJ, Kyriakos M, Zhu X, et al: Malignant peripheral nerve sheath tumors with T(X;18). A pathologic and molecular genetic study. Mod Pathol 2000;13:1336–1346.
67. Ladanyi M, Woodruff JM, Scheithauer BW, et al: Letter to editor. Re: O'Sullivan MJ, Kyriakos M, Zhu X, et al: Malignant peripheral nerve sheath tumors with T(X;18). A pathologic and molecular genetic study. Mod Pathol 2000;13:1336–1346. Mod Pathol. 2001;14: 733–737.
68. Mandahl N, Limon J, Mertens F, et al: Nonrandom secondary chromosome aberrations in synovial sarcomas with t(X;18). Int J Oncol 1995;7:495–499.
69. Szymanska J, Serra M, Skytting B, et al: Genetic imbalances in 67 synovial sarcomas evaluated by comparative genomic hybridization. Genes Chromosomes Cancer 1998;23:213–219.

Epithelioid Sarcoma

70. Enzinger FM: Epithelioid sarcoma—A sarcoma simulating a granuloma or a carcinoma. Cancer 1970;26: 1029–1041.
71. Prat J, Woodruff JM, Marcove RC: Epithelioid sarcoma. An analysis of 22 cases indicating the prognostic significance of vascular invasion and regional lymph node metastasis. Cancer 1978;41:1472–1487.
72. Chase DR, Enzinger FM: Epithelioid sarcoma. Diagnosis, prognostic indicators, and treatment. Am J Surg Pathol 1985;9:241–263.
73. Bos GD, Pritchard DJ, Reiman HM, Dobyns JH, Ilstrup DM, Landon GC: Epithelioid sarcoma. An analysis of fifty-one cases. J Bone Joint Surg A 1988; 70:862–870.
74. Halling AC, Wollen PC, Pritchard DJ, Vlasak R, Nascimento AG: Epithelioid sarcoma. A clinicopathologic review of 55 cases. Mayo Clin Proc 1996;71: 636–642.
75. Mirra JM, Kessler S, Bhuta S, Eckardt J: The fibroma-like variant of epithelioid sarcoma. A fibrohistiocytic/myoid cell lesion often confused with benign and malignant spindle cell tumors. Cancer 1992;69:1382–1395.
76. von Hochstetter AR, Meyer VE, Grant JW, Honegger HP, Schreiber A: Epithelioid sarcoma mimicking angiosarcoma: The value of immunohistochemistry in the differential diagnosis. Virchows Arch A Pathol Anat Histopathol 1991;418:271–278.
77. Guillou L, Wadden C, Coindre J-M, Krausz T, Fletcher CDM: "Proximal-type" epithelioid sarcoma, a distinctive aggressive neoplasm showing rhabdoid features. Clinicopathological, immunohistochemical and ultrastructural study of a series. Am J Surg Pathol 1997;21:130–146.
78. Chase DR, Weiss SW, Enzinger FM, Langloss JM: Keratin in epithelioid sarcoma. An immunohistochemical study. Am J Surg Pathol 1984;8:435–441.
79. Mukai M, Torikata C, Iri H, et al: Cellular differentiation of epithelioid sarcoma. An electron microscopic, enzyme histochemical, and immunohistochemical study. Am J Pathol 1985;119:44–56.
80. Daimaru Y, Hashimoto H, Tsuneoshi M, Enjoji M: Epithelial profile of epithelioid sarcoma. An immunohistochemical analysis of eight cases. Cancer 1987;59: 131–141.
81. Manivel JC, Wick MR, Dehner LP, Sibley RK: Epithelioid sarcoma. An immunohistochemical study. Am J Clin Pathol 1987:319–326.
82. Meis JM, Mackay B, Ordonez NG: Epithelioid sarcoma—An immunohistochemical and ultrastructural study. Surg Pathol 1988;1:13–31.
83. Arber DA, Kandalaft PL, Mehta P, Battifora H: Vimentin-negative epithelioid sarcoma. The value of an immunohistochemical panel that includes CD34. Am J Surg Pathol 1993;17:302–307.
84. Miettinen M, Fanburg-Smith JC, Virolainen M, Shmookler BM, Fetsch JF: Epithelioid sarcomas: An immunohistochemical analysis of 112 of classical and variant cases and a discussion of the differential diagnosis. Hum Pathol 1999,30:934–942.
85. Gerharz CD, Moll R, Meister P, Knuth A, Gabbert H: Cytoskeletal heterogeneity of an epithelioid sarcoma with expression of vimentin, cytokeratins, and neurofilaments. Am J Surg Pathol 1990;14:274–283.
86. Gerharz CD, Moll R, Ramp U, Mellin W, Gabbert HE: Multidirectional differentiation in a newly established human epithelioid sarcoma cell line (GRU-1) with co-expression of vimentin, cytokeratin and neurofilament proteins. Int J Cancer 1990;45:143–152.
87. Sirgi KE, Wick MR, Swanson PE: B72.3 and CD34 immunoreactivity in malignant epithelioid soft tissue tumors. Adjuncts in the recognition of endothelial neoplasms. Am J Surg Pathol 1993;17:177–185.
88. Smith MEF, Brown JI, Fisher C: Epithelioid sarcoma: Presence of vascular-endothelial cadherin and lack of epithelial cadherin. Histopathology 1998;33:425–431.
89. Wick MR, Manivel JC: Epithelioid sarcoma and isolated necrobiotic granuloma: A comparative immunocytochemical study. J Cutan Pathol 1986;13:253–260.

Epithelioid Sarcoma—Genetics

90. Stenman S, Kindblom LG, Willems J, Angervall L: A cell culture, chromosomal and quantitative DNA analysis of a metastatic epithelioid sarcoma. Cancer 1990;65:2006–2013.
91. Cordoba JC, Parham DM, Meyer WH, Dauglas EC: A new cytogenetic finding in an epithelioid sarcoma t(8;22)(q22;q11). Cancer Genet Cytogenet 1994;72: 151–154.
92. Iwasaki H, Ohjimi Y, Ishiguro M, et al: Epithelioid sarcoma with an 18q aberration. Cancer Genet Cytogenet 1996;91:46–52.
93. Debiec-Rychter M, Sciot R, Hagemeijer A: Common chromosome aberrations in the proximal type of epithelioid sarcoma. Cancer Genet Cytogenet 2000; 123:133–136.
94. Quezado MM, Middleton LP, Bryant B, Lane K, Weiss SW, Merino MJ: Allelic loss on chromosome 22q in epithelioid sarcomas. Hum Pathol 1998;29:604–608.
95. Lushnikova T, Knuutila S, Miettinen M: DNA copy number changes in epithelioid sarcoma and its variants: A comparative genomic hybridization study. Mod Pathol 2000;13:1092–1096.

Myoepithelioma/Mixed Tumor of Soft Tissues

96. Kilpatrick SE, Hitchcock MG, Kraus MD, Calonje E, Fletcher CD: Mixed tumors and myoepitheliomas of soft tissue: A clinicopathologic study of 19 cases with a unifying concept. Am J Surg Pathol 1997;21:13–22.
97. Michal M, Miettinen M: Myoepitheliomas of skin and soft tissues. Virchows Arch 1999;434:393–400.

Parachordoma

98. Dabska M: Parachordoma—A new clinical entity. Cancer 1977;40:1586–1592.
99. Fisher C, Miettinen M: Parachordoma: Clinicopathologic and immunohistochemical study of four cases of an unusual soft tissue neoplasm. Ann Diagn Pathol 1997;1:3–10.

100. Folpe AL, Agoff SN, Willis J, Weiss SW: Parachordoma is immunohistochemically and cytogenetically distinct from axial chordoma and extraskeletal myxoid chondrosarcoma. Am J Surg Pathol 1999;23: 1059–1067.

Chordoma

101. Chambers PW, Schwinn CP: Chordoma. A clinicopathologic study of metastasis. Am J Clin Pathol 1979;72:765–776.
102. Su WPD, Louback JB, Gagne EJ, Scheithauer BW: Chordoma cutis: A report of nineteen patients with cutaneous involvement of chordoma. J Am Acad Dermatol 1993;29:63–66.
103. Suster S, Moran C: Chordomas of the mediastinum: Clinicopathologic, immunohistochemical, and ultrastructural study of six cases presenting as posterior mediastinal masses. Hum Pathol 1995;26: 1354–1362.
104. O'Hara BJ, Paetau A, Miettinen M: Keratin subsets and monoclonal antibody HBME-1 in chordoma—Immunohistochemical differential diagnosis between tumors simulating chordoma. Hum Pathol 1998;29:119–126.

Ectopic Hamartomatous Thymoma

105. Rosai J, Limas C, Husband EM: Ectopic hamartomatous thymoma: A distinctive benign lesion of lower neck. Am J Surg Pathol 1984;8:501–513.
106. Fetsch JF, Weiss SW: Ectopic hamartomatous thymoma: Clinicopathologic, immunohistochemical, and histogenetic considerations in four new cases. Hum Pathol 1990;21:662–668.
107. Chan JK, Rosai J: Tumors of the neck showing thymic or related branchial pouch differentiation: A unifying concept. Hum Pathol 1991;22:349–367.
108. Michal M, Zamecnik M, Gogora M, Mukensnabl P, Neubauer L: Pitfalls in the diagnosis of ectopic hamartomatous thymoma. Histopathology 1996;29: 549–555.

Mesothelioma and Related Tumors

109. Weiss SW, Tavassoli FA: Multicystic mesothelioma. An analysis of pathological findings and biologic behavior in 37 cases. Am J Surg Pathol 1988;12: 737–746.
110. Goepel JR: Benign papillary mesothelioma of the peritoneum: A histological, histochemical and ultrastructural study of six cases. Histopathology 1981; 5:21–30.
111. Daya D, McCaughey WTE: Well-differentiated papillary mesothelioma of the peritoneum. A clinicopathologic study of 22 cases. Cancer 1990;65: 292–296.
112. Craighead JE: Current pathogenetic concepts of diffuse malignant mesothelioma. Hum Pathol 1987;18: 544–557.
113. Battifora H, McCaughey WTE: Tumors of the Serous Membranes. Washington, DC: Armed Forces Institute of Pathology; 1995.
114. Attanoos RL, Gibbs AR: Pathology of malignant mesothelioma. Histopathology 1997;30:403–418.
115. Kannerstein M, Churg A: Peritoneal mesothelioma. Hum Pathol 1977;8:83–94.
116. Sussman J, Rosai J: Lymph node metastasis as the initial manifestation of malignant mesotheliomas: Report of six cases. Am J Surg Pathol 1990;14:819–828.
117. Crotty TB, Myers JL, Katzenstein AL, Tazelaar HD, Swensen SJ, Churg A: Localized malignant mesothelioma. A clinicopathologic and flow cytometric study. Am J Surg Pathol 1994;18:357–363.
118. Nascimento AG, Keeney GL, Fletcher CDM: Deciduoid peritoneal mesothelioma: An unusual phenotype affecting young females. Am J Surg Pathol 1994;18: 439–445.
119. Shanks JH, Harris M, Banerjee SS, et al: Mesotheliomas with deciduoid morphology. A morphologic spectrum and a variant not confined to young females. Am J Surg Pathol 2000;24:285–294.
120. Ordonez NG: Epithelial mesothelioma with deciduoid features. A report of four cases. Am J Surg Pathol 2000;24:816–823.
121. Cantin R, Al-Jabi M, McCaughey WTE: Desmoplastic diffuse mesothelioma. Am J Surg Pathol 1982;6: 215–222.
122. Churg A, Colby TV, Cagle P, et al: The separation of benign and malignant mesothelial proliferations. Am J Surg Pathol 2000;24:1183–1200.
123. Mangano WE, Cagle PT, Churg A, Vollmer RT, Roggli VL: The diagnosis of desmoplastic malignant mesothelioma and its distinction from fibrous pleurisy: A histologic and immunohistochemical analysis of 31 cases including p53 immunostaining. Am J Clin Pathol 1998;110:191–199.

Immunohistochemistry and Differential Diagnosis of Mesothelioma

123A. Carella R, Deleonardi G, D'Errico A, et al: Immunohistochemical panels for differentiating epithelial malignant mesothelioma from lung adenocarcinoma. A study with logistic regression analysis. Am J Surg Pathol 2001;25:43–50.
124. Wick MR, Loy T, Mills SE, Legier JF, Manivel JC: Malignant epithelioid pleural mesothelioma versus peripheral pulmonary adenocarcinoma: A histochemical, ultrastructural, and immunohistologic study of 103 cases. Hum Pathol 1990;21:759–766.
125. Sheibani K, Shin SS, Kezirian J, Weiss LM: Ber-Ep4 antibody as a discriminant in the differential diagnosis of malignant mesothelioma versus adenocarcinoma. Am J Surg Pathol 1991;15:779–784.
126. Amin KM, Litzky LA, Smythe WR, et al. Wilms' tumor 1 susceptibility (WT1) gene products are selectively expressed in malignant mesothelioma. Am J Pathol 1995;146:344–356.

127. Dei Tos AP, Doglioni C: Calretinin: A novel tool for diagnostic immunohistochemistry. Adv Anat Pathol 1998;5:61–66.
128. Attanoos RL, Goddard H, Gibbs AR: Mesothelioma-binding antibodies: Thrombomodulin, OV 632 and HBME-1 and their use in the diagnosis of malignant mesothelioma. Histopathology 1996;29:209–215.
129. Riera, JR, Astengo-Osuna C, Longmate JA, Battifora H: The immunohistochemical diagnostic panel for epithelial mesothelioma. A reevaluation after heat-induced epitope retrieval. Am J Surg Pathol 1997;21: 1409–1417.
130. Ordonez NG: The immunohistochemical diagnosis of epithelial mesothelioma. Hum Pathol 1999;30: 313–323.
131. Cury PM, Butcher DN, Fisher C, Corrin B, Nicholson AG: Value of the mesothelium-associated antibodies thrombomodulin, cytokeratin 5/6, calretinin, and CD44H in distinguishing epithelioid pleural mesothelioma from adenocarcinoma metastatic to pleura. Mod Pathol 2000;13:107–112.
132. Blobel GA, Moll R, Franke WW, Kayser KW, Gould VE: The intermediate filament cytoskeleton of malignant mesotheliomas and its diagnostic significance. Am J Pathol 1985;121:235–247.
133. Moll R, Dhouailly D, Sun TT: Expression of keratin 5 as a distinctive feature of epithelial and biphasic mesotheliomas. An immunohistochemical study using monoclonal antibody AE14. Virchows Arch B Cell Pathol 1989;58:129–145.
134. Ordonez NG. Value of cytokeratin 5/6 immunostaining in distinguishing epithelial mesothelioma of the pleura from lung adenocarcinoma. Hum Pathol 1999;22:1215–1221.
135. Bolen JW, Hammar SP, McNutt MA: Reactive and neoplastic serosal tissue: A light microscopic, ultrastructural, and immunocytochemical study. Am J Surg Pathol 1986;10:34–47.
136. Epstein JI, Budin RE: Keratin and epithelial membrane antigen immunoreactivity in nonneoplastic fibrous pleural lesions: Implications for the diagnosis of desmoplastic mesothelioma. Hum Pathol 1986;17:514–519.
137. Shimizu M, Toki T, Konishi I, Fuji S: Immunohistochemical detection of the Wilms' tumor gene (WT1) in epithelial ovarian tumors. Int J Gynecol Pathol 2000;19:158–163.
138. Goldstein NS, Bassi D, Uzieblo A: WT1 is an integral component of an antibody panel to distinguish pancreaticobiliary and some ovarian epithelial neoplasms. Am J Clin Pathol 2001;116:246–252.
139. Oury TD, Hammar SP, Roggli VL: Ultrastructural features of diffuse malignant mesotheliomas. Hum Pathol 1998;29:1382–1392.
140. Lin BT, Colby T, Gown AM, et al: Malignant vascular tumors of the serous membranes mimicking mesothelioma. A report of 14 cases. Am J Surg Pathol 1996;20:1431–1439.
141. PJ, Livolsi VA, Brooks JJ: Malignant epithelioid vascular tumors of the pleura: Report of a series and literature review. Hum Pathol 2000;31:29–34.

Merkel Cell Carcinoma

142. Toker C: Trabecular carcinoma of the skin. Arch Dermatol 1972;105:107–110.
143. Sibley RK, Dehner LP, Rosai J: Primary neuroendocrine (Merkel cell) carcinoma of the skin. I. A clinicopathologic and ultrastructural study. Am J Surg Pathl 1985;9:95–108.
144. Gould VE, Moll R, Moll I, Lee I, Franke WW: Neuroendocrine (Merkel) cells of the skin: Hyperplasias, dysplasias and neoplasms. Lab Invest 1985;52: 334–353.
145. Haag ML, Glass LF, Fenske NA: Merkel cell carcinoma. Diagnosis and treatment. Dermatol Surg 1995;21:669–683.
146. Tai PT, Yu E, Tonita J, Gilchist J: Merkel cell carcinoma of the skin. J Cutan Med Surg 2000;4:186–195.
147. Skelton HG, Smith KJ, Hitchcock CL, McCarthy WF, Lupton GP, Graham JH: Merkel cell carcinoma: Analysis of clinical, histologic, and immunohistologic features of 132 cases with relation to survival. J Am Acad Dermatol 1997;37:734–739.
148. Penn I, First MR: Merkel cell carcinoma in organ recipients: Report of 41 cases. Transpalantation 1999;68:1717–1721.
149. Eusebi V, Capella C, Cossu A, Rosai J: Neuroendocrine carcinoma within lymph nodes in the absence of a primary tumor, with a special reference to Merkel cell carcinoma. Am J Surg Pathol 1992;16: 658–666.
150. Foschini MP, Eusebi V: Divergent differentiation in endocrine and nonendocrine tumors of the skin. Sem Diagn Pathol 2000;17:162–168.
151. Moll R, Lowe A, Leufer J, Franke WW: Cytokeratin 20 in human carcinomas. A new histodiagnostic marker detected by monoclonal antibodies. Am J Pathol 1992;140:427–447.
152. Chan JK, Suster S, Wenig BM, Tsang WY, Chank JB, Lau AL: Cytokeratin 20 immunoreactivity distinguishes Merkel cell (primary cutaneous neuroendocrine) carcinomas and salivary gland small cell carcinomas from small cell carcinomas of various sites. Am J Surg Pathol 1997;21:226–234.
153. Byrd-Gloster AL, Khoor A, Glass LF, et al: Differential expression of thyroid transcription factor I in small cell lung carcinomas and Merkel cell tumor. Hum Pathol 2000;31:58–62.
154. Hernett PR, Kearsley JH, Hayward NK, Dracopoli NC, Kefford R: Loss of allelic heterozygosity on distal chromosome 1p in Merkel cell carcinoma. A marker for neural crest origin? Cancer Genet Cytogenet 1991;54:109–113.
155. van Gele M, van Roy N, Ronan SG, et al: Molecular analysis of 1p breakpoints in two Merkel cell carcinomas. Genes Chromosomes Cancer 1998;23:67–71.

Miscellaneous Soft Tissue Tumors of Unknown Histogenesis

CHAPTER 20

This group contains three unrelated tumors and tumor groups that have not been not included elsewhere. Common to them is incompletely resolved histogenesis, and in some cases, lack of resemblance to any normal cell type; this is especially true for the enigmatic alveolar soft part sarcoma.

Tenosynovial Giant Cell Tumor

The many synonyms reflect in part clinicopathologic heterogeneity, in part historical differences in understanding of the nature of this tumor. It is also called giant cell tumor of tendon sheath, nodular tenosynovitis, pigmented villonodular synovitis, fibroxanthoma, and fibrous histiocytoma. The four clinicopathologic variants of tenosynovial giant cell tumor are (1) localized, (2) diffuse extra-articular, (3) diffuse intra-articular (diffuse pigmented villonodular synovitis), and (4) malignant. The common presence of clonal chromosomal changes and the occurrence of metastasizing tumors support neoplastic nature of these lesions, which once were considered reactive. Furthermore, similarities in the genetic changes in different types support their mutual relationship.

Tenosynovial Giant Cell Tumor—Localized Type

This is defined as a circumscribed lesion that is microscopically not infiltrating in fat or skeletal muscle. The tumor most commonly occurs in the fingers and may be extra-articular or intra-articular, or both.

Clinical Features

This is by far the most common subtype; its population incidence was estimated as 2/100,000 in one study.[1] This tumor is usually diagnosed in young to middle-age adults between ages 20 and 50, with a 2:1 female predominance. Occurrence in children and elderly is also possible.

Based on five large series,[1–5] this tumor most commonly occurs in the fingers (70–75%), slightly more often in the first to third ones and in the proximal parts, and more often in the right hand. Less

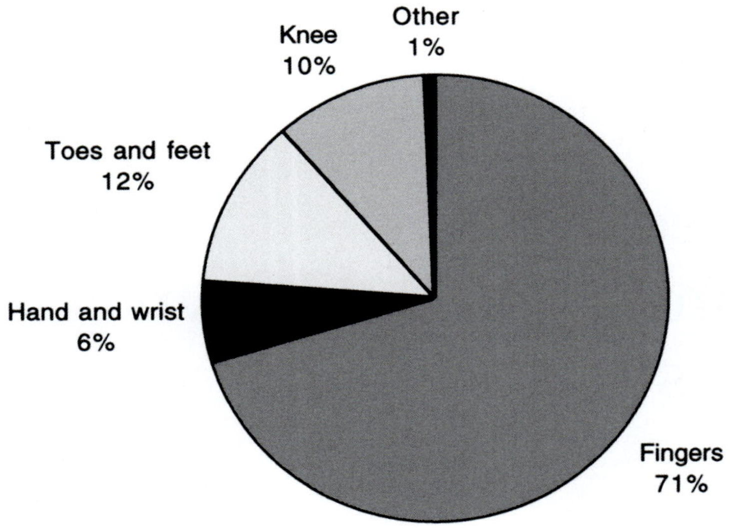

Figure 20–1. Anatomic distribution of localized tenosynovial giant cell tumor according to five series.[1–5]

common is occurrence in hands and wrists, toes, feet, ankles, knees, and rare in the hip (Fig. 20–1). The tumor typically presents as a slowly growing painless mass varying from 0.5 to 4.0 cm (average <2 cm). Bone erosion is occasionally noted. Lesions of the knee are usually intra-articular and may cause pain and joint effusion.

Following local excision, the digital tumors have some tendency to recur (10–20%), but the intra-articular ones in the knee joint recur with a greater frequency.[6]

Pathology

Grossly, the localized tumors are typically lobulated, irregularly oval nodules. They are often partly demarcated by the synovial space or bone. When involving synovia of the large joints, such as the knee, the intra-articular tumor may be pedunculated and become infarcted and sometimes detached by torsion. On sectioning, the tumor is firm and homogenous and varies from yellowish to brown, often with darker streaks.

Microscopically, the localized tumors are often partly surrounded by a band of dense fibrosis and lobulated by fibrous septa. The lobules are composed of ovoid and epithelioid mononuclear and multinucleated histiocyte-like cells set in varying amounts of dense collagenous stroma, sometimes in a trabecular pattern (Fig. 20–2*A* and *B*). The mononuclear cells have varying amounts of cytoplasm and large, round, sometimes grooved nuclei with a single prominent nucleolus. The multinucleated giant cells have an osteoclast-like appearance, vary in numbers, and are less prominent in highly cellular lesions. The giant cells have a widely varying number of nuclei from a few to over 50. Their cytoplasm varies from mildly basophilic to eosinophilic (Fig. 20–2*C*), and some giant cells may develop into apoptotic bodies.[1] Foci of xanthoma cells with foamy cytoplasm are usually present, often in the periphery of the lesion and accompanied by prominent, branching capillaries (Fig. 20–2*D*). Hyalinized areas also occur, and foci of hemosiderin deposition are seen especially in the fibrous septa. Touton-type giant cells and cholesterol crystals are occasional findings.

Some mitotic activity is almost always present and it varies from 2 to over 10/10 high-power field (HPF; average 5/10 HPF), depending on the degree of cellularity.[1,5] The higher degree of mitotic activity did not associate with development of recurrence.[1] Atypical mitoses and nuclear atypia are not present.

Immunohistochemical Features and Histogenesis

The osteoclast-like component shows phenotypic features similar to osteoclasts and is positive for CD68[6–8] and expresses calcitonin receptor.[8] The mononuclear component is positive for histiocyte-specific markers, such as CD14, whereas only the giant cells are positive for CD45 (leukocyte common antigen).[6,8] A desmin-positive and actin-negative subpopulation of spindled dendritic tumor cells of unknown significance has been reported both in the localized and diffuse types.[9] Based on the extensive content of histiocytes, some consider these tumors histiocytic neoplasms.

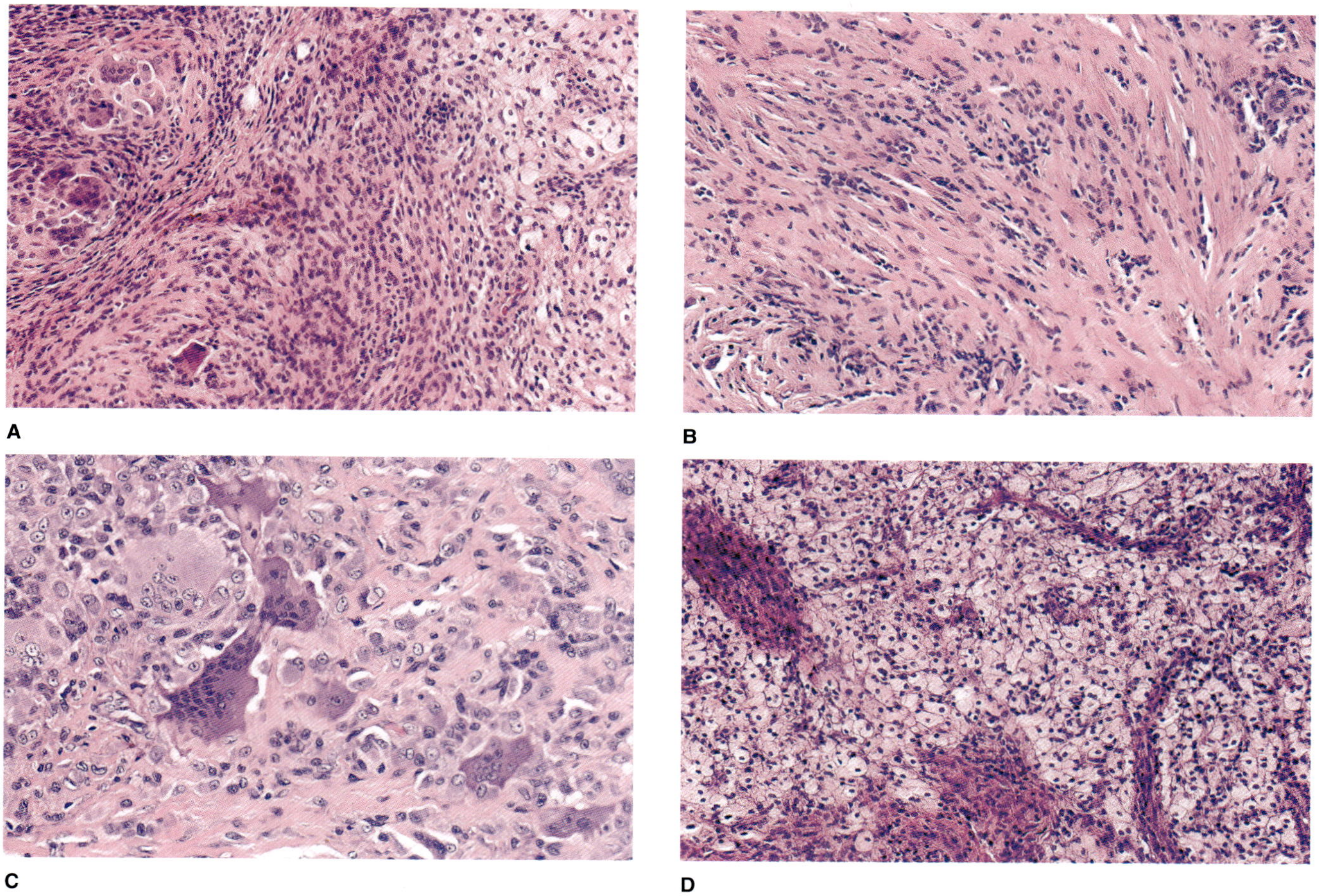

Figure 20–2. Histologic spectrum of localized tenosynovial giant cell tumor. *A*, Tumor with a vague lobulation. *B*, Trabecular pattern with extensive sclerosis. *C*, Osteoclast-like giant cells with basophilic and eosinophilic cytoplasm. *D*, Foci of xanthoma cells and prominent capillaries.

Tenosynovial Giant Cell Tumor—Diffuse Type, Extra-articular

The diffuse extra-articular type is defined by microscopic evidence of invasion to fat or skeletal muscle; this type may have a concomitant intra-articular component.

Clinical Features

Both the diffuse extra-articular and articular tumors present predominantly in young adults with a female predominance, similar to the localized tumors.[10,11] These types overlap because the tumors predominantly forming an extra-articular mass may also have an intra-articular component and vice versa. The diffuse tumors typically occur more proximally than the localized ones and are rare in the digits. In a recent large series, wrist, knee, thigh, and foot were the most common locations, and together comprised 60% of cases of extra-articular tumors.[11] These tumors vary from a small nodule to a mass larger than 10 cm. The recurrence rate is much higher than that of the localized tumors and was estimated as 33% in one study.[11] Therefore, wide excision would be optimal, whenever possible.

Pathology

The diffuse extra-articular tumors are typically grossly yellowish to brown and may appear circumscribed or infiltrative. On sectioning, they are usually softer than the localized examples, and larger tumors may have cystic change.

Histologically typical and diagnostic is infiltration in the adjacent adipose tissue and sometimes in the skeletal muscle. The diffuse tumors are in general more cellular and less sclerotic than the localized ones. Other features more commonly seen in the diffuse variant are hemosiderin-pigmented epithelioid tumor cells and microscopic cysts lined by the lesional cells (Fig. 20–3). Some tumors contain large

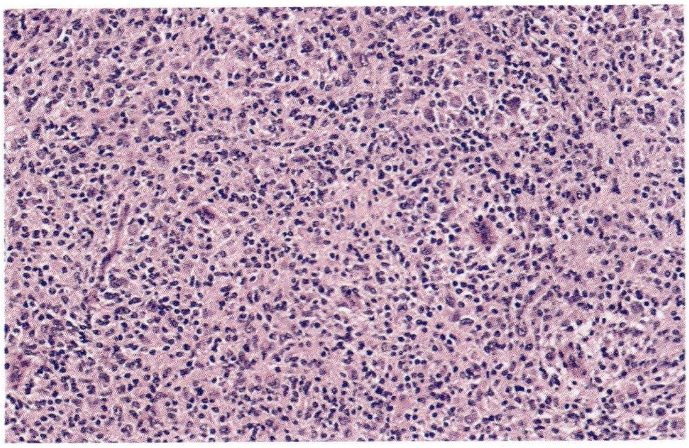

A

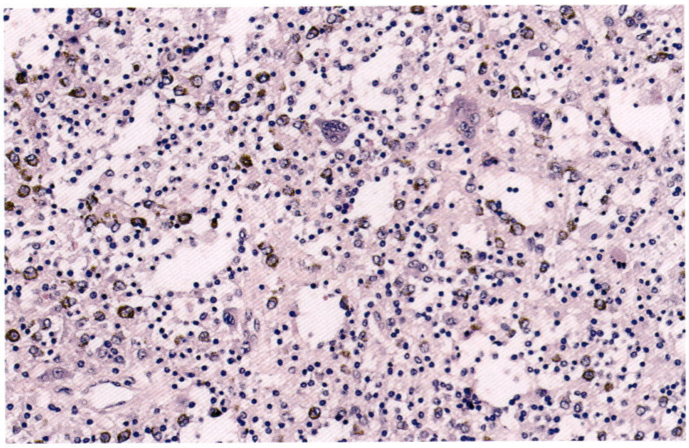

B

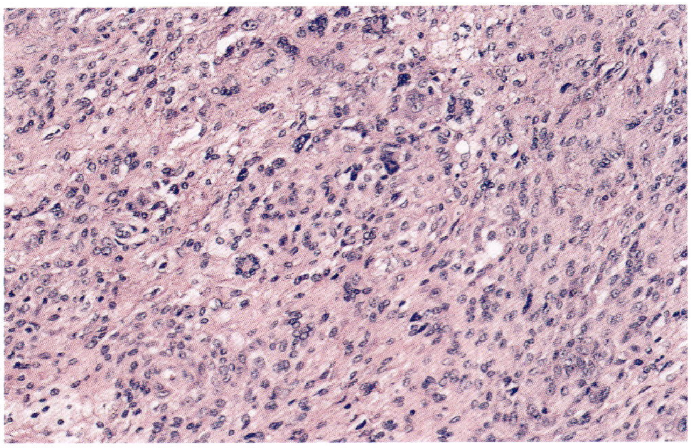

C

Figure 20–3. Diffuse extra-articular tenosynovial giant cell tumor. *A,* An example displaying a highly cellular, uniform pattern with scant giant cells. *B,* Pseudoglandular spaces and hemosiderin-pigmented cells. *C,* Touton-like giant cells and spindled cells in a fibrosing stroma.

numbers of xanthoma cells, and others have lymphocytes and plasma cells, often concentrated in the tumor periphery. The mitotic rate varies in a wide range, and is generally in a similar range as in the localized type, varying between 1 and 10/10 HPF.[11]

Tenosynovial Giant Cell Tumor—Diffuse Type, Intra-articular

This locally aggressive disease (also called diffuse pigmented villonodular synovitis [PVNS]) of large joints most commonly occurs in the knee. Note that some use PVNS synonymously with tenosynovial giant cell tumor in general, whereas others use it to indicate a diffuse intra-articular process.

Clinical Features

The diffuse intra-articular giant cell tumor occurs in younger patients than the localized type and also has a 2:1 female predominance. It usually presents as painful monoarticular swelling or effusion of a large joint, most commonly in the knee, and sometimes in the hip or shoulder and rarely in the elbow or ankle.[12–14] The diffuse nature is best highlighted by magnetic resonance imaging studies. The proliferative synovial process may cause extensive cartilage damage and cystic changes in the adjacent bones, especially when involving the hip and shoulder.[15,16] The clinical course is often lingering, and recurrences develop cumulatively in 30% to 40% of patients, sometimes 20 years or more after the first surgery. Knee lesions recur more often than those in the other large joints.[14,16] Total synovectomy is advocated for treatment, but recurrences may nevertheless develop. In some cases, extensive cartilage destruction requires total arthroplasty and prosthetic joint, especially in the hip lesions. Radiation treatment was historically used to control recurrent disease.[12–16]

Pathology

Grossly, the diffuse intra-articular variant transforms the synovia diffusely into villous, brown proliferation discolored by hemosiderin deposition. The villous proliferation may coexist with solid, yellow-to-tan tumor nodules and form complex masses, and extra-articular extension is also possible (Fig. 20–4).

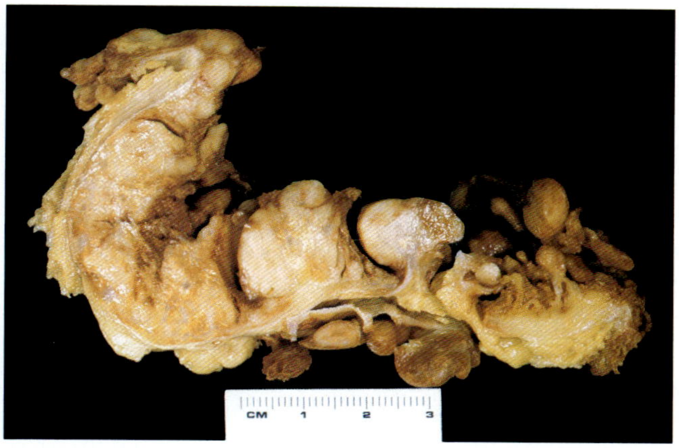

Figure 20–4. Diffuse intra-articular tenosynovial giant cell tumor (pigmented villonodular synovitis) in the knee joint forms a complex mass with multiple polypoid protrusions into the joint space.

Histologically, the villous component is lined by proliferative synovial cells that may involve most of the villi. The villi may also be extensively fibrous with rather nonspecific microscopic appearance, except the presence of solid areas of tumor (Fig. 20–5*A* to *C*). The specific diagnostic elements are often easier to find in the solid tumor areas and the nonvillous component in the base of the synovium. Their composition is generally similar to the localized tumors, except that there is more variation, often with greater fibrosis.

Differential Diagnosis

Granulomatous inflammation of the synovia contains epithelioid histiocytes forming clusters and aggregates. The giant cell nuclei are often in horseshoe configuration, and there is typically an accompanying

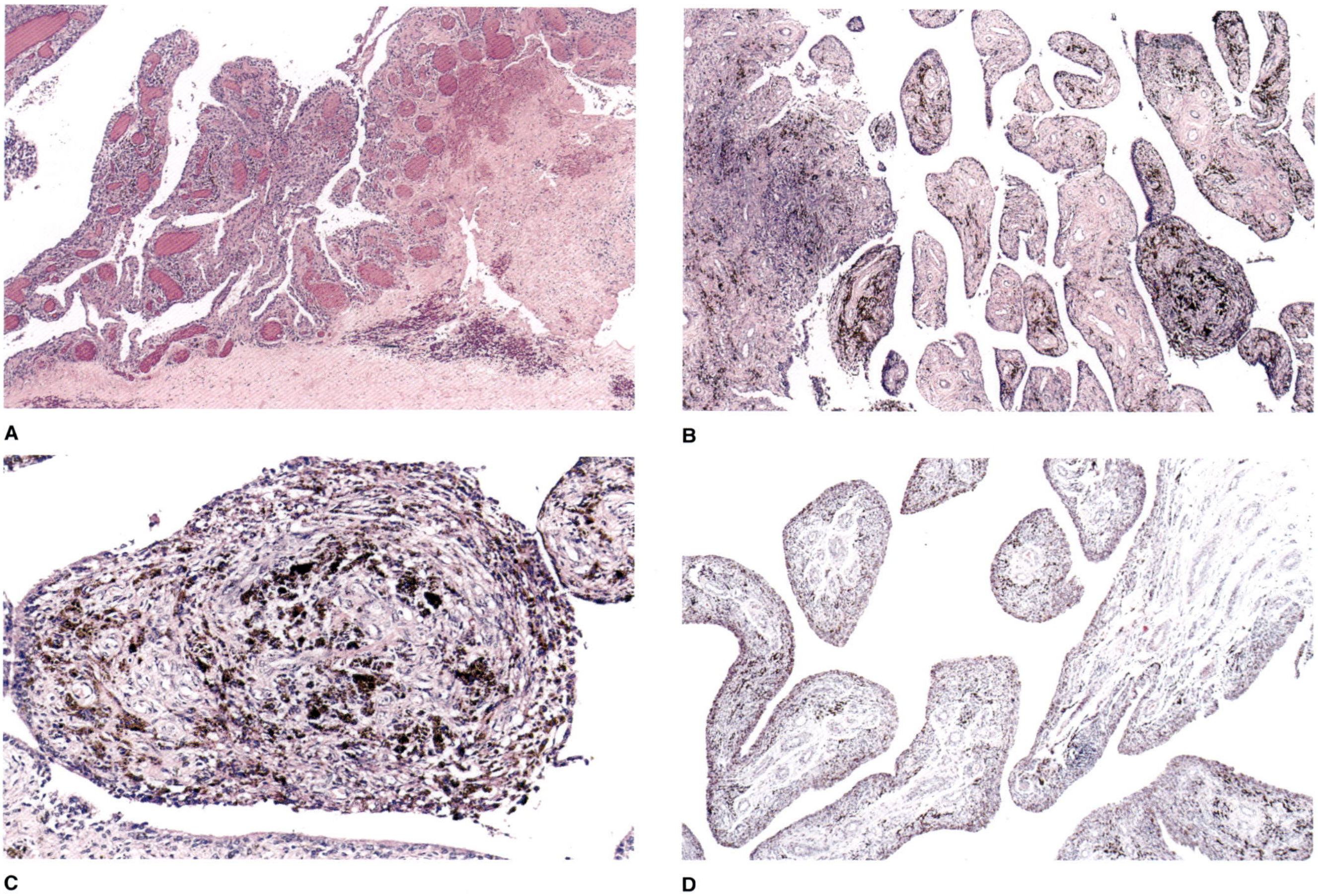

Figure 20–5. Histologic features of diffuse intra-articular tenosynovial giant cell tumor. *A,* Multiple villous processes and a larger necrotic villus. *B,* A villous pattern with giant cell tumor on the left. *C,* Higher magnification of a villus with synovial hyperplasia and giant cell tumor in the core. *D,* In comparison, hemosiderotic synovitis has a similar villous pattern with equal pigmentation, but the villi are thin and have paucicellular cores.

lymphoid population. The process usually lacks the circumscription typical of giant cell tumors.

True xanthoma has no typical osteoclasts and is composed of histiocytes and prominent cholesterol crystals; the latter are rare in giant cell tumors.

Giant cell tumor of soft tissues is a rare tumor that by the presence of osteoclast-like cells has some resemblance to tenosynovial giant cell tumor (see Chapter 7). However, these tumors are typically more homogeneously cellular and less collagenous. They may have foci of metaplastic bone and do not occur in tenosynovial locations.

Extra-osseous extension of giant cell tumor of bone may be seen near the large joints, especially the knee. These tumors are histologically similar to giant cell tumors of soft tissue, being more homogenous and richer in giant cells; radiologic studies reveal the parent tumor as a lytic bone lesion.

Epithelioid sarcoma may simulate localized tenosynovial giant cell tumors when containing numerous osteoclastic giant cells, but it also contains an atypical, eosinophilic epithelioid cell population that can be identified as positive for keratins and epithelial membrane antigen (EMA); this differential diagnosis is especially relevant in the digital lesions.

Hemosiderotic synovitis resulting from chronic, repetitive intra-articular hemorrhage, most often in hemophilia, may grossly simulate diffuse villonodular synovitis as a brown, villous process. Similar to it the synovial cells contain extensive hemosiderin deposition. However, the villous projections are narrow and stroma is paucicellular, fibrous, and hemosiderotic, and does not have the cellular infiltration (Fig. 20–5*D*).

Foreign body reaction to a prosthetic device may cause diffuse villous synovial hyperplasia. However, this process contains birefringent foreign body material and often has an inflammatory mononuclear component.

Rheumatoid synovium may be extensively villous, but it typically contains extensive perivascular lymphoplasmacytic infiltration.

Genetics

Clonal cytogenetic changes have been detected in over half the localized examples, whereas most diffuse tumors have shown aberrations. The most common recurrent changes in the localized tumors have been translocations involving chromosome 1, t(1;2)(p11;q36-37) in particular.[17–19] Alternative translocations seem to also involve 1p11, suggesting that this region contains a gene important in the pathogenesis. Some diffuse tumors have also shown 1p11 alterations. Some diffuse tumors have shown trisomy of chromosomes 5 and 7,[19–21] and a subgroup has been identified with involvement of 16q24.[22] More complex changes have been seen occasionally in both localized and diffuse variants.[21] In one study the localized tumors were reported as diploid in DNA flow cytometric analysis, but diffuse tumors had aneuploidy with an elevated DNA index.[23] This might reflect the more common occurrence of trisomies in the diffuse tumors, as observed in the subsequent cytogenetic studies.[19] Although the clonal genetic aberrations in general support neoplastic nature, a point has been made that also rheumatoid synovia can have clonal chromosomal changes, such as trisomy 7.[17]

Failure to detect a clonality in the HUMARA assay in one study[24] probably reflects the heterogeneous cellular composition of these tumors that may dilute the neoplastic population below the limit of clonality detection in this assay.

Malignant Tenosynovial Giant Cell Tumor

This occurrence is extremely rare, but a small number of well-documented cases have been reported. In some cases, the tumors have been defined based on the observed malignant behavior, and in others on sarcomatous histologic features.[25–31]

The reported tumors have occurred in average in older patients than the benign counterparts, and have represented the diffuse variants with adipose tissue or skeletal muscle infiltration. Most common location has been the knee joint, and local recurrence has developed in the majority of cases and metastases in over half of the patients, half of which had died of the tumor. In some cases, the malignant evolution has been slow, occurring over a span of 20 years.[26,29] Some patients have developed multiple soft tissue metastases in the adjacent regions.[28]

In one series, some tumors arose from a pre-existing PVNS and some de novo.[29] Histologically typical is multinodular pattern of growth, high cellularity, and relative paucity of giant cells and collagen and the common presence of significant necrosis (Fig. 20–6). Although the mitotic rate is often over 10/10 HPF, some tumors have counts similar to those in benign tumors. Some metastasizing tumors have spindle cell sarcomatous patterns, and others have the features of conventional diffuse tenosynovial giant cell tumor but nevertheless metastasize. Some patients have received radiation for PVNS, which could have played a role in the sarcomatous transformation.

In our series of 27 cases, malignant tenosynovial giant cell tumors occurred in a wide age range with

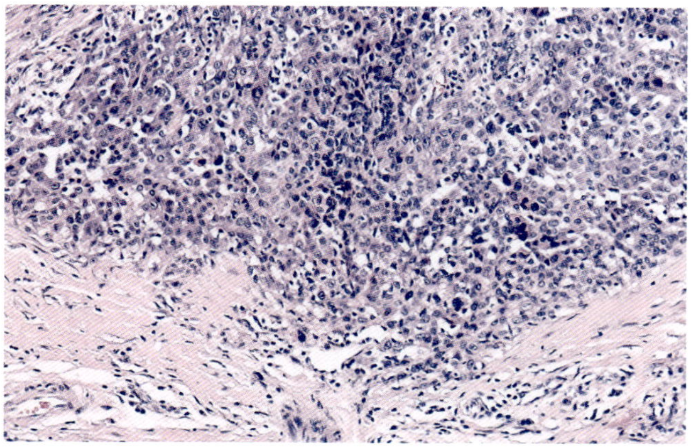

Figure 20–6. Malignant tenosynovial giant cell tumor with a nodular pattern is composed of large, slightly epithelioid cells.

a mild female predominance 15:12. The most common location was the knee. Some tumors had a strikingly histiocytic phenotype with diffuse positivity for histiocytic markers; spindle cell sarcomatous features were rare. The best criterion for malignancy was the combination of the following factors: diffuse infiltrative growth, scant number of giant cells, tumor cell dyscohesion, pleomorphism, increased nucleocytoplasmic ratio and large cell size, extremely large nucleoli, mitotic rate over 10/10 HPF, and coagulation necrosis. In cases with six or more of these factors, the tumor-related death occurred in 38% patients who often developed pulmonary metastases.[31]

Differential Diagnosis

Several specific tumor types potentially occurring in similar locations have to be ruled out. They especially include epithelioid sarcoma, which has deeply eosinophilic epithelioid cells and is positive for epithelial markers (see Chapter 19), clear cell sarcoma of tendons and aponeuroses, which has a melanoma-like immunophenotype (see Chapter 16), and malignant lymphomas.

Angiomatoid (Malignant) Fibrous Histiocytoma

Angiomatoid fibrous histiocytoma (AFH) is a histologically distinctive childhood neoplasm composed of small, round or spindled cells with common desmin positivity and relatively indolent behavior with rare lymph node metastasis. Histogenesis is unknown.

Clinical Features

This tumor, originally described as angiomatoid malignant fibrous histiocytoma by Enzinger,[32] has more recently been renamed as AFH because of very infrequent malignant behavior.[33]

The tumor typically presents in the superficial soft tissues of children and young adults. The median age in three largest recent series has varied from 12 to 18 years, and 80% of patients are under age 20, and only 6% are over age 40. Some series have shown a mild female predominance, 55%.[32–35] The lesions occur in the subcutis of extremities, trunk, or less commonly head and neck as a painless nodule clinically usually thought of a cyst or a benign tumor. As many as half of the tumors occur in major lymph node regions, such as axilla, inguinal region antecubital fossa, and head and neck. A minority of patients have larger tumors and constitutional symptoms, such as anemia and, occasionally weight loss and polyclonal gammopathy.[32]

Recurrence is rare following a local excision (<10%), but factors indicating increased risk for this are infiltrative border, deep fascial or periosteal, or head and neck location. However, atypia and mitotic activity do not seem to correlate with increased risk for recurrence. Lymph node metastases have been reported in 1% of cases, but in more recent series, distant metastases have been exceedingly rare if they occur.[33,34] The reported metastatic tumors have had some usual features, such as deep intramuscular location and large tumor size over 10 cm,[32,36] and some of such cases might now be reclassifiable as other entities. However, rare fatal cases continue to be reported, including one of a 9-year-old girl, whose foot tumor caused massive metastases to liver and lung and killed the patient in 14 months.[37] Wide excision is considered an optimal treatment.

Histopathology

The tumor usually measures 1 to 3 cm in diameter, but is occasionally much larger. It varies grossly from a tan homogeneous nodule to a hemorrhagic, cystic mass.[32–34,37]

Histologically typical is a peripheral band of dense fibrosis and a cuff of lymphoplasmacytic infiltration, which often contains germinal centers; this may lead into initial consideration of lymph node metastasis (Fig. 20–7*A* and *B*). The tumor may also contain diffuse lymphoplasmacytic infiltration. An exceptional case was reported with extensive lymphadenopathy simulating Castleman disease accompanying the tumor.[38]

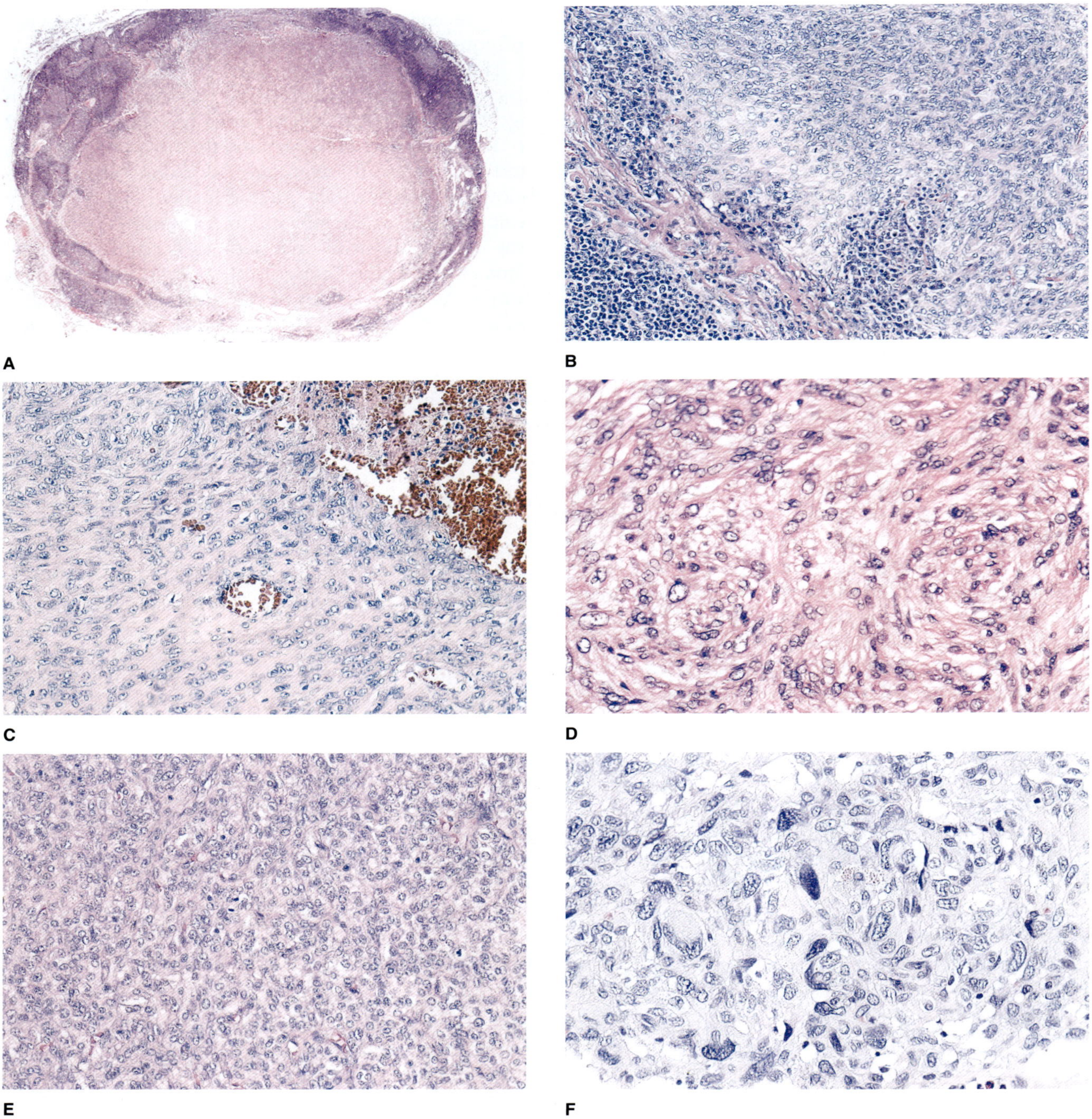

Figure 20–7. Histologic spectrum of angiomatoid fibrous histiocytoma. *A,* Low magnification showing a lymphoid cuff around the tumor. *B,* Higher magnification of tumor cells with a uniform, oval appearance. *C,* A tumor with hemorrhagic cysts. *D,* A storiform spindle cell pattern. *E,* A tumor with round cell pattern. *F,* Focal pleomorphism occurs in a minority of cases.

Some tumors contain multiple hemorrhagic cysts directly lined by tumor cells, and focal hemosiderin deposition is common in these variants (Fig. 20–7C). The tumor cells are often arranged in a storiform pattern, sometimes in a "cannonball" fashion surrounded by lymphoplasmacytic infiltration. Some tumors are arranged in diffuse sheets and some have a trabecular pattern with myxoid stroma. Hyalinized areas may occur.

Cytologically, the tumors are equally often composed of spindled and oval to round cells, or a mixture of them, often seen in a storiform pattern (Fig. 20–7*D* and *E*). The tumor cells have poorly delineated borders with a moderate amount of pale eosinophilic cytoplasm. The nuclei are usually uniform with a pale or vesicular chromatin and a small nucleolus, but some tumors contain moderate atypia (Fig. 20–7*F*), sometimes with nuclear pseudoinclusions. Mitotic rate is usually low, but some cases have 5 or more mitoses per 10 HPF; this is not an alarming feature and has no further significance.

Immunohistochemistry

The tumor cells are usually positive for vimentin and calponin and variably for CD68, CD99, and desmin in 50% of the cases.[35,39,40] They are occasionally positive for true smooth muscle markers, such as h-caldesmon and smooth muscle actins, but are negative for the skeletal muscle specific transcriptional regulators MyoD1 and myogenin. The desmin-positive round tumor cells associated with lymphoid tissue have some analogy with the myoid cells of lymphoid tissue, but a direct histogenetic link has yet to be proven.[35]

The tumor cells are negative for endothelial cell markers and CD34, keratins, S-100 protein and CD21 and CD35, markers for dendritic reticulum cells.[35] Some examples have been positive for EMA.[41]

Differential Diagnosis

Lymph node metastases of melanoma, primary tumors of lymphoid tissue, such as the rare dendritic reticulum cell sarcoma have to be considered. However, AFH does not have a sinus system thus differing from a lymph node; usually metastatic melanoma has greater cytologic atypia and is recognizable by immunohistochemical markers. The hemorrhagic examples of AFH differ from true vascular tumors by the lack of vasoformation by tumor cells, practically always evident in true endothelial neoplasms. The hemorrhagic, highly malignant giant cell malignant fibrous histiocytomas (MFHs) in older patients should not be confused with angiomatoid MFHs.[42]

The desmin-positive examples of AFH should not be confused with childhood rhabdomyosarcoma. The clinical presentation in superficial soft tissues and lack of rhabdomyoblastic differentiation are the most significant differences. Similarly, the CD99 positivity should not lead to confusion with Ewing sarcoma; the latter is typically composed of densely packed small round cells with a lesser amount of cytoplasm.

Genetics

Translocation t(12,16)(q13,p11) leading to the fusion of *ATF1* and *FUS* genes and expression of the fusion transcript has been reported in one case.[43] This may be the primary pathogenetic event in AFH but needs to be confirmed in a larger series.

Alveolar Soft Part Sarcoma

This histologically distinctive sarcoma with a predilection to children and young adults was originally described by Christopherson, Foote, and Stewart in 1952.[44] In earlier times, these tumors were considered peripheral examples of nonchromaffin paragangliomas or organoid malignant granular cell tumors.

Clinical Features

Alveolar soft part sarcoma (ASPS) is a very rare tumor comprising less than 1% of all soft tissue sarcomas. Based on Armed Forces Institute of Pathology statistics of over 200 cases, 39% of the cases occur in individuals below the age of 20 years (Fig. 20–8). According to a recent review, childhood tumors have a female predominance, whereas those in adulthood have a male predominance.[45]

The tumor occurs in a wide variety of locations. Most common are deep muscles of the thigh, buttocks, and other extremity-based locations. In children, orbit and tongue are possible sites. A small number of cases has been reported in the retroperitoneum, female genital tract (uterine corpus, cervix and vagina), and stomach.[45–54] Primary bone origin in femur, fibula, and ilium,[55] and tumors considered primary in the lung have also been reported.[56] However, the possibility of occult primary tumor should be ruled out in the case of pulmonary or osseous presentation, because these tumors may present with metastatic disease.

Clinically, some tumors may be pulsatile due to high vascularization, and for this reason the tumor may also bleed massively during surgery. Pulmonary and less commonly brain metastases develop in a high percentage of patients in long-term follow-up. For example, the 5-year survival rate in a Memorial Sloan-

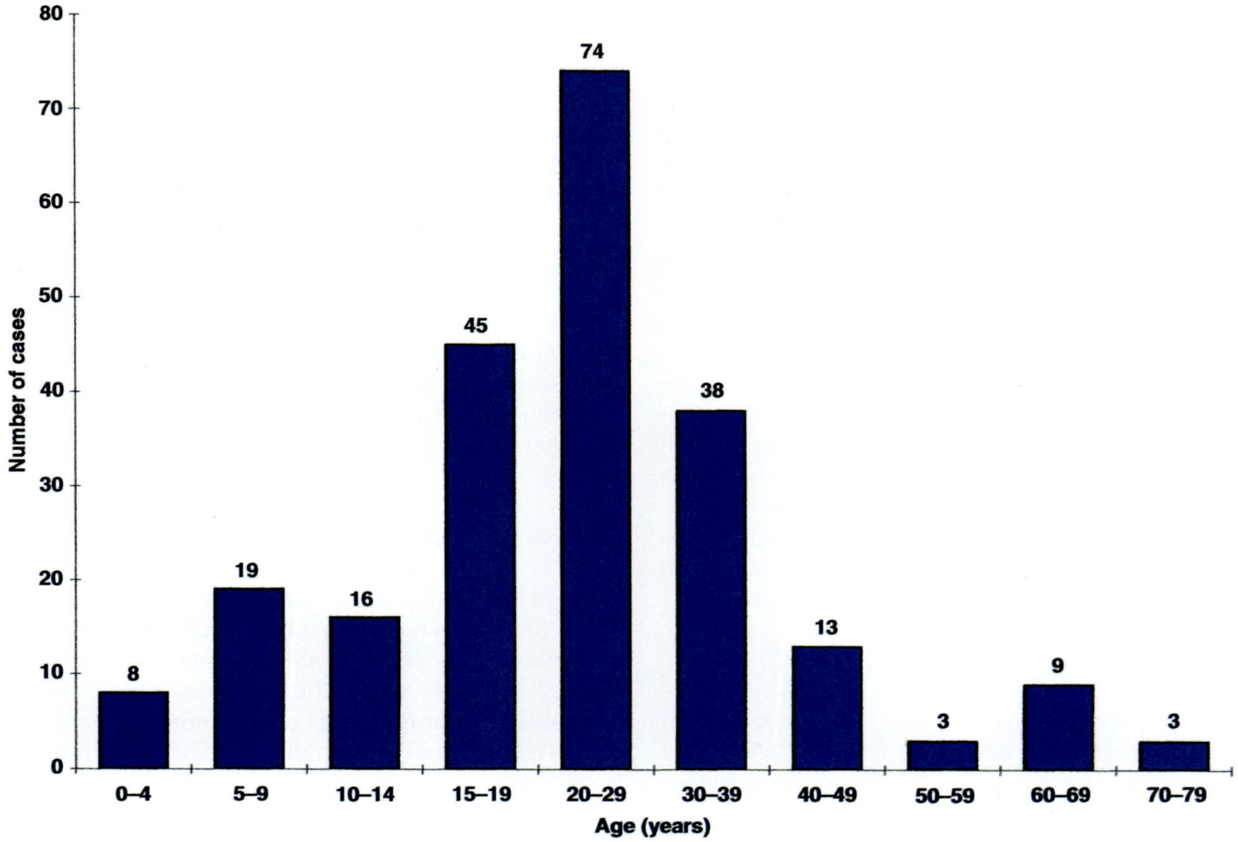

Figure 20–8. Age distribution of alveolar soft part sarcoma according to data of the Armed Forces Institute of Pathology.

Kettering series was 38%, but 20-year survival fell to 15%, reflecting continuous development of metastases.[49] In one case, brain metastasis developed 33 years after surgery.[51] A recent series from M. D. Anderson Hospital suggested that localized tumors at presentation (stage 1) have a better prognosis.[54] Aggressive surgery is generally believed to be the most important part of the treatment. This includes treatment of metastatic disease, because many patients live long after metastases developed.[49] Small tumor size (<5 cm) is a favorable prognostic factor, and one study showed a better prognosis in children.[53]

Pathology

Grossly, the tumor is circumscribed and soft and varies from yellow to brownish and may be colored by hemorrhage. The tumors in the head and neck are typically smaller (1–3 cm), compared to those located deep in the extremities, which often reach the size of 10 cm or more.[44–49]

Histologically highly distinctive is a compartmental pattern, often with central alveolar spaces (Fig. 20–9*A* to *C*). The compartments are typically separated by delicate thin-walled, sometimes gaping capillaries that may be empty or less often hyperemic. Larger numbers of compartments are often separated by thick fibrous septa creating a microlobular pattern. Some tumors are composed of very small compartments resulting in a nearly solid appearance, but clusters of tumor cells are separated by fine capillary network in this variant as well (Fig. 20–9*D*). The solid variant may be more common in head and neck of children and have a better prognosis.[49] Some cases show extensive degenerative changes, such as hyalinization and reactive vascular proliferation, but coagulative necrosis is uncommon. Vascular invasion is a frequent finding (Fig. 20–9*E*).

Cytologically, the tumor cells have abundant cytoplasm that varies from clear or pale granular to deeply eosinophilic, "oncocytic" (Fig. 20–9*F*). The cytoplasm is rich in glycogen. Distinctive periodic acid-Schiff (PAS)-positive, diastase-resistant cytoplasmic crystals are found in 70% to 80% of cases, and some tumor cells are diffusely PAS positive (Fig. 20–9*G*). The nuclei are usually round and uniform with a delicate

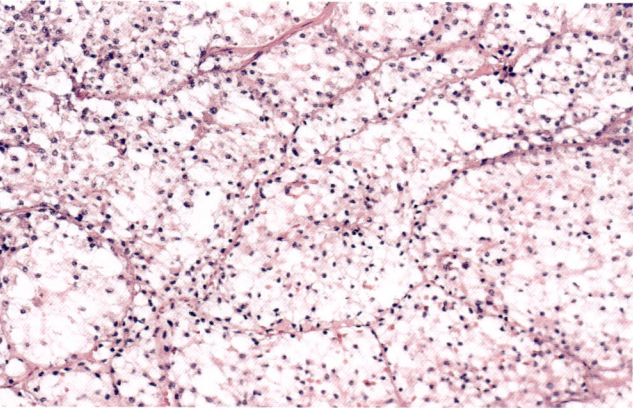

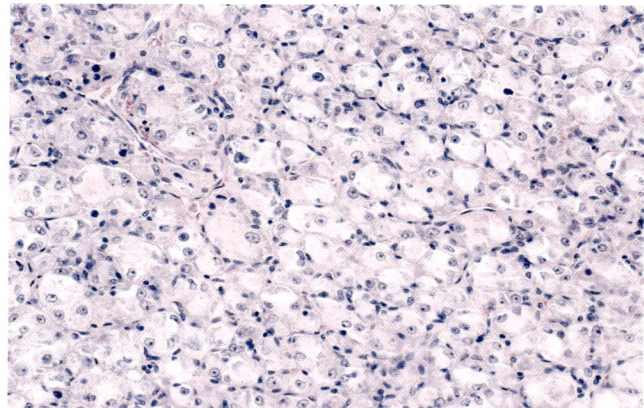

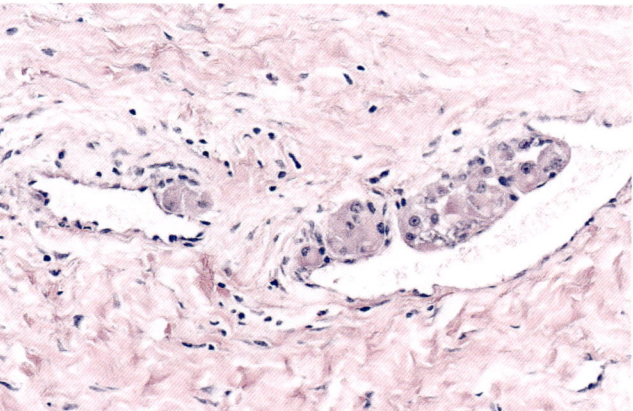

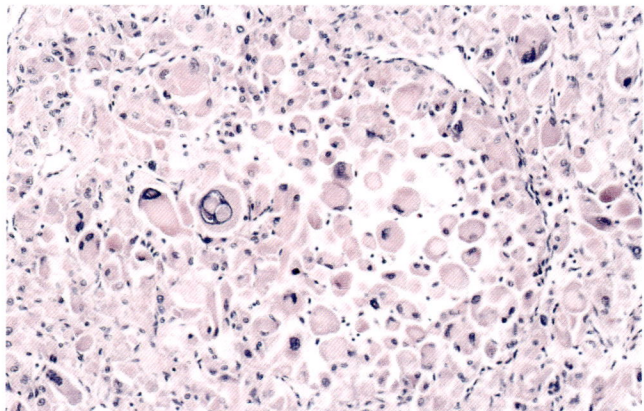

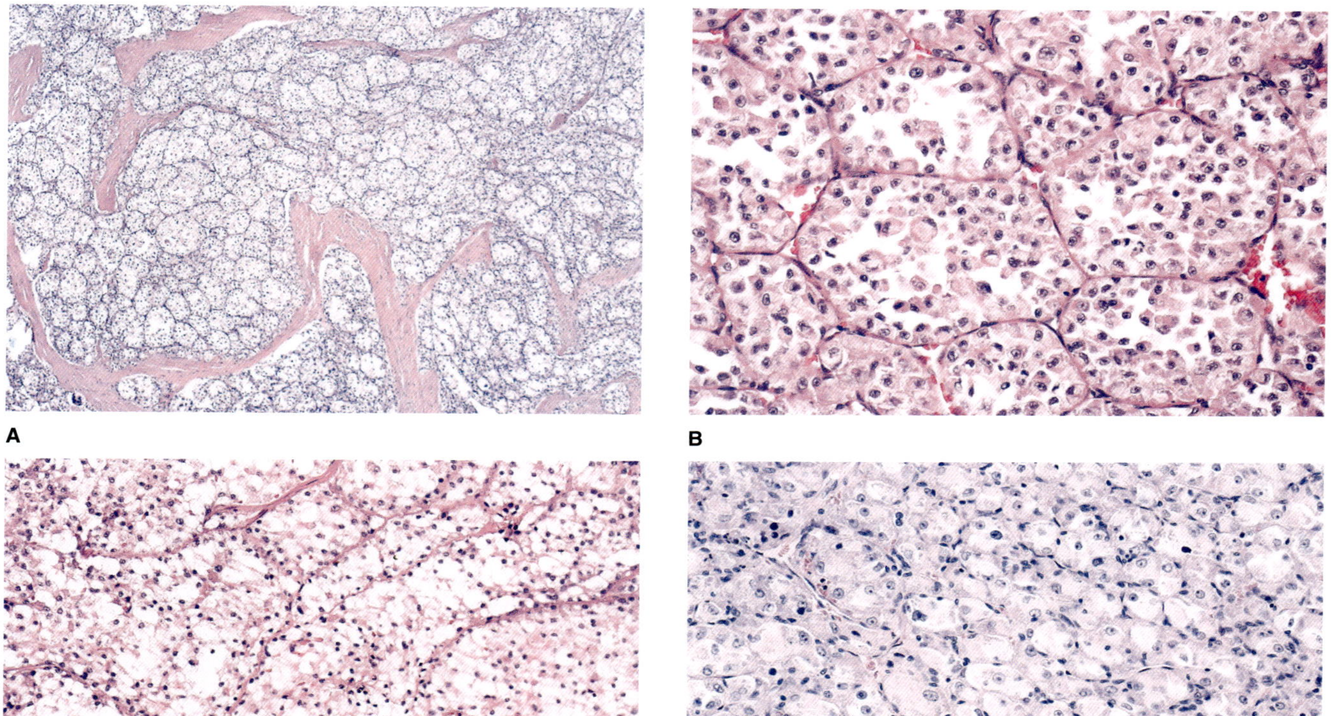

Figure 20–9. Histologic spectrum of alveolar soft part sarcoma. *A,* Compartmental pattern with lobulation by fibrous septa. *B,* A typical compartmental pattern with central alveolar spaces. *C,* A clear cell variant simulating a renal cell carcinoma. *D,* A solid variant often occurring in head and neck of children. *E,* Vascular invasion is a typical feature. *F,* Oncocytic features and focal nuclear atypia.

Illustration continued on following page

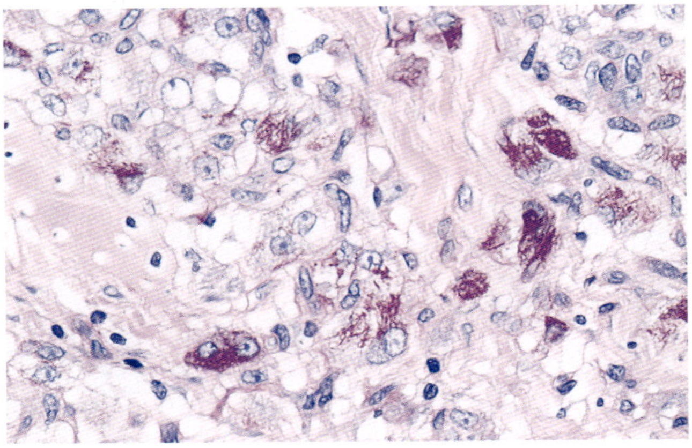

G

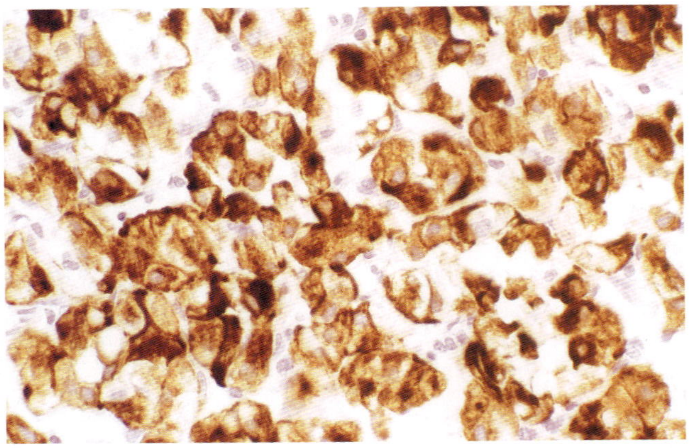

H

Figure 20–9. *Continued G,* PAS+ needle-shaped cytoplasmic crystals are seen in most cases. *H,* Desmin positivity is common and may be extensive.

chromatin pattern and a single prominent nucleolus. Rarely, there is significant nuclear pleomorphism with hyperchromasia or nuclear complexity with pseudoinclusions. Mitoses and necrosis are distinctly rare in this tumor, except in rare variants with nuclear atypia; these tumors may have a worse prognosis.[47]

Immunohistochemistry

Variable desmin positivity has been observed in over half of the cases (Fig. 20–9*H*). The percentage of positive cases in various series have ranged from 0% to 100%,[57–63] which probably reflects historical problems in desmin detection in formalin-fixed tumors with some antibodies, because desmin has been more consistently demonstrated in frozen sections of these tumors using various antibodies.[58] Positivity for muscle actin has been detected in some cases, and sarcomeric actins have been reported. The expression of muscle markers has raised the question of skeletal muscle relationship, and this tumor has even been suggested to be related with rhabdomyosarcoma. Although an initial observation based on one case seemed to indicate MyoD1 positivity and expression by Western blotting,[64] larger series have not confirmed MyoD1 and myogenin, the skeletal muscle cell transcriptional regulators, in the tumor cell nuclei. However, cytoplasmic MyoD1 positivity seems to be quite common,[62,63] raising the possibility of aberrant cytoplasmic expression of these proteins.

In contrast to most other sarcomas, the tumor cells show only limited if any vimentin positivity. They may be positive for S-100 protein, but have been almost uniformly negative for chromogranin, synaptophysin, neurofilaments, various neuropeptides, and keratins.[45]

Ultrastructure

Cytoplasmic membrane-bound rhomboid crystals with internal 70Å periodicity are a characteristic feature seen in most cases.[65,66] These crystals seem to be formed from large granules containing filamentous structures, possibly actin-related.[67] Myofilaments, as expected in true myosarcomas, are not features of this tumor. Electron microscopic studies have also ruled out relationship with paraganglioma and granular cell tumor.[66]

Histogenesis

The histogenesis of this tumor remains obscure, but relationship with skeletal muscle cells has been suggested based on expression of desmin and that of myogenic regulators and possibly sarcomeric actin.[61] Carstens noted similar crystals in muscle spindles, but was cautious to invoke a histogenetic relationship.[68] It is also possible that the unique genetic makeup of this tumor (gene fusion, see later discussion) has created an unparalleled phenotypic pattern in this tumor not comparable to any normal cell type. Older theories on the relationship with granular cell tumor or paraganglioma have not been supported by special studies.

Differential Diagnosis

Other tumors with compartmental or granular cell pattern that must be differentiated include metastatic melanoma, paraganglioma, renal carcinoma, and granular cell tumor. Melanoma usually shows a more variable histology, less developed compartmental pattern, and expression of multiple melanoma markers. Paraganglioma may enter in the differential diagnosis in the head and neck area. It typically has a bimodal chief and sustentacular cell population and is uniformly positive for neuroendocrine markers chromogranin and synaptophysin. Renal carcinoma is typically positive for keratin and EMA. Granular cell tumors, especially the malignant ones, have a more solid architecture and a tendency for spindling.

Genetics

Rearrangement of 17q25 was the initially detected recurrent chromosomal aberration.[69–71] Subsequently, a nonbalanced translocation t(X;17) (p11.2q25) was identified with loss of one copy of the terminal 17q and gain of Xp.[72,73] Cloning of this translocation revealed fusion of the *TFE3* transcription factor gene in Xp11 with a new widely expressed gene named *ASPL* (alveolar soft part sarcoma locus) in 17q25.[74] Also recurrent gains in 1q, 8q, and 12q were seen by comparative genomic hybridization; these probably represent secondary chromosomal changes.[75]

Detection of the t(X;17) translocation may become a new gold standard for the definition of this tumor. However, a variant of childhood renal carcinoma shows a similar but balanced (reciprocal) translocation t(X;17)(p11.2q25).[76]

REFERENCES

Tenosynovial Giant Cell Tumor—Clinicopathologic and Immunohistochemical Studies

1. Monaghan H, Salter DM, Al-Nafussi A: Giant cell tumour of tendon sheath (localised nodular tenosynovitis): Clinicopathological features of 71 cases. J Clin Pathol 2001;54:404–407.
2. Jones FE, Soule EH, Coventry MB: Fibrous xanthoma of synovium (giant cell tumor of tendon sheath, pigmented nodular synovitis): A study of one hundred and eighteen cases. J Bone Joint Surg Am 1969;51:76–86.
3. Myers BW, Masi AT, Feigenbaum SL: Pigmented villonodular synovitis and tenosynovitis: A clinical and epidemiologic study of 166 cases and literature review. Medicine 1980;59:223–238.
4. Rao AS, Vigorita VJ: Pigmented villonodular synovitis (giant cell tumor of the tendon sheath and synovial membrane). J Bone Joint Surg Am 1984;66:76–94.
5. Ushijima M, Hashimoto H, Tsuneyoshi M, Enjoji M: Giant cell tumor of tendon sheath (nodular tenosynovitis). A study of 207 cases to compare the large joint group with the common digit group. Cancer 1986;57:875–884.
6. Wood GS, Beckstead JH, Medeiros LJ, Kempson RL, Warnke RA: The cells of giant cell tumor of tendon sheath resemble osteoclasts. Am J Surg Pathol 1988;12:444–452.
7. O'Connell JX, Fanburg JC, Rosenberg AE: Giant cell tumor of tendon sheath and pigmented villonodular synovitis: Immunophenotype suggests a synovial cell origin. Hum Pathol 1995;26:771–775.
8. Darling JM, Goldring SR, Harada Y, Handel ML, Glowacki J, Gravallese EM: Multinucleated cells in pigmented villonodular synovitis and giant cell tumor of tendon sheath express features of osteoclasts. Am J Pathol 1997;150:1383–1393.
9. Folpe AL, Weiss SW, Fletcher CDM, Gown AM: Tenosynovial giant cell tumors: Evidence for a desmin-positive dendritic cell subpopulation. Mod Pathol 1998;11:939–944.
10. Rowlands CG, Roland B, Hwang WS, Sevick RJ: Diffuse variant tenosynovial giant cell tumor: A rare and aggressive lesion. Hum Pathol 1994;25:423–425.
11. de Aubain Somerhausen N, Fletcher CDM: Diffuse-type giant cell tumor: Clinicopathologic and immunohistochemical analysis of 50 cases with extraarticular disease. Am J Surg Pathol 2000;24:479–492.
12. Granowitz SP, D'Antonio J, Mankin HL: The pathogenesis and long-term end results of pigmented villonodular synovitis. Clin Orthop 1976;114:335–351.
13. Ushijima M, Hashimoto H, Tsuneyoshi M, Enjoji M: Pigmented villonodular synovitis. A clinicopathologic study of 52 cases. Acta Pathol Jpn 1986;36:317–326.
14. Schwartz HS, Unni KK, Pritchard DJ: Pigmented villonodular synovitis. A retrospective review of affected large joints. Clin Orthop 1989;247:243–255.
15. Dorwart RH, Genant HK, Johnston WH, Morris JM: Pigmented villonodular synovitis of synovial joints: Clinical, pathologic, and radiologic features. Am J Roentgenol 1984;143:877–885.
16. Gonzalez Della Valle A, Piccaluga F, Potter HG, Salvati EA, Pusso R: Pigmented villonodular synovitis of the hip: 2- to 23-year followup study. Clin Orthop 2001;388:187–199.

Tenosynovial Giant Cell Tumor—Genetics

17. Mertens FM, Örndal C, Mandahl N, et al: Chromosome aberrations in tenosynovial giant cell tumors and nontumorous synovial tissue. Genes Chromosomes Cancer 1993;6:212–217.
18. Dal Cin P, Sciot R, Samson I, et al: Cytogenetic characterization of tenosynovial giant cell tumors (nodular tenosynovitis). Cancer Res 1994;54:3986–3987.
19. Sciot R, Rosai J, Dal Cin P, de Wever I, et al: Analysis of 35 cases of localized and diffuse tenosynovial giant cell tumor. A report from the Chromosomes and Morphology (CHAMP) Study Group. Mod Pathol 1999;12:576–579.
20. Ray RA, Morton CC, Lipinski KK, Corson JM, Fletcher JA: Cytogenetic evidence for clonality in a case of pigmented villonodular synovitis. Cancer 1991;67:121–125.
21. Fletcher JA, Henkle C, Atkins L, Rosenberg AE, Morton CC: Trisomy 5 and trisomy 7 are nonrandom aberrations in pigmented villonodular synovitis: Confirmation of trisomy 7 in uncultured cells. Genes Chromosomes Cancer 1992;4:264–266.

22. Dal Cin P, Sciot R, De Smet L, van Damme B, van den Berghe H: A new cytogenetic subgroup in tenosynovial giant cell tumors (nodular tenosynovitis) is characterized by involvement of 16q24. Cancer Genet Gytogenet 1996;87:85–87.
23. Abdul-Karim FW, el-Naggar AK, Joyce MJ, Makley JT, Carter JR: Diffuse and localized tenosynovial giant cell tumor and pigmented villonodular synovitis: A clinicopathologic and flow cytometric DNA analysis. Hum Pathol 1992;23:729–735.
24. Vogrincic GS, O'Connell JX, Gilks CB: Giant cell tumor of tendon sheath is a polyclonal cellular proliferation. Hum Pathol 1997;28:815–819.

Malignant Tenosynovial Giant Cell Tumor

25. Kahn LB: Malignant giant cell tumor of the tendon sheath. Arch Pathol 1973;95:203–208.
26. Cartens PHB, Howell RS: Malignant giant cell tumor of tendon sheath. Virchows Arch A Pathol Anat Histol 1979;382:237–243.
27. Lynge-Nielsen A, Kiaer T: Malignant giant cell tumor of synovium and locally destructive pigmented villonodular synovitis: Ultrastructural and immunohistochemical study and review of the literature. Hum Pathol 1989;20:765–771.
28. Choong PFM, Willen H, Nilbert M, et al: Pigmented villonodular synovitis. Monoclonality and metastasis—A case for neoplastic origin? Acta Orthop Scand 1995;66:64–68.
29. Bertoni F, Unni KK, Beabout JW, Sim FH: Malignant giant cell tumor of tendon sheaths and joints (malignant pigmented villonodular synovitis). Am J Surg Pathol 1997;21:153–163.
30. Layfield LJ, Meloni-Ehrig A, Liu K, Shepard R, Harrelson JM: Malignant giant cell tumor of synovium (malignant pigmented villonodular synovitis). A histopathological and fluorescence in situ hybridization analysis of 2 cases and review of the literature. Arch Pathol Lab Med 2000;124:1636–1641.
31. Fanburg-Smith JC, Miettinen M: Malignant giant cell tumors of tendon sheath: Histologic classification with clinical correlation [abstract]. Clin Exp Pathol 1998; 46:16A.

Angiomatoid (Malignant) Fibrous Histiocytoma

32. Enzinger FM: Angiomatoid malignant fibrous histiocytoma. A distinct fibrohistiocytic tumor of children and young adults simulating a vascular neoplasm. Cancer 1979;44:2147–2157.
33. Costa MJ, Weiss SW: Angiomatoid malignant fibrous histiocytoma. A follow-up study of 108 cases with evaluation of possible histologic predictors of outcome. Am J Surg Pathol 1990;14:1126–1132.
34. Leu HJ, Makek M: Angiomatoid malignant fibrous histiocytoma. Virchows Arch A Pathol Anat Histopathol 1982;395:99–107.
35. Fanburg-Smith JF, Miettinen M: Angiomatoid "malignant" fibrous histiocytoma. A clinicopathologic study of 158 cases and further exploration of the myoid phenotype. Hum Pathol 1999;30:1336–1343.
36. Pettinato G, Manivel JC, De Rosa G, Petrella G, Jaszcz W: Angiomatoid malignant fibrous histiocytoma: Cytologic, immunohistochemical, ultrastructural, and flow cytometric study of 20 cases. Mod Pathol 1990;3: 479–487.
37. Chow LT, Allen PW, Kumta SM, Griffith J, Li CK, Leung PC: Angiomatoid malignant fibrous histiocytoma: Report of an unusual case with highly aggressive clinical course. J Foot Ankle Surg 1998;37:235–238.
38. Seo IS, Frizerra G, Coates TD, Mirkin LD, Cohen MD: Angiomatoid malignant fibrous histiocytoma with extensive lymphadenopathy simulating Castleman's disease. Pediatr Pathol 1986;6:233–247.
39. Fletcher CDM: Angiomatoid "malignant fibrous histiocytoma": An immunohistochemical study indicative of myoid differentiation. Hum Pathol 1991;22:563–568.
40. Smith MEF, Costa MJ, Weiss SW: Evaluation of CD68 and other histiocytic antigens in angiomatoid malignant fibrous histiocytoma. Am J Surg Pathol 1991;15:757–763.
41. Hasegawa T, Seki K, Ono K, Hirohashi S: Angiomatoid (malignant) fibrous histiocytoma: A peculiar low-grade tumor showing immunophenotypic heterogeneity and ultrastructural variations. Pathol Int 2000;50:731–738.
42. Costa MJ, McGlothlen L, Pierce M, Munn R, Vogt PJ: Angiomatoid features in fibrohistiocytic sarcomas. Immunohistochemical, ultrastructural, and clinical distinction from vascular neoplasms. Arch Pathol Lab Med 1995;119:1065–1071.
43. Waters BL, Panagopoulos I, Allen EF: Genetic characterization of angiomatoid fibrous histiocytoma identifies fusion of the FUS and ATF-1 genes induced by a chromosomal translocation involving bands 12q13 and 16p11. Cancer Genet Cytogenet 2000;121:109–116.

Alveolar Soft Part Sarcoma—Clinicopathological Studies

44. Christopherson WM, Foote FW, Stewart FW: Alveolar soft-part sarcomas. Structurally characteristic tumors of uncertain histogenesis. Cancer 1952;5:100–111.
45. Ordonez NG: Alveolar soft part sarcoma: A review and update. Adv Anat Pathol 1999;6:125–139.
46. Font RL, Jurco S 3d, Zimmerman, LE: Alveolar soft-part sarcoma of the orbit: A clinicopathologic analysis of seventeen cases and a review of the literature. Hum Pathol 1982;13:569–579.
47. Evans HL: Alveolar soft-part sarcoma. A study of 13 typical examples and one with a histologically atypical component. Cancer 1985;55:912–917.
48. Auerbach HE, Brooks JJ: Alveolar soft part sarcoma. A clinicopathologic and immunohistochemical study. Cancer 1987;60:66–73.
49. Lieberman PH, Brennan MF, Kimmel M, Erlandson RA, Garin-Chesa P, Flehinger BY: Alveolar soft-part sarcoma. A clinico-pathologic study of half a century. Cancer 1989;63:1–13.
50. Matsuno Y, Mukai K, Itabashi M, et al: Alveolar soft-part sarcoma. A clinicopathologic and immunohistochemical study of 12 cases. Acta Pathol Jpn 1990;40:199–205.

51. Lillehei KO, Kleinschmidt-DeMasters B, Mitchell DH, Spector E, Kruse CA: Alveolar soft-part sarcoma: An unusually long interval between presentation and brain metastasis. Hum Pathol 1993;24:1030–1034.
52. Nielsen GP, Oliva E, Young RH, Rosenberg AE, Dickersin GR, Scully RE: Alveolar soft-part sarcoma of the female genital tract: A report of nine cases and review of the literature. Int J Gynecol Pathol 1995;14:283–292.
53. Pappo AS, Parham DM, Cain A, et al: Alveolar soft part sarcoma in children and adolescents: Clinical features and outcome of 11 patients. Med Pediatr Oncol 1996;26:81–84.
54. Portera CA Jr, Ho V, Patel SR, et al: Alveolar soft part sarcoma. Clinical course and patterns of metastasis in 70 patients treated at a single institution. Cancer 2001; 91:585–591.
55. Park YK, Unni KK, Kim YW, et al: Primary alveolar soft part sarcoma of bone. Histopathology 1999;35:411–417.
56. Sonobe H, Ro JY, Mackay B, Ordonez NG, Rundell MM, Ayala AG: Primary pulmonary alveolar soft part sarcoma. Report of a case. Int J Surg Pathol 1994;2: 57–62.

Alveolar Soft Part Sarcoma—Immunohistochemistry, Ultrastructure, and Histogenesis

57. Persson S, Willems JS, Kindblom LG, Angervall L: Alveolar soft part sarcoma. An immunohistochemical, cytologic and electron-microscopic study and a quantitative DNA analysis. Virchows Arch A Pathol Anat Histopathol 1988;412:499–513.
58. Mukai M, Torikata C, Shimoda T, Iri H: Alveolar soft-part sarcoma. Assessment of immunohistochemical demonstration of desmin using paraffin sections and frozen sections. Virchows Arch A Pathol Anat Histopathol 1989;414:503–509.
59. Miettinen M, Ekfors T: Alveolar soft part sarcoma. Immunohistochemical evidence for muscle cell differentiation. Am J Clin Pathol 1990;93:32–38.
60. Hirose T, Kudo E, Hasegawa T, Abe JI, Hizawa K: Cytoskeletal properties of alveolar soft-part sarcoma. Hum Pathol 1990;21:204–211.
61. Foschini MP, Eusebi V: Alveolar soft-part sarcoma: A new type of rhabdomyosarcoma? Semin Diagn Pathol 1994;11:58–68.
62. Wang NP, Bacchi CE, Jiang JJ, McNutt MA, Gown AM: Does alveolar soft-part sarcoma exhibit skeletal muscle differentiation? An immunocytochemical and biochemical study of myogenic regulatory protein expression. Mod Pathol 1996;9:496–506.
63. Gomez JA, Amin MB, Ro JY, Linden MD, Lee MW, Zarbo RJ: Immunohisto-chemical profile of myogenin and Myo D1 does not support skeletal muscle lineage in alveolar soft part sarcoma. A study of 19 tumors. Arch Pathol Lab Med 1999;123:503–507.
64. Rosai J, Dias P, Parham DM, Shapiro DN, Houghton P: MyoD1 protein expression in alveolar soft part sarcoma as confirmatory evidence of its skeletal muscle nature. Am J Surg Pathol 1991;15:974–981.
65. Shipkey FH, Lieberman PH, Foote FW Jr, Stewart FW: Ultrastructure of alveolar soft-part sarcoma. Cancer 1964;17:821–830.
66. Mukai M, Torikata C, Iri H, et al: Alveolar soft part sarcoma. An elaboration of a three-dimensional configuration of the crystalloids by digital image processing. Am J Pathol 1984;116:398–406.
67. Ordonez NG, Ro JY, Mackay B: Alveolar soft part sarcoma. An ultrastructural and immunocytochemical investigation of its histogenesis. Cancer 1989;63: 1721–1736.
68. Carstens PHB: Membrane-bound cytoplasmic crystals, similar to those in alveolar soft part sarcoma, in a human muscle spindle. Ultrastruct Pathol 1990;14: 423–428.

Alveolar Soft Part Sarcoma—Genetics

69. Cullinane C, Thorner PS, Greenberg ML, Ng YK, Kumar M, Squire J: Molecular genetic, cytogenetic, and immunohistochemical characterization of alveolar soft-part sarcoma. Implications for cell of origin. Cancer 1992;70:2444–2450.
70. Sciot R, Dal Cin P, De Vos R, et al: Alveolar soft-part sarcoma: Evidence for its myogenic origin and for the involvement of 17q25. Histopathology 1993;23:439–444.
71. van Echten J, van den Berg E, van Baarlen J, et al: An important role for chromosome 17, band q25, in the histogenesis of alveolar soft part sarcoma. Cancer Genet Cytogenet 1995;82:57–61.
72. Heimann P, Devalck C, Debusscher C, Sariban E, Vamos E: Alveolar soft-part sarcoma: Further evidence by FISH for the involvement of chromosome band 17q25. Genes Chromosomes Cancer 1998;23:194–197.
73. Joyama S, Ueda T, Shimizu K, et al: Chromosome rearrangement at 17q25 and Xp11.2 in alveolar soft-part sarcoma. A case report and review of the literature. Cancer 1999;86:1246–1250.
74. Ladanyi M, Lui MY, Antonescu CR, et al: The der(17)t(X;17)(p11;q25) of human alveolar soft part sarcoma fuses the TFE3 transcription factor gene to ASPL, a novel gene at 17q25. Oncogene 2001;20:48–57.
75. Kiuru-Kuhlefelt S, El-Rifai W, Sarlomo-Rikala M, Knuutila S, Miettinen M: DNA copy number changes in alveolar soft part sarcoma: A comparative genomic hybridization study. Mod Pathol 1998;11:227–231.
76. Argani P, Antonescu CR, Illei PB, et al: Primary renal neoplasms with the ASPL-TFE3 gene fusion of alveolar soft part sarcoma: A distinctive tumor entity previously included among renal cell carcinomas of children and adolescents. Am J Pathol 2001;159:179–192.

John K. C. Chan

Lymphoid, Myeloid, and Histiocytic Neoplasms Involving Soft Tissues

CHAPTER 21

Hematolymphoid cells comprise myeloid cells, erythroid cells, megakaryocytes and platelets, lymphocytes (B, T, or natural killer [NK]), and monocytes/histiocytes. Reactive or neoplastic accumulations of one or more of these cellular elements can occur in the somatic soft tissues, resulting in tumors or tumor-like lesions, albeit uncommonly (Table 21–1). The immunohistochemical markers that are helpful for demonstration of the various cell types are listed in Table 21–2.

Tumors and Tumor-like Lesions of Lymphoid Cells

The spectrum of lymphoid neoplasms occurring in the soft tissues includes various types of non-Hodgkin lymphomas of B, T, or NK lineage and plasmacytoma, whereas Hodgkin lymphoma practically never presents in such a way. A variety of reactive lymphoid infiltrates can also affect the soft tissues, ranging from well-defined clinicopathologic entities to nonspecific lymphoid infiltrates.

Primary Malignant Lymphoma of Somatic Soft Tissues

Definition

Involvement of somatic soft tissues by malignant lymphoma usually represents systemic lymphoma with soft tissue involvement or contiguous involvement by a nodal or cutaneous lymphoma. Strict criteria have to be applied in rendering a diagnosis of primary soft tissue lymphoma: (1) presentation as a soft tissue mass in the absence of identifiable lymph node structures, that is, excluding nodal lymphoma with extensive perinodal tissue involvement; (2) absence of lymphadenopathy or other sites of disease on staging; and (3) exclusion of cases with predominant involvement of the skin or bone. Some studies even exclude cases occurring in lymph node-rich areas, such as the neck, axilla, groin, and retroperitoneum,[1] but this is too restrictive.

Clinical Presentation

Primary soft tissue lymphomas are uncommon. Most reports in the literature have included only a single case or a few cases; there are few substantial series on this subject. According to the series of Meister, primary soft tissue lymphomas account for only slightly over 1% of soft tissue tumors in a consultation practice.[2] At the Armed Forces Institute of Pathology (AFIP), only 75 cases were identified over a 20-year period, and many of these cases have not been thoroughly worked up to exclude systemic lymphoma.[3]

Clinically, primary soft tissue lymphoma can affect any age group, but most patients are over the age of 50 years.[1,3–5] There is no sex predilection. The patients present with a soft tissue mass, swelling, or pain. The most common sites of involvement are, in

Table 21–1. Classification of Hematolymphoid Lesions of Soft Tissues

Cell Types	Tumors	Tumor-like Lesions
Lymphoid cells	• Malignant lymphoma • Plasmacytoma	• Localized lymphoid hyperplasia unspecified • Inflammatory pseudotumor • Inflammatory fibrosclerosing lesions • Kimura disease • Hyaline-vascular Castleman disease
Myeloid and hematopoietic cells	• Extramedullary myeloid tumor (granulocytic sarcoma) • Mast cell disease	• Extramedullary hematopoietic tumor, including the sclerosing variant
Monocytic-phagocytic cells	• Histiocytic sarcoma • Extramedullary monocytic tumor • Erdheim-Chester disease*	• Rosai-Dorfman disease • Mycobacterial spindle cell pseudotumor, and histoid leprosy • Miscellaneous histiocytic reactions mimicking neoplasm (e.g., xanthogranulomatous inflammation, malakoplakia, reaction to foreign material, granular histiocytic reaction, granulomatous reaction) • Xanthogranulomatous inflammation masking an underlying malignancy (e.g., Hodgkin lymphoma) • Xanthoma or xanthelasma • Crystal storing histiocytosis mimicking adult rhabdomyoma
Dendritic cells	• Langerhans cell histiocytosis • Follicular dendritic cell sarcoma • Interdigitating dendritic cell sarcoma • Fibroblastic reticular cell sarcoma • Indeterminate cell tumor • Dendritic cell sarcoma not otherwise specified	• Follicular dendritic cell overgrowth in setting of Castleman disease • Thymoma-like follicular dendritic cell hyperplasia • Indeterminate cell histiocytosis
Uncertain relationship to monocytes/phagocytes and dendritic cells	• Juvenile xanthogranuloma* • Reticulohistiocytoma*	• Multicentric reticulohistiocytosis

*Unclear whether the disease is a neoplastic disorder.

order of frequency, the thigh, trunk, arm, and leg.[3,4] Exceptionally, the lymphoma can show exclusive localization to a major nerve.[6]

Usually only limited types of non-Hodgkin lymphomas occur as primary soft tissue lymphomas, as summarized in Table 21–3.[4,7–9] The clinical features of the more common and distinctive types are listed in Table 21–4.

Little is known about the etiology of primary soft tissue lymphoma. The predisposing factors identified in a small proportion of cases include postmastectomy lymphedema, chronic suppurative inflammation, chronic autoimmune-mediated inflammatory lesion (juxta-articular soft tissue lymphoma arising in patients with long-standing rheumatoid arthritis), previous radiation therapy, and site of prior trauma or surgery (particularly joint replacement).[4,10–13] In those cases associated with chronic suppuration, the lymphoma cells are shown to harbor Epstein-Barr virus (EBV).[12] Lymphoma occurring in patients with acquired immunodeficiency syndrome (AIDS) may also show primary localization in the soft tissues.[14]

Table 21-2. Paraffin Section-Reactive Immunohistochemical Markers Helpful for Diagnosis of Hematolymphoid Neoplasms

Immunohistochemical Marker	Immunoreactivity	Main Applications
CD45 (leukocyte common antigen)	All leukocytes, including monocytes and histiocytes	Confirming the hematolymphoid nature of a neoplasm
CD20, e.g., L26	B cells, except plasma cells	Confirming the B-cell lineage of a lymphoma; plasma cell neoplasms are typically CD20$^-$
CD79a	B cells, including plasma cells	"Back-up" B-cell lineage marker when B-cell neoplasm is suspected but CD20 is negative (e.g., B-lymphoblastic lymphoma). Approximately 50% of plasmacytomas are positive.
Immunoglobulin	B cells	Monotypic immunoglobulin helps to distinguish plasmacytoma or B-cell lymphoma from reactive lymphoid hyperplasia.
CD138 (syndecan-1)	Plasmablasts and plasma cells; many different types of epithelial cells	Aiding in diagnosis of plasmacytoma in the appropriate setting (note that many other tumor types are also CD138$^+$)
CD3	T cells	Confirming the T or NK cell lineage of a lymphoma
CD43	T cells, monocytes/histiocytes, myeloid cells	Coexpression of CD43 in a B-cell proliferation strongly favors a diagnosis of lymphoma over lymphoid hyperplasia.
CD30, e.g., BerH2	Activated lymphoid cells	Diagnosis of anaplastic large cell lymphoma
CD56 (neuronal cell adhesion molecule N-CAM)	NK cells, some cytotoxic T cells	Confirming a diagnosis of NK/T-cell lymphoma
Terminal deoxynucleotidyl transferase (TdT)	Precursor lymphoid cells	Confirming diagnosis of lymphoblastic lymphoma/leukemia
CD68 (e.g., PGM1, KP1)	Monocytes/histiocytes; activated dendritic cells; myeloid cells (stained by KP1 only, but not PGM1); cells rich in lysosomes	Diagnosis of histiocytic sarcoma
S-100 protein	Immune accessory cells (dendritic cells); nerve sheath cells; melanocytes; and some other cell types such as myoepithelium	Diagnosis of Langerhans cell histiocytosis, Rosai-Dorfman disease, and interdigitating dendritic cell sarcoma. Many other tumor types are also S-100 protein positive, such as melanoma and nerve sheath tumor
CD1a	Langerhans cells; precursor T cells	Diagnosis of Langerhans cell histiocytosis
CD21 or CD35	Follicular dendritic cells	Diagnosis of follicular dendritic cell sarcoma
Factor XIIIa (tissue transglutaminase)	Dermal and interstitial dendritic cells	Diagnosis of lesions believed to be related to dermal dendritic cells (such as xanthogranuloma)
Myeloperoxidase	Myeloid cells	Diagnosis of myeloid leukemia/tumor

Table 21–3. Frequency of Primary Soft Tissue Lymphomas (Various Types According to the New WHO Classification)

Histologic Type of Lymphoma	Frequency
Diffuse large B-cell lymphoma	21/37 (56.8%)
Extranodal marginal zone B-cell lymphoma of mucosa-associated lymphoid tissue type	4/37 (10.8%)
Unclassifiable B-cell lymphoma	3/37 (8.1%)
Peripheral T-cell lymphoma unspecified	3/37 (8.1%)
Anaplastic large cell lymphoma	2/37 (5.4%)
Extranodal NK/T-cell lymphoma, nasal type	2/37 (5.4%)
Follicular lymphoma	1/37 (2.7%)
Burkitt-like lymphoma	1/37 (2.7%)

(Modified from series by Goodlad et al.[4])

Clinical Course

The clinical outcome depends on the type of lymphoma (see Table 21–4). According to the AFIP series, for stage I disease showing no additional sites of disease within 3 months, the prognosis is favorable (>80% disease-free survival at median follow-up of 6 years) after treatment by surgical excision with or without radiotherapy or chemotherapy.[3] On the other hand, if additional sites of disease appear within 3 months (perhaps indicating that it was probably disseminated lymphoma from the start), most patients die from disease, with a median survival of only 4 months.[3] Relapses can develop in other soft tissue sites. According to the Mayo Clinic series, 39% of patients died of disease, 44% were alive and well, and 17% died of unrelated disease; there was no apparent relationship of disease stage with the outcome.[1]

Key Histologic Findings

Soft tissue lymphoma typically exhibits a highly infiltrative growth, with destruction of the normal structures and permeation of the surrounding tissues (Fig. 21–1). Invasion of skeletal muscle can result in atrophy and destruction of muscle fibers; sometimes there is even colonization of the cytoplasm of the skeletal muscle fibers. Occasionally drop-out of individual muscle fibers leaves empty spaces (Fig. 21–1*B*). Invasion of blood vessel walls can be seen, and this phenomenon can occur in B-cell, T-cell, or NK cell lymphomas. The central portion of the lymphoma can undergo coagulative necrosis. Broad or delicate sclerotic bands sometimes traverse the tumor. The architectural and cytologic features of the various types of lymphomas involving soft tissues are detailed in Table 21–4 and shown in Figures 21–2 through 21–9.[1,3–5,7,9,15–30]

Unusual Histologic Findings and Deceptive Appearances

The morphologic appearances that can be assumed by lymphomas are protean—some patterns previously considered incompatible with a diagnosis of lymphoma are now recognized to be within its accepted morphologic spectrum.

Myxoid Pattern

Rare lymphomas grow in the form of isolated or cords of neoplastic cells suspended in abundant myxoid stroma, mimicking myxoid chondrosarcoma, myxofibrosarcoma, or other sarcomas with myxoid change (Fig. 21-10*A*).[31–33]

Spindle Cell Growth

Some lymphomas feature many neoplastic spindly cells, mimicking sarcoma (Fig. 21–10*B*). Nevertheless, well-formed fascicles are rarely formed. Usually this growth pattern results from the presence of a fibrous stroma, whereby lymphoma cells insinuate between the pre-existing collagen fibers and thus assume a spindly morphology. However, spindling of lymphoma cells can also occur in the absence of a fibrous component.[34,35]

Fibrillary Matrix or Rosette Formation

Rare lymphomas are accompanied by an appreciable amount of fibrillary material, sometimes with rosette formation, mimicking peripheral primitive neuroectodermal tumor (PNET; Fig. 21–10*C*). The fibrillary material is not stromal matrix but is formed by interdigitating long cell processes of the lymphoma cells. Because this material is composed mostly of cell membranes, it shows immunoreactivity for the various cell surface leukocyte antigens expressed by the lymphoma, such as CD20 (for B-lineage lymphomas) and CD45.[36,37]

Intravascular Growth

Intravascular lymphoma is a rare form of lymphoma characterized by exclusive or predominant growth of lymphoma cells within blood vessels (Fig. 21–10*D*). Practically all cases are large B-cell lymphomas; of interest, some cases express the T cell-associated

Text continued on page 516

Table 21–4. More Common or Distinctive Types of Primary Soft Tissue Lymphoma

Lymphoma Type	Main Clinical Features and Behavior	Salient Histologic Features	Immunogenetics	Comments
Diffuse large B-cell lymphoma	The patients, usually adults with a median age of 64 y, present with mass lesion in the soft tissues. The overall survival is approximately 50%.	Diffuse infiltration of large or medium-sized lymphoid cells. Lymphoma cells have round, folded or multilobated nuclei and distinct nucleoli. Cytoplasm is amphophilic. Necrosis is common. Rare cases can exhibit unusual growth patterns or cytologic features, such as myxoid change, spindly cells (see text).	B-lineage markers positive. Those related to follicular center cells often express CD10 and bcl-6. Some cases can express CD30.	Gene expression profile as studied by DNA microarray technique holds promise for predicting the response to treatment and clinical outcome.
Extranodal marginal zone B-cell lymphoma of mucosa-associated lymphoid tissue type	The patients, usually adults with a median age of 60 y, present with mass lesion in the soft tissues. This lymphoma type is indolent.	The background often shows sclerotic bands. Medium-sized pale cells resembling monocytoid B cells grow around pre-existing lymphoid follicles and sometimes colonize them. There can be some interspersed large transformed cells with nucleoli. Patches of plasma cells (part of the neoplasm) are commonly present.	This is a B-cell neoplasm with no distinctive positive identifying immunohistochemical markers so far ($CD20^+$, $CD5^-$, $CD23^-$, cyclin $D1^-$). 30–40% of cases show t(11;18) translocation, implicating the *API2* and *MLT* genes.	In contrast to extranodal marginal zone B-cell lymphomas of other sites, the diagnosis is more difficult to make because lymphoepithelial lesions are not found, due to absence of epithelial structures in soft tissues.
B-lymphoblastic lymphoma	This lymphoma type most commonly involves skin, lymph node, bone, and soft tissues. It usually affects children and young adults (median age 20 y). The prognosis is quite favorable when treated aggressively and is superior to that of T-lymphoblastic lymphoma.	Monotonous medium-sized cells with delicate nuclear membranes, fine chromatin, and inconspicuous nucleoli. Cytoplasm is typically scanty, such that the nuclei appear crowded.	B-lineage markers are positive ($CD79a^+$, CD20 variable). TdT is the defining marker. CD10 is often positive.	Main differential diagnosis is blastoid mantle cell lymphoma ($CD5^+$, cyclin $D1^+$). B-lymphoblastic lymphoma can also be mistaken for small cell lymphoma in suboptimally prepared histologic materials.

Table continued on following page

Table 21–4. More Common or Distinctive Types of Primary Soft Tissue Lymphoma (*Continued*)

Lymphoma Type	Main Clinical Features and Behavior	Salient Histologic Features	Immunogenetics	Comments
Anaplastic large cell lymphoma, primary systemic form	There is bimodal age distribution. The soft tissue involvement may or may not be accompanied by lymphadenopathy or other sites of involvement. If treated with aggressive chemotherapy, a high cure rate can be achieved.	The lymphoma cells are large or very large, with oval, reniform or embryo-like nuclei, multiple distint nucleoli, abundant amphophilic cytoplasm, and a distinct paranuclear Golgi zone. Some cases are composed of uniform cells, imparting a monotonous apappearance. Rare cases may show sarcomatoid growth pattern, with spindly cells or myxoid change.	By definition, B-lineage markers should be negative. T-lineage markers are positive (T-cell type) or negative (null cell type). $CD30^{+}$; $EMA^{+/-}$; $ALK^{+/-}$. In a significant proportion of cases, there is chromosomal translocation involving the *ALK* gene on chromosome 2p23.	The cases showing ALK immunoreactivity are associated with a much better survival (~75%) compared with the ALK^{-} cases (~35%).
Subcutaneous panniculitis-like T-cell lymphoma	Patients present with solitary or multiple subcutaneous nodules, most commonly involving the limbs. Dissemination to lymph nodes or other organs is uncommon. When complicated by hemophagocytic syndrome at presentation or during the clinical course, the disease is associated with a poor outcome. Cases not complicated by hemophagocytic syndrome often pursue an indolent course.	Lacelike pattern of involvement of the subcutaneous tissue with no or little involvement of the dermis. The lymphoma cells are often small to medium-sized cells, with minimal to mild cytologic atypia. Characteristically, the lymphoma cells rosette around individual fat cells. Apoptotic bodies are often prominent. There are commonly interspersed histiocytes with phagocytosed cell debris.	This is a cytotoxic T-cell lymphoma ($CD3^{+}$) most commonly expressing CD8 and cytotoxic markers (such as TIA1, granzyme B). Occasional cases can express CD56. Most cases express αβ T-cell receptor, but some cases express γδ T-cell receptor.	There is no association with EBV, and this is a feature that can be used for distinguishing the $CD56^{+}$ cases from NK/T-cell lymphoma.

Lymphoma Type	Main Clinical Features and Behavior	Salient Histologic Features	Immunogenetics	Comments
Peripheral T-cell lymphoma unspecified	This lymphoma type usually occurs in adults, presenting as a mass lesion. The disease is aggressive.	The cytologic features are variable: predominance of medium-sized cells, large cells, or mixture of cell types. The nuclei are often irregularly folded. Some cells can have clear cytoplasm. There can be admixed plasma cells and eosinophils.	This is a "waste-basket" category, and thus there are no distinctive immunophenotypic features. T-lineage markers are positive. Most cases express cytotoxic molecules. There is commonly loss of one or more pan-T markers, such as CD2, CD5, or CD7.	Peripheral T-cell lymphoma is often found on staging to represent part of disseminated disease, i.e., not primary soft tissue lymphoma.
Extranodal NK/T-cell lymphoma	This putative NK cell lymphoma typically presents in extranodal sites, including soft tissues and skin, among others. The mass lesions are often multiple and may undergo ulceration and necrosis. The disease often progresses very rapidly, with dissemination to other sites. The prognosis is poor.	Common findings are prominent coagulative necrosis, apoptosis, and angiocentric-angiodestructive growth. The lymphoid cells range from small cells to large cells. Nuclei are often irregularly folded.	The typical immunophenotype is surface $CD3/Leu4^-$, cytoplasmic $CD3^+$, $CD56^+$, cytotoxic molecules positive. T-cell receptor genes are in germline configuration.	There is a strong association with EBV, and its demonstration can aid in the diagnosis of difficult cases.

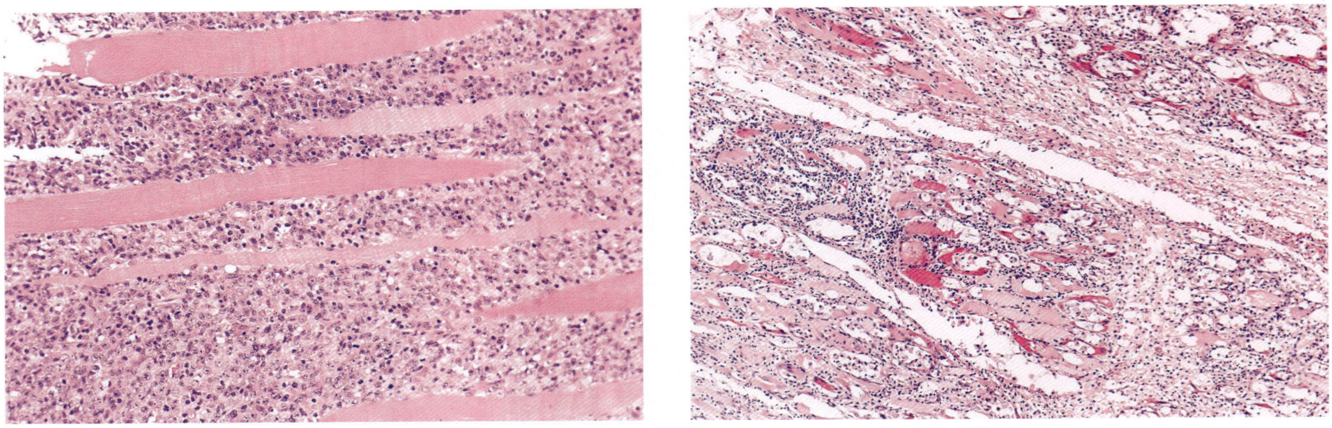

A B

Figure 21–1. Primary malignant lymphoma of soft tissue. *A*, The lymphoma cells permeate between the skeletal muscle fibers in this example of large B-cell lymphoma. *B*, The skeletal muscle shows extensive destruction by the lymphomatous infiltrate (NK/T-cell lymphoma). Many empty spaces are left behind after dissolution of the individual muscle fibers.

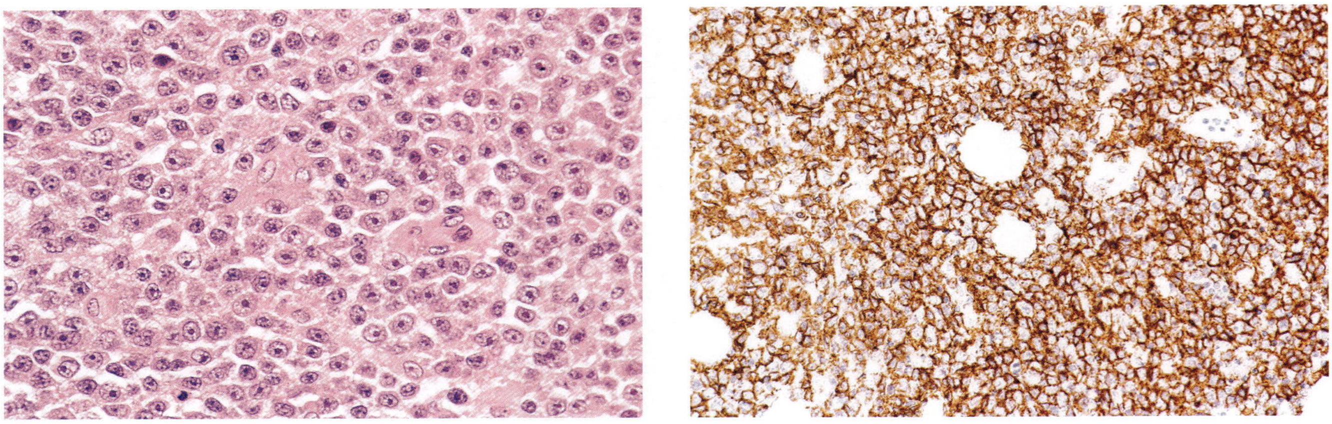

A B

Figure 21–2. Diffuse large B-cell lymphoma of soft tissue. *A*, The large lymphoma cells possess round vesicular nuclei and distinct nucleoli. *B*, All the cells show strong immunostaining for CD20, indicating B lineage.

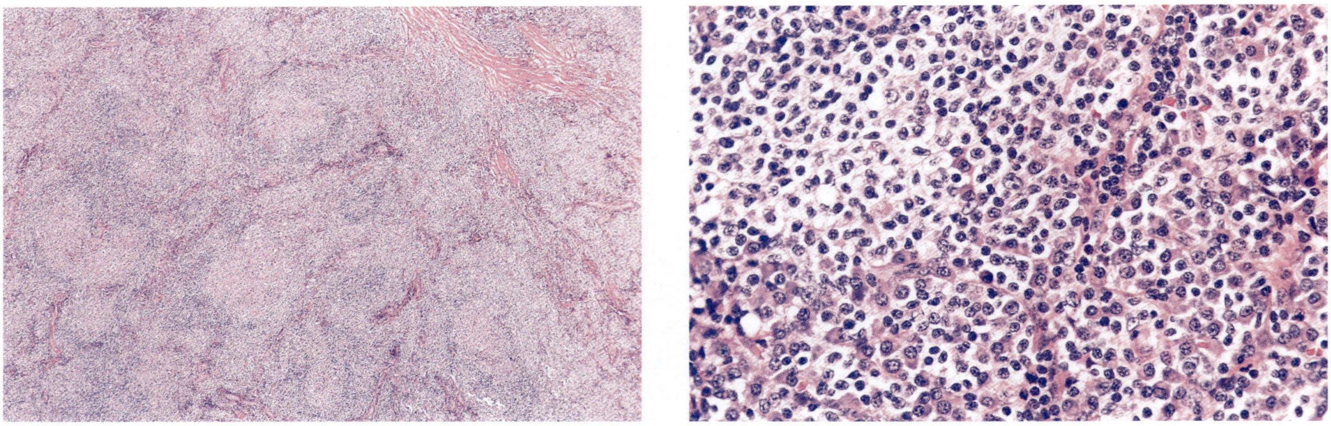

A B

Figure 21–3. Primary soft tissue extranodal marginal zone B-cell lymphoma of mucosa-associated lymphoid tissue type. *A*, Coalescent bands of pale-staining cells grow around and between reactive lymphoid follicles. Sclerotic bands are characteristically present *(right upper field)*. *B*, The left field shows lymphoma cells resembling monocytoid B cells. The right field shows large clusters of plasma cells, which are commonly found in this lymphoma type.

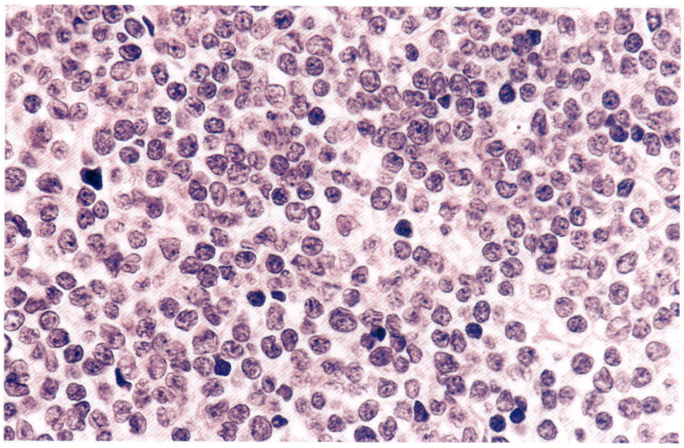

A

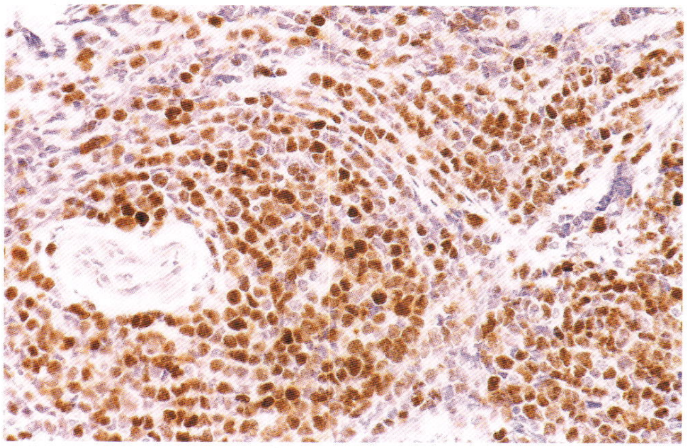

B

Figure 21–4. Precursor B-lymphoblastic lymphoma of soft tissue. *A*, The medium-sized lymphoma cells typically appear monotonous, with fine chromatin and scanty cytoplasm. *B*, Nuclear staining for terminal deoxynucleotidyltransferase (TdT), a marker for precursor lymphoid cells, is the immunohistochemical hallmark of this lymphoma type.

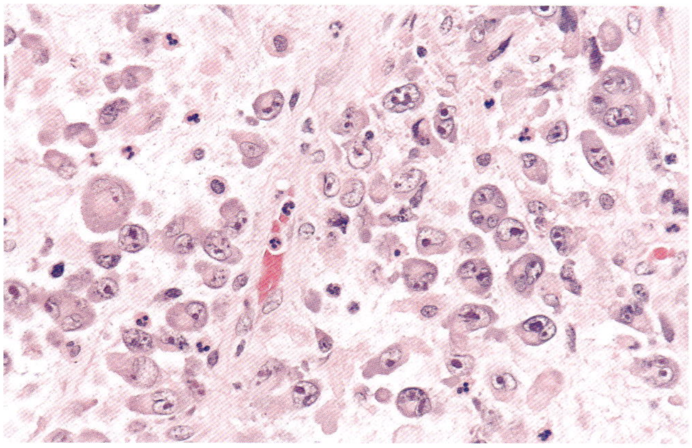

A

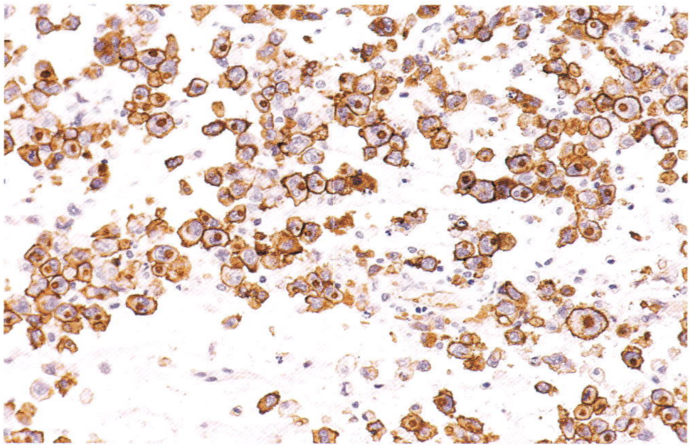

B

Figure 21–5. Anaplastic large cell lymphoma, T cell, anaplastic lymphoma kinase (ALK) negative. *A*, The lymphoma cells are very large, with reniform or embryo-like nuclei, distinct nucleoli, voluminous amphophilic cytoplasm, and prominent pale-staining Golgi zone. The nuclei are arranged in the form of a wreath in the multinucleated tumor cells. This case is unusual in that a myxoid stroma is present. *B*, The neoplastic cells are immunoreactive for CD30 in a cell membrane and Golgi pattern.

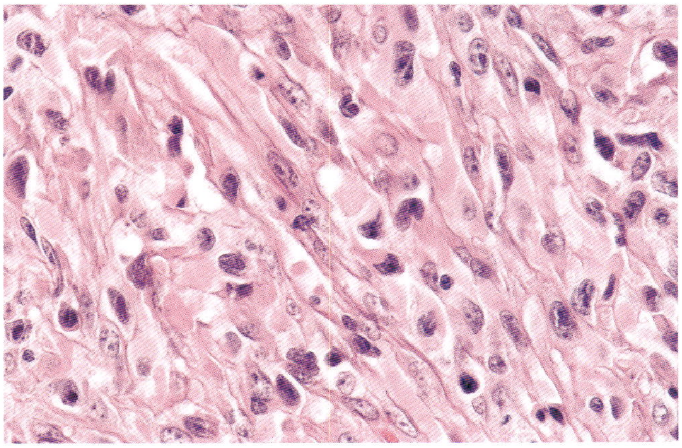

Figure 21–6. Anaplastic large cell lymphoma with sarcomatoid appearance. The presence of many plump spindly tumor cells results in mimicry of spindle cell sarcoma.

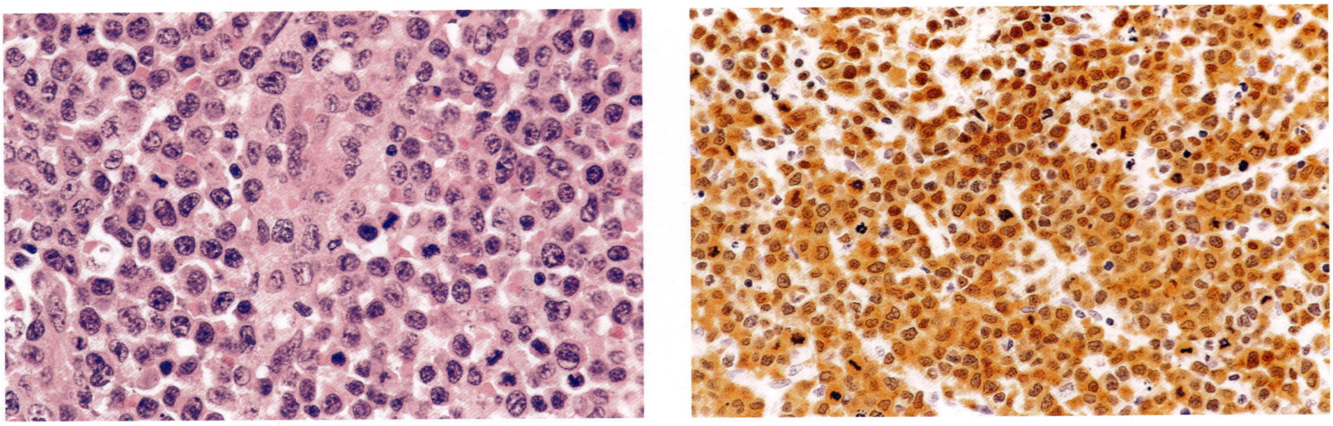

A B

Figure 21-7. Anaplastic large cell lymphoma, positive for T-cell markers and ALK. *A*, In this example, the large to medium-sized lymphoma cells appear monotonous. As a result, the initial impression is usually not that of an anaplastic large cell lymphoma. However, in a young patient, this possibility must be considered. *B*, The neoplastic cells show nuclear and cytoplasmic staining for ALK, indicating the presence of t(2;5) translocation. CD30 is also strongly positive (result not shown).

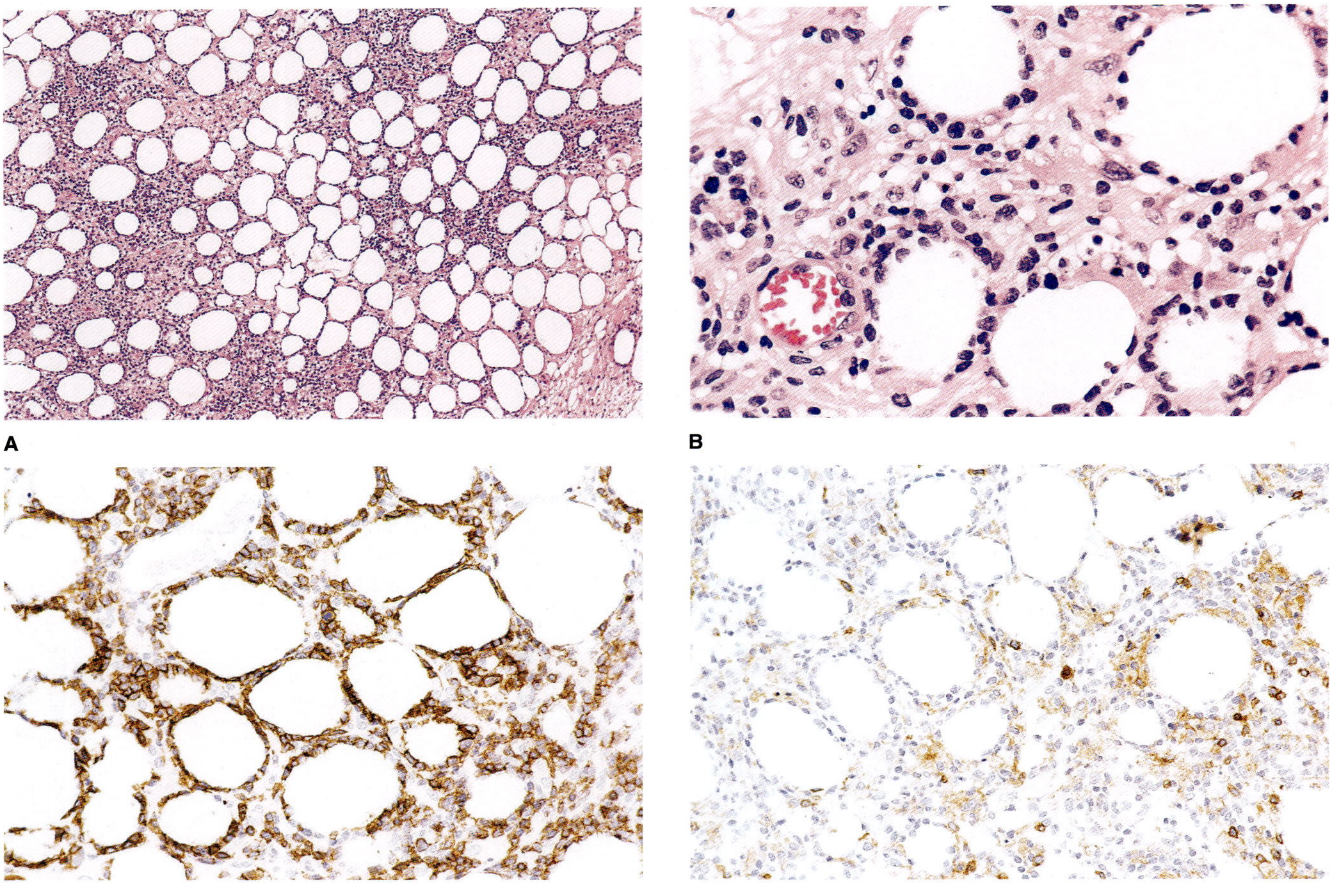

A B C D

Figure 21-8. Subcutaneous panniculitis-like T-cell lymphoma. *A*, Interstitial infiltration of the subcutaneous tissue by lymphoma cells produces a lace-like pattern. There is no involvement of the overlying dermis (not shown). *B*, In addition to infiltration of the spaces between the adipose cells, the neoplastic cells also form rosettes around the individual adipose cells, a characteristic but not pathognomonic feature of this lymphoma type. In this case, a diagnosis of lymphoma is not too difficult to make because there is definite cytologic atypia. Note also the typical admixed karyorrhectic debris. *C*, Immunostaining for CD8 highlights large numbers of lymphoid cells, especially those that rosette around the adipose cells. *D*, In contrast, immunostaining for CD4 highlights only occasional lymphoid cells in the interstitium and some weakly stained histiocytes.

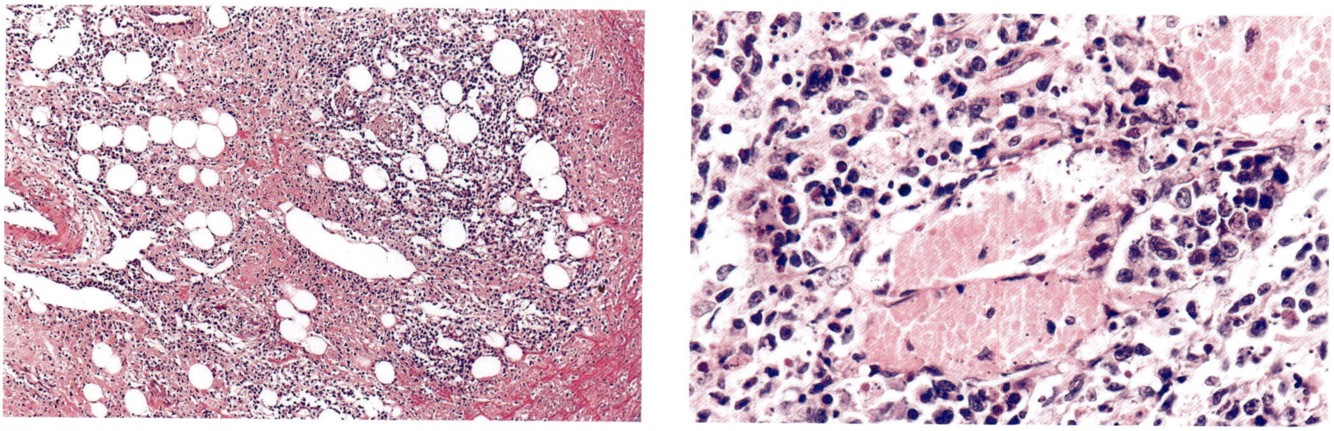

Figure 21-9. Extranodal NK/T-cell lymphoma involving soft tissue. *A,* The lymphoma is highly permeative. There is coagulative necrosis *(right field)* and angiocentric-angioinvasive growth *(center field* and *left field). B,* The lymphoma cells are medium-sized and show irregular nuclear foldings. Note the presence of numerous apoptotic cells. The skeletal muscle fibers are necrotic, and some are colonized by lymphoma cells *(right field).*

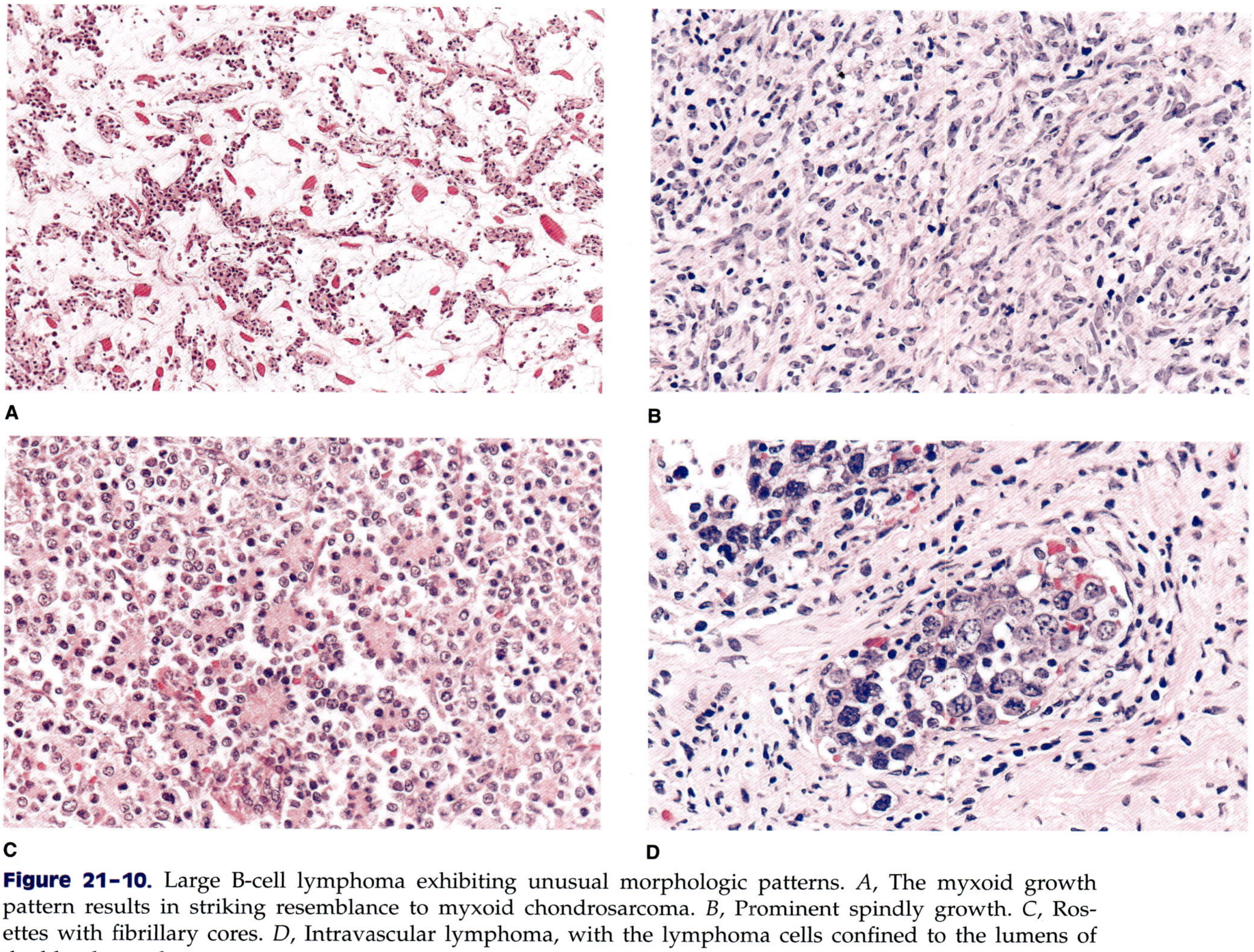

Figure 21-10. Large B-cell lymphoma exhibiting unusual morphologic patterns. *A,* The myxoid growth pattern results in striking resemblance to myxoid chondrosarcoma. *B,* Prominent spindly growth. *C,* Rosettes with fibrillary cores. *D,* Intravascular lymphoma, with the lymphoma cells confined to the lumens of the blood vessels.

marker CD5.[38,39] The tissue can undergo infarction as a result of vascular occlusion by lymphoma cells. Sometimes the neoplastic cells are apparently palisaded along the luminal side of the blood vessels, mimicking angiosarcoma.[34,40]

Immunohistochemical Profile and Genetic Features

The immunohistochemical profile varies according to type of lymphoma (see Table 21–4). B-cell lymphomas greatly outnumber T-cell or NK-cell lymphomas, and account for 81% to 95% of all cases.[1,4] Diffuse large B-cell lymphoma is the most common (see Fig. 21–2). The most informative B-lineage marker is CD20, although this marker may be negative in B-lymphoblastic lymphoma. In such circumstance, CD79a positivity, in combination with CD3 negativity, would support the B lineage. Among the T-cell–associated markers, CD3 is the most sensitive and specific for the T and NK lineage (see Table 21–2). For a lymphoma shown to be $CD3^+$, further work-up should include at least immunostaining for CD30 and CD56 to rule out anaplastic large cell lymphoma (good prognosis) and NK/T-cell lymphoma, (usually fatal), respectively.

There is no known association of soft tissue lymphoma with EBV, except for extranodal NK/T-cell lymphoma[1,4,15] and cases associated with chronic suppuration.[12]

Differential Diagnosis

It is important to make a correct diagnosis of lymphoma versus *sarcoma*, because this tumor type is potentially curable by chemotherapy and radiotherapy even if disseminated, and radical excisions are generally not required. The various deceptive growth patterns that lymphoma can assume are discussed in a previous section.

The possibility of *extramedullary myeloid tumor* should always be considered whenever the morphologic impression is that of a soft tissue malignant lymphoma. The following findings would strongly suggest the former diagnosis: (1) fine granules in the cytoplasm; (2) interspersed eosinophilic myelocytes; and (3) a $CD43^+$ only immunophenotype ($CD20^-$, $CD3^-$). The diagnosis of myeloid tumor can be confirmed by a positive Leder (chloroacetate esterase) stain or immunoreactivity for myeloperoxidase.

Occasional cases of large B-cell lymphomas can show a deceptively cohesive growth, forming a sharp interface with the fibrous stroma, mimicking *undifferentiated carcinoma* (Fig. 21–11). The following features would favor the former diagnosis: (1) permeative growth at least in some areas; (2) amphophilic cytoplasm; and (3) frequent presence of multilobated or irregularly folded nuclei. If in doubt, immunohistochemical staining ($CD45^+$, cytokeratin negative) can provide an unequivocal support for a diagnosis of lymphoma over carcinoma.

Ectopic thymomas of lymphocyte-rich type (B1 or B2 thymoma) occurring in the soft tissues of the neck can potentially be mistaken for small cell lymphoma. Clues to the correct diagnosis include jigsaw puzzle-like lobulation and presence of some unexplained large cells with pale-staining nuclei and indistinct cell borders (epithelial component).[41]

Lobular panniculitis is an important differential diagnosis of subcutaneous panniculitis-like T-cell lymphoma. The following features would favor the latter diagnosis: definite cytologic atypia or predominance of medium-sized lymphoid cells (if present), rosetting of lymphoid cells around individual fat cells, and predominance of $CD3^+$ T cells expressing CD8 or TIA1 around fat cells. In panniculitis, the T cells represent a mixture of $CD4^+$ and $CD8^+$ lymphocytes, there are few $TIA1^+$ cytotoxic cells, and some nodular aggregates of B cells are present.[21]

Differential diagnosis with *reactive lymphoid infiltrates* is addressed in a later section, "Approach to Diagnosis of Lymphoid Infiltrates in the Soft Tissues."

Localized Lymphoid Hyperplasia

Clinical Presentation

Localized collections of lymphoid tissue sometimes occur in the soft tissues. In some instances, they show features of specific entities, such as inflammatory pseudotumor, inflammatory fibrosclerosing lesion, Kimura disease, or hyaline-vascular Castleman disease. However, in most instances, the histologic

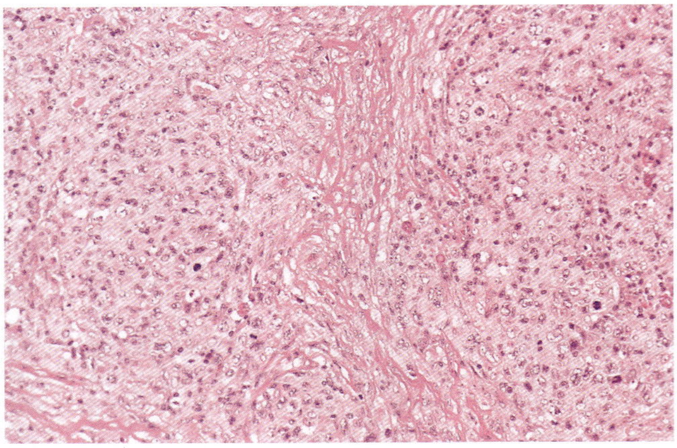

Figure 21–11. Large B-cell lymphoma showing deceptively cohesive growth, forming a sharp interface with the fibrous stroma, mimicking carcinoma.

features do not conform to the preceding entities, and the descriptive term "localized lymphoid hyperplasia unspecified" can be applied. This nomenclature is preferred to the once popular term "pseudolymphoma," which has been indiscriminately used and is nonspecific. *Localized lymphoid hyperplasia unspecified* is not a specific disease entity, but represents the limited morphologic response of the immune system to a variety of stimuli, such as infection, hypersensitivity, and foreign substance. The clinical features have not been well characterized due to lack of specificity of the histologic findings. The presentation is usually that of a mass or swelling in the somatic soft tissues.

Inflammatory pseudotumor (inflammatory myofibroblastic tumor) is discussed in a separate chapter on fibroblastic lesions. In essence, the lesion forms a discrete mass and is histologically composed of an admixture of spindly myofibroblastic cells, lymphocytes, plasma cells, and collagen fibers.

Inflammatory fibrosclerosing lesion (tumefactive fibroinflammatory lesion) is discussed in a separate chapter on fibroblastic lesions. This is a family of disorders presenting in different sites (such as retroperitoneal fibrosis, sclerosing mesenteritis, sclerosing mediastinitis, Riedel thyroiditis) but sharing similar morphologic features, including tumor-like infiltrative process, prominent sclerosis, patchy aggregates of chronic inflammatory cells, and phlebitis.

Kimura disease is an idiopathic inflammatory-allergic condition affecting predominantly Orientals, but people of other races can also be occasionally affected.[42–44] It occurs mostly in young and middle-aged men, who present with nontender subcutaneous or deep soft tissue masses in the head and neck region, with or without regional lymphadenopathy. The overlying skin is normal or shows erythema. The peripheral blood typically shows eosinophilia, and the serum IgE level is elevated. The lesion often grows slowly, and then achieves a stable size or shows slight regression. If a firm diagnosis can be made from fine-needle aspiration or incisional biopsy, the lesion need not be removed except for aesthetic purposes. Even if surgery is performed, recurrences are common. Renal involvement due to immune complex deposition (most commonly minimal change disease or membranous glomerulopathy), manifesting as proteinuria or nephrotic syndrome, may be a complication in a small proportion of patients.[45,46]

Key Histologic Features

Kimura disease is characterized by a constellation of histologic features, none of which individually is pathognomonic.[42,44] The lesion is deep-seated, involving subcutaneous tissue or deeper structures. There is a prominent lymphoid infiltrate including many florid reactive follicles with germinal centers commonly showing deposits of proteinaceous precipitate or necrosis (Fig. 21–12). Some germinal centers are penetrated by several venules (vascularization of germinal centers), a process almost always accompanied by eosinophil infiltration of the germinal centers. The eosinophils in the germinal centers can form abscesses and be associated with necrosis (eosinophil folliculolysis). The interfollicular lymphoid tissue consists of small lymphocytes admixed with plasma cells, mast cells, and numerous eosinophils, sometimes with formation of eosinophil abscess. High endothelial venules are increased; the endothelial cells have pale, nonvacuolated cytoplasm. Polykaryocytes are commonly identified in the germinal centers and interfollicular tissues. Sclerosis is common, often breaking up the tissue into nodules. The sclerosis apparently commences in the perivenular zone and is often found even in early lesions. To render a diagnosis of Kimura disease, in addition to tissue eosinophilia, the characteristic lymphoid reaction must be seen—reactive lymphoid follicles, with at least some showing vascularization of germinal center or eosinophil infiltration.

Localized lymphoid hyperplasia unspecified is characterized by a dense infiltrate of lymphoid cells, in which small lymphocytes and plasma cells usually predominate. However, there can be variable numbers of intermingled immunoblasts (Fig. 21–13). In some cases, there are interspersed reactive lymphoid follicles. Sclerotic bands can be present in the background.

Immunohistochemical Profile

The immunohistochemical profile of localized lymphoid hyperplasia unspecified varies. In most cases, immunostaining demonstrates nodules of $CD20^+$ cells, which correspond to the reactive lymphoid follicles or primary follicles not evident in the histologic sections (Fig. 21–14). There are at most small clusters or isolated $CD20^+$ cells in between, which is generally heavily populated by $CD3^+$ T cells. In other cases, sheets of $CD3^+$ are present, with few interspersed $CD20^+$ B cells.

Differential Diagnosis

The most important differential diagnosis of localized lymphoid hyperplasia is *malignant lymphoma*. See subsequent section "Approach to Diagnosis of Lymphoid Infiltrates in the Soft Tissues."

Kimura disease is most often confused with *angiolymphoid hyperplasia with eosinophilia (epithelioid*

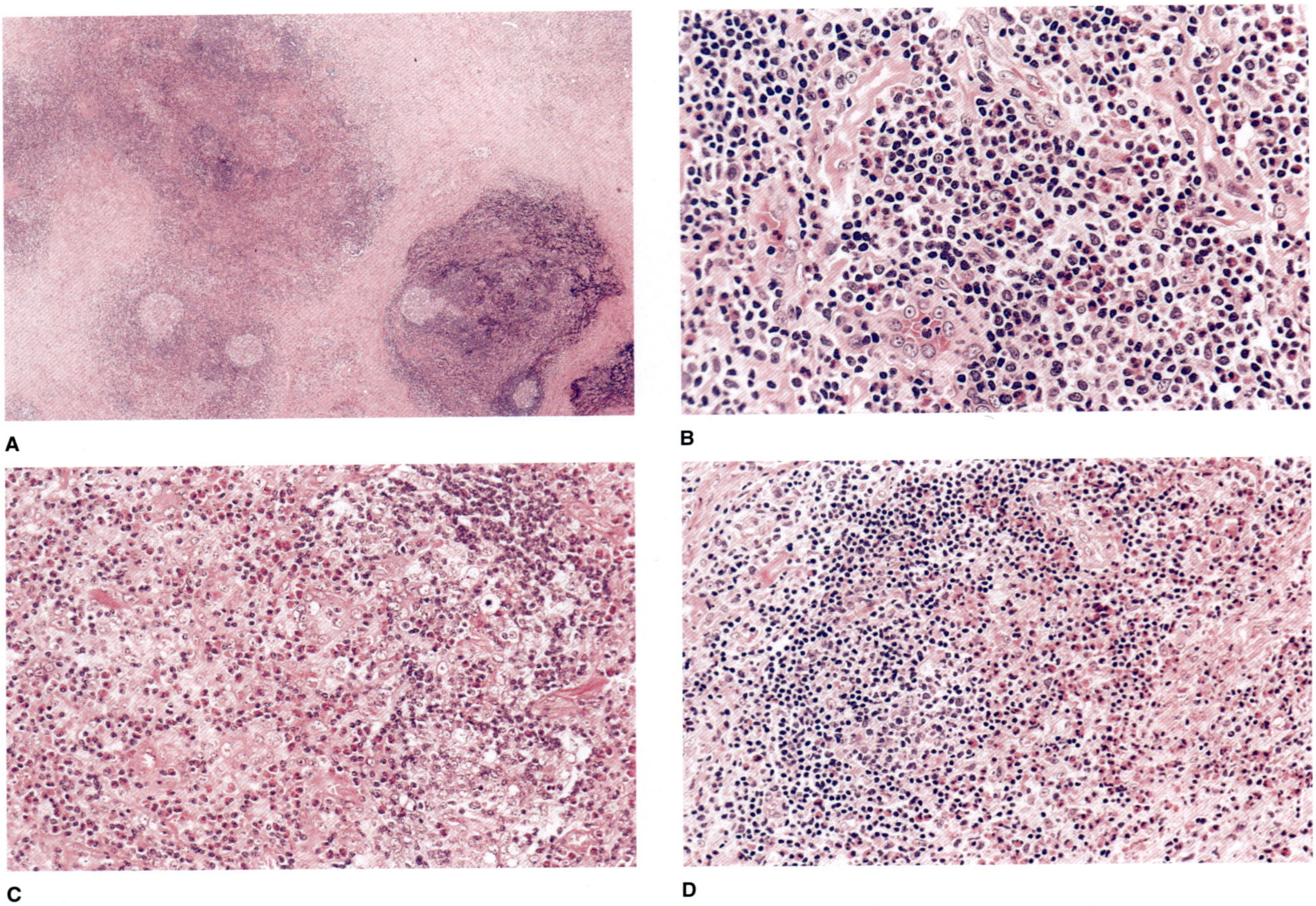

Figure 21–12. Kimura disease involving soft tissues. *A*, The dense lymphoid infiltrate occurs in a sclerotic stroma, and lymphoid follicles are evident. Some areas appear eosinophilic *(left field)* because of presence of large numbers of eosinophils. *B*, The tissue between the follicles comprises venules (some with perivenular sclerosis), small lymphocytes, plasma cells, and eosinophils. *C*, This lymphoid follicle shows vascularization and heavy infiltration by eosinophils. Some polykaryocytes are also seen. Residual follicular center cells are evident in the right field. *D*, Although this appears to be an eosinophil abscess in the interfollicular region, closer scrutiny shows that this is actually centered on a destroyed lymphoid follicle. A group of residual follicle center cells is seen near the lower left field.

hemangioma). Angiolymphoid hyperplasia with eosinophilia is a tumor or tumor-like condition characterized by proliferation of blood vessels lined by plump, oval to hobnail endothelial cells with abundant eosinophilic hyaline cytoplasm harboring occasional sharp vacuoles, and often but not necessarily accompanied by reactive lymphoid cells and eosinophils. In many cases, connection of the proliferated vessels with an adjacent damaged muscular artery or vein can be demonstrated. The distinctive epithelioid (histiocytoid) appearance of the endothelial cells lining the proliferated vessels is the most important distinguishing feature.[42] In contrast, the cells lining the proliferated venules of Kimura disease have scanty pale cytoplasm. Heavy eosinophil infiltration and eosinophil abscesses are usually more prominent in Kimura disease than angiolymphoid hyperplasia with eosinophilia.

Hyaline-Vascular Castleman Disease

Clinical Presentation and Clinical Course

Hyaline-vascular Castleman disease is a distinctive form of lymphoid proliferation that can affect patients of a wide age range, but most often young adults.[47–50] The most common sites of involvement are the mediastinum, neck, and retroperitoneum, but many other sites can be involved, such as skeletal muscle, axilla, and pelvic soft tissues. The patients present with a mass lesion. In contrast to the

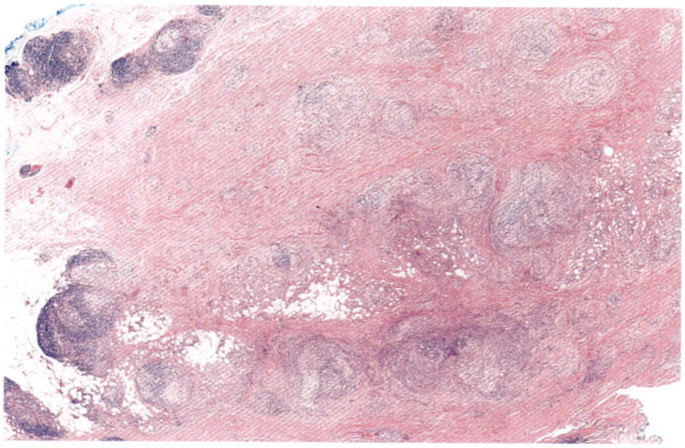

A

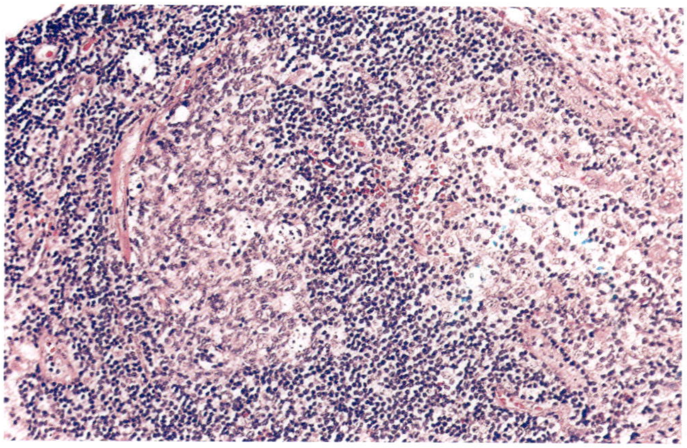

B

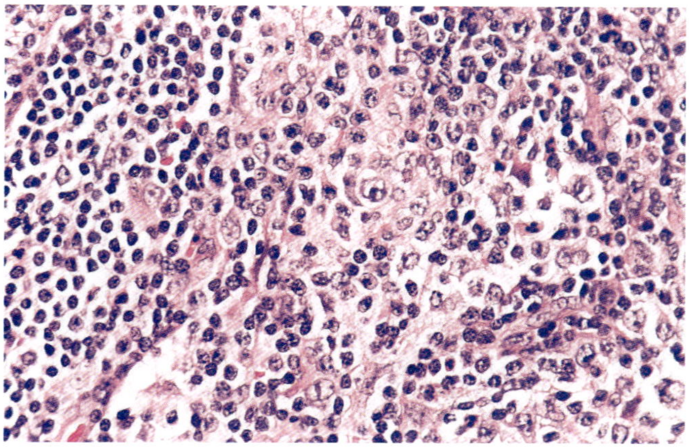

C

Figure 21–13. Reactive lymphoid hyperplasia unspecified of soft tissue. *A*, Lymphoid aggregates occur in a sclerotic stroma. *B*, Lymphoid follicles with germinal centers are identified, but they are not as well formed as those commonly encountered in lymph nodes. *C*, Outside the follicles, there is a mixture of small lymphocytes, and large activated lymphoid cells.

plasma cell and multicentric types, systemic symptoms are very rare. This is a totally benign condition that is curable by local excision, although the surgical procedure may be difficult because of profuse bleeding.

Key Histologic Findings

The essential diagnostic features include abnormal hyaline-vascular follicles, hypervascular interfollicular zone, and lack of nodal sinuses within the main lesion (although sinuses may sometimes be found in

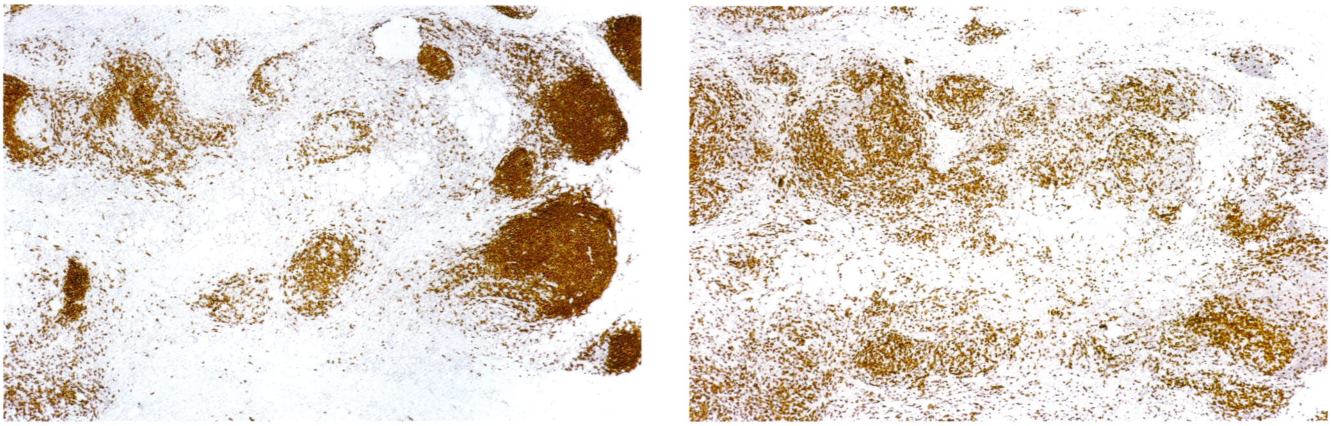

A B

Figure 21–14. Reactive lymphoid hyperplasia unspecified of soft tissue, immunohistochemical staining (same case as Fig. 21–13). *A*, Nodules of $CD20^+$ lymphoid cells are present. There are few $CD20^+$ cells between the nodules. *B*, Many $CD3^+$ lymphoid cells are present in between.

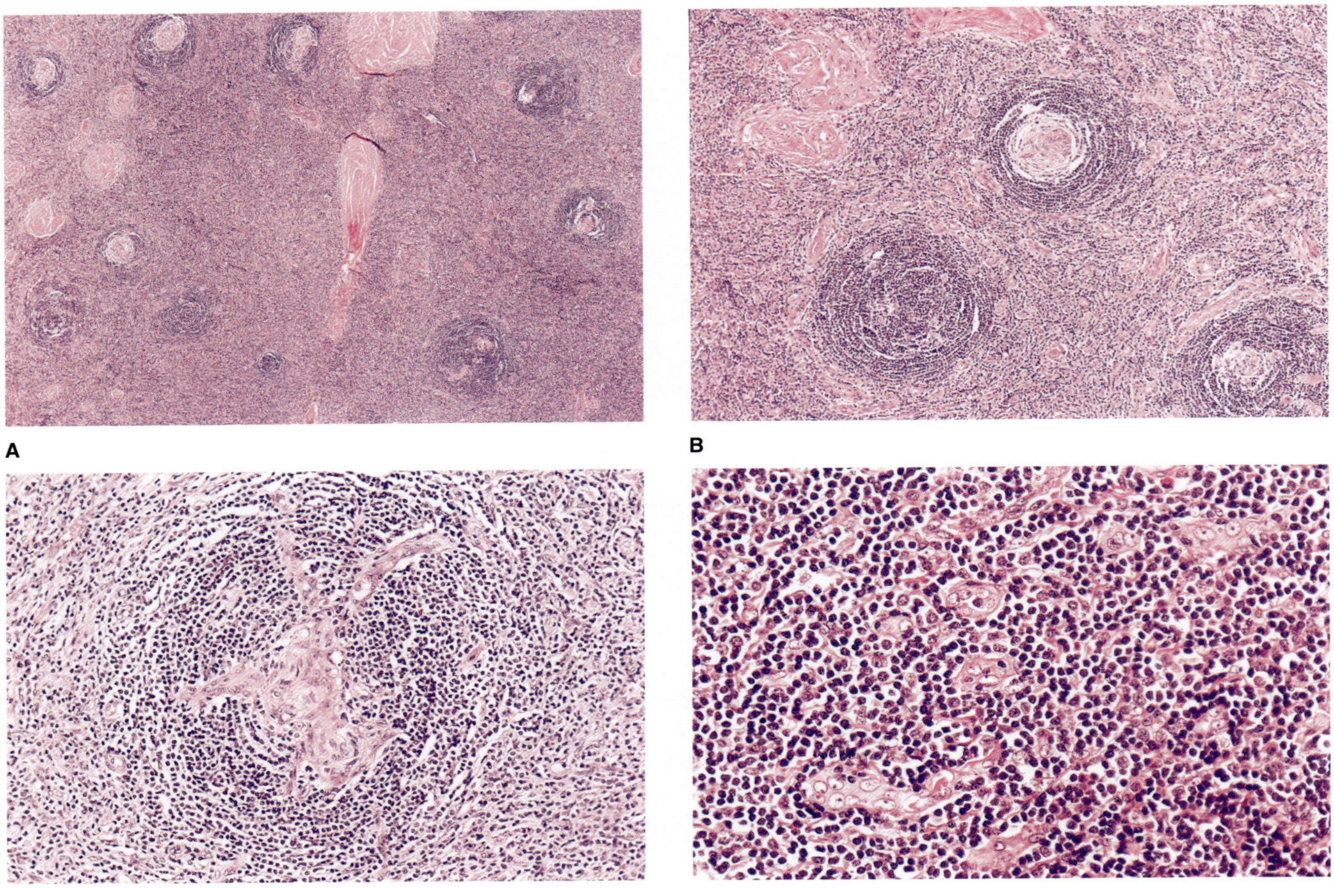

A B C D

Figure 21–15. Hyaline-vascular Castleman disease exhibiting classical histologic features. *A*, Typical hyaline-vascular follicles are separated by a moderate amount of interfollicular tissue. *B*, The follicles have whorled centers and are surrounded by concentric rings of small lymphocytes. Note the absence of sinuses. *C*, Follicle penetrated by multiple hyalinized venules. The germinal center is depleted of follicular center lymphoid cells. *D*, The interfollicular zone is rich in high endothelial venules and small lymphocytes.

the periphery of the lesion; Fig. 21–15).[47] The last feature has led to controversies as to whether hyaline-vascular Castleman disease originates in extranodal tissue or lymph node. The percentage areas occupied by the follicles and the interfollicular zone are highly variable from case to case.

In the typical example, the follicles have small germinal centers depleted of lymphoid cells and composed mostly of follicular dendritic cells and endothelial cells, surrounded by thick mantles with concentric disposition of the small lymphocytes (see Fig. 21–15). Some follicular dendritic cells can have enlarged hyperchromatic or bizarre nuclei (so-called follicular dendritic cell dysplasia; Fig. 21–16).[51,52] The follicles are penetrated by one or more hyalinized venules, producing a lollipop-like appearance. The interfollicular zone is rich in high endothelial venules and densely populated by small lymphocytes, with few large lymphoid cells or plasma cells.

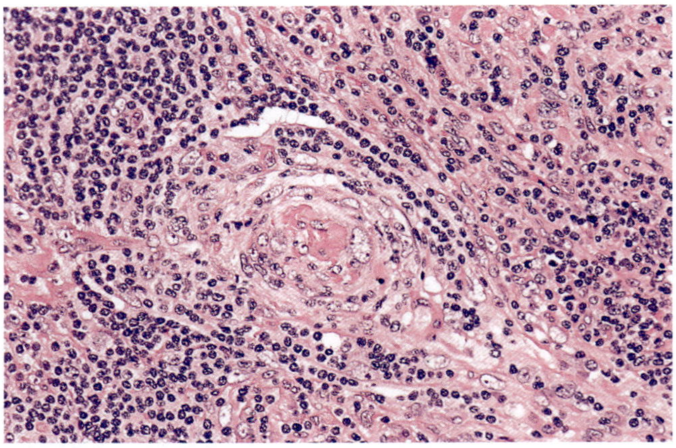

Figure 21–16. Hyaline-vascular Castleman disease. Occasional follicles can harbor isolated large bizarre cells (predominantly follicular dendritic cells). The significance of this cytologic change is not known.

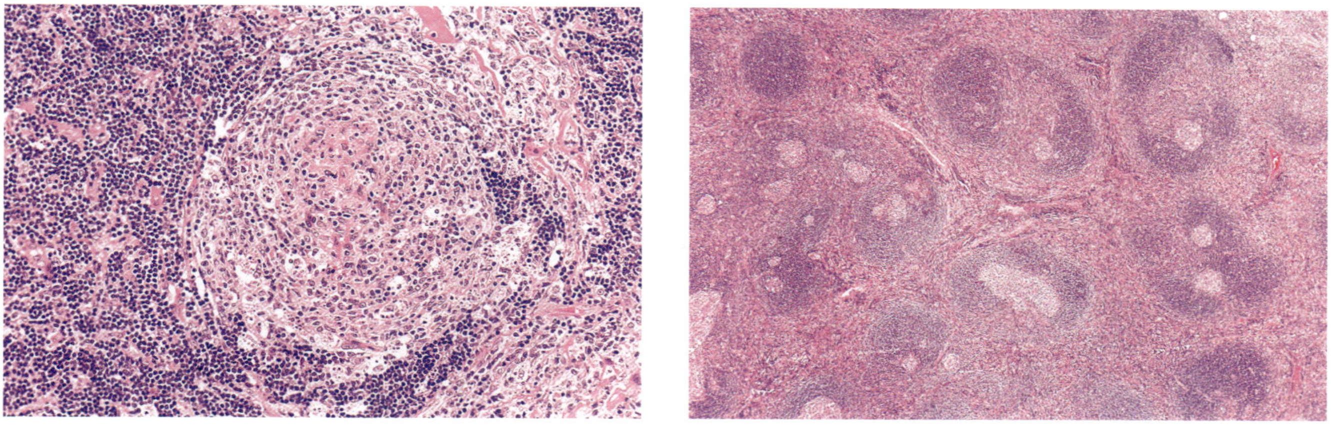

A B

Figure 21-17. Hyaline-vascular Castleman disease. *A*, Follicles can have large germinal centers, but they are whorled and contain hyalinized venules. *B*, Some follicles have multiple whorled germinal centers, a feature characteristic of hyaline-vascular Castleman disease if present.

Perivenular sclerosis can be present. There are commonly some clusters of plasmacytoid monocytes, which are medium-sized cells with eccentrically placed round nuclei, amphophilic cytoplasm, and frequent apoptotic bodies. Rare large bizarre cells can also be found in the interfollicular zone in some cases.[51]

In a significant proportion of cases, the diagnosis of hyaline-vascular Castleman disease may not be so classical.[51] The follicles can have large germinal centers, resembling usual reactive follicles, but they can be distinguishable from the latter by the whorled arrangement of germinal center cells, lack of polarity, lower cell density, and focal presence of hyalinized venules in the germinal centers (Fig. 21-17). Some follicles are large and composed almost exclusively of small lymphocytes, but contain multiple small and whorled germinal centers; such follicles are practically pathognomonic of hyaline-vascular Castleman disease when found (Fig. 21-17*B*). Some follicles can be very large, being devoid of germinal centers and decorated by multiple venules. It may be difficult to recognize the follicles because their outlines can be poorly defined and merge into the interfollicular zone. On immunostaining for CD20, these nodules stand out remarkably, and they are typically traversed by nonstaining streaks due to the presence of penetrating venules (Fig. 21-18). In some cases, the interfollicular zone is very broad (so-called stroma-rich variant, defined by an interfollicular zone occupying >50% of the lesional area), such that the diagnostic hyaline-vascular follicles are widely scattered or inconspicuous.[53]

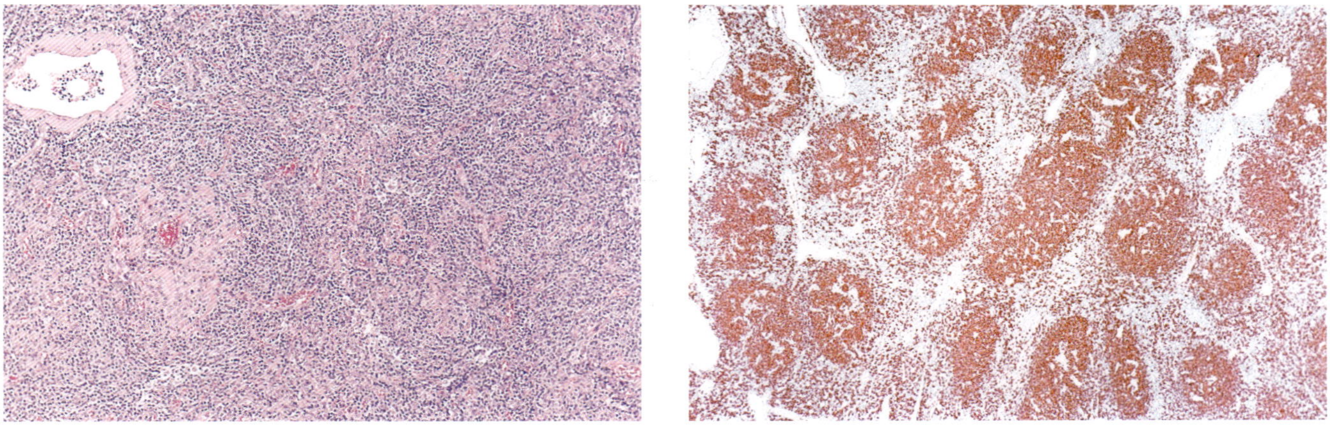

A B

Figure 21-18. Hyaline-vascular Castleman disease, difficult case. *A*, The dense lymphoid infiltrate is apparently diffuse, but careful examination reveals a vague nodular pattern. A large follicle actually occupies the left field. *B*, Immunostaining for CD20 shows up a surprising follicular architecture. Note the multiple nonstaining streaks in the follicles created by the presence of penetrating venules.

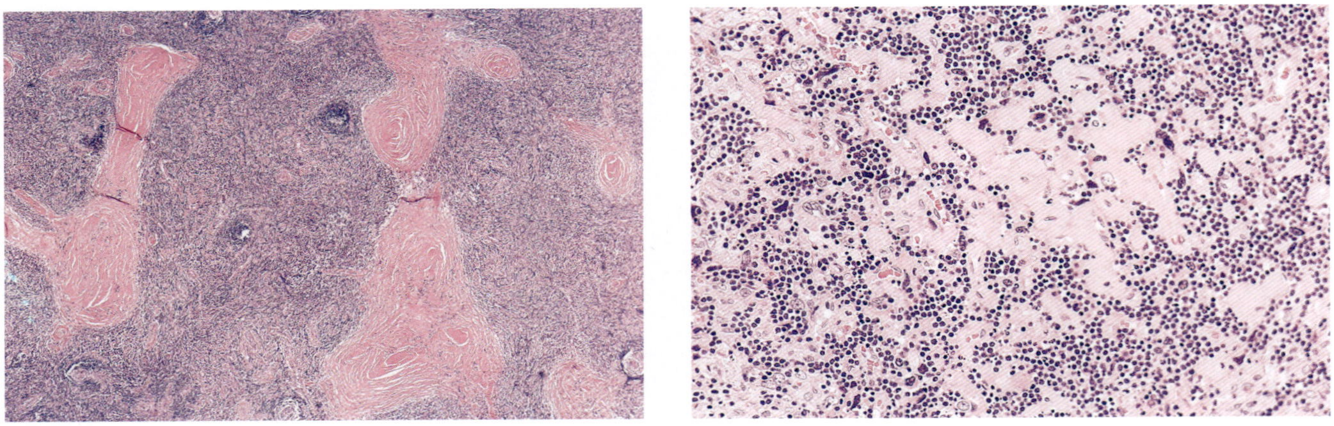

A B

Figure 21–19. Hyaline-vascular Castleman disease. *A*, Sclerotic bands are not uncommon in Castleman disease. *B*, Perivenular sclerosis can be very extensive, such that the venules may no longer be evident.

Sclerosis can also be prominent, particularly in long-standing lesions and those occurring in the retroperitoneum (Fig. 21–19). The sclerosis takes the form of extensive perivenular sclerosis merging into broad sclerotic bands or large sclerotic nodules, which can show central calcification (Fig. 21–19).

Immunohistochemical Profile

The lymphoid follicles possess thick mantles composed mostly of CD20$^+$ B cells, but the germinal centers often contain few CD20$^+$ lymphocytes.[53] Within the follicles, CD21$^+$ follicular dendritic cells form expanded and disrupted meshworks or multiple tight concentric collections.[54] The interfollicular zone is rich in CD3$^+$ T lymphocytes as well as venules, which can be highlighted by CD31, CD34, or factor VIII-related antigen. There are also scattered CD68$^+$ histiocytes with a dendritic appearance and aggregates of CD68$^+$ plasmacytoid monocytes.

Differential Diagnosis

The main differential diagnosis is *malignant lymphoma* (see subsequent section "Approach to Diagnosis of Lymphoid Infiltrates in the Soft Tissues"). When the lesion is stroma-rich, differential diagnosis with various *soft tissue tumors* can also be raised.

Associated Lesions and Supervening Neoplasms

Angiolipomatous hamartoma, characterized by blood vessels interspersed within fibroadipose tissue, occasionally accompanies hyaline-vascular Castleman disease.[34,55–57] The hamartoma can form a mass contiguous with the Castleman lesion, or form a main bulk within which nodules of the Castleman lesion are found.

Hyaline-vascular Castleman disease can be complicated by a *vascular neoplasm*, which apparently evolves from interfollicular vascular hyperplasia. The vascular neoplasm can be morphologically benign or malignant.[57–59] In some of the reported cases, the endothelial nature of the neoplasm has not been proven beyond doubt.[58,60]

A variety of *stromal proliferative lesions (stromal overgrowths)* can occur in the interfollicular zone of hyaline-vascular Castleman disease, ranging from lesions that merge well into the interfollicular tissue to discrete expansile nodules. The former may represent hyperplastic, dysplastic, or neoplastic proliferations, whereas the latter signifies the development of a supervening neoplasm. (1) Angiomyoid proliferations comprise poorly canalized blood vessels and haphazardly disposed spindly cells, usually without cellular atypia. The outcome of the reported cases has been benign. The blood vessels can be highlighted by immunostaining for CD34, and immunostaining for smooth muscle actin highlights the spindly cells and the pericytes of the blood vessels (Fig. 21–20).[60] Occasionally there can be many admixed CD68$^+$ histiocytes with a dendritic morphology.[53] (2) Follicular dendritic cell overgrowth comprises extrafollicular proliferations of spindly follicular dendritic cells (CD21$^+$), which form storiform arrays and fascicles, often accompanied by variable degrees of cellular atypia (Fig. 21–21). The process probably begins as a hyperplastic condition, and evolves to a frank neoplasm, although it is difficult to tell at which point in time the lesion should be considered neoplastic (i.e., follicular dendritic

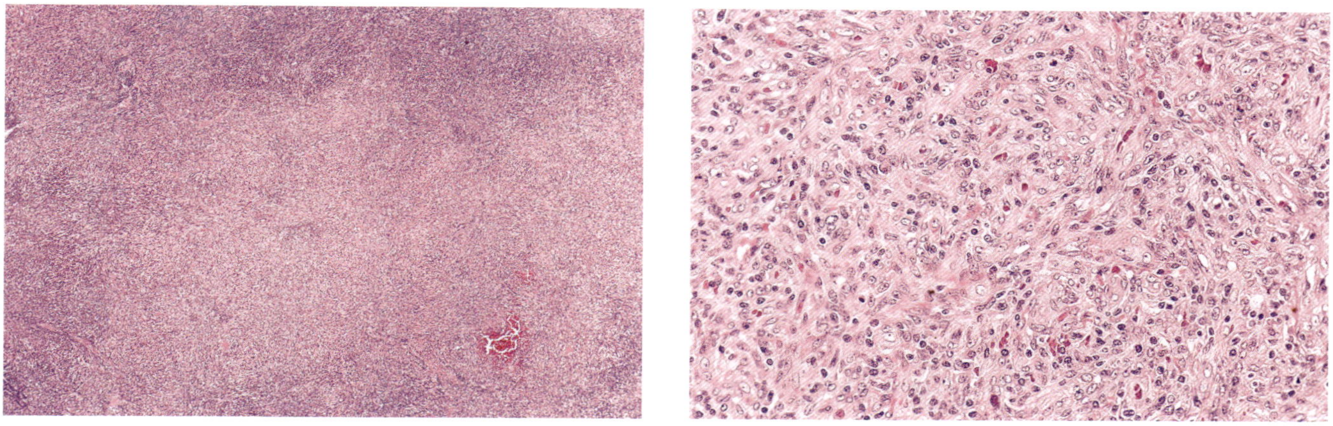

A B

Figure 21-20. Hyaline-vascular Castleman disease with interfollicular angiomyoid proliferation. *A,* There are broad diffuse areas with barely discernible small hyaline-vascular follicles. *B,* Intersecting short fascicles of spindly cells and barely canalized venules are present. There is no cytologic atypia.

cell sarcoma).[61,62] This lesion is potentially malignant because recurrence or metastasis occurs in at least 60% of cases on follow-up.[60] (3) Atypical stromal overgrowth unspecified refers to interfollicular proliferations of atypical spindle cells with haphazard, storiform, or fascicular pattern, and whose nature defies elucidation despite extensive immunohistochemical evaluation (Fig. 21–22).[63] The clinical behavior of this group is currently unknown.

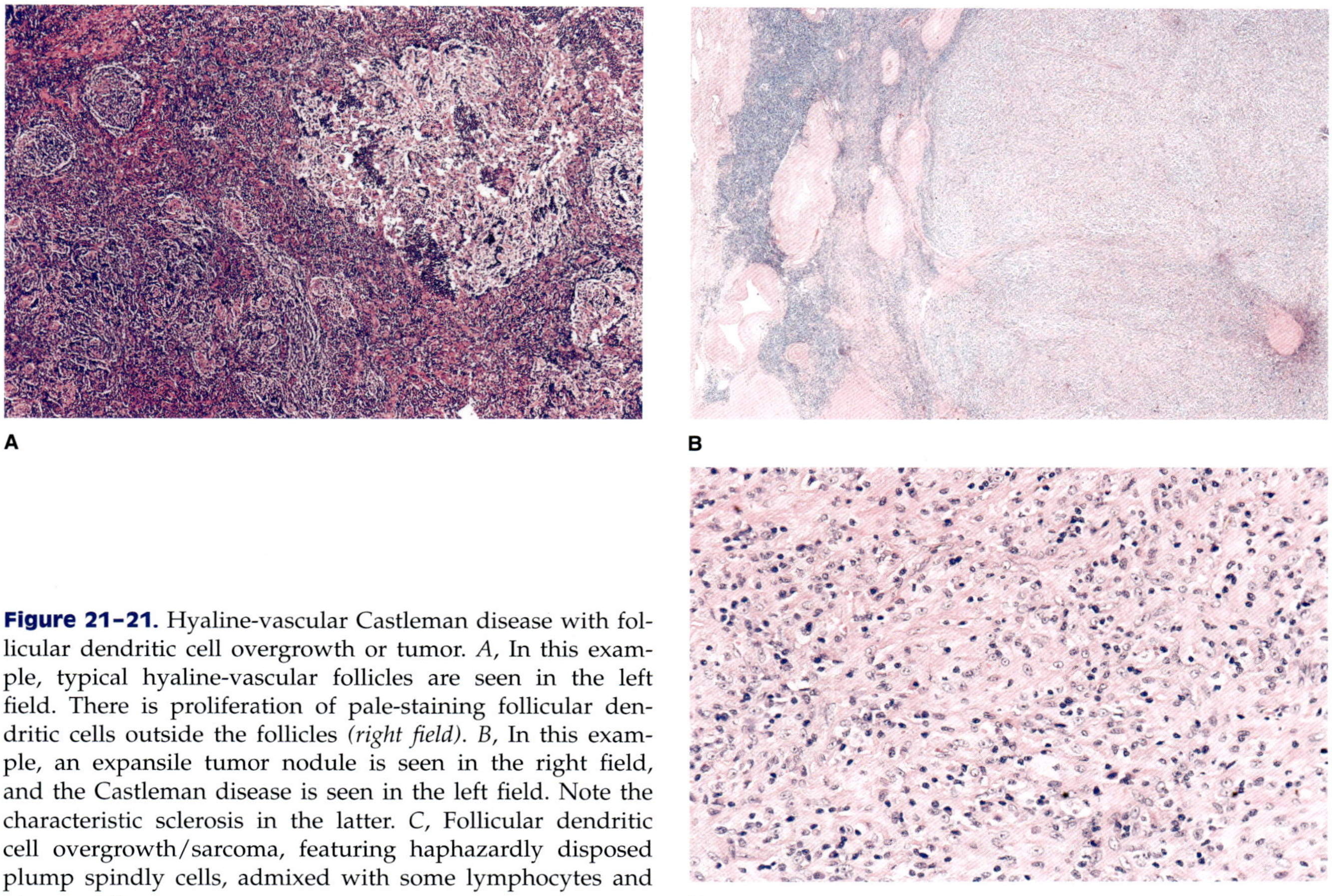

A B C

Figure 21-21. Hyaline-vascular Castleman disease with follicular dendritic cell overgrowth or tumor. *A,* In this example, typical hyaline-vascular follicles are seen in the left field. There is proliferation of pale-staining follicular dendritic cells outside the follicles *(right field). B,* In this example, an expansile tumor nodule is seen in the right field, and the Castleman disease is seen in the left field. Note the characteristic sclerosis in the latter. *C,* Follicular dendritic cell overgrowth/sarcoma, featuring haphazardly disposed plump spindly cells, admixed with some lymphocytes and plasma cells.

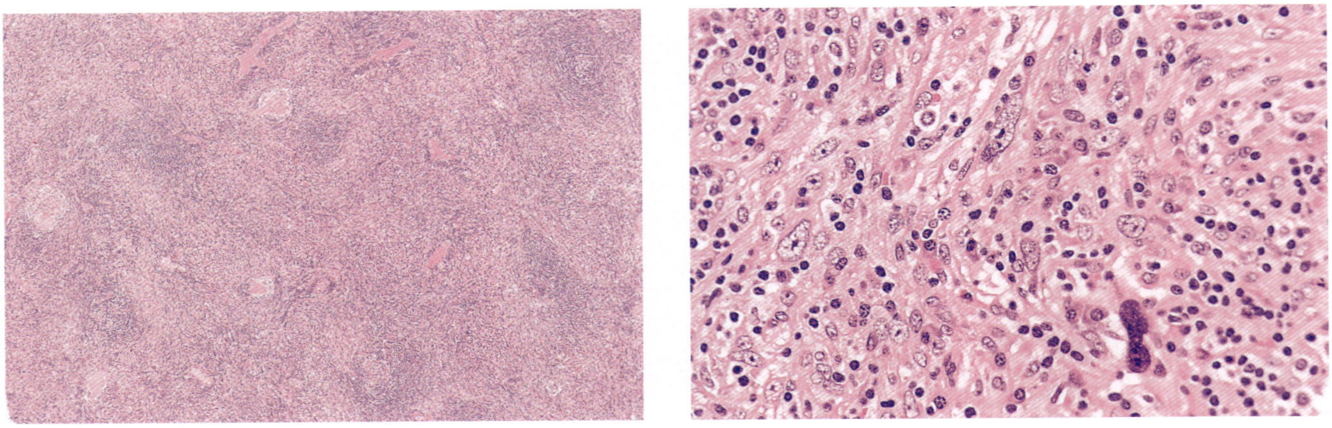

A B

Figure 21-22. Hyaline-vascular Castleman disease with atypical stromal overgrowth of uncertain nature. *A*, The broad interfollicular zone constitutes more than 90% of the lesional tissue. A few scattered hyaline-vascular follicles are seen. *B*, In the interfollicular zone, there are intersecting short fascicles of plump spindly cells with large atypical nuclei. The nature of these atypical cells remains uncertain even after immunohistochemical evaluation (immunohistochemically inert except for vimentin).

Plasmacytoma Involving Soft Tissues

Clinical Presentation and Clinical Course

Plasmacytoma, a tumorous lesion composed of neoplastic (monoclonal) plasma cells, can involve soft tissues, most commonly the paravertebral region.[34,64,65] It can develop in patients with documented or previously undiagnosed multiple myeloma as part of the disseminated disease process or occur as a sole lesion. In any case, if the patient is not known to have multiple myeloma, the diagnosis should prompt staging work-up to look for evidence of multiple myeloma, such as serum immunoglobulin levels, serum and urine immunoelectrophoresis, and marrow examination. For solitary plasmacytoma, multiple myeloma eventually supervenes in 10% to 20% of patients.[34]

Key Histologic Findings

In most cases, the diffuse neoplastic infiltrate is readily recognizable as being plasmacytic in nature by virtue of the eccentrically placed nuclei with clock-face chromatin, amphophilic cytoplasm, and distinct Golgi zone (Fig. 21–23*A*). The plasma cells are often slightly larger than normal plasma cells and exhibit slightly less condensed chromatin. Some cells can contain intracytoplasmic inclusion globules (Russell bodies) or crystals, or intranuclear inclusions (Dutcher bodies).

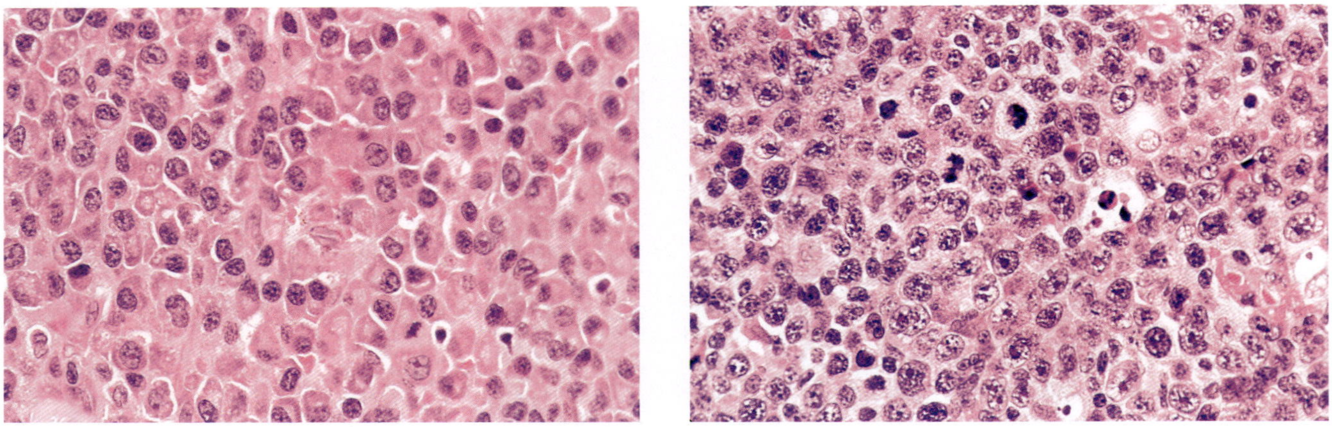

A B

Figure 21-23. Soft tissue plasmacytoma. *A*, In this example, the neoplastic cells are obviously plasma cells with mild atypia. *B*, In plasmablastic/anaplastic plasmacytoma, distinction from a large cell lymphoma can be difficult. Note the coarsely clumped chromatin in some cells and resemblance to immature plasma cells in rare cells.

The plasmablastic/anaplastic variant comprises large cells with vesicular or coarse chromatin and prominent nucleoli (Fig. 21–23*B*). The Golgi zone may be inconspicuous in the amphophilic cytoplasm of the cells. Mitotic figures are often easy to find.

Unusual Histologic Findings

There can be irregular masses of amyloid interspersed among the tumor cells; the amyloid deposits are frequently surrounded by foreign body giant cells. Prominent hemorrhage can result in the formation of blood lakes. Exceptionally, accumulation of abundant mucosubstance in the stroma can occur, resulting in mimicry of myxoid sarcomas.

Immunohistochemical Profile

Plasmacytoma characteristically shows a $CD20^-$, $CD3^-$, immunoglobulin-positive, $CD138^+$ immunophenotype. Staining for CD45, CD79a, CD43, CD56, or epithelial membrane antigen is variable.[34] A $CD20^-$, $CD43^+$ immunophenotype can potentially lead to a misinterpretation of the process as a T-cell lymphoma. The occasional immunoreactivity for cytokeratin, frequently in a punctate pattern, can lead to a misdiagnosis of carcinoma.[66]

Differential Diagnosis

For plasmacytoma composed of mature plasma cells, the differential diagnoses of *nonspecific chronic inflammation* and *plasma cell granuloma (inflammatory pseudotumor)* have to be considered. Reactive lesions typically exhibit a more mixed cell population, including lymphocytes and myofibroblasts. Presence of large numbers of Dutcher bodies, if present, favors a diagnosis of a neoplastic process. The problem can be easily solved by immunostaining for immunoglobulin, with light chain restriction supporting a diagnosis of plasmacytoma.

Extranodal marginal zone B-cell lymphoma of mucosa-associated lymphoid tissue type can have a rich component of plasma cells, but it can be distinguished from plasmacytoma by the presence of small lymphocytes and cells resembling monocytoid B cells, which tend to show localization around residual lymphoid follicles.

The plasmablastic/anaplastic variant of plasmacytoma can pose considerable difficulties in differential diagnosis from *carcinoma*, *melanoma*, or *large B-cell lymphoma*. Presence of coarsely clumped clock-face chromatin in some cells, marked basophilia of the cytoplasm with a pale Golgi zone, and presence of interspersed atypical plasma cells provide the most important morphologic clues to the correct diagnosis. Plasmacytoma is almost invariably $CD20^-$, which contrasts with the almost invariable CD20 positivity in large B-cell lymphomas. Although CD138 immunoreactivity supports the presence of plasmacytic differentiation, it has to be interpreted in context because many nonlymphoid tumors, including carcinomas, can be $CD138^+$.

Approach to Diagnosis of Lymphoid Infiltrates in the Soft Tissues

When there is a dense lymphoid infiltrate comprising large atypical cells, a diagnosis of lymphoma is usually obvious, although the differential diagnosis with various nonlymphoid malignancies such as carcinoma, melanoma, or sarcoma can also be raised. Immunohistochemical studies can readily confirm the diagnosis, as well as provide information for cell lineage assignment and classification.

When the lymphoid infiltrate comprises predominantly small cells or a mixture of small and large cells, it can be difficult to determine whether the process represents malignant lymphoma or reactive lymphoid hyperplasia (specific and nonspecific types) because of morphologic overlap. Figure 21–24 outlines the features that favor a diagnosis of lymphoma. Usually two or more features have to be present to support the diagnosis; some caveats are listed in Table 21–5. Immunohistochemical staining is most helpful for confirming or refuting a diagnosis of lymphoma. In a reactive lymphoid infiltrate, T cells predominate or T cells occur between nodules of B cells. When sheets of B cells are demonstrated, a diagnosis of B-cell lymphoma is favored (Fig. 21–25). On the other hand, presence of sheets of T cells is not diagnostic of either lymphoid hyperplasia or lymphoma (Fig. 21–26); the latter diagnosis would be supported if there is loss of expression of one or more pan-T markers or abnormal expression of CD56 or TIA1.[40,51,67]

If the findings remain inconclusive after immunohistochemical evaluation, molecular detection of clonal rearrangements of the immunoglobulin or T-cell receptor genes will support a diagnosis of lymphoma. Southern blot is the gold standard technique, but it is time-consuming and requires the use of fresh or frozen tissue. Currently, the polymerase chain reaction (PCR) technique is more popular because of applicability to routine paraffin-embedded tissues, but caution has to be exercised in interpretation of the results (see Table 21–5).[68] For cases that remain inconclusive after

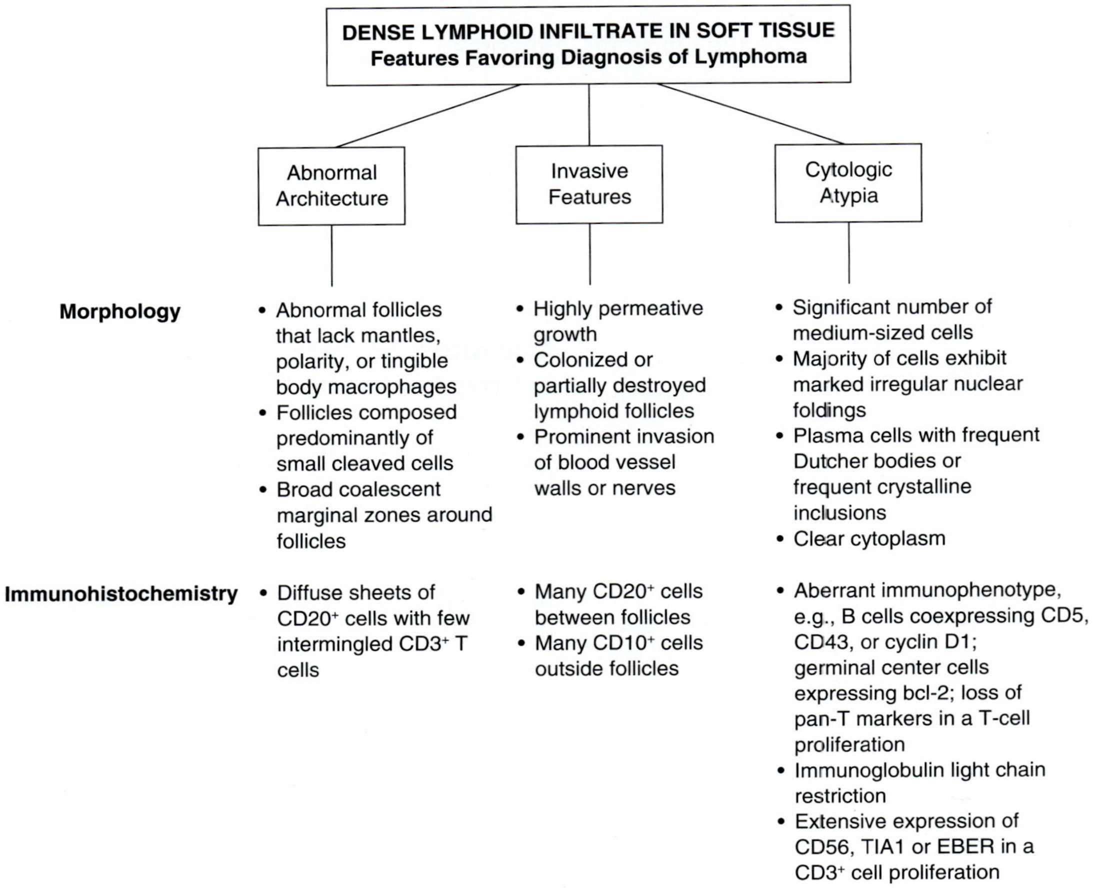
DENSE LYMPHOID INFILTRATE IN SOFT TISSUE
Features Favoring Diagnosis of Lymphoma
Abnormal Architecture
Invasive Features
Cytologic Atypia
Morphology
• Abnormal follicles that lack mantles, polarity, or tingible body macrophages
• Follicles composed predominantly of small cleaved cells
• Broad coalescent marginal zones around follicles
• Highly permeative growth
• Colonized or partially destroyed lymphoid follicles
• Prominent invasion of blood vessel walls or nerves
• Significant number of medium-sized cells
• Majority of cells exhibit marked irregular nuclear foldings
• Plasma cells with frequent Dutcher bodies or frequent crystalline inclusions
• Clear cytoplasm
Immunohistochemistry
• Diffuse sheets of CD20+ cells with few intermingled CD3+ T cells
• Many CD20+ cells between follicles
• Many CD10+ cells outside follicles
• Aberrant immunophenotype, e.g., B cells coexpressing CD5, CD43, or cyclin D1; germinal center cells expressing bcl-2; loss of pan-T markers in a T-cell proliferation
• Immunoglobulin light chain restriction
• Extensive expression of CD56, TIA1 or EBER in a CD3+ cell proliferation

Figure 21–24. Schematic chart to show features that would support a diagnosis of lymphoma over reactive lymphoid infiltrate in the soft tissues.

extensive evaluation, the term "atypical lymphoid hyperplasia" can be applied. If the difficulties in diagnosis are due to the small size of the tissue sample, a larger biopsy should be obtained for assessment. If the entire lesion has already been removed, the patient should be closely followed up, and further biopsies should be taken when the lesion recurs.[51]

Tumors and Tumor-like Lesions of Hematopoietic Cells

Extramedullary Hematopoietic Tumor

Clinical Presentation and Clinical Course

Extramedullary hematopoietic tumor is a nonneoplastic mass-forming lesion produced by accumulation of hematopoietic cells in extramedullary sites. It typically occurs in the setting of severe anemia (such as thalassemia, hemoglobinopathies, congenital hemolytic anemia), chronic myeloproliferative disorders (especially agnogenic myeloid metaplasia), bone disease with compromised marrow volume (such as Gaucher disease, marble bone disease), and treatment with granulocyte colony-stimulating factor.[69–75] It can occur in various sites, including soft tissues, in particular the paraspinal and intrathoracic regions. The mass lesion can reach an alarming size, clinically and radiologically mimicking a malignant neoplasm.

Key Histologic Findings

The lesion is typically noncircumscribed or partly circumscribed. It is highly cellular, comprising a mixture of cell types from the megakaryocytic, myeloid, and erythroid series in different stages of maturation. Erythroid cells (normoblasts) occur in clusters or are intimately admixed with other hematopoietic cell elements (Fig. 21–27). The mature myeloid cells of the neutrophil or eosinophil series, metamyelocytes (with eccentrically placed and dark-staining indented nuclei) and myelocytes (with eccentrically placed oval

Table 21-5. Caveats in Diagnosis of Lymphoid Lesions in Soft Tissues

- Do not lightly discard the possibility of lymphoma when an unusual-looking malignant soft tissue neoplasm is encountered.
- Presence of reactive lymphoid follicles does not rule out the possibility of lymphoma. Lymphoid follicles are commonly found in extranodal marginal zone B-cell lymphoma of mucosa-associated lymphoid tissue type.
- In the soft tissues, the presence of angiocentric-angioinvasive growth per se is not specific for NK/T-cell lymphoma. It can sometimes be seen in peripheral T-cell lymphomas and large B-cell lymphomas, and even rarely in inflammatory lesions (such as syphilitic gumma).
- Although the presence of dense sheets of B cells ($CD20^+$) supports a diagnosis of lymphoma (B-cell lymphoma), the presence of sheets of T cells ($CD3^+$) can either be due to a reactive lymphoid lesion or a T-cell lymphoma.
- Lack of immunoglobulin gene or T-cell receptor gene rearrangement by PCR technique does not totally rule out the possibility of lymphoma because there is a significant false-negative rate of 30–40%.
- Do not accept reports on PCR of immunoglobulin or T-cell receptor gene rearrangement at face value. The results must be repeatable and must come from a trustworthy laboratory.

nuclei) can be recognized by the presence of eosinophilic cytoplasmic granules, which are brightly eosinophilic and larger for those of the eosinophil series. The myeloblasts and promyelocytes, with vesicular nuclei and distinct nucleoli, are scattered or form small clusters. The megakaryocytes, which are haphazardly interspersed throughout the lesion, are characterized by large irregular-shaped and hyperchromatic nuclei and voluminous eosinophilic cytoplasm. Some can exhibit bizarre nuclei, especially in the setting of agnogenic myeloid metaplasia.

Unusual Variant: Sclerosing Extramedullary Hematopoietic Tumor

Sclerosing extramedullary hematopoietic tumor is an unusual morphologic variant characterized by a prominent sclerotic to myxoid stroma with thick collagen fibers, and thus the cellularity is much lower than that of conventional extramedullary

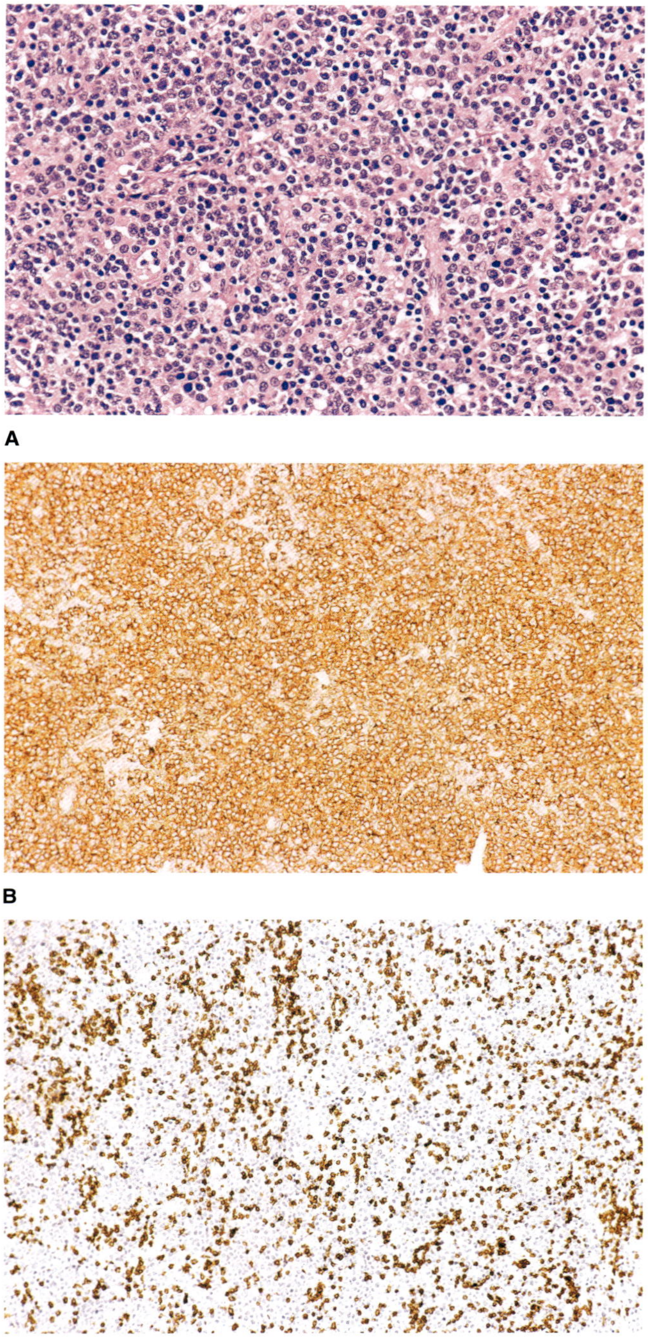

A

B

C

Figure 21-25. Worrisome small lymphoid cell infiltrate in soft tissue caused by small B-cell lymphoma. *A*, Histologically, there is a dense infiltrate of small lymphoid cells with no definite cytologic atypia. *B*, Immunostaining for CD20 shows diffuse sheets of positive cells, supporting a diagnosis of lymphoma. *C*, Immunostaining for CD3 shows few positive cells.

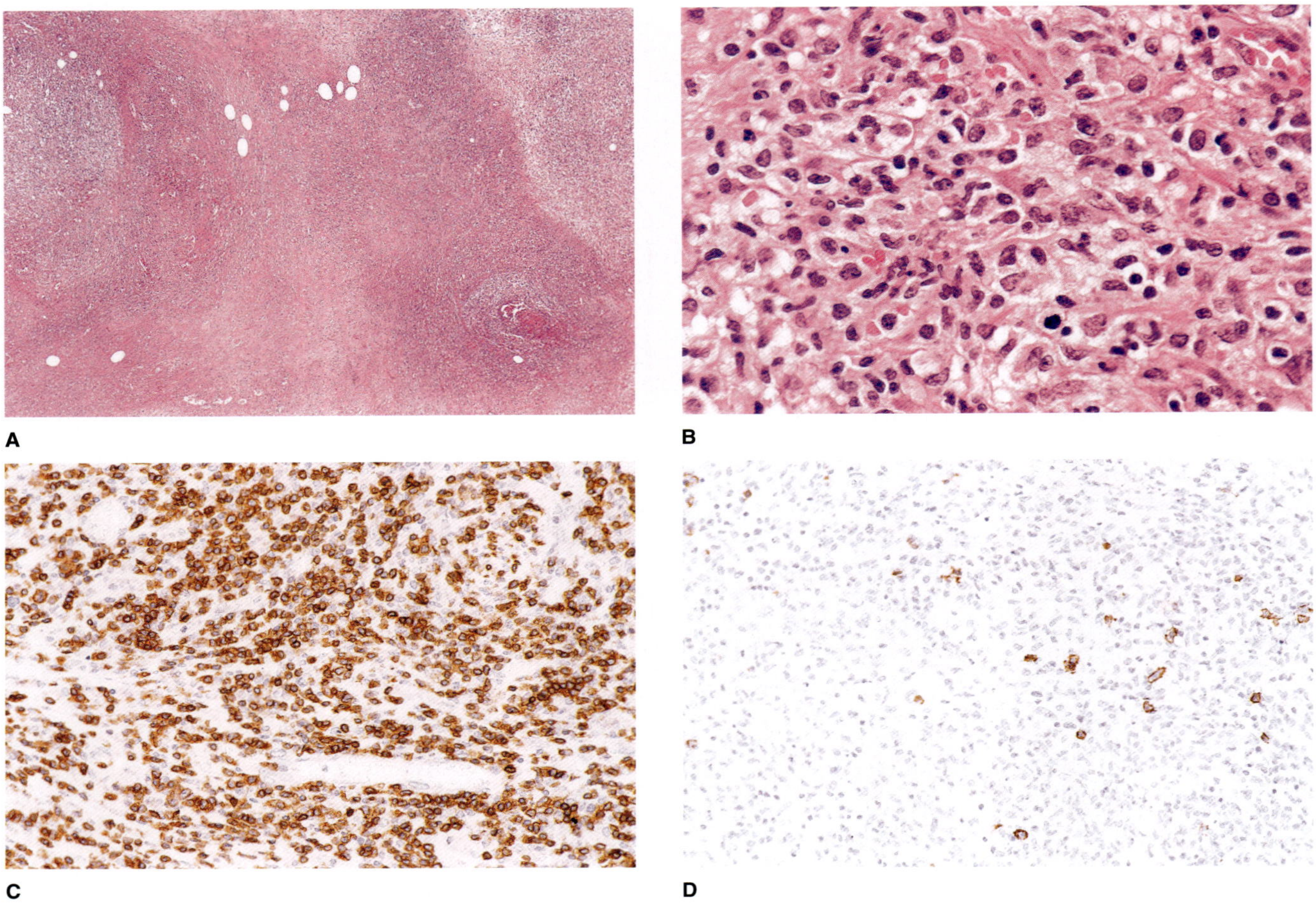

Figure 21–26. Worrisome lymphoid cell infiltrate caused by syphilitic gumma. *A*, There is heavy lymphoid infiltration with coagulative necrosis and angiocentric growth, raising a serious concern for malignant lymphoma. *B*, Cytologically the infiltrate comprises a mixture of small and large cells, with some showing mild nuclear atypia. *C*, Immunostaining for CD3 shows numerous T cells, but this per se is not sufficient to support a diagnosis of lymphoma. *D*, Few $CD20^+$ B cells are present.

hematopoietic tumor (Fig. 21–28).[76] The peculiar stromal component is probably induced by fibrogenic factors secreted by the megakaryocytes. There can be some admixed adipose cells. Blood vessels were usually prominent and thick-walled. Because of the unusual stromal changes and the presence of large atypical cells (megakaryocytes), the lesion is not uncommonly misdiagnosed as Hodgkin lymphoma, myxoid sarcoma, or sclerosing liposarcoma.

Differential Diagnosis

The presence of megakaryocytes, with their large and somewhat pleomorphic nuclei, commonly invites a misdiagnosis of malignant neoplasm, such as *malignant histiocytosis, histiocytic sarcoma, large cell lymphoma, or Hodgkin lymphoma*. The clues suggesting that the large cells are probably megakaryocytes and not malignant cells include the presence of immature myeloid cells, in particular myelocytes with recognizable cytoplasmic granules, and the presence of normoblasts, often in the form of clusters. Late normoblasts differ from lymphocytes in having perfectly round nuclei, markedly condensed chromatin, and a broader rim of amphophilic or eosinophilic cytoplasm. The clusters of immature myeloid cells or early normoblasts can also be alarming because of the high nuclear-cytoplasmic ratio and vesicular nuclei, and can lead to a misdiagnosis of malignant lymphoma. The diagnosis of extramedullary hematopoietic tumor can be readily confirmed by immunohistochemical staining for: (1) megakaryocytes, such as CD31, CD34, CD41 (glycoprotein IIb), CD42b (glycoprotein Ib), CD61 (glycoprotein IIIb), factor VIII-related antigen; (2) mature and immature myeloid cells, such as myeloperoxidase; and

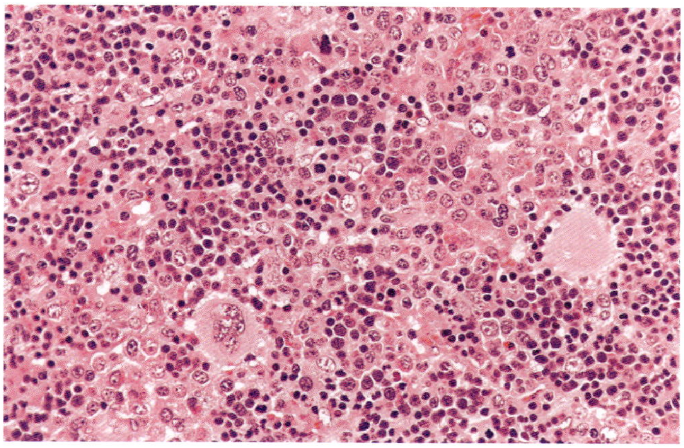

Figure 21–27. Extramedullary hematopoietic tumor involving retroperitoneal soft tissue. There is a dense infiltrate of cells with variable sizes and appearances. The islands of cells with dark round nuclei represent normoblasts. The interspersed large cells represent megakaryocytes, which can potentially be mistaken for malignant cells. The immature myeloid cells and early normoblasts can be mistaken for lymphoma cells because of their vesicular nuclei.

(3) erythroid cells, such as glycophorin A or hemoglobin (Fig. 21–29).

Extramedullary Myeloid Tumor

Clinical Presentation and Clinical Course

Extramedullary myeloid tumor, also known as granulocytic sarcoma or chloroma, is a mass-forming lesion comprising primitive myeloid cells.[34] It can occur in practically any site in the body, including somatic soft tissues.[77,78]

Extramedullary myeloid tumor can represent the first manifestation of leukemia or can occur in patients known to have acute myeloid leukemia or chronic myeloproliferative disorder during the active phase of the disease or as the first evidence of relapse. When myeloid tumor is the presenting feature, there may or may not be evidence of leukemia in the peripheral blood or bone marrow on work-up. Even if the disease is localized at presentation, systemic involvement will usually ensue within 1 to 2 years if systemic therapy is not given.[34]

Gross Findings

The freshly cut surfaces usually exhibit a greenish hue, which is the reason for its original designation "chloroma." The green color is often lost after prolonged formalin fixation and can be restored by immersing the tissue in hydrogen peroxide.

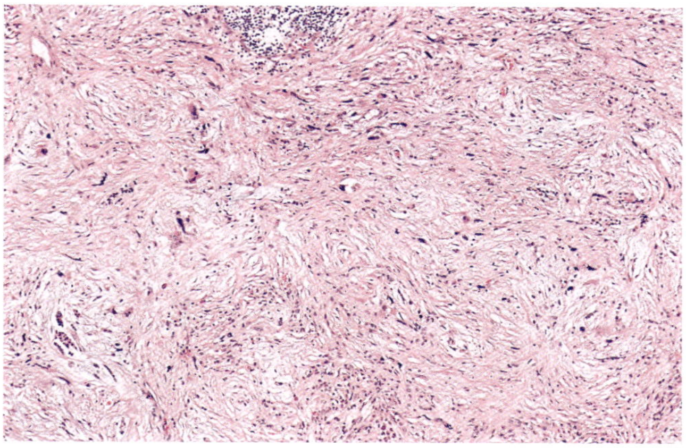

A

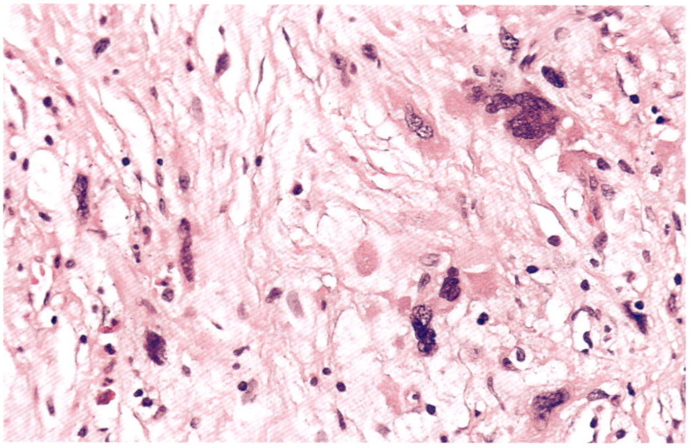

B

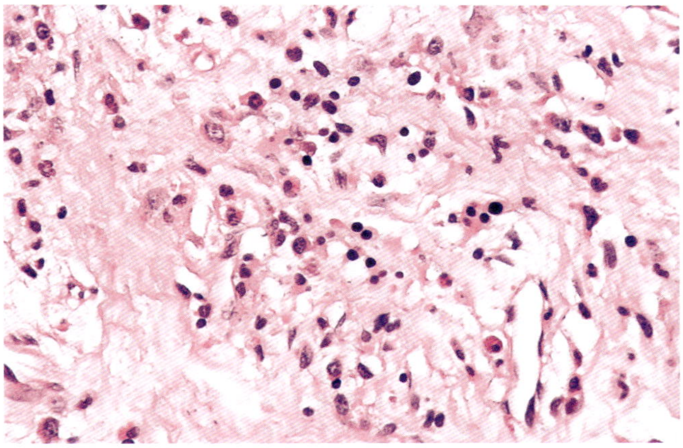

C

Figure 21–28. Sclerosing extramedullary hematopoietic tumor. *A*, Large cells with hyperchromatic nuclei are dispersed in a stroma comprising collagen fibers and myxoid matrix. *B*, The large cells with hyperchromatic nuclei are megakaryocytes. Their occurrence in a fibromyxoid background results in a striking resemblance to various soft tissue sarcomas. *C*, The small islands of normoblasts (cells with dark round nuclei) and immature myeloid cells provide the best clue to the correct diagnosis.

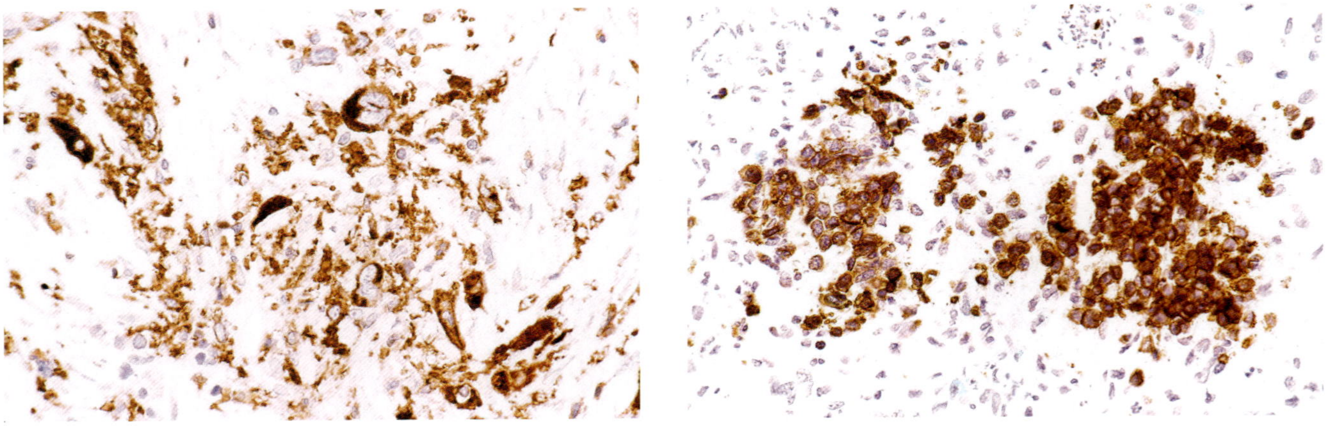

A B

Figure 21–29. Extramedullary hematopoietic tumor, immunohistochemical staining. *A*, The megakaryocytes can be highlighted by immunostaining for CD31. *B*, The islands of normoblasts are best highlighted by immunostaining for glycophorin A.

Key Histologic Findings

The neoplastic infiltrate appears monotonous and noncohesive, permeating and destroying the soft tissues. At the peripheral portion, there is commonly a single-file pattern of infiltration produced by insinuation of individual cells between the collagen fibers (Fig. 21–30). The neoplastic cells are medium-sized, with oval or indented nuclei, thin nuclear membrane, vesicular chromatin, and small distinct nucleoli. They possess a rim of lightly eosinophilic cytoplasm, which may contain fine eosinophilic granules. Admixed eosinophilic myelocytes (recognized by their indented

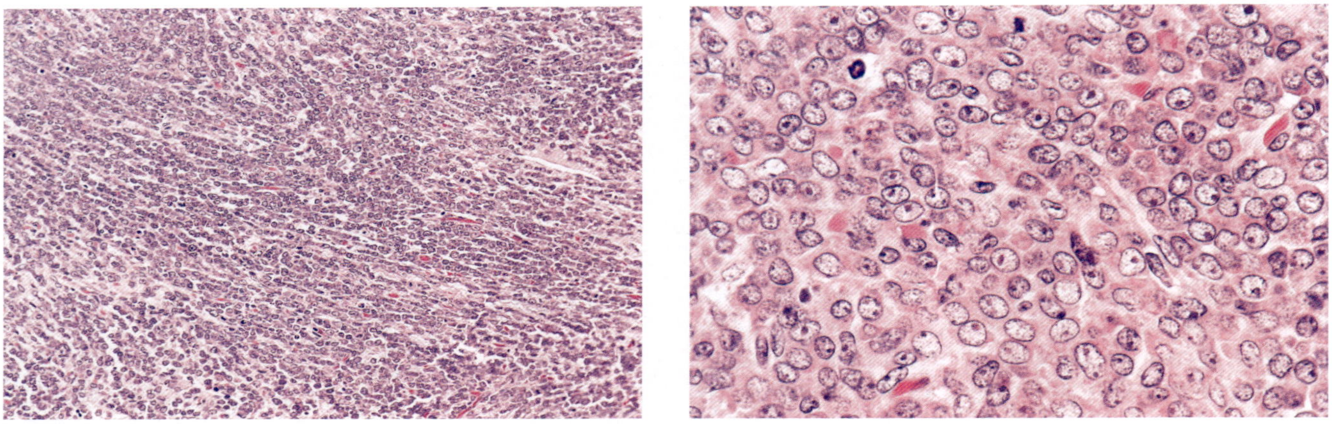

A B

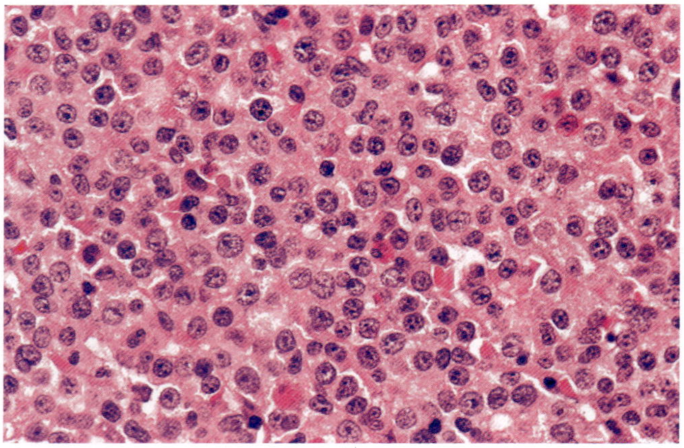

C

Figure 21–30. Extramedullary myeloid tumor involving soft tissue. *A*, A characteristic single-file growth pattern is seen. *B*, The cells are medium-sized and have a blastic look. The cytoplasm shows an eosinophilic hue. *C*, Another example showing medium-sized cells with a moderate amount of eosinophilic cytoplasm. An important clue to diagnosis is the presence of interspersed eosinophilic myelocytes with brightly eosinophilic granules.

nuclei and brightly eosinophilic cytoplasmic granules), if present (found in ~45% of cases), can provide an important clue to the correct diagnosis.[79]

Histochemical and Immunohistochemical Profile

A diagnosis of myeloid tumor can be supported by a positive Leder (chloroacetate esterase) stain, but this histochemical stain has a limited sensitivity of about 70%, staining only the more differentiated examples and usually only in subpopulations of neoplastic cells.[78–80]

The most sensitive and specific immunohistochemical marker is myeloperoxidase, which is positive in more than 95% of cases, with a cytoplasmic granular pattern.[77,79,81] On paraffin sections, the polyclonal antiserum works much better than monoclonal antibodies. Neutrophil elastase is another specific but less sensitive marker (positive in ~40% of cases).[80] CD117 (c-kit) is positive in 87% of cases.[77] Lysozyme is commonly positive (60–90%), but its specificity is low.[77–80] Myeloid tumor is negative for CD20 and CD3, and can show variable staining for CD34, CD15, and KP1 (CD68). PGM1 (CD68) is negative except for the monocytic and myelomonocytic type of leukemia. The frequent positive staining for CD43 and CD45RO may lead an erroneous diagnosis of T-cell lymphoma.

Differential Diagnosis

Extramedullary myeloid tumor is commonly misdiagnosed as *malignant lymphoma*, and a correct diagnosis requires a high index of suspicion. In contrast to lymphoblastic lymphoma, the neoplastic cells possess a greater amount of cytoplasm, the cytoplasm often exhibits an eosinophilic hue, and nucleoli are readily identifiable. In contrast to large cell lymphoma, the neoplastic cells often show a smaller size, more delicate nuclear membranes, and eosinophilic rather than amphophilic cytoplasm. The identification of eosinophilic cytoplasmic granules provides the strongest histologic clue to the correct diagnosis, which can be readily confirmed by histochemical or immunohistochemical studies.

Mast Cell Disease

Systemic mast cell disease (systemic mastocytosis) can rarely involve the somatic soft tissues. Extremely rarely, mast cell disease occurs as a solitary tumor mass in the absence of systemic or cutaneous disease, and the term mast cell sarcoma (with atypical mast cells and destructive growth) or extracutaneous mastocytoma (with mature mast cells and nondestructive growth) is applied.[82–86]

Mast cells often occur in groups and sheets, and they are not uncommonly mistaken for monocytes or monocytoid B cells because of the indented nuclei, pale cytoplasm, and inconspicuous cytoplasmic granules. The mast cells are almost invariably accompanied by sclerosis and eosinophils, which provide important clues to the correct diagnosis. The diagnosis of mast cell disease can be confirmed by a positive Leder (chloroacetate esterase) stain, or positive immunostaining for CD117 (c-kit) in a cell membrane pattern or tryptase in a cytoplasmic pattern.

Tumors and Tumor-like Lesions of Histiocytes

Histiocytes comprise two major groups of cells (1) monocytes-phagocytes (macrophages) and (2) dendritic (immune accessory) cells.[87–90]

Monocytes-phagocytes (macrophages) are derived from bone marrow and serve both antigen-processing and effector functions in the immune response. They include blood monocytes, sinus histiocytes, and tingible-body macrophages in lymph nodes, tissue macrophages, and epithelioid histiocytes. They are rich in lysosomal enzymes, and the best immunohistochemical marker is CD68 (PGM1).[91] These cells are usually immunoreactive for CD4, CD11c, CD14, CD45, and HLA-DR.

Dendritic (immune accessory) cells are nonphagocytic antigen-presenting cells and are derived from bone marrow CD34$^+$ stem cells except follicular dendritic cells, for which the origin remains unclear. These cells characteristically have dendritic cell processes and are often highly motile. They usually lack or contain only small amounts of lysosomal enzymes and richly express HLA-DR. They are negative for CD68 (except when activated), CD11c, and CD14. They include indeterminate cells (in skin), Langerhans cells (in skin, especially epidermis), veiled cells (in lymphatics), interdigitating dendritic cells (in paracortex of lymph node), follicular dendritic cells (within lymphoid follicles), and dermal dendritic cells (in the dermis). It is believed that indeterminate cells, Langerhans cells, veiled cells, and interdigitating dendritic cells represent sequential stages of development of a single cell type rather than different cell types,[88,92] although it has also been suggested that indeterminate cells represent members of the epidermal/dermal dendritic cell system during their passage from skin to lymph node.[93] Fibroblastic reticular cells in lymph nodes probably only serve a supporting but not an antigen-presenting function, and their origin is unclear.[88]

Although monocytes-phagocytes and dendritic cells represent two distinct cell types, they are closely related and show overlaps. For example, under extreme conditions, mature monocytes can differentiate into Langerhans cells. The main characteristic of these cells are listed in Table 21–6.

The histiocytic proliferative disorders constitute a complicated subject, which is not unexpected given the marked heterogeneity of the cell types within the histiocyte family. The terminology is confusing because of the plethora of terms that have been invented, especially in the dermatology literature, and lack of proof of the histiocytic nature of some entities christened "histiocytosis" (such as malignant histiocytosis and regressing atypical histiocytosis). In fact, most cases diagnosed in the past as "histiocytic lymphoma" or "malignant histiocytosis" represent lymphomas of B- or T-cell type.[34,94] There are usually only a handful of reported cases for many of the esoteric "histiocytosis," which are often defined more on clinical than pathologic grounds; their relationship with the better defined entities remains unclear. There have been attempts to group the non-malignant histiocytic disorders into (1) Langerhans cell histiocytosis or formerly histiocytosis X and (2) non-Langerhans cell histiocytosis or non-X histiocytosis. The latter includes juvenile xanthogranuloma, benign cephalic histiocytosis, papular xanthoma, multicentric reticulohistiocytosis, xanthoma disseminatum, reticulohistiocytoma, Rosai-Dorfman disease, self-healing reticulohistiocytosis, progressive nodular histiocytosis, necrobiotic xanthogranuloma, and indeterminate cell histiocytosis.[95–101] The proposed classification of the Histiocyte Society is listed in a simplified form in Table 21–7 and compared with the new World Health Organization (WHO) classification.[89,102,103] The latter consists of a much shorter list because reactive disorders are not included.

Tumors of histiocytes (including dendritic cells) are totally unrelated histogenetically with benign or malignant fibrous histiocytoma. The former, with the exception of follicular dendritic cell or fibroblastic reticular cell tumors, are neoplasms of mononuclear-phagocytic cells (within the leukocyte family), which have an origin from bone marrow cells, whereas the latter are mesenchymal neoplasms composed of undifferentiated cells, fibroblastic cells, and myofibroblasts.

Table 21–6. Characteristics of the Various Types of Histiocytes

Cell Type	Characteristic Enzyme or Immunohistochemical Profile	Ultrastructure
Monocyte-phagocyte	$CD68^+$, $S\text{-}100^-$, $CD1a^-$, $CD45^+$, acid phosphatase positive, nonspecific esterase positive	Short cell processes; lysosomes; no Birbeck granules
Follicular dendritic cell	$CD21^+$, $CD35^+$, $S100^{-/+}$, $CD45^-$	Elongated cell processes connected by desmosomes; no Birbeck granules
Interdigitating dendritic cell	$S\text{-}100^+$, $CD1a^-$, $CD45^+$, ATPase positive	Elongated and complex cell processes with interdigitations; no well-formed desmosomes; no Birbeck granules
Langerhans cell	$S\text{-}100^+$, $CD1a^+$, $CD45^+$, ATPase positive	Birbeck granules; no desmosomes
Indeterminate cell	$S\text{-}100^+$, $CD1a^+$, $CD45^+$, ATPase positive	No Birbeck granules
Veiled cell	$S\text{-}100^+$, $CD1a^-$, $CD45^+$, ATPase positive	No Birbeck granules
Dermal dendritic cell (dermal dendrocyte)	Factor $XIIIa^+$, $CD68^+$, $S\text{-}100^-$, $CD45^-$, $CD4^-$	Long dendritic cell processes; no Birbeck granules

ATPase, adenosine triphosphatase.

Table 21–7. Classification of the Histiocytic Proliferations (According to the Histiocyte Society and WHO Classifications[89,102])

Histiocyte Society Classification	New WHO Classification
Disorders of Varied Biologic Behavior 1. Dendritic cell–related • Langerhans cell histiocytosis • Secondary dendritic cell processes (reactive collections of Langerhans cells associated with other diseases) • Juvenile xanthogranuloma and related disorders • Solitary histiocytoma of various dendritic cell phenotypes (e.g., indeterminate cell histiocytosis) 2. Macrophage-related • Hemophagocytic syndromes • Rosai-Dorfman disease • Solitary histiocytoma with macrophage phenotype (e.g., reticulohistiocytoma, multicentric reticulohistiocytosis) *Malignant Disorders* 1. Monocyte-related • Leukemias (acute monocytic, acute myelomonocytic, chronic myelomonocytic) • Extramedullary monocytic tumor 2. Dendritic cell–related histiocytic sarcoma • Follicular dendritic cell sarcoma • Interdigitating dendritic cell sarcoma 3. Macrophage-related histiocytic sarcoma • Histiocytic sarcoma (localized or disseminated)	*Dendritic Cell Neoplasms* • Langerhans cell histiocytosis • Langerhans cell sarcoma • Interdigitating dendritic cell sarcoma or tumor • Follicular dendritic cell sarcoma or tumor • Dendritic cell sarcoma, not otherwise specified *Macrophage or Histiocytic Neoplasm* • Histiocytic sarcoma

Extranodal Rosai-Dorfman Disease

Definition

Rosai-Dorfman disease, also known as sinus histiocytosis with massive lymphadenopathy (SHML), is a nonclonal histiocytic proliferation characterized by large histiocytes with a distinctive morphology and commonly exhibiting emperipolesis.[104,105] Although this disease is generally considered a macrophage-related disease,[102] some authors consider the cell lineage uncertain or a possible relationship with sinus dendritic cell.[89,101,106]

Clinical Presentation and Clinical Course

Rosai-Dorfman disease can affect any age group, but most commonly children and young adults. There is a slight male predominance. Most patients present with lymphadenopathy, but extranodal involvement occurs in 43% of patients as the sole manifestation or in association with nodal disease or other extranodal sites of disease.[104] Among the 423 cases of Rosai-Dorfman disease recorded in the SHML Registry, soft tissue involvement occurs in 38 cases (9%).[104] For this group, the mean age is 43 years, and there is no sex predilection. The preferential sites of involvement are the proximal limbs and trunk.[104,107] The size ranges from 0.5 to 10 cm.[104]

The lesions are usually treated by surgical excision. Approximately half of the patients have persistent disease or develop recurrence, but disease-associated mortality is extremely rare.[104,107,108]

Key Histologic Findings

In soft tissues involved by Rosai-Dorfman disease, as in other extranodal sites involved by this disease, a highly characteristic sinusoid-like pattern is observed even though true sinusoids do not exist: pale-staining bands of cells (rich in histiocytes) alternate with darkstaining bands (rich in lymphocytes and plasma cells) as shown in Figure 21–31. Examination of the pale-staining areas at high magnification reveals the distinctive histiocytes of Rosai-Dorfman disease. The histiocytes are much larger than conventional histiocytes; their diameter is usually in the range of

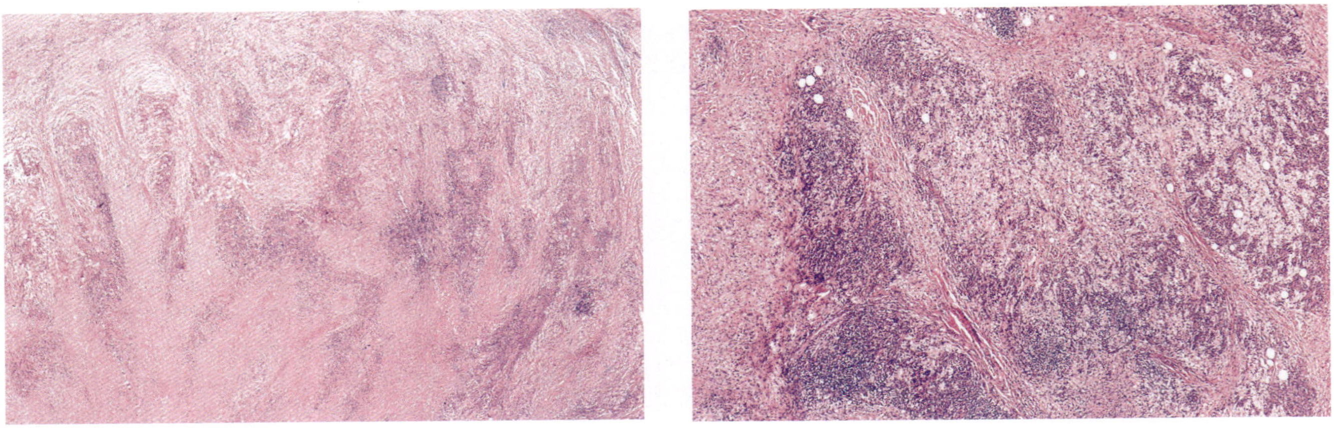

A B

Figure 21–31. Rosai-Dorfman disease of soft tissue. *A* and *B*, Two different examples illustrating the highly characteristic low-magnification appearance of blue stripes alternating with whitish/pinkish stripes.

6 to 12 times that of a lymphocyte nucleus (compared with 3–6 times for conventional histiocytes). The large size of the histiocytes is attributable to the presence of voluminous pale cytoplasm. The histiocytes possess centrally or eccentrically located round nuclei with vesicular chromatin and a central distinct nucleolus (Figs. 21–32 and 21–33). Occasional cells may display atypical enlarged or hyperchromatic nuclei (Fig. 21–33*B*). The pale and delicate cytoplasm of the histiocytes can impart a reticulated to fibrillary appearance, reminiscent of neural tissue. Some cells contain apparently intact lymphocytes or plasma cells in the cytoplasm, a phenomenon often referred to as emperipolesis or lymphophagocytosis. Although emperipolesis is a characteristic feature of Rosai-Dorfman disease, it is not worth spending too much time looking for this phenomenon, which is often difficult owing to problems in defining the cell borders of the histiocytes. It will be much easier to identify the histiocyte cell bodies and emperipolesis in a slide immunostained for S-100 protein. Rarely, small foci of suppuration or necrosis can be present. Plasma cells are always abundant. If they are difficult to find, the presumptive diagnosis of Rosai-Dorfman disease is probably wrong.

In the late involutional phase, the distinctive histiocytes are reduced in number, and conventional histiocytes, foamy histiocytes, and myofibroblasts are often increased, accompanied by fibrosis. The Rosai-Dorfman disease histiocytes entrapped in the fibrous tissue sometimes assume a spindly configuration (Fig. 21–33*C*). In this stage, the histologic features

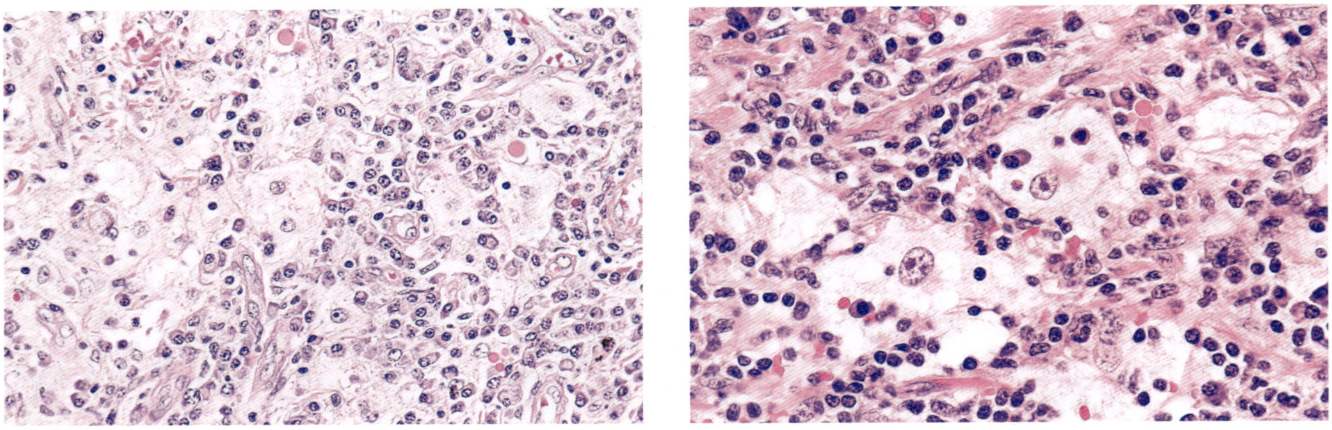

A B

Figure 21–32. Rosai-Dorfman disease of soft tissue, cytologic features of histiocytes. *A*, Typically, groups of pale-staining histiocytes are found among clusters or bands of plasma cells. *B*, The histiocytes are typically very large, usually more than eight times the diameter of a lymphocyte nucleus. The nuclei are often centrally placed, round and vesicular, with a distinct central nucleolus. The cytoplasm is very pale and almost "watery." Some histiocytes contain intracytoplasmic lymphocytes or plasma cells (emperipolesis).

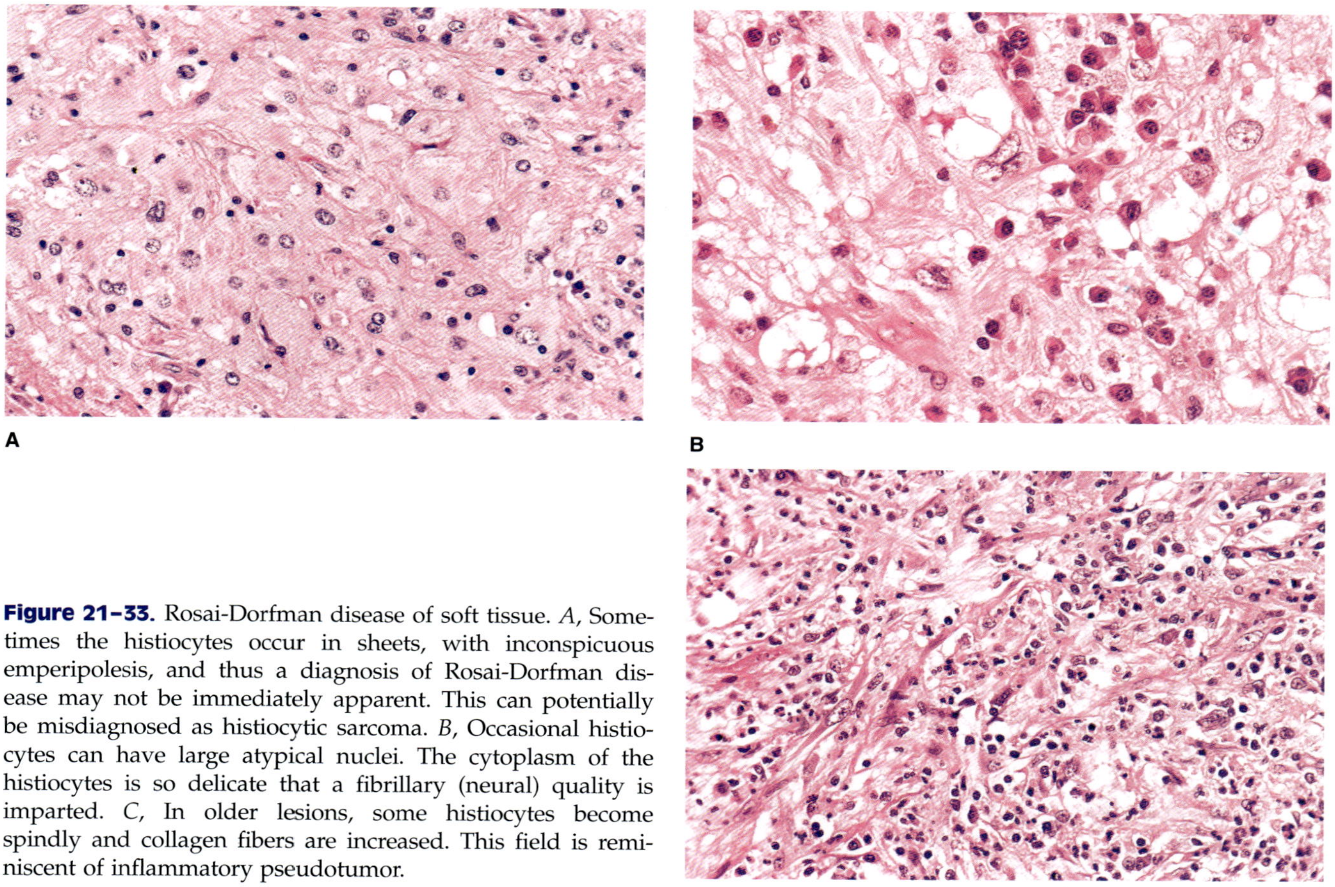

Figure 21–33. Rosai-Dorfman disease of soft tissue. *A*, Sometimes the histiocytes occur in sheets, with inconspicuous emperipolesis, and thus a diagnosis of Rosai-Dorfman disease may not be immediately apparent. This can potentially be misdiagnosed as histiocytic sarcoma. *B*, Occasional histiocytes can have large atypical nuclei. The cytoplasm of the histiocytes is so delicate that a fibrillary (neural) quality is imparted. *C*, In older lesions, some histiocytes become spindly and collagen fibers are increased. This field is reminiscent of inflammatory pseudotumor.

may mimic inflammatory pseudotumor or fibrous histiocytoma.

Immunohistochemical Profile

A diagnosis of Rosai-Dorfman disease can be readily confirmed by immunostaining for S-100 protein, whereby both the nucleus and cytoplasm of the large histiocytes are intensely stained (Fig. 21–34).[104] The phenomenon of emperipolesis is much easier to appreciate in this immunostain because the cell bodies of the individual histiocytes are highlighted, whereas the nuclei of the lymphocytes and plasma cells within the cytoplasm of the histiocytes stand out because of negative staining. CD68 is positive, but is not required for diagnosis. CD1a is negative.

Differential Diagnosis

Rosai-Dorfman disease of the soft tissues is most often misdiagnosed as *inflammatory pseudotumor, fibrohistiocytic tumor*, or *nonspecific chronic inflammation*, especially in the later phases of the lesion. The strongest clues to the correct diagnosis are the characteristic alternating pale and dark bands, which recapitulate the dilated sinusoid-like pattern in lymph nodes. Whenever this pattern is seen (irrespective of site), the possibility of Rosai-Dorfman disease must be seriously considered. The diagnosis can be confirmed by finding the diagnostic histiocytes and by performing an S-100 protein immunostain.

In some cases, scattered histiocytes in Rosai-Dorfman disease may exhibit nuclear atypia or hyperchromasia, raising the differential diagnosis of *histiocytic sarcoma*. In contrast to the latter, cytologic atypia is seen in only a minority of cells and the histiocytes characteristically occur in bands and islands separated by collections of plasma cells.

Histiocytic Sarcoma

Definition and Nomenclature

Histiocytic sarcoma is a malignant neoplasm showing macrophage differentiation.[103,109] It is also known as true histiocytic lymphoma; the prefix "true" is applied to emphasize its distinction from "histiocytic

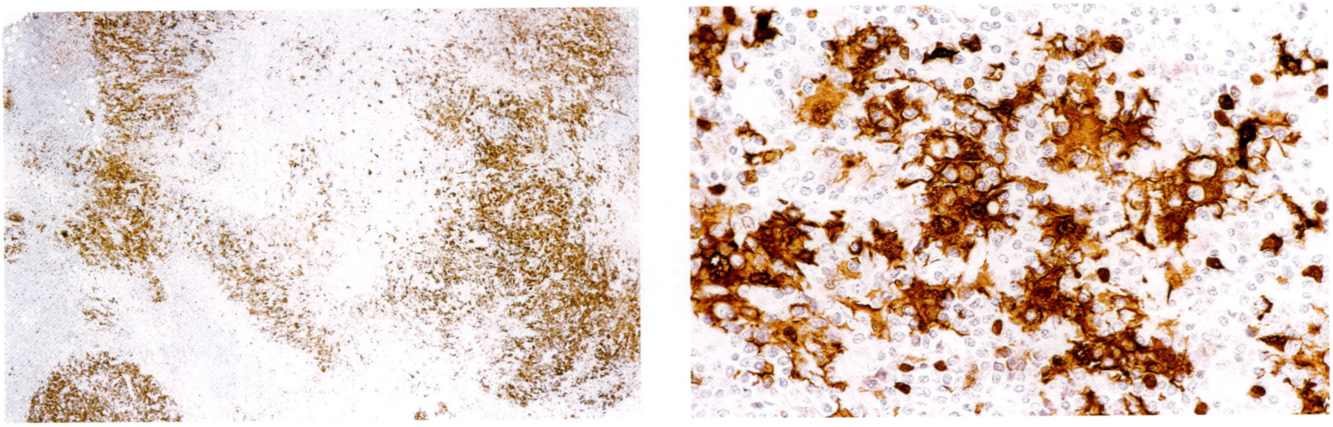

A B

Figure 21–34. Rosai-Dorfman disease of soft tissue, immunostained for S-100 protein. *A*, Characteristically, the positive cells occur in the form of bands, accentuating the sinusoid-like pattern. *B*, The individual histiocytes are well highlighted because the cell bodies are positively stained. The nuclei are also stained. The emperipolesis phenomenon becomes obvious in the form nonstaining "holes" in the cytoplasm of the histiocytes.

lymphoma" as used in the older literature, which, in fact, represents conventional large cell lymphoma of B or T lineage. The term "histiocytic sarcoma" is preferred to "histiocytic lymphoma" even though the clinical presentation and initial morphologic impression of this tumor is often that of a large cell lymphoma, because this is a disease of histiocytes and not lymphoid cells.

Clinical Presentation and Clinical Course

Histiocytic sarcoma is very rare. It can occur over a wide age range, with a mean age of 44 years.[110–113] The disease presents in lymph nodes or extranodal sites, such as soft tissue. Most patients have high-stage disease at presentation. In rare cases, the histiocytic sarcoma develops within a few years of a diagnosis of lymphoblastic lymphoma/leukemia or mediastinal germ cell tumor; limited molecular analysis suggests that the histiocytic lymphoma is clonally related to the prior malignancy.[114–121]

Histiocytic sarcoma is aggressive, with most patients dying from disseminated disease within 2 years. According to a series of 12 patients (including cases from various sites), 7 (58%) died of disease and 2 (17%) were alive with disease.[110]

Key Histologic Findings

The neoplasm is permeative, with destruction and replacement of normal tissues. The neoplastic cells are typically very large, with abundant eosinophilic cytoplasm that may show fine vacuoles (Fig. 21–35). The nuclei are eccentrically placed, with round, oval, irregular, or grooved contour and delicate or coarse chromatin. Nucleoli are often small and multiple. Some neoplastic cells can be spindly or multinucleated. The degree of cellular pleomorphism is highly variable from case to case. Phagocytosis of red cells or lymphocytes is very rare. There can be variable admixtures of lymphocytes, plasma cells, neutrophils, and eosinophils, sometimes to the extent that the neoplastic cells are masked.[122] In rare cases, a myxoid or spindly cell (sarcomatoid) growth pattern can be observed.[123]

Immunohistochemical Profile

The neoplastic cells are immunoreactive for the histiocyte/monocyte-associated antigens CD68 and lysozyme, in a granular pattern (Fig. 21–35*D*).[110] Among the CD68 antibodies, PGM1 is more specific than KP1 because myeloid cells are not stained.[124] The neoplastic cells should be negative for T-cell, B-cell, myeloid cell, and follicular dendritic cell markers, as well as CD1a. Nonetheless, the T-cell–associated markers CD43 and CD45RO are frequently positive, which is not surprising because these markers are also normally positive in histiocytes. The neoplastic cells show variable expression of histiocyte/monocyte-associated markers such as CD4, CD11c, CD14, and CD15. CD45 (leukocyte common antigen) staining is variable. Some cases can be S-100 protein positive, but the staining is often focal or weak.[109,110]

Ultrastructurally Important Diagnostic Features

Ultrastructurally, the neoplastic cells show short villous cell processes, but do not exhibit interdigitating cell processes or cell junctions. The Golgi apparatus is prominent, and many primary and secondary

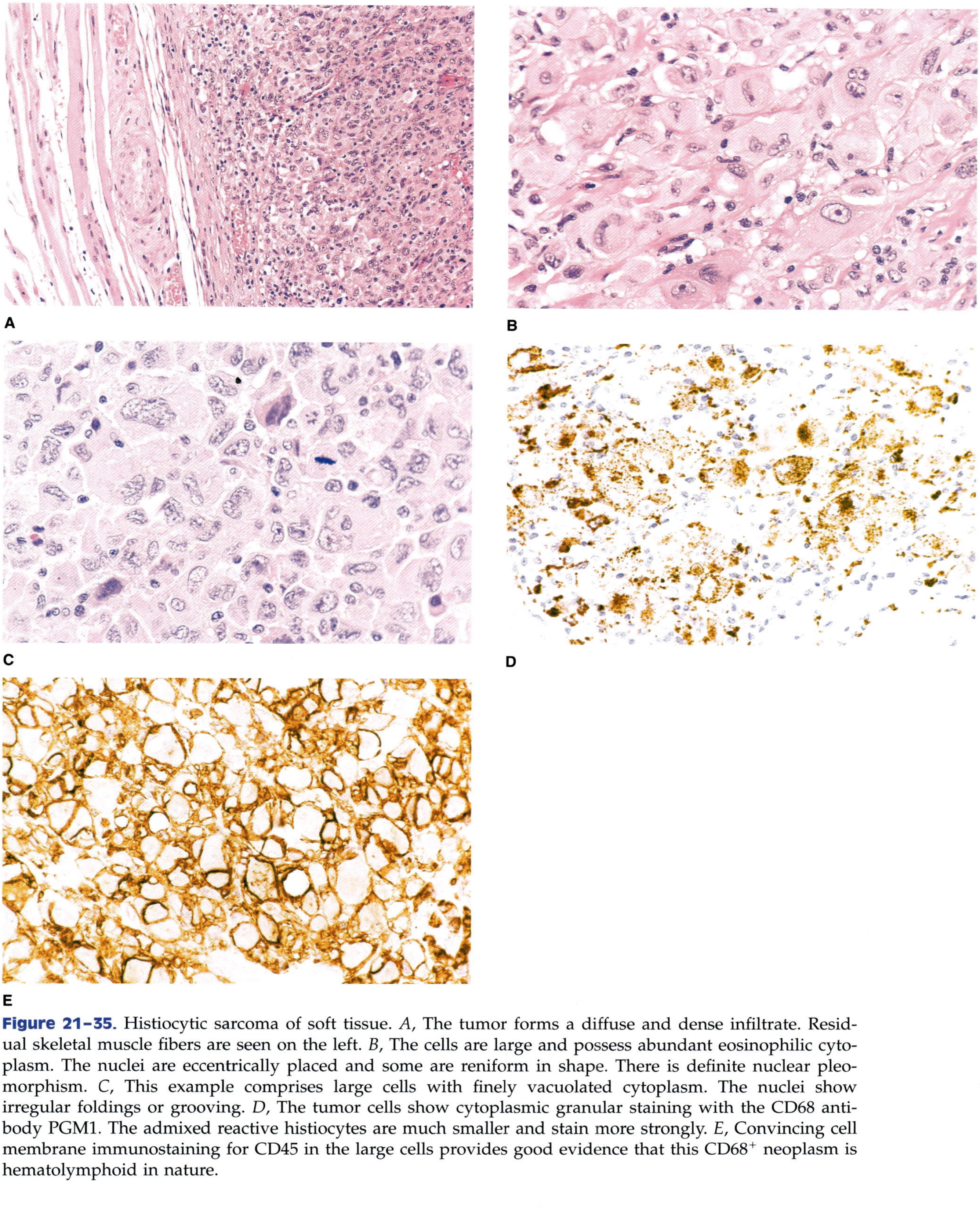

Figure 21–35. Histiocytic sarcoma of soft tissue. *A*, The tumor forms a diffuse and dense infiltrate. Residual skeletal muscle fibers are seen on the left. *B*, The cells are large and possess abundant eosinophilic cytoplasm. The nuclei are eccentrically placed and some are reniform in shape. There is definite nuclear pleomorphism. *C*, This example comprises large cells with finely vacuolated cytoplasm. The nuclei show irregular foldings or grooving. *D*, The tumor cells show cytoplasmic granular staining with the CD68 antibody PGM1. The admixed reactive histiocytes are much smaller and stain more strongly. *E*, Convincing cell membrane immunostaining for CD45 in the large cells provides good evidence that this $CD68^+$ neoplasm is hematolymphoid in nature.

lysosomes are present. Besides some mitochondria and occasional lipid droplets, other organelles are rare.

Genetic Changes

Molecular studies show no rearrangements of the immunoglobulin and T-cell receptor genes. So far, no specific cytogenetic or molecular aberrations have been found. There is no known association with EBV.

Differential Diagnosis

It can be difficult to distinguish between histiocytic sarcoma and *large cell lymphoma* on morphologic grounds, and immunohistochemical studies are required. The former should be suspected whenever the neoplastic cells exhibit voluminous eosinophilic rather than amphophilic cytoplasm.

Extramedullary monocytic tumor is a localized tumor of acute monocytic leukemia and can sometimes be the first manifestation of the leukemia. The distinction from histiocytic sarcoma is not always sharp because both are composed of monocytes/histiocytes with an identical immunophenotype. Nonetheless, the former often shows a more monotonous population of smaller neoplastic cells (Fig. 21–36).

For cases that express S-100 protein, the differential diagnosis of *interdigitating dendritic cell sarcoma* has to be considered. Histiocytic sarcoma is predominantly composed of ovoid cells, while interdigitating dendritic cell sarcomas are usually composed of spindly cells (although some can be composed of ovoid cells). Additional features favoring the latter diagnosis include presence of long dendritic cell processes as shown on S-100 protein immunostaining or ultrastructural examination, more diffuse and strong staining for S-100 protein, and variable and often weaker staining for CD68.

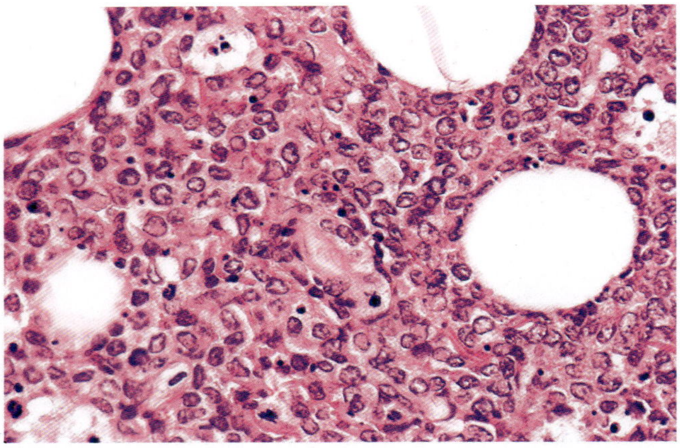

Figure 21–36. Extramedullary monocytic tumor of soft tissue (localized presentation of acute monocytic leukemia). Compared with histiocytic sarcoma (Fig. 21–35), the neoplastic cells appear more monotonous and smaller. The nuclei have a blastic appearance.

Although positive staining for CD68 is characteristic of histiocytic sarcoma, this is not entirely specific. Because CD68 antibodies stain lysosome-related proteins, *nonhistiocytic tumors* containing lysosomes can also be positive, such as granular cell tumor, malignant melanoma, and angiomatoid fibrous histiocytoma.[125–127] Thus, a diagnosis of histiocytic sarcoma is not secure enough based on CD68 immunoreactivity alone. It is important to confirm that the neoplastic cells are indeed hematolymphoid in lineage (such as by looking for CD45, CD43, or CD4 expression), exclude other forms of histiocytic neoplasms, and exclude myeloid leukemia (see Fig. 21–35*E*).[122]

Mycobacterial Spindle Cell Pseudotumor and Histoid Leprosy

Clinical Presentation

Mycobacterial spindle cell pseudotumor is a tumor-like lesion characterized by accumulation of spindly histiocytes engorged with mycobacterial microorganisms, most commonly *Mycobacterium aviumintracellulare* complex.[128] This disease is seen most often in immunocompromised patients, especially those with AIDS, who present with a mass lesion in the soft tissues, skin, lymph node, or other sites.[129,130]

Histoid leprosy is an uncommon variant of lepromatous leprosy believed to be related to secondary or primary resistance of dapsone therapy.[131] It is clinically characterized by the presence of multiple nodules in the subcutis or dermis.

Key Histologic Findings

Mycobacterial spindle cell pseudotumor is noncircumscribed and comprises spindly cells disposed haphazardly or in short fascicles. The spindly cells possess uniform oval to elongated nuclei with fine chromatin and a moderate amount of eosinophilic cytoplasm that often exhibits a fibrillary or granular quality (Fig. 21–37). They are histiocytes and are thus immunoreactive for CD68. There are usually few admixed lymphocytes or plasma cells. In touch preparations stained with Giemsa, a highly characteristic appearance is the nonstaining streaks in the

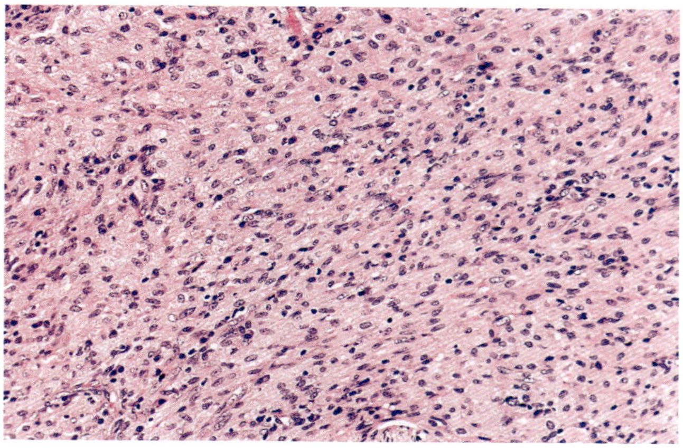

Figure 21–37. Mycobacterial spindle cell pseudotumor. Spindly histiocytes with eosinophilic cytoplasm form fascicles, mimicking smooth muscle, fibrohistiocytic, or dendritic cell tumor.

cytoplasm of the spindly cells created by the intracytoplasmic mycobacteria.[132] The diagnosis is readily confirmed by a Ziehl-Neelsen stain, whereby myriads of acid-fast bacilli are found within the spindly cells.

Histoid leprosy comprises spindly histiocytes forming an expansile nodule. The histiocytes are engorged with the leprosy bacilli.[133] Thus, in a broad sense it is also a form of mycobacterial spindle cell pseudotumor, the only difference being that the bacilli represent *Mycobacterium leprae* and are thus usually positive with Wade-Fite stain but not Ziehl-Neelsen stain.

Differential Diagnosis

Because of the compact arrangement of the spindly cells and the eosinophilia of the cytoplasm, the lesion can potentially be misdiagnosed as a *smooth muscle tumor*. To complicate matters, the spindly cells can show immunoreactivity for desmin.[134] A high index of suspicion for an infective etiology should always be held for an immunocompromised host, and an acid-fast stain permits the correct diagnosis to be reached. Of note, smooth muscle tumors occurring in immunocompromised hosts are associated with EBV, whereas mycobacterial spindle cell pseudotumor is not.[135]

Demonstration of the histiocytic nature of the spindly cells (CD68$^+$) and large numbers of acid-fast bacilli also rule out *inflammatory myofibroblastic tumor*, *fibrous histiocytoma*, and *Kaposi sarcoma*. Mycobacterial spindle cell pseudotumor can also be potentially mistaken for the *follicular dendritic cell sarcoma or interdigitating dendritic cell sarcoma*.

Malakoplakia

Nature of Disease and Clinical Presentation

Malakoplakia is an uncommon and apparently ineffective form of histiocytic reaction to an infection, mostly commonly *Escherichia coli*, and sometimes *Klebsiella, Staphylococcus aureus, Rhodococcus equi*, or other bacteria. The bacteria ingested by the histiocytes are only partially digested and thus accumulate in the lysosomes.[136,137]

Malakoplakia most commonly involves the urogenital tract and alimentary tract, but any site of the body can be affected, including somatic soft tissue, subcutaneous tissue, and retroperitoneum. In the soft tissues, the presentation is usually that of chronic suppuration leading to formation of sinus tract.[136,138–142] The disease can often be successfully controlled by antibiotics with or without surgical excision.[143]

Key Histologic Findings

The lesion is noncircumscribed and comprises diffuse sheets of large round or oval histiocytes (so-called von Hansemann cells) with abundant eosinophilic cytoplasm that contains remarkable numbers of variable-sized eosinophilic granules, which are positive for diastase-periodic acid Schiff (PAS) and which ultrastructurally correspond to phagolysosomes (some containing partially digested bacteria).[136] Some cells can be vacuolated. The diagnostic hallmark of malakoplakia is the Michaelis-Gutmann bodies, which are basophilic targetoid inclusions found within the cytoplasm of the histiocytes or extracellularly; they may mimic nuclei at medium magnification (Fig. 21–38). Michaelis-Gutmann bodies are calcospherites that contain calcium and phosphate; they can be highlighted by stains for calcium (such as von Kossa) or iron (such as Perl). Lymphocytes, plasma cells, and neutrophils are usually found in the background.

Differential Diagnosis

Malakoplakia is distinguished from *xanthogranulomatous inflammation* by predominance of histiocytes with coarse eosinophilic granules rather than foamy histiocytes, and presence of Michaelis-Gutmann bodies. *Granular cell tumor* differs from malakoplakia in showing a nested growth pattern, polygonal appearance of the cells, lack of inflammatory component, and lack of Michaelis-Gutmann bodies.

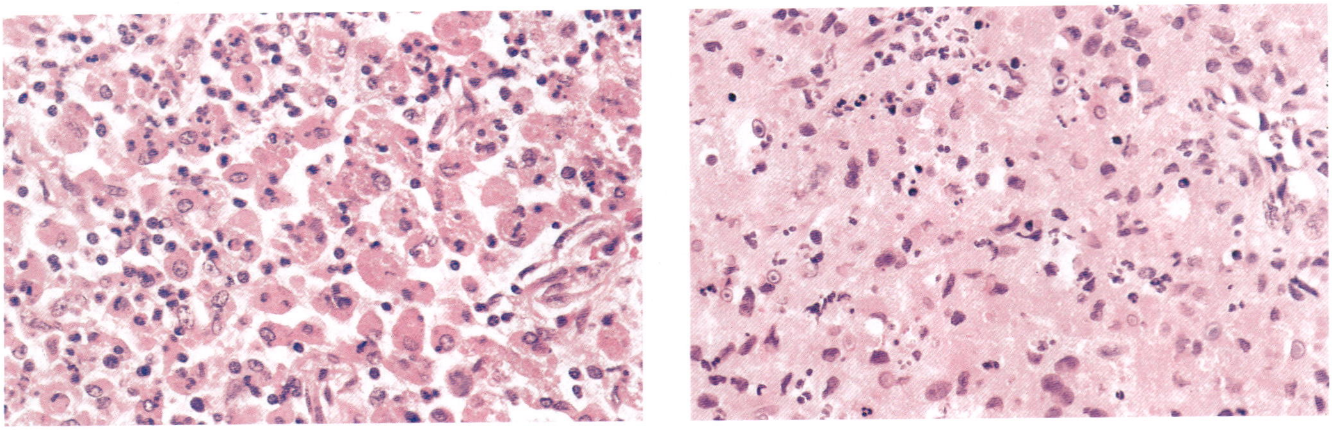

A B

Figure 21–38. Malakoplakia involving soft tissue. *A*, There are many histiocytes with coarsely granular cytoplasm. Many inflammatory cells are interspersed. *B*, In this field, many diagnostic Michaelis-Gutmann bodies are seen: These are basophilic bodies with a targetoid appearance, mimicking nuclei. Note presence of neutrophils among the granular histiocytes.

Histiocytic Reaction to Foreign Materials

Clinical Presentation

Prominent histiocytic reaction to "foreign materials" can result in the formation of mass lesions in the soft tissues. The "foreign materials" can be derived from different routes: (1) endogenous substances released from normal cells, such as lipid extruded from adipose cells (lipogranuloma), or abnormally deposited locally, such as urate (gouty tophus), amyloid (amyloidoma), and cholesterol (cholesterol granuloma); (2) exogenous substances introduced locally, such as joint prosthesis, silicone implants, silica, paraffin implants, hemostatic agents (such as aluminium chloride or oxidized regenerated cellulose);[144,145] (3) exogenous substances introduced via a systemic route, such as polyvinylpyrrolidone (PVP); or through ingestion, such as clofazimine.[146–151] PVP was previously widely used as a plasma expander or "blood tonic" as well as in many intravenous preparations, especially in areas of Asia.[152,153] This is a high-molecular-weight polymer that accumulates in the body after injection because it cannot be excreted or metabolized. PVP histiocytosis (PVP storage disease) is usually an incidental finding, particularly in the reticuloendothelial system, but it can also produce a mass lesion, usually after local injection.[154–156]

Key Histologic Findings

The histologic features differ according to the type of foreign material (Fig. 21–39). Mononuclear histiocytes predominate in some circumstances, whereas foreign body-type giant cells predominate in others. The histiocytes can have nondescript eosinophilic, foamy, eosinophilic granular, or basophilic granular cytoplasm.

Silica reaction in soft tissue results from the now obsolete practice of injection therapy for hernias. Histologically, it can mimic fibrous histiocytoma because the histiocytes are admixed with large amounts of collagen. The histiocytes can sometimes exhibit some degree of nuclear atypia. Birefringent silica particles can be identified in the histiocytes.[157]

Polyvinylpyrrolidone storage disease is characterized by the accumulation of bubbly histiocytes with single or multiple discrete vacuoles having blue-gray rims. The nuclei are often displaced to the periphery, resulting in a signet ring appearance. Sometimes the histiocytes lie in pools of lightly basophilic extracellular PVP (Fig. 21–40). There are usually few or no inflammatory cells in the background. The PVP

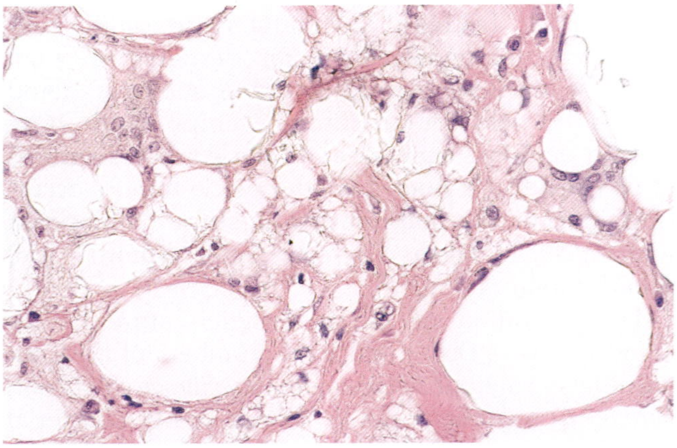

Figure 21–39. Histiocytic reaction to silicone implant. Histiocytes surround apparently empty spaces, which in fact contain films of refractile material characteristic of silicone. Some histiocytes are vacuolated and contain ingested silicone.

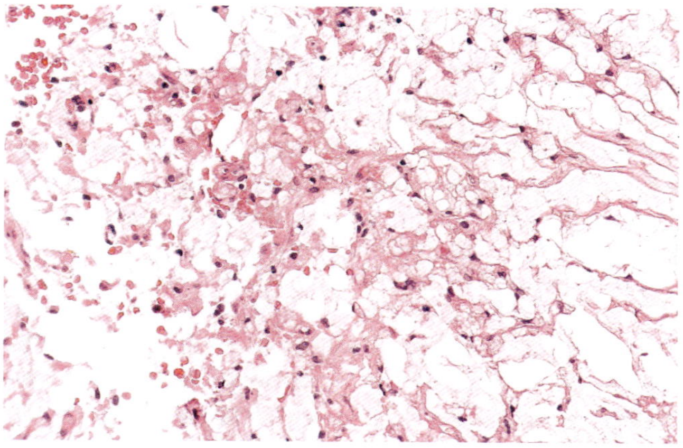

Figure 21–40. Histiocytic reaction to PVP. "Bubbly" histiocytes are suspended in pools of lightly basophilic PVP material.

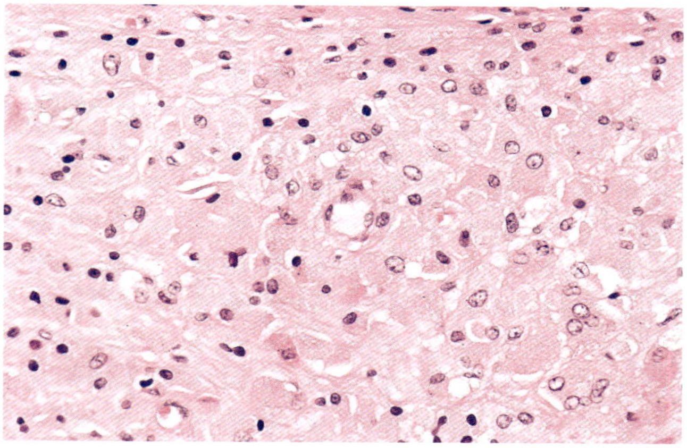

Figure 21–41. Granular histiocytic reaction in the vicinity of a joint prosthesis. There are sheets of histiocytes with bland-looking nuclei and abundant eosinophilic granular cytoplasm.

shows positive histochemical reaction to mucicarmine (hence also known as "mucicarminophilic histiocytosis" and further heightening the mimicry of signet ring cell carcinoma), colloidal iron, Congo red and Sirius red, but not PAS and Alcian blue.[152]

Clofazimine-induced crystal-storing histiocytosis is characterized by clear crystals in the cytoplasm of the histiocytes. The crystals appear clear in conventional histologic sections because they have been dissolved by alcohol and xylene during tissue processing. The crystals appear red in frozen section and show bright-red birefringence.[151]

Diagnosis

On encountering a prominent histiocytic infiltrate, besides the possibility of an infective process, the possibility of histiocytic reaction to foreign materials must be considered. The foreign material is sometimes obvious at the light microscopic level, such as amyloid, urate crystals, and dark-staining metallic granules. If foreign materials are not obvious, closing the condenser of the microscope may reveal refractile materials, such as silicone. Examination under polarizing light will reveal other foreign materials, such as silica and stitch material. Histochemical stains can aid in identifying PVP (see preceding section). The different types of metals can be identified using energy-dispersive x-ray microanalysis.

Granular Histiocytic Reaction

Clinical Presentation

There are two main settings for the occurrence of granular histiocytic reaction: (1) in areas of prior surgical trauma,[158,159] and (2) in the soft tissues adjacent to an implanted prosthesis.[147–150] In the latter circumstance, the histiocytes are recruited to ingest the wear debris derived from the prosthesis materials, such as polyester, polyethylene, and polyformaldehyde.

Key Histologic Findings

Granular histiocytic reaction in the soft tissues is characterized by accumulation of histiocytes with abundant coarsely granular eosinophilic cytoplasm. The granularity results from the presence of large numbers of lysosomes and phagolysosomes (Fig. 21–41).[158,159] The granules are often well highlighted by PAS stain. In cases associated with prosthesis, the histiocytes may in addition contain needle-shaped birefringent particles of polyethylene or birefringent black granules of metal. The histiocytes sometimes surround collections of eosinophilic granular debris. They are immunoreactive for CD68, but not S-100 protein.[148] Granular histiocytic reaction differs from malakoplakia in an inconspicuous inflammatory background and absence of Michaelis-Gutmann bodies.

Xanthogranulomatous Inflammation

Clinical Presentation

Xanthogranulomatous inflammation can occur in various tissues, most commonly the kidney and gallbladder. Rarely, somatic soft tissues or the retroperitoneum can be involved.[160,161] It is usually caused by chronic bacterial infection.

Key Histologic Findings

Xanthogranulomatous inflammation is characterized by a dense infiltrate of foamy histiocytes with abundant pale-staining, finely vacuolated cytoplasm. The

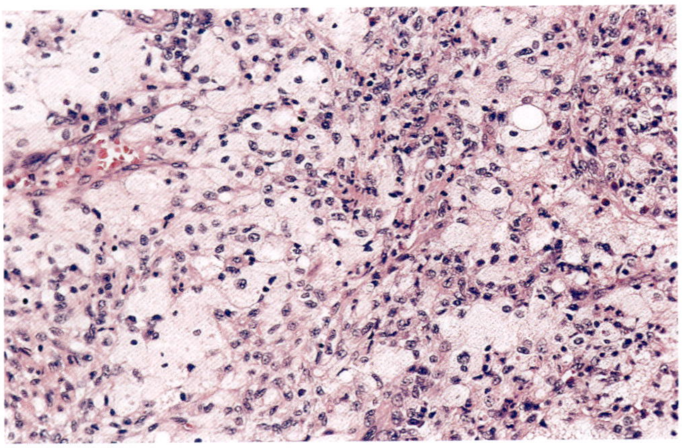

Figure 21–42. Xanthogranulomatous inflammation of soft tissue, characterized by numerous foamy histiocytes admixed with mixed inflammatory cells.

nuclei of the histiocytes are centrally or eccentrically located and are small. There are often some admixed histiocytes with eosinophilic or granular cytoplasm, especially in the early stages (Fig. 21–42).[160] Michaelis-Gutmann bodies are not found. There are frequently admixed lymphocytes, plasma cells and neutrophils, sometimes with abscess formation. Fibrosis is commonly present, especially in long-standing lesions.

Differential Diagnosis

For any unexplained xanthogranulomatous process, the possibility of *Erdheim-Chester disease* must be excluded (see later discussion). It is also prudent to scrutinize the histologic sections for an underlying neoplasm, especially *Hodgkin lymphoma*, which can be masked by a prominent component of foamy cells.[162] *Inflammatory malignant fibrous histiocytoma* is often rich in foamy histiocytes, but it can be recognized by the presence of many large atypical ovoid cells with prominent nucleoli.[163–165]

Erdheim-Chester Disease

Clinical Presentation and Clinical Course

This is an uncommon systemic disorder characterized by symmetrical osteosclerosis of the diaphysis and metaphysis of the long bones and xanthogranulomatous infiltration in bones and various tissues.[166–168] The cause for this disease is not known, and postulations have included primary metabolic (lipid storage) disease or a reactive nonspecific inflammatory condition. A recent molecular study using X-chromosome inactivation pattern has found this disease to be a clonal (neoplastic) disorder, perhaps representing the macrophage counterpart of Langerhans cell histiocytosis.[168]

The disease affects adults, usually over the age of 40 years. The most common presenting symptom is bone pain, and x-ray shows bilateral symmetrical osteosclerosis affecting the metaphyseal and diaphyseal regions of long bones, in particular the distal femur, proximal tibia, and proximal fibula. Extraosseous lesions are common, such as the hypothalamus and posterior pituitary (presenting as diabetes insipidus), orbit (proptosis), eyelid (xanthoma-like lesion), lung (dyspnea), brain, dura, retroperitoneum, perirenal tissue, pericardium, and pleura. Systemic symptoms such as fever, malaise, and weight loss can also be present. Over half of the patients die from the disease, some within 6 months.[169]

Key Histologic Findings

Erdheim-Chester disease is characterized by accumulation of foamy histiocytes with round or oval nuclei and abundant finely vacuolated cytoplasm. Scattered Touton-type giant cells are often present. Granuloma is not formed. The background shows variable numbers of lymphocytes and plasma cells, and frequently fibrosis (Fig. 21–43).

Immunohistochemical Profile

The proliferated histiocytes are immunoreactive for CD68. S-100 protein is usually negative, but can occasionally be positive, whereas CD1a is consistently negative.[166,167] The findings suggest that the

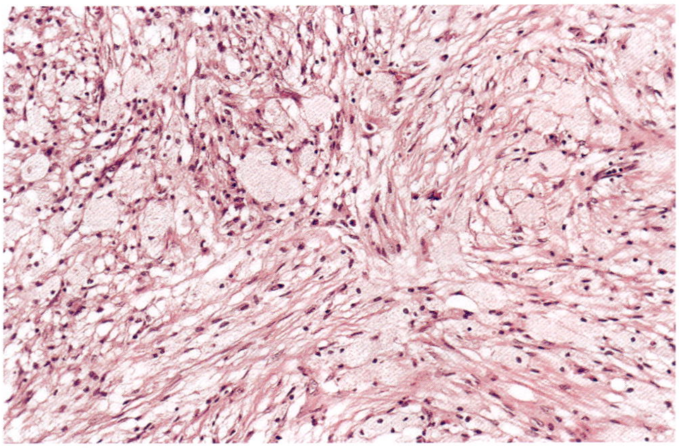

Figure 21–43. Erdheim-Chester disease. This disease is characterized by foamy histiocytes admixed with delicate collagen fibers and some lymphocytes.

histiocytes belong to the monocyte-phagocyte rather than dendritic cell series.[166]

Differential Diagnosis

Although there is clinical overlap with *Langerhans cell histiocytosis* in that diabetes insipidus and exophthalmos can constitute a component of the syndrome, Erdheim-Chester disease is distinguished by occurrence in an older age group, predominantly osteosclerotic rather than osteolytic lesions, a different morphology of the histiocytes, and an S-100/CD1a-immunophenotype.

Erdheim-Chester disease can be distinguished from other *xanthogranulomatous inflammatory processes* by the clinical findings, in particular the presence of osteosclerotic bone lesions.

Crystal-Storing Histiocytosis Mimicking Adult Rhabdomyoma

Clinical Presentation

In rare cases of immunoglobulin-secreting B-cell neoplasms, such as lymphoplasmacytic lymphoma, extranodal marginal zone B-cell lymphoma or plasmacytoma/myeloma, the secreted immunoglobulin molecules crystallize to form needle-shaped structures, which are then phagocytosed by histiocytes. Accumulation of the crystals in the histiocytes result in a remarkable resemblance to skeletal muscle cells.[170] The clinical features and outcome vary according to the underlying neoplastic B-cell proliferation. Many different sites can be involved, such as lymph node, head and neck mucosal sites, lung, skin, and soft tissue.[170-175]

Key Histologic Findings

The clusters and sheets of crystal-containing histiocytes often mask the underlying lymphoma.[170-175] They are spindly ("straplike") or polygonal, and contain a single bland-looking eccentrically placed nucleus or multiple nuclei. The abundant cytoplasm contains sheaves of brightly eosinophilic, rod-shaped crystals with pointed ends. The packed crystals result in a remarkable resemblance to the striations seen in adult rhabdomyoma cells (Fig. 21–44). The crystals can be readily highlighted by diastase-PAS or phosphotungstic acid hematoxylin stain. The histiocytes are immunoreactive for CD68 and monotypic immunoglobulin, but not myoid markers such as desmin and myoglobin.

Intimately admixed with the histiocytes or forming separate aggregates are neoplastic B cells, which usually comprise small lymphocytes, lymphoplasmacytoid cells, and mature plasma cells. Some plasma cells can contain Dutcher bodies or cytoplasmic crystals. The lymphoid cells and plasma cells can be shown on immunostaining to express monotypic immunoglobulin and variably B-lineage markers.

Differential Diagnosis

Crystal-storing histiocytosis shows many morphologic similarities with *adult rhabdomyoma*. The distinguishing features include presence of a monoclonal lymphoid/plasmacytic infiltrate, cytoplasmic striations produced by PAS^+ crystals instead of PAS^-

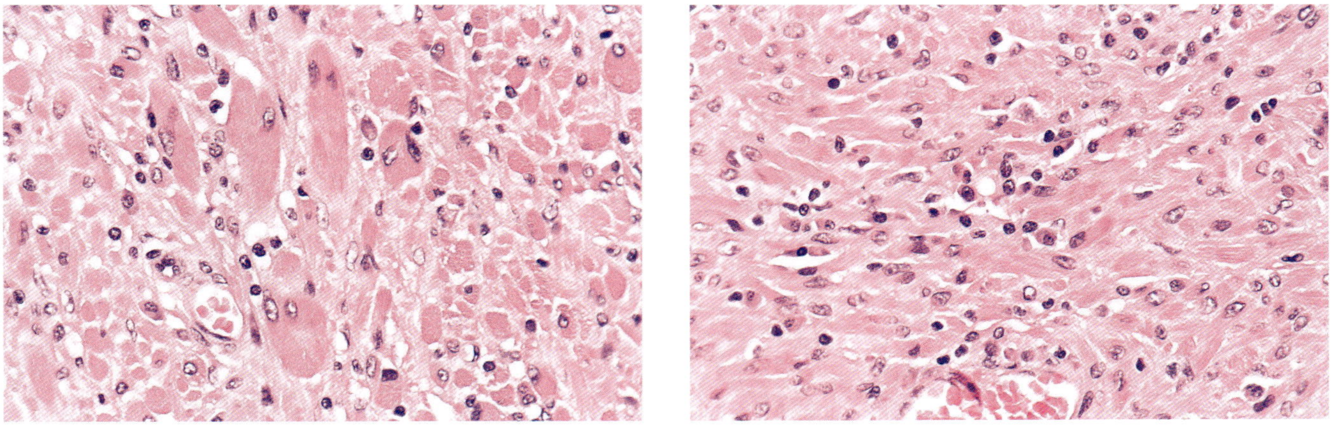

A B

Figure 21–44. Crystal storage histiocytosis associated with lymphoplasmacytic lymphoma, resembling adult rhabdomyoma. *A*, The multinucleated giant cells containing crystals result in a striking resemblance to rhabdomyoma cells. *B*, Most crystal-containing histiocytes resemble strap cells with striations. Some neoplastic lymphocytes and plasma cells are intermingled with the histiocytes.

myoid filaments, lack of glycogen-rich granular or vacuolated cytoplasm as typical of rhabdomyoma cells, and cells demonstrating a histiocytic rather than myoid immunophenotype.[170]

Xanthoma

Clinical Presentation

Xanthoma is a nonneoplastic collection of lipid-laden macrophages, but lacking features of other defined tumor types or inflammatory processes that are rich in foamy cells.[163,176,177] It usually occurs in a setting of primary hyperlipidemia or secondary hyperlipidemia (such as diabetes, primary biliary cirrhosis), but some cases do not show such an association. Many different forms of xanthoma are recognized, and they differ in the clinical presentation and association with specific types of hyperlipidemia:

1. Tuberous xanthoma, characterized by nodular masses around the elbows, knees, or fingers
2. Tendinous xanthoma, characterized by involvement of the extensor tendons of the hands, knees, elbows and Achilles tendon
3. Eruptive xanthoma, characterized by myriads of small yellow papules over the extensor sufaces of the limbs and the buttock
4. Xanthelasma, characterized by small yellow patches in the eyelids
5. Plane xanthoma, characterized by involvement of the skin folds, such as the palm

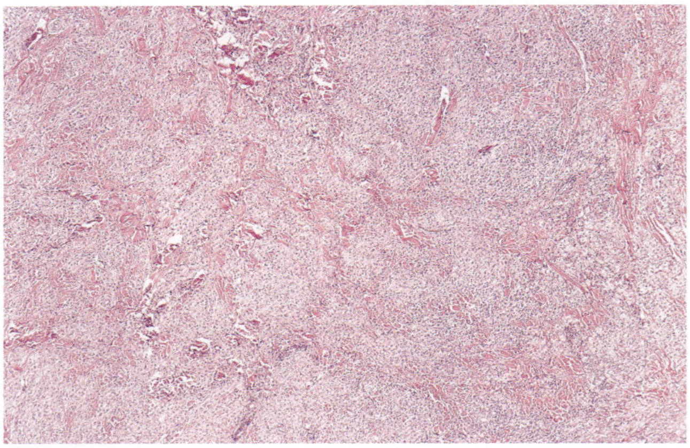

A

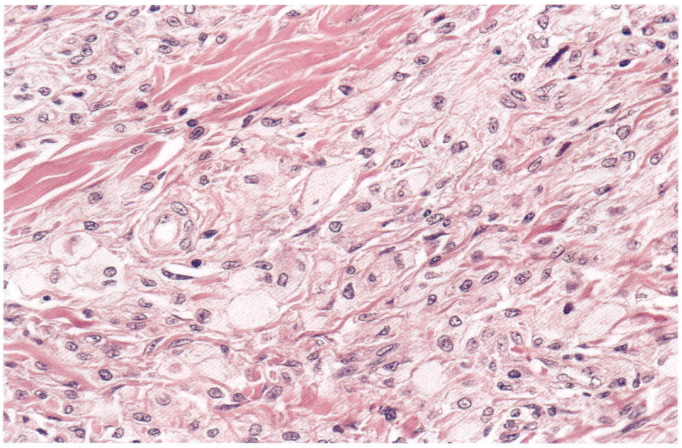

B

Figure 21–45. Tuberous xanthoma. *A*, Large collections of foamy histiocytes are traversed by thin sclerotic bands. *B*, Note the uniform appearance of the foamy histiocytes and paucity of inflammatory cells.

Key Histologic Findings

Xanthoma is characterized by tumorous accumulation of lipid-laden macrophages with finely vacuolated clear to pale cytoplasm. Some nonfoamy macrophages may be present in the early lesions. There can be interspersed multinucleated histiocytes, but inflammatory cells are usually scanty (Fig. 21–45). In tuberous and tendinous xanthoma, commonly collections of cholesterol crystals are admixed with eosinophilic extracellular material, surrounded by foreign body giant cells (Fig. 21–46). Xanthoma is commonly decorated by variable amounts of fibrous tissue, except xanthelasma. In eruptive xanthoma, the foamy histiocytes are accompanied by nonfoamy histiocytes, lymphocytes, neutrophils, and eosinophils. Exceptionally, xanthoma may exhibit a plexiform growth pattern; all such reported cases have so far lacked association with hyperlipidemia (Fig. 21–47).[178,179]

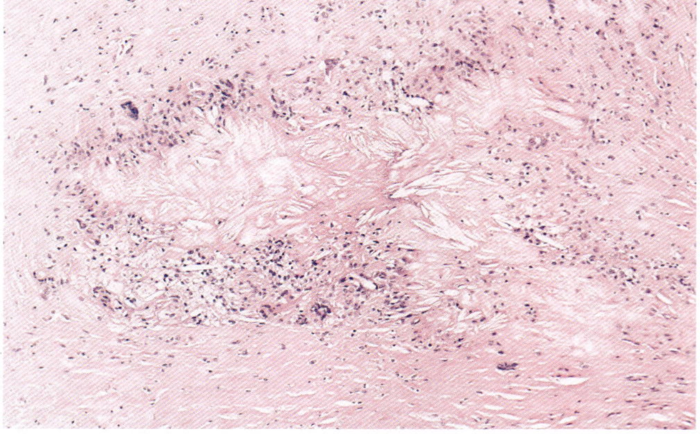

Figure 21–46. Tendinous xanthoma. In xanthomas, there are frequently extracellular deposits of cholesterol crystals, associated with foreign body giant cell reaction around.

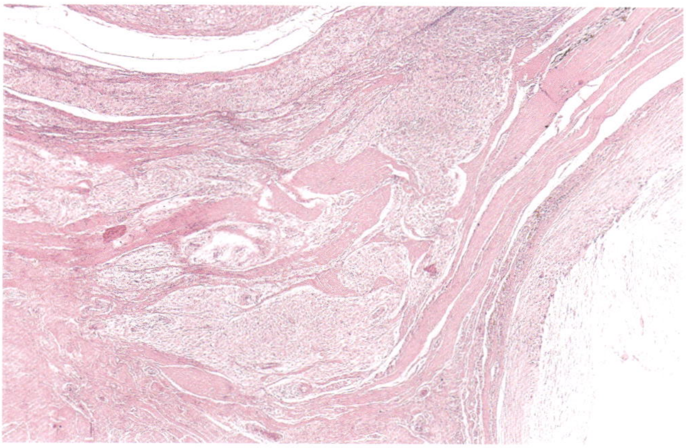

Figure 21-47. Plexiform xanthoma. A plexiform growth pattern is evident in this xanthoma. Note also the presence of extracellular cholesterol crystals *(right field)*.

Differential Diagnosis

The main differential diagnoses include *juvenile xanthogranuloma* and the lipidized form of *benign fibrous histiocytoma*. The distinguishing features of some cutaneous histiocytic proliferations are shown in Table 21–8.

Langerhans Cell Histiocytosis

Clinical Presentation

Langerhans cell histiocytosis (histiocytosis X; eosinophilic granuloma), a monoclonal proliferation of Langerhans cells, can rarely involve soft tissues.[96,180–184] Although it can occur in patients of any age, it is seen most frequently in children.[89,185] Localized or multifocal unisystem disease is associated with a highly favorable prognosis, whereas multisystem disease is associated with significant mortality.

The entity "congenital self-healing reticulohistiocytosis" (Hashimoto-Pritzker disease) is probably a variant of Langerhans cell histiocytosis.[186–191] The patients develop solitary or multiple skin nodules, which spontaneously regress within a few months.

Key Histologic Findings

Proliferated Langerhans cells occur in sheets and clusters.[89,192–194] They typically exhibit oval, deeply grooved, or contorted nuclei, delicate nuclear membrane, fine chromatin, inconspicuous nucleoli, and an appreciable amount of lightly eosinophilic cytoplasm (Fig. 21–48). In contrast to the markedly dendritic appearance of the normal Langerhans cells, they usually have an oval contour. There are commonly interspersed multinucleated giant cells with nuclei morphologically similar to those of the mononuclear cells. Eosinophils are usually present in large numbers, sometimes forming abscesses. Foci of necrosis can be present, particularly in areas with heavy eosinophil infiltration. In long-standing lesions, the number of Langerhans cells is usually decreased, often accompanied by an increase in foamy macrophages and fibrous stroma.

Variant: Langerhans Cell Sarcoma (Sarcomatous Langerhans Cell Histiocytosis)

Langerhans cell sarcoma is characterized by malignant cytologic features and high mitotic activity in the proliferated Langerhans cells, often accompanied by few or no eosinophils (Fig. 21–49). The neoplastic cells show the same immunophenotype of classical Langerhans cell histiocytosis. This variant affects an older age group (mean 40 years) and is more aggressive, with a mortality rate of at least 50%.

Immunohistochemical Profile

The diagnostic immunophenotypic markers for Langerhans cell histiocytosis are S-100 protein and CD1a. The former immunostain decorates the nuclei and cytoplasm of the neoplastic cells, whereas the latter produces cell membrane staining.[34,195–197] The immunophenotype corresponds to that of activated Langerhans cells, and thus some markers not expressed or only expressed in subpopulations of normal Langerhans cells are expressed in this condition (such as macrophage-associated markers).[198] Commonly positive markers are CD4, CD68, HLA-DR, placental alkaline phosphatase, and peanut lectin agglutinin, but it is usually unnecessary to demonstrate these markers for diagnostic purposes.[199–202]

Ultrastructurally Important Diagnostic Features

The pathognomonic organelle of Langerhans cell histiocytosis is the Birbeck granule. It has a tennis-racquet or zipper-like appearance, measuring 200 to 400 nm long and 33 nm wide, with a central striated line and double outer sheath.[194]

Differential Diagnosis

See Table 21–8 for differential diagnosis.

Indeterminate Cell Tumor and Indeterminate Cell Histiocytosis

A small number of cases of indeterminate cell tumor have been reported in the literature. The patients are adults who present with single or multiple skin lesions.[34,88,203–208] Some patients have an antecedent low-grade B-cell neoplasm.

Table 21–8. Distinguishing Features of Some Cutaneous Histiocytic Proliferations

	Langerhans Cell Histiocytosis	Juvenile Xanthogranuloma	Reticulohistiocytoma	Tuberous or Tendinous Xanthoma	Benign Fibrous Histiocytoma, Including Lipidized Form
Age group	Usually children; sometimes adults	Mostly children; sometimes adults	Adults	Adults	Adults
Predilection sites	Skin lesions in scalp, face, neck and trunk	Head and neck, trunk	No predilection site	Around joints	Lower limbs; ankle for the lipidized form
Appearance of histiocytes	Histiocytes with deeply grooved nuclei; foamy histiocytes may be seen in late phase	Foamy histiocytes commonly present; early lesions are rich in nonlipidized histiocytes	Large histiocytes with abundant eosinophilic cytoplasm; usually no foamy histiocytes	Usually uniform population of foamy cells	Many foamy histiocytes in lipidized form
Touton giant cells	Absent	Often prominent	Absent	Absent	Often present
Eosinophils	Common, often abundant and may form abscesses	Common	Common	Absent	Usually absent
Overlying epidermis	Often invaded by histiocytes (epidermotropism)	No epidermotropism; no hyperplasia	No epidermotropism; no hyperplasia	No epidermotropism; no hyperplasia	Hyperplastic
S-100 protein	Positive	Usually negative (positive in up to 30% of cases)	Negative	Negative	Negative
Birbeck granules	Present (by definition)	Absent	Absent	Absent	Absent
Other features	$CD1a^+$	The histiocytes sometimes appear spindly; skin adnexae are often entrapped in the lesion	Rich in multinucleated giant cells, which have randomly arranged nuclei and no lipid vacuoles	Extracellular cholesterol crystal deposits common; association with hyperlipidemia	Storiform pattern, with some admixed fibroblast-like cells; "curl around collagen" pattern at the edges; no entrapped skin adnexae within lesion

Histologically, the tumor cells show oval or deeply grooved nuclei and abundant eosinophilic cytoplasm, similar to Langerhans cell histiocytosis or Langerhans cell sarcoma (Fig. 21–50). They are immunoreactive for S-100 protein and CD1a, but lack Birbeck granules on ultrastructural examination. The clinical course of the disease is highly variable, ranging from disease-free after excisional biopsy to progressive disease and systemic dissemination.

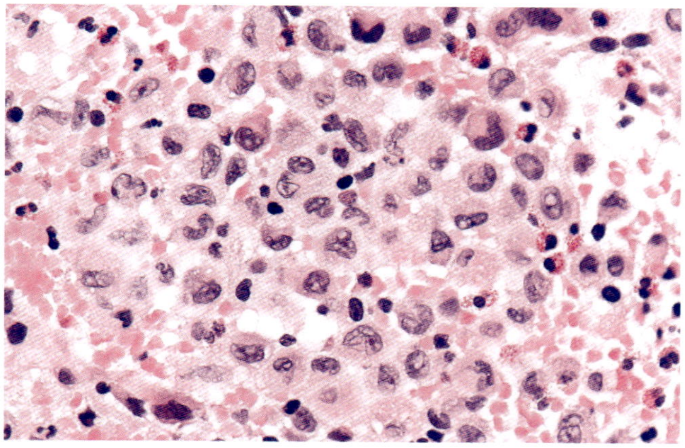

A

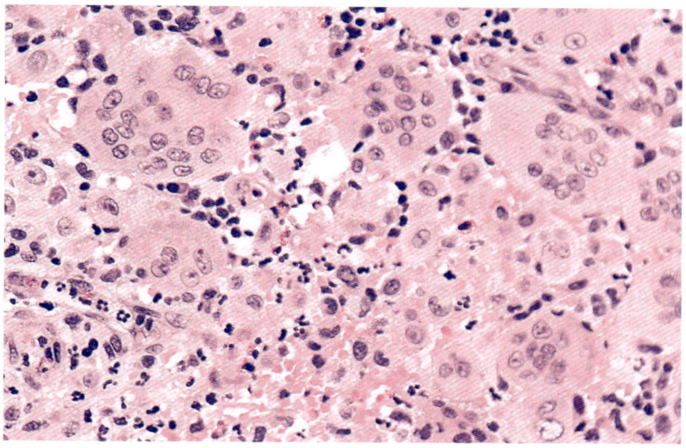

B

Figure 21–48. Langerhans cell histiocytosis involving soft tissue. *A*, Sheets of ovoid cells with deeply grooved nuclei are admixed with eosinophils. Note the well-defined contours of the individual cells. *B*, Multinucleated giant cells are almost always found.

Indeterminate cell histiocytosis, a reactive proliferation of indeterminate cells usually with a benign clinical course, has also been rarely reported in the literature.[95,100,176,208,209] The patients are usually adults, but children can also be affected. They present with numerous small reddish brown papules or nodules, predominantly over the trunk and limbs. Solitary lesions have also been described. Histologically, mononuclear histiocytes with round or grooved nuclei predominate, and giant cells are absent. Some lymphocytes may be intermingled. The histiocytes are immunoreactive for S-100 protein and CD1a, but lack Birbeck granules on ultrastructural examination. The distinction from a neoplasm of indeterminate cells is not sharp, but the lesions tend to be small and superficial.

Follicular Dendritic Cell Sarcoma

Definition

Follicular dendritic cell sarcoma, also known as follicular dendritic cell tumor or dendritic reticulum cell sarcoma/tumor, is a malignant neoplasm showing morphologic, immunohistochemical, and ultrastructural evidence of follicular dendritic cell differentiation.[61,210,211] This diagnosis must be confirmed by special studies.

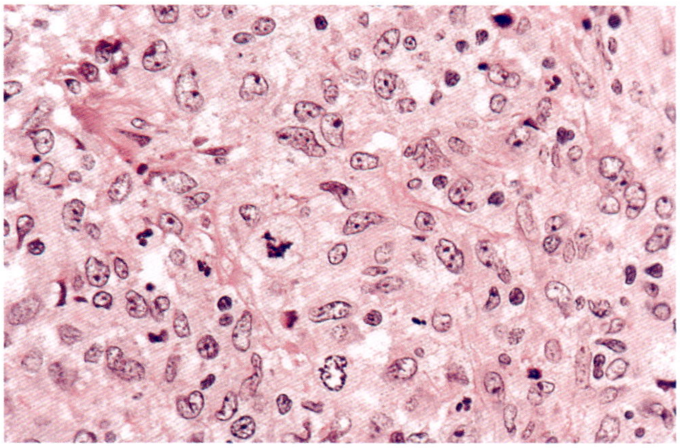

Figure 21–49. Langerhans cell sarcoma. Many tumor cells still show grooved nuclei, reminiscent of Langerhans cells. However, there is definite nuclear pleomorphism, mitotic figures are easily found, and there are no admixed eosinophils.

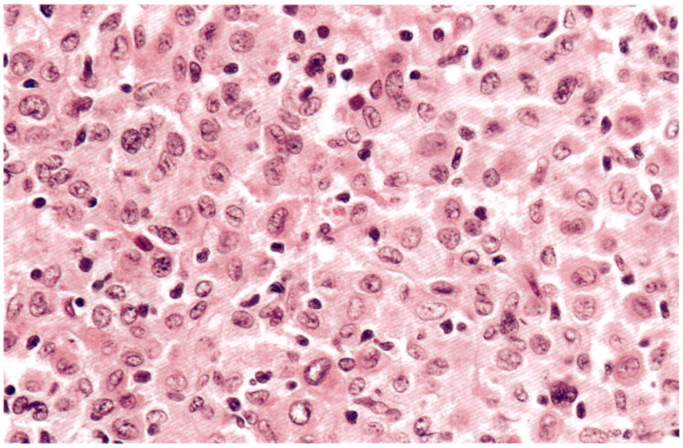

Figure 21–50. Indeterminate cell tumor forming multiple skin nodules. On morphologic grounds, it is not possible to distinguish this tumor from Langerhans cell sarcoma. However, Birbeck granules are not found ultrastructurally (not shown).

Clinical Presentation

Follicular dendritic cell sarcoma affects mostly adults with a mean age of 44 years. There is no sex predilection. Approximately two thirds of patients present as lymphadenopathy, and one third present in extranodal sites, which include, among others, somatic soft tissues.[61,212,213] The tumor usually manifests as a slow-growing mass, which can reach a large size (mean size 7 cm).

Clinical Outcome

As a group, follicular dendritic cell sarcoma often pursues an indolent protracted course, with recurrence occurring in approximately half of the patients, and metastasis in about one third of patients on long-term follow-up. The relapse is not uncommonly delayed, sometimes occurring more than 10 years after the initial diagnosis. Of note, relapses can be repeated and may still be compatible with long sur-

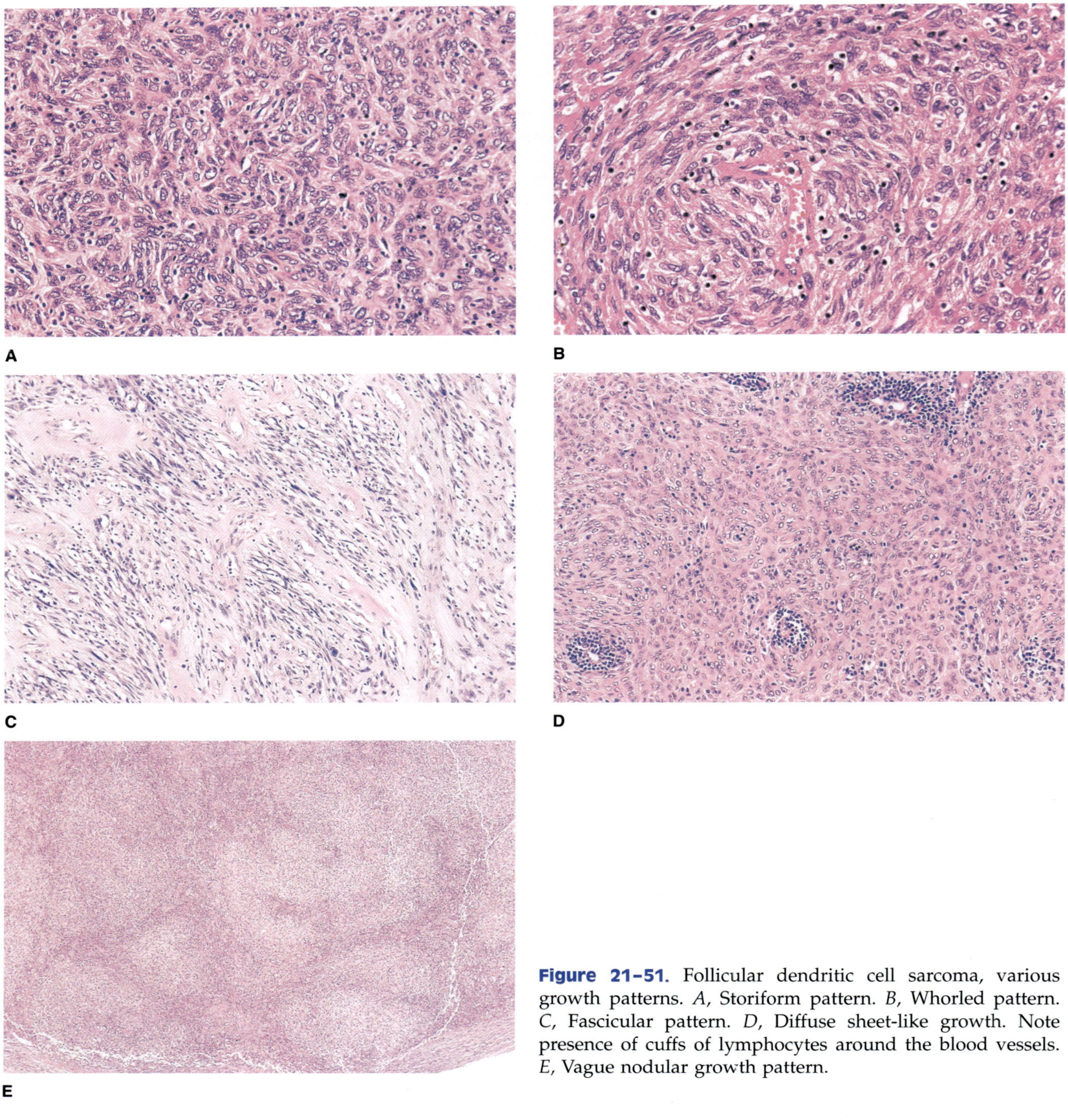

Figure 21–51. Follicular dendritic cell sarcoma, various growth patterns. *A*, Storiform pattern. *B*, Whorled pattern. *C*, Fascicular pattern. *D*, Diffuse sheet-like growth. Note presence of cuffs of lymphocytes around the blood vessels. *E*, Vague nodular growth pattern.

vivals. The lung represents the most common site of distant metastasis.[213] Thus the behavior and pattern of spread are more reminiscent of those of a sarcoma than a lymphoma.[61,214] Occasional cases, particularly those showing "aggressive" histologic features (significant cellular atypia, coagulative necrosis, and frequent mitoses) or those occurring in intra-abdominal sites, can pursue a rapidly fatal course.[61,213–215]

Total surgical excision is the treatment of choice. The value of adjuvant radiotherapy or chemotherapy is still not well defined because of the rarity of this tumor type.

Key Histologic Findings

The tumor typically has smooth borders, invading the tissues in broad fronts. The tumor cells are spindly, plump spindly, or ovoid, forming storiform arrays, circular whorls, fascicles, diffuse sheets, and vague nodules (Fig. 21–51). Occasionally, there are interspersed irregular cleftlike or cystic spaces, mimicking the architectural features of vascular tumors.

The tumor cells characteristically have poorly defined cell borders at the light microscopic level attributable to the presence of numerous interdigitating villous cell processes, which also explain the fibrillary quality observed in the eosinophilic cytoplasm. The tumor cell nuclei often appear uniform and are oval or elongated (Fig. 21–52). The nuclear membranes are typically thin. The chromatin is usually vesicular, but sometimes coarsely granular. Nucleoli are small but distinct. Some multinucleated forms are commonly present. Nuclear pseudoinclusions can be present. However, some cases may show significant nuclear pleomorphism, coagulative necrosis, and frequent mitoses. Recurrent tumors may be morphologically identical to the original tumors or can show increased cellular atypia and mitotic activity.[213]

The tumors are characteristically diffusely sprinkled with small lymphocytes. In some cases, the lymphocytes also form cuffs around the blood vessels (see Figs. 21–51 and 21–52). Plasma cells are sparse except in rare cases.

Unusual Histologic Findings

Uncommon histologic features include polygonal tumor cells with hyaline cytoplasm, oncocytic tumor cells, myxoid change, neuroendocrine tumor-like vasculature, presence of perivascular spaces, and presence of interspersed osteoclastic giant cells.[212,216] In some cases, the tumor can be traversed by sclerotic septa, breaking up the tumor into irregular-shaped lobules. This feature, coupled with the presence of perivascular spaces, can result in a striking mimicry of ectopic thymoma or carcinoma showing thymus-like element (Fig. 21–53).[213] In fact, some cases diagnosed as carcinoma showing thymus-like element in the past have been reinterpreted as follicular dendritic cell sarcomas.[213]

For tumors occurring in the liver or spleen, there is often a heavy infiltrate of lymphocytes and plasma cells, mimicking the histologic features of inflammatory pseudotumor.[217] Such tumors show a consistent association with EBV.

Predisposing Factors and Precursor Lesions

Slightly over 10% of cases of follicular dendritic cell sarcoma show an association with Castleman disease, most commonly the hyaline-vascular type, and rarely the plasma cell type.[212] In most cases, the Castleman disease lesion occurs side-by-side with the follicular dendritic cell sarcoma,[59,61,218–221] but some cases show temporal evolution from Castleman disease to follicular dendritic cells sarcoma over time.[61,62] The intermediary lesion is characterized by patchy proliferation of follicular dendritic cells in the interfollicular zone, but it is unclear whether so-called follicular dendritic cell dysplasia is a precursor lesion (see section, "Hyaline-Vascular Castleman Disease").

Rare cases of follicular dendritic sarcoma have been reported in patients with schizophrenia.[219,222] Whether this association is significant or fortuitous remains to be clarified.

Thymoma-like follicular dendritic cell hyperplasia of the soft tissues is another possible but rare precursor lesion.[213] It is characterized by B lymphocyte-rich lobules separated by sclerotic septa. Scattered throughout are occasional large cells with vesicular nuclei and indistinct cell borders, which prove on immunohistochemical studies to represent follicular dendritic cells rather than epithelial cells (Fig. 21–54).

Immunohistochemical Profile

A diagnosis of follicular dendritic cell sarcoma must be confirmed by immunohistochemical staining. The neoplastic cells express one or more follicular dendritic cell markers, such as CD21, CD23, CD35, R4/23, and KiM4p.[61,212] The most commonly used ones are CD21 and CD35, which stain almost all cases; these two antibodies can be combined as a cocktail to increase the intensity of immunostaining

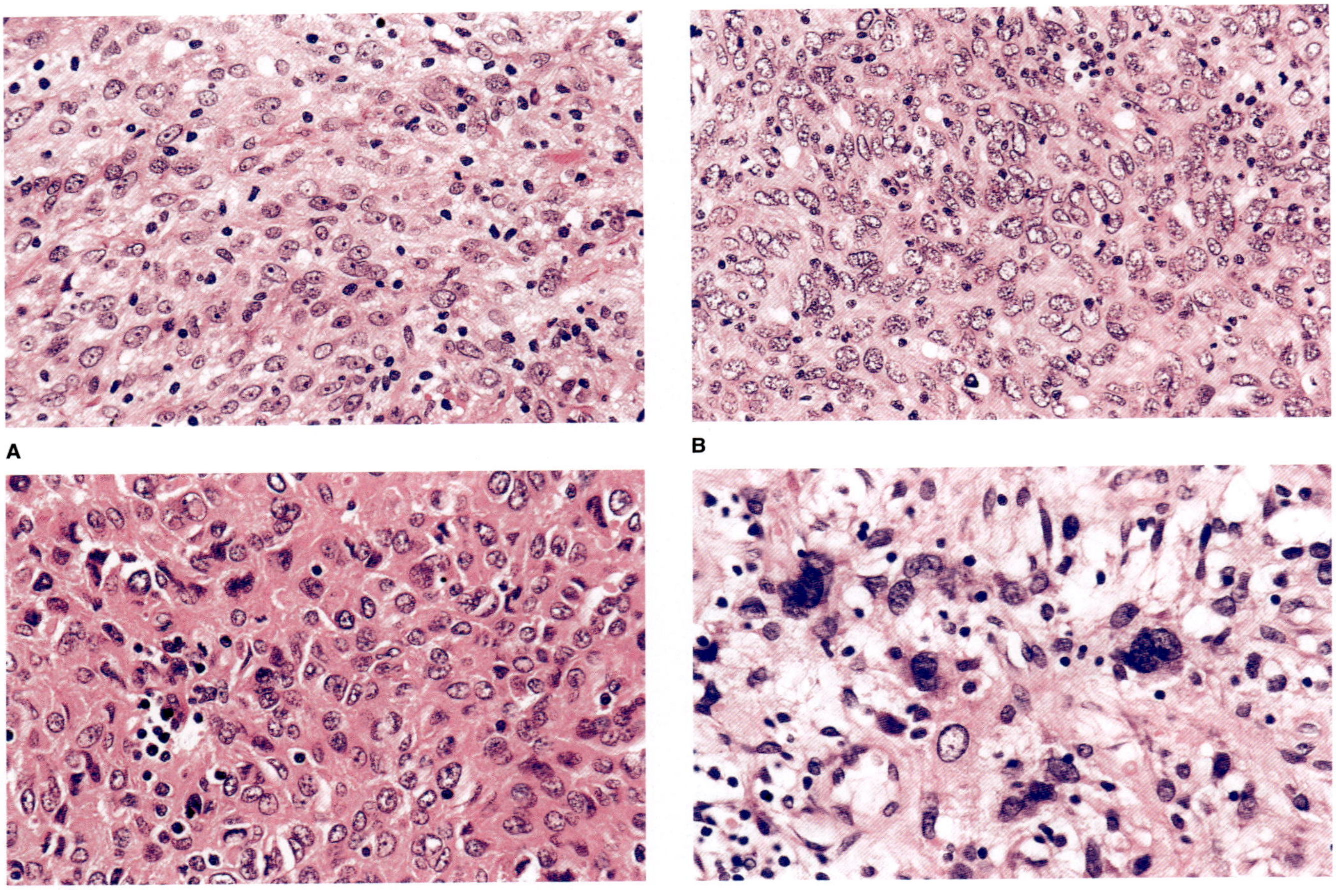

A B C D

Figure 21–52. Follicular dendritic cell sarcoma, cytologic spectrum. Note also the sprinkling of small lymphocytes throughout the tumor. *A*, Typical example comprising spindly cells with indistinct cell borders, vesicular nuclei, thin nuclear membranes, and distinct nucleoli. *B*, In this example, the chromatin is slightly more stippled. Note the characteristic syncytial quality of the cytoplasm. *C*, Tumor cells appear ovoid. Some nuclei contain intranuclear pseudoinclusions *(left upper field)*. *D*, Large hyperchromatic nuclei can be seen in some cases.

(Fig. 21–55). CD23 stains only approximately 60% of cases. The follicular dendritic cell-associated marker CNA.42 is sensitive but less specific. The immunostains typically highlight the delicate cytoplasmic processes of the tumor cells, which form complex meshworks. Occasionally a multinodular pattern, not obvious on routine histologic sections, may be observed, recapitulating the ability of the neoplastic cells to form follicle structures.

The tumor is negative for cytokeratin, CD45, B-lineage markers, T-lineage markers, CD1a, and lysozyme. There can be variable immunoreactivity for S-100 protein, CD68, and muscle-specific actin. The occasional immunoreactivity for epithelial membrane antigen can potentially lead to a misdiagnosis of carcinoma, ectopic meningioma, or perineurial cell tumor.[61,212]

Ultrastructurally Important Diagnostic Features

Similar to their normal counterparts, follicular dendritic cell sarcomas ultrastructurally exhibit long complex interdigitating cytoplasmic processes connected by desmosomes. Cytoplasmic organelles are often sparse.

Genetic Changes

There are no rearrangements of the immunoglobulin and T-cell receptor genes. EBV is negative except for the inflammatory pseudotumor-like variant occurring in the liver and spleen.[61,217] Little is known about the cytogenetic or molecular alterations in follicular dendritic cell sarcomas.

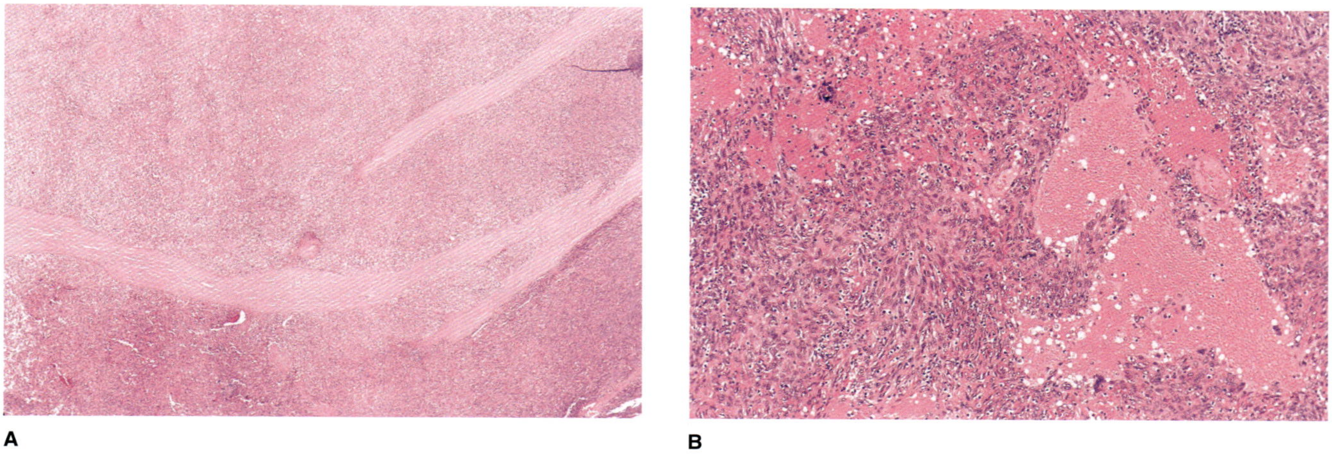

Figure 21–53. Follicular dendritic cell sarcoma mimicking thymoma. *A,* There are broad sclerotic bands, resulting in a jigsaw puzzle-like lobulation, reminiscent of thymoma. *B,* The presence of perivascular spaces filled with blood further heightens the morphologic similarities with thymoma.

Differential Diagnosis

Follicular dendritic cell sarcoma can mimic *thymoma, thymic carcinoma* (including carcinoma showing thymus-like element), *meningioma, angiomatoid fibrous histiocytoma, malignant fibrous histiocytoma, angiosarcoma, undifferentiated carcinoma, malignant melanoma, lymphoepithelioma-like carcinoma,* or *gastrointestinal stromal tumor,* and vice versa. A high index of suspicion is required for rendering the correct diagnosis. The most important clues to diagnosis are syncytial-appearing spindly cells with storiform or whorled growth pattern, usually thin nuclear membrane and vesicular chromatin, and sprinkling of small lymphocytes throughout the tumor. *Mycobacterial spindle cell pseudotumor* can also be mistaken for a dendritic cell tumor, but the spindly cells are histiocytes ($CD68^+$) lacking definite nuclear atypia and containing many acid-fast bacilli. *Fibrohistiocytic variant of nodular sclerosis Hodgkin lymphoma* can potentially mimic dendritic cell tumor because of the presence of fascicles of spindly histiocytes and myofibroblasts. It can be recognized by the presence of scattered large ovoid cells with inclusion-like nucleoli and the presence of eosinophils, and the diagnosis can be confirmed by immunostaining for CD30 and CD15.[40]

Interdigitating Dendritic Cell Sarcoma

Clinical Presentation and Clinical Outcome

Interdigitating dendritic cell sarcoma (also known as interdigitating reticulum cell sarcoma) is an uncommon dendritic cell neoplasm usually affecting adults,

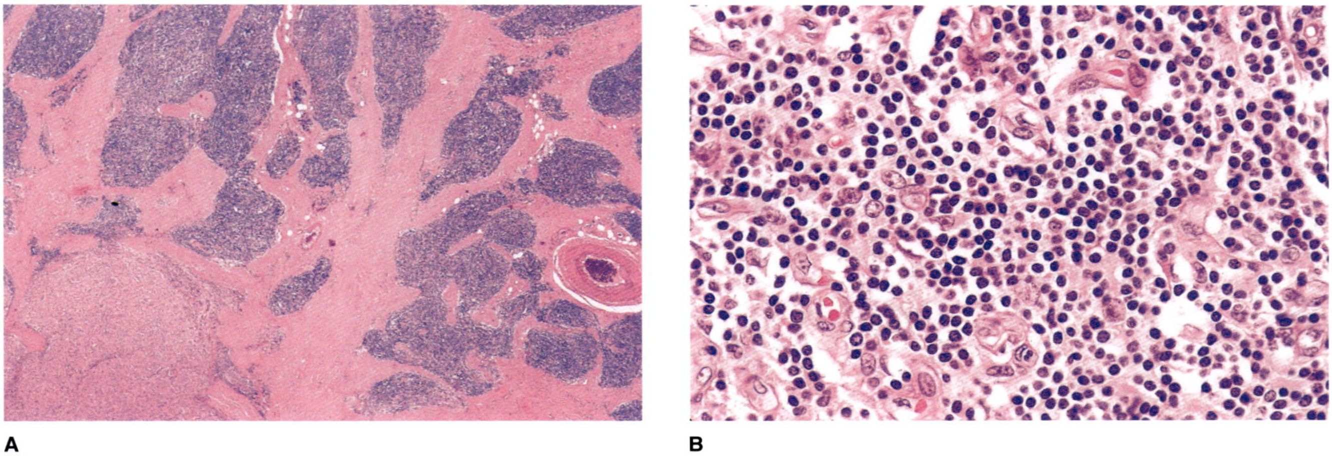

Figure 21–54. Thymoma-like follicular dendritic cell hyperplasia. *A,* Lymphoid cell lobules are separated by a dense fibrous stroma. This lesion is contiguous with a frank follicular dendritic cell sarcoma *(left lower field). B,* The lesion is composed mostly of small lymphocytes, interspersed with isolated large cells with indistinct cell borders and distinct nucleoli. Immunostaining for CD21 shows that these large cells are follicular dendritic cells forming complex meshworks (not shown).

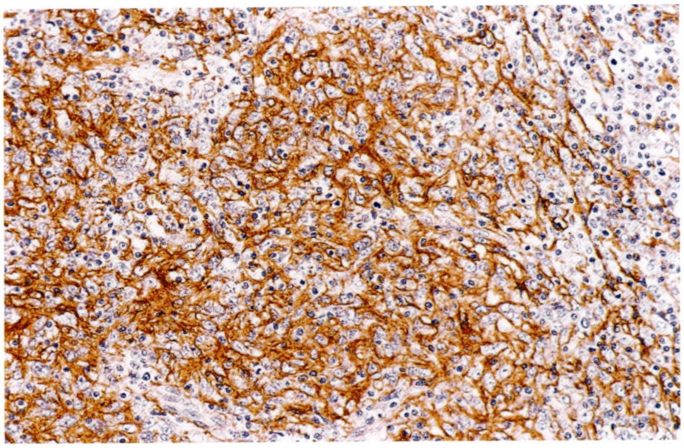

Figure 21–55. Follicular dendritic cell sarcoma. Immunostaining for CD21 highlights the complex anastomosing cell processes of the tumor cells, forming meshworks.

who present with lymphadenopathy or extranodal disease, such as in the gastrointestinal tract and somatic soft tissues. Most patients have advanced stage disease at presentation, and systemic symptoms are common.[110,203,211,218,223–229]

Interdigitating dendritic cell sarcomas are generally aggressive, and response to chemotherapy is often only partial or transient. The limited follow-up data indicate that at least one third of patients die from widespread disease at 1 week to 3 years. The overall median survival is about 15 months.[88]

Key Histologic Findings

The histologic features are highly variable. Most cases are morphologically indistinguishable from or very similar to follicular dendritic cell sarcoma, with predominance of spindly cells. Some cases are composed of large round to ovoid cells with voluminous cytoplasm and multiple deep notches in the nuclei, reminiscent of Langerhans cell sarcoma (Fig. 21–56). Rare cases are composed of large pleomorphic cells, resembling histiocytic sarcoma or large cell lymphoma. An

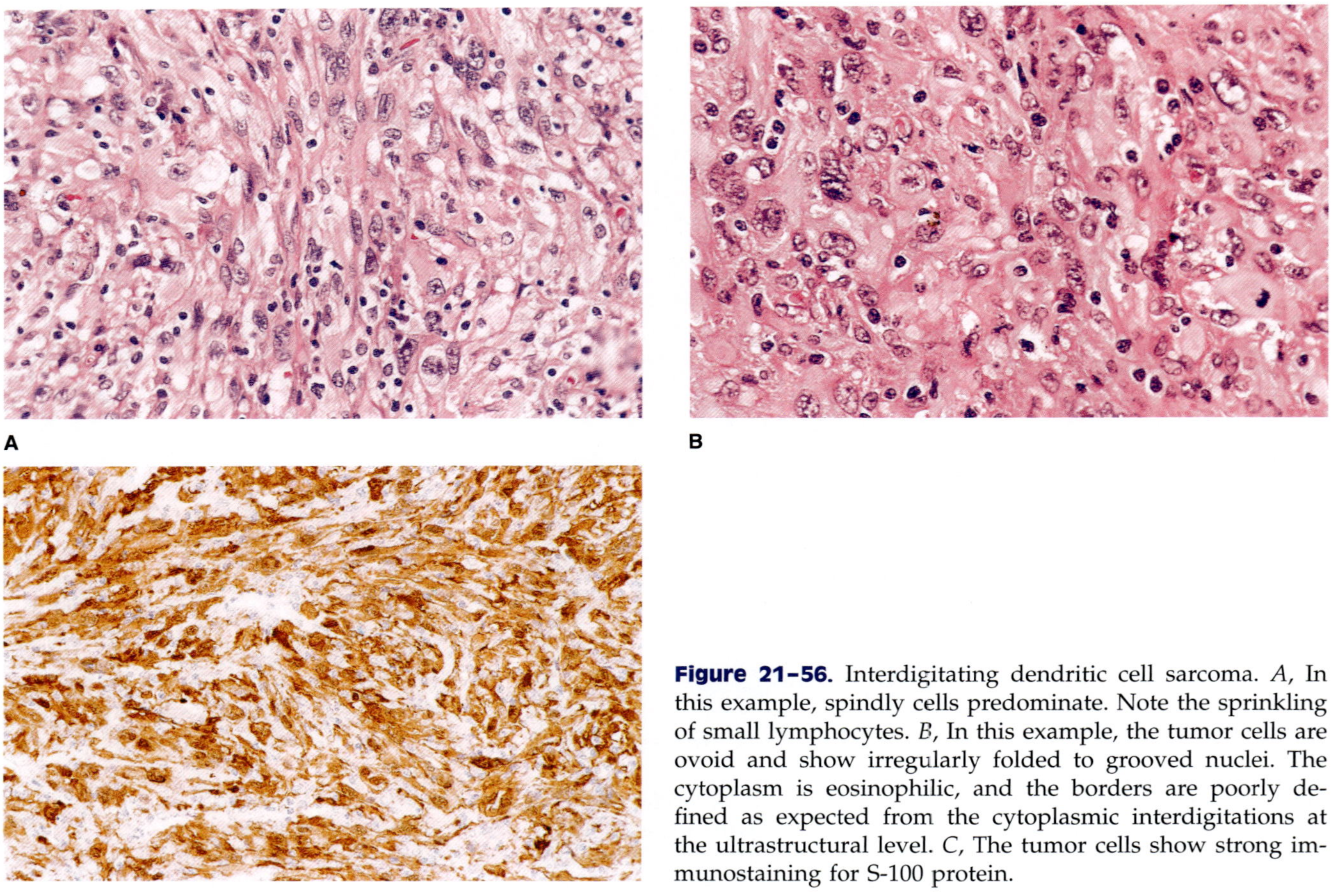

A

B

C

Figure 21–56. Interdigitating dendritic cell sarcoma. *A*, In this example, spindly cells predominate. Note the sprinkling of small lymphocytes. *B*, In this example, the tumor cells are ovoid and show irregularly folded to grooved nuclei. The cytoplasm is eosinophilic, and the borders are poorly defined as expected from the cytoplasmic interdigitations at the ultrastructural level. *C*, The tumor cells show strong immunostaining for S-100 protein.

individual case may comprise cells with different morphologic features in different parts of the same tumor.

Immunohistochemical Profile

The immunohistochemical hallmark of interdigitating dendritic cell sarcoma is S-100 protein immunoreactivity (Fig. 21–56C), coupled with negative staining for CD1a, follicular dendritic cell markers, B-cell markers, and T-cell markers. There is often weak immunoreactivity for CD68, CD45, and CD4.

Ultrastructurally Important Diagnostic Features

Because morphologic and immunophenotypic features overlap between interdigitating dendritic cell sarcoma and histiocytic sarcoma, the definitive diagnosis is best supported by ultrastructural findings, which include long and complex interdigitating cytoplasmic processes but no desmosomes or Birbeck granules.

Differential Diagnosis

In addition to histiocytic sarcoma and Langerhans cell sarcoma, the same differential diagnoses listed for follicular dendritic cell sarcoma also apply.

Fibroblastic Reticular Cell Sarcoma

Clinical Presentation and Clinical Outcome

Fibroblastic reticular cell tumor is very rare, and "cytokeratin-positive interstitial reticulum cell tumor" probably represents a subset of this tumor type. It occurs in adolescents and adults.[218,230–232] Among the nine reported cases, seven involve lymph node, one involves the posterior mediastinum, and one involves soft tissue of the proximal forearm. Among six patients with follow-up information, five were alive and well at 1 to 12 years, and one died of disease at 9 months.[218,230,231]

Key Histologic Findings

Fibroblastic reticular cell sarcomas are morphologically similar to follicular dendritic cell sarcomas or interdigitating dendritic cell sarcomas, but lack the immunophenotypic profile of these tumor types (such as CD21, CD35, S-100 protein). The spindly or plump cells show mild to moderate nuclear pleomorphism. In addition, there are often interspersed delicate collagen fibers (Fig. 21–57).

Immunohistochemical Profile

The neoplastic cells are strongly immunoreactive for vimentin and show inconsistent immunoreactivity for smooth muscle actin, desmin, cytokeratin (in a dendritic pattern), and CD68. Positive staining for cytokeratin is not surprising because nodal reticular cells have long been known to be cytokeratin positive, but this immunophenotype can certainly lead to an erroneous diagnosis of metastatic carcinoma (Fig. 21–57*B*).[232]

There are many architectural and cytologic similarities of angiomatoid fibrous histiocytoma with fibroblastic reticular cell sarcomas, and both tumors not uncommonly express desmin.[126] Their relationship, if any, remains to be clarified.

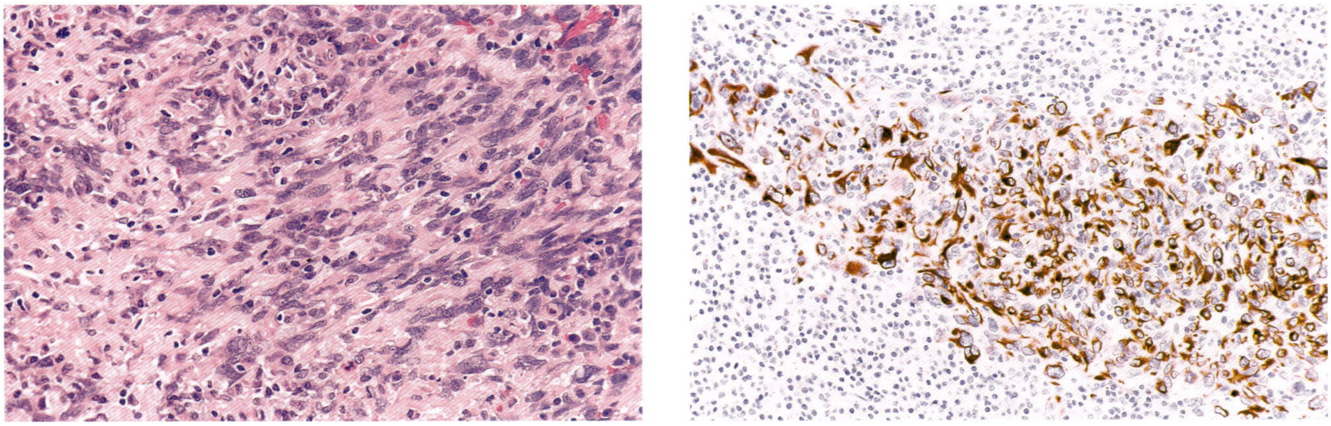

A B

Figure 21–57. Fibroblastic reticular cell sarcoma. *A*, Short fascicles of spindly cells are admixed with collagen fibers and small lymphocytes. *B*, In this example, the spindly cells are strongly immunoreactive for desmin. Note that the delicate cell processes are well highlighted.

Ultrastructurally Important Diagnostic Features

The spindly cells show delicate cytoplasmic extensions and features reminiscent of myofibroblasts (filaments with occasional fusiform densities, well-developed desmosomal attachments, rough endoplasmic reticulum, basal lamina-like material).[218]

Dendritic Cell Sarcoma Not Otherwise Specified

The designation "dendritic cell sarcoma not otherwise specified" is reserved for those spindle cell neoplasms showing histologic similarities to follicular dendritic cell, interdigitating dendritic cell, or fibroblastic reticular cell sarcoma, but lacking immunoreactivity for follicular dendritic cell markers, S-100 protein, cytokeratin, actin, and desmin.[218] This designation is also appropriate for dendritic cell sarcomas showing hybrid or equivocal features of two or more types of dendritic cell tumors on evaluation by various techniques.[233] The same differential diagnoses for follicular dendritic cell sarcoma should also be considered for this tumor type.

Juvenile Xanthogranuloma

Clinical Presentation and Clinical Course

Juvenile xanthogranuloma typically occurs in infants and children, but up to 15% to 20% of cases occur in adults. Some lesions are already present at birth, and most appear by the age of 2 years.[163,234–238] There is no sex predilection. Although the prefix "juvenile" may be objectionable when the lesion occurs in adults, use of the unqualified term "xanthogranuloma" is not desirable either because it is too nonspecific and has been applied for many other unrelated lesions. An alternative is to use the term "juvenile-type xanthogranuloma" when the lesion occurs in adults.

Juvenile xanthogranuloma usually presents as a solitary yellow-red papule or nodule, but the lesions are multiple in about one third of cases. Approximately 5% of cases arise in the deep tissues, such as skeletal muscle.[90,163,234,236–246] The head and neck and upper trunk are the most commonly involved locations. Other sites, such as the eye, liver, spleen, lymph node, lung, bone, and nerve, can also be occasionally involved. There is no association with hyperlipidemia. Rare cases have been associated with von Recklinghausen neurofibromatosis and juvenile myelomonocytic leukemia.[247–252]

Juvenile xanthogranuloma is a benign lesion that usually involutes spontaneously within 1 year. However, in adults, the lesion often persists.

Nature of Disease

It is still unclear whether juvenile xanthogranuloma is a neoplasm or a reactive process.[253–255] The nature of the proliferated cells in juvenile xanthogranuloma is also controversial. This lesion is generally considered a neoplasm of dermal dendritic cell in view of a factor XIIIa^{+}, CD68^{+} immunophenotype.[89,95] Nonetheless, a recent study challenges this view because of frequent CD4 expression, and a relationship with plasmacytoid monocytes is proposed.[90]

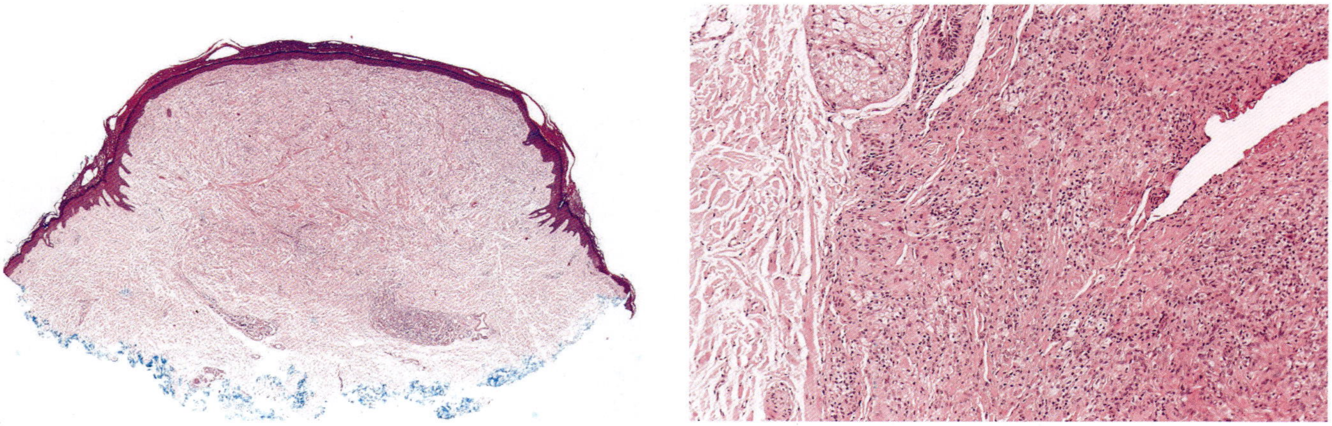

A B

Figure 21–58. Juvenile xanthogranuloma of skin. *A*, It is a dermal-based nodule stretching the overlying epidermis. *B*, The lateral border does not show a "curl around collagen" pattern as typical of benign fibrous histiocytoma (dermatofibroma).

Key Histologic Findings

The cutaneous lesion usually measures less than 1 cm. The overlying epidermis is normal or atrophic and is not invaded by the lesional cells (Fig. 21–58). The lesion is noncircumscribed, abutting the base of the epidermis, and sometimes extending to the subcutis. There are often entrapped skin appendages within the lesion. The morphologic features vary according to the stage of evolution.

In the early phase, there are monotonous sheets of nondescript ovoid cells with oval and occasionally grooved nuclei, fine chromatin, and a moderate amount of eosinophilic cytoplasm (Fig. 21–59).[256] Mitotic figures are occasionally present in considerable numbers.[236] The xanthomatous nature of the lesion can be difficult to appreciate at this stage because foamy cells and Touton giant cells are rare or absent.

In the fully evolved lesion, the mononuclear cells show fine lipid vacuoles in the cytoplasm, and there are clusters of admixed foamy cells. Scattered Touton giant cells with a ringlike arrangement of nuclei, central eosinophilic cytoplasm, and peripheral vacuolated cytoplasm are present (Fig. 21–60). In some cases, spindly cells predominate (so-called spindle cell xanthogranuloma) or cells with serrated contour predominate (so-called scalloped cell xanthogranuloma).[257,258] Eosinophils are usually admixed and can be abundant. There can also be intermingled small lymphocytes, plasma cells, and neutrophils.

In the regressing lesion, there is fibrosis and a reduction in the number of histiocytes. The intermingling of spindly histiocytes with fibroblasts can produce a vague storiform growth pattern, reminiscent of benign fibrous histiocytoma (Fig. 21–61).

The deep-seated lesions differ from the cutaneous lesions in the following aspects: (1) usually larger; (2) more circumscribed, although the edges can

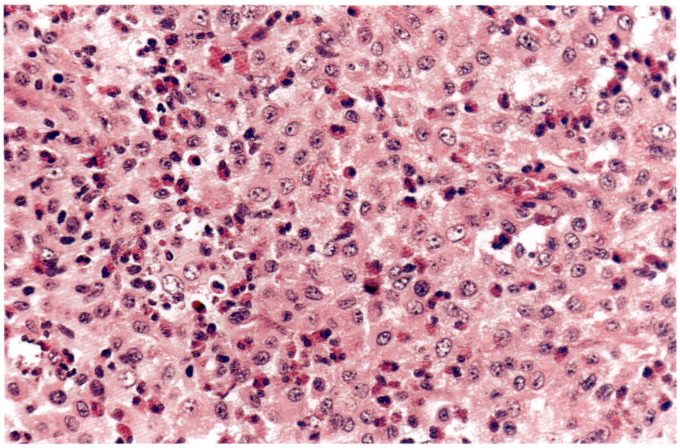

Figure 21–59. Juvenile xanthogranuloma of skin, early lesion. Nondescript mononuclear cells predominate; foamy cells and Touton giant cells are not found. Although most cells have oval nuclei, some have grooved nuclei. Coupled with the presence of eosinophils, the lesion can be mistaken for Langerhans cell histiocytosis.

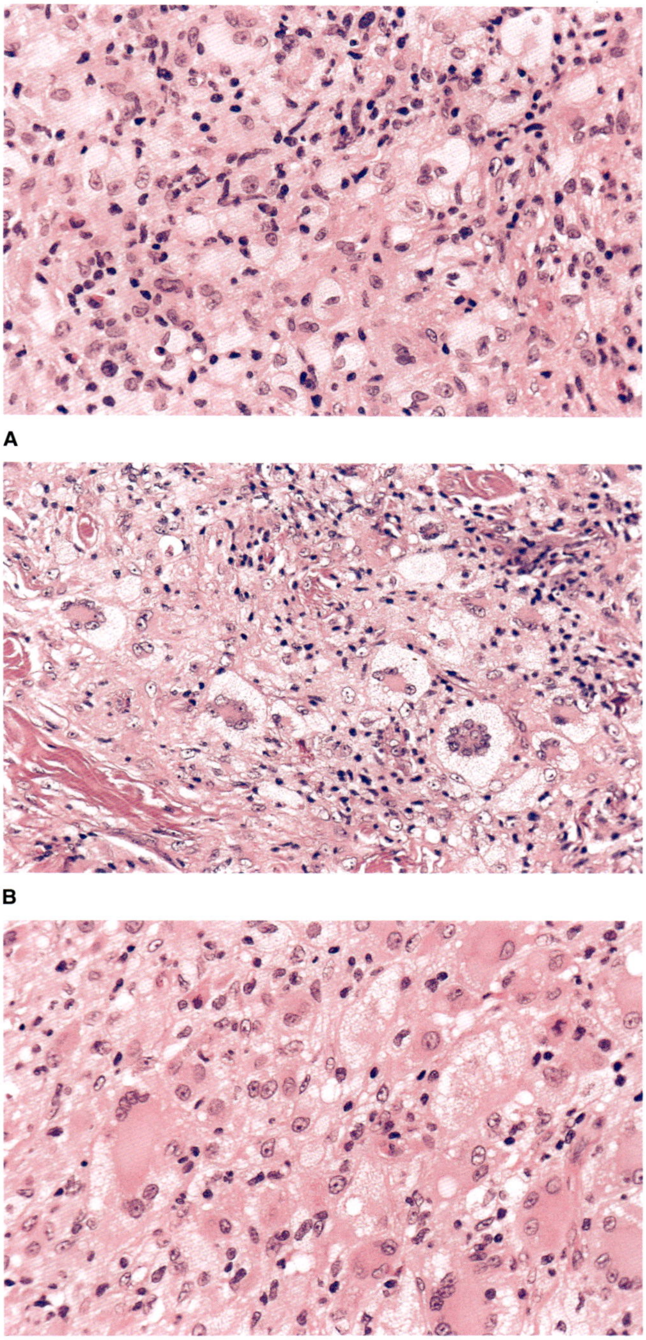

C

Figure 21–60. Juvenile xanthogranuloma of skin, well-developed lesion. *A*, Usually the cytologic composition is polymorphous, including foamy cells, histiocytes, and chronic inflammatory cells. *B*, Many Touton giant cells are seen. *C*, Sometimes there are multinucleated giant cells that do not conform to the definition of Touton giant cells.

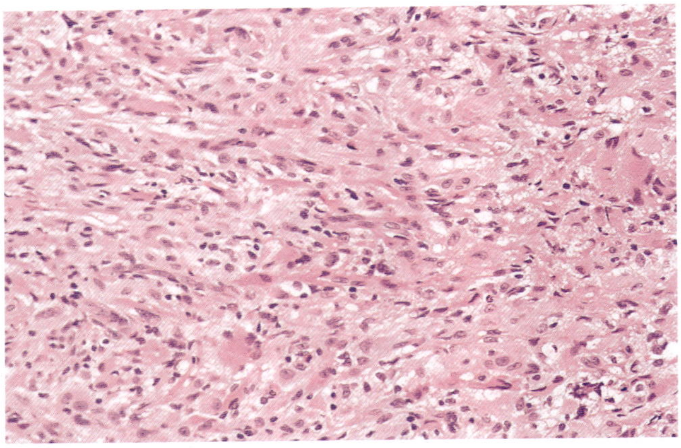

Figure 21-61. Juvenile xanthogranuloma, late phase. Spindly cells and collagen fibers are intermingled with the foamy cells and mononuclear cells.

merge into the normal structures; (3) more monotonous cell composition; (4) fewer lipidized cells; and (5) fewer Touton giant cells (Fig. 21–62).[243,259]

Possible Variants of Juvenile Xanthogranuloma

Benign cephalic histiocytosis is characterized by multiple skin eruptions over the face, affecting children younger than 3 years. The lesions usually regress after a few years.[260–268] Histologically, the dermis is infiltrated by histiocytes with eosinophilic cytoplasm, sometimes in the form of a lichenoid band. Eosinophils are common, but foamy cells are rare.

Progressive nodular histiocytosis (histiocytoma) is characterized by myriads of lesions, including superficial small xanthomatous papules (rich in foamy cells and Touton giant cells) and slightly larger deep nodules that morphologically resemble spindle cell

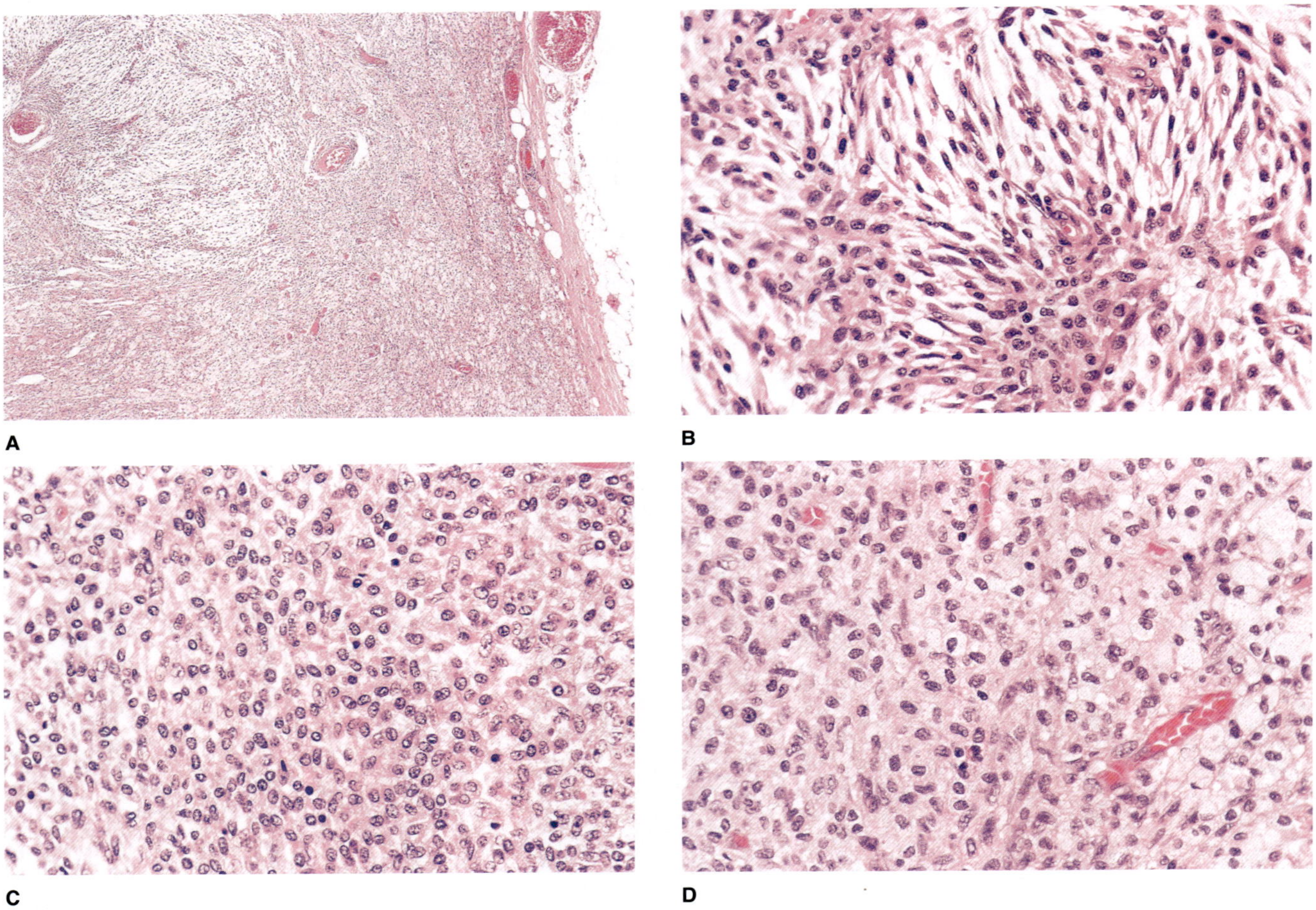

Figure 21-62. Deep juvenile xanthogranuloma occurring in the fascia. *A*, This cellular lesion is largely circumscribed. *B*, In focal areas, spindly cells and ovoid cells are separated by edematous stroma. *C*, In most areas, sheets of nondescript, uniform, ovoid cells are seen. There are practically no admixed inflammatory cells. *D*, In some areas, the ovoid cells merge imperceptibly into clusters of foamy cells. That is, the nuclei of both cell types are similar. This feature provides an important clue to diagnosis of juvenile xanthogranuloma.

juvenile xanthogranuloma. The lesions usually do not regress.[257,269–272]

Xanthoma disseminatum is characterized by numerous papules in skin and mucous membrane.[89] It is predominantly a disease of adults, and some patients can develop diabetes insipidus.[273–281]

Generalized eruptive histiocytoma is characterized by the development of recurrent crops of symmetrical small papules over the skin, trunk, and arms. The disease usually resolves spontaneously after several years. Both adults and children can be affected.[282–285] The exact relationship with other non-Langerhans cell histiocytosis is still unclear, but some reports suggest a relationship with xanthoma disseminatum or benign cephalic histiocytosis.[283,286]

Immunohistochemical Profile

The lesional cells are often immunoreactive for CD68, factor XIIIa, fascin, and muscle-specific actin (Fig. 21–63).[287] Staining for lysozyme (23% of cases) or CD4 (78% of cases) is variable, whereas smooth muscle actin and CD1a are negative.[90,288] S-100 protein is generally considered to be negative, but a recent study reports positive staining in 30% of cases.[90,288,289]

Differential Diagnosis

For differential diagnosis with *Langerhans cell histiocytosis, xanthoma,* and *benign fibrous histiocytoma,* see Table 21–8. The deep form of juvenile xanthogranuloma can potentially be mistaken for sarcoma because of the high cellularity and fascicular architecture. The bland cytology and the focal presence of foamy cells that merge into the mononuclear cells should provide the strongest clues to the correct diagnosis, which can be further confirmed by immunohistochemistry.[234]

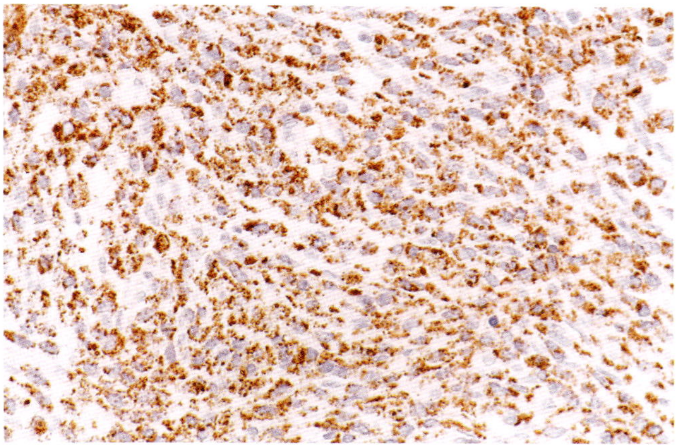

Figure 21–63. Juvenile xanthogranuloma, immunostained for CD68 (PGM1). Most cells are positive.

Reticulohistiocytoma

Clinical Presentation and Clinical Course

Reticulohistiocytoma is an uncommon disorder affecting young or middle-aged adults, with female predominance. The patients present with solitary, sometimes multiple, yellow-brown cutaneous nodules. There is no particular site predilection, but multicentric reticulohistiocytosis has to be seriously considered if the lesions are found on acral sites.[163,186,290–296]

Local excision of the lesion is usually curative. Lesions that are not excised may regress spontaneously.

Key Histologic Findings

The lesions usually measure less than 1 cm. In the dermis, there are dense sheets of large histiocytes with voluminous, eosinophilic, glassy to finely granular cytoplasm that is positive for PAS and resistant to diastase (Fig. 21–64). Characteristically, there are multinucleated giant cells with randomly oriented nuclei, but no Touton giant cells. The nuclei are round, oval, or occasionally grooved, and can be mildly atypical. Some mitotic figures can be seen. There are frequently some scattered lymphocytes and eosinophils.

Immunohistochemical Profile and Nature of Disease

In most cases, the histiocytes are positive for CD68, factor XIIIa, and muscle-specific actin, but negative for S-100 protein and smooth-muscle actin. Staining for lysozyme is variable.[296] It remains controversial whether reticulohistiocytoma should be considered a macrophage-related or dendritic cell-related proliferation.[89,95,102]

Differential Diagnosis

For differential diagnosis with *juvenile xanthogranuloma,* see Table 21–8. Reticulohistiocytoma can be distinguished from *malignant fibrous histiocytoma* by its small size, paucity of mitotic figures, and inconspicuous cellular spindling. It can be distinguished from *atypical fibroxanthoma* by the paucity of spindly cells and much lower degree of cellular pleomorphism. *Malignant melanoma* is an important differential diagnosis given the presence of large cells with

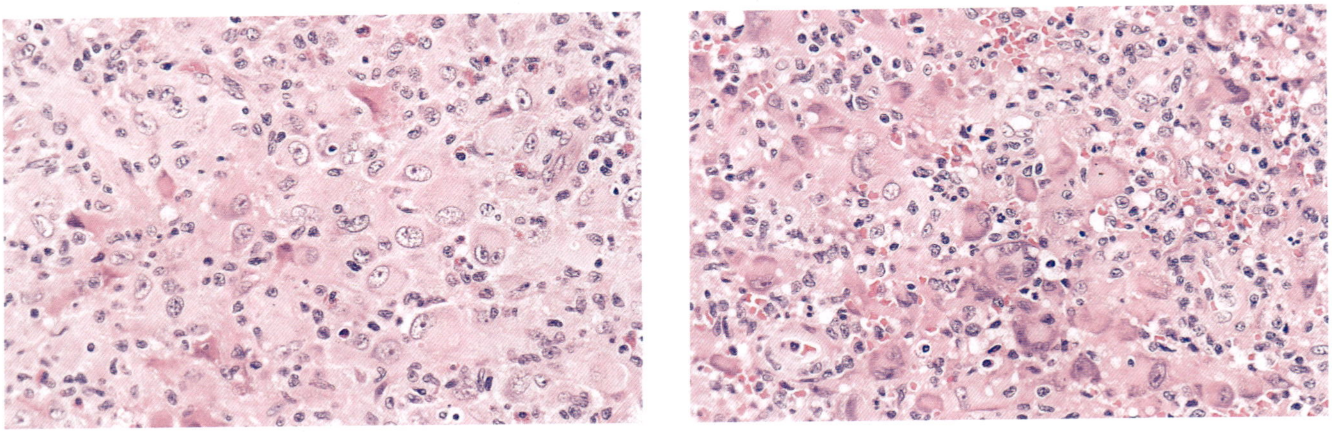

A B

Figure 21–64. Solitary reticulohistiocytoma of skin. *A*, There are sheets of large ovoid cells with mildly atypical vesicular nuclei and abundant glassy eosinophilic cytoplasm, sprinkled with some lymphocytes and eosinophils. *B*, There are interspersed multinucleated cells with randomly oriented nuclei.

eosinophilic cytoplasm; melanoma usually shows a junctional component, epidermal invasion, nested growth pattern, and S-100 immunoreactivity.

Multicentric Reticulohistiocytosis

Clinical Presentation and Clinical Course

Multicentric reticulohistiocytosis is clinically different from solitary reticulohistiocytoma, and there are also some histologic and immunohistochemical differences.[292,294,296–303] It occurs in adults, with female predominance. The most striking feature is destructive polyarthritis, which usually ends up with crippling deformities. The joints of the hands are most commonly affected, but the knee, ankle, elbow, wrist, and shoulder can also be affected. Multiple yellow-brown papules or nodules affecting acral sites (such as hand, forearm, face) can appear before or after the development of arthritis. The patients can also have intermittent pyrexia. In more than one third of patients, there is an associated underlying disease, such as malignancy, thyroid disease, tuberculosis, diabetes, dermatomyositis, and systemic lupus erythematosus. Thus it has been postulated that multicentric reticulohistiocytosis is a manifestation of a disturbed immune system.

Key Histologic Findings

Large histiocytes with abundant eosinophilic cytoplasm can be found in many sites of the body, such as skin, soft tissue, synovium, and bone. The histiocytes form aggregates or are dispersed (Fig. 21–65). In the skin, they show a more interstitial distribution between collagen fibers, and usually fewer and smaller-sized multinucleated cells compared with solitary reticulohistiocytoma.

Immunohistochemical Profile

The histiocytes are immunoreactive for CD68, lysozyme, CD45 (leukocyte common antigen), and CD4, but not S-100 protein, factor XIIIa, and muscle-specific actin.[288,296,304]

Approach to Diagnosis of Histiocytic Proliferative Lesions

Tables 21–8 and 21–9 outline the approach to diagnosis of histiocytic proliferative disorders,[95] and lesions rich in foamy histiocytes are listed in Table 21–10. In some cases, the diagnosis is straight-

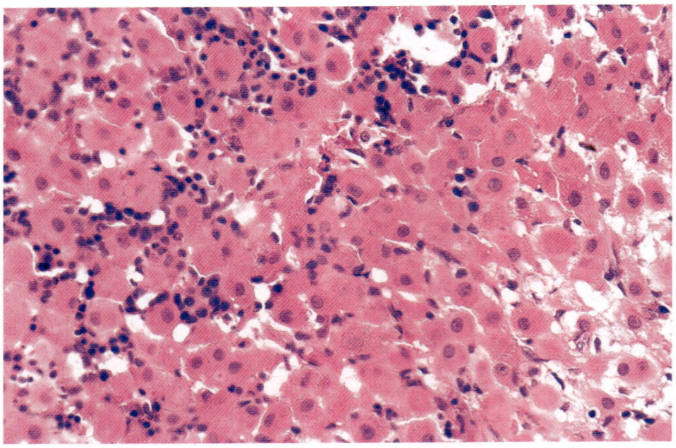

Figure 21–65. Multicentric reticulohistiocytosis involving bone/bone marrow of patient with destructive arthropathy. Note the presence of many large cells with abundant eosinophilic hyaline cytoplasm.

Table 21–9. Approach to Diagnosis of Histiocytic Proliferations

	Morphologic Clues	Caveats
Is this a histiocytic proliferation?	Abundant eosinophilic cytoplasm, which may sometimes be finely vacuolated. It is not necessary to find phagocytosis, which is in fact very uncommon.	Megakaryocytes can also have abundant eosinophilic cytoplasm. The histiocytic nature can be confirmed by the appropriate immunohistochemical markers, such as CD68 for monocytes-phagocytes, CD21 for follicular dendritic cells, and S-100 protein for other dendritic cells.
What is the shape of the histiocytes?	Histiocytes are usually ovoid. If spindle cells predominate, consider: • Dendritic cell tumors (various types) • Mycobacterial spindle cell pseudotumor and histoid leprosy • Spindle cell juvenile xanthogranuloma	In the late (burned out) phases of histiocytic proliferations, such as Rosai-Dorfman disease, juvenile xanthoma and Langerhans cell histiocytoma, spindly histiocytes may be present.
What is the nuclear morphology?	If nuclear grooves are prominent, consider: • Langerhans cell histiocytosis • Interdigitating dendritic cell, indeterminate cell, or fibroblastic reticular cell sarcoma • Histiocytic sarcoma (some cases) Large cells with round nuclei, vesicular chromatin, and distinct central nucleoli are characteristic of Rosai-Dorfman disease.	Some nuclear grooves can also be seen in various other histiocytic lesions, such as follicular dendritic cell sarcoma, juvenile xanthogranuloma, and reticulohistiocytoma.
Are the cells cytologically malignant?	Highly atypical cells are observed in the following: • Histiocytic sarcoma • Langerhans cell sarcoma • Follicular dendritic cell sarcoma (some cases) • Interdigitating dendritic cell sarcoma (some cases)	Scattered large atypical nuclei can sometimes be seen in Rosai-Dorfman man disease and reticulohistiocytoma.
Other accompanying features?	Eosinophils are often prominent in Langerhans cell histiocytosis, juvenile xanthogranuloma, and reticulohistiocytoma; and plasma cells are prominent in Rosai-Dorfman disease. Entities rich in foamy cells are listed in Table 21–10. Touton giant cells are a feature of juvenile xanthogranuloma and its possible variants, as well as Erdheim-Chester disease.	Touton giant cells can also be found in benign fibrous histiocytoma.
Clinical features?	The age of patient, extent of disease (solitary, localized, generalized, or systemic), site of involvement, and size of lesions are important in defining the various types of cutaneous histiocytoses.	Some cases may remain unclassifiable after consideration of all the features.

forward based on the morphologic or immunophenotypic features, such as Rosai-Dorfman disease, follicular dendritic cell sarcoma, and juvenile xanthogranuloma. Other cases, in particular the cutaneous histiocytic syndromes, require correlation with the clinical features in formulating a diagnosis. Some cases may show overlapping features of two clinicopathologic entities[95] or may not be readily classifiable.

The difficulties in classification of histiocytic proliferative disorders are compounded by the dynamic nature of histiocytes, which can change in morphology, immunophenotype, and functional state according to factors in the environment.[101]

Table 21-10. Foamy Cell-Rich Soft Tissue Lesions

Xanthoma/xanthelasma

Juvenile xanthogranuloma

Erdheim-Chester disease

Common component in some tumor types:
- Benign fibrous histiocytoma, especially the lipidized type
- Schwannoma, especially cellular schwannoma
- Giant cell tumor of tendon sheath (nodular tenosynovitis)
- Inflammatory malignant fibrous histiocytoma

Burned out phase of histiocytic proliferative lesions
- Late phase of Langerhans cell histiocytosis
- Late phase of Rosai-Dorfman disease

Foamy histiocyte inflammatory reaction:
- Xanthogranulomatous inflammation
- Foamy histiocytic reaction in association with Hodgkin lymphoma
- Foamy histiocytic reaction in areas of tissue breakdown or necrosis in a variety of tumor types

REFERENCES

Tumors and Tumor-like Lesions of Lymphoid Cells

Primary Malignant Lymphoma of Somatic Soft Tissues

1. Salamao DR, Nascimento AG, Lloyd RV, et al: Lymphoma in soft tissue: A clinicopathologic study of 19 cases. Hum Pathol 1996;27:253–237.
2. Meister HP: Malignant lymphomas of soft tissues. Verh Dtsch Ges Pathol 1992;76:140–145.
3. Lanham GR, Weiss SW, Enzinger FM: Malignant lymphoma: A study of 75 cases presenting in soft tissue. Am J Surg Pathol 1989;13:1–10.
4. Goodlad JR, Fletcher CDM, Chan JKC, et al: Primary soft tissue lymphoma: An analysis of 37 cases [abstract]. J Pathol 1996;179(suppl):42A.
5. Travis WD, Banks PM, Reiman HM: Primary extranodal soft tissue lymphoma of the extremities. Am J Surg Pathol 1987;11:359–366.
6. Eusebi V, Bondi A, Cancellieri A, et al: Primary malignant lymphoma of sciatic nerve. Report of a case. Am J Surg Pathol 1990;14:881–885.
7. Lin P, Jones D, Dorfman DM, et al: Precursor B-cell lymphoblastic lymphoma: A predominantly extranodal tumor with low propensity for leukemic involvement. Am J Surg Pathol 2000;24:1480–1490.
8. Neth O, Seidemann K, Jansen P, et al: Precursor B-cell lymphoblastic lymphoma in childhood and adolescence: Clinical features, treatment, and results in trials NHL-BFM 86 and 90. Med Pediatr Oncol 2000;35:20–27.
9. Maitra A, McKenna RW, Weinberg AG, et al: Precursor B-cell lymphoblastic lymphoma. A study of nine cases lacking blood and bone marrow involvement and review of the literature. Am J Clin Pathol 2001;115:868–875.
10. d'Amore ES, Wick MR, Geisinger KR, et al: Primary malignant lymphoma arising in postmastectomy lymphedema. Another facet of the Stewart-Treves syndrome. Am J Surg Pathol 1990;14:456–463.
11. Goodlad JR, Hollowood K, Smith MA, et al: Primary juxtaarticular soft tissue lymphoma arising in the vicinity of inflamed joints in patients with rheumatoid arthritis. Histopathology 1999;34:199–204.
12. Copie-Bergman C, Niedobitek G, Mangham DC, et al: Epstein-Barr virus in B-cell lymphomas associated with chronic suppurative inflammation. J Pathol 1997;183:287–292.
13. Radhi JM, Ibrahiem K, al-Tweigeri T: Soft tissue malignant lymphoma at sites of previous surgery. J Clin Pathol 1998;51:629–632.
14. Smith KJ, Skelton HG, Ruiz N, et al: Malignant lymphoma of soft tissue in an HIV-1+ patient. A rare site for primary malignant lymphoma with implications for treatment. Military Medical Consortium for the Advancement of Retroviral Research. Am J Dermatopathol 1995;17:403–406.
15. Chan JK, Sin VC, Wong KF, et al: Nonnasal lymphoma expressing the natural killer cell marker CD56: A clinicopathologic study of 49 cases of an uncommon aggressive neoplasm. Blood 1997;89:4501–4513.
16. Chan JK: Natural killer cell neoplasms. Anat Pathol 1998;3:77–145.
17. Gonzalez CL, Medeiros LJ, Braziel RM, et al: T-cell lymphoma involving subcutaneous tissue. A clinicopathologic entity commonly associated with hemophagocytic syndrome. Am J Surg Pathol 1991;15:17–27.
18. Salhany KE, Macon WR, Choi JK, et al: Subcutaneous panniculitis-like T-cell lymphoma: Clinicopathologic, immunophenotypic, and genotypic analysis of alpha/beta and gamma/delta subtypes. Am J Surg Pathol 1998;22:881–893.
19. Jaffe ES: Subcutaneous panniculitis-like T cell lymphoma. In Mason DY, Harris NL (eds): Human Lymphoma: Clinical Implications of the REAL Classification. London, Springer, 1999, pp 34.1–34.4.
20. Craig AJ, Cualing H, Thomas G, et al: Cytophagic histiocytic panniculitis—A syndrome associated with benign and malignant panniculitis: Case comparison and review of the literature. J Am Acad Dermatol 1998;39:721–736.
21. Kumar S, Krenacs L, Medeiros J, et al: Subcutaneous panniculitic T-cell lymphoma is a tumor of cytotoxic T lymphocytes. Hum Pathol 1998;29:397–403.
22. Soslow RA, Baergen RN, Warnke RA: B-lineage lymphoblastic lymphoma is a clinicopathologic entity distinct from other histologically similar aggressive lymphomas with blastic morphology. Cancer 1999;85:2648–2654.

23. Bueso-Ramos CE, Pugh WC, Butler JJ: Anaplastic large cell lymphoma presenting as a soft-tissue mass mimicking sarcoma. Mod Pathol 1994;7:497–500.
24. Chan JK: Anaplastic large cell lymphoma: Redefining its morphologic spectrum and importance of recognition of the ALK-positive subset. Adv Anat Pathol 1998;5:281–313.
25. Falini B, Bigerna B, Fizzotti M, et al: ALK expression defines a distinct group of T/null lymphomas ("ALK lymphomas") with a wide morphological spectrum. Am J Pathol 1998;153:875–886.
26. Benharroch D, Meguerian-Bedoyan Z, Lamant L, et al: ALK-positive lymphoma: A single disease with a broad spectrum of morphology. Blood 1998;91: 2076–2084.
27. Pelstring RJ, Essell JH, Kurtin PJ, et al: Diversity of organ site involvement among malignant lymphomas of mucosa-associated tissues. Am J Clin Pathol 1991;96:738–745.
28. Ngan BY, Warnke RA, Wilson M, et al: Monocytoid B-cell lymphoma: A study of 36 cases. Hum Pathol 1991;22:409–421.
29. Alizadeh AA, Eisen MB, Davis RE, et al: Distinct types of diffuse large B-cell lymphoma identified by gene expression profiling. Nature 2000;403:503–511.
30. Shipp MA, Ross KN, Tamayo P, et al: Diffuse large B-cell lymphoma outcome prediction by gene-expression profiling and supervised machine learning. Nat Med 2002;8:68–74.
31. Chan JK, Buchanan R, Fletcher CD: Sarcomatoid variant of anaplastic large-cell Ki-1 lymphoma. Am J Surg Pathol 1990;14:983–988.
32. Tse CC, Chan JK, Yuen RW, et al: Malignant lymphoma with myxoid stroma: A new pattern in need of recognition. Histopathology 1991;18:31–35.
33. Fung DT, Chan JK, Tse CC, et al: Myxoid change in malignant lymphoma. Pathogenetic considerations. Arch Pathol Lab Med 1992;116:103–105.
34. Warnke RA, Weiss LM, Chan JK, et al: Tumors of the Lymph Nodes and Spleen, Atlas of Tumor Pathology, 3rd series, Fascicle 14. Washington DC, Armed Forces Institute of Pathology, 1995.
35. Wang J, Sun NC, Nozawa Y, et al: Histological and immunohistochemical characterization of extranodal diffuse large-cell lymphomas with prominent spindle cell features. Histopathology 2001;39:476–481.
36. Tsang WY, Chan JK, Tang SK, et al: Large cell lymphoma with fibrillary matrix. Histopathology 1992;20: 80–82.
37. Koo CH, Shin SS, Bracho F, et al: Rosette-forming non-Hodgkin's lymphomas. Histopathology 1996;29: 557–563.
38. Khalidi HS, Brynes RK, Browne P, et al: Intravascular large B-cell lymphoma: The CD5 antigen is expressed by a subset of cases. Mod Pathol 1998;11:983–988.
39. Estalilla OC, Koo CH, Brynes RK, et al: Intravascular large B-cell lymphoma. A report of five cases initially diagnosed by bone marrow biopsy. Am J Clin Pathol 1999;112:248–255.
40. Chan JKC: Tumors of the lymphoreticular system, including spleen and thymus. In Fletcher CDM (ed): Diagnostic Histopathology of Tumors, 2nd ed. London, Churchill Livingstone, 2000, pp 1099–1316.
41. Chan JK, Rosai J: Tumors of the neck showing thymic or related branchial pouch differentiation: A unifying concept. Hum Pathol 1991;22:349–367.

Localized Lymphoid Hyperplasia

42. Chan JK, Hui PK, Ng CS, et al: Epithelioid haemangioma (angiolymphoid hyperplasia with eosinophilia) and Kimura's disease in Chinese. Histopathology 1989;15:557–574.
43. Kung IT, Gibson JB, Bannatyne PM: Kimura's disease: A clinico-pathological study of 21 cases and its distinction from angiolymphoid hyperplasia with eosinophilia. Pathology 1984;16:39–44.
44. Hui PK, Chan JK, Ng CS, et al: Lymphadenopathy of Kimura's disease. Am J Surg Pathol 1989;13:177–186.
45. Akosa AB, Sherif A, Maidment CG: Kimura's disease and membranous nephropathy. Nephron 1991;58: 472–474.
46. Matsumoto K, Katayama H, Hatano M: Minimal-change nephrotic syndrome associated with subcutaneous eosinophilic lymphoid granuloma (Kimura's disease). Nephron 1988;49:251–254.
47. Frizzera G: Castleman's disease and related disorders. Semin Diagn Pathol 1988;5:346–364.
48. Castleman B, Iverson L, Menendez VP: Localized mediastinal lymph node hyperplasia resembling thymoma. Cancer 1956;9:822–830.
49. Tung KS, McCormack LJ: Angiomatous lymphoid hamartoma. Report of five cases with a review of the literature. Cancer 1967;20:525–536.
50. Keller AR, Hochholzer L, Castleman B: Hyaline-vascular and plasma-cell types of giant lymph node hyperplasia of the mediastinum and other locations. Cancer 1972;29:670–683.
51. Chan JK, Tsang WY: Reactive lymphadenopathies. In Weiss LM (ed): Pathology of Lymph Nodes. Contemporary Issues in Surgical Pathology, vol 21. New York: Churchill Livingstone, 1996, pp 81–167.
52. Ruco LP, Gearing AJ, Pigott R, et al: Expression of ICAM-1, VCAM-1 and ELAM-1 in angiofollicular lymph node hyperplasia (Castleman's disease): Evidence for dysplasia of follicular dendritic reticulum cells. Histopathology 1991;19:523–528.
53. Danon AD, Krishnan J, Frizzera G: Morpho-immunophenotypic diversity of Castleman's disease, hyaline-vascular type: With emphasis on a stroma-rich variant and a new pathogenetic hypothesis. Virchows Arch A Pathol Anat Histopathol 1993;423:369–382.
54. Nguyen DT, Diamond LW, Hansmann ML, et al: Castleman's disease. Differences in follicular dendritic network in the hyaline vascular and plasma cell variants. Histopathology 1994;24:437–443.
55. Madero S, Onate JM, Garzon A: Giant lymph node hyperplasia in an angiolipomatous mediastinal mass. Arch Pathol Lab Med 1986;110:853–855.
56. Al-Jabi M, Tolnai G, McCaughey WT: Angiofollicular lymphoid hyperplasia in an angiolipomatous mass. Arch Pathol Lab Med 1980;104:313–315.

57. Tsang WY, Chan JK, Dorfman RF, et al: Vasoproliferative lesions of the lymph node. Pathol Annu 1994;29: 63–133.
58. Gerald W, Kostianovsky M, Rosai J: Development of vascular neoplasia in Castleman's disease. Report of seven cases. Am J Surg Pathol 1990;14:603–614.
59. Chan JK, Tsang WY, Ng CS: Follicular dendritic cell tumor and vascular neoplasm complicating hyaline-vascular Castleman's disease. Am J Surg Pathol 1994; 18:517–525.
60. Lin O, Frizzera G: Angiomyoid and follicular dendritic cell proliferative lesions in Castleman's disease of hyaline-vascular type: A study of 10 cases. Am J Surg Pathol 1997;21:1295–1306.
61. Chan JK, Fletcher CD, Nayler SJ, et al: Follicular dendritic cell sarcoma. Clinicopathologic analysis of 17 cases suggesting a malignant potential higher than currently recognized. Cancer 1997;79:294–313.
62. Chan AC, Chan KW, Chan JK, et al: Development of follicular dendritic cell sarcoma in hyaline-vascular Castleman's disease of the nasopharynx: Tracing its evolution by sequential biopsies. Histopathology 2001; 38:510–518.
63. Chan JK, Luk SC, Ho PL: Stroma-rich Castleman's disease with superimposed Kikuchi's lymphadenitis-like changes. Int J Surg Pathol 1997;4:197–202.

Plasmacytoma Involving Soft Tissues

64. Bhat RV, Iyengar KR: Soft tissue plasmacytoma diagnosed by fine needle aspiration cytology. Acta Cytol 2001;45:481–483.
65. Sanyal B, Pant GC, Sahni K, et al: Extramedullary plasmacytoma: Simulating a soft tissue sarcoma of the chest wall. J Surg Oncol 1980;14:147–151.
66. Wotherspoon AC, Norton AJ, Isaacson PG: Immunoreactive cytokeratins in plasmacytomas. Histopathology 1989;14:141–150.

Approach to Diagnosis of Lymphoid Infiltrates in the Soft Tissues

67. Chan JK: Peripheral T-cell and NK-cell neoplasms: An integrated approach to diagnosis. Mod Pathol 1999; 12:177–199.
68. Medeiros LJ, Carr J: Overview of the role of molecular methods in the diagnosis of malignant lymphomas. Arch Pathol Lab Med 1999;123:1189–1207.

Tumors and Tumor-like Lesions of Hematopoietic Cells

Extramedullary Hematopoietic Tumor

69. Wu JH, Shih LY, Kuo TT, et al: Intrathoracic extramedullary hematopoietic tumor in hemoglobin H disease. Am J Hematol 1992;41:285–288.
70. Koudieh MS, Afzal M, Rasul K, et al: Intrathoracic extramedullary hematopoietic tumor in hemoglobin C disease. Arch Pathol Lab Med 1996;120:504–506.
71. Dewar G, Leung NW, Ng HK, et al: Massive, solitary, intrahepatic, extramedullary hematopoietic tumor in thalassemia. Surgery 1990;107:704–707.
72. Newton KL, McNeeley SG Jr, Novick M: Extramedullary hematopoiesis presenting as a pelvic mass in a patient with beta-thalassemia intermedia. JAMA 1983;250:2178–2179.
73. Redmond J 3rd, Kantor RS, Auerbach HE, et al: Extramedullary hematopoiesis during therapy with granulocyte colony-stimulating factor. Arch Pathol Lab Med 1994;118:1014–1015.
74. de Morais JC, Spector N, Lavrado FP, et al: Spinal cord compression due to extramedullary hematopoiesis in the proliferative phase of polycythemia vera. Acta Haematol 1996;96:242–244.
75. Hsu FI, Filippa DA, Castro-Malaspina H, et al: Extramedullary hematopoiesis mimicking metastatic lung carcinoma. Ann Thorac Surg 1998;66: 1411–1413.
76. Remstein ED, Kurtin PJ, Nascimento AG: Sclerosing extramedullary hematopoietic tumor in chronic myeloproliferative disorders. Am J Surg Pathol 2000;24: 51–55.

Extramedullary Myeloid Tumor

77. Chen J, Yanuck RR III, Abbondanzo SL, et al: c-Kit (CD117) reactivity in extramedullary myeloid tumor/ granulocytic sarcoma. Arch Pathol Lab Med 2001;125: 1448–1452.
78. Neiman RS, Barcos M, Berard C, et al: Granulocytic sarcoma: A clinicopathologic study of 61 biopsied cases. Cancer 1981;48:1426–1437.
79. Wong KF, Chan JKC: Antimyeloperoxidase: Antibody of choice for labeling of myeloid cells including diagnosis of granulocytic sarcoma. Adv Anat Pathol 1995; 2:65–68.
80. Hutchison RE, Kurec AS, Davey FR: Granulocytic sarcoma. Clin Lab Med 1990;10:889–901.
81. Pinkus GS, Pinkus JL: Myeloperoxidase: A specific marker for myeloid cells in paraffin sections. Mod Pathol 1991;4:733–741.

Mast Cell Disease

82. Valent P, Horny HP, Li CY, et al: Mastocytosis. In Jaffe ES, Harris NL, Stein H, et al (eds): Pathology and Genetics. Tumours of the Haematopoietic and Lymphoid Tissues. World Health Organization Classification of Tumours. Lyon, France: IARC Press, 2001, pp 293–302.
83. Longley BJ, Metcalfe DD: A proposed classification of mastocytosis incorporating molecular genetics. Hematol Oncol Clin North Am 2000;14:697–701, viii.
84. Valent P, Horny HP, Escribano L, et al: Diagnostic criteria and classification of mastocytosis: A consensus proposal. Leuk Res 2001;25:603–625.
85. Kojima M, Nakamura S, Itoh H, et al: Mast cell sarcoma with tissue eosinophilia arising in the ascending colon. Mod Pathol 1999;12:739–743.

86. Horny HP, Parwaresch MR, Kaiserling E, et al: Mast cell sarcoma of the larynx. J Clin Pathol 1986;39: 596–602.

Tumors and Tumor-like Lesions of Histiocytes

87. Foucar K, Foucar E: The mononuclear phagocyte and immunoregulatory effector (M-PIRE) system: Evolving concepts. Semin Diagn Pathol 1990;7:4–18.
88. Weiss LM: Histiocytic and dendritic cell proliferations. In Knowles DM (ed): Neoplastic Hematopathology, 2nd ed. Philadelphia. Lippincott Williams & Wilkins, 2001, pp 1815–1845.
89. Jaffe R: The histiocytoses. Diagn Pediatr Hematol 1999;19:135–155.
90. Kraus MD, Haley JC, Ruiz R, et al: "Juvenile" xanthogranuloma: An immunophenotypic study with a reappraisal of histogenesis. Am J Dermatopathol 2001;23:104–111.
91. Lasser A: The mononuclear phagocytic system: A review. Hum Pathol 1983;14:108–126.
92. Wood GS, Turner RR, Shiurba RA, et al: Human dendritic cells and macrophages. In situ immunophenotypic definition of subsets that exhibit specific morphologic and microenvironmental characteristics. Am J Pathol 1985;119:73–82.
93. Romani N, Schuler G: The immunologic properties of epidermal Langerhans cells as a part of the dendritic cell system. Springer Semin Immunopathol 1992;13: 265–279.
94. Wilson MS, Weiss LM, Gatter KC, et al: Malignant histiocytosis. A reassessment of cases previously reported in 1975 based on paraffin section immunophenotyping studies. Cancer 1990;66:530–536.
95. Zelger BW, Sidoroff A, Orchard G, et al: Non-Langerhans cell histiocytoses. A new unifying concept. Am J Dermatopathol 1996;18:490–504.
96. Zelger B. Langerhans cell histiocytosis: A reactive or neoplastic disorder? Med Pediatr Oncol 2001;37: 543–544.
97. Zelger BW, Cerio R: Xanthogranuloma is the archetype of non-Langerhans cell histiocytoses. Br J Dermatol 2001;145:369–370.
98. Winkelmann RK. Cutaneous syndromes of non-X histiocytosis: A review of the macrophage-histiocyte diseases of the skin. Arch Dermatol 1981;117:667–672.
99. Gianotti F, Caputo R. Histiocytic syndromes: A review. J Am Acad Dermatol 1985;13:383–404.
100. Sidoroff A, Zelger B, Steiner H, et al: Indeterminate cell histiocytosis—A clinicopathological entity with features of both X- and non-X histiocytosis. Br J Dermatol 1996;134:525–532.
101. Wechsler J: Reactive and neoplastic histiocytic skin disorders. In Kirkham N, Lemoine NR (eds). Progress in Pathology, vol 5. London, Greenwich Medical Media, 2001, pp 27–43.
102. Favara BE, Feller AC, Paulli M, et al: Contemporary classification of histiocytic disorders. The WHO Committee on Histiocytic/Reticulum Cell Proliferations. Reclassification Working Group of the Histiocyte Society. Med Pediatr Oncol 1997;29:157–166.
103. Jaffe ES: Histiocytic and dendritic cell neoplasms. In Jaffe ES, Harris NL, Stein H, et al (eds): Pathology and Genetics. Tumours of Haematopoietic and Lymphoid Tissues. World Health Organization Classification of Tumours. Lyon, France: IARC Press, 2001, pp 273–277.

Extranodal Rosai-Dorfman Disease

104. Foucar E, Rosai J, Dorfman R: Sinus histiocytosis with massive lymphadenopathy (Rosai-Dorfman disease): Review of the entity. Semin Diagn Pathol 1990;7:19–73.
105. Paulli M, Bergamaschi G, Tonon L, et al: Evidence for a polyclonal nature of the cell infiltrate in sinus histiocytosis with massive lymphadenopathy (Rosai-Dorfman disease). Br J Haematol 1995;91:415–418.
106. Wacker HH, Frahm SO, Heidebrecht HJ, et al: Sinus-lining cells of the lymph nodes recognized as a dendritic cell type by the new monoclonal antibody Ki-M9. Am J Pathol 1997;151:423–434.
107. Montgomery EA, Meis JM, Frizzera G: Rosai-Dorfman disease of soft tissue. Am J Surg Pathol 1992;16: 122–129.
108. Foucar E, Rosai J, Dorfman RF: Sinus histiocytosis with massive lymphadenopathy. An analysis of 14 deaths occurring in a patient registry. Cancer 1984;54: 1834–1840.

Histiocytic Sarcoma

109. Weiss LM, Grogan TM, Muller-Hermelink K, et al: Histiocytic sarcoma. In Jaffe ES, Harris NL, Stein H, et al (eds): Pathology and Genetics. Tumours of Haematopoietic and Lymphoid Tissues. World Health Organization Classification of Tumours. Lyon, France: IARC Press, 2001, pp 278–279.
110. Pileri SA, Grogan TM, Banks PM, et al: Tumors of histiocytes and accessory dendritic cells, a proposed classification from the International Lymphoma Study Group based on comprehensive analysis of 61 cases. Histopathology 2002. In press.
111. Copie-Bergman C, Wotherspoon AC, Norton AJ, et al: True histiocytic lymphoma: A morphologic, immunohistochemical, and molecular genetic study of 13 cases. Am J Surg Pathol 1998;22:1386–1392.
112. Hanson CA, Jaszcz W, Kersey JH, et al: True histiocytic lymphoma: Histopathologic, immunophenotypic and genotypic analysis. Br J Haematol 1989;73: 187–198.
113. Kamel OW, Gocke CD, Kell DL, et al: True histiocytic lymphoma: A study of 12 cases based on current definition. Leuk Lymphoma 1995;18:81–86.
114. Soslow RA, Davis RE, Warnke RA, et al: True histiocytic lymphoma following therapy for lymphoblastic neoplasms. Blood 1996;87:5207–5212.

115. Bouabdallah R, Abena P, Chetaille B, et al: True histiocytic lymphoma following B-acute lymphoblastic leukaemia: Case report with evidence for a common clonal origin in both neoplasms. Br J Haematol 2001; 113:1047–1050.
116. van der Kwast TH, van Dongen JJ, Michiels JJ, et al: T-lymphoblastic lymphoma terminating as malignant histiocytosis with rearrangement of immunoglobulin heavy chain gene. Leukemia 1991;5:78–82.
117. Ladanyi M, Roy I, Landanyi M: Mediastinal germ cell tumors and histiocytosis. Hum Pathol 1988;19: 586–590.
118. Zon R, Orazi A, Neiman RS, et al: Benign hematologic neoplasm associated with mediastinal mature teratoma in a patient with Klinefelter's syndrome: A case report. Med Pediatr Oncol 1994;23:376–379.
119. Nichols CR, Roth BJ, Heerema N, et al: Hematologic neoplasia associated with primary mediastinal germ-cell tumors. N Engl J Med 1990;322:1425–1429.
120. DeMent SH, Eggleston JC, Spivak JL: Association between mediastinal germ cell tumors and hematologic malignancies. Report of two cases and review of the literature. Am J Surg Pathol 1985;9:23–30.
121. deMent SH: Association between mediastinal germ cell tumors and hematologic malignancies: An update. Hum Pathol 1990;21:699–703.
122. Cheuk W, Walford N, Lou J, et al: Primary histiocytic lymphoma of the central nervous system: A neoplasm frequently overshadowed by a prominent inflammatory component. Am J Surg Pathol 2001;25:1372–1379.
123. Strauchen JA: Sarcomatoid neoplasm of monocytic lineage. Am J Surg Pathol 1991;15:1206–1207.
124. Falini B, Flenghi L, Pileri S, et al: PG-M1: A new monoclonal antibody directed against a fixative-resistant epitope on the macrophage-restricted form of the CD68 molecule. Am J Pathol 1993;142:1359–1372.
125. Tsang WY, Chan JK: KP1 (CD68) staining of granular cell neoplasms: Is KP1 a marker for lysosomes rather than the histiocytic lineage? Histopathology 1992;21: 84–86.
126. Fanburg-Smith JC, Miettinen M: Angiomatoid "malignant" fibrous histiocytoma: A clinicopathologic study of 158 cases and further exploration of the myoid phenotype. Hum Pathol 1999;30:1336–1343.
127. Pernick NL, DaSilva M, Gangi MD, et al: "Histiocytic markers" in melanoma. Mod Pathol 1999;12:1072–1977.

Mycobacterial Spindle Cell Pseudotumor and Histoid Leprosy

128. Wood C, Nickoloff BJ, Todes-Taylor NR: Pseudotumor resulting from atypical mycobacterial infection: A "histoid" variety of Mycobacterium avium-intracellulare complex infection. Am J Clin Pathol 1985;83: 524–527.
129. Logani S, Lucas DR, Cheng JD, et al: Spindle cell tumors associated with mycobacteria in lymph nodes of HIV-positive patients: "Kaposi sarcoma with mycobacteria" and "mycobacterial pseudotumor." Am J Surg Pathol 1999;23:656–661.
130. Chen KT: Mycobacterial spindle cell pseudotumor of lymph nodes. Am J Surg Pathol 1992;16:276–281.
131. Kontochristopoulos GJ, Aroni K, Panteleos DN, et al: Immunohistochemistry in histoid leprosy. Int J Dermatol 1995;34:777–781.
132. Wolf DA, Wu CD, Medeiros LJ: Mycobacterial pseudotumors of lymph node. A report of two cases diagnosed at the time of intraoperative consultation using touch imprint preparations. Arch Pathol Lab Med 1995;119:811–814.
133. Sehgal VN, Srivastava G, Beohar PC: Histoid leprosy—A histopathological reapparel. Acta Leprol 1987;5:125–131.
134. Umlas J, Federman M, Crawford C, et al: Spindle cell pseudotumor due to Mycobacterium avium-intracellulare in patients with acquired immunodeficiency syndrome (AIDS). Positive staining of mycobacteria for cytoskeleton filaments. Am J Surg Pathol 1991;15: 1181–1187.
135. Lee ES, Locker J, Nalesnik M, et al: The association of Epstein-Barr virus with smooth-muscle tumors occurring after organ transplantation. N Engl J Med 1995; 332:19–25.

Malakoplakia

136. Damjanov I, Katz SM: Malakoplakia. Pathol Annu 1981;16:103–126.
137. Kwon KY, Colby TV: *Rhodococcus equi* pneumonia and pulmonary malakoplakia in acquired immunodeficiency syndrome. Pathologic features. Arch Pathol Lab Med 1994;118:744–748.
138. Moore WM 3rd, Stokes TL, Cabanas VY: Malakoplakia of the skin: Report of a case. Am J Clin Pathol 1973;60:218–221.
139. Colby TV: Malakoplakia. Two unusual cases which presented diagnostic problems. Am J Surg Pathol 1978;2:377–382.
140. Douglas-Jones AG, Rodd C, James EM, et al: Prediagnostic malakoplakia presenting as a chronic inflammatory mass in the soft tissues of the neck. J Laryngol Otol 1992;106:173–177.
141. Kogulan PK, Smith M, Seidman J, et al: Malakoplakia involving the abdominal wall, urinary bladder, vagina, and vulva: Case report and discussion of malakoplakia-associated bacteria. Int J Gynecol Pathol 2001;20:403–406.
142. Palou J, Torras H, Baradad M, et al: Cutaneous malakoplakia. Report of a case. Dermatologica 1988;176: 288–292.
143. van Furth R, van't Wout JW, Wertheimer PA, et al: Ciprofloxacin for treatment of malakoplakia. Lancet 1992;339:148–149.

Histiocytic Reaction to Foreign Materials

144. Barr RJ, Alpern KS, Jay S: Histiocytic reaction associated with topical aluminum chloride (Drysol reaction). J Dermatol Surg Oncol 1993;19:1017–1021.
145. Kershisnik MM, Ro JY, Cannon GH, et al: Histiocytic reaction in pelvic peritoneum associated with oxidized

regenerated cellulose. Am J Clin Pathol 1995;103: 27–31.
146. Albores-Saavedra J, Vuitch F, Delgado R, et al: Sinus histiocytosis of pelvic lymph nodes after hip replacement. A histiocytic proliferation induced by cobalt-chromium and titanium. Am J Surg Pathol 1994;18: 83–90.
147. Hicks DG, Judkins AR, Sickel JZ, et al: Granular histiocytosis of pelvic lymph nodes following total hip arthroplasty. The presence of wear debris, cytokine production, and immunologically activated macrophages. J Bone Joint Surg Am 1996;78:482–496.
148. Zaloudek C, Treseler PA, Powell CB: Postarthroplasty histiocytic lymphadenopathy in gynecologic oncology patients. A benign reactive process that clinically may be mistaken for cancer. Cancer 1996;78:834–844.
149. Gray MH, Talbert ML, Talbert WM, et al: Changes seen in lymph nodes draining the sites of large joint prostheses. Am J Surg Pathol 1989;13:1050–1056.
150. O'Connell JX, Rosenberg AE: Histiocytic lymphadenitis associated with a large joint prosthesis. Am J Clin Pathol 1993;99:314–316.
151. Sukpanichnant S, Hargrove NS, Kachintorn U, et al: Clofazimine-induced crystal-storing histiocytosis producing chronic abdominal pain in a leprosy patient. Am J Surg Pathol 2000;24:129–135.
152. Kuo TT, Hsueh S: Mucicarminophilic histiocytosis. A polyvinylpyrrolidone (PVP) storage disease simulating signet-ring cell carcinoma. Am J Surg Pathol 1984;8:419–428.
153. Kuo TT, Hu S, Huang CL, et al: Cutaneous involvement in polyvinylpyrrolidone storage disease: A clinicopathologic study of five patients, including two patients with severe anemia. Am J Surg Pathol 1997;21:1361–1367.
154. Kossard S, Ecker RI, Dicken CH: Povidone panniculitis. Polyvinylpyrrolidone panniculitis. Arch Dermatol 1980;116:704–706.
155. Hizawa K, Inaba H, Nakanishi S, et al: Subcutaneous pseudosarcomatous polyvinylpyrrolidone granuloma. Am J Surg Pathol 1984;8:393–398.
156. Reske-Nielsen E, Bojsen-Moller M, Vetner M, et al: Polyvinylpyrrolidone-storage disease. Light microscopical, ultrastructural and chemical verification. Acta Pathol Microbiol Scand [A] 1976;84:397–405.
157. Weiss SW, Enzinger FM, Johnson FB: Silica reaction simulating fibrous histiocytoma. Cancer 1978;42: 2738–2743.

Granular Histiocytic Reaction

158. Sobel HJ, Avrin E, Marquet E, et al: Reactive granular cells in sites of trauma. A cytochemical and ultrastructural study. Am J Clin Pathol 1974;61:223–234.
159. Sobel HJ, Marquet E: Granular cells and granular cell lesions. Pathol Annu 1974;9:43–79.

Xanthogranulomatous Inflammation

160. Cozzutto C, Carbone A: The xanthogranulomatous process. Xanthogranulomatous inflammation. Pathol Res Pract 1988;183:395–402.
161. Shalev E, Zuckerman H, Rizescu I: Pelvic inflammatory pseudotumor (xanthogranuloma). Acta Obstet Gynecol Scand 1982;61:285–286.
162. Variakojis D, Strum SB, Rappaport H: The foamy macrophages in Hodgkin's disease. Arch Pathol 1972; 93:453–456.
163. Weiss SW, Goldblum JR: Enzinger and Weiss's Soft Tissue Tumors. St. Louis, Mosby, 2001.
164. Khalidi HS, Singleton TP, Weiss SW: Inflammatory malignant fibrous histiocytoma: Distinction from Hodgkin's disease and non-Hodgkin's lymphoma by a panel of leukocyte markers. Mod Pathol 1997;10: 438–442.
165. Kyriakos M, Kempson RL: Inflammatory fibrous histiocytoma. An aggressive and lethal lesion. Cancer 1976;37:1584–1606.

Erdheim-Chester Disease

166. Kenn W, Eck M, Allolio B, et al: Erdheim-Chester disease: Evidence for a disease entity different from Langerhans cell histiocytosis? Three cases with detailed radiological and immunohistochemical analysis. Hum Pathol 2000;31:734–739.
167. Egan AJ, Boardman LA, Tazelaar HD, et al: Erdheim-Chester disease: Clinical, radiologic, and histopathologic findings in five patients with interstitial lung disease. Am J Surg Pathol 1999;23:17–26.
168. Chetritt J, Paradis V, Dargere D, et al: Chester-Erdheim disease: A neoplastic disorder. Hum Pathol 1999;30:1093–1096.
169. Veyssier-Belot C, Cacoub P, Caparros-Lefebvre D, et al: Erdheim-Chester disease. Clinical and radiologic characteristics of 59 cases. Medicine (Baltimore) 1996; 75:157–169.

Crystal Storing Histiocytosis Mimicking Adult Rhabdomyoma

170. Kapadia SB, Enzinger FM, Heffner DK, et al: Crystal-storing histiocytosis associated with lymphoplasmacytic neoplasms. Report of three cases mimicking adult rhabdomyoma. Am J Surg Pathol 1993;17:461–467.
171. Harada M, Shimada M, Fukayama M, et al: Crystal-storing histiocytosis associated with lymphoplasmacytic lymphoma mimicking Weber-Christian disease: Immunohistochemical, ultrastructural, and gene-rearrangement studies. Hum Pathol 1996;27:84–87.
172. Prasad ML, Charney DA, Sarlin J, et al: Pulmonary immunocytoma with massive crystal storing histiocytosis: A case report with review of literature. Am J Surg Pathol 1998;22:1148–1153.
173. Thorson P, Hess JL: Transformation of monocytoid B-cell lymphoma to large cell lymphoma associated with crystal-storing histiocytes. Arch Pathol Lab Med 2000;124:460–462.
174. Jones D, Bhatia VK, Krausz T, et al: Crystal-storing histiocytosis: A disorder occurring in plasmacytic tumors expressing immunoglobulin kappa light chain. Hum Pathol 1999;30:1441–148.

175. Friedman MT, Molho L, Valderrama E, et al: Crystal-storing histiocytosis associated with a lymphoplasmacytic neoplasm mimicking adult rhabdomyoma, a case report and review of the literature. Arch Pathol Lab Med 1996;120:1133–1136.

Xanthoma

176. Peters MS, Farmer ER: Histiocytic and Langerhans cell reactions. In Farmer ER, Hood AF (eds): Pathology of the Skin, 2nd ed. New York, McGraw-Hill, 2000, pp 399–424.
177. Parker F: Xanthomas and hyperlipidemias. J Am Acad Dermatol 1985;13:1–30.
178. Beham A, Fletcher CD: Plexiform xanthoma: An unusual variant. Histopathology 1991;19:565–567.
179. Michal M: Plexiform xanthomatous tumor. A report of three cases. Am J Dermatopathol 1994;16:532–536.

Langerhans Cell Histiocytosis

180. Willman CL, Busque L, Griffith BB, et al: Langerhans'-cell histiocytosis (histiocytosis X)—A clonal proliferative disease [see comments]. N Engl J Med 1994;331:154–160.
181. Yu RC, Chu C, Buluwela L, et al: Clonal proliferation of Langerhans cells in Langerhans cell histiocytosis. Lancet 1994;343:767–768.
182. de Graaf JH, Egeler RM: New insights into the pathogenesis of Langerhans cell histiocytosis. Curr Opin Pediatr 1997;9:46–50.
183. Henck ME, Simpson EL, Ochs RH, et al: Extraskeletal soft tissue masses of Langerhans' cell histiocytosis. Skeletal Radiol 1996;25:409–412.
184. al-Abbadi M, Masih A, Braylan RC, et al: Soft tissue Langerhans' cell histiocytosis in an adult. A case presentation with flow cytometric analysis and literature review. Arch Pathol Lab Med 1997;121:169–172.
185. Malpas JS: Langerhans cell histiocytosis in adults. Hematol Oncol Clin North Am 1998;12:259–268.
186. Hashimoto K, Pritzker MS: Electron microscopic study of reticulohistiocytoma. An unusual case of congenital, self-healing reticulohistiocytosis. Arch Dermatol 1973;107:263–270.
187. Tay YK, Friednash MM, Weston WL, et al: Solitary congenital nodule in an infant. Solitary congenital self-healing reticulohistiocytosis (CSHR). Arch Dermatol 1998;134:627–630.
188. Schaumburg-Lever G, Rechowicz E, Fehrenbacher B, et al: Congenital self-healing reticulohistiocytosis—A benign Langerhans cell disease. J Cutan Pathol 1994; 21:59–66.
189. Chun SI, Song MS: Congenital self-healing reticulohistiocytosis—Report of a case of the solitary type and review of the literature. Yonsei Med J 1992;33: 194–198.
190. Ofuji S, Tachibana S, Kanato M, et al: Congenital self-healing reticulohistiocytosis (Hashimoto-Pritzker): A case report with a solitary lesion. J Dermatol 1987;14: 182–184.
191. Divaris DX, Ling FC, Prentice RS: Congenital self-healing histiocytosis. Report of two cases with histochemical and ultrastructural studies. Am J Dermatopathol 1991;13:481–487.
192. Favara BE, Jaffe R: Pathology of Langerhans cell histiocytosis. Hematol Oncol Clin North Am 1987;1: 75–97.
193. Lieberman PH, Jones CR, Steinman RM, et al: Langerhans cell (eosinophilic) granulomatosis. A clinicopathologic study encompassing 50 years [see comments]. Am J Surg Pathol 1996;20:519–552.
194. Schmitz L, Favara BE: Nosology and pathology of Langerhans cell histiocytosis. Hematol Oncol Clin North Am 1998;12:221–246.
195. Emile JF, Wechsler J, Brousse N, et al: Langerhans' cell histiocytosis. Definitive diagnosis with the use of monoclonal antibody O10 on routinely paraffin-embedded samples. Am J Surg Pathol 1995;19: 636–641.
196. Fartasch M, Vigneswaran N, Diepgen TL, et al: Immunohistochemical and ultrastructural study of histiocytosis X and non-X histiocytoses. J Am Acad Dermatol 1990;23:885–892.
197. Azumi N, Sheibani K, Swartz WG, et al: Antigenic phenotype of Langerhans cell histiocytosis: An immunohistochemical study demonstrating the value of LN-2, LN-3, and vimentin. Hum Pathol 1988;19: 1376–1382.
198. Emile JF, Fraitag S, Leborgne M, et al: Langerhans' cell histiocytosis cells are activated Langerhans' cells. J Pathol 1994;174:71–76.
199. Hage C, Willman CL, Favara BE, et al: Langerhans' cell histiocytosis (histiocytosis X): Immunophenotype and growth fraction. Hum Pathol 1993;24:840–845.
200. Weiss LM, Grogan TM, Muller-Hermelink HK, et al: Langerhans cell histiocytosis. In Jaffe ES, Harris NL, Stein H, et al (eds): Pathology and Genetics. Tumours of Haematopoietic and Lymphoid Tissues. World Health Organization Classification of Tumours. Lyon, France: IARC Press, 2001, pp 280–282.
201. Ornvold K, Ralfkiaer E, Carstensen H: Immunohistochemical study of the abnormal cells in Langerhans cell histiocytosis (histiocytosis X). Virchows Arch A Pathol Anat Histopathol 1990;416:403–410.
202. Ruco LP, Pulford KA, Mason DY, et al: Expression of macrophage-associated antigens in tissues involved by Langerhans' cell histiocytosis (histiocytosis X). Am J Clin Pathol 1989;92:273–279.

Indeterminate Cell Tumor and Indeterminate Cell Histiocytosis

203. Chan WC, Zaatari G: Lymph node interdigitating reticulum cell sarcoma. Am J Clin Pathol 1986;85: 739–744.
204. Segal GH, Mesa MV, Fishleder AJ, et al: Precursor Langerhans cell histiocytosis. An unusual histiocytic proliferation in a patient with persistent non-Hodgkin lymphoma and terminal acute monocytic leukemia. Cancer 1992;70:547–553.

205. Kolde G, Brocker EB: Multiple skin tumors of indeterminate cells in an adult. J Am Acad Dermatol 1986;15:591–597.
206. Berti E, Gianotti R, Alessi E: Unusual cutaneous histiocytosis expressing an intermediate immunophenotype between Langerhans' cells and dermal macrophages. Arch Dermatol 1988;124:1250–1253.
207. Bonetti F, Knowles DM 2nd, Chilosi M, et al: A distinctive cutaneous malignant neoplasm expressing the Langerhans cell phenotype. Synchronous occurrence with B-chronic lymphocytic leukemia. Cancer 1985;55:2417–2425.
208. Jaffe ES, Harris NL, Diebold J, et al: World Health Organization Classification of lymphomas: A work in progress. Ann Oncol 1998;9:S25–30.
209. Wood GS, Hu CH, Beckstead JH, et al: The indeterminate cell proliferative disorder: Report of a case manifesting as an unusual cutaneous histiocytosis. J Dermatol Surg Oncol 1985;11:1111–1119.

Follicular Dendritic Cell Sarcoma

210. Monda L, Warnke R, Rosai J: A primary lymph node malignancy with features suggestive of dendritic reticulum cell differentiation. A report of 4 cases. Am J Pathol 1986;122:562–572.
211. Weiss LM, Berry GJ, Dorfman RF, et al: Spindle cell neoplasms of lymph nodes of probable reticulum cell lineage. True reticulum cell sarcoma? Am J Surg Pathol 1990;14:405–414.
212. Chan JK: Proliferative lesions of follicular dendritic cells: An overview, including a detailed account of follicular dendritic cell sarcoma, a neoplasm with many faces and uncommon etiologic associations. Adv Anat Pathol 1997;4:387–411.
213. Choi PC, To KF, Lai FM, et al: Follicular dendritic cell sarcoma of the neck, report of two cases complicated by pulmonary metastases. Cancer 2000;89:664–672.
214. Perez-Ordonez B, Erlandson RA, Rosai J: Follicular dendritic cell tumor: Report of 13 additional cases of a distinctive entity. Am J Surg Pathol 1996;20:944–955.
215. Perez-Ordonez B, Rosai J: Follicular dendritic cell tumor: Review of the entity. Semin Diagn Pathol 1998;15:144–154.
216. Fisher C, Magnusson B, Hardarson S, et al: Myxoid variant of follicular dendritic cell sarcoma arising in the breast. Ann Diagn Pathol 1999;3:92–98.
217. Cheuk W, Chan JK, Shek TW, et al: Inflammatory pseudotumor-like follicular dendritic cell tumor: A distinctive low-grade malignant intra-abdominal neoplasm with consistent Epstein-Barr virus association. Am J Surg Pathol 2001;25:721–731.
218. Andriko JW, Kaldjian EP, Tsokos M, et al: Reticulum cell neoplasms of lymph nodes: A clinicopathologic study of 11 cases with recognition of a new subtype derived from fibroblastic reticular cells. Am J Surg Pathol 1998;22:1048–1058.
219. Katano H, Kaneko K, Shimizu S, et al: Follicular dendritic cell sarcoma complicated by hyaline-vascular type Castleman's disease in a schizophrenic patient. Pathol Int 1997;47:703–706.
220. Lee IJ, Kim SC, Kim HS, et al: Paraneoplastic pemphigus associated with follicular dendritic cell sarcoma arising from Castleman's tumor. J Am Acad Dermatol 1999;40:294–297.
221. Saiz AD, Chan O, Strauchen JA: Follicular dendritic cell tumor in Castleman's disease, a report of two cases. Int J Surg Pathol 1997;5:25–30.
222. Masunaga A, Nakamura H, Katata T, et al: Follicular dendritic cell tumor with histiocytic characteristics and fibroblastic antigen. Pathol Int 1997;47:707–712.

Interdigitating Dendritic Cell Sarcoma

223. Fonseca R, Yamakawa M, Nakamura S, et al: Follicular dendritic cell sarcoma and interdigitating reticulum cell sarcoma: A review. Am J Hematol 1998;59:161–167.
224. Banner B, Beauchamp ML, Liepman M, et al: Interdigitating reticulum-cell sarcoma of the intestine: A case report and review of the literature. Diagn Cytopathol 1997;17:216–222.
225. Hammar SP, Rudolph RH, Bockus DE, et al: Interdigitating reticulum cell sarcoma with unusual features. Ultrastruct Pathol 1991;15:631–645.
226. Nakamura S, Hara K, Suchi T, et al: Interdigitating cell sarcoma. A morphologic, immunohistologic, and enzyme-histochemical study. Cancer 1988;61:562–568.
227. Nakamura S, Koshikawa T, Kitoh K, et al: Interdigitating cell sarcoma: A morphologic and immunologic study of lymph node lesions in four cases. Pathol Int 1994;44:374–386.
228. Rousselet MC, Francois S, Croue A, et al: A lymph node interdigitating reticulum cell sarcoma. Arch Pathol Lab Med 1994;118:183–188.
229. Gaertner EM, Tsokos M, Derringer GA, et al: Interdigitating dendritic cell sarcoma. A report of four cases and review of the literature. Am J Clin Pathol 2001;115:589–597.

Fibroblastic Reticular Cell Sarcoma

230. Chan AC, Serrano-Olmo J, Erlandson RA, et al: Cytokeratin-positive malignant tumors with reticulum cell morphology: A subtype of fibroblastic reticulum cell neoplasm? Am J Surg Pathol 2000;24:107–116.
231. Gould VE, Warren WH, Faber LP, et al: Malignant cells of epithelial phenotype limited to thoracic lymph nodes. Eur J Cancer 1990;26:1121–1126.
232. Gould VE, Bloom KJ, Franke WW, et al: Increased numbers of cytokeratin-positive interstitial reticulum cells (CIRC) in reactive, inflammatory and neoplastic lymphadenopathies: Hyperplasia or induced expression? Virchows Arch 1995;425:617–629.

Dendritic Cell Sarcoma not Otherwise Specified

233. Jones D, Amin M, Ordonez NG, et al: Reticulum cell sarcoma of lymph node with mixed dendritic and fibroblastic features. Mod Pathol 2001;14:1059–1067.

Juvenile Xanthogranuloma

234. Coffin CM: Fibrohistiocytic tumors. In Coffin CM, Dehner LP, O'Shea PA (eds): Pediatric Soft Tissue Tumors, A Clinical, Pathological, and Therapeutic Approach. Baltimore, Williams & Wilkins, 1997, pp 179–213.
235. Helwig EB, Hackney VC: Juvenile xanthogranuloma (nevoxantho-endothelioma). Am J Pathol 1954; 30:625–626.
236. Sonoda T, Hashimoto H, Enjoji M: Juvenile xanthogranuloma. Clinicopathologic analysis and immunohistochemical study of 57 patients. Cancer 1985;56: 2280–2286.
237. Tahan SR, Pastel-Levy C, Bhan AK, et al: Juvenile xanthogranuloma. Clinical and pathologic characterization. Arch Pathol Lab Med 1989;113:1057–1061.
238. Cohen BA, Hood A: Xanthogranuloma: Report on clinical and histologic findings in 64 patients. Pediatr Dermatol 1989;6:262–266.
239. Chang MW: Update on juvenile xanthogranuloma: Unusual cutaneous and systemic variants. Semin Cutan Med Surg 1999;18:195–205.
240. Cusick EL, Spicer RD: Juvenile xanthogranuloma with extra-cutaneous lesions—A case report. Eur J Pediatr Surg 1994;4:368–369.
241. de Graaf JH, Timens W, Tamminga RY, et al: Deep juvenile xanthogranuloma: A lesion related to dermal indeterminate cells. Hum Pathol 1992;23:905–910.
242. George DH, Scheithauer BW, Hilton DL, et al: Juvenile xanthogranuloma of peripheral nerve: A report of two cases. Am J Surg Pathol 2001;25:521–526.
243. Janney CG, Hurt MA, Santa Cruz DJ: Deep juvenile xanthogranuloma. Subcutaneous and intramuscular forms. Am J Surg Pathol 1991;15:150–159.
244. Malcic I, Novick WM, Dasovic-Buljevic A, et al: Intracardiac juvenile xanthogranuloma in a newborn. Pediatr Cardiol 2001;22:150–152.
245. Sanchez Yus E, Requena L, Villegas C, et al: Subcutaneous juvenile xanthogranuloma. J Cutan Pathol 1995;22:460–465.
246. Torok E, Daroczy J: Juvenile xanthogranuloma: An analysis of 45 cases by clinical follow-up, light- and electron microscopy. Acta Derm Venereol 1985;65: 167–169.
247. Tan HH, Tay YK: Juvenile xanthogranuloma and neurofibromatosis 1. Dermatology 1998;197:43–44.
248. Gutmann DH, Gurney JG, Shannon KM: Juvenile xanthogranuloma, neurofibromatosis 1, and juvenile chronic myeloid leukemia. Arch Dermatol 1996;132: 1390–1391.
249. Zvulunov A: Juvenile xanthogranuloma, neurofibromatosis, and juvenile chronic myelogenous leukemia. Arch Dermatol 1996;132:712–713.
250. van Leeuwen RL, Berretty PJ, Knots E, et al: Triad of juvenile xanthogranuloma, von Recklinghausen's neurofibromatosis and trisomy 21 in a young girl. Clin Exp Dermatol 1996;21:248–249.
251. Zvulunov A, Barak Y, Metzker A: Juvenile xanthogranuloma, neurofibromatosis, and juvenile chronic myelogenous leukemia. World statistical analysis. Arch Dermatol 1995;131:904–908.
252. Cooper PH, Frierson HF, Kayne AL, et al: Association of juvenile xanthogranuloma with juvenile myeloid leukemia. Arch Dermatol 1984;120:371–375.
253. Kobayashi K, Imai T, Adachi S, et al: Juvenile xanthogranuloma with hematologic changes in dizygotic twins: Report of two newborn infants. Pediatr Dermatol 1998;15:203–206.
254. Herbst AM, Laude TA: Juvenile xanthogranuloma: Further evidence of a reactive etiology. Pediatr Dermatol 1999;16:164.
255. Herbst AM, Laude TA: Juvenile xanthogranuloma: Further evidence of a reactive etiology [letter; comment]. Pediatr Dermatol 1999;16:164.
256. Newman CC, Raimer SS, Sanchez RL: Nonlipidized juvenile xanthogranuloma: A histologic and immunohistochemical study. Pediatr Dermatol 1997;14: 98–102.
257. Zelger BW, Staudacher C, Orchard G, et al: Solitary and generalized variants of spindle cell xanthogranuloma (progressive nodular histiocytosis). Histopathology 1995;27:11–19.
258. Zelger BG, Orchard G, Rudolph P, et al: Scalloped cell xanthogranuloma. Histopathology 1998;32:368–374.
259. Nascimento AG: A clinicopathologic and immunohistochemical comparative study of cutaneous and intramuscular forms of juvenile xanthogranuloma. Am J Surg Pathol 1997;21:645–652.
260. Gianotti R, Alessi E, Caputo R: Benign cephalic histiocytosis: A distinct entity or a part of a wide spectrum of histiocytic proliferative disorders of children? A histopathological study. Am J Dermatopathol 1993;15: 315–319.
261. Barsky BL, Lao I, Barsky S, et al: Benign cephalic histiocytosis. Arch Dermatol 1984;120:650–655.
262. de Luna ML, Glikin I, Golberg J, et al: Benign cephalic histiocytosis: Report of four cases. Pediatr Dermatol 1989;6:198–201.
263. Eisenberg EL, Bronson DM, Barsky S: Benign cephalic histiocytosis. A case report and ultrastructural study. J Am Acad Dermatol 1985;12:328–331.
264. Khoo BP, Tay YK: Benign cephalic histiocytosis in Singapore—A review of 8 cases. Singapore Med J 1999;40:697–699.
265. Pena-Penabad C, Unamuno P, Garcia-Silva J, et al: Benign cephalic histiocytosis: Case report and literature review. Pediatr Dermatol 1994;11:164–157.
266. Rodriguez-Jurado R, Duran-McKinster C, Ruiz-Maldonado R: Benign cephalic histiocytosis progressing into juvenile xanthogranuloma: A non-Langerhans cell histiocytosis transforming under the influence of a virus? Am J Dermatopathol 2000;22:70–74.
267. Weston WL, Travers SH, Mierau GW, et al: Benign cephalic histiocytosis with diabetes insipidus. Pediatr Dermatol 2000;17:296–298.
268. Zelger BG, Zelger B, Steiner H, et al: Solitary giant xanthogranuloma and benign cephalic histiocytosis—Variants of juvenile xanthogranuloma. Br J Dermatol 1995;133:598–604.

269. Burgdorf WH, Kusch SL, Nix TE Jr, et al: Progressive nodular histiocytoma. Arch Dermatol 1981;117: 644–649.
270. Gonzalez Ruiz A, Bernal Ruiz AI, Aragoneses Fraile H, et al: Progressive nodular histiocytosis accompanied by systemic disorders. Br J Dermatol 2000;143:628–631.
271. Taunton OD, Yeshurun D, Jarratt M: Progressive nodular histiocytoma. Arch Dermatol 1978;114:1505–1508.
272. Torres L, Sanchez JL, Rivera A, et al: Progressive nodular histiocytosis. J Am Acad Dermatol 1993;29:278–280.
273. Kuligowski M, Gorkiewicz-Petkow A, Jablonska S: Xanthoma disseminatum. Int J Dermatol 1992;31: 281–283.
274. Giller RH, Folberg R, Keech RV, et al: Xanthoma disseminatum. An unusual histiocytosis syndrome. Am J Pediatr Hematol Oncol 1988;10:252–257.
275. Gallant CJ, From L: Juvenile xanthogranulomas and xanthoma disseminatum—Variations on a single theme. J Am Acad Dermatol 1986;15:108–109.
276. Davies CW, Marren P, Juniper MC, et al: Xanthoma disseminatum with respiratory tract involvement and fatal outcome. Thorax 2000;55:170–172.
277. Caputo R, Veraldi S, Grimalt R, et al: The various clinical patterns of xanthoma disseminatum. Considerations on seven cases and review of the literature. Dermatology 1995;190:19–24.
278. Levine HL, Taylor JS: Xanthoma disseminatum of the head and neck. Ear Nose Throat J 1979;58:340–344.
279. Mishkel MA, Cockshott WP, Nazir DJ, et al: Xanthoma disseminatum. Clinical, metabolic, pathologic, and radiologic aspects. Arch Dermatol 1977;113: 1094–1100.
280. Szekeres E, Tiba A, Korom I: Xanthoma disseminatum: A rare condition with non-X, non-lipid cutaneous histiocytopathy. J Dermatol Surg Oncol 1988;14: 1021–1024.
281. Zelger B, Cerio R, Orchard G, et al: Histologic and immunohistochemical study comparing xanthoma disseminatum and histiocytosis X. Arch Dermatol 1992;128:1207–1212.
282. Winkelmann RK, Muller SA: Generalized eruptive histiocytoma: A benign papular histiocytic reticulosis. Arch Dermatol 1963;88:586–595.
283. Umbert IJ, Winkelmann RK: Eruptive histiocytoma. J Am Acad Dermatol 1989;20:958–964.
284. Wee SH, Kim HS, Chang SN, et al: Generalized eruptive histiocytoma: A pediatric case. Pediatr Dermatol 2000;17:453–455.
285. Caputo R, Ermacora E, Gelmetti C, et al: Generalized eruptive histiocytoma in children. J Am Acad Dermatol 1987;17:449–454.
286. Repiso T, Roca-Miralles M, Kanitakis J, et al: Generalized eruptive histiocytoma evolving into xanthoma disseminatum in a 4-year-old boy. Br J Dermatol 1995;132:978–982.
287. Misery L, Boucheron S, Claudy AL: Factor XIIIa expression in juvenile xanthogranuloma. Acta Derm Venereol 1994;74:43–44.
288. Zelger B, Cerio R, Orchard G, et al: Juvenile and adult xanthogranuloma. A histological and immunohistochemical comparison. Am J Surg Pathol 1994;18: 126–135.
289. Tomaszewski MM, Lupton GP: Unusual expression of S-100 protein in histiocytic neoaplasms. J Cutan Pathol 1998;25:129–135.

Reticulohistiocytoma

290. Caputo R, Grimalt R: Solitary reticulohistiocytosis (reticulohistiocytoma) of the skin in children: Report of two cases [letter]. Arch Dermatol 1992;128:698–699.
291. Hunt SJ, Shin SS: Solitary reticulohistiocytoma in pregnancy: Immunohistochemical and ultrastructural study of a case with unusual immunophenotype. J Cutan Pathol 1995;22:177–181.
292. Oliver GF, Umbert I, Winkelmann RK, et al: Reticulohistiocytoma cutis—Review of 15 cases and an association with systemic vasculitis in two cases. Clin Exp Dermatol 1990;15:1–6.
293. Ornvold K, Vidar Jacobsen S, Nielsen MH: Congenital self-healing reticulohistiocytoma. A clinical, histological and ultrastructural study. Acta Paediatr Scand 1985;74:143–147.
294. Perrin C, Lacour JP, Michiels JF, et al: Reticulohistiocytomas versus multicentric reticulohistiocytosis. Am J Dermatopathol 1995;17:625–626.
295. Van Hecke E, Kint A: Reticulohistiocytoma. Dermatologica 1980;161(suppl 1):144–149.
296. Zelger B, Cerio R, Soyer HP, et al: Reticulohistiocytoma and multicentric reticulohistiocytosis. Histopathologic and immunophenotypic distinct entities [see comments]. Am J Dermatopathol 1994;16:577–584.

Multicentric Reticulhistiocytosis

297. Barrow MV, Holubar K: Multicentric reticulohistiocytosis. A review of 33 patients. Medicine (Baltimore) 1969;48:287–305.
298. Gorman JD, Danning C, Schumacher HR, et al: Multicentric reticulohistiocytosis: Case report with immunohistochemical analysis and literature review. Arthritis Rheum 2000;43:930–938.
299. Lotti T, Santucci M, Casigliani R, et al: Multicentric reticulohistiocytosis. Report of three cases with the evaluation of tissue proteinase activity. Am J Dermatopathol 1988;10:497–504.
300. Morris-Jones R, Walker M, Hardman C: Multicentric reticulohistiocytosis associated with Sjogren's syndrome. Br J Dermatol 2000;143:649–650.
301. Napoli J: Multicentric reticulohistiocytosis (lipoid dermatoarthritis). J Manipulative Physiol Ther 1994; 17:621.
302. Perrin C, Lacour JP, Michiels JF, et al: Multicentric reticulohistiocytosis. Immunohistological and ultrastructural study: A pathology of dendritic cell lineage. Am J Dermatopathol 1992;14:418–425.
303. Uhl M, Gutfleisch J, Rother E, et al: Multicentric reticulohistiocytosis. A report of 3 cases and review of literature. Bildgebung 1996;63:126–129.
304. Salisbury JR, Hall PA, Williams HC, et al: Multicentric reticulohistiocytosis. Detailed immunophenotyping confirms macrophage origin. Am J Surg Pathol 1990;14:687–693.

Index

Page numbers followed by f indicate figures; those followed by t indicate tables.